TRAUMA

EMERGENCY SURGERY
AND CRITICAL CARE

TRAUMA
EMERGENCY SURGERY AND CRITICAL CARE

Edited by

John H. Siegel, M.D.

Professor of Surgery
University of Maryland School of Medicine
Professor of Surgery
Johns Hopkins University School of Medicine
Director, MIEMSS Clinical Center
Deputy Director, Maryland Institute for
Emergency Medical Services Systems
Baltimore, Maryland

Churchill Livingstone
New York, Edinburgh, London, Melbourne   1987

Library of Congress Cataloging-in-Publication Data

Trauma: emergency surgery and critical care.

   Includes bibliographies and index.
   1. Wounds and injuries—Surgery. 2. Shock.
3. Surgical emergencies. 4. Critical care medicine.
I. Siegel, John H., date. [DNLM: 1. Critical
Care. 2. Emergencies. 3. Shock. 4. Surgery,
Operative. 5. Wounds and Injuries. WO 700 T77565]
RD93.T687   1987   617'.1026   86–20788
ISBN 0–443–08330–4

Distributed in the United Kingdom by Churchill Livingstone,
Robert Stevenson House, 1-3 Baxter's Place, Leith Walk, Edinburgh
EH1 3AF, and by associated companies, branches, and representatives
throughout the world.

Accurate indications, adverse reactions, and dosage schedules for
drugs are provided in this book, but it is possible that they
may change. The reader is urged to review the package information
data of the manufacturers of the medications mentioned.

Sponsoring Editor: *Linda Panzarella*
Copy Editor: *Ozzievelt Owens*
Production Designer: *Rosalie Marcus*
Production Supervisor: *Sharon Tuder*

Printed in the United States of America

First published in 1987

This book is dedicated to three individuals whose contributions to my life and career have made it possible.

To my father, the late *Dr. Isadore A. Siegel, M.D.,* Emeritus Professor of Obstetrics and Gynecology at the University of Maryland, who encouraged me to go into medicine and provided me with a role model of a compassionate and academically oriented practitioner of surgery.

To *Dr. R. Adams Cowley, M.D.,* Professor of Cardiothoracic Surgery and Director of MIEMSS, who founded and fathered that magnificent instrument of comprehensive trauma care known as the Maryland Institute for Emergency Medical Services Systems, and who has given me the support and experience that has made it possible for me to understand the disease of trauma and its therapy.

To my wife, *Carol Siegel,* whose love, support, and at times, tolerant forbearance of my medical preoccupations over more than 30 years have permitted me the time to study, comprehend, and write about pathophysiology, trauma, and critical illness.

CONTRIBUTORS

Frederick Alexander, M.D.
Formerly, Surgical Resident, Department of Surgery, Brigham and Women's Hospital, Boston, Massachusetts; Presently, Resident in Surgery, Children's Hospital, University of Cincinnati College of Medicine, Cincinnati, Ohio

Lindsay Staubus Alger, M.D.
Assistant Professor of Obstetrics and Gynecology, Division of High Risk Obstetrics, University of Maryland School of Medicine, Baltimore, Maryland

Mark M. Applefeld, M.D.
Associate Professor of Medicine, University of Maryland School of Medicine; Director, Division of Cardiology, Mercy Hospital, Baltimore, Maryland

Donald C. Arthur, M.A., M.D.
Commander, Medical Corps, U.S. Navy; Senior Medical Officer, USS Kitty Hawk (CU 63), San Francisco, California; Resident, Department of Emergency Medicine, Naval Hospital Balboa, San Diego, California

William R. Beisel, M.D.
Formerly, Deputy for Science, U.S. Army Institute for Infectious Diseases, Fort Detrick, Maryland; Presently, Senior Associate, Department of Immunology and Infectious Disease, The Johns Hopkins School of Hygiene and Public Health, Baltimore, Maryland

George L. Blackburn, M.D., Ph.D.
Associate Professor of Surgery and Chief, Nutrition/Metabolism Laboratory, Harvard Medical School; Director of Nutrition Support Service, New England Deaconess Hospital, Boston, Massachusetts

Ulf Borg, B.S.
Senior Research Fellow, Pulmonary Function Laboratory, Maryland Institute for Emergency Medical Services Systems (MIEMSS), Baltimore, Maryland

David Bregman, M.D.
Associate Clinical Professor of Surgery, Columbia University College of Physicians and Surgeons, New York, New York; Chairman, Department of Surgery, St. Joseph's Hospital and Medical Center, Paterson, New Jersey

Andrew R. Burgess, M.D.
Assistant Professor of Surgery, University of Maryland School of Medicine; Director of Orthopedic Services, Maryland Institute for Emergency Medical Services Systems (MIEMSS), Baltimore, Maryland

Michael D. Burton, M.S., D.O.
Lieutenant Commander, Medical Corps, U.S. Navy Reserve; Head, Acute Care Division, Branch Clinic, Parris Island, Naval Hospital Beaufort, Beaufort, South Carolina; Medical Officer, Naval Medical Clinic, Key West, Florida

Ellis S. Caplan, M.D.
Associate Professor of Medicine, University of Maryland School of Medicine; Director of Infectious Disease Services, Maryland Institute for Emergency Medical Services Systems (MIEMSS), Baltimore, Maryland

Mark P. Carol, M.D.
Assistant Professor of Surgery, Division of Neurosurgery, University of South Florida College of Medicine, Tampa, Florida

Vincent D. Chang, M.D.
Surgical Resident, Department of Surgery, University of Rochester School of Medicine and Dentistry, Rochester, New York

Bart Chernow, M.D.
Associate Professor, Department of Anaesthesiology, Harvard Medical School; Associate Director, Respiratory Surgical Intensive Care Unit, Massachusetts General Hospital, Boston, Massachusetts

Bill Coleman, Ph.D.
Assistant Professor of Pathology, University of Maryland School of Medicine; Director of Mathematical and Statistical Research, Maryland Institute for Emergency Medical Services Systems (MIEMSS), Baltimore, Maryland

Everard F. Cox, M.D.
Associate Professor of Surgery, University of Maryland School of Medicine; Director of Surgery (Retired), Maryland Institute for Emergency Medical Services Systems (MIEMSS), Baltimore, Maryland

M. Carlyle Crenshaw, Jr., M.D.
Professor and Chairman, Department of Obstetrics and Gynecology, Division of High Risk Obstetrics, University of Maryland School of Medicine, Baltimore, Maryland

R. Ben Dawson, M.D.
Professor of Pathology, Associate Professor of Medicine, University of Maryland School of Medicine; Formerly, Director, Blood Bank, Division and Transfusion Service, University of Maryland Hospital; Director, Blood Research Lab, University of Maryland School of Medicine, Baltimore, Maryland

William R. Drucker, M.D.
Professor and Chairman, Department of Surgery, University of Rochester School of Medicine and Dentistry, Rochester, New York

Thomas B. Ducker, M.D.
Professor of Neurosurgery, University of Maryland School of Medicine; Formerly, Director, Neurotrauma Service, Maryland Institute for Emergency Medical Services Systems (MIEMSS), Baltimore, Maryland

C. Michael Dunham, M.D.
Assistant Professor of Surgery, University of Maryland School of Medicine; Attending Surgeon, Maryland Institute for Emergency Medical Services Systems (MIEMSS), Baltimore, Maryland

Glenn W. Geelhoed, M.D.
Professor of Surgery, Director of Surgical Research, George Washington University Medical Center, Washington, D.C.

Fred H. Geisler, M.D., Ph.D.
Assistant Professor of Neurosurgery, University of Maryland School of Medicine; Neurotrauma Service, Maryland Institute for Emergency Medical Services Systems (MIEMSS), Baltimore, Maryland

Steven A. Gould, M.D.
Associate Professor of Surgery, The University of Chicago Pritzker School of Medicine; Director, Blood Flow Laboratory, Michael Reese Hospital and Medical Center, Chicago, Illinois

Lazar J. Greenfield, M.D.
Professor and Chairman, Department of Surgery, Medical College of Virginia, Virginia Commonwealth University, Richmond, Virginia

Frank E. Gump, M.D.
Professor of Surgery, Columbia University College of Physicians and Surgeons, Columbia-Presbyterian Medical Center, New York, New York

Herbert B. Hechtman, M.D.
Professor of Surgery, Harvard Medical School and Brigham and Women's Hospital, Boston, Massachusetts

Robert J. Henning, M.D.
Associate Professor of Medicine, Case Western Reserve University School of Medicine; Chief, Medical Intensive Care Unit, University Hospitals of Cleveland, Cleveland, Ohio

Peter Kaskel, B.A.
Consultant in Circulatory Assistance, Department of Surgery, St. Joseph's Hospital and Medical Center, Paterson, New Jersey

Marvin M. Kirsh, M.D.
Professor of Thoracic Surgery, University of Michigan Medical School, Ann Arbor, Michigan

Marc E. Lanser, M.D.
Assistant Professor of Surgery, Harvard Medical School; Associate Director, Longwood Area Trauma Center at the Beth Israel, Brigham and Women's, and Children's Hospitals, Boston, Massachusetts

Shlomo Lelcuk, M.D.
Formerly, Surgical Fellow, Department of Surgery, Brigham and Women's Hospital, Boston, Massachusetts; Presently, Assistant Professor of Surgery, Hadassah University Hospital, Tel Aviv, Israel

Steven E. Linberg, Ph.D.
Clinical Research Scientist, Department of Clinical Medicine, Burroughs-Wellcome Company, Research Triangle Park, North Carolina; Assistant Professor of Pathology, University of Maryland School of Medicine; Research Associate, Maryland Institute for Emergency Medical Services Systems (MIEMSS), Baltimore, Maryland

Bert R. Mandelbaum, M.D.
Orthopedic Fellow, Orthopedic Services, Maryland Institute for Emergency Medical Services Systems (MIEMSS), Baltimore, Maryland

Paul N. Manson, M.D.
Associate Professor of Plastic Surgery, Johns Hopkins University; Director, Maxillo-Facial and Plastic Surgical Service, Maryland Institute for Emergency Medical Services Systems (MIEMSS), Baltimore, Maryland

Robert A. Margulies, M.D., M.P.H.
Captain, Medical Corps, U.S. Navy; Executive Officer, Naval Hospital Beaufort, Beaufort, South Carolina; Commanding Officer, Naval Hospital Camp Lejuene, Jacksonville, North Carolina

Louis L. Marzella, M.D., Ph.D.
Associate Professor of Pathology, University of Maryland School of Medicine; Director of Hyperbaric Research, Maryland Institute for Emergency Medical Services Systems (MIEMSS), Baltimore, Maryland

Gerald S. Moss, M.D.
Professor of Surgery, The University of Chicago Pritzker School of Medicine; Chief, Department of Surgery, Michael Reese Hospital and Medical Center, Chicago, Illinois

Roy A. M. Myers, M.D.
Assistant Professor of Surgery, University of Maryland School of Medicine; Director, Hyperbaric Chamber, Maryland Institute for Emergency Medical Services Systems (MIEMSS), Baltimore, Maryland

Richard M. Peters, M.D.
Professor of Surgery and Bioengineering, University of California, San Diego, School of Medicine, San Diego, California

Basil A. Pruitt, Jr., M.D.
Commander and Director, U.S. Army Institute for Surgical Research, Brooke Army Medical Center, Fort Sam Houston, Texas

Sheldon Randall, M.D.
Assistant Professor of Surgery, Harvard Medical School; Assistant Director, Nutrition/ Metabolism Laboratory, New England Deaconess Hospital, Boston, Massachusetts

Charles L. Rice, M.D.
Professor and Vice Chairman of Surgery, University of Washington School of Medicine; Surgeon-in-Chief, Harborview Medical Center, Seattle, Washington

Michael Salcman, M.D.
Professor and Head of Neurosurgery, Department of Surgery, University of Maryland School of Medicine; Director of Neurotrauma Service, Maryland Institute for Emergency Medical Services Systems (MIEMSS), Baltimore, Maryland

William Schumer, M.D.
Professor and Chairman, Department of Surgery; Professor, Department of Biochemistry, University of Health Sciences/Chicago Medical School, North Chicago, Illinois

Steven Sharpe, M.D.
Instructor in Medicine, Uniformed Services University of the Health Sciences School of Medicine, Bethesda, Maryland

David Shepro, Ph.D.
Professor of Physiology, Boston University, Boston, Massachusetts

John H. Siegel, M.D.
Professor of Surgery, University of Maryland School of Medicine; Professor of Surgery, Johns Hopkins University School of Medicine; Director, MIEMSS Clinical Center; Deputy Director, Maryland Institute for Emergency Medical Services Systems (MIEMSS), Baltimore, Maryland

William M. Stahl, M.D.
Professor and Vice Chairman, Department of Surgery, New York Medical College, Valhalla, New York; Director, Department of Surgery, Lincoln Medical and Mental Health Center, Bronx, New York

John K. Stene, M.D., Ph.D.
Assistant Professor of Anesthesiology, University of Maryland School of Medicine; Director of Anesthesiology, Maryland Institute for Emergency Medical Services Systems (MIEMSS), Baltimore, Maryland

Joan C. Stoklosa, B.S.
Director, Pulmonary Function Laboratory, Maryland Institute for Emergency Medical Services Systems (MIEMSS), Baltimore, Maryland

H. Harlan Stone, M.D.
Professor of Surgery and Chief, Division of General Surgery, University of Maryland School of Medicine, Baltimore, Maryland

Benjamin F. Trump, M.D.
Professor and Chairman, Department of Pathology and Research Programs, University of Maryland School of Medicine, Baltimore, Maryland

Thomas C. Vary, Ph.D.
Assistant Professor of Physiology, University of Maryland School of Medicine; Director of Biochemical Research, Maryland Institute for Emergency Medical Services Systems (MIEMSS), Baltimore, Maryland

Charles E. Wiles III, M.D.
Assistant Professor of Surgery, University of Maryland School of Medicine; Surgical Director, Critical Care Medicine, Maryland Institute for Emergency Medical Services Systems (MIEMSS), Baltimore, Maryland

PREFACE

Trauma, and in particular the high-velocity blunt trauma associated with motor vehicle and industrial accident injury, has become the major cause of death and disability for the working age population in the United States and other industrialized nations of the world. Presently, in the United States alone, the total cost of injury and long-term disability has been estimated in excess of 100 billion dollars per year. While the dollar equivalent cost of posttrauma medical care is less in most European and in all Latin American and Asian countries, it nevertheless represents a significant source of economic resource diversion in all modern societies, especially those that offer a package of health care benefits to their citizens.

In the past, the trauma patient was viewed as having a malfortuitous collection of injuries, each to be dealt with by a specialist in that particular anatomic system. The orthopedist set the bones, the neurosurgeon decompressed the traumatized brain or spinal cord, the general surgeon treated hemorrhage, shock, and visceral injuries, and the plastic surgeon attempted to recreate a cosmetic appearance that approximated a normal human physiogomy. The trauma-interested general surgeon was supposed to be captain of the team, but every general surgeon was assumed to be a trauma specialist regardless of the extent of his or her previous trauma experience, and no one discipline really devoted itself to teaching the organization and leadership skills needed for comprehensive care of the injured patient. Fortunately for present trauma victims, this view is changing. Recent developments in the study of physiologic, biochemical, and immunologic responses to shock and trauma, as well as clinical observations and classifications of injury patterns, have led to the conclusion that trauma, and especially blunt polytrauma, is a disease. The disease entity of trauma, like the disease that we call cancer, is in reality a set of related pathologies that have similar etiologies and that induce a similar set of host defense responses that determine the nature, extent, and severity of the disease process. As a result of this understanding, modern trauma care is predicated on a comprehensive knowledge of the basic mechanisms of cellular and organ injury and the integrated host response. This knowledge in turn mandates a protocol for timely resuscitation, diagnosis, emergency surgery, and critical care of the severely injured patient. Also, because of the magnitude of the impacting forces that induce the various types and patterns of multiple injuries, it is essential that a coordinated plan for multispecialty-multidisciplinary care be established from the very beginning of the therapeutic intervention and that this program be directed by a trauma surgeon who is an accomplished student of the trauma process and who is knowledgeable of the potential complications of this disease and its therapies.

The purpose of this book is not to provide an encyclopedic textbook that covers every conceivable topic in trauma care. Rather, it is to present a coordinated and interrelated set of chapters that are in themselves comprehensive indepth monographs. These address the major trauma surgical and critical care problems seen in adults. These subjects are approached by the contributors from a shared view about the nature and therapy of posttraumatic injury and its complications. However, this does not imply that every author has been chosen because he or she marches in lockstep with all of the others. The reader will find differences of opinion concerning the relative importance of a particular injury mechanism or host response and the value of certain specific therapeutic measures, but should also be impressed with the range of fundamental agreements on basic mechanisms, resuscitative and diagnostic goals, and priorities. It is our hope that the reader will achieve an understanding of the common philosophy that underlies state-of-the-art research-derived emergency surgery and critical care of the trauma patient. While the basic science and clinical science chapters have been authored by a group of individuals with international reputations as authorities in their respective fields of endeavor, the majority of chapters on the clinical approach to the multiple injury patients are derived from the experience of the staff of the Maryland Institute for Emergency Medical Services Systems. This has been done intentionally in order to present an example of how a particular comprehensive, coordinated, multispecialty-multidisciplinary institute's approach has been applied to reduce the mortality and morbidity of a large trauma patient population with severe multiple system injuries.

My colleagues and I sincerely hope that the readers of this book will find in it sufficient new information and innovative approaches to trauma care to justify their efforts. The strengths of this book lie in the depth of knowledge and extensive trauma-related experience of the contributors. Any weaknesses lie in my choices of topics and editorial direction, as reflected in the basic science emphasis of many of the chapters. I accept in advance all criticisms as mine and trust that the light of knowledge shed by my distinguished colleagues will shine through any murkiness imposed by my organizational and editorial inadequacies.

John H. Siegel, M.D.

ACKNOWLEDGMENT

I would like to acknowledge the important contribution to the construction and organization of the manuscripts that make up this book of Ms. Lynn Eminizer and Ms. Marie Armstrong who carried out many of the secretarial and coordinating tasks required and of Ms. Linda Panzarella of Churchill Livingstone who supported, encouraged, and suffered through its birth. I would also like to sincerely thank Mr. Miklos Fabian who has assisted me for more than 25 years in carrying out much of the experimental work reported in my portions of this book.

CONTENTS

SECTION VIII. Selected Problems in Trauma Care

TRAUMA

EMERGENCY SURGERY AND CRITICAL CARE

Trauma, the Disease of the 20th Century

John H. Siegel
C. Michael Dunham

Thou'rt slave to fate, chance, kings and desperate men

John Donne, Holy Sonnets, III

Trauma and its handmaiden, death, have stalked 20th century America, summoned in John Donne's words as the slaves to fate, chance, kings, and desperate men. Between 1980 and 1984 in the United States, there were between 140,000 and 150,000 fatal injuries yearly. This is equivalent in numbers to the death of every man, woman, and child in a moderate-sized American city such as Bridgeport, Connecticut; Raleigh, North Carolina; Newport News, Virginia; or Stockton, California, *each year!* In 1984, 44,241 deaths alone were related to motor vehicle accidents on the highways, including both occupants and pedestrians. This represented a 3.9 percent increase[10] over 1983. While exact figures for all causes of death in the United States are not yet available for 1984, complete data for the 147,884 fatalities occurring in 1982 have been analyzed by the National Center for Health Statistics[14]

(Table 1-1). The year 1982 had a comparable number of motor vehicle deaths, 44,786 (43,945 by the Fatal Accident Report System, FARS[10]), accounting for 30 percent of the total mortality from injury. In addition there were 13,013 deaths (9 percent) related to falls and jumps and 5,904 deaths (4 percent) due to fires or burns. Most disturbing were the 32,988 fatalities (22 percent) caused by firearms, because of these *only 5 percent were unintentional injuries*, while 93 percent were the result of either suicide (50 percent) or homicide (43 percent). Indeed, of the total mortality from injury for the 1982 year, 22,348 deaths (15 percent) were related to homicide or manslaughter (including 276 due to "legal intervention") and 28,242 deaths (19 percent) were caused by self-inflicted injury resulting in death. Viewed in another way, blunt trauma including motor vehicle, industrial, and farm accidents and other types of transportation injuries accounted for 43 percent of all deaths, penetrating trauma for 26 percent, drowning or suffocation for 9 percent, poisonings from solids or liquids, and

TABLE 1-1 Major Categories of Injury Deaths in 1982 in the United States

Injury Category	Unintentional	Suicide	Homicide	Undetermined	Total
Motor vehicles (traffic)	44,713	57	*a*	16	44,786
Firearms	1,756	16,575	14,117[b]	540	32,988
Falls and jumps	12,077	797	12	127	13,013
Drowning	6,351	530	85	387	7,353
Poisoning by solids or liquids	3,474	2,943	22	787	7,226
Fires and burns	5,364[c]	147	242	151	5,904
Suffocation, hanging, and strangulation	881	4,061	977	81	6,000
Cutting	118	409	4,365	36	4,928
Poisoning by motor vehicle carbon monoxide	596	2,032	*a*	163	2,791
Other	18,752[d]	691	2,528	924	22,895
Total	94,082	28,242	22,348	3,212	147,884

[a] Not separately identified in mortality statistics.

[b] Includes 276 firearm deaths termed "legal intervention."

[c] Includes 4,200 deaths from housefires, primarily attributable to carbon monoxide poisoning rather than burns.

[d] Includes about 2,600 deaths from surgical and medical complications and misadventures, 1,700 from airplane crashes, 1,400 deaths from machinery, 1,100 deaths from nontraffic motor vehicle crashes, 1,000 electrocutions, and 1,000 deaths caused by falling objects.

Data from National Center for Health Statistics. Motor vehicle deaths differ slightly from 1982 figures (43,945) obtained from Fatal Accident Reporting System (FARS) because of methodologic differences.

(Injury in America; A continuing public health problem. National Academic Press, Washington, D.C.; 1985, p. 23.)

burns and electrocutions for 5 percent each, and carbon monoxide toxic deaths for 2 percent of the total mortality.

Over the 10 years from 1975 to 1984, 470,512 Americans died on the nation's highways and there were more than 300,000 fatalities due to firearms. Considering that America's most reviled armed conflict, the Vietnamese War, resulted in the death of only 57,000 Americans over the immediately preceding 10 year period and produced a national crisis of confidence in America's leadership and governmental institutions, it remains a source of constant surprise and sorrow that contemporary America has accepted so passively a level of carnage, increasing year by year, by means that, to a significant extent, are preventable.

The injuries that produce these deaths are, of course, much more numerous than the fatal cases. It has been estimated that each year approximately 70 million Americans are injured severely enough to require medical treatment.[14] In 1984, 3.6 million were injured in motor vehicle accidents alone.[21] The numbers of individuals who sustain long-term disability following trauma is staggering. It has been estimated that each year 75,000 Americans receive brain injuries severe enough to produce long-term disability.[15] More than 6,000

injured individuals per year sustain spinal cord trauma sufficient to cause paraplegia or quadriplegia.[16] Trauma has been estimated to result in an annual loss of over 4 million years of future work life, compared to only 2.1 million years of lost work life due to heart disease and 1.7 million caused by cancer.[14] The total cost to society of these injuries has been estimated as between 75 to 100 billion dollars, resulting from both the direct hospital costs of injury and the estimated costs of disability, loss of income, and social services to the injured patient, or to his or her family.[14,26]

Trauma as classically described in the Smith Papyrus,[5] the treatise of Ambrose Paré,[23] and the works of John Hunter[13] and Theodor Billroth[4] was the medical science of wounds and the causes of these wounds. As stated by Paré in his famous *Apologie and Treatise*[23] published in 1585:

all things which may outwardly assayle the body with force and violence, may be counted the cause of wounds; which are called greene and properly bloody. These things are either animate, or inanimate. The animate, as the bitings, and prickings of beasts, the inanimate, as the stroake of an arrow, sword, clubb, gunne, stone, a dagger and all such like things.

For more than 300 years after Paré's remarkable dissertation on the causes of injury, the major preoccupation of surgeons concerned with trauma was the study of the mechanisms and treatments of penetrating injury. These studies produced many extremely important surgical advances. However, what appears to separate the practice of modern trauma surgery from that of the past, as the nations of the first and second worlds have moved from a state of perpetual wars between countries to that of civil "peace" interrupted by sporadic violence, has been the advent of major high-velocity blunt trauma as the primary cause of civilian injuries.

Blunt trauma was recognized in the past, primarily as the consequence of falls, or low-velocity explosions such as might occur with gunpowder or cannon balls. However, the pathophysiology and pattern of multiple system and organ injuries characteristic of 20th century trauma has followed the evolution of the modern industrial age with the development of the automobile, the motorcycle, and the airplane, and the creation of explosive compounds capable of producing enormous compression forces upon impact on the human body. These new inventions and their societal impact have opened a new era in the surgery of trauma and forced surgeons and critical care specialists with an interest in these problems to recognize a new and different set of patterns of injury pathophysiology that must be recognized and treated.

It is to the art of diagnosis and the science of the physiologic therapy of the multiply injured patient with blunt trauma that this book is primarily directed. Although important aspects of penetrating trauma are considered, as they must be, the purpose of this book is to focus on the polytraumatized patient with multiple organ and system injury. In these patients, critical care and surgical expertise must be combined in proper measure to effect a successful outcome, both in improving survival and reducing the disability that results from the unsuccessfully treated morbidity of multiple injury.

Since every experience is particular and peculiarly relevant to the population from which it is drawn, it is worth considering the patient population from which the Maryland

Institute for Emergency Medical Services Systems (MIEMSS) draws its case material, since this represents the major population group from which the clinical experience reported here is developed. Important chapters in this book are directed at issues related to the biochemical, physiologic, and immunologic aspects of trauma and critical care. Although, contributed by individuals with different clinical experiences, the material presented is of a general nature and the similarity of conclusions regarding basic science information serves to reinforce the universal nature of these observations. However, in contrast to these general issues, the specific clinical problems presented by the multiply injured patient are mainly elucidated by considering the prototypes seen in the large experience of the MIEMSS Systems.

MARYLAND SYSTEM FOR TRAUMA AND EMERGENCY MEDICAL SERVICES

Facilities and Population

The Maryland Institute for Emergency Medical Services Systems is a state agency embedded in a major state university with responsiblity for the organization and coordination of trauma and emergency services in a defined geopolitical population area. The state of Maryland, a geographic entity of 10,577 square miles, has divergent geographic areas ranging from largely rural mountainous regions in the Appalachian chain in the western part of the state to an agricultural tide-water area in the east, divided by a large bay from an heavily urbanized and industrially developed coastal plain in the central portion of the state. There are two major metropolitan areas, the city of Baltimore with its environs and the heavily populated suburbs surrounding Washington, D.C., which between them contain more than 3 million of the state's total 4.3 million popula-

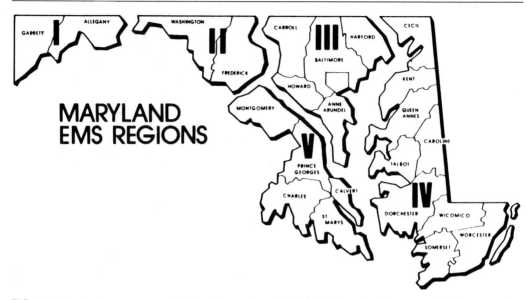

FIG. 1-1 Maryland emergency medical services regions. Each region has at least one areawide trauma center.

tion. The state is divided into five emergency medical services (EMS) regions (Fig. 1-1) in which there are nine regional trauma centers, five in the major EMS regions of the state and four within the city of Baltimore, the major metropolitan area. There are 5 specialty centers and approximately 20 other specialized functional units for EMS services. The central unit for the treatment of adults is the Maryland Institute for Emergency Medical Services Systems Clinical Center, located in Baltimore, which maintains a hospital facility of 89 beds. It is administratively part of and connected to the University of Maryland Medical System hospital for general medical and surgical care. A specialized center for pediatric trauma is located at the Children's Medical Center of the Johns Hopkins University Hospital which is linked to the EMS network and coordinated and controlled by the MIEMSS state system.

In the MIEMSS system, each of the regional trauma centers (Fig. 1-2) is assigned a well-defined geographic area for primary admissions. The MIEMSS Clinical Center and the Children's Medical Center accept patients from the entire state, as well as a small number of patients transported from the border areas of the four surrounding states. In addition, the MIEMSS Clinical Center also has an area of primary responsibility: the five counties surrounding the physical limits of Baltimore City. This particular designation of primary responsibility also plays a role in defining a major aspect of the patient population admitted to the MIEMSS Clinical Center. Through this corridor run the major highway systems connecting Washington and Baltimore with Philadelphia and New York. Consequently, a large percentage of the motor vehicle traffic of the state and region passes through this primary area; this accounts for the disproportionately large number of motor vehicle accidents admitted to the MIEMSS Clinical Center, with their associated high velocity multisystem injury pattern.

In coordinating the trauma and emergency medical services of the entire state, the MIEMSS system has developed an *echelons of care* protocol.[6] Under this protocol, patients with relatively minor traumatic injuries may be admitted to the nearest hospital, which is frequently one of the 74 community hospitals in the state. Patients with a more severe second level of injury are admitted to the regional trauma centers, or as primary cases to the MIEMSS Clinical Center from its area of responsibility. Cases representing specialty problems of a particular nature are referred to specialty centers. In the case of the Children's Medical Center, all major cases of trauma occurring in children below the age of

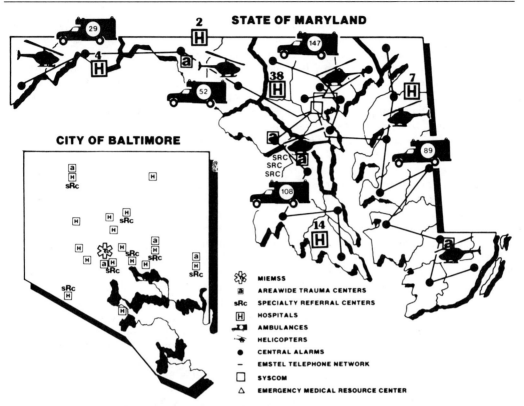

FIG. 1-2 The State of Maryland communications network and system of areawide centers, specialty referral centers, community hospitals, ambulances, helicopters and other emergency medical resources. The MIEMSS Clinical Center is located in the city of Baltimore and serves as the central adult unit for the entire state as well as the center for the communications network.

14 are transported directly to that facility. The MIEMSS Clinical Center is also a trauma specialty center and receives the majority of patients with major spine or spinal cord injury, significant head injury, and patients with major polytrauma, especially if they demonstrate severe physiologic instability, or shock, in the field.

The entire network of trauma centers, community hospitals, ambulances, and helicopters is linked by a communication system run by MIEMSS[22] (Fig. 1-2). It coordinates the activities of the more than 12,000 emergency medical technicians (EMTs) who are organized in either volunteer rescue squads or full-time county or municipal fire companies. The MIEMSS system is responsible for the maintenance of the communication network, for setting the standards for EMT training, for training the primary trainers of the EMTs, and for pre-paring and administering the certification examination for the EMTs at various levels. It is also responsible for programs of postgraduate education for physicians, nurses, and paramedical personnel involved in trauma and emergency medical services.

This organized and coordinated system of EMS care established by R. A. Cowley[6] has links to other agencies of the state. The most important is the legally mandated cooperation with the Maryland State Police, who provide the physical resources and manpower of the helicopter retrieval system. The medical aspects of this helicopter transport system are coordinated by MIEMSS.[7] The regulations demand a priority for medical retrieval over all other activities of surveillance and traffic monitoring, save armed pursuit of violent criminals (in which case a back-up helicopter would be available). The state police helicopter service provides rapid transport for injured patients from the site of injury to a regional trauma center, the specialized center for adults (MIEMSS), or, for children, to the JHU Children's Medical Center, as well as other specialized units such as a regional burn center, a center for neurologic injuries (also at MIEMSS Clinical Center), a hand surgical center, and an eye center. A second major area of interrelationship with another state agency is with the Maryland Institute for Fire and Rescue, which establishes training for the many local fire department's personnel who are often involved in rescue operations.

The MIEMSS legal mandate to coordinate these activities, as well to serve in a consultant relationship to the State Legislature regarding EMS legislation, has allowed the development of a comprehensive system for trauma and emergency medical services throughout the state of Maryland. It has also ensured the rapid transport of injured patients to an appropriate center within the briefest possible period, "the golden hour," so that the physiologic derangements produced by the injury or secondary hypovolemia can be corrected in the shortest possible time. In addition, the MIEMSS system coordinates and facilitiates interhospital transfers from either community hospitals or regional trauma centers to the MIEMSS Clinical Center or one of the other specialty centers, should a patient have a more serious problem than originally recognized by the field provider. This feature allows for triage and resuscitation of certain types of cases at the nearest qualified center with immediate transfer on stabilization to a definitive center, which can then provide all appropriate diagnostic and therapeutic facilities.

MIEMSS Clinical Center

The MIEMSS Clinical Center has evolved over more than 20 years from a two-bed shock research unit into a full-fledged institute that presently admits more than 2,300 adult patients per year.[19,20] The professional staff includes 33 full- or major part-time faculty members of the University of Maryland and/or the Johns Hopkins University, in the fields of general and thoracic surgery, orthopedic surgery, neurosurgery, plastic surgery, oral surgery, critical care medicine, anesthesiology, infectious disease, hyperbaric medicine, and psychiatry. There are also 23 clinical Fellows in the fields of general surgery, critical care medicine, orthopedics, neurosurgery, anesthesiology, infectious disease, plastic surgery, and hyperbaric medicine as well as a variable number of research Fellows. All of the clinical Fellows have finished their board eligibility requirements for certification by the American Board of Surgery, Orthopedic Surgery, Neurologic Surgery, Medicine, Emergency Medicine, or Anesthesiology with a full level of residency training in a recognized American or Canadian institution. The Institute also serves as a training ground for residents who rotate through the general and specialty surgery, critical care medicine, emergency medicine, plastic surgery, anesthesiology, and psychiatry services from more than 28 different residency training programs, primarily on the east coast and in the central United States, as well as from the United States military services. It also provides experience in trauma medicine and surgery to fourth-year medical students from the University of Maryland and for students from other academic institutions on elective rotations. The Institute has its own cadre of 250 nurses, and maintains its own trauma admitting area and operating rooms, as well as bed units for acute and stepdown critical care and neurotrauma care. The nursing staff for these areas functions under a system of primary nursing care responsiblity and is organized into homogeneous level of care units supervised by a dedicated MIEMSS Nursing Director. In addition, there are specialized paramedical professional services in the areas of family services, speech pathology, respiratory therapy, physiotherapy, and psychology. The MIEMSS Clinical Director reports to the Director of the statewide MIEMSS system, who is in turn responsible to the Chancellor of the University of Maryland at Baltimore.

The Institute also coordinates the activities of a major trauma rehabilitation unit of 50 beds at an affiliated institution with professional rehabilitation physicians who serve both at the rehabilitation facility and as consultants to the MIEMSS Clinical Center. This facility serves as the acute rehabilitation unit for victims of major spinal cord and head injury, as well as for patients with major orthopedic injury who require late secondary or tertiary procedures. All secondary reconstructive procedures are done at the MIEMSS Clinical Center by the same staff of medical professionals who began the patient's primary care, so that a comprehensive program of medical, surgical, and rehabilitative care can be established and carried to completion.

DEMOGRAPHICS AND COSTS OF INJURY

Obtaining the comprehensive demographics of injury has been difficult in the United States[3,14] as well as in other western countries and is nearly impossible to estimate in less developed countries. However, because of the overlapping systems of trauma reporting in the state of Maryland, it is possible to obtain information from a variety of sources, which, together, demonstrate with a reasonable degree of accuracy the pattern of injury in a modern industrialized state. This rate is shown for motor vehicle accidents in Table 1-2, which summarizes incidents reported from the field as

developed by the Maryland Automated Accident Reporting System (MAARS) in which the number of motor vehicle accidents and the incidence of injury of various severities is reported.[8] As demonstrated in this table, the number of accidents from 1980 to 1983 remained relatively constant, as did the incidence of the various severities of injury resulting from these accidents. However, there was a drop in the fatality rate from 1980 to 1983 even though the incidence of the more severe class of injuries increased slightly during this period. As is also demonstrated from this table, on the average 10,698 motor vehicle accident victims had injuries whose severity was either incapacitating or fatal. These severe injuries occurred in 8.8 percent of all motor vehicle accidents, or 23 percent of motor vehicle accidents producing any injury, and, except in those instances where death was apparent on the roadway, were serious enough to require admission to a hospital. Both the incidence of serious motor vehicle accident (MVA) injury and the mortality rate showed a seasonal variation, being highest in the summer months and lowest in the winter.[8] The trend in MVA deaths is similar to that in the United States as a whole,[10] where the mortality declined from 51,091 in 1980 to 42,584 in 1983. However, of concern is the finding, in many states and nationally, that in 1984 and 1985 the death rate has either not fallen, or has actually risen. More ominous for the future is the fact that the percent increase of fatalities in accidents involv-

TABLE 1-2. Motor Vehicle Accidents and Injuries: State of Maryland, 1980–1983

Year	Damage Only		Possible Injury		Nonincapac-itating		Incapaci-tating		Fatal		Total
	N	%	N	%	N	%	N	%	N	%	
1980	75,530	62.4	20,486	16.9	14,839	12.3	9,586	7.9	704	0.6	121,145
1981	73,636	61.6	20,535	17.2	14,651	12.3	10,118	8.5	701	0.6	119,641
1982	74,422	62.4	20,322	17.0	14,108	11.8	9,858	8.3	595	0.5	119,305
1983	75,731	61.5	21,774	17.7	14,486	11.8	10,620	8.6	613	0.5	123,224
Total	299,317	61.9	83,117	17.2	58,084	12.0	40,182	8.3	2,613	0.5	483,313
Mean	74,829	61.9	20,779	17.2	14,521	12.0	10,045	8.3	653	0.5	120,828

10,698
(23% of all injuries)

(Dischinger PC, Shankar BS, Kochesfani D et al: Automotive collisions involving serious injury or death: an analysis of trends over time (1980–1983) in Maryland. Amercan Association for Automotive Medicine, 29th Proceedings, 1985, p. 287.)

TABLE 1-3.   Increase in Trauma as a Cause of Hospitalization: State of Maryland, 1980–1983

Date	Year				% Change in 3 years (1980–1983)
	1980	1981	1982	1983	
All hospital discharges	579,089	591,357	614,406	626,809	8.21
All trauma discharges	31,183	33,301	33,718	33,466	7.32
Severe trauma (ISS ≥ 13)	4,182	4,469	4,572	4,745	13.46
Population	4,216,975	4,242,436	4,267,897	4,293,359	1.81
Incidence of severe trauma per 100,000 pop.	99.2	109.6	107.1	110.5	11.39

(Shanker BS, Dischinger PC, Cowley RA: Am J Public Health, submitted 1986)

ing compact or smaller cars has risen by nearly 40 percent as these types of automobiles have become a larger proportion of the total vehicles in service.[10,11]

With regard to the incidence of all trauma during this period, Shankar and his colleagues[24] have compared the increase in total trauma discharges as well as severe trauma discharges (injury severity scores, ISS $\geq$ 13) to the increase in all hospital discharges, as a function of the growth in population in the state of Maryland. These data, presented in Table 1-3, clearly show that trauma, and especially severe trauma, has increased, both absolutely and relative to the rate of population growth, disproportionate to the rise in other diseases requiring hospitalization. In the case of severe trauma (ISS $\geq$ 13) this rise was 1.6 times the rate of increase in all discharges, 1.8 times the rate of rise in all hospitalized trauma, and 7.4 times the rate of increase in population growth. These data strongly suggest that traumatic injury is rising as cause of disease requiring medical care.

Cost of Trauma Care

Looking only at the more serious types of injuries to put in perspective the nature, pattern, and cost of causes of trauma, Shankar (unpublished data, 1985) studied the Health Services Cost Review Commission data of 1984 for 21,685 Maryland trauma admissions to hospital in which the cause of trauma was identified. This group of serious injuries represented about 65 percent of all patients hospitalized

for trauma in the state. Of these injuries 5,046 (23 percent) were caused by motor vehicle accidents; 7,614 (35 percent) represented injuries secondary to falls; 208 (1 percent) represented burn injuries; 4,614 (21 percent) represented injuries secondary to industrial, farm, or construction accidents; 224 (1 percent) represented suicide attempts; and 1,713 (7.9 percent) represented the consequence of a violent crime or homicide attempt in which the patient survived to reach the hospital. These data are roughly in keeping with those reported for other major metropolitan areas in the United States.

It is of importance in understanding the fiscal impact of trauma care to consider the in-hospital cost of caring for these injuries. The total bill for the 21,685 Maryland patients with traumatic injuries studied was $157,835,106. Of this $39,531,000, or 25 percent of the total cost, was incurred by patients with motor-vehicle-related injuries. Injuries related to falls incurred costs of $38,368,000 (24.3 percent), costs of $31,738,000 (20.1 percent) were due to industrial and farm-related injuries, trauma caused by violent crime resulted in costs of $15,593,000 (9.9 percent), burns and suicide, respectively, accounted for $2.4 million (1.5 percent) and $972,000 (1 percent) of total costs.

These dollar values represent only a fraction of the total cost of care, since, as indicated by studies of MVA injuries,[12,25] the consequences of prolonged rehabilitation care out of the acute hospital, the loss of job income, and the requirements for social services, such as aid to dependent children, unemployment compensation, and the cost of long-term disability compensated for by workers' compensation, or other disability insurance, will increase this bill by several times. Consider that

TABLE 1-4. Summary of Societal Costs of Motor Vehicle Accidents, 1980[a] (Millions of Dollars)

	AIS Injury Level[b]						
	1	2	3	4	5	Fatality	Total
Medical Costs	543	622	631	335	1,125	70	3,326
Productivity Losses	319	251	313	451	801	12,102	14,237
Property Loss	2,656	612	424	100	33	174	3,999
Other Losses	3,933	590	684	640	245	1,384	7,476
Total	7,451	2,075	2,052	1,526	2,204	13,730	29,038

[a] Government costs are not included in this table as they are not additive with the other cost categories.

[b] Injury level represents the maximum AIS level survivors. All fatalities are shown in the Fatality column, no matter what the injury level prior to death. 1, minor; 2, moderate; 3, serious; 4, severe; 5, critical.

(Adapted from *The Economic Cost to Society of Motor Vehicle Accidents.* National Highway Traffic Safety Administration: U.S. Department of Transportation, Washington, D.C., Report DOT HS 806 342, 1983.)

Maryland includes approximately 1.8 percent of the population of the United States and assume that its incidence of injury is approximately the same as for the rest of the United States and that the same cost can be extrapolated to the remaining Maryland trauma admissions. This total cost of hospitalization of injury, $157.8 million for 22 thousand trauma victims, is therefore roughly equivalent to $13.5 billion of direct hospital costs in the United States for the 1984 year, with 3.4 billion of these medical care costs due to MVA. This figure for MVA is of the same order of magnitude as that obtained by a different methodology by the National Highway Traffic Safety Administration (NHTSA) for 1980 using the National Accident Sampling System (NASS) data[21,25] (Table 1-4).

The estimates of indirect costs are harder to come by for all injuries. However, the NHTSA studies for 1980 of the societal costs of 4,023,000 injuries resulting from motor vehicle accidents (Table 1-4) showed that the $3.3 billion in medical costs generated a staggering $29 billion in total costs, or an indirect cost factor of *7.7 times* the cost of direct medical care.[25] Legal and court costs (Table 1-5) for the average case ranged from 8 percent of $97.023 for an abbreviated injury scale[1] (AIS) category 5 injury, to 320 percent of $166 for an AIS category 1 injury, with an incredible 978 percent of the direct medical cost for the average fatal accident and insurance costs similarly scaled. These figures make the outrageous legal fees and court costs incurred by the unfortunate victims of the Chancery Court

TABLE 1-5. Legal and Insurance Costs and Productivity Loss as Percent of Average Medical Cost Per Case (1980)

	AIS Injury Level					
	1	2	3	4	5	Fatality
Medical costs ($)	**166**	**1,377**	**3,153**	**9,598**	**97,020**	**1,370**
% Legal and court costs	320	99	85	54	8	978
% Insurance expense	320	39	17	131	13	914
% Productivity loss	59	40	50	135	71	17,289
% All other costs (excluding property loss)	184	57	106	106	101	185
% All costs (excluding property damage)	883	235	258	426	193	19,366

(Data from *The Economic Cost to Society of Motor Vehicle Accidents* National Highway Traffic Safety Administration: U.S. Department of Transportation, Washington, D.C., Report DOT HS 806 342, 1983.)

described in Charles Dickens' great novel of societal abuse, *Bleak House,* seem trivial compared to today's expenses. These data strongly suggest that a closer look at these aspects of the cost of injury, which alone account for 2.2 times the cost of direct medical care, may be a more cost- and quality-effective means of reducing the societal cost of injury than are financial strictures limiting the scope of diagnostic and therapeutic options for the injured.

Finally, applying the factors in Table 1-4 and 1-5, excluding property damage (which may not be applicable) to the remaining 10.1 billion estimated direct medical cost for non-MVA injuries gives a 1984 estimated figure of $102 billion for all direct and indirect costs of injury, except associated property damage: a figure large enough to fund most of this nation's social welfare programs for the poor, or nearly one-third of the proposed 1987 defense budget of the United States.

The MIEMSS Experience

The Maryland Institute for Emergency Medical Services Systems admits approximately 5 percent of the hospitalized injured patients in the state of Maryland. As shown in Figure 1-3, over the past 12 years the number of total admissions has increased from slightly under 1000 in 1973 to 1954 in 1984, with more than 2,100 during the 1985 fiscal year.[19,20] This is related in part to an increase in compliance with the echelons of care protocols of the system. However, in recent years (as shown in Table 1-3) it has clearly reflected the increase in serious injuries in the state relative to the incidence of hospitalizations for other types of disease.

The pattern of causes of injuries (Fig. 1-4) treated by the MIEMSS trauma center has remained extremely constant, with MVA-related injuries (automobile, motorcycle, pedestrian) representing between 52 and 58 percent of the total admissions. On the average there has been a greater than 85 percent incidence of blunt trauma and an occurrence of between 12 and 15 percent of penetrating trauma injuries of the more severe type.[9,19,20]

The age distribution (Fig. 1-5) is consistent with national data indicating that the bulk of cases occur in persons younger than 40, with the mean age being approximately 26 years. However, there is a second smaller rise in patients admitted over the age of 60, which reflects the increased incidence of falls and the vulnerability of this older population to crime.

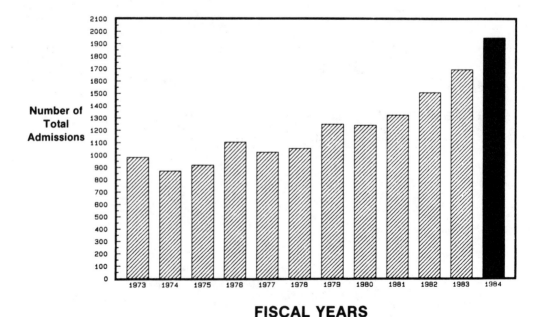

FISCAL YEARS

FIG. 1-3 The MIEMSS Clinical Center total admissions by fiscal year (June–July) from 1973 to 1984, showing the progressive increase in numbers of admissions to the central unit MIEMSS of the Maryland state system.

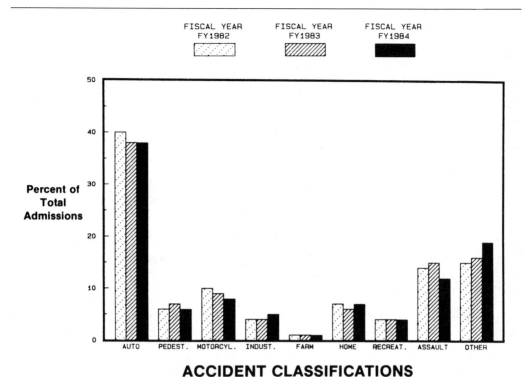

ACCIDENT CLASSIFICATIONS

FIG. 1-4 The MIEMSS Clinical Center accident classification for fiscal years 1982, 1983, and 1984 by type of injury or injury location.

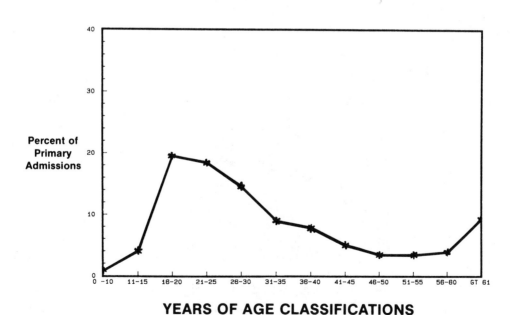

YEARS OF AGE CLASSIFICATIONS

FIG. 1-5 The MIEMSS Clinical Center patient age distribution for fiscal year 1984, as percent of primary admissions. Peak admissions are in the 16 through 20 age range. There is a secondary peak in the greater-than-60 age range.

In 1984 to 1985, for example, 42 percent of patients admitted to MIEMSS were under 25, 74 percent were under 40, and only 6.5 percent of the patients were in the over-60 range. This preponderance of young patients shows the importance of an organized trauma system in treating a young population with a high potential for complete recovery, or for rehabilitation with limited disability. The potential for reducing the death rate is also high, since trauma is the leading cause of death[14] in the United States for persons under 44 years of age. On the average, three quarters of MIEMSS patients were male and the vast majority were employed and were often the major wage earner in a young and growing family.

The pattern of injury distribution of patients without head or spinal cord injury compared to that of the nine areawide trauma centers (AWTC) is shown in Figure 1-6, which demonstrates that the clinical center admits a patient population whose injury distribution is skewed to the higher end of the injury severity score (ISS).[2] Even patients with lower ISS scores (1 to 12) admitted to MIEMSS generally have a more severe class of injury, based on their potential for disability, for example, a compound, comminuted fracture of the tibia with tissue loss or disruption.

The MIEMSS Clinical Center also admits about 15 percent of patients who do not have traumatic injury, including those with smoke inhalation, or those with anaerobic infections who are admitted for hyperbaric oxygen therapy. The diagnosis and therapy of these extremely ill types of patients are discussed in Chapter 37. Some desperately sick patients are transferred from other critical care units because of severe respiratory insufficiency or sepsis.

Over the past 3 years approximately 85 percent of the total MIEMSS admissions have involved some form of serious trauma, as shown in Figure 1-7. This figure also demon-

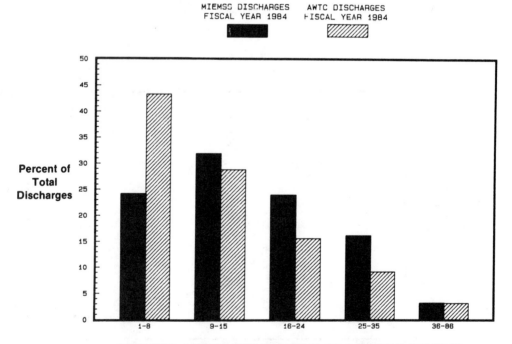

Injury Severity Score > 0

INJURY SEVERITY SCORE CLASSIFICATIONS

FIG. 1-6 The MIEMSS trauma discharges compared to those of areawide trauma centers for fiscal year 1984, by injury severity score.

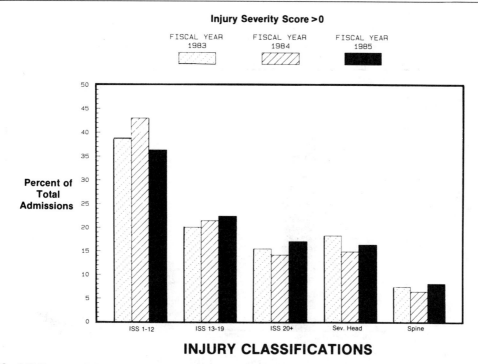

Injury Severity Score >0

INJURY CLASSIFICATIONS

FIG. 1-7 Pattern of distribution of injury severity scores, severe head injuries, and spinal cord injuries on admittance into MIEMSS Clinical Center over 3 fiscal years (1983, 1984, and 1985).

strates the ISS distribution of polytrauma patients without major neurologic injury as well as the percent admitted with severe head or spinal cord injuries who were admitted to MIEMSS because of its designation as the spinal cord and head injury center for the state. As can be seen, the distribution and percentage of admissions in each of these areas has remained relatively constant over the past 3 years. There has been a slight increase in percent of the nonneurologic polytrauma injuries with higher ISS scores, as increased compliance with the echelons of care system has tended to select out those cases with a more severe set of injuries for admission to MIEMSS, in preference to the areawide trauma centers.

As shown in Figure 1-8, approximately 70 percent of MIEMSS trauma admissions were brought direct from the site of injury and approximately 25 percent of the admissions were triaged first at a community hospital or regional trauma center. Approximately 75 percent of all patients were transported by helicopter (79 percent of the direct trauma admissions) and the remaining patients were brought by land transport. In addition, a small but increasing percentage of admissions were readmissions of former patients for delayed reconstructive procedures, generally of a plastic surgical or orthopedic nature.

To provide a picture of the pattern of injures represented in the patient population, data from the last completely analyzed year (June 1983 to July 1984; FY1984) has been used to show the types of injuries and outcomes. In fiscal year 1984, of the 1,954 total admissions 1,651 represented those admitted for trauma. This percentage is almost identical to that in 1985, during which 1,768 trauma admissions occurred out of 2,104 total admissions.

Of the 1,651 trauma admissions in 1984 (Table 1-6), it can be seen that blunt trauma accounted for 1,448 or 87.7 percent, with 54.4 percent being MVA-related and 7.9 percent pedestrian accidents. Falls accounted for 14 percent of all trauma admissions, violent crime accounted for 15.9 percent of injuries, with penetrating injuries representing 12 percent of

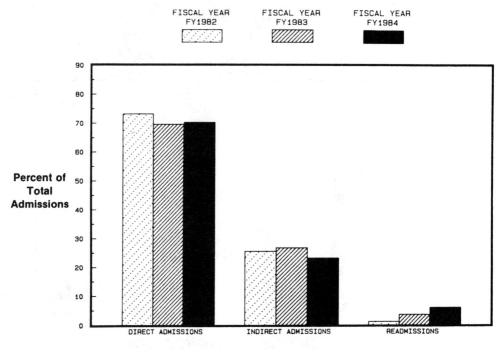

ADMISSION TYPES

FIG. 1-8 Distribution of direct versus indirect admissions for fiscal years 1982, 1983, and 1984. Direct admissions are those retrieved from the field. Indirect admissions are triaged first at a community hospital, or an areawide trauma center, prior to transfer to MIEMSS. Readmissions are previous trauma patients who are readmitted for secondary reconstructive procedures.

TABLE 1-6.   Types of Injuries in 1,651 MIEMSS Trauma Patients, 1983–1984

	Number of Patients with Injury		% of Patients
Trauma			
Blunt	1448		87.7
Penetrating	198		12.0
Both	5		0.3
Blunt trauma (n = 1448)		% Blunt	
Vehicle	728	50.3	44.1
Motorcycle	170	11.7	10.3
Pedestrian	130	9.0	7.9
Bicycle	17	1.2	1.0
Fall	231	16.0	14.0
Crush	87	6.0	5.3
Beating	64	4.4	3.9
Diving	21	1.5	1.3
Penetrating trauma (n = 198)		% Penetrating	
Gunshot only	120	60.6	7.3
Shotgun	16	8.1	1.0
Knife only	43	21.7	2.6
Gunshot and knife	2	1.0	0.1
Other	17	8.6	1.0

trauma admissions; of these 70 percent involved gunshot wounds. Of the total patients, 74.3 percent were male and 79.9 percent were white. The demographics of age showed that 75.7 percent of admitted patients were between the ages of 13 and 40, 15.5 percent were between 41 and 60, and only 8.3 percent were older than 60. However, 18.7 percent of all trauma patients had some form of chronic illness prior to their acute injury.

PATTERNS OF INJURY

Tables 1-7 and 1-8 demonstrate the numbers of patients sustaining various types of major organ injuries, major soft tissue, or osseous injuries. As can be seen in Table 1-7, 43.4 percent of all patients had injury to the central nervous system (34.7 percent to the brain and 8.7 percent to the spinal cord), 10.1 percent had injuries to the thoracic viscera, 17.4 percent

sustained injuries to the intra-abdominal or retroperitoneal structures, and only 3.4 percent sustained peripheral arterial or major venous vascular injury, including injuries of the abdominal aorta.

In soft tissue and osseous trauma (Table 1-8), injuries to the head can be seen to represent the largest single category, with 14.7 percent of patients having fractures of the skull and 19.8 percent injuries to the maxillofacial bones or jaw. Spinal column fractures accounted for 12.3 percent of patients (7.2 percent involving the cervical spine) and 75.2 percent of all patients sustained a significant soft tissue laceration of head or face. Other than soft tissue contusions and lacerations of the body or extremities, which appeared in 81.1 percent of all patients, lower extremity injuries were the most common form of orthopedic problem, accounting for 32.8 percent of all patients' injuries. Pelvic fractures were present in 6.2 percent of patients and osseous injuries to the thoracic torso (ribs or sternal fractures) occurred in 11.1 percent of patients. Upper extremity injuries were present in 23.3 percent of trauma admissions. There was a total of 1,227 major organ injuries (21.2 percent) and

TABLE 1-7. Organ Injuries in 1,651 MIEMSS Trauma Patients, 1983–1984

Major Organ Injuries	Number of Patients with Injury		% of Patients	
Brain	573		34.7	
(severe brain injury)	(279)	717	(16.9)	43.4
Spinal cord	144		8.7	
Heart	34		2.1	
Thoracic great vessels	19	167	1.2	10.1
Lung	114		6.9	
Diaphram	18		1.1	
Esophagus and stomach	7		0.4	
Duodenum	6		0.4	
Small bowel	20		1.2	
Colon and rectum	31		1.9	
Pancreas	9	287	0.5	17.4
Spleen	62		3.8	
Liver	75		4.5	
Kidney	32		1.9	
Ureter, bladder, and urethra	6		0.4	
Vena cava, hepatic, mesenteric, renal veins	21		1.3	
Peripheral arterial (including abdominal aorta)	52	56	3.2	3.4
Femoral vein	4		0.2	
Brachial plexus and peripheral nerve	33		2.0	
Total	1,227			

TABLE 1-8. Soft Tissue and Osseous Injuries in 1,651 MIEMSS: Trauma Patients, 1983–1984

Soft Tissue and Osseous Injuries	Number of Patients with Injury	% of Patients
Skull fractures	243	14.7
Basilar	(109)	(6.6)
Calvarium	(181)	(11.0)
Maxillofacial and jaw fractures	326	19.8
Head and face soft tissue laceration	1241	75.2
Rib or sternal fractures	183	11.1
Spinal column fractures	203	12.3
Cervical	(118)	(7.2)
Thoracic	(42)	(2.5)
Lumbar	(33)	(2.0)
Cervical and thoracic	(7)	(0.4)
Thoracic and lumbar	(3)	(0.2)
Pelvic fractures	102	6.2
Upper extremity (fracture, dislocation, amputation)	384	23.3
Clavicle or Scapula Fractures	(87)	(5.3)
Humerus fractures	(54)	(3.3)
Radius fractures	(25)	(1.5)
Ulnar fractures	(32)	(2.0)
Wrist, hand, digital fractures	(124)	(7.5)
Lower extremity (fracture, dislocation, amputation)	541	32.8
Femur fractures	(122)	(7.4)
Tibia fractures	(123)	(7.5)
Ankle fractures	(61)	(3.7)
Foot fractures	(44)	(2.7)
Other soft tissue injuries (body or extremities)	1339	81.8
Total	4,562[a]	

[a] Total of all injuries (Tables 1-7 and 1-8): 5,789 or 3.5 injuries/patient: 21.2% visceral organ injuries, 78.8% osseous or soft tissue injuries. Numbers in parentheses are not included in the total.

4,562 soft tissue or osseous injuries (78.8 percent) out of a total of 5,785 injuries in the 1,651 patients, *for an average of 3.5 injuries per patient.* As will be noted later this is consistent with the need for a multidisciplinary, multispecialty service that can organize resuscitative care and whose members can plan and carry out simultaneous operative procedures at the time of initial injury.

Resuscitative Problems

PREADMISSION

In this group of 1,651 trauma patients, 77.2 percent were brought to the MIEMSS Clinical Center directly from the scene of accident and of these direct admissions 74.1 percent were transported by helicopter. Of all trauma patients seen in 1984, 64 (3.9 percent) were noted to have had a cardiac arrest in the field and 12.6 percent had a blood pressure of less than 90 mmHg reported from the field. Other patients became hypotensive during transport and as a result 17.4 percent of all admissions were brought in by the field providers in military anti-shock trousers (MAST) or suit. Cardiac arrest on admission was present in 62 (3.8 percent) of patients and of these 95.2 percent died in the admitting area. The fact that there was very little difference between the numbers of patients who had a preadmission cardiac arrest and those who were in arrest on admission suggests that the immediacy of field resuscitation by trained EMT teams and the rapidity of field transport following acute trauma life support (ATLS) protocols is an efficient and effective way of reducing the acute postinjury hypovolemic mortality to a minimum.

ADMISSION

The basic principles of the MIEMSS approach to the acutely injured patient are to resuscitate first, to prevent maneuvers or delays that may further harm the already traumatized patient, and to carry out x-ray studies and other diagnostic procedures during the stable periods between the critical resuscitative measures. This philosophy and its practical considerations are outlined in Chapter 26.

The rationale for this protocol approach is seen in the analysis of resuscitation problems. Following admission to the MIEMSS Clinical Center admitting area, 46.4 percent of the entire group of trauma patients required intubation, and of these 49.9 percent were intubated in the first 30 minutes, 8.9 percent in the second 30 minutes, and 41.2 percent after the first hour. This need for early intubation focuses on the value of a close coordination between the surgical admitting team and an anesthesiologist experienced in treating trauma, *all physically present* in the admitting area, as is discussed in Chapter 27.

Hypotension was found on admission in 15.7 percent of the patients (excluding those with cardiac arrest), indicating the need for rapid volume resuscitation measures. Major external hemorrhage was present in 8.5 percent of all admissions and the total blood volume given within the first 24 hours is shown in Table 1-9 for 1,478 of the trauma patients (excluding those with cardiac arrest, or with a Glasgow coma scale score less than 5, where the major life-threatening problem was generally related to the lethality of the head injury). In this group it can be seen that 22.3 percent of patients required more than 500 ml blood and 8.5 percent required more than 2,000 ml blood. The role of acute coagulation disorders in trauma patients with intravascular volume losses of these magnitudes is of great importance. The diagnosis and treatment of coagulation in the setting of acute trauma are presented in Chapter 23. As also shown in this figure, the percent mortality for these patients was directly related to the volume of blood required for resuscitation in the first 24 hours.

A related observation (Table 1-10) shows the magnitude of the intraoperative hemorrhage in those patients receiving blood during surgery; the magnitude of this blood loss is also seen to be directly related to the increase in eventual mortality. The physiologic mechanisms related to the establishment of cardiovascular compensation for intraoperative hemorrhage, the need for volume replacement and the type of volume to be administered, and the use of vasodilator or inotropic support in shock resuscitation and during the intraoperative and post hemorrhage periods are discussed in Chapters 6 to 9.

A particularly difficult group of patients to resuscitate and to treat after serious traumatic injury are pregnant women who are near term. These women have a particular sensitivity to acute hemorrhagic volume loss and posi-

TABLE 1-9. Resuscitative Blood Requirements in the Initial 24 Hours

Total Blood Given (ml packed red cells)[a]	Number of Patients (n = 1,478)	% Patients	% Mortality
0	1047	70.8	1.4
1–500	98	6.6	2.0
501–1,000	104	7.0	2.9
1,001–2,000	103	7.0	7.8
2,000–3,000	41	2.8	14.6
3,000–4,000	33	2.2	15.2
4,001–5,000	23	1.6	30.4
5,001–10,000	23	1.6	39.1
>10,000	6	0.1	50.0

[a] Excludes patients with cardiac arrest or Glasgow coma scale ≤5.

TABLE 1-10. Magnitude of Intraoperative Blood Loss

	Number of Patients (n = 1,478)	% Mortality
Major external hemorrhage	141	8.5
Operative blood loss for all trauma (ml)*a*		
0	967	2.0
1–500	216	3.2
501–1,000	105	3.8
1,001–2,000	74	8.1
2,001–3,000	49	10.2
3,001–4,000	18	5.6
4,001–5,000	14	21.4
>5,000	35	37.1

a Excludes patients with cardiac arrest or Glasgow coma scale ≤5.

tional changes. Also, the trauma surgeon who is not an obstetrician must be concerned simultaneously with the salvage of two lives, mother and baby, and with protecting the fetus from hypoxemia during resuscitation and surgery and from radiation injury during diagnostic studies. On rare occasions, it is necessary for the trauma surgeon to perform an emergency caesarean section in the case of maternal death. These decisions and the technique for postmortem caesarean delivery are discussed in Chapter 35.

Other important resuscitation problems are presented by patients with major body burns either from thermal or caustic injuries. While the Maryland state EMS system coordinated by MIEMSS includes an excellent regional burn unit, perhaps the unique and most varied national experience in acute burn management is available from the Brooke Army Hospital Burn Unit. For that reason we have chosen to complement the chapters on the MIEMSS trauma experience with that of the burn program at Brooke presented by Dr. Basil Pruitt in Chapter 36.

Though less frequent as civilian trauma admissions, important thermally related environmental injuries are produced by acute hypothermia with local cold injury or by acute hyperthermia with associated dehydration. In these areas as well the military experience is the most comprehensive available and is discussed by the Navy group in Chapter 20.

The relationship of shock, direct contusion injury to the lung, and the volume and type of resuscitation fluids given as mechanisms un-

derlying the development of the posttraumatic adult respiratory distress syndrome (ARDS) are discussed in Chapters 18 and 19. The incidence of this troublesome and often fatal syndrome was studied in a similar group of 1,768 MIEMSS trauma patients seen in the 1984 to 1985 fiscal year. This group had an almost identical incidence of blunt versus penetrating trauma as the 1983 to 1984 patients. It was found that 19.0 percent of trauma patients were considered to be at risk for ARDS and of those at risk 34.1 percent actually developed the full-blown ARDS syndrome with an eventual 39.1 percent mortality (Chap. 19). The use of advanced computer-based methodologies of evaluation that can be used for the guidance of therapy for ARDS is also discussed in Chapter 19, as is the relationship between ARDS and the development of sepsis.

Neurologic Injury

As shown in Table 1-7, because of the echelons of care system that directs the field triage of suspected head- and spinal cord-injured victims to the MIEMSS Clinical Center, the incidence of neurologic injury in the MIEMSS trauma patient population is quite high (43.4 percent) with severe injury to the brain being manifested in 16.9 percent of all trauma patients and 8.7 percent having injury to the spinal cord. However, some form of brain concussion with complete, partial, or transient loss

TABLE 1-11. Status and Survival of Head-Injuried Patients (n = 1,589)

A. Neurologic Status of All Head-Injured Patients by Glasgow Coma Scale (Excluding Cardiac Arrests)

Glasgow Coma Scale	Number of Patients	% of Total
3	60	3.8
4–8	124	7.8
9–12	95	6.0
13–14	294	18.5
15 and TLC[a]	359	22.6
15 and no TLC	656	41.3
Missing	1	<0.1
Total	1,589	100.0

B. Survival of Head-Injured Patients with Blunt Trauma by Glasgow Coma Score (Excluding Cardiac Arrests)

Glasgow Coma Score	Blunt Trauma		Total Trauma	
	No.	% Mortality	No.	% Mortality
3	30	80	60	80
4	16	31	28	46
5	15	40	22	46
6	18	22	27	26
7	18	6	23	4
8	17	6	24	13
9	12	0	21	0
10–14	266	5	369	7
15±TLC	668	2	1,015	2
Total	1,060		1,589	

[a] TLC, Transient loss of consciousness.

of consciousness was noted in 932 trauma patients (58.6 percent), excluding those with cardiac arrest on admission. This can also be seen from Table 1-11A, which shows that 573 (36.1 percent), excluding those with cardiac arrest) of the trauma patients had some degree of reduction in Glasgow coma scale on admission and based on AIS scores and discharge diagnoses, 279 (49 percent) of these head-injured individuals had a severe brain injury. Table 1-11B shows the relationship of the Glasgow coma score (GCS) to percent mortality for the total trauma group and for the blunt trauma cases alone. It demonstrates that while there is a low mortality in the cases whose GCS is 7 or above, due largely to the interaction with the other organ injuries in the polytraumatized patient, at GCS of 6 or below the mortality of the head-injured patient rises substantially, independent of the effect of other injuries. These data also indicate the need for careful neurologic evaluation and early computerized tomographic (CT) examination in the evaluation of such patients.

Table 1-12 reports the findings in those cases where a CT scan was performed on admission, prior to any surgical procedure, in patients with either a trauma history or clinical examination compatible with head injury. There was an increasing percentage of CT abnormality directly proportional to the Glasgow coma scale reading. Also, in many of the patients with an initially normal scan, subsequent repeat scanning during their clinical course demonstrated the later appearance of abnormal brain findings, or progression in the original abnormalities. The criteria for the early diagnosis and management of the head-injured patient, as well as the pathophysiologic mechanisms for the evolution and progression of central nervous system dysfunction after trauma to the brain, are discussed in Chapter 31. This chapter also covers the modalities of therapy and provides information relevant to the prediction of outcome after head injury. The recognition and prompt treatment of brain injury are of particular importance, since the mortality for the 245 blunt trauma severely brain-injured patients in this series was 25.3 percent (11.5 percent of all blunt brain injuries) and 17 per-

TABLE 1-12.   Frequency Table for Glasgow Coma Scale Scores (Excluding Cardiac Arrests) Abnormalities by Admission CT Scan

Glasgow Coma Scale	CT Not Done	CT Scan Performed		Total Patients
		Normal	Abnormal (%)	
3	23[a]	3	34(92%)	60
4–8	15[a]	21	88(81%)	124
9–12	5[a]	41	49(54%)	95
13–14	78[a]	156	60(28%)	294
15 and TLC	229	108	22(17%)	359
15 and no TLC	614	39	3(7%)	656
Missing	0	0	1	1
Total Number	964	368	257	1,589
% of CT Scans Done	—	58.9%	41.1%	100%

[a] Admission CT scan pre-empted by emergency surgical procedure, TLC, transient loss of consciousness.

cent of all surviving brain-injured patients had sufficient neurologic disability to require subsequent inpatient rehabilitation therapy at a trauma rehabilitation unit following their acute course at the MIEMSS Clinical Center.

A significant number of spinal-cord-injured patients have an incomplete deficit (Table 1-13). This reflects the incidence of central cord lesions, or partial motor or sensory preservation below the site of cord injury. These data focus attention on the importance of proper spinal column and spinal cord management in the spine-injured patient, either to prevent injury or to salvage the maximum available neurologic function remaining. A discussion of the problems of spinal cord and spinal column injury is presented in Chapter 32, which also deals specifically with the modalities of diagnosis, stabilization, and surgical and medical therapy for spinal cord lesions.

Cranial and Maxillofacial Injuries

Trauma to the soft tissues and bony architecture of the head and face represents one of the most common injuries seen in this population (Table 1-8). Fractures of the calvarium occurred in 11.0 percent and maxillofacial or jaw fractures were present in 19.8 percent of patients. Often these injuries were multiple and complex craniofacial reconstructive proce-

dures were necessary. In addition, fully 75.2 percent of MIEMSS trauma admissions sustained a severe laceration or soft tissue injury to the head or face. The diagnosis and surgical therapy of this particularly difficult set of problems are discussed in Chapter 33.

Special Problems of Thoracic Trauma

The diagnosis of thoracic visceral or intra-abdominal organ injury in blunt or penetrating trauma presents a significant diagnostic problem, especially in patient with multiple injuries or who has sustained a head or spinal cord injury in association with possible abdominal or pelvic trauma, in which one or more visceral organs may be injured. As indicated in Chapter 26, the MIEMSS resuscitation and diagnosis protocol is designed to prevent the failure to recognize a potentially life-threatening injury in these circumstances. Injuries to the thoracic viscera occurred in 10.1 percent of trauma patients in this series (Table 1-7). The most common organ injured was the lung (6.9 percent) either by a penetrating missile, laceration from a rib fracture, or by blunt compression injury resulting from impact or blast. However injuries to the heart and great vessels accounted for 3.3 percent of all injuries. While the majority of cardiac injuries were due to knife or missile penetration, nearly all of the thoracic aortic

TABLE 1-13. Spinal Cord Trauma with or without Spinal Column Fracture

Spinal Cord Function (Excluding Cardiac Arrests)	Number of Patients (n = 1,589)	Cord Injury (%)	% of all Patients
All normal	1445		90.9
Incomplete deficit	87	60.4	5.5
Complete deficit	57	39.6	3.6
Total	1589	100.0	100.0

injuries represented an acute aortic rupture with pseudoaneurysm formation secondary to blunt deceration impact, usually due to a motor vehicle accident or fall. The management of these injuries is discussed in Chapter 28 by Dr. Kirsh whose experience and knowledge of these injuries is considerable and whose approach, though from another institution, has significantly influenced the present MIEMSS care protocols for thoracic trauma.

Special Problems of Abdominal Trauma

In the multiply injured patient suspected of having sustained blunt abdominal injury, the MIEMSS protocol mandates that peritoneal lavage be done when intra-abdominal visceral injury cannot be explicitly ruled out. This is of particular importance in the patient with a severe head injury or spinal cord deficit and in the patient who may have to undergo extensive extra-abdominal surgery for several hours under anesthesia where serial abdominal examinations will be impossible to perform. Peritoneal lavage (Table 1-14) was carried out in patients with blunt trauma in 39.8 percent of the patients for the reasons indicated above. It was negative in 54.9 percent of these cases, making it possible to proceed with other modes of therapy with a reasonable assurance that no intra-abdominal organ injury existed since the present false-negative rate in our hands is less than 0.5 percent (Chap. 29). In 22 percent of the cases, there was a lavage of less than 50,000 cells/ml^3 and in these cases the lavage was either repeated, or CT scan or other diag-

nostic modality, such as angiography, was carried out to clarify the situation. In the remaining 23.1 percent of cases the lavage was diagnostic of an intra-abdominal injury and resulted in exploration. The false-positive rate in these cases remains slightly over 2 percent, as in the previously reported MIEMSS experience (Chap. 29). However, in all other instances a significant injury was found which justified the exploration. The technique and rationale behind this are discussed in Chapters 26 and 29, and a review of the outcomes of the MIEMSS experience with blunt abdominal trauma is presented in Chapter 29. A companion chapter (Chap. 30) on major intra-abdominal vascular trauma, representing the experience from another trauma service, extends this discussion to a less common, but extremely difficult to treat, set of injuries.

Orthopedic Injuries

Trauma to the bony skeleton including the spine, pelvis, and extremities occurred in 74.8 percent of all patients in this series, with 62.5 percent sustaining major pelvic or limb fractures (Table 1-8). Frequently these osseous injuries are compounded by extensive soft tissue damage and multiple fractures are the rule rather than the exception in such a population, where 72.2 percent of patients were injured as a result of motor vehicle, bicycle, or pedestrian accidents. Among the most difficult subset of orthopedic injuries are the severe pelvic fractures; these frequently also have a serious intra-abdominal or retroperitoneal organ injury. Another particularly challenging group are

TABLE 1-14.   Results of Peritoneal Lavage in Trauma in 1,651
Patients

Peritoneal Lavage by Type of Trauma	Number of Patients	% of Total	
Blunt only (n = 1,448)			
Not done[a]	872	60.2	
Done	576	39.8	
Clear	316	54.9	(of total done)
<50,000	127	22.0	
50,000–100,000	25	4.3	
>100,000	14	2.4	
Grossly bloody	94	16.3	
Penetrating only(n = 198)			
Not done[a]	181	91.4	
Done[b]	17	8.6	
Clear	8	47.1	(of total done)
<50,000	2	11.8	
50,000–100,000	0	0	
>100,000	0	0	
Grossly bloody	7	41.2	
Blunt and penetrating (n = 5)			
Not done[a]	4	80.0	
Done	1	20.0	
Clear	1	100.0	(of total done)
<50,000	0	0	
50,000–100,000	0	0	
>100,000	0	0	
Grossly bloody	0	0	

[a] Either no abdominal trauma or indications for exploration precluded need for diagnostic lavage.
[b] Equivocal penetration of peritoneal cavity.

those patients with compound tibial fractures where proper early management by an experienced multidisciplinary team of orthopedic, vascular, and plastic surgeons may be the key to limb salvage and reduction of subsequent disability. These problems are discussed in Chapter 34.

Surgical Therapy

The multiply injured nature of the trauma population admitted to the MIEMSS institute (Tables 1-7 and 1-8) is reflected in the nature and complexity of the surgical procedures performed by category of injury. This is shown in Table 1-15. In Table 1-16, patients with severe visceral, osseous, or soft tissue injuries, but without severe head injury, are categorized by ISS score. Patients with severe head injury,

or with spinal column fractures with spinal cord deficits, are categorized separately and excluded from those listed with ISS scores, so that all categories are mutually exclusive. As is noted in Table 1-7, 34.7 percent of all patients admitted had some form of mild or severe brain injury. As also can be seen in Table 1-16, there were 699 patients with ISS scores from 1 to 12. Of this group 16.7 percent underwent emergency surgery and 22.2 percent required a surgical procedure at some time during their hospital course. Of the patients operated on in this category (see Table 1-18), 5.4 percent required some form of minor neurologic surgery (generally insertion of an intracranial device to monitor intracranial pressures, ICP, during surgery for some other condition). Nearly 17 percent (16.7 percent) of the patients in the ISS 1 to 12 category required a general surgical procedure, and there were a small number of thoracic (2 percent), or craniofacial (7.9 percent) procedures, but 12.6 percent of patients re-

TABLE 1-15.   MIEMSS Trauma Admissions, Emergency Surgery and Mortality (1983–1984)

Category	Number	% Total	% Emergency Operations	% Any Surgery	% Mortality of Category
All trauma	1,651	100			11.4
Admission cardiac arrest (CA)	62	3.8			95.2
Trauma (−fatal CA)	1,592	96.4			8.1
Admission GCS = 3	60	3.6			80.0
Trauma (−Fatal CA and GCS=3)	**1,544**	**93.5**	**40.9**	**54.6**	**5.3**

TABLE 1-16.   Total Trauma Admissions: Blunt and Penetrating (Excluding Admission Cardiac Arrests) by Category of Injury (1983–1984)

	Number	% Total	% Emergency Operation	% Any Surgery	% Mortality of Category
ISS 1–12	699	42.3	16.7	22.2	0.6
ISS 13–19	209	12.7	53.1	63.2	3.4
ISS ≥ 20	228	13.8	77.2	86.8	11.8
Severe brain injury	279	16.9	49.1	61.3	29.8[a]
Spinal cord deficit	132	8.0	25.0	50.0	3.0
Multiple neurologic injury (brain and spinal cord)	9	0.5	44.4	66.6	33.3

[a] 14.5% mortality for all brain injury (573 patients).

quired an orthopedic operation and more than one third (35.1 percent) required some form of plastic or soft tissue surgery. The majority of nonoperated patients in this category were admitted to rule out a head or spine injury since MIEMSS is the spinal cord and major head injury center for the state.

In the ISS 13 to 19 category (Tables 1-16 and 1-17), which consisted of 209 patients, 53.1 percent required emergency surgery and 63.2 percent required surgery at some time during the hospital course. In this group also (Table 1-18) 12.4 percent required some minor neurosurgical procedure. As also can be seen from Table 1-18, there was an increase in the percentages of surgical procedures in all specialty categories, with the largest percentages being in general surgery (35.9 percent) and in orthopedic surgery (46.4) percent. Nearly half of all patients required some form of soft tissue surgery or debridement (45.5 percent). In the most severe category of injury (ISS ≥ 20) there were 228 patients (Table 1-16). Of these, 77.2 percent required emergency surgery and 86.8 percent had some form of surgical therapy during their hospital course. As would be expected, the percentage of more serious visceral injuries increased in this group. Thoracic surgery was shown to increase from 2.0 percent of the ISS 1 to 12 group to 37.2 percent in the ISS ≥ 20 group, while general surgical procedures increased from 16.7 percent of the 1 to 12 ISS patients, to 64.5 percent of the ISS ≥ 20 group (Table 1-18).

TABLE 1-17.   Blunt Trauma Admissions (Excluding Admission Cardiac Arrests) by Category of Injury (1983–1984)

	Number	(% Blunt)	% Emergency Operation	% Any Surgery	% Mortality of Category
ISS 1–12	640	(45.6)	14.1	19.7	0.6
ISS 13–19	179	(12.8)	53.0	63.7	3.9
ISS ≥ 20	185	(13.2)	76.8	88.1	11.4
Severe brain injury	245	(17.5)	49.0	62.0	25.3[a]
Spinal cord deficit	113	(8.1)	23.9	50.4	2.7
Multiple neurologic injury (brain and spinal cord)	9	(0.6)	44.4	66.6	33.3

[a] 11.5% mortality for all blunt brain injury.

TABLE 1-18.   Percentages of Types of Surgery Done in all Operated Patients by Trauma Category (1983–1984)

Procedure Type	ISS 1–12	ISS 13–19	ISS≥20	Severe Brain Injury	Spinal Fracture with Cord Deficit
Neurosurgery	5.4[a]	12.4[a]	20.2[a]	65.6	53.0
Craniofacial	7.9	14.8	19.7	18.6	6.1
Thoracic surgery	2.0	15.8	37.3	18.3	15.9
General surgery	16.7	35.9	64.5	56.6	28.8
Orthopedic surgery	12.6	46.4	49.6	18.3	19.7
Plastic reconstructure debridement (including craniofacial)	35.1	45.5	43.0	28.0	14.4

[a] Minor neurologic surgery (eg., ICP bolt, etc.).

When the 279 patients with severe brain injuries were considered, it can be seen not all of the major problems in these cases could be attributed to their life-threatening neurologic injury (Table 1-18). Although 65.6 percent of these patients required some sort of a neurosurgical procedure (49.1 percent as emergencies, including intracranial pressure monitoring), there were also a large fraction (18.6 percent) of patients requiring craniofacial procedures, reflecting the magnitude of the impact forces on the head and face. There was a marked reduction in the percent of patients needing thoracic surgical procedures (18.3 percent) compared to the ISS ≥ 20 group (37.3 percent), but 56.6 percent of the severe head-injured patients required a general surgical procedure and 18.3 percent needed an orthopedic procedure.

Similarly, the 132 pure spinal trauma patients who also had a spinal cord deficit could not be classified as having a simple single system injury. Of these patients 53.0 percent had some form of neurosurgical procedure for stabilization of the spinal column or decompression of the spinal cord (25.0 percent as emergencies), but there was a major component of other surgical procedures required. The largest percent of patients (28.8 percent) had general surgical operations, with orthopedic procedures not far behind (19.7 percent of patients), but 15.9 percent had a thoracic surgical procedure and 14.4 percent required craniofacial surgery. As might be expected, the percentage of soft tissue injuries was reduced in the spinal-cord-injured patient group.

Since such a large percent of the total trauma population seen at MIEMSS have blunt trauma (87 percent of admissions) the relative ratio of emergency to total patients requiring surgery and the distribution of types of operations are very similar for this group (Table 1-17) compared to the total group (Table 1-16). The point Tables 1-15 to 1-18 make is that a population of injured patients with largely blunt trauma is characterized by a multiplicity of injuries that complicate even the neurologic surgical cases. This fact makes for a somewhat different approach to surgery in which all of the major life- or organ-saving, or limb salvage or stabilization surgical procedures are done at the initial emergency operation, with multiple secondary debridements, or procedures designed to deal with posttraumatic or septic complications, being carried out later. This requires a multidisciplinary, multispecialty team approach to the initial surgery involving general and thoracic surgeons, neurosurgeons, orthopedic surgeons, and plastic surgeons together with a trauma-trained anesthesiologist group. This is especially important since although the average length of surgery for the different injury groups varied from less than 30 minutes to more than 8 hours, depending on the severity of the case and the complexity of procedures, many cases required more than 12 hours of anesthesia to complete all of the major surgical operations done as primary procedures. This was particularly true when a major craniofacial injury was one of the features of the trauma pattern. Close team coordination in prioritizing the types of surgery and the ability of the surgical specialty teams to operate either simultaneously, or in tandem, without interfering with each other, or compromising the patient's survival, becomes important in this circumstance. Equally important to outcome is coordination and cooperation in preoperative resuscitation, intraoperative management and comprehensive postoperative critical care.

On the average (Table 1-15 excluding fatal cardiac arrests and brain dead patients only), those patients who required surgery made 2.1 separate trips to operating room. Overall, 40.9 percent of all patients operated upon required primary emergency surgery and 54.6 percent of all patients had surgery at some time during their hospital course. Viewed in another way, 38.8 percent of all the trips to the operating room were for surgical procedures done as an emergency and the remaining 61.2 percent of operating room procedures were for some form of follow-up surgery related to secondary procedures to deal with complications of the injury or surgery.

To help us understand the complexity of the operative procedures, Table 1-19 shows the mean duration of the emergency and follow-up procedures by type and severity of injury with respect to the eventual outcome of the patients. It also can be seen that there is an important difference between the duration of both the emergency and the follow-up procedures in those patients who were discharged directly to home and those who were subsequently discharged to a rehabilitation facility. The duration of surgery was directly proportional to the severity of illness of injury in both circumstances. However, the length of either the emergency or follow-up surgical procedures (reflecting the complexity of the problems) was greater in those patients who eventually required extensive rehabilitation services. This was primarily due to the increased number of difficult orthopedic and neurosurgical procedures in this class of patient. The patients who died did not on the whole show any significant

differences in the duration of their surgeries, except in the case of spinal cord injury where the procedures in fatal cases tended to be more complex, reflecting the severity of injury and, in the case of the severe head-injured patients, where the procedures tended to be shorter reflecting the decision of the neurosurgeon that decompression of an otherwise fatal head injury was the only justifiable approach.

OUTCOMES OF THERAPY IN THE MULTIPLY INJURED PATIENT

Trauma surgery is the art of the possible. Success or failure is measured in terms of what can be done to resuscitate the otherwise fatally injured patient or to salvage the remaining functional potential of a damaged organ, limb, or face. By applying the resuscitative and diagnostic protocols and research-derived therapeutic programs described in this book, the mortality has steadily declined from 1976 to the present (Fig. 1-9). The mortality rates of the MIEMSS 1984 experience are also shown in Table 1-15. The overall death rate for these 1,651 trauma patients was 11.4 percent. There were 62 patients admitted in full cardiac arrest of whom 95.2 percent died (a 4.8 percent survival of this dead on arrival, DOA, class of patients). In addition 60 patients were admitted with a GCS of 3, showing no brain function. Forty-eight of these (80 percent) died but 12 patients (20 percent) were saved, some with surprisingly good late function (Table 1-11B).

TABLE 1-19. Duration of Surgery in Hours by Type and Severity of Injury and by Outcome

Outcome		Spinal Cord Injury	Severe Head Injury	ISS 1–12	ISS 13–19	ISS ≥20	Total
Discharged to home	Emergency	0.23	2.48	0.48	1.73	3.13	1.2
	follow-up	0.86	1.33	0.66	1.22	2.15	1.0
Discharged to rehabilitation facility	Emergency	1.28	3.56	4.25	5.16	6.23	3.95
	follow-up	4.95	2.35	3.90	8.47	6.75	5.38
Fatal cases (in-hospital deaths)	Emergency	1.97	1.30	1.10	1.00	2.68	1.65
	follow-up	1.17	0.48	1.73	1.80	1.35	1.18

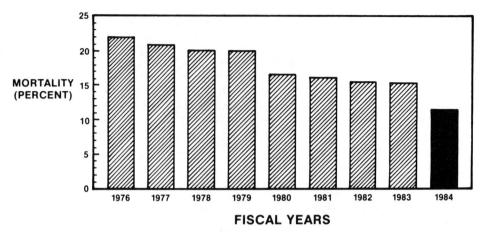

FISCAL YEARS

FIG. 1-9 Pattern of reduction in mortality at the MIEMSS Shock Trauma Clinical Center 1976 to 1984. The major decrease in trauma mortality occurring between 1979 and 1980 fiscal was related to definitive organization of care protocols. Improvement in retrieval system between 1983 and 1984 reflects introduction of advanced physiologic techniques for patient evaluation and management using computer-based methodologies. These advances in care have continued to sustain a low mortality (12.4%) in the 1985 fiscal year.

If one excludes the fatal cardiac arrest group as being already dead on admission, there was an 8.1 percent mortality rate for 1,592 patients and if one excludes both the fatal cardiac arrests and the patients with brain death on admission (fatal GCS-3) there were 1,544 patients who had only a 5.3 percent mortality rate, in spite of the multiplicity of the injuries received and the surgical procedures required (Table 1-15).

If one looks carefully at the breakdown of the various injury groups and takes into consideration the severity of the injuries and the complexities of surgery, it can be seen (Table 1-15) that in the ISS 1 to 12 group there was a 0.6 percent mortality due largely to complications of multiple injuries, age, or intercurrent disease; in the ISS 13 to 19 group a 3.4 percent mortality; and in the ISS $\geq$ 20 group there was a 11.8 percent mortality. In the severely brain-injured group there was a mortality of 29.8 percent (14.5 percent of all 573 brain-injured patients died), but these were 25.3 percent and 10.8 percent, respectively, for the blunt-head-injury group alone. Patients with spinal column fractures and a spinal cord deficit had a mortality rate of 3.0 percent. This mortality was largely related to the presence of other major injuries in the patients with a serious spinal cord injury, primarily at the cervical level,

since, as shown in Table 1-3, the vast majority of spinal column injuries involved the cervical spine. These figures indicate that in spite of the severity of injury in this population, if one excludes only those patients who arrive DOA with a fatal cardiac arrest and those who had verifiable brain death on admission, the comprehensive protocol-based system of trauma and critical care used at MIEMSS and presented in this book resulted in a nearly 95 percent survival for potentially salvageable patients.

In analyzing the causes of trauma mortality further, Table 1-20 shows the percent of total trauma mortality occurring in each of the specialized areas. As can be seen 4.6 percent of all trauma admissions, 40.4 percent of all trauma deaths, were either DOA (representing patients with cardiac arrest resuscitated in the field and admitted to MIEMSS), or died in the admitting area (representing patients who had a cardiac arrest following admission or who were brain dead and died in the resuscitation area). Of all trauma patients 1.8 percent died in the operating room and such deaths accounted for 15.4 percent of the trauma mortality, due largely to uncontrollable hemorrhage and/or coagulation defects and hypothermia, shock, and acidosis. Deaths in the critical care unit occurred in 2.4 percent of all trauma cases

TABLE 1-20. **Hospital Unit Locations of Death in Fatal Trauma Cases as Percent of Trauma (1983–1984)**

Location	% All Trauma Admissions	% Trauma Deaths
DOA in admitting area	4.6	40.4
Operating room	1.8	15.4
Critical care recovery unit	2.4	21.3
Neurotrauma unit and wards	2.6	22.9
Total	11.4	100.0

and accounted for 21.3 percent of the trauma mortality (primarily of the late complications of head injury or of sepsis, with ARDS and multiple organ failure syndromes predominating). Finally, 22.9 percent of all trauma deaths occurred in the neurotrauma unit, or the other step-down units, due to late head injury, or complications such as bronchopneumonia, pulmonary embolus, myocardial infarction, and other conditions.

These numbers point out to us the areas where advances in care may possibly result in increased patient salvage. As is evident from the preceding numbers, these deaths fall in to three different categories which are addressed in various sections of this book. There are the immediate acute cardiovascular complications produced by hypovolemic, hemorrhagic shock which require decisions regarding fluid resuscitation (Chap. 7), the choice of volume support (Chap. 8), the management of cardiovascular shock (Chap. 9), including newer pharmacologic approaches (Chap. 6), and the therapy of acute coagulation defects (Chap. 23). The early and critical care management of severe head injury (Chap. 31) and spinal cord trauma (Chap. 32) is essential if mortality is to be reduced. The third major cause of morbidity and mortality in this population is related to the factors predisposing to sepsis (Chap. 14), prevention of which includes the understanding of the humoral mediators of the septic insult (Chap. 3) and the metabolic consequences of these insults (Chaps. 4 and 15). From a therapeutic point of view the management of posttrauma sepsis requires an understanding of the proper choice and use of antibiotics (Chap. 16) as well as the therapy of established sepsis and the septic multiple organ failure syndrome (Chap. 15).

In treating this class of patients, the critical care specialist also must be aware of the factors influencing the development of the posttraumatic and septic ARDS (Chap. 18) and the cardiorespiratory management of ARDS (Chap. 19). Problems created by pre-existing diabetes mellitus and its management (Chap. 24) must be understood as well as the role of pre-existing or acutely acquired endocrine dysfuntions (Chap. 25). Finally, the management of trauma and sepsis demands a working comprehension of the principles of nutritional support after injury (Chap. 17) and their modification by severe sepsis (Chap. 15).

Other less common, though still potentially preventable, causes of death after trauma are related to acute pulmonary embolization (Chap. 13), myocardial infarction with cardiogenic shock (Chaps. 10 and 11), hypertensive crises (Chap. 12), fluid and electrolyte disorders (Chap. 21), including renal failure (Chap. 22), and a variety of environmental (Chap. 20), toxic gas (Chap. 37), or drug toxicities (Chap. 6). All of these issues are discussed in greater detail in the appropriate chapters as indicated above.

PATIENT DISPOSITION: OUTCOMES OF CARE

In the final analysis, the success of a trauma system must be measured not only on the basis of the reduction in fatal outcomes but also with regard to its effectiveness in reducing functional disability and enhancing the return to work, or pretrauma activity, in the surviving patients. The posthospital disposition of the trauma population at the MIEMSS Clinical Center is shown in Figure 1-10. Nearly 60 percent of the discharges from the Institute are directly to home. Another 15 percent are transferred to the physically adjacent larger University Hospital because of a longer than average length of stay required for extensive reconstructive surgical procedures. (This number was increased to 19 percent in 1985 because of the MIEMSS average occupancy of 97.9 percent, forcing a larger number of long-stay patients to be transferred into the general hospital.) Between 17 and 18 percent of patients, primarily head- and spinal-cord-injured patients, required longer-term acute rehabilitation care (at Montebello Rehabilitation Trauma Service or other rehabilitation hospital).

In a recent study of 597 trauma patients between the ages of 16 to 45 who were discharged from either the Johns Hopkins Hospital (a regional trauma center in the Maryland system) (187 patients), or the Maryland Institute for Emergency Medical Services Systems Clinical Center (MIEMSS) (286 patients), MacKenzie, et al.[17] showed that the functional disability of the patients without brain injury was primarily related to spinal cord, pelvis, and lower extremity injuries. Injuries with the greatest threat to life, those with the highest ISS scores, had relatively little impact on late disability after 6 months to 1 year. In a companion study[18] in a subset of 266 individuals who were working full-time prior to sustaining the injury, her group also demonstrated that at 1 year 56 percent were employed full-time and an additional 5 percent were working part-time. As shown in Figure 1-11, which demonstrates the cumulative percent distribution of the time between injury and full time employment, the functional return at 60 weeks is least

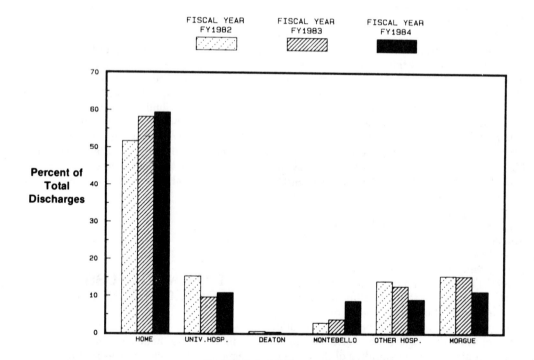

DISPOSITION LOCATIONS

FIG. 1-10 Disposition of MIEMSS Clinical Center patients by institution. University Hospital: University of Maryland General Hospital. Deaton, Montebello, and Other Hospitals are rehabilitation units for discharge of patients requiring longer-term acute rehabilitation therapy.

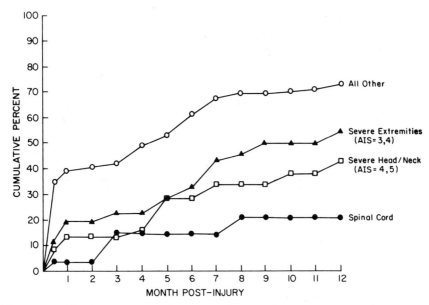

FIG. 1-11 Cumulative percent return to work of patients with various types of injuries, 60 months after injury. (MacKenzie EJ, Shapiro S, Smith RT et al: Factors influencing return to work following traumatic injury. Am J Public Health 1986 (in press).)

in patients with spinal cord injury, where it remained at 21 percent. Patients with severe head injury (AIS 4, and 5) had a somewhat better early and long-term capability of returning to work, with a 43 percent recovery being achieved at 60 weeks. Patients with severe pelvis or lower extremity injuries (AIS 3, and 4), while showing a major functional disability comparable to head and spinal cord injury at 15 weeks postinjury, had a gradual and steady progressive increase in the ability to return to work, so that by 60 weeks nearly 54 percent had returned to gainful employment. Patients with other types of injuries including soft tissue injuries and visceral trauma showed a 74 percent return to full-time employment by 60 weeks.

It is of interest to examine the patient characteristics reflected in this study that influenced the ability of the non-head-injured patient to return to gainful employment.[17] Age, sex, racial characteristics, and marital status were of no significance in influencing return to work. However the level of responsibilities, as designated by being the head of the house-

hold; the degree of education; the type of work prior to injury (blue collar or white collar); and the patient's level of income prior to injury are all significant factors, with a positive correlation between a greater level of education, white collar employment, and higher income as both motivating and empowering factors enabling early employment after injury. Another important factor demonstrated to be significant was related to the number of supporting individuals in the home or in the network of family and friends who could provide physical and emotional support for the patient recovering from serious traumatic injury. This factor also had a significant correlation with the return to employment. The information demonstrated by this analysis is obviously of great importance in designing programs to facilitate and maximize the capability of the injured patient to return to productive life following injury. It offers many points of tangency that can be explored by imaginative programs in education, job retraining, and family therapy to maximize the rehabilitation potential of the trauma victim.

THE ROLE OF RESEARCH IN IMPROVING THE OUTCOME AFTER SERIOUS INJURY

Research is the lifeblood of progress in improving the care of the injured patient. The reduction in mortality is related to the introduction of cardiovascular and respiratory physiologically guided therapy to the care of the critically ill (Chaps. 9 and 19). This approach has been shown to be highly significant in trauma patients (Fig. 1-12). Also, as demonstrated in Chapter 19, support of the patient using physiologically directed techniques can permit a substantial return of function after the acute phase of critical illness has passed, thus not only improving survival but also maximizing the degree and rate of recovery to normal function. The role of basic studies in immunology and host defense mechanisms in elucidating the pathophysiology and therapy of sepsis and ARDS is covered in Chapters 14 and 18, respectively. The application of computer techniques to cardiovascular and metabolic support is presented in Chapters 9 and 15, and the influence of computer-based methods in the physiologically guided management of ventilatory dysfunction in ARDS is discussed in Chapter 19.

TRAUMA: ICU MORTALITY

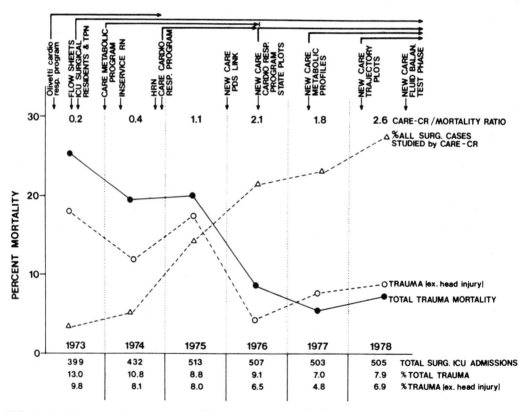

FIG. 1-12 Influence of introduction of computer-based physiologic cardiorespiratory assessment system (CARE-CR) on trauma mortality as a function of percentage cases (CARE-CR) in whom physiologic patterns were used or guidelines for adjustment of therapy. (Siegel JH, Cerra FB, Moody EA: The affect on survival of critically ill and injured patients of an ICU teaching service organized about a computer-based physiologic CARE system. J Trauma 20:558, © 1980 the Williams & Wilkins Co., Baltimore.)

Five chapters also discuss practical applications of basic science work in the fundamental mechanisms of cell injury (Chap. 2), the biochemical basis (Chaps. 4 and 7), and humoral control mechanisms (Chaps. 3 and 14) underlying the response to trauma and ARDS (Chap. 18). Fundamental research studies are presented in Chapter 6 to demonstrate the application of pharmacologic methods in revealing the mechanisms behind the development of shock and in designing a polypharmacologic therapeutic program to reverse the shock state. Specific basic science and human investigative work related to the immunobiologic aspects of septic disease in the posttrauma state is discussed at length in Chapter 14 and the role of altered metabolic control and nutritional support in sepsis is covered in Chapters 15, 17, and 36.

Undoubtedly the most troublesome area for the traumatologist is the head- and spinal-cord-injured patient. A basic understanding of the pathophysiology of central nervous system disease and a review of research applications to the therapy of the brain and spinal cord injuries are presented in Chapters 31 and 32. Other important research-related efforts underlie the therapy of acute burns; these studies are discussed in Chapters 14 and 36. Finally, a careful explanation of the use and interpretation of statistics used to evaluate clinical research data is presented in Chapter 5.

At a more directly clinical level, research in newer limb salvage and stabilization techniques described in Chapter 34 has played a major role in facilitating the recovery of patients with extremity injuries and in enabling a earlier return to gainful employment. The newer maxillofacial reconstructive surgical techniques described in Chapter 33 represent an evolution in posttrauma reconstructive cosmetic surgery that has enabled badly disfigured patients to regain a positive self-image. This aggressive approach increases their ability to sustain the social interactions required in employment and in social encounters.

In no other area of medicine does the research into basic biochemical and physiologic mechanisms, biomechanics, and computer technology offer more rapid practical applications in effecting changes to increase the survival rate and enhance the recovery from an acute disease state. In each of these areas, much work needs to be done and it is hoped that the stimulation provided by this book will encourage others to explore the application of basic science and clinical research to surgical and critical care problems in the field of trauma.

REFERENCES

1. Joint Committee on Injury Scaling of the American Medical Association. American Association for Automotive Medicine and Society of Automotive Engineers: Abbreviated Injury Scale (AIS). 1980 Revision
2. Baker SP, O'Neill B: The injury severity score. An update. J Trauma 16: 882, 1976
3. Baker SP, O'Neill B, Karpf RS: The Injury Fact Book. D.C. Health, Lexington Books, Lexington, MA 1984, p. 312
4. Billroth T: General Surgical Pathology and Therapeutics. Translated by CE Hackley. D. Appleton & Co., New York, 1871
5. Breasted JH: The Edwin Smith Surgical Papyrus. University of Chicago Press, Chicago, 1930, p. 596
6. Cowley RA: A total emergency medical systems for the state of Maryland. Maryland State Med J 24: 37, 1975
7. Cowley RA, Hudson F, Scanlan E et al: An economical and proved helicopter program for transporting the emergency critically ill and injured patient in Maryland. J Trauma 13: 1029, 1973
8. Dischinger PC, Shankar BS, Kochesfahani D et al: Automotive collisions involving serious injury or death: an analysis of trends over time (1980–1983) in Maryland. American Association for Automotive Medicine, 29th Proceedings, 1985, pp. 287–297
9. Dunham CM, Gens DR, Ramzy AI et al: Trauma registry: criteria, implementation, and initial results. J Trauma (submitted) 1986
10. Fatal Accident Reporting System 1984, U.S. Department of Transportation, National Highway Traffic Safety Administration, National Center for Statistics and Analysis, Washington, D.C.
11. Haddon W: Small car deaths, injuries worst: models vary greatly. Status Report vol. 17, No. 20. Insurance Institute for Highway Safety Administration. Washington, D.C., 1982

12. Hartunian NS, Simart CN, Thompson MS: The incidence and economic costs of major health impairments. D.C. Health, Lexington Books, 1981, pp. 255–337
13. Hunter J: Treatise on the blood, inflammation, and gun-shot wounds. John Richardson, London, 1794, pp. 521–565
14. Injury in America: A continuing public health problem. National Academic Press, Washington, D.C., 1985, pp. 1–47
15. Kraus JF, Black MA, Hessol N et al: The incidence of acute brain injury and serious impairment in a defined population. Am J Epidemiol 119: 186, 1984
16. Kraus JF, Franti CE, Riggins RS et al: Incidence of traumatic spinal cord lesions. J Chron Dis 28: 471, 1975
17. MacKenzie EJ, Shapiro S, Moody M et al: Predicting post-trauma functional disability for individuals without severe brain injury. Med Care 24:377 1986
18. MacKenzie EJ, Shapiro S, Smith RT et al: Factors influencing return to work following traumatic injury. Am J Public Health (in press) 1986
19. MIEMSS: Annual Report, 1984
20. MIEMSS: Annual Report, 1985
21. National Accident Sampling System, 1984: U.S. Department of Transportation, National Highway Traffic Safety Administration Report DOT HS 806 867, 1985, p. 64
22. Neat RL, Cowley RA: The Maryland emergency services communications system. Emergency Med Services 11: 28, 1982
23. Paré A: Apologie and treatise and selections from the surgical writings. G. Keynes, ed. Falcon Educational Books, London, pp. 117–142, 1951
24. Shankar BS, Dischinger PC, Cowley RA: Am J Public Health (submitted 1986).
25. National Highway Traffic Safety Administration: The Economic Cost to Society of Motor Vehicle Accidents. U.S. Department of Transportation, Washington, D.C., Report DOT HS 806 342, 1983, p. 262
26. Trunkey DD: Trauma. Sci Am 249: 28, 1983

SECTION I

BASIC SCIENCE FOUNDATIONS

2

Cell Injury and Its Meaning in Shock and Resuscitation

Louis L. Marzella

Benjamin F. Trump

CELL INJURY

Definition

Cell injury is defined as an alteration of normal homeostasis that leads to unfavorable consequences for the organism. Different degrees of severity of cell injury are recognized at the morphologic and biochemical levels. If the insulting agent is successfully handled by host defenses, the cell may revert to its normal state. The injury is said to have been reversible. Cell injury states may also persist chronically. In this case the cell may maintain the altered homeostasis by the expenditure of metabolic energy and by undergoing structural and functional modifications. If the insult is severe or prolonged the cell may become irreversibly injured and die. Many of the alterations that follow the initial injury have been defined mor-

phologically and biochemically. However, the precise sequence of events leading to cell death is not known. It is hypothesized that the loss of key membrane functions is an important event and may constitute a common final pathway towards cell death. The abilities to regulate the distribution of ions, particularly calcium, and to generate high-energy phosphate compounds are likely to be key functions whose loss leads to irreversible injury.

Different organs and different cells within the same organ manifest different susceptibility to cell injury. Particularly in the context of shock and anoxia, tissues with high oxygen consumption are more susceptible to injury and death. Oxygen consumption is not related to tissue mass but to metabolic rates. Therefore, cells with the highest metabolic rates are most susceptible to injury and death. Energy in the form of adenosine triphosphate (ATP) is one of the most important by-products of oxidative metabolism. This energy is necessary to maintain the stable internal environment in the cell.

In addition, energy is necessary for the cell to perform the many complex tasks necessary for its own function and that of the whole organism. Adequate blood flow is necessary to maintain a steady supply of oxygen and metabolites and to remove metabolic by-products. Some of the highest rates of oxygen consumption occur in the kidney and brain. Biochemically and physiologically specialized regions of these organs exist where cells manifest different metabolic rates.

Application of the Concept of Cell Injury to the Study, Diagnosis, and Treatment of Illness

Some types of insults, particularly if severe enough, can lead immediately to clinical sequelae. This is often the case in mechanical trauma. Various insults can also quickly induce an altered physiologic state and obvious clinical manifestations. Acute severe blood loss, for example, causes circulatory collapse and the clinical manifestations of shock. In other cases, the insulting agent, whether infectious, toxic, or metabolic, manifests itself slowly. Altered cellular function becomes then the first manifestation of injury. If cellular protective mechanisms fail, the injury may disrupt a variety of complex cell functions and lead to subtle alterations in the physiologic state. In time, as these alterations become more severe, they become apparent clinically. This pathophysiologic sequence of events is illustrated in Figure 2-1.

The concept that the status of the critically ill patient is most meaningfully expressed in terms of cellular function is obvious. This concept has important diagnostic, therapeutic, and prognostic implications. It is well recognized that subtle changes in hemodynamics and oxygen consumption are key physiologic manifestations of sepsis which require prompt diagnostic and therapeutic measures. However, in addition to nutritional, antibiotic, and surgical interventions, it is necessary to counter the profound metabolic cellular disturbances. It is clear, therefore, that improved cellular function is the fundamental criterion for successful therapeutic intervention. Improved methods of early diagnosis of cellular dysfunction are necessary for earlier and more successful interventions. It is also important to emphasize that somatic death in the setting of acute trauma often occurs at a time when cells in many organs remain biologically viable. These reversibly injured cells are able to recover and replicate if placed in an appropriate environment. Somatic death, therefore, may occur due to loss of coordinated cell function at a time when many cells in most tissues are reversibly injured; they can be rescued if placed in an appropriate environment. This point is illustrated in Table 2-1, which shows the typical viability of human epithelial cell populations after somatic death due to trauma. These tissues

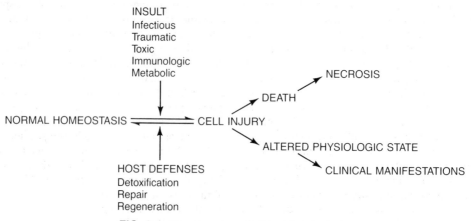

FIG. 2-1 Consequences of altered homeostasis.

TABLE 2-1. Viability[a] of Human Epithelial Cells in Postmortem Tissue

| | Hours Postmortem | | | | | |
	1	2	4	8	12	16
Liver	3	1	0	—	—	—
Pancreas	2	1	0	—	—	—
Bladder	3	2	1	0	—	—
Esophagus	4	3	3	0	—	—
Bronchus	3	3	3	2	1	0
Kidney	3	2	2	2	1	0
Prostate	4	3	3	3	2	1

[a] Viability is defined as ability to maintain the cell in culture. Success in rescuing the tissue at each time point is rated on an arbitrary scale of 0 to 4.

were obtained from routine or immediate autopsies.[25] Viability of the epithelia is defined as the capacity of the cells to be maintained in culture with or without cellular replication. As can be seen in Table 2-1, cells in many organs remain viable hours after somatic death. These results have important implications for harvesting of tissues for organ transplantation and for study.[25,140,141] Most importantly, studies aimed at enhancing survival of these tissues hold the promise that further progress can be made in the resuscitation of patients.

Necrosis follows cell death and is an active process of clearing away the dead cells from injured organs. This function is largely accomplished by macrophages that ingest the dead cells. Dead cells begin to break up under the stress of mechanical factors and from the digestive action of enzymes released from the dead cell itself as well as from macrophages. This cellular debris is a potent activator of inflammatory reaction and has a toxic and depressant effect on organ function.

MECHANISMS: ALTERED CELL FUNCTIONS

In this section we will outline disturbances in basic cell function of particular importance in the critically ill surgical patient.

Infectious Agents

Bacterial peptides bind to specific receptors on the cell surface of macrophages, neutrophils, and other mature cells of the myeloid series.[118,129] This binding initiates a series of responses directed at defending the host against the bacterial infection. These responses include chemotaxis (the accumulation of acute inflammatory cells at the site of bacterial invasion), production of superoxide (highly reactive oxygen species), and release of lytic enzymes from the neutrophils.[81]

Several biologic actions of endotoxin and other bacterial products are therefore mediated by inflammatory cells.[64] These responses, although overall beneficial to the host, produce tissue damage. The release of these inflammatory mediators from activated leukocytes is in part responsible for cell injury induced by endotoxin.[147] For example, it has been shown that activated leukocytes in vitro can affect the function of cell membranes (sarcoplastic reticulum) responsible for the excitation–contraction coupling of heart muscle. This injury is due to free-radical-mediated processes.[80] Local vascular factors are often invoked to explain differences in the severity of injury induced by endotoxin in various tissues.[112] Endotoxin also causes activation of coagulation and kinin cascades.[66,123] Disseminated intravascular coagulation and depletion of platelets occur in sepsis.

Endotoxin is also known to suppress some inflammatory responses. This effect is due in part to decreased chemotactic and degranulation responses to complement-derived peptides found in the extravascular space.[115] Endotoxin may also induce the release of an anti-inflammatory factor from polymorphonuclear leukocytes (PMN) and of prostaglandins from macrophages.[68] Prostaglandins are known to inhibit the movement of PMN from the vasculature. The well-known increased adherence of PMN in response to endotoxin may also contribute to anti-inflammatory effects.[29] Endotoxin also inhibits phagocytosis mediated by the binding of immunoglobulins to plasma membrane Fc receptors.[145]

Infectious agents are also responsible for inducing the initiation of tissue repair mechanisms. Monocytes, macrophages, and platelets release a growth-promoting factor with stimulatory effects on mesenchymal cells including fibroblasts, smooth muscle, and endothelial cells.[12,84,117] This growth-promoting activity contributes to fibrosis and vascular proliferation[133] seen in tissue repair and normal healing. The release of growth factor can be stimulated by endotoxin and other bacterial products.[46] Increased amounts of fibronectin are deposited at sites of tissue repair and inflammation.[21,48] At these sites fibronectin binds to collagen, fibrin, and actin. Fibronectin also binds to receptors on the cell surface of monocytes and promotes the spreading and adhesion of monocytes. Fibronectin also stimulates the synthesis and release of growth factors from the monocytes.[10,83]

Immunologic Responses

The activation of the complement system initiates a series of immune responses designed to block the spread of infections and to clear the bloodstream of toxic agents and necrotic debris. The activation of this system also causes damage to host tissues. In general these responses lead to phagocytic uptake, inactivation, and degradation of toxic materials and of tissue debris. For example, cytoskeletal components and intracellular membranes activate complement.[42,75] Thus, the phagocytosis of necrotic debris by macrophages is enhanced.

Antigen–antibody complexes bind and activate the first component of the complement system. In addition, many other substances bind C1, the first component of the complement system, and trigger the activation of the classic pathway of the complement system in the absence of antibodies. Examples of these substances are bacteria, endotoxin, some cellular membranes, and C-reactive protein (CRP) complexes. The CRP is synthesized and released by the liver in response to stimuli such as sepsis.[23] Activation of complement through the classic pathway is thus an important means of neutralizing a variety of pathogens.[51,96] Bacterial products can also activate the alternative pathway.

Clearance of endotoxin from the bloodstream occurs primarily in the liver macrophages, namely the Kupffer cells.[97,116] Impaired clearance by the liver and/or increased entry of endotoxin in the portal circulation may lead to entry of the endotoxin in the systemic circulation. Here endotoxin can activate both the classic and alternative complement cascades and can thus lead to the formation of lesions on the surface membranes of cells.[94] The complement lesions can be visualized by electron microscopy as hollow cylindrical structures that span the surface membrane bilayer of cells.[136] This channel-like lesion is created by the insertion of complement proteins (C5b through C9) on the cell surface membrane.[107] The lesion is called the *membrane attack complex*. Electrolytes and small molecules thus flow into the cell through the channel lesions. It is thought to be less likely that the membrane attack complex of complement can damage cells independently of channel formation. This damage had been postulated to occur through the disruption of membrane phospholipid adjacent to the membrane attack complex.[11] Swelling and lysis of cells due to colloid osmotic forces follow the formation of channel lesions. This has been demonstrated in classic experiments with erythrocytes. Nucleated cells, on the other hand, are usually more resistant than erythrocytes to lysis induced by complement lesions. In sepsis and in extensive trauma and burns, a decrease in serum complement components is seen.[3] This decrease is associated with the development of bacteremia. Removal of necrotic tissue and drainage of infected sites are associated with a restoration of serum complement levels.[52]

With intravital microscopy, the leukocytes have been directly seen to block capillaries during hypotension in skeletal muscle,[7] and after myocardial ischemia.[33] Endothelial and perivascular cell swelling, interstitial hemorrhage, as well as immunologic activation are all factors contributing to the capillary plugging. An incomplete return of blood flow, after long periods of ischemia, has been reported also for brain and kidney.[4,38] Aggregation and accumulation of neutrophils in pulmonary vasculature occur during hemodialysis and cardiac bypass.[14,26] Complement activation is responsible for this aggregation. Sequestration of neutrophils in the lungs is also induced by endotoxin.[148] When chemotactic and other inflammatory factors induce the neutrophils to migrate out of the vascular bed into the interstitial and alveolar space, edema as well as hemorrhage and tissue damage occur.[122]

Free Radicals

Several cellular enzymes and organelles generate free radicals during normal functioning. The free radicals are very unstable, reactive species capable of inducing cell injury by damaging proteins, lipids, and nucleic acids and by inducing lipid peroxidation. Exposure to a great variety of exogenous agents or drugs such as, for example, x rays, antibiotics, and anesthetics, can also generate free radicals. In this case the free radicals are generated during the metabolism of the drugs by a specialized membrane (endo-plasmic reticulum) in the cell.

The endoplasmic reticulum of the liver is responsible for several key functions such as synthesis of proteins and lipids, detoxification of endogenous and exogenous substances, and calcium regulation. In particular, the cytochrome P-450 system in liver endoplasmic reticulum is responsible for the initial oxidation of many drugs. The drugs are subsequently acted upon by a second group of enzymes. The collective function of these enzymes is to make the drugs more water soluble and more easily excreted from the body.

During detoxification reactions a number of highly reactive chemical intermediates, including free radicals, are created from the original drugs. These intermediate products are able to form stable chemical bonds with cellular enzymes and nucleic acids. The resultant malfunctions or inactivations can induce cell injury and death. Binding of reactive intermediates to membrane phospholipids can also occur. The properties of the phospholipids are thus altered and cell membrane permeability and functions are damaged.

Superoxide radical (O_2^-) is produced in the endoplasmic reticulum by the detoxification reactions.[69] The radical is also produced during other metabolic or inflammatory processes. Superoxide radical is highly reactive and damaging to cells. The enzyme *superoxide dismutase* transforms superoxide radicals into molecular oxygen (O_2) and hydrogen peroxide (H_2O_2). Hydrogen peroxide is less toxic and is inactivated by cellular enzyme systems such as *catalase, peroxidase,* and *glutathione peroxidase.*

Radical species are able to attack the unsaturated fatty acids in cellular membranes. A self-sustaining cycle of lipid peroxidation is thus initiated. Lipid peroxidation induces severe damage to cellular membranes. Figure 2-2 shows the results of free radical attack on a liver cell caused by intoxication with carbon tetrachloride. Hyperbaric oxygen treatment is one of the therapies effective in inhibiting cell injury caused by this particular toxin.[87] Free radical injury is usually caused when antioxidant defense systems present in the cell's cytosol are overwhelmed.[108] The most important cellular protective system against oxidative stress is glutathione. Glutathione can inactivate toxic drug metabolites by making stable chemical bonds with these toxic molecules. Glutathione can also inactivate hydroperoxides.[67] The initiation of cell damage by these drug metabolites may be mediated by calcium. It has been shown that hydroperoxides impair the ability of mitochondria to retain calcium because of the reduction of NADPH.[78] Hydroperoxides can also impair the sequestration of calcium in the endoplasmic reticulum by inhibiting the calcium pump present in these membranes.[101] Loss of calcium homeostasis can thus result from damage to mitochondria and endoplasmic reticulum. A typical reaction to calcium imbalance caused by this injury is the formation of blebs on the cell surface membrane.[60] Surface membrane blebs are prominent manifestations of cell injury induced by many other agents including sepsis and hemorrhagic shock.

Ion Regulation

Several ions such as sodium, potassium, calcium, and magnesium are present in the extracellular fluid as well as inside the cell, where they are confined inside special compartments. The levels and the location of these ions are tightly regulated by the cell. The maintenance of this control requires the presence of intact

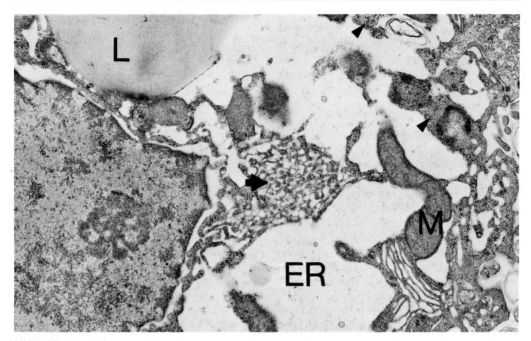

FIG. 2-2 Free radical injury. Intoxication with carbon tetrachloride administered 24 hours previously to a rat. There is marked dilatation of endoplasmic reticulum (ER). The ribosomes (arrowheads) are dispersed. Some ER membranes are aggregated in discrete clumps (arrow). A large lipid droplet is seen (L). Damage begins in the ER with this type of toxin. Note relative sparing of mitochondria (M) ($\times$ 13,000).

membranes and the expenditure of metabolic energy. Tight control is necessary because changes in the levels and in the location of these ions have profound influences on a great number of cellular functions. The controlled modulation of these ions allows such diverse phenomena as cell division, nerve impulse conduction, muscular contraction, alteration in cell shape, endocytosis, secretion, and changes in enzyme activity. Loss of ion regulation can thus be expected to induce cell injury. Calcium regulation appears to be particularly important for normal cell function. In addition, accumulation of calcium inside the cell appears to have adverse effects on the function of many cell processes.[138,139]

The plasma membrane functions as a physical barrier between the cell and the extracellular environment. Membrane pumps, driven by energy, function to exchange ions between these two environments. The mitochondria provide the metabolic energy for these pumps. In the case of calcium, an intracellular membrane compartment, namely the

endoplasmic reticulum, is active in taking up calcium from the cytosol and releasing it back as needed. This calcium regulation is most refined in contractile tissues such as the heart. It is known that following an insult such as ischemia or chronic injury, the ability of the endoplasmic reticulum to take up and release calcium is impaired.[35,103] When levels of intracellular calcium begin to rise to abnormal levels, the mitochondria begin also to take up calcium. Massive accumulation of calcium inside the mitochondria can result.[100,142] In Figure 2-3, the consequences of loss of calcium regulation are illustrated in muscle cells of mouse diaphragm. The diaphragms were incubated in vitro in the presence of a drug (ionophore) that causes the cell membranes to become permeable to calcium. The cells shown are irreversibly injured.

Thus damage to cellular membranes (surface, mitochondrial, and endoplasmic), as well as energy loss, result in loss of ion regulation and accumulation of calcium within the cell. After injury such as hemorrhagic or septic

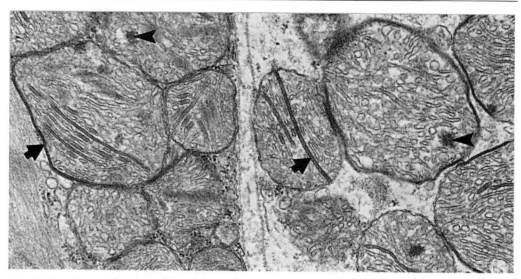

FIG. 2-3 Injury induced by loss of calcium homeostasis in the mouse diaphragm. Injury induced by in vitro incubation with A23187 (a calcium ionophore) for 2 hours. Note swelling of cytosol. The mitochondria show dense opacities in their cristae (intracristal densities) and in the intermembranous spaces (arrows). Note the flocculent densities (arrowheads) ($\times$ 25,000).

shock, cells lose potassium and gain sodium, chloride, and water.[126,137] The consequences of in vivo loss of ion regulation on the cell are readily seen ultrastructurally. In Figure 2-4, swelling of the endoplasmic reticulum and of mitochondria and marked increase in size and number of lysosomes are demonstrated in a human hepatocyte.

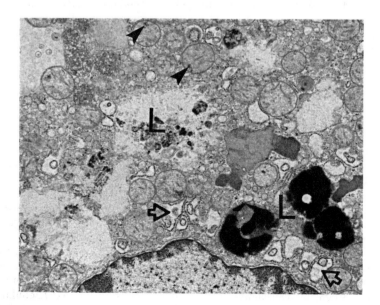

FIG. 2-4 Human liver in sepsis. This hepatocyte shows vesiculation and dilatation of endoplasmic reticulum (arrows). The number and size of the lysosomes (L) are markedly increased. The mitochondria (arrowheads) are swollen and show flocculent densities. From immediate autopsy ($\times$ 10,000).

An important result of the loss of ion regulation is the modification of the cellular cytoskeleton. The cellular cytoskeleton is made up of proteins responsible for the maintenance of cell shape and for the locomotion of cells as well as the movement of organelles within the cell. The cytoskeleton is made up of an organized system of rigid tubules and filaments as well as contractile filaments. The whole makes up a miniature musculoskeletal system essential for the proper function of the cell. The alteration of cytoskeletal organization involved by the loss of ion regulation is illustrated by Figure 2-5. The structural consequences of alterations of the cytoskeletal system are illustrated in Figure 2-6. Hepatocytes from a dog in hemorrhagic shock are seen. Profound changes in the cell surface membrane are shown (Fig. 2-6). Deep infoldings (the white clear areas) and outpouching (arrows) of cell surface membranes are seen. It is hypothesized that the stimulation of lysosomal protein catabolism seen in injury may also be a consequence of similar structural alterations of intracellular membranes. These alterations may cause the trapping of cellular parts inside autophagic vacuoles such as the one illustrated in Figure 2-7. As will be discussed later in this chapter the autophagic vacuoles are important for the catabolism of intracellular proteins.

Ion regulation is thus a cellular process of fundamental importance and is disturbed early in cell injury. The primary and secondary effects of loss of ion regulation may play an important role in the evolution of cell injury towards irreversible stages.[137] In particular, the loss of calcium regulation may represent a final common pathway towards cell death.[139]

Figure 2-8 summarizes current concepts about the role of calcium deregulation in cell injury and death. The regulation of cellular calcium levels depends on the transport activity of three key cell organelles, namely the plasma membranes, the mitochondria, and the endoplasmic reticulum. The calcium transport activity of each of these three organelles is governed by different regulatory mechanisms. However, all three systems function to transport calcium actively out of the cytosol. This active transport is necessary to maintain intracellular calcium levels very low relative to extracellular calcium (10,000-fold concentration difference).

Figure 2-8 indicates how agents that interfere with plasma membrane integrity or with energy metabolism ultimately cause an increase in levels of cytosolic calcium. In fact, calcium accumulation of massive proportions is seen in necrotic tissue caused by many pathologic conditions. In addition to (or in the absence of) increased influx of calcium into the cell, loss of transport capacity by the mitochondria or endoplasmic reticulum may raise cytosolic calcium levels. In such case, total intracellular calcium levels may remain constant. However, the redistribution of the available intracellular calcium from one cellular location to another would induce dysfunction. Figure 2-8 summarizes the structural alterations induced by the loss of calcium regulation. These changes are illustrated in the figures indicated: intracristal mitochondrial densities (Fig. 2-3), dilatation of mitochondria and endoplasmic reticulum (Fig. 2-4), cytoskeletal modifications (Fig. 2-5), disruption of gap junctions and formation of blebs and toxic vacuoles (Fig. 2-6), and increase in the number and size of autophagic vacuoles and lysosomes (Figs. 2-4, and 2-7). Figure 2-8 indicates how loss of calcium regulation may enhance the degradation of lipids within membranes. The by-products of this degradation or their metabolites may in turn promote further calcium influx into the cell. Calcium deregulation may therefore serve as the final common pathway towards cell death.

Intermediary Metabolism

Overproduction of lactate by muscle, liver, and kidney occurs in septic, hemorrhagic, and cardiogenic shock. A concomitant underutilization of lactate by the liver occurs because of decreased blood perfusion to the liver.[102] In livers of septic rats, increased lactate accumulation and decreased ratio of pyruvate to lactate are observed.[98] Changes in metabolic pathways, discussed in Chapter 15, may be responsible for these alterations. As a result, systemic acidosis develops. Acidosis per se is not injurious to cells. In fact extracellular acidosis has been found to protect cells against injury.[104,105] This protection is probably related to an effect on calcium fluxes. Of course the underlying

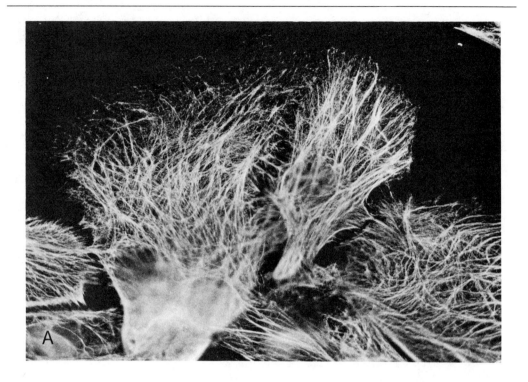

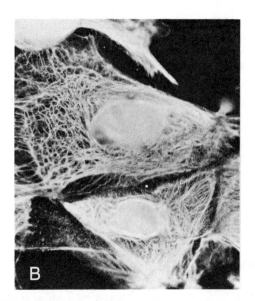

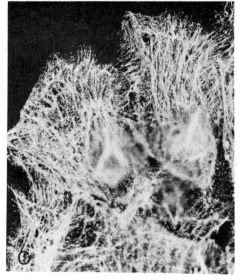

FIG. 2-5 Organization of actin filaments in normal and in injured hamster trachea cells. **(A)** Normal cells showing a complex interwoven arrangement of actin filaments. **(B)** Cells injured by a calcium ionophore (A 23187, 10^{-5} M, 48 hours) show a compact irregular network arrangement of the actin. **(C)** Cells injured by amphotericin B (12 μg/ml, 2 hours) show actin filaments with indistinct "defective" borders ($\times$ 420). (Trump BF, Berezesky IK, Phelps PC et al: Ion regulation and the cytoskeleton in preneoplastic and neoplastic cells. p. 35. In Harris C, Autrup H (ed): Human Carcinogenesis. Academic Press, New York, 1983.)

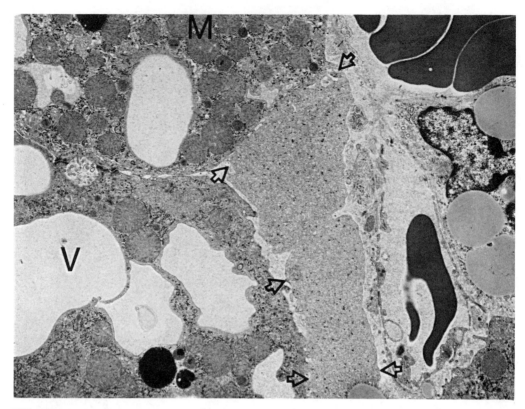

FIG. 2-6 Dog liver in severe hemorrhagic shock. The hepatocyte mitochondria (M) are swollen. Note large clear vacuoles (V) due to infolding of cell surface membrane. Blebbing of plasma membrane in the space of Disse (arrows) is evident (× 7,500).

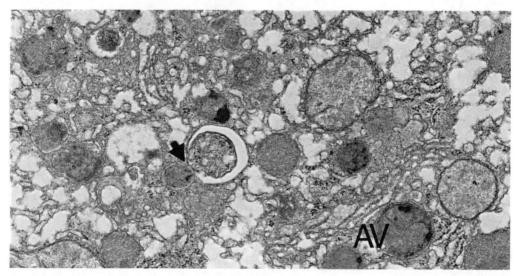

FIG. 2-7 Stimulation of autophagy by systemic insults. Hepatocyte from a rat with a sterile abscess; several autophagic vacuoles (AV) contain cellular parts undergoing digestion. Fusion between an autophagic vacuole and a lysosome is seen (arrow). The lysosome supplies the enzymes necessary for the digestion of membranes and cytosol in the autophagic vacuole (× 25,000).

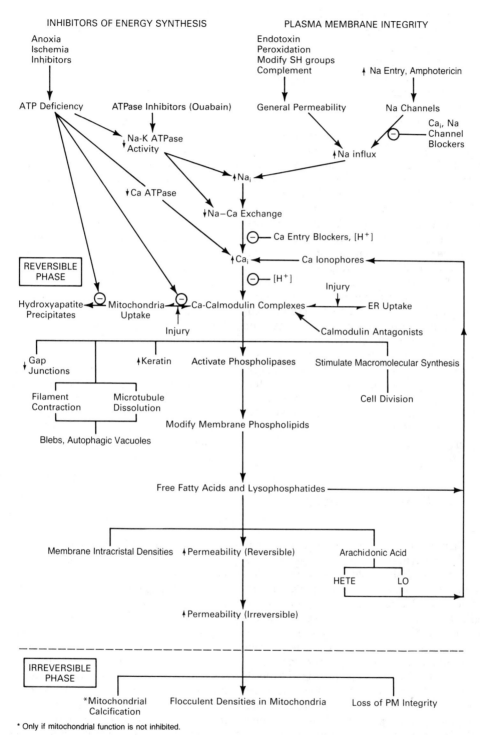

FIG. 2-8 Calcium deregulation and cell injury and death. This flow diagram outlines our concept of how loss of ion regulation, particularly calcium, is related to the pathogenesis of cell injury and death. See text for further details. (Trump BF, Berezesky IK: Role of sodium and calcium regulation in toxic cell injury. p. 261. In Mitchell JR, Horning MG (ed): Drug Metabolism and Drug Toxicity. Raven Press, New York, 1984.)

cause(s) of the acidosis must be promptly treated and the acidosis itself must be corrected because of its arrhythmogenic potential, among other reasons.

Experimental endotoxin injection and sepsis cause a decrease in liver glycogen and an initial increase followed by a decrease in blood glucose. The disturbance in gluconeogenesis is caused by disturbances in substrate and hormone levels as discussed in Chapter 15. The activities of key glycolytic enzymes are also altered.[76] The preterminal hypoglycemia seems to be due to a defect in the ability of the liver to synthesize glucose. Stimulation of pyruvate carboxylase and phosphoenolpyruvate carboxykinase as well as an influx of alanine and lactate from skeletal muscle, drive the synthesis of glucose in the hepatocytes.[125] Incomplete glucose utilization has been reported to occur in sepsis due to decreased entry of pyruvate into the Krebs cycle. Inhibition of pyruvate dehydrogenase activity may be responsible.[9] Impaired oxidation of fatty acids occurs in sepsis and can be induced by the administration of endotoxin.[77] This impairment leads to the accumulation of triglyceride in the cytosol. Fat droplets are commonly seen in injured cells in many tissues.

Protein Synthesis

Disturbances of protein synthesis are seen in many types of cell injury. Disaggregation of polysomes is in fact one of the earliest manifestations of cell injury visible at the light microscopic level due to loss of basophilia of the cell cytoplasm. It has been shown that inhibition of protein synthesis over the short run does not influence survival of injured cells. In some cases cells are actually more resistant to injury in the presence of protein synthesis inhibitors.[111] These protective effects are short-lived and are probably due to shunting of metabolic energy from protein synthesis to other critical energy-requiring cell functions.

A reprioritization of protein synthesis is seen in sepsis. This response is probably indirectly induced by inflammatory mediators. Typically in the liver, the synthesis and secretion of acute phase reactants such as C-reactive protein, ceruloplasmin, and fibrinogen are stimulated. On the other hand, albumin, prealbumin, and transferrin show a decrease in biosynthesis.[61,79] Blocks in protein synthesis can be rapidly reversed. This suggests that reversible inactivation of the synthetic machinery is involved. The synthetic machinery reutilizes amino acids derived from catabolism, particularly of skeletal muscle. Degradation of hepatocyte cytoplasm inside autophagic vacuoles is a characteristic ultrastructural feature of cell injury such as occurs in sepsis (Fig. 2-7). Amino acids derived from the degradation of the cytoplasmic proteins may be also reutilized for new protein synthesis in the hepatocytes.

New classes of proteins, collectively referred to as "heat shock" proteins, are synthesized by cells exposed to a variety of stresses. These proteins may enhance the resistance of cells to repetitive injurious stimuli. For example, the exposure of cells to elevated temperature, hypoxia, toxic agents, or deprivation of amino acids causes an inhibition of protein synthesis. However, a selected number of proteins show increased synthesis and accumulate in the cells under these conditions.[62,71,72] The mechanism of this response includes the activation of transcription of few specific genes and preferential translation. Typically in these cells, a concomitant decline in general protein synthesis occurs. It has been proposed that a decline in cellular ATP levels triggers the synthesis of "heat shock" proteins.[37] The synthesis of these new proteins has been shown to increase the resistance of cells to lethal injury induced by hyperthermia. This type of "protective" protein has yet to be identified in sepsis.

Newly synthesized proteins destined for export to the extracellular space follow an intracellular pathway (see Fig. 2-9). The export pathway ferries these secretory proteins from the site of their synthesis to the plasma membrane where discharge to the extracellular space occurs. The pathway is tightly regulated. In many cells, blocks in the export of secretory proteins have been identified in pathologic conditions.[44] As a result of these blocks, a portion of the newly synthesized secretory proteins are degraded intracellularly instead of being exported to the blood stream.[111]

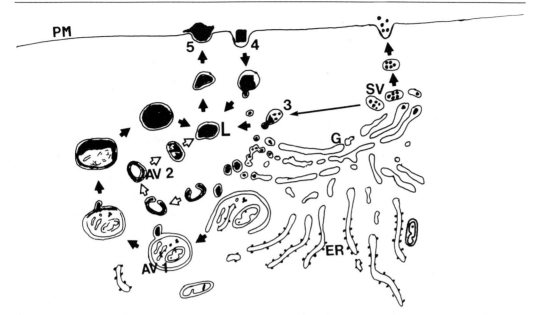

FIG. 2-9 Lysosomal pathways of degradation in a typical cell. Note that all the degradation pathways converge into the lysosome (L). Pathways 1 to 3 serve to degrade intracellular material, namely, membranes (1), cytosol (2), and secretory products (3). The autophagic vacuole (AV) is the first stage in the degradation pathways 1 and 2. Pathway 4 serves to degrade extracellular material internalized via the plasma membrane (PM) by endocytosis. Pathway 5 indicates that lysosomal contents are extruded from the cell in certain situations. The diagram also outlines the secretory pathway, namely, endoplasmic reticulum (ER) → Golgi apparatus (G) → secretory vacuole (SV) → plasma membrane (PM) → extracellular space.

The inhibition of protein synthesis in the liver may cause a block in the export of triglycerides and cholesterol to the bloodstream because a protein moiety is necessary for packaging the lipids. Such a block causes the accumulation of lipid particles inside the endoplasmic reticulum. An accumulation of triglycerides in the cell's cytosol is also frequently seen in injured cells. In sepsis the failure of fatty acid oxidation seems to be also responsible for triglyceride accumulation. Hormone-mediated effects on parenchymal organs and adipose tissue may also contribute.

Alteration in hepatic bile flow is a common event in septic patients and results in accumulation of bile within hepatocytes. Impairment in bile conjugation and transport, drugs, and hyperalimentation mixtures may all contribute to the cholestatic picture. The precise cellular mechanism of this disturbance remains to be elucidated.

Protein Catabolism

The loss of protein mass is a characteristic feature of many pathologic processes. This loss of protein results from the alteration of catabolic and biosynthetic pathways that regulate the turnover of proteins.[43,106] If persistent, these alterations induce atrophy of cells. Host responses to inflammatory, ischemic, and traumatic stimuli are known to stimulate protein catabolism in muscles.[8,22,73] These responses are mediated by inflammatory substances released from phagocytic cells. One of these substances, interleukin-1, acts by stimulating the release of prostaglandin from cellular membranes. The prostaglandin in turn activates lysosomal catabolic pathways.[8] Calcium influx into skeletal muscle cells can also stimulate protein degradation. The signal appears to be an increase in prostaglandin synthesis.[114] Several types of cellular and systemic perturbations modulate protein catabolism at least in part through the action of glucagon and insulin. Glucagon stimulates, while insulin inhibits, protein degradation. These hormones ultimately activate lysosomal catabolic pathways. The liver parenchymal cells are particularly sensitive to modulation of proteolysis by these two hormones.[90,99,149] Insulin also inhibits proteolysis in cardiac and skeletal muscle.[40] In the livers of rats with streptozoticin-induced diabetes the molar ratio of glucagon to insulin is elevated and the fractional volume of lysosomes increases. Insulin treatment reduces the fractional volume of the lysosomes.[5,17] In traumatic shock and burns and in life-threatening bacterial infections the glucagon to insulin molar ratio is elevated.[113,124] Not surprisingly, therefore, the rate of protein degradation, is elevated. The rates of protein degradation in liver and skeletal muscle are increased by the administration of thyroid hormones and decreased by thyroidectomy. These hormonal effects appear to be modulated by changes in the levels of proteolytic enzymes, particularly in the lysosomes.[32] Since the early studies of Green and Miller[47] and Marsh,[82] glucagon and insulin have been known to have profound influences on the synthesis of plasma proteins by the liver.

It is clear then that the lysosomes play an important role in the degradation of proteins both in normal and in pathologically altered conditions. It is thought that the lysosomes are responsible for at least 40 to 50 percent of the normal cellular protein breakdown. The lysosomes preferentially degrade membrane proteins and "longer-lived" proteins. It is generally accepted that the predominant if not the entire extent of stimulated protein degradation that occurs during nutrient deprivation in isolated cells,[121] in glucagon administration and amino acid deprivation in perfused liver,[95] and in injury states[8] results from an activation of the lysosomal pathway of degradation. The lysosomes are intracellular collections of digestive enzymes enclosed in membrane sacs. Electron microscopic studies have helped to show how the lysosomes can digest selected cellular structures without damaging the entire cell.[85] This sequence of degradative steps is outlined schematically in Figure 2-9. The first step in

the degradation is the formation of membrane pockets that gradually surround and enclose cellular membranes and cytosol. At this stage the material to be digested is isolated from the remainder of the cell within a closed membranous sac. This structure is called the autophagic vacuole. The lysosomes next fuse with the autophagic vacuoles and infuse into it the necessary digestive enzymes. At this point degradation begins. The final degradation products (amino acids, sugars, and fatty acids) permeate or are transported through the autophagic vacuole membranes back into the cytosol where they can be reutilized for biosynthetic reactions.[55,86] This catabolic process is termed *autophagocytosis* (or *autophagy* for short) to differentiate it from ordinary phagocytosis. Mechanistically, phagocytosis and autophagocytosis are analogous in some respects. In a wide variety of pathologic states such as ischemia, anoxia, and tissue involution an increase in the number of autophagic vacuoles is seen.[88,89] Examples of the ultrastructural appearance of the autophagic vacuoles induced by systemic insults are shown in Figures 2-4 and 2-7. In Figure 2-7, autophagic vacuoles at different stages of formation are seen. Note the coalescing of an autophagic vacuole and a lysosome (Fig. 2-7, arrow).

The stimulation of protein catabolism is thought to be a protective response designed to provide amino acids for gluconeogenesis and energy production and for the synthesis of proteins necessary for host defense. The coupling between enhanced catabolism and increased synthesis of new proteins is exemplified by the effects of interleukin-1. This substance stimulates muscle catabolism as well as the synthesis of acute phase proteins in the liver.[8,131] The lysosomes are also involved in the degradation of newly synthesized secretory proteins. Some of these proteins fail to be exported outside of the cell and are instead digested intracellularly (Fig. 2-9). This phenomenon occurs in normal cells but appears to be stimulated in cell injury; it has been demonstrated in several cell types, for example, in hepatocytes and pancreatic acinar cells.[44,111] The finding that stimulation of lysosomes is responsible for the enhanced catabolism in injury opens the way for pharmacologic intervention to block lysosomal stimulation. For example, blockers of prostaglandin synthesis have been shown in vitro to block protein catabolism. Indomethacin at concentrations compatible with therapeutic levels was shown to protect muscle from the stimulation of protein catabolism induced by leukocytic pyrogen.[8]

In addition to the lysosomal catabolic pathways described above, a nonlysosomal pathway of protein catabolism is operative inside cells. The nonlysosomal catabolic pathway preferentially degrades abnormal cellular proteins and "short-lived" proteins. Some proteins to be degraded in this pathway are tagged by the addition of a small protein called ubiquitin. Energy in the form of ATP is required for this coupling. The cellular proteins tagged with ubiquitin become susceptible to degradation by proteolytic enzymes.[20] Other cellular proteins are directly attacked and degraded by protease enzymes that are ATP-dependent.[132] In sum, the extralysosomal pathway seems to be more specific in that it selectively degrades abnormal proteins resulting from chromosomal aberrations, errors in proteins synthesis, or postsynthetic denaturation.

PHARMACOLOGIC INTERVENTIONS

Cytotoxicity due to administration of therapeutic agents is a constant risk. For example, renal damage occurs from immunologically mediated cell injury induced by the β-lactam class of antibiotics. Methicillin is the principal offender and it induces interstitial nephritis.[6] Acute tubulointerstitial nephropathy due to the direct toxic action of antibiotics, particularly those of the aminoglycoside class, is another well-known phenomenon. Lysosomal dysfunction has been demonstrated after the administration of aminoglycosides.[63] The necrosis of cells in the proximal tubules seems to be induced by the uptake of aminoglycosides into the lysosomes without transtubular secretion.[63,127] Therapeutic agents normally well tolerated may be lethal to injured tissues.

For example, therapy with catecholamines may induce myocardial cell necrosis in conditions of hypoxia and/or ischemia.[41] The necrosis may result from the stimulation of the slow inward calcium currents by the catecholamines and consequent accumulation of calcium in the myocardial cells.[49] Trunkey et al. demonstrated a decrease in the levels of serum calcium during experimental hemorrhagic and septic shock.[143,144] This suggests that increased influx of calcium occurs in injured tissues. Pharmacologic approaches designed to modulate calcium levels may be of use. For example, agents that block the entry of calcium (calcium blockers) inside cells have been tried. Calcium blockers have been shown to increase the survival of injured cells in myocardium and brain.[28,56]

Blockers of the slow calcium channel can also inhibit the pulmonary vessel vasoconstriction induced by hypoxic states.[91,130] These observations suggest that influx of calcium into vascular smooth muscle cells occurs as a result of decreased energy levels. This influx then triggers contraction of the cells and causes vasoconstriction.[92] Vasoactive phenomena are also induced by increased plasma levels of catecholamines and other mediators. This neuroendocrine hyperactivity is responsible for the development of various circulatory shock syndromes. The end result of these vascular events is a maldistribution of blood volume and flow and inadequate perfusion of multiple organs.[1,54]

Attempts to bolster the intracellular levels of high-energy metabolites have met with some success. Beneficial effects of adenine nucleotides combined with magnesium chloride have been reported in ischemic injury.[19,45] These effects may be mediated by vasoactive phenomena. Administration of ribose has been shown to restore ATP levels to normal in ischemic myocardium due to stimulation of adenosine resynthesis.[150] In an attempt to stabilize cellular membranes,[57] corticosteroids have been used and have proven to be beneficial. However, corticosteroid therapy can delay wound healing and interfere with immunologic defense systems.

As discussed previously, in vitro antioxidant therapy also protects against lethal cell injury.[39] It is interesting that exposure to low doses of endotoxin protects cells against the effects of injurious agents.[58,134] At these doses endotoxin may help to stabilize cellular membranes against injury.[30]

INTERACTION OF CELL INJURY AND CELL REPAIR MECHANISMS

Cell injury and repair mechanisms interact in complex ways to result in tissue healing or organ failure. The type and severity of the injury play a role in the eventual outcome. The interplay of the injury and repair mechanisms is best illustrated by the evolution of endothelial cell injury in the lung.

Endothelial injury can be caused by a long list of mediators such as superoxide radicals, metabolites of arachidonic acid, and vasoactive peptides.[53] Some microbial components are directly cytotoxic to endothelial cells[36] and endotoxin can injure endothelial cells in the presence of complement.[34] Finally, polymorphonuclear leukocytes stimulated by endotoxin are cytotoxic to endothelial cells.[59] Figure 2-10 shows a lung capillary from a dog in shock. A polymorphonuclear leukocyte is seen adjacent to a lung capillary endothelial cell. Bleb formation due to cell injury is seen in the figure.

Mild acute endothelial cell injury can be repaired without sequelae by proliferation of cells to cover the denuded areas left by cells that have died and sloughed off.[16] Some agents, such as endotoxin, injure endothelial cells and at the same time induce regeneration.[110] More severe injury, with a delay in regeneration, will stimulate smooth muscle proliferation and fibrosis in the vascular wall.[50,109] Damage to collagen components of basement membranes may also induce proliferation of interstitial fibroblasts that secrete types I and III collagen. Endothelial cells are induced to proliferate further by this type of collagen substrate.

The importance of endothelial cell injury in the pathogenesis of organ failure can be demonstrated in adult respiratory distress syndrome (ARDS). In lung capillaries, endothelial cell injury leads to increased vascular permeability[120] with subsequent interstitial and alveolar hemorrhage, edema, and vascular micro- and macrothrombi. Some of these capillary thrombi may originate peripherally due to a hypercoagulable state caused by trauma and shock.[13,24] In addition, the pulmonary endothelial injury can directly lead to localized intravascular coagulation in the lung.[15,119] Clinically, at this initial stage of tissue injury hypoxemia,

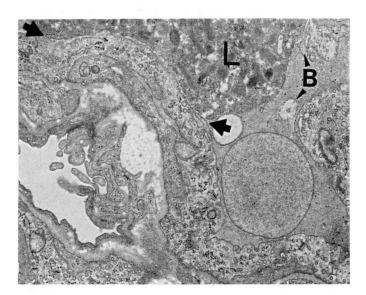

FIG. 2-10 Endothelial cell injury in canine hemorrhagic shock. Polymorphonuclear leukocyte (L) is in close approximation to the endothelial cell of a lung capillary (arrows). Blebs (B) are present in the lumen of the capillary ($\times$ 12,500).

decreased pulmonary compliance, and diffuse interstitial and alveolar infiltrates are demonstrable on radiographs.

The stage of edema and hemorrhage in the lung is often further complicated by additional toxic insults such as hyperoxia from high inspired oxygen concentration[31] and infection. A proliferative phase follows the initial stage of injury with obliteration of arteries, veins, and lymphatics in the lung by replicating mesenchymal cells and by collagen deposition. In the late stage, vascular remodeling occurs. Hypertrophy of muscle cells in arteries and obliteration of capillaries are seen; the remaining capillaries dilate. Dense fibrosis of lung parenchyma is the end result.[128,135] Inflammatory cells, particularly macrophages and lymphocytes, also play a role in the stimulation of fibroblast proliferation and secretion of collagen.[74,146] The inflammatory cells, particularly neutrophils and eosinophils, are responsible for collagen degradation and remodeling.[70] Thus, in the lung, a severe initial injury to endothelium causes a loss in the normal endothelium–fibroblast control system. Extensive cell proliferation and collagen deposition occur.

Work with experimental models of lung injury has shown that damage to the cells (epithelial) lining the alveoli can also result in lung fibrosis by disturbing normal epithelial–mesenchymal cell relationships.[2,18] The role of injury to epithelial cells in the pathogenesis of ARDS is, however, not established. Type II epithelial cells are usually the source of renewal of alveolar lining cells.[65]

The therapeutic implications to be derived from understanding the pathogenesis of ARDS are that interventions directed toward treating the interstitial edema, thromboembolism, and pulmonary vasoconstriction during the early stages may be beneficial. Development of new pharmacologic interventions to salvage endothelial cells in the pulmonary blood vessels is necessary. Early treatment of infections is an obvious necessity. Both hypoxia and hyperoxia cause hypertrophy of the wall of pulmonary arteries[93] and must be avoided by careful respiratory management. High oxygen levels, in particular, are very toxic to endothelial cells. The damage is probably mediated by toxic oxygen species. Endothelial cells can be made more resistant to oxygen-induced injury by increasing the levels of antioxidant defense systems inside the cell. *Superoxide dismutase,* for example, has been shown in vitro to protect endothelial cells.[39] Exposure of animals to 85 percent oxygen for a few days causes adaptive changes in pulmonary endothelial cells. As a result,[27] the animals are able to survive exposure to 100 percent oxygen. Exposure of non-adapted animals to 100 percent oxygen is usually lethal in 2 to 3 days. The later vascular and fibrotic changes of ARDS are largely irreversible.

REFERENCES

1. Adams HR: Pharmacologic problems in circulation research: alpha adrenergic blocking drugs. Circ Shock 10: 215, 1983
2. Adamson IYR, Bowden DH: Pulmonary injury and repair: organ culture studies of murine lung after oxygen. Arch Pathol 100: 640, 1976
3. Alexander JW, McClennan MA, Ogle CK et al: Consumptive opsonopathy: possible pathogenesis in lethal and opportunistic infections. Ann Surg 184: 672, 1976
4. Ames A, Wright RL, Kowada M et al: Cerebral ischemia: II. The no reflow phenomenon. Am J Pathol 52: 437, 1968
5. Amherdt M, Harris V, Renold AE et al: Hepatic autophagy in uncontrolled experimental diabetes and its relationship to insulin and glucagon. J Clin Invest 54: 188, 1974
6. Appel GB, Neu HC: The nephrotoxicity of antimicrobial agents. N Engl J Med 296: 663, 1977
7. Bagge U, Ammundson B, Lauritzen C: White blood cell deformability and plugging of skeletal muscle capillaries in hemorrhagic shock. Acta Physiol Scand 108: 159, 1980
8. Baracos V, Rodermann PH, Dinarello CA, Goldberg AL: Stimulation of muscle protein degradation and prostaglandin E_2 release by leukocytic pyrogen (interleukin-1). A mechanism for the increased degradation of muscle proteins during fever. N Engl J Med 308: 553, 1983
9. Batenburg JJ, Olson MS: Regulation of pyruvate dehydrogenase by fatty acid in isolated rat liver mitochondria. J Biol Chem 251: 1364, 1976
10. Bevilacqua MP, Amrani D, Mosessan MW, Bianco C: Receptors for cold-insoluble globulin

(plasma fibronectin) on human monocytes. J Exp Med 153: 42, 1981

11. Biesecker G: Membrane attack complex of complement as a pathologic mediator. Lab Invest 49: 237, 1983

12. Bitterman PB, Rennard SI, Hunninghake GW, Crystal RG: Human alveolar macrophage growth factor for fibroblasts. J Clin Invest 70: 806, 1982

13. Blaisdell FW, Lim RC, Stallone RJ: The mechanism of pulmonary damage following traumatic shock. Surg Gynecol Obstet 130: 15, 1970

14. Bolanowski PJP, Bawer J, Machiedo G, Neville WE: Prostaglandin influence on pulmonary artery intravascular leukocytic aggregation during cardiopulmonary bypass. J Thorac Cardiovasc Surg 73: 221, 1977

15. Bone RC, Francis PB, Pierce AK: Intravascular coagulation associated with the adult respiratory distress syndrome. Am J Med 61: 585, 1976

16. Bowden DH, Adamson IYR: Endothelial regeneration as a marker of the differential vascular responses in oxygen-induced pulmonary edema. Lab Invest 30: 350, 1974

17. Brekke IB, Danielsen H, Reith A: Normalization of hepatic lysosomal autophagy in streptozotocin diabetic rats after pancreatic transplantation. Virchows Arch [Cell Pathol] 43: 189, 1983

18. Brody AR, Soler P, Basset F et al: Epithelial-mesenchymal associations of cells in human pulmonary fibrosis and in BHT-oxygen induced fibrosis in mice. Exp Lung Res 2: 207, 1981

19. Chaudry IH, Clemens MG, Ohkawa M et al: Restoration of hepatocellular function and blood flow following hepatic ischemia with ATP-MgCl₂. Adv Shock Res 8: 177, 1982

20. Ciechanover A, Elias S, Heller H et al: Characterization of the heat stable polypeptide of the ATP-dependent proteolytic system from reticulocytes. J Biol Chem 255: 7525, 1980

21. Clark RAF, Quinn JH, Winn HJ et al: Fibronectin is produced by blood vessels in response to injury. J Exp Med 156: 646, 1982

22. Clowes GHA, George BC, Villee CA, Saravis CA: Muscle proteolysis induced by a circulating peptide in patients with sepsis or trauma. N Engl J Med 308: 545, 1983

23. Cooper NR: Activation and regulation of the first complement component. Fed Proc 42: 134, 1983

24. Costabella PM, Lindquist O, Kapanci Y, Saldeen T: Increased vascular permeability in the delayed microembolism syndrome, experimental and human findings. Microvasc Res 15: 275, 1978

25. Cowley RA, Mergner WJ, Fischer RS, et al: The subcellular pathology of shock in trauma patients: studies using the immediate autopsy. Am Surg 45: 255, 1979

26. Craddock PR, Fehr J, Brigham KL et al: Complement and leucocyte-mediated pulmonary dysfunction in hemodyalisis. N Engl J Med 296: 769, 1977

27. Crapo JD, Barry BE, Foscue HA, Shelburne J: Structural and biochemical changes in rat lungs occurring during exposures to lethal and adaptive doses of oxygen. Am Rev Respir Dis 122: 123, 1980

28. Daenen W, Flameng W: Myocardial protection by lidoflazine during one-hour normothermic global ischemia. Angiology 32: 543, 1981

29. Dahinden C, Galanos C, Fehr J: Granulocyte activation by endotoxin: I. Correlation between adherence and other granulocyte functions, and role of endotoxin structure on biologic activity. J Immunol 130: 857, 1983

30. Davies M, Stewart-Tull DES, Jackson DM: The binding of lipopolysaccharide from *Escherichia coli* to mammalian cell membranes and its effect on liposomes. Biochim Biophys Acta 508: 260, 1978

31. Davies WB, Rennard SI, Bitterman PB, Crystal RG: Pulmonary oxygen toxicity. Early reversible changes in human alveolar structures induced by hyperoxia. N Engl J Med 309: 878, 1983

32. DeMartino GN, Goldberg AL: Thyroid hormones control lysosomal enzyme activities in liver and skeletal muscle. Proc Natl Acad Sci USA 75: 1369, 1978

33. Engler RL, Schmid-Schonbein GW, Pavelec RS: Leukocyte capillary plugging in myocardial ischemia and reperfusion in the dog. Am J Pathol 111: 98, 1983

34. Evensen SA, Pickering RJ, Batbouta J, Sherpo D: Endothelial injury induced by bacterial endotoxin: effect of complement depletion. Eur J Clin Invest 5: 463, 1975

35. Feher JJ, Briggs FN, Hess ML: Characterization of cardiac SR from ischemic myocardium: comparison of isolated SR with fractionated homogenates. J Mol Cell Cardiol 12: 427, 1980

36. Fillit HM, Jaffe EA, Zabriskie JB: *In vitro* correlates of endothelial injury and repair. Lab Invest 46: 1, 1982

37. Findly RC, Gilles RJ, Shulman RG: In vivo phosphorus-31 nuclear magnetic resonance reveals lowered ATP during heat shock of tetrahymena. Science 219: 1223, 1983

38. Flores J, DiBona DR, Beck CH, Leaf A: The role of cell swelling in ischemia renal damage and the protective effect of hypertonic solute. J Clin Invest 51: 118, 1972

39. Freeman BA, Young SL, Crapo JD: Liposome-mediated augmentation of superoxide dismutase in endothelial cells prevents oxygen injury. J Biol Chem 258: 12534, 1983

40. Fulks RM, Li JB, Goldberg AL: Effects of insulin, glucagon, and amino acids on protein turnover in rat diaphragm. J Biol Chem 250: 290, 1975

41. Gauduel Y, Karagueuzian HS, DeLeiris J: Deleterious effects of endogenous catecholamines on hypoxic myocardial cells following reoxygenation. J Mol Cell Cardiol 11: 717, 1979

42. Giclas PC, Pinckard RN, Olson MS: *In vitro* activation of complement by isolated human heart subcellular membranes. J Immunol 122: 146, 1979

43. Glaumann H, Ericsson JLE, Marzella L: Mechanisms of intralysosomal degradation with special reference to autophagocytosis and heterophagocytosis of cell organelles. Int Rev Cytol 73: 149, 1981

44. Glaumann H, Sandberg PO, Marzella L: Degradation of secretory content in Golgi enriched fractions from rat liver after vinblastine administration. Exp Cell Res 140: 201, 1982

45. Glazier WB, Siegel NJ, Chaudry IH et al: Enhanced recovery from severe ichemic renal injury with adenosine triphosphate-magnesium chloride: administration after the insult. Surg Forum 29: 82, 1978

46. Glenn KC, Ross R: Human monocyte-derived growth factor(s) for mesenchymal cells: activation of secretion by endotoxin and concanavalin A. Cell 25: 603, 1981

47. Green M, Miller LL: Protein catabolism and protein synthesis in perfused livers of normal and alloxan-diabetic rats. J Biol Chem 235: 3202, 1960

48. Grinell F, Billingham RE, Burgess L: Distribution of fibronectin during wound healing in vivo. J Invest Dermatol 76: 181, 1981

49. Harding DP, Poole-Wilson PA: Calcium exchange in rabbit myocardium during and after hypoxia: effect of temperature and substrate. Cardiovasc Res 14: 435, 1980

50. Haudenschild CC, Schwartz SM: Endothelial regeneration: II. Restitution of endothelial continuity. Lab Invest 41: 407, 1979

51. Heideman M: Complement activation *in vitro* induced by endotoxin and injured tissue. J Surg Res 26: 670, 1979

52. Heideman M, Saravis C, Clowes GHA: Effect of nonviable tissue and abscesses on complement depletion and the development of bacteremia. J Trauma 22: 527, 1982

53. Hempel FG, Lenfant CJM: Current and future research on adult respiratory distress syndrome. Semin Respir Med 11: 165, 1981

54. Hinshaw LB, Beller-Todd BK, Archer LT: Current management of the septic shock patient: experimental basis for treatment. Circ Shock 9:543–553, 1982

55. Hirsimaki P, Arstila AV, Trump BF, Marzella L: Autophagocytosis. p. 201. In Trump BF, Arstila AV (eds): Pathobiology of Cell Membranes III. Academic Press, New York, 1983

56. Hoffmeister F, Kazda S, Krause HP: Influence of nimodipine on the postischemic changes of brain function. Acta Neurol Scand 60 (suppl) 72: 358, 1979

57. Hoffstein S, Weismann G, Fox AC: Lysosomes in myocardial infarction: Studies by means of cytochemistry and subcellular fractionation with observations of methyl prednisolone. Circulation 53 (suppl) 1: 33–40, 1976

58. Hollinger MA, Patwell SW, Zucherman JE: Effect of endotoxin in thiourea-induced pulmonary edema and pleural effusion. Res Commun Chem Pathol Pharmacol 31: 217, 1981

59. Jacob HS, Craddock PR, Hammerschmidt DE, Moldoso CF: Complement induced granulocyte aggregation: an unsuspected mechanism of disease. N Engl J Med 307: 789, 1980

60. Jewell SA, Bellomo G, Thor H et al: Bleb formation in hepatocytes during drug metabolism is caused by alterations in intracellular thiol and Ca^+ hemeostasis. Science 217: 1257, 1982

61. Johansson BG: Plasma proteins as diagnostic aids. Methods and clinical applications. p. 309. In Blombäck B, Hanson LÅ (eds): Plasma Proteins. Wiley, New York, 1979

62. Johnston D, Opperman H, Jackson J, Levinson W: Induction of four proteins in chick embryo cells by sodium arsenite. J Biol Chem 255: 6975, 1980

63. Kaloyanides GJ, Pastoriza-Munoz E: Aminoglycoside nephrotoxicity. Kidney Int 18: 571, 1980

64. Kampschmidt RF, Pulliam LA, Upchurch HF: The activity of partially purified leucocytic endogenous mediator in endotoxin resistant C3H/HeJ mice. J Lab Clin Med 95: 616, 1980

65. Kawanami O, Ferrans VJ, Crystal RG: Structure of alveolar epithelial cells in patients with fibrotic lung disorders. Lab Invest 46: 39, 1982

66. Kimball HR, Melman KL, Wolff SM: Endotoxin-induced kinin production in man. Proc Soc Exp Biol Med 139: 1078, 1972

67. Kosower NS, Kosower EM: The glutathione status of cells. Int Rev Cytol 54: 109, 1978

68. Kurland JI, Bockman RS: Prostaglandin E production by human blood monocytes and mouse peritoneal macrophages. J Exp Med 147: 952, 1978

69. Kuthan H, Tsuji H, Graf H, et al: Generation of superoxide anion as a source of hydrogen peroxide in a reconstituted monooxygenase system. FEBS Lett 91: 343, 1978

70. Lazarus GS, Daniels JR, Lian J, Burleigh MC: Role of granulocyte collagenases in collagen degradation. Am J Pathol 68: 565, 1972

71. Levinson W, Kravitz S, Jackson J: Amino acid

deprivation induces synthesis of four proteins in chick embryo cells. Exp Cell Res 130: 459, 1980

72. Li G, Werb Z: Correlation between synthesis of heat shock proteins and development of thermotolerance in Chinese hamster fibroblasts. Proc Natl Acad Sci USA 79: 3218, 1982

73. Libby P, Goldberg AL: The control and mechanism of protein breakdown in striated muscle: studies with selective inhibitors. p. 201. In Wildenthal K (ed): Degradative Processes in Heart and Skeletal Muscle. Elsevier/North Holland, Amsterdam, 1980

74. Liebovich SJ, Ross RA: A macrophage dependent factor that stimulates the proliferation of fibroblasts *in vitro*. Am J Pathol 84: 501, 1979

75. Linder E, Lehto BP, Stenman S: Activation of complement by cytoskeletal intermediate filaments. Nature 278: 176, 1979

76. Liu MS, Sharma C: Glycolytic enzyme activities in normal and diabetic dog livers during endotoxic shock. Am J Physiol 240: R10, 1981

77. Liu MS, Spitzer JJ: In vitro effects of *E. coli* endotoxin on fatty acid and lactate oxidation in canine myocardium. Circ Shock 4: 181, 1977

78. Lotscher HR, Winterhalter KH, Carofoli E, Richter C: Hydroperoxide-induced loss of pyridine nucleotides and release of calcium from rat liver mitochondria. J Biol Chem 255: 9325, 1980

79. MacIntyre SS, Schultz D, Kushner I: Bio-synthesis of C-reactive protein. Ann NY Acad Sci 389: 76, 1982

80. Manson NH, Hess ML: Interaction of oxygen free radicals and cardiac sarcoplastic reticulum: proposed role in the pathogenesis of endotoxin shock. Circ Shock 10: 205, 1983

81. Marasco WA, Fantone JC, Freer RJ, Ward PA: Characterization of rat neutrophil formyl peptide chemotaxis receptor. Am J Pathol 111: 273, 1983

82. Marsh JB: Effects of fasting and alloxan diabetes on albumin synthesis by perfused rat liver. Am J Physiol 201: 55, 1961

83. Martin BA, Gimbrone MA, Majeau GR et al: Stimulation of human monocyte/macrophage-derived growth factor (MDGF) production by plasma fibronectin. Am J Pathol 111: 367, 1983

84. Martin BA, Gimbrone MA, Unanue ER, Cotran RS: Stimulation of nonlymphoid mesenchymal cell proliferation by a macrophage-derived growth factor. J Immunol 126: 1510, 1981

85. Marzella L, Ahlberg J, Glaumann H: Autophagy, heterophagy microautophagy and crinophagy as the means of intracellular degradation. Virchows Arch [Cell Pathol] 36: 219, 1981

86. Marzella L, Ahlberg J, Glaumann H: Isolation of autophagic vacuoles from rat liver. Morpho-

logical and biochemical characterization. J Cell Biol 93: 144, 1982

87. Marzella L, Bernacchi AS, Mayers R, Trump BF: Protection of hepatocytes by hyperbaric oxygen against CCl₄ toxicity. Fed Proc 43: 384, 1984

88. Marzella L, Glaumann H: Increased degradation in rat liver induced by vinblastine. II. Morphological characterization. Lab Invest 42: 18, 1980

89. Marzella L, Glaumann H: Effects of in vivo liver ischemia on microsomes and lysosomes. Virchows Arch [Cell Pathol] 36: 1, 1981

90. Marzella L, Sandberg PO, Glaumann H: Autophagic degradation in rat liver after vinblastine treatment. Exp Cell Res 128: 291, 1980

91. McMurtry IF, Davidson AB, Reeves JT, Grover RF: Inhibition of hypoxic pulmonary vasoconstriction by calcium antagonists in isolated rat lungs. Circ Res 38: 99, 1976

92. McMurtry IF, Rounds S, Stanbrook HS: Studies on the mechanism of hypoxic pulmonary vasoconstriction. Adv Shock Res 8: 21, 1982

93. Meyrick B, Reid L: The effect of continued hypoxia on rat pulmonary artery circulation: An ultrastructural study. Lab Invest 38: 188, 1978

94. Morrison DC, Kline LF: Activation of the classical and properdin pathways of complement by bacterial lipopolysaccharides (LPS). J Immunol 118: 362, 1977

95. Mortimore GE, Schworer CM: Induction of autophagy by amino acid deprivation in perfused rat liver. Nature 270: 174, 1977

96. Muller-Eberhard HJ, Schreiber RD: Molecular biology and chemistry of alternative pathway of complement. Adv Immunol 29: 1, 1980

97. Munford RS: Endotoxin(s) and the liver. Gastroenterology 75: 532, 1978

98. Nakatani T, Sato T, Marzella L et al: Hepatic and systemic response to an intraabdominal abscess in a highly reproducible rat model. Circ Shock 13: 271, 1984

99. Neely AN, Cox JR, Fortney JA et al: Alterations of lysosomal size and density during rat liver perfusion. Suppression by insulin and amino acids. J Biol Chem 252: 6948, 1977

100. Nicholls DG, Crompton M: Mitochondrial calcium transport. FEBS Letts 111: 261, 1980

101. Orrenius S, Ormstad K, Thor H, Jewell SA: Turnover and functions of glutathione studied with isolated hepatic and renal cells. Fed Proc 42: 3177, 1983

102. Park R, Arieff AI: Lactic acidosis. Adv Intern Med 25: 33, 1980

103. Penpargkul S, Fein F, Sonnenblick EH, Scheuer J: Depressed cardiac sarcoplasmic reticulum function from diabetic rats. J Mol Cell Cardiol 13: 303, 1981

104. Penttila A, Glaumann H, Trump BF: Studies on the modification of the cellular response to in-

jury. IV. Protective effect of extracellular acidosis against anoxia, thermal and p-chloromercuribenzene sulfonic acid treatment of isolated liver cells. Life Sci 18: 1419, 1976

105. Penttila A, Trump BF: Extracellular acidosis protects Ehrlich ascites tumor cells and rat renal cortex against anoxic injury. Science 185: 277, 1974

106. Pfeifer U: Kinetic and subcellular aspects of hypertrophy and atrophy. Int Rev Exp Pathol 23: 1, 1982

107. Podack ER, Kolb WP, Muller-Eberhard HJ: The C5b-9 complex: subunit composition of the classical and alternative pathway-generated complex. J Immunol 116: 1431, 1976

108. Recknagel RO, Glende EA, Waller RL, Lowrey K: Lipid peroxidation: biochemistry, measurement, and significance in liver cell injury. p. 213. In Plaa G, Hewitt WR (eds): Toxicology of the Liver. Raven Press, New York, 1982

109. Reidy MA, Schwartz SM: Endothelial regeneration: III. Time course of intimal changes after small defined injury to aortic endothelium. Lab Invest 44: 301, 1981

110. Reidy MA, Schwartz SM: Endothelial injury and regeneration: IV. Endotoxin a non-denuding injury to aortic endothelium. Lab Invest 48: 25, 1983

111. Resau J, Marzella L, Trump BF, Jones RT: Lysosomal degradation of zymogen granules in cultured pancreatic explants. Am J Pathol 115: 139, 1984

112. Richman AV, Gerber LI, Balis JU: Peritubular capillaries: a major site of endotoxin-induced vascular injury in the primate kidney. Lab Invest 43: 327, 1980

113. Rocha D, Santeusanio F, Faloona GR, Unger RH: Abnormal pancreatic alpha-cell function in bacterial infections. N Engl J Med 288: 700, 1973

114. Rodemann HP, Waxman L, Goldberg AL: The stimulation of protein degradation in muscle by Ca^{2+} is mediated by prostaglandin E_2 and does not require the calcium-activated protease. J Biol Chem 257: 8716, 1982

115. Rosenbaum JT, Hartiala KT, Webster RO et al: Anti-inflammatory effects of endotoxin. Inhibition of rabbit polymorphonuclear leukocyte responses to complement (C5)-derived peptides *in vivo* and *in vitro*. Am J Pathol 113: 291, 1983

116. Ruiter DJ, Van Der Meulen J, Brower A et al: Uptake by liver cells of endotoxin following its intravenous injection. Lab Invest 45: 38, 1981

117. Rutherford RB, Ross R: Platelet factors stimulate fibroblast and smooth muscle cells quiescent in plasma serum to proliferate. J Cell Biol 69: 196, 1976

118. Schiffman E, Corcoran BA, Wahl SM: N-formyl-methionyl peptides as chemoattractants for leucocytes. Proc Natl Acad Sci USA 72: 1059, 1975

119. Schneider RC, Zapol WM, Carvalho AC: Platelet consumption and sequestration in severe acute respiratory failure. Am Rev Respir Dis 122: 445, 1980

120. Schnells G, Voigt WH, Redl H et al: Electron microscopic investigation of lung biopsies in patients with post traumatic respiratory insufficiency. Acta Chir Scand (S) 449: 9, 1980

121. Seglen PO, Grinde B, Solheim AE: Inhibition of the lysosomal pathway of protein degradation in isolated hepatocytes by ammonia, methylamine, chloroquine and leupeptin. Eur J Biochem 95: 215, 1979

122. Shaw JO, Henson PM, Henson J, Webster RO: Lung inflammation induced by complement-derived chemotactic fragments in the alveolus. Lab Invest 42: 547, 1980

123. Shen SM-C, Rapaport SI, Feinstein DI: Intravascular clotting after endotoxin in rabbits with impaired intrinsic clotting produced by a factor VIII antibody. Blood 42: 523, 1980

124. Shuck JM, Eaton RP, Shuck LW et al: Dynamics of insulin and glucagon secretion in severely burned patients. J Trauma 17: 706, 1977

125. Siegel JH, Cerra FB, Coleman B et al: Physiological and metabolic correlations in human sepsis. Surgery 86: 163, 1979

126. Silver IA: Ion movements induced by endotoxin in cultured cells. Circ Shock 5: 221, 1978

127. Silverblatt FJ, Kuehn C: Autoradiography of gentamycin uptake by the rat proximal tubule cell. Kidney Int 15: 335, 1979

128. Snow RL, Davies P, Pontoppidan H et al: Pulmonary vascular remodelling in adult respiratory distress syndrome. Am Rev Respir Dis, 126: 887, 1982

129. Snyderman R, Fudman EJ: Demonstration of a chemotactic factor receptor on macrophages. J Immunol 124: 2754, 1980

130. Suggett AJ, Mohammed FH, Barer GR: Angiotensin, hypoxia, verapamil and pulmonary vessels. Clin Exp Pharmacol Physiol 7: 263, 1980

131. Sztein MB, Vogel SN, Sipe JD et al: The role of macrophages in the acute phase response: SAA inducer is closely related to lymphocyte activating factor and endogenous pyrogen. Cell Immunol 63: 164, 1981

132. Tanaka K, Waxman L, Goldberg AL: ATP serves two distinct roles in protein degradation in reticulocytes, one requiring and one independent of ubiquitin. J Cell Biol 96: 1580, 1983

133. Thakral KK, Goodson WH, Hunt TK: Stimulation of wound blood vessel growth by macrophages. J Surg Res 26: 430, 1979

134. Thet LA, Wrobel DJ, Crapo JD, Shelburne JD: Morphologic aspects of the protection by endo-

toxin against acute and chronic oxygen-induced lung injury in adult rats. Lab Invest 48: 448, 1983

135. Tomashefski JF, Davies P, Boggis C et al: The pulmonary vascular lesions of the adult respiratory distress syndrome. Am J Pathol 112: 112, 1983

136. Tranum-Jensen J, Bhakdi S, Bhakdi-Lehnen B et al: Complement lysis: the ultrastructure and orientation of the C5b-9 complex on target sheep erythrocyte membranes. Scand J Immunol 7: 45, 1978

137. Trump BF, Berezesky IK, Chang SH et al: The role of ion shifts in cell injury. Scan Electron Microsc 3: 1, 1979

138. Trump BF, Berezesky IK, Cowley RA: The cellular and subcellular characteristics of acute and chronic injury with emphasis on the role of calcium. p. 6. In Cowley RA, Trump BF (eds): Pathophysiology of Shock, Anoxia and Ischemia. William and Wilkins, Baltimore, 1982

139. Trump BF, Berezesky IK, Phelps PC: Sodium and calcium regulation and the role of the cytoskeleton in the pathogenesis of disease. Scan Electron Microsc 2: 435, 1981

140. Trump BF, Harris CC: Human tissues in biomedical research. Hum Pathol 10: 245, 1979

141. Trump BF, Mergner WJ, Jones RT, Cowley RA: The use and application of autopsy in research. Am J Clin Pathol 69: 230, 1978

142. Trump BF, Mergner WJ, Kahng MW, Saladino

AJ: Studies on the subcellular pathophysiology of ischemia. Circulation 53 (suppl. 1):17–26, 1976

143. Trunkey D, Holcroft J, Carpenter MA: Calcium flux during hemorrhagic shock in baboons. J Trauma 16: 633, 1976

144. Trunkey D, Holcroft J, Carpenter MA: Ionized calcium and magnesium: The effect of septic shock in baboons. J Trauma 18: 166, 1978

145. Vogel SN, Marshall ST, Rosenstreich DL: Analysis of the effects of lipopolysaccharide on macrophages: differential phagocytic responses of C_3H/HeN and C_3H/HeJ macrophages in vitro. Infect Immun 25: 328, 1979

146. Wahl SM, Wahl LM, McCarthy LB: Lymphocyte-mediated activation of fibroblast proliferation and collagen production. J Immunol 121: 942, 1978

147. Weissmann G, Smolen JE, Korchak HM: Release of inflammatory mediators from stimulated neutrophils. N Engl J Med 303: 27, 1980

148. Wittels EH, Coalson JJ, Welch MH, Guenter CA: Pulmonary intravascular leukocyte sequestration. A potential mechanism of lung injury. Am Rev Respir Dis 109: 502, 1974

149. Woodside KH, Ward WF, Mortimore GE: Effects of glucagon on general protein degradation and synthesis in perfused rat liver. J Biol Chem 249: 5458, 1974

150. Zimmer HG: Normalization of depressed heart function in rats by ribose. Science 220: 81, 1983

3

Humoral Mediators of Cellular Response and Altered Metabolism*

William R. Beisel

INTRODUCTION

When insulted by trauma, infection, or surgical stress, the body is able to call upon a number of physiologic mechanisms to initiate and coordinate an array of defensive responses.[12,13,35,45,53,55,58,67,68,90,94] These defenses include fever, immune system activation, leukocytic and reticuloendothelial cell changes, metabolic effects, responses by the brain and autonomic nervous system, the release of various hormones, and sometimes the activation of the coagulation, complement, and kinin systems. In addition, localized cell injury or death provokes immediate reactions by other cells in the area, stimulating them to release factors with unique biologic activities. Some of these factors initiate a localized inflammatory reaction, recruit a variety of mobile

cells, or help in the healing process, while other locally produced soluble factors, or mediators, are carried via the blood to distant sites in the body where they function as a hormonelike system of messenger substances.

The system of mediators to be discussed in this chapter is of the latter variety. Although normally quiescent in periods of health, this messenger system, comprised of locally produced endogenous mediators, provides the body with a unique alarm mechanism. This mechanism serves in a manner analogous to the alarm system of a city fire department. These endogenous mediators, now collectively termed interleukin-1 (IL-1),[44,81] give the body an additional, quickly responsive, humoral coordinating mechanism for initiating and modulating a number of important but diverse host responses as needed to defend against the initiating insult.[9,12,13,27,35,53,55,90,94] When released by activated monocytic phagocytes and macrophages, the IL-1 mediators stimulate metabolic, physiologic, and immunologic responses in distant cells and tissues.

---

* The views of the author do not purport to reflect the positions of the Department of the Army or the Department of Defense.

The IL-1 mediators show little detectable activity under conditions of normal health. However, any one of a diverse variety of activating stimuli can cause the IL-1 mediators to be synthesized and released. This response occurs whenever monocytic phagocytes are activated or stimulated by some acute pathologic process or suitable chemical or immunologic stimulus. The magnitude of the IL-1 response seems proportional to the severity of the initiating insult or stimulus and the number of phagocytic cells activated. Because IL-1 type mediators are produced in response to diverse stimuli, their effects are considered to be nonspecific in nature.[12,90] Combinations of host responses initated by IL-1 mediators can be anticipated during virtually all types of major acute injuries and illnesses. In fact, these IL-1-induced responses help to characterize the patterns and progression of illness seen clinically.[6,12,13,20,94]

INTERLEUKIN-1-TYPE MEDIATORS

It has become evident that several incompletely characterized, biologically active, humoral substances are, in reality, closely related or identical endogenous mediators. When released, these IL-1 mediators serve as a rapidly responsive, broad mechanism for activating many defensive responses of the body.[12,35,36,43,45,53,55,78] The control mechanism represented by this unique array of mediators is functionally independent of other major coordinating mechanisms of the body, such as the central nervous system, the endocrine system, or the immune system.[13,35] While these three major control mechanisms routinely serve to coordinate and regulate body functions during normal health, each one of them can be influenced and activated by the IL-1 mediators during acute illness or injury. The IL-1 mediators can also influence some aspects of the complement and coagulation systems.

Interleukin-1-type mediators are released whenever the body is invaded by pathogenic microorganisms or whenever inflammatory reactions are generated. These IL-1 mediators have diverse functions and stimulate many different cell populations.[13] Interleukin-1-type mediators are responsible for triggering febrile reactions,[35] for initiating leukocytic responses,[53,55] for accelerating general metabolic activity and oxygen consumption by body cells,[12,94] for stimulating the liver to accumulate free amino acids, zinc, and iron from plasma pools,[55,59,90] and also for stimulating the liver to produce a number of intracellular proteins (enzymes and metallothioneins)[108] as well as a large variety of "acute-phase" glycoproteins for secretion into the plasma.[20,45,58,90,94,95,113,121]

In other locations, the IL-1 mediators stimulate the pancreatic islet cells to secrete both insulin and glucagon.[41] These mediators activate lysosomal enzymes in both neutrophils and skeletal muscle cells.[6] Through the latter mechanism, IL-1 initiates active proteolysis, which serves to break down the contractile proteins of muscle to their constituent amino acids.[6,27] These free amino acids can then be metabolized as direct forms of energy by muscle cells, or made available for gluconeogenesis in the liver and kidneys. The free amino acids can also be reutilized elsewhere in the body for synthesis of new proteins that support generalized host defensive measures. Because IL-1 appears to stimulate fibroblast proliferation in vitro,[103] it may also function in the healing of wounds.

Another important role of the IL-1 mediators is to activate and modulate various functions of both T- and B-lymphocytes.[43,67] This role led to the selection of the name, interleukin-1, for this group of mediators.[81] Although this recently defined immunologic role of IL-1 is also nonspecific, IL-1 serves to stimulate and enhance the development of specific immunity against foreign antigens that may be involved in the pathogenesis of an acute illness.

Because of the apparent multiplicity and diversity of IL-1 actions, the existence of a number of different endogenous mediators was postulated initially.[12,13,43,45,53,59,85,94,116] Investigators working in different fields first described these mediators and conferred a variety of names on them according to their biologic activities. Unfortunately, because IL-1 mediators existed in only ultratrace quantities and were exceedingly difficult to purify or assay, their exact molecular nature has yet to be characterized.[13,35] Nevertheless, as it became evident that these mediators were small proteins with similar structures and a similar array of functions, a new system of nomenclature was developed.[81] Table 3-1 represents an attempt to assemble the names of mediators that can now be grouped under the term interleukin-1.

This chapter will describe the apparent actions of the IL-1 mediators, discuss their assay methods and apparent molecular structures, and attempt to evaluate their role and importance in acute surgical illnesses and the complications of those illnesses.

HISTORICAL ASPECTS OF THE IL-1 CONCEPT

The release of biologically active substances by cells engaged in phagocytic activity has long been recognized, as has the concept that some of these substances initiate purposeful physiologic responses in distant cells and tissues. Until recently, work in this area tended to focus on individual mediators, but emerging evidence has now indicated that commonalities exist among them. Table 3-2 lists chronologically the experimental findings that led slowly to our current understandings of the IL-1 mediators.

Menkin is generally credited for introducing the concept that endogenously produced substances, released from areas of localized tissue necrosis or inflammation, served to trigger generalized defensive body responses.[77] Menkin supported this concept by demonstrating that a leukocytosis-promoting factor could be recovered from inflammatory exudates.[76] However, Menkin's claims to have discovered an endogenous pyrogen are generally discounted,[9,35] because he failed to exclude contaminating bacterial lipopolysaccharide endotoxin from his fever-producing preparations. Then, after Beeson[7] demonstrated that an endotoxin-free endogenous pyrogen of leukocytic origin actually did exist, Atkins and Wood[3] began, in 1955, an extended series of comprehensive studies into the nature, source, and actions of endogenous pyrogen. Such studies are still being conducted by students and colleagues

TABLE 3-1. Endogenous Mediators Now Named Interleukin 1

Response Induced	Putative Mediator
Fever	Endogenous pyrogen (EP)
	Leukocytic pyrogen (LP)
	Granulocytic pyrogen (GP)
Leukocytosis	Leukocytosis-promoting factor (LPF)
	Leukocytosis-inducing factor (LIF)
	?? Colony-stimulating factor (CSF)
Metabolic changes	Leukocytic endogenous mediator (LEM)
	Proteolysis-inducing factor (PIF)
	Serum amyloid A inducer (SAA Inducer)
	Serum amyloid A stimulating factor (SAASF)
	Mononuclear cell factor (MCF)
	Fibroblast proliferating factor (FPF)
	Macrophage insulin-releasing activity (MIRA)
Lympphocyte activation	Lymphocyte-activating factor (LAF)
	Interleukin-1 (IL-1)
	Helper peak-1 (HP-1)
	T-cell replacing factor III (TRF-III)
	T-cell replacing factor $_{M\phi}$ (TRF$_{M\phi}$)
	B-cell activating factor (BAF)
	B-cell differentiation factor (BDF)

TABLE 3-2.   Investigations of Interleukin 1-Type Endogenous Mediators

Year	Investigator(s)	Noteworthy Discovery of Event
1940	Menkin[76]	Demonstrated a leukocytosis-promoting factor in inflammatory exudates
1948	Beeson[7]	Demonstrated the release of EP from peritoneal exudate cells. Attributed EP to neutrophils
1955	Atkins and Wood[3]	Initiated comprehensive research into EP
1966	Katz et al.[60]	Partially purified LIF
1967	Bodel and Atkins[18]	Demonstrated production of EP by human monocytes
1969	Kampschmidt & Upchurch[56]	Found that EP caused plasma iron levels to decline
1971	Murphy et al.[84]	Achieved a major advance in purification of EP
	Pekarek and Beisel[88]	Found that LEM caused plasma zinc levels to decline
	Vane[117]	Reported that aspirin-like drugs inhibited the synthesis of prostaglandins (PGs)
1972	Pekarek et al.[89]	Showed that LEM caused plasma copper and ceruloplasmin levels to increase
	Wannemacher et al.[118,119]	Demonstrated that LEM caused an increased uptake of plasma free amino acids by the liver, that LEM caused the liver to synthesize and release acute phase plasma proteins, and that LEM-like substances appeared de novo in the plasma of febrile patients with infectious diseases
	Kampschmidt et al.[54]	Showed that EP had LIF activity
	Clark and Coldwell[26]	Found that aspirin blocked induction of fever by EP when both were given ICV
	Gery and Waksman[42]	Demonstrated that macrophages were the source of LAF
1973	Powanda et al.[95]	Demonstrated that LEM had effects on muscle protein metabolism and induced systemic metabolic changes typical of infection
1976	Bailey et al.[5]	Showed that ICV injection of minute doses of LEM produced the systemic effect of large IV doses
1977	Sobocinski et al.[108]	Demonstrated that LEM induced the hepatocellular synthesis of zinc-binding metallothionein
	George et al.[41]	Found that LEM caused the secretion of pancreatic insulin and glucagon
	Kampschmidt and Upchurch[57]	Demonstrated that LEM had CSF activity
	Dinarello et al.[33]	Developed a radioimmunoassay for human EP
	Merriman et al.[78]	Showed that highly purified EP and LEM had similar in vivo activities
	Blyden and Handschumacher[16]	Achieved a 500-fold purification of LAF
1978	Bodel[17]	Discovered a spontaneous, continuing release of EP by several tumor cell lines
	Klempner et al.[64]	Showed that EP induced the release of lysosomal enzymes in neutrophils
1979	Rupp and Fuller[100]	Showed that EP induced the synthesis of fibrinogen in cultured hepatocytes
	Sipe et al.[106]	Discovered that mouse macrophages produce serum amyloid A stimulating factor
	Mizel and Farrar[81]	2nd International Lymphokine Worshop agreed to rename LAF and its synonyms "Interleukin 1"
1980	Hanson et al.[47]	Excluded neutrophils as a source for EP
1981	Dinerello and Bernheim[31]	Demonstrated direct stimulation of EP of PGE_2 synthesis in vitro by brain tissue
	Murphy et al.[83]	Purified two distinct forms of EP
	Mizel et al.[80]	Found that IL-1 stimulated the synthesis of PGs and collagenase by synovial cells
1982	Schmidt et al.[103]	Demonstrated that IL-1 caused cultured fibroblasts to proliferate
1983	Clowes et al.[27] & Baracos et al.[6]	Reported simultaneously that PIF/EP/IL-1 induced proteolysis of skeletal muscle in vitro

of these original investigators.[2,4,17-19,47,83-85]

Investigators studying some specific aspect of generalized host responses during acute illness often discovered that an endogenous mediator was involved in initiating and controlling the response. The name they applied to a mediator substance generally reflected the biological activity under study. Initial work was restricted to mediators that caused either fever or leukocytosis. In the early 1970s, workers at the U.S. Army Medical Research Institute of Infectious Diseases began an extensive series of investigations into the actions of a factor they termed leukocytic endogenous mediator (LEM).[5,8,9-14,41,71,87-91,94,95,114,118-121] Their studies centered on the biochemical and metabolic responses of the liver during generalized infections, that is, responses involving protein synthesis and the release of acute-phase glycoproteins by the liver, the accelerated hepatic uptake of free amino acids from the plasma, and the hepatic accumulation of iron and zinc. It was also found that LEM could stimulate the release of insulin and glucagon from pancreatic islet cells and thereby influence the metabolism of hepatic carbohydrates and lipids as well as proteins.

During the same years, Kampschmidt and his colleagues also investigated the nonpyrogenic actions of endogenous pyrogen, including those that induced leukocytosis, altered trace metal distribution, or contributed to the hepatic actions attributed to LEM.[5,53,55-59,78,79] The studies by all these research teams were based on the original assumption of Beeson[7] that activated neutrophils were the primary source of the endogenous mediators. This concept began to change with the findings of Bodel and Atkins[17,18] that endogenous pyrogen could be produced by human monocytes, as well as by certain tumor cell lines that could grow continuously in culture. It became increasingly evident that blood monocytes, mobile tissue macrophages, and fixed macrophage-life cells in various tissues were the primary sources for IL-1-type mediators. The final exclusion of the neutrophil as a likely source of endogenous pyrogen came through studies of Murphy and his group.[23,47,83-85,122]

The immunologists entered the IL-1 picture with the discovery by Gery and Waksman[42] that macrophages were the source of a lymphocyte-activating factor. This finding coincided with other major advances in immunologic technology that quickly led to the discovery of several additional monokines (factors produced by monocytes) and lymphokines (factors produced by lymphocytes) with special biologic properties. These newly recognized, immunologically active substances also generated a confusing array of overlapping names and claimed functions. As described by Gillis,[43] the precise characterization of these activities was nebulous during the late 1970s, because the lymphokines and monokines, as then described, were all present in the same kinds of conditioned media, which typically were generated by mitogen stimulation of cultured mouse spleen cells or human peripheral blood leukocytes.

Some welcome order has emerged from this chaos. Recent technologic advances in immunology, molecular biology, and genetic engineering have been combined to provide new clarity and understanding.[43,66,67] The development of rapid, sensitive, small-volume bioassays led the way; these were based on the use of cultures of clearly identified, isolated, cloned lymphocyte subset populations. A major breakthrough emerged when T-cell growth factor (TCGF) was isolated and characterized, both biochemically and functionally.[43] This lymphokine is now termed interleukin-2 (IL-2). It then became evident that the monokine, lymphocyte-activating factor (LAF), now termed IL-1, was required to induce the synthesis of IL-2 by T-lymphocytes. These two interleukins are thereby coordinated functionally to form an amplification mechanism for T cell growth.

The subsequent development of monoclonal anti-IL-2 antibodies, the creation of IL-2 hybridomas, and the in vitro translation of mRNA by the IL-2 gene have recently been reported.[43] Findings such as these are now giving individual lymphokines and monokines an identity and a biologic purpose that can be recognized and accepted by all.[66] We hope that these accomplishments will lead the way for future similar advances in IL-1 biology. Unlike IL-2, however, the stimulatory activities IL-1 are not restricted to the immunoregulatory system alone, but, rather, as previously noted, IL-1 type mediators influence a broad array of host defensive responses.

SOURCES OF IL-1 MEDIATORS

The earliest source of IL-1 mediators was the noncellular fluids of purulent exudates.[35,76,90] For several decades, sterile exudates were produced in the peritoneal cavity of rabbits by the use of injected irritants such as sterile shellfish glycogen. When collected, cells in these exudates were endotoxin-free and fully activated. Mediator substances could be recovered from the supernatant fluid following incubation of these exudate cells in normal saline. Most of the original studies of endogenous pyrogens (EP) and LEM employed crude preparations of this nature.[7,35,59,90,121]

Leukocytes from the buffy coat of peripheral blood could be induced to produce similar mediators in vitro, but only if the cells were first activated by a stimulus (such as heat-killed staphylococci) that caused them to initiate phagocytosis.[45] Because neutrophils were the predominant phagocytic cells in the exudate or buffy coat preparations, mediator production was at first attributed to them, and the possible contribution of monocytic phagocytes was not given much attention. Although the crude supernatant fluids originally studied undoubtedly contained many biologically active factors, the functions attributed to crude preparations of EP and LEM have generally been retained by more highly purified preparations.

With the advent of cell culture techniques and observations that monocyte and macrophage populations could be isolated by their propensity to adhere to surfaces and to remain viable for prolonged periods, these latter cells were found to produce EP and LAF when suitably activated.[115] Then, after the development of highly sensitive assay systems for identifying IL-1, other varieties of normal tissue cells were also identified as sources for this mediator. These tissue cells resemble macrophages in some of their characteristics and include reticuloendothelial system cells, rat glomerular mesangial cells, skin keratinocytes, tissue fibroblasts, and neuronal glial cells and astrocytes.[40,46,50,73,74,86,101]

A number of tumor cell lines were observed to produce these mediators spontaneously when grown in culture. These cell lines include cultured human histiocytic lymphoma cells, Hodgkin's disease cells, CM-S cells, renal carcinoma cells, and mouse histiocytic and myelomonocytic tumor cell lines.[17,21,35]

The cellular production of EP has been studied in some detail. It is well established that the mediator does not exist in a preformed state in normal monocytes or macrophages, but, rather, the cells must be activated before they begin their production and release of the protein mediators. The cells can be activated by any one of a large variety of microorganisms or chemically defined substances.[35] These include certain viruses, gram-positive bacteria, mycobacteria, spirochetes, and a number of fungi and their products. Bacterial lipopolysaccharide endotoxins can activate producer cells as can the phagocytosis of latex or quartz particles. When complexed with antibody, a number of nonmicrobial antigens can activate monocytes and macrophages, as can certain of the lymphokines.[2,82] Pyrogenic adrenal and testicular androgenic steroids, double-stranded synthetic RNA, bleomycin, colchicine, and the synthetic adjuvant, muramyl dipeptide, are all chemicals of known structure that can serve as activating stimuli.

Following their activation, the producer cells exhibit a period of latency before mediator proteins are produced and released.[35] Direct and indirect evidence indicates that production must begin with the synthesis of mRNA from a nuclear DNA genome; this step can be blocked by the pretreatment of cells with actinomycin D. Mediator production can also be blocked by inhibitors of either mRNA translation or protein synthesis. The same is true for tumor cell lines that produce mediators continuously. The synthesis of mediators can also be halted by inhibiting cellular energy expenditure with fluoride. The necessity for continued in vitro protein synthesis of EP has been confirmed by using radioactively tagged amino acids; these free amino acids are taken up by producer cells and incorporated into the mediator during its synthesis.[35] Certain disease processes, such as systemic lupus erythematosus, appear to reduce the capacity of blood monocytes to produce IL-1.[70]

The most recent source of cells used for producing relatively large amounts of human IL-1 has been the blood monocytes that adhere to the inner surface of plastic plasmapheresis bags that are normally discarded following use.[66] When blood monocytes are first collected, purified, and placed in culture medium, small amounts of IL-1 are produced on an apparently spontaneous basis. This production, however, may be due to the activation or stimulation of some cells caused by the techniques used for monocyte separation and purification, or possibly, early mediator production may be stimulated by trace contamination of commercial culture media with bacterial endotoxin.

After the first day in culture, blood monocytes produce very little IL-1 spontaneously. However, they can readily be activated by the addition of bacterial endotoxin, quartz silica particles, zymozan, or phorbol myristic acetate.[1] Each of these factors stimulates a somewhat different pattern of response by the cells, in terms of the duration and amounts of IL-1 produced.[75] A T-cell lymphokine, macrophage-activating factor, can augment the output of IL-1 from activated cells. As cultured monocytes become older, they have a diminished capacity to produce IL-1.[16] When produced by these methods, highly purified IL-1 shows some microheterogeneity in both its isoelectric focusing points and molecular weights.[66,75,86]

Placental macrophages have also been identified[39] as another readily available source of human cells. These could possibly be harvested and used for the production of large quantities of IL-1.

MOLECULAR CHARACTERIZATION OF IL-1 MEDIATORS

Despite almost three decades of continuing effort by numerous investigators, no IL-1-type mediator has been purified in sufficient quantity to allow an exact definition of its molecular structure. All evidence indicates that IL-1 is a low molecular weight protein, but it is not yet known if it is a single-chain simple protein, or if IL-1 is initially produced as a precursor molecule that must be cleaved or modified to render it active. We do not know which amino acids are in terminal positions on the molecule, and there are no data on the amino acid composition or sequence of products produced in vitro. Some evidence suggests that IL-1 species may circulate in plasma as dimers or trimers.[35]

New techniques for protein separation and purification have been applied with some success to IL-1 studies, although final answers are not yet available. An unusual number of difficult obstacles have slowed progress in purifying these mediators: IL-1 type mediators exist in only ultratrace quantities in biological fluids; their production in vitro requires meticulous care to avoid contamination by all too ubiquitous bacterial endotoxins; current methods also require purified populations of living cells, grown in tissue culture; and mediator yields in supernatant fluids are small at best,[36] and losses of over 95 percent of mediator activities are experienced with the available purification methods.[66]

Methods must be selected and used with care so that the native mediator molecules will not be denatured or altered. Until recently, bioassays have been based on relatively crude in vivo methods in experimental animals. Such assays consume inordinate amounts of scarce material. Bioassays must be conducted without the benefits of acceptable quantitative standards for making comparisons. Purified fractions of any mediator preparation also require testing after heat inactivation to rule out the possible presence of contaminating endotoxin that could influence bioassay results.

Despite these obstacles, progress has been made. Biologic effects of the mediators have increased in their specific activity with sequential steps of purification, thereby indicating that the effects were not due to impurities or contaminants in the starting material. Assays are becoming more rapid and precise, therefore requiring smaller samples. Antibodies are being raised against the mediators and these can now be used for affinity purification techniques. Producer cells are becoming more available, and cell-activating methods are being studied for their ability to stimulate the greatest yields. The advances in genetic engineering also hold promise for offering alternative choices for producing the IL-1 mediators in desirable quantities.

Because the most highly purified IL-1 type mediators have demonstrated molecular microheterogeniety,[15,23,86] information is not yet available to answer the theoretical question of whether the multiple biologic activities attributed to IL-1 are all stimulated by a single molecular species or, alternatively, if each type of biologic activity is produced by one of a closely related family of IL-1 mediators. This question can only be addressed in full when a single, large, homogeneous lot of purified mediator becomes available for testing in all assay systems heretofore used to demonstrate the various biologic actions claimed for IL-1-type endogenous mediators. This question has some clinical importance for, ultimately, purified IL-1 preparations may become available for therapeutic use. A product with effects limited to well-defined immunostimulatory actions would certainly have a different clinical value than a mediator preparation that could only stimulate fever.

The best current molecular characterizations have been reported for EP and IL-1.[15,16,35,66,67,83] Mouse and human IL-1 preparations have some differences.[15] Mouse IL-1 is slightly larger, has lower isoelectric points, and is sensitive to chymotrypsin digestion, whereas human IL-1 resists proteolysis with either trypsin or chymotrypsin. Activity is not lost after treatment with neuraminidase, periodate, sulfhydral reagents, or ribonuclease.[15,16] Human IL-1 is stable through a wide pH range and at temperatures below 56°C. It can be inactivated by pronase, cyanogen bromide, urea, and possibly by zinc chelators. IL-1 can be eluted from cationic resins but not from ion exchange resins.

Endogenous pyrogen is also thought to be a small protein with a molecular weight of 13,000 to 15,000 daltons, which may circulate as a dimer or trimer molecule of larger size.[35] As little as 30 to 50 ng of purified EP can produce a 1.0°C rise in temperature in a test rabbit when injected IV. However, pyrogenic fractions have been purified to the point where they no longer exhibit a chemical reaction for protein. Endogenous pyrogen is thought to have three sulfhydryl groups. It can be inactivated by boiling or high pH. Purified preparations do not lose their activity when subjected to procedures that would remove lipid or carbohydrate moieties from the molecule. Unlike endotoxin, EP does not produce tolerance on repeated administration. It is not species-specific, and it is only poorly antigenic. In addition to molecular microheterogeneity with respect to its isoelectric focusing points,[23,59,83] purified EP shows some heterogeneity in its antibody-binding sites.[83]

Following its partial purification from plasma by means of ultrafiltration and chromatography, proteolysis-inducing factor (PIF) was found to be a peptide and thought to contain sialic acid. The protein chain was characterized as having 33 amino acids and a molecular weight of approximately 4274 daltons.[27] Although purified EP of cell culture origin appears to have identical in vitro activities in rat skeletal muscle assays with those of PIF of plasma origin,[6,27] the differences in molecular characterization (i.e., a much lower molecular weight and the presence of carbohydrate in PIF) between these two products require further exploration.

The other named mediators in the IL-1 group have been even less well characterized. Leukocyte-inducing factor is thought to be a heat-labile, small protein that resembles weakly ionic α globulins.[60] Leukocytic endogenous mediator is also characterized as a heat labile proteinaceous substance that is precipitated by ammonium chloride.[90,121] The active components of LEM can be destroyed by pronase and trypsin but not by lipase. Its biologic activities lack species specificity, but there may be inconsistencies from batch to batch when various biologic effects are compared quantitatively. Like other IL-1 mediators, LEM is also stable over a wide pH range and in storage, and it can be inactivated by heating.

ASSAY OF IL-1-TYPE MEDIATORS

Although most of the available information concerning the activities of the IL-1-type endogenous mediators has been gained through the use of relatively crude bioassay systems, these data-based concepts have generally remained valid as more sensitive assays were developed. The in vitro cell culture bioassays that measure immune system activities of IL-1 are currently the most sensitive and probably the most useful.

Interleukin-1 Assays

Interleukin-1 was first assayed by its comitogenic effects on mouse thymocytes, but it can be measured equally well by its ability to heighten the in vitro plaque-forming cell response to an antigen such as sheep red blood cells. It can also be assayed because of its ability to replace living macrophages when measuring in vitro responses by lymphocytes that have been stimulated by recall antigens.[15,66]

The thymocyte mitogenic bioassay for IL-1 is usually conducted by culturing mouse thymocytes along with suboptimal concentrations of a polyclonal T-cell activator and different amounts of an IL-1 standard. The IL-1 concentration determines the magnitude of the proliferative response after several days in culture.[15] Unfortunately, sensitive immunologic assays such as these have not as yet been used to test for the presence of IL-1 type mediators in the blood or plasma of patients with surgical or septic illnesses.

Endogenous Pyrogen Assays

The pyrogenic aspects of IL-1 or EP preparations were traditionally assayed by their fever-producing effects in rabbits.[35] This form of bioassay is subject to many difficult-to-control variables and is quite costly in terms of the large amounts of a sample required. Mice may also be used as bioassay animals, but although less sample is required per animal, sufficient numbers of mice must be used to ensure statistical validity.[19] The lateral ventricle of the brain of an assay rat can be cannulated and fever can be produced by very small EP doses.[29,116] Although the cannulated rats can be used repeatedly, the necessity for precise surgical procedures and maintenance of sterility makes this a difficult bioassay to employ.

A radioimmunoassay for EP was developed by Dinneralo et al.[33] This assay had reasonable sensitivity and specificity, and avoided many of the problems of bioassays, but was of limited availability and usefulness because of the difficulty in producing both highly purified EP for isotope tagging and specific high-titer anti-EP immunoglobulin for binding the EP in samples tested with the assay.

Proteolysis-Inducing Factor Bioassays

A new form of in vitro bioassay was used to detect the proteolytic activity of IL-1/PIF[6,27] in rat skeletal muscle. The soleus muscles from the hind legs of fasting rats were dissected free and placed in culture medium. Serum or fluids containing PIF (or an IL-1 type mediator) were then added to the muscle from one leg, while the muscle from the other leg served as a control. Linear accumulation of tyrosine in the media permitted quantitation of the proteolytic activity in IL-1/PIF.[27] Human skeletal muscle obtained at surgery served equally well for assay purposes, thereby demonstrating the lack of species specificity of PIF.

Leukocytic Endogenous Mediator Bioassays

Because of the multiple biologic activities ascribed to LEM, in vivo bioassays are usually performed by measuring a number of different biochemical parameters in each of six rats.[18,119] Following injection of LEM-containing specimens into the peritoneal cavity, there occurs a dose-related decrease in plasma concentrations of iron, zinc, and amino acids;[88,90,119,121] a rapid flux of iron, zinc, and amino acids into the liver;[90,121] and a stimulation (at a slower rate) of a protein synthetic response by the liver.[89,90] This last response includes an initial transcription of hepatic RNA species, followed closely by an accelerated synthesis and release of acute-phase reactant plasma glycoproteins.[20] The synthesis of other intracellular proteins and the pancreatic release of insulin and glucagon can also be measured.[38,41] As controls, six other rats must be given a similar volume of heat-inactivated LEM material to demonstrate that the observed biologic responses are not due to contamination of the sample with endotoxin.

For practical bioassay purposes (as opposed to research studies), trace metal fluxes induced by LEM are evaluated by the decline in plasma zinc, only a few plasma free amino acids are measured, a radioactively tagged nonmetabolizable amino acid, α-amino-isobutyric acid, is used to measure the hepatic uptake of free amino acids, and the production of acute-phase proteins is quantitated by the increase in plasma copper, or in rats, and by the appearance of a highly responsive, unique rat protein, α-2-macrofetoprotein.[89,90] Serum amyloid A is an analogous acute-phase reactant in mice.[106]

Much smaller amounts of LEM can be assayed by intracerebroventricular (ICV) administration in the rat[5] or rabbit.[116] Along with fever, ICV injections stimulate the occurrence of the other systemic effects generally seen with intraperitoneal injections of LEM. This observation could imply that all systemic effects of LEM are mediated via the central nervous system, but such a hypothesis would appear to be at variance with other data showing that LEM stimulates direct effects in certain cells maintained in culture.[57,100] It also seems possible that LEM effects after ICV injection in vivo could be amplified by activation of several varieties of brain cells now known to produce IL-1-like mediators. Locally produced mediators could circulate following their endogenous release from brain tissue to stimulate other known actions of LEM in distant tissues.

Bioassay of the Other IL-1 Mediators

Granulocytopoiesis has generally been assumed to be regulated, in part, by two humoral agents, leukocytosis-inducing factor (LIF) and colony-stimulating factor (CSF).[25] Assays for LIF are based on the in vivo increase of the neutrophil count in animals given an IL-1-type mediator,[54,55,60] or on the in vitro stimulation of colonies in bone marrow cultures.[57] Other IL-1 actions that stimulate cell multiplication or the production or secretion of cellular products are assayed by using in vitro cultures of fibroblasts[46,102,103] or synovial cells.[80]

GENERAL ASPECTS OF HOST DEFENSIVE RESPONSES

To evaluate the role of IL-1 type mediators in clinical illnesses, it is necessary to define and understand the nature of the generalized host biochemical and physiologic responses that are typical components of a disease process or trauma.

Depending on the severity of illness, a surgical patient may exhibit a varying array of metabolic, physiologic, and nutritional responses to the combined effects of trauma, surgical stress, and the possible presence of superimposed infectious complications. On the one hand, simple, clean, elective surgery should elicit virtually no inflammatory response or generalized symptoms, and the healing process should proceed rapidly and in the absence of a troublesome postoperative illness. On the other hand, severely traumatized patients who develop sepsis may face complicated problems of severe illness, the wasting away of body tissues and nutrient stores, and ultimately, the heightened possibility of cardiovascular shock, multiorgan failure, and death. The role of endogenous IL-1 mediators in initiating or modulating physiologically based responses has been demonstrated, but a potential role, if any exists, has not been defined for the IL-1 mediators with respect to complications of acute surgical illnesses associated with a dysfunction of the molecular mechanisms within the cells of various organs and tissues.

Responses to Surgery and Trauma

Acute surgical illnesses appear to include a purposeful array of metabolic and physiologic responses initiated by the body to assist in the recovery process.[24,28,104,105] These initial responses, although quite complex, involve a general acceleration of body metabolism, sometimes accompanied by fever, a catabolic degradation of skeletal muscle protein, the generation of necessary extra energy substrates from endogenous sources already present within the body, the production of new body cells and molecular products as needed for host defense and the healing process, certain transient derangements in electrolyte and water metabolism, a redistribution of certain minerals and trace elements, a need for the elimination of toxic waste products and metabolites, and the direct participation of body cells in defensive mechanisms such as inflammatory processes, immune responses, and tissue repair.

Responses to Sepsis

A comparable pattern of generalized host responses and fever is also induced by sepsis due to different kinds of pathogenic microorganisms, or by other disease processes characterized by severe inflammatory reactions in the absence of infection.[8,9,28] Host defensive mechanisms generally include the mobilization of neutrophilic leukocytes and the secretion of many hormones.[10] Hepatic cells begin to synthesize an altered variety of intracellular and extracellular proteins.[20,58] Even before the onset of fever, the liver begins to take up free amino acids from plasma, some of which are made available by an accelerated catabolism of skeletal muscle protein. Trace element redistribution involves the early hepatic accumulation of iron and zinc. The iron is deposited as ferritin or hemosiderin granules, and the zinc forms complexes with newly made hepatic metallothioneins.[108]

Copper is excreted from the liver as a component of ceruloplasmin during this period.[89] The accelerated synthesis of ceruloplasmin typifies that of other plasma acute-phase reactant glycoproteins produced in large quantities during acute infections, inflammation, or surgical illness. In addition to ceruloplasmin, the acute-phase reactants include fibrinogen, C-reactive protein, the third component of complement, orosomucoid, α-1-antitrypsin, and haptoglobin in humans.[20,58] Animal species may produce other forms of acute-phase proteins that are not made by the human liver,

such as α-2-macrofetoprotein in the rat or amyloid A in the mouse.

During these generalized responses, priorities for the use of certain metabolic pathways within body cells appear to be changed in a purposeful manner. To meet the increased cellular demands for energy-yielding substrates, glycogen stores are utilized and the rates of gluconeogenesis are accelerated within the liver.[14] Needed substrates for glucose production are obtained, in part, from two free amino acids, alanine and glutamine.[14] Lactate and pyruvate are also used, as is the glycerol made available by the lipolysis of stored triglycerides. Additional gluconeogenic amino acids are formed de novo in skeletal muscle through the increased use of transamination reactions. These employ components of branched-chain amino acids that had previously undergone in situ oxidation in muscle as direct sources of energy.[14] This entire process has been colorfully termed "septic autocannibalism."[24] Skeletal muscle protein is thereby degraded to provide amino acid and glucose fuels in support of the hypermetabolic responses of acute surgical illnesses and sepsis.[8,9,11,14,27]

The combined metabolic and physiologic responses to severe surgical illness and sepsis appear to be purposeful and ultimately beneficial, although nutritional wasting occurs as a transient cost. Recovery should take place unless untoward complications, or the overwhelming severity of the disease process, cause a functional breakdown of the essential molecular machinery of individual body cells. Failure of intracellular metabolic processes may lead, in turn, to a functional failure of multiple organs and, ultimately, to death.

Responses to Complex Problems of Surgery, Trauma, and Sepsis

Siegel and his colleagues[104,105] have defined a number of response patterns in patients with surgical or septic stress. These are termed prototype patterns A, B, C and D. Each pattern or state is characterized by the development of a unique set of metabolic, hormonal, and physiologic data measurements that differ from those of the normal reference (or R) state. After uncomplicated, clean surgery, the postoperative patient should recover without any appreciable deviations from the R state.

The A state is viewed as an expected, typical, physiologically generated stress response in most patients who experience well-compensated major trauma, postsurgical illness, or sepsis. The A state response is characterized by increased body oxygen consumption and accelerated amino acid and carbohydrate metabolism as described in preceding paragraphs. Many of the responses typical of the A state are initiated by IL-1-type mediators. These responses are accompanied by cardiovascular changes including an increase in cardiac output and a more rapid flow of blood through the lungs to permit the increase in oxygen consumption and to help prevent metabolic acidosis.[104] The cardiovascular responses cannot be ascribed to IL-1 mediators.

In contrast, the B state is viewed as a pathophysiologic one, represented by an unbalanced hyperdynamic cardiovascular response to sympathetic stimuli. Despite an increased cardiac index and heart rate, and a decreased cardiac ejection time, the arteriovenous oxygen difference is narrowed. This reflects an absolute reduction in body oxygen consumption, often accompanied by a fall in the mixed venous pH which is indicative of generalized metabolic acidosis. The C state is seen when the severe respiratory insufficiency is superimposed upon B state abnormalities.[105] It is manifested by a combination of both severe respiratory and metabolic acidosis, and may be accompanied by hypotensive shock. The D state is typified by severe cardiogenic decompensation and shock. Greater details about these classifications[104,105] and their value for estimating prognosis and planning therapy are discussed in Chapters 8 and 15. No data suggest that IL-1 mediators contribute to, or cause, transition of a patient's condition from a physiologic A state to a pathologic B, C, or D state.

Interleukin-1 Mediation of Febrile Responses

It is not known how IL-1/EP crosses the blood–brain barrier, or precisely where or how it interacts with neurons in the temperature-regulating center in the hypothalamic area. Traditional explanations for EP activity suggest that it "turns up" a theoretical thermostat within the center, allowing all heat-regulating functions to proceed normally, but at a higher baseline of body temperature.[35,10] Most current theories about the molecular nature of the hyperthermic action of EP are based on findings that EP stimulates brain prostaglandin synthesis,[31] and that the pyrogenic responses of EP can be inhibited by drugs such as aspirin or ibuprofen that inhibit the cyclooxygenase enzymes needed for prostaglandin E (PGE) synthesis. Accordingly, the effects of EP on neurons are thought to be indirect, mediated locally via secondary neuroactive or neurotransmitter substances released within the brain itself.[35]

Endogenous pyrogen stimulates the local formation of PGE from their arachidonic acid precursor.[31] It has also been suspected that other products of arachidonic acid metabolism, such as the thromboxanes and prostacyclines, could serve as key neurotransmitter substances for fever production. These biologically active substances are thought to stimulate the activity of adenylate cyclase enzymes in key neurons or, alternatively, to change the local intracellular neuronal ratios of calcium and sodium ions. As a net result, neural impulses are initiated that serve to reduce dermal heat loss, and, simultaneously, to stimulate body heat production.

Endogenous pyrogen has been shown by bioassay to be present in the bloodstream of febrile patients.[4] In experimental animals, EP initiates fever about 15 minutes after its IV injection, but in a much shorter time after intracarotid artery injection. Mapping studies show that EP is most active when injected into the preoptic area of the anterior hypothalamus, although some secondary sites of thermoregulatory activity may exist in the medulla oblongata.[35] Depletion of brain monoamines prevents EP-induced fevers, so these neurotransmitters must be ascribed a role in temperature regulation. During naturally occurring and EP-induced fevers, the concentration of prostaglandins in the cerebrospinal fluid has been shown to increase.[35]

There is no current evidence to suggest that either the mononuclear cells or macrophages of infants[34] or the elderly[52,61] have a reduced ability to synthesize or release IL-1/EP. Rather, the apparent inability of newborn infants or extremely aged persons to generate a fever in response to typically pyrogenic infections would seem to be related to noncentral factors of body temperature regulation. Because of an increase in the ratio of body surface area to body weight, heat loss may be greater than normal in the elderly. Infants and some aged persons lack the skeletal muscle protein needed to provide amino acid substrates that can be used for body heat production.

On the other hand, severe protein malnutrition can be associated with a reduced ability of macrophages and monocytes to produce IL-1 or EP[48,61] as well as a deficit in the amino acids substrates needed to accelerate basal metabolism. If patients with severe disease exhibit marked protein depletion, it can be assumed that their cells do not have the nutritional factors necessary to allow them to synthesize and release IL-1 mediator proteins in a normal manner. A deficit in heat-producing capabilities can also be assumed.

Interleukin-1 Mediation of Leukocytosis

These mediators play an active role in the generation of leukocytic responses.[54,55,57] Interleukin-1/LIF is believed to accelerate the mobilization and transport of mature neutrophils from bone marrow reserves into the blood while, in contrast, CSF is believed to stimulate the proliferation and differentiation of the stem cells, myeloblasts, promyelocytes, and myelocytes in the marrow.[25] Relationships between these two substances are not clear, for although LIF and CSF may be differentiated by certain subtle differences in the timing and patterns of their actions,[25] some studies suggest that IL-1-type mediators can induce both effects.[54,57,79] Schlick et al.[102] have shown that CSF-life myelopoietic growth factors are produced by monocytes and macrophages under the same general conditions that allow for IL-1 production.

Kampschmidt and his co-workers[54,55] have shown that IL-1-type mediators induce the prompt appearance of an increased number of neutrophils in the circulating blood, and that repeated inoculations cause an increased cellularity in the bone marrow. Their in vitro studies demonstrate that the addition of LEM to adher-

ent rat bone marrow colony cells cultured in the presence of rat serum cause the cells to proliferate.[57] Klempner et al.[64,65] have shown further that IL-1/EP stimulates oxygen-dependent metabolism and lysosomal enzyme release in the neutrophils.

Despite this experimental evidence, it remains unclear why some forms of viral disease fail to exhibit a mobilization of neutrophils, or, as in the sandfly and dengue fevers, why patients develop a characteristic neutropenia. Certain viruses may have a propensity to invade either the producer cells of IL-1 mediators (monocytes and macrophages) or the responding marrow neutrophils. Viruses could thus prevent either producer or responder cells from making, or responding to, IL-1/EP. A similar line of reasoning would show that patients with severe protein malnutrition associated with starvation or severe disease may be unable to generate a leukocytic response to a bacterial infection. Again, it is uncertain if intracellular nutritional or energy deficits might prevent mediator formation by producer cells, or alternatively, if nutritional deficits might inhibit the production of mediator-responding neutrophils by the marrow.[48] Both mechanisms could be operating in combination.

Interleukin-1 Interactions with Endocrine Responses

Trauma, surgical stress, and sepsis are all accompanied by a relatively stereotypic array of endocrine responses.[11,24,104,105] An ACTH-mediated increase in adrenal glucocorticoid production is typical, and is more extensive with trauma or surgery than with infectious processes. The tendency for the body to retain excess salt and water is mediated by mineralocorticoids and antidiuretic hormones after surgery or trauma. In infectious diseases, such responses are most common if the infection is complicated by a hemorrhagic diathesis or an intracranial localization.[8,9,11] Catecholamine increases are usually minimal unless hypotensive shock intervenes, but then the catecholamines have a prominent influence on cardiovascular and metabolic responses. In contrast, thyroidal hormones do not appear to play an important role in influencing host responses. All of the endocrine responses mentioned in this paragraph appear to be independent of IL-1 mediator stimulation.

On the other hand, the IL-1 mediators do stimulate the release of two hormones (insulin and glucagon) that play a highly important role in the host metabolic responses to the stress of trauma, surgery, or sepsis.[41,62] Interleukin-1 mediators could themselves be categorized as hormones, in that they are produced by uniquely stimulated cells, they circulate via the blood stream, and they exert their stimulative biologic effects on distant tissues. Roth et al.[99] have placed these mediators in a special category termed "nonhormone messengers that are very hormone-like in structure or function."

The IL-1-induced, simultaneous release of both insulin and glucagon from pancreatic islet cells is somewhat unusual, since typically these two glucoregulatory hormones act in a check-and-balance manner. During acute surgical stress, however, their simultaneous release (with a relatively greater increase in glucagon concentrations, as shown by a depressed ratio molar of insulin to glucagon) contributes importantly to the augmented use of glucose as a fuel,[14,62] to the accelerated use of amino acids as substrates for gluconeogenesis, and to the somewhat inhibited production of ketone fuels by the liver. The modest excess of insulin may serve to inhibit lipolysis and the liberation of free fatty acids from peripheral fat depots.[8,10,11,14,62,71,87,91,114,120]

The elevated concentrations of insulin and glucagon in plasma, known to appear at the onset of fever in acute infections,[14] were shown by George et al.[41] and Keenen et al.[62] to be a response to LEM administration. Filkins and Yelich[38] subsequently showed that these bihormonal actions of LEM could be demonstrated in isolated pancreas preparations. Accordingly, LEM appears to act directly on pancreatic islet cells without the mediation of other hormones or central nervous system stimuli.

Interleukin-1 Mediation of Metabolic Responses

Aside from the glucoregulatory effects of IL-1 mediators described in the preceding paragraphs, the predominant direct metabolic actions of IL-1/LEM take place in the liver[13,58,124]

and skeletal muscle.[6,27,124] Recent publications[46,102-124] indicate that other somatic tissues may be influenced as well.

The majority of the hepatic effects of IL-1/LEM are centered about the induction of synthesis of new proteins and the apparent reprioritization of the kinds of new proteins the liver will make.[20,79,90,100,108,113] All molecular aspects of protein synthesis are stimulated in the hepatocytes. The liver accelerates its uptake of plasma free amino acids.[119,121] Nucleic acid metabolism is stimulated within hepatocyte nuclei to produce the mRNAs for the many different proteins that will be produced. Other forms of ribosomal RNA are also made to create the ribosomes needed for synthesis of individual proteins. Some of the proteins produced by the liver, such as enzymes and metallothioneins, are for intrahepatic use. A 30-hour infusion of IL-1/LEM in rats causes a doubling of the hepatic synthesis of these nonsecretory proteins.[124] Other proteins produced by the liver after IL-1/LEM stimulation are destined for transport to the plasma. Many of the latter group are acute-phase glycoproteins and require the addition of sugar moieties before they are secreted. This is accomplished through glycosylation mechanisms that take place in the smooth endoplasmic reticulum and Golgi apparatus of the hepatocytes. Eventual transport of the acute-phase glycoproteins to the plasma occurs via the Golgi apparatus.

A partial stimulation of accelerated hepatic protein synthesis by IL-1/LEM can take place in animals that lack pituitary and/or adrenal glands. Increased synthesis of acute-phase proteins that normally are produced in small amounts, such as haptoglobin, can be stimulated by LEM in the absence of adrenal hormones.[114] However, the increased do novo production of several acute-phase proteins by the liver, such as alpha-2-macrofetoprotein in the rat, requires the permissive presence of physiologic quantities of adrenal glucocorticoid hormones.[90] Thompson et al[90,114] used an isolated perfused liver system to show that LEM acted directly on liver cells. However, the permissive presence of glucocorticoids was necessary for LEM to stimulate the incorporation of orotate into RNA and, thus, to form new ribosomes for the synthesis of new proteins.

In contrast to the accelerated production of many kinds of proteins by the liver in response to IL-1,[90,95,124] the same mediator simultaneously stimulates an accelerated catabolism of skeletal muscle protein.[6,27,124] An increase in the urinary excretion of both methylhistidine and hydroxyproline in rats given IL-1/LEM indicates that collagen as well as muscle protein is being broken down.[124] Although the latter phenomenon results clinically in a wasting away of muscle and somatic protein mass and a negative nitrogen balance, the process appears to have ultimate (albeit temporary) benefit because it provides a balanced supply of free amino acids that can be used wherever necessary to support host defensive mechanisms.[14,27,72] However, the stores of "labile" nitrogen in somatic proteins are finite, and are generally depleted by 1 to 3 weeks of severe illness. Thereafter, in the absence of new exogenous sources of amino acids, the body reestablishes a new, relatively steady state of nitrogen equilibrium, but at a dangerously low, cachectic level that may fail to meet the cellular requirements of vital organs.

The recent studies of Clowes et al.[27] showed that the content of IL-1/PIF in the serum of patients, as bioassayed in vitro in rat skeletal muscle, correlated well with in vivo estimates of the rates of release of free amino acids from skeletal muscle in patients with trauma or sepsis. Baracos et al.[6] found that IL-1-induced proteolysis in rat skeletal muscle appeared to require both a mediation by prostaglandins formed in situ, as well as an activation of muscle lysosomal proteases.

Additional metabolic effects of IL-1/LEM that stimulate the hepatic accumulation of zinc and iron and cause hepatic copper secretion as a component of ceruloplasmin have been mentioned in preceding paragraphs. Metabolic effects are also produced in cultured human fibroblasts stimulated to proliferate[61,103] and to secrete plasminogen.[46] Mitogenic stimulation is only seen in nonconfluent cultures.[61] It is not known if IL-1 stimulates the production of fibronectin (cold-insoluble globulin) by fibroblasts and other cells, although plasma concentrations of fibronectin are altered by surgery or sepsis. Interleukin-1 does, however, stimulate synovial cells to produce prostaglandins and collagenase.[80,93] The direct in vitro addition of purified IL-1 to brain tissue activates microsomal (Na + K)-dependent ATPase enzymes.[96]

Interleukin-1 Mediation of Immunologic Responses

Interleukin-1 is now recognized to be one of the most important of the monokines or lymphokines that stimulate immune system cells. In combination, these factors serve a major amplifying role in immunologic responses by stimulating cellular proliferation and differentiation, as well as by maximizing the functional capacities of individual lymphocytes.[15,30,42,43,86,97,108] The molecular mechanisms used by IL-1 to activate or stimulate individual lymphocytes have not, as yet, been determined, and cell surface receptors for IL-1 have not been described.

Interleukin-1 is considered to be a potent monokine with stimulatory effects on thymocytes, T lymphocytes, and B lymphocytes, but it appears to have no primary function in cellular proliferation.[15,37,42,43,86,92,97,108] In this regard, monocytes and macrophages exert a fine control on the lymphoid system, not only by binding, processing, and presenting antigens in an immunogenic form to T cells, but also by secreting monokines that initiate lymphocyte growth and differentiation. In some immunologic assays, IL-1 can completely fulfill the requirements for live macrophages, or it can greatly reduce the number of macrophages needed for a measurable response.[111] However, IL-1 cannot replace the functional properties of macrophages in processing antigens or in presenting them to T lymphocytes. Neither can IL-1 substitute for the necessary role of histocompatibility antigens found on the surface of macrophages.

A major function of IL-1 is to induce the biosynthesis and secretion of the T-helper-cell-produced lymphokine, IL-2.[15,43,97,107] Unlike IL-1, IL-2 stimulates lymphocyte proliferation,[63] thereby creating a feedback loop to amplify the system for producing T cells and their products. The fever-producing effects of IL-1 may also contribute indirectly to this immunostimulatory feedback phenomena, because higher in vitro temperatures appear also to favor lymphocyte proliferation[36] and a similar effect may occur in vivo. Effects of IL-1 on lymphocytes have not been shown to require the intermediary production of PGE species.[32]

Because it is a macrophage product, IL-1 has the unique ability to replace macrophages in certain immunologic assays based on the induction of T-cell proliferation by mitogenic lectins (or antigens) together with IL-2.[15,30,97,108] Along with IL-2 and a lectin (or antigen), the presence of macrophages (or IL-1) is the third factor required for inducing replication in T cells.[51,98] The potency of IL-1 is very high in such systems, with activities demonstrated in the 10^{-10} to 10^{-12} molar concentric range. IL-1 may also influence the phenotypic characteristics of proliferating thymocyte subpopulations.[97] However, in the presence of certain specific antigens, IL-1 alone cannot influence T-cell activation. Under such experimental conditions,[97] T-cell activation requires the presence of macrophages that can make contact with lymphocytes. Interleukin-1 appears to amplify this response. These actions of IL-1 can be blocked by antibodies prepared against purified EP.[44]

Interleukin-1 enhances antibody production by human and mouse B cells and plasma cells.[37,43,49,66,69,86,92] This action may not be direct, but may be mediated through T-cell effects. In either event, IL-1 can readily be shown to augment the in vitro production of immunoglobulin by B cells. When given in vivo, IL-1 enhances the secondary antibody response of mice to protein antigens.[112]

CLINICAL ROLE OF IL-1 MEDIATORS

Evidence continues to accumulate indicating that the IL-1 mediators play a major clinical role in acute disease processes by initiating and coordinating a number of important host defensive responses. Bioassay data demonstrate that these mediators appear in human plasma during infectious and noninfectious fevers, severe inflammatory states, and after major trauma.[18,27,29,53,64,110,120] Quantitative data, where available, indicate that the amount of mediator activity that can be measured in plasma varies in direct proportion to the severity of the inciting illness or trauma. Interleukin-1 mediators then disappear from the plasma when the disease process is terminated. Assay systems used thus far have not clearly shown the presence of IL-1 mediators in normal plasma, but small amounts of IL-1 are detectable in the plasma during severe physical exercise.[22]

In terms of acute surgical illness and sepsis, the IL-1 mediators would appear responsible, in large part, for initiating many of the clinical phenomena associated with the transition of a patient from the R, or reference, state to the A state, as categorized by Siegel et al.[104,105] Production of IL-1 mediators in early disease or trauma, and the host responses they initiate, should be regarded as important physiological processes that are not inherently pathologic. Similarly, the A state is viewed as a typically normal response to surgical stress in patients with well-compensated major trauma or sepsis.

On the other hand, there is no evidence to indicate that the IL-1 mediators play any role in the possible subsequent transition of a patient's condition to a pathologic B, C, or D state. Unfortunately, no assay data are currently available to indicate the status of IL-1-type mediators in the plasma of patients categorized clinically as being in one of these latter pathologic states. It is not known if IL-1 mediator concentrations in plasma are high, low, or nonmeasurable in patients with these severe problems. It may be, on the basis of the severe protein malnutrition that often typifies these patients, or on the basis of a widespread breakdown in intracellular molecular functions, that the cells of such patients are simply unable to produce IL-1 mediators.[100] On the other hand, an infusion of large doses of crude IL-1/LEM in monkeys led to hypotension, tachycardia, and vasodilitation.[71] Based on such evidence, high plasma values of IL-1, if demonstrated to be present in the plasma of such severely ill patients, could be exerting untoward cardiovascular effects.

The actions of IL-1 mediators, although diverse, cannot explain all of the metabolic and physiologic adaptive responses to acute surgical illness or sepsis. Many of the hormonal responses to these stresses are independent of IL-1 stimulation, as are the important cardiovascular and pulmonary adaptations. Although IL-1 does not influence activation of the kinin, complement, or coagulation systems, it may have an influence on the latter two systems because it helps to stimulate production of important protein components of these systems that are synthesized by the liver as acute-phase reactants. Too little information is available for us to evaluate the possible role of IL-1 in wound healing and fibroblast activity.

Based on data discussed in previous paragraphs, it is possible to conclude that IL-1 has a direct role in fever production, neutrophil mobilization, skeletal muscle proteolysis, hepatic protein synthesis, pancreatic islet cell output of hormones, trace element sequestration and/or redistribution, and immune system responsiveness. Through these primary actions on numerous target tissues of the host, IL-1 appears to induce a secondary increase of generalized body metabolism and metabolism of amino acids, carbohydrates, and possibly lipids.

A recent publication by Sobrado et al[109] is instructive in this regard. These investigators administered IL-1/EP continuously to guinea pigs in doses sufficient to cause a febrile response of 0.6 to 0.8°C temperature elevation in 4 hours. As anticipated, leukocytosis was induced, zinc and iron values declined in the serum, rates of whole body amino acid appearance, oxidation, and incorporation into protein were all increased, as were the fractional hepatic rates for protein and seromucoid synthesis. If the animals were pretreated with ibuprofen, a specific cyclooxygenase inhibitor, fever was controlled, overall increases in whole body amino acid kinetics were minimized, but the other actions of IL-1/EP were unchanged. These results are in keeping with previous data[6] showing that PGE formation is an important local mediator of IL-1/EP actions in fever production and muscle proteolysis, and clinical observations that aspirin administration during febrile disease can reduce both the elevated temperature and the rates of nitrogen loss from the body. The other actions of IL-1-type mediators would not seem to require PGE synthesis as an intermediary step.

POSSIBLY HARMFUL CLINICAL EFFECTS OF THE IL-1 MEDIATORS

Although IL-1 production may be viewed essentially as a physiologic mechanism for initiating the prompt onset of generalized nonspecific host defense reactions and for enhancing and amplifying antigen-specific host defense reactions and for enhancing and amplifying antigen-specific immunologic responses, IL-1 mediated effects are not without their costs. Skeletal muscle proteolysis, if protracted, can lead to muscle wasting, body nitrogen losses, and an eventual severe depletion of body protein.

As an additional, but unstudied, concern, it is not known if the proteolysis induced by IL-1 in skeletal muscle also involves the striated muscle of the heart. Further, it is not known if plasma concentrations of IL-1 become high enough in humans to exert potentially toxic effects.

Febrile reactions induced by IL-1/EP, if sufficiently severe, can lead to convulsive seizures (especially in children) and even to permanent brain damage. The generalized hypermetabolic state associated with fever can consume, or lead to sizable losses, of body nutrients such as the vitamins, minerals, and trace elements in addition to those of nitrogen. Iron sequestration induced by IL-1/LEM, if prolonged, can lead to anemia.[68]

Finally, IL-1 may produce harmful local effects, especially in joint spaces. It has been shown to accumulate or to be produced in inflamed or arthritic joint spaces.[123] Fibroblasts and synovial cells stimulated by IL-1 to produce proteinases, collagenases,[46,80,93] and PGE[80] may be contributing to the destruction of joint tissues in arthritic diseases.

SUMMARY

The interleukin-1 mediators are endogenous products of activated monocytes and macrophages that are released at the onset of trauma, surgical stress, or sepsis. Interleukin-1 stimulates and modulates a variety of host defensive responses in widespread organs and cells. Known previously by names such as endogenous pyrogen, leukocytosis-inducing factor, leukocytic endogenous mediator, or lymphocyte-activating factor, these hormonelike mediators constitute a unique mechanism that becomes activated during certain pathologic states. This mechanism appears to serve in a coordinating role that is independent of, but may work through, the central nervous system and the endocrine system. It also has important immunostimulatory functions.

Known characteristics of the interleukin-1 system are as follows:

The system is rapidly responsive and can be activated with relative ease.

Activation of IL-1 release is proportional to the magnitude of the stimulus.

IL-1 producer cells are monocytes, macrophages, and macrophage-like cells.

Producer cells can be activated by many different stimuli, such as certain microorganisms and their products, particulate matter, and certain chemicals, antigen–antibody complexes, and biologically active factors.

IL-1-type mediators are thought to be small proteins. They are difficult to purify, characterize, and assay. They are poorly antigenic.

The most pure IL-1 preparations exhibit some molecular microheterogeneity, so that it is not yet known if IL-1 is a single substance, or a closely related family of similar substances.

IL-1 mediators stimulate fever, apparently by initiating PGE synthesis within neuronal cells of the hypothalamic temperature-regulating center.

IL-1 mediators stimulate the production and release of neutrophils by bone marrow.

IL-1 mediators initiate proteolysis in skeletal muscles, apparently by stimulating PGE synthesis and activating lysosomal enzymes.

IL-1 mediators stimulate the hepatocellular synthesis of acute-phase plasma reactant glycoproteins and other intrahepatic proteins.

IL-1 mediators stimulate the hepatocellular accumulation of iron, zinc, and free amino acids.

IL-1 mediators stimulate pancreatic islet cells to produce insulin and glucagon.

Primary actions of IL-1 mediators in stimulating fever, muscle proteolysis, and glucoregulatory hormone release lead directly to important secondary effects on generalized body oxygen consumption and the metabolism of amino acids, carbohydrates, and lipids.

IL-1 activates lymphoid series cells, causing helper T cells to produce the lymphokine IL-2, assisting in thymocyte and T-cell differentiation and proliferative responses, and stimulating (directly or indirectly) the production of immunoglobulins by B lymphocytes and plasma cells.

IL-1 stimulates the formation of new fibroblasts and the production of biologically active products by fibroblasts and synovial cells.

The actions of IL-1 mediators incur certain costs in terms of body stores of nitrogen and other nutrients. In addition, IL-1 mediators may have some potentially harmful effects, especially in the synovial spaces of joints.

REFERENCES

1. Arenzana-Seisdedos F, Virelizier JL: Interferons as macrophage-activating factors. II. Enhanced secretion of interleukin 1 by lipopolysaccharide-stimulated human monocytes. Eur J Immunol 13: 437, 1983.

2. Atkins E, Francis L: Pathogenesis of fever in delayed hypersensitivity: Factors influencing release of pyrogen-inducing lymphokines. Infect. Immun., 21: 806, 1978.

3. Atkins E, Wood WB, Jr.: Studies on the pathogenesis of fever. I. The presence of transferable pyrogen in the blood stream following the injection of typhoid vaccine. J Exp Med 101: 519, 1955

4. Atkins E, Wood WB, Jr.: Studies on the pathogenesis of fever. II. Identification of an endogenous pyrogen in the blood stream following the injection of typhoid vaccine. J Exp Med, 102: 499, 1955

5. Bailey PT, Abeles FB, Hauer EC et al: Intracerebroventricular administration of leukocytic endogenous mediators (LEM) in the rat. Proc Soc Exp Biol Med 153: 419, 1976

6. Baracos V, Rodemann HP, Dinarello CA et al: Stimulation of muscle protein degradation and prostaglandin E_2 release by leukocytic pyrogen (interleukin-1). A mechanism for the increased degradation of muscle proteins during fever. N Engl J Med 308: 553, 1983

7. Beeson PB: Temperature-elevating effect of a substance obtained from polymorphonuclear leukocytes. J Clin Invest 27: 524, 1948

8. Beisel WR: Metabolic and nutritional consequences of infection. p. 125. In Draper HH (ed):

Advances in Nutritional Research, Vol. 1. Plenum Press, New York, 1977.

9. Beisel WR: Infectious Diseases: effects on food intake and nutrient requirements. p. 329. In Hodges RE (ed): Human Nutrition—A Comprehensive Treatise, Vol. 4. Metabolic and Clinical Applications. Plenum Press, New York, 1979

10. Beisel WR: Endogenous pyrogen physiology. Physiologist 23: 38, 1980

11. Beisel WR: Alterations in hormone production and utilization during infection. p. 7. In Powanda MC, Canonico PG (eds): Infection. The Physiologic and Metabolic Responses of the Host. Elsevier/North Holland, Amsterdam, 1981

12. Beisel WR: Editorial. Mediators of fever and muscle proteolysis. N Engl J Med 308: 586, 1983

13. Beisel WR, Sobocinski PZ: Endogenous mediators of fever-related metabolic and hormonal responses. p. 39. In Lipton JM (ed): Fever. Raven Press, New York, 1980

14. Beisel WR, Wannemacher RW, Jr.: Gluconeogenesis, ureagenesis, and ketogenesis during sepsis. JPEN, 4: 277, 1980

15. Bendtzen K: Biological properties of interleukins. Allergy 38: 219, 1983

16. Blyden G, Handschumacher RE: Purification and properties of human lymphocyte activating factor (LAF). J Immunol 118: 1631, 1977

17. Bodel P: Spontaneous pyrogen production by mouse histiocytic and myelomonocytic tumor cell lines in vitro. J Exp Med 147: 1503, 1978

18. Bodel P, Atkins E: Release of endogenous pyrogen by human monocytes. N Engl J Med 276: 1002, 1967

19. Bodel P, Miller H: A new sensitive method for detecting human endogenous (leukocyte pyrogen. Inflammation 3: 103, 1978

20. Bornstein DL: Leukocyte pyrogen: a major mediator of the acute phase reaction. Ann NY Acad Sci 389: 323, 1982

21. Butler RH, Revoltella RP, Musiani P et al: Constitutive production of interleukin-1 by the human continuous cell line, CM-S. Cell Immunol 78: 368, 1983

22. Cannon JG, Kluger MJ: Endogenous pyrogen activity in human plasma after exercise. Science 220: 617, 1983

23. Cebula TA, Hanson DF, Moore DM et al: Synthesis of four endogenous pyrogens by rabbit macrophages. J Lab Clin Med 94: 95, 1979

24. Cerra FB, Siegel JH, Coleman B et al: Septic autocannibalism. A failure of exogenous nutritional support. Ann Surg 192: 570, 1980

25. Chikkappa G, Chanana AD, Chandra P et al: Granulocytopoiesis: studies on leukocytosis-inducing and colony-stimulating factors. Proc Soc Exp Biol Med 154: 192, 1977

26. Clark WG, Coldwell BA: Competitive antagonism of leukocytic pyrogen by sodium salicylate and acetaminophen. Proc Soc Exp Biol Med 141: 669, 1972

27. Clowes GHA, Jr., George BC, Villee CA, Jr. et al: Muscle proteolysis induced by a circulating peptide in patients with sepsis or trauma. N Engl J Med 308: 545, 1983

28. Clowes GHA, Jr., Randall HT, Cha C-J: Amino acid and energy metabolism in septic and traumatized patients. JPEN 4: 195, 1980

29. Critz WJ: Intracerebroventricular injection of rats: a sensitive assay method for endogenous pyrogen circulating in rats. Proc Soc Exp Biol Med 166, 6, 1981

30. de Vries JE, Vyth-Dreese FA, Figdor CG et al: Induction of phenotypic differentiation, interleukin 2 production, and PHA responsiveness of "immature" human thymocytes by interleukin 1 and phorbol ester. J Immunol 131: 201, 1983

31. Dinarello CA, Bernheim HA: Ability of human leukocytic pyrogen to stimulate brain prostaglandin synthesis in vitro. J Neurochem 37: 702, 1981

32. Dinarello CA, Marnoy SO, Rosenwasser LJ: Role of arachidonate metabolism in the immunoregulatory function of human leukocytic pyrogen/lymphocyte-activating factor/interleukin 1. J Immunol 130: 890, 1983

33. Dinarello CA, Renfer L, Wolff SM: Human leukocytic pyrogen: purification and development of a radioimmunoassay. Proc Natl Acad Sci 74: 4624, 1977

34. Dinarello CA, Shparber M, Kent EF, Jr., et al: Production of leukocytic pyrogen from phagocytes of neonates. J Infect Dis 144: 337, 1981

35. Dinarello CA, Wolff SM: Molecular basis of fever in humans. Am J Med 72: 799, 1982

36. Duff GW, Durum SK: The pyrogenic and mitogenic actions of interleukin-1 are related. Nature 304: 449, 1983

37. Falkoff RJM, Muraguchi A, Hong JX et al: The effects of interleukin 1 on human B cell activation and proliferation. J Immunol 131: 801, 1983

38. Filkins JP, Yelich MR: Mechanism of hyperinsulinemia after reticuloendothelial system phagocytosis. Am J Physiol 242: E115, 1982

39. Flynn A, Finke JH, Hilfiker ML: Placental mononuclear phagocytes as a source of interleukin-1. Science 218: 475, 1982

40. Fontana A, Kristensen F, Dubs R et al: Production of prostaglandin E and interleukin-1 like factor by cultured astrocytes and C_6 glioma cells. J Immunol 129: 2413, 1982

41. George DT, Abeles FB, Mapes CA et al: Effect of leukocytic endogenous mediators on endocrine pancreas secretory responses. Am J Physiol 233: E240, 1977

42. Gery I, Waksman BH: Potentiation of the T-lymphocyte response to mitogens. II. The cellular source of potentiating mediators(s). J Exp Med 136: 143, 1972

43. Gillis S: Interleukin biochemistry and biology: summary and introduction. Fed Proc 42: 2635, 1983

44. Gilman SC, Rosenberg JS, Feldman JD: Inhibition of interleukin synthesis and T cell proliferation by a monoclonal anti-Ia antibody. J Immunol 130: 1236, 1983

45. Gordon AH, Limaos EA: Human blood and rabbit peritoneal-leucocytes as sources of endogenous mediators. Br J Exp Pathol 60: 441, 1979

46. Hamilton JA, Zabriskie JB, Lachman LB et al: Streptococcal cell walls and synovial cell activation. Stimulation of synovial fibroblast plasminogen activator activity by monocytes treated with group A streptococcal cell wall sonicates and muramyl dipeptide. J Exp Med 155: 1702, 1982

47. Hanson DF, Murphy PA, Windle BE: Failure of rabbit neutrophils to secrete endogenous pyrogen when stimulated with staphylococci. J Exp Med 151: 1360, 1980

48. Hoffman-Goetz L, McFarlane D, Bistrian BR et al: Febrile and plasma iron responses of rabbits injected with endogenous pyrogen from malnourished patients. Am J Clin Nutr 34: 1109, 1981

49. Howard M, Mizel SB, Lachman L et al: Role of interleukin 1 in anti-immunoglobulin-induced B cell proliferation. J Exp Med 157: 1529, 1983

50. Iribe H, Hoga T, Kotani S et al: Stimulating effect of MDP and its adjuvant-active analogues on guinea pig fibroblasts for the production of thymocyte-activating factor. J Exp Med 157: 2190, 1982

51. Jakway JP, Shevach EM: Stimulation of T-cell activation by UV-treated, antigen-pulsed macrophages: evidence for a requirement for antigen processing and interleukin 1 secretion. Cell Immunol 80: 151, 1983

52. Jones PG, Kauffman CA, Kluger MJ: Endogenous pyrogen production by monocytes from elderly persons. Clin Res 31: 366A, 1983

53. Kampschmidt RF: Metabolic alterations elicited by endogenous pyrogens. p. 49. In Lipton JM (ed): Fever. Raven Press, New York, 1980

54. Kampschmidt RF, Long RD, Upchurch HF: Neutrophil releasing activity in rats injected with endogenous pyrogen. Proc Soc Exp Biol Med 139: 1224, 1972

55. Kampschmidt RF, Pulliam LA, Merriman CR: Further similarities of endogenous pyrogen and leukocytic endogenous mediator. Am J Physiol 235: C118, 1978

56. Kampschmidt RF, Upchurch H: Lowering of plasma iron concentration in the rat with leukocytic extract. Am J Physiol 216: 1287, 1969

57. Kampschmidt RF, Upchurch HF: Possible involvement of leukocytic endogenous mediator in granulopoiesis. Proc Soc Exp Biol Med 155: 89, 1977

58. Kampschmidt RF, Upchurch HF, Pulliam LA: Characterization of a leukocyte-derived endogenous mediator responsible for increased plasma fibrinogen. Ann NY Acad Sci 389: 338, 1982

59. Kampschmidt RF, Upchurch HF, Worthington ML, III: Further comparisons of endogenous pyrogens and leukocytic endogenous mediators. Infect Immun 41: 6, 1983

60. Katz R, Gordon AS, Lapin DM: Mechanisms of leukocyte production and release. VI. Studies on the purification of the leukocytosis-inducing factor (LIF). J Reticuloendothel Soc 3: 103, 1966

61. Kauffmann CA, Jones PG, Kluger MJ: Aging and nutrition: effects on leukocytic pyrogen production by monocytes. Clin Res 31: 773A, 1983

62. Keenan RA, Moldawer LL, Sakamoto A et al: Effect of leukocyte endogenous mediator(s) on insulin and substrate profiles in the fasted rat. J Surg Res 33: 151, 1982

63. Klein B, Rey A, Jourdan M et al: The role of interleukin 1 and interleukin 2 in human T colony formation. Cell Immunol 77: 348, 1983

64. Klempner MS, Dinarello CA, Gallin JI: Human leukocytic pyrogen induces release of specific granule contents from human neutrophils. J Clin Invest 61: 1330, 1978

65. Klempner MS, Dinarello CA, Henderson WR et al: Stimulation of neutrophil oxygen-dependent metabolism by human leukocytic pyrogen. J Clin Invest 64: 996, 1979

66. Lachman LB: Human interleukin 1: purification and properties. Fed Proc 42: 2639, 1983

67. Lachman LB, Maizel AL: Human immunoregulatory molecules: interleukin 1, interleukin 2, and B-cell growth factor. Contemp Topics Mol Immunol 9: 147, 1983

68. Lee GR: The anemia of chronic disease. Semin Hematol 20: 61, 1983

69. Leibson HJ, Endres R, Roehm N et al: B cell helper factors. Fed Proc 42: 1072, 1983

70. Linker-Israeli M, Bakke AC, Kitridou RC et al: Defective production of interleukin 1 and interleukin 2 in patients with systemic lupus erythematosus (SLE). J Immunol 130: 2651, 1983

71. Liu CT, Sanders RP, Hadick CL et al: Effects of intravenous injection of leukocytic endogenous mediator on cardiohepatic functions in rhesus macaques. Am J Vet Res 40: 1035, 1979

72. Long CL, Jeevanadam M, Kim BM et al: Whole body protein synthesis and catabolism in septic man. Am J Clin Nutr 30: 1340, 1977

73. Lovett DH, Ryan JL, Sterzel RB: A thymocyte-activating factor derived from glomerular mesangial cells. J Immunol 130: 1796, 1983

74. Luger TA, Sztein MB, Schmidt JA et al: Properties of murine and human epiderman cell-derived thymocyte-activating factor. Fed Proc 42: 2772, 1983

75. McKernan LN, Largen MT: Identification of multiple-molecular-weight forms of thymocyte comitogenic activity from the monocyte/macrophage cell line RAW 264.7. Cell Immunol 80: 84, 1983

76. Menkin V: Studies on inflammation. XVIII. On the mechanism of leukocytosis with inflammation. Am J Pathol 16: 13, 1940

77. Menkin V: Chemical factors and their role in inflammation. Arch Pathol 41: 376, 1946

78. Merriman CR, Pulliam LA, Kampschmidt RF: Comparison of leukocytic pyrogen and leukocytic endogenous mediator. Proc Soc Exp Biol Med 154: 224, 1977

79. Merriman CR, Upchurch HF, Kampschmidt RF: Effects of leukocytic endogenous mediator on hemopexin, transferrin, and liver catalase. Proc Soc Exp Biol Med 157: 669, 1978

80. Mizel SB, Dayer J-M, Krane SM et al: Stimulation of rheumatoid synovial cell collagenase and prostaglandin production by partially purified lymphocyte-activating factor (interleukin 1). Proc Natl Acad Sci 78: 2474, 1981

81. Mizel SB, Farrar JJ: Letter to the Editor. Revised nomenclature for antigen-nonspecific T-cell proliferation and helper factors. Cell Immunol 48: 433, 1979

82. Moore RN, Steeg PS, Mergenhagen SE: Mediator interactions regulating macrophage secretion of interleukin 1 and interferon. Adv Exp Med Biol 162: 121, 1983

83. Murphy PA, Cebula TA, Levin J et al: Rabbit macrophages secrete two biochemically and immunologically distinct endogenous pyrogens. Infect Immun 34: 177, 1981

84. Murphy PA, Chesney PJ, Wood WB, Jr.: Purification of an endogenous pyrogen with an appendix on assay methods. p. 59. In Wolstenholme GEW, Birch J (eds): Ciba Foundation Symposium on Pyrogens and Fever. Churchill Livingstone, Edinburgh, 1971

85. Murphy PA, Simon PL, Willoughby WF: Endogenous pyrogens made by rabbit peritoneal exudate cells are identical with lymphocyte-activating factors made by rabbit alveolar macrophages. J Immunol 124: 2498, 1980

86. Oppenheim JJ, Stadler BM, Siraganian RP et al: Lymphokines: their role in lymphocyte responses. Properties of interleukin 1. Fed Proc 41: 257, 1982

87. Pekarek R, Wannemacher R, Powanda M et al: Further evidence that leukocytic endogenous mediator (LEM) is not endotoxin. Life Sci 14: 1765, 1974

88. Pekarek RS, Beisel WR: Characterization of the endogenous mediator(s) of serum zinc and iron depression during infection and other stresses. Proc Soc Exp Biol Med 138: 728, 1971

89. Pekarek RS, Powanda MC, Wannemacher RW, Jr.: The effect of leukocytic endogenous mediator (LEM) on serum copper and ceruloplasmin concentrations in the rat. Proc Soc Exp Biol Med 141: 1029, 1972

90. Pekarek RS, Wannemacher RW, Jr.: A mediator for triggering non-specific host defense mechanisms. Army Sci Conf III: 129, 1972

91. Pekarek RS, Wannemacher RW, Jr., Chapple FE, III et al: Further characterization and species specificity of leukocytic endogenous mediator (LEM). Proc Soc Exp Biol Med 141: 643, 1972

92. Phillips R, Rabson AR: The effect of interleukin 1 (IL-1) containing supernatants on murine thymocyte maturation. J Clin Lab Immunol 11: 101, 1983

93. Postlethwaite AE, Lachman LB, Mainardi CL et al: Interleukin 1 stimulation of collagenase production by cultured fibroblasts. J Exp Med 157: 801, 1983

94. Powanda MC, Beisel WR: Hypothesis: leukocyte endogenous mediator/endogenous pyrogen/lymphocyte-activating factor modulates the development of nonspecific and specific immunity and affects nutritional status. Am J Clin Nutr 35: 762, 1982

95. Powanda MC, Pekarek RS, Cockerell GL et al: Mediator of alterations in protein synthesis during infection and inflammation. Fed Proc 32: 953, 1973

96. Riley RS, Rafter GW: Activation of rabbit brain microsomal ($Na^+ + K^+$)-dependent ATPase by leukocytic product. Biochim Biophys 381: 120, 1975

97. Rosenberg SA, Lipsky PE: The role of monocytes in pokeweed mitogen-stimulated human B cell activation: separate requirements for intact monocytes and a soluble monocyte factor. J Immunol 126: 1341, 1981

98. Rosenwasser LJ, Dinarello CA, Rosenthal AS: Adherent cell function in murine T-lymphocyte antigen recognition. IV. Enhancement of murine T-cell antigen. Recognition by human leukocytic pyrogen. J Exp Med 150: 709, 1979

99. Roth J, Roith DL, Shiloach J et al: Intercellular communication: an attempt at a unifying hypothesis. Clin Res 31: 354, 1983

100. Rupp RG, Fuller GM: The effects of leucocytic and serum factors on fibrogen biosynthesis in cultured hepatocytes. Exp Cell Res 118: 23, 1979

101. Sauder DN, Noonan FP, DeFabo EC et al: Ultra-

violet radiation inhibits alloantigen presentation by epidermal cells: partial reversal by the soluble epidermal cell product, epidermal cell-derived thymocyte-activating factor (ETAF). J Invest Dermatol 80: 485, 1983

102. Schlick E, Hartung K, Piccoli M et al: The capacity of biological response modifiers (BRM) to induce the secretion of colony stimulating factor(s) by murine macrophages and human monocytes. Fed Proc 42: 1221, 1983

103. Schmidt JA, Oliver CN, Green I et al: Silica stimulated macrophages (MΦ) release a fibroblast proliferation factor identical to interleukin-1 (IL-1). Fed Proc 41: 438A, 1982

104. Siegel JH, Cerra FB, Peters D et al: The physiologic recovery trajectory as the organizing principle for the quantification of hormonometabolic adaptation to surgical stress and severe sepsis. p. 177. In Schumer W, Spitzer JJ, Marshall BE (eds): Advances in Shock Research, Vol. 2. Alan R Liss, New York, 1979

105. Siegel JH, Giovannini I, Coleman B: Ventilation: perfusion maldistribution secondary to the hyperdynamic cardiovascular state as the major cause of increased pulmonary shunting in human sepsis. J Trauma 19: 432, 1979

106. Sipe JD, Vogel SN, Ryan JL et al: Detection of a mediator derived from endotoxin-stimulated macrophages that induces the acute phase serum amyloid A response in mice. J Exp Med 150: 597, 1979

107. Smith KA, Lachman LB, Oppenheim JJ et al: The functional relationship of the interleukins. J Exp Med 151: 1551, 1980

108. Sobocinski PZ, Canterbury WJ, Mapes CA: Induction of hepatic zinc-binding proteins by endotoxin and leukocytic endogenous mediators (LEM). Fed Proc 36: 1100, 1977

109. Sobrado J, Moldawer LL, Bistrian BR et al: Effect of ibuprofen on fever and metabolic changes induced by continuous infusion of leukocytic pyrogen (Interleukin 1) or endotoxin. Infect Immun 42: 997, 1983

110. Solomons NW, Elson CO, Pekarek RS et al: Leukocytic endogenous mediator in Crohn's diseases. Infect Immun 22: 637, 1978

111. Souvannanvong V, Rimsky L, Adam A: In vitro immune response to sheep erythrocytes in macrophage depleted cultures. Restoration with interleukin 1 or a monokine from resident macrophages and stimulation by N-acetyl-muramyl-L-alanyl-D-isoglutamine (MDP). Biochem Biophys Res Commun 114: 721, 1983

112. Staruch MJ, Wood DD: The adjuvanticity of interleukin 1 *in vivo*. J Immunol 130: 2191, 1983

113. Sztein MB, Vogel SN, Sipe JD et al: The role of macrophages in the acute-phase response: SAA inducer is closely related to lymphocyte activating factor and endogenous pyrogen. Cell Immunol 63: 164, 1981

114. Thompson WL, Abeles FB, Beall FA et al: Influence of the adrenal glucocorticoids on the stimulaiton of synthesis of hepatic ribonucleic acid and plasma acute-phase globulins by leucocytic endogenous mediator. Biochem J 156: 25, 1976

115. Togawa A, Oppenheim JJ, Mizel SB: Characterization of lymphocyte-activating factor (LAF) produced by human mononuclear cells: biochemical relationship of high and low molecular weight forms of LAF. J Immunol 122: 2112, 1979

116. Turchik JB, Bornstein DL: Role of the central nervous system in acute-phase responses to leukocytic pyrogen. Infect Immun 30: 439, 1980

117. Vane JR: Inhibition of prostaglandin synthesis as a mechanism of action for aspirin-like drugs. Nature 231: 232, 1971

118. Wannemacher RW, Jr., Pekarek RS, Beisel WR: An endogenous mediator(s) of plasma amino acid flux and trace metal depression during experimentally induced infection in man. Am J Clin Nutr 25: 461, 1972

119. Wannemacher RW, Jr., Pekarek RS, Beisel WR: Mediator of hepatic amino acid flux in infected rats. Proc Soc Exp Biol Med 139: 128, 1972

120. Wannemacher RW, Jr., Pekarek RS, Klainer AS et al: Detection of a leukocytic endogenous mediator-like mediator of serum amino acid and zinc depression during infectious illnesses. Infect Immun 11: 873, 1975

121. Wannemacher RW, Jr., Pekarek RS, Thompson WL et al: A protein from polymorphonuclear leukocytes (LEM) which affects the rate of hepatic amino acid transport and synthesis of acute-phase globulins. Endocrinology 96: 651, 1975

122. Windle BE, Murphy PA, Cooperman S: Rabbit polymorphonuclear leukocytes do not secrete endogenous pyrogens or interleukin 1 when stimulated by endotoxin, polyinosine:polycytosine, or muramyl dipeptide. Infect Immun 39: 1142, 1983

123. Wood DD, Ihrie EJ, Dinarello CA et al: Isolation of an interleukin-1-like factor from human joint effusions. Arthritis Rheum 26: 975, 1983

124. Yang RD, Moldawer LL, Sakamoto A et al: Leukocyte endogenous mediator alters protein dynamics in rats. Metabolism 32: 654, 1983

4

Biochemical Disorders in Hypovolemia and Sepsis

William Schumer

BIOCHEMICAL DISORDERS IN HYPOVOLEMIA

The crucial factor and common denominator of all types of hypovolemic shock is cellular hypoperfusion. This occurs first in the nonvital tissues of the gastrointestinal tract, muscle, connective tissue, and skin and subsequently in the vital tissues of the brain, heart, lung, liver, and kidney. The result is cellular anoxia and starvation. Under these conditions, the minimal amounts of substrates available for passage through the cell membrane into the energy pathways are blocked by anoxia. More profound hypovolemia may compound this cellular injury. Consequently, it is in the cell's energy pathways that the most profound metabolic effects of hypovolemic shock occur.

Energy-Producing Pathways

Ordinarily, substrates such as glucose, glucogenic α-amino acids (alanine), and glycerol are actively transported into the liver cell by a transfer system requiring adenosine nucleotides. Energized adenosine nucleotides can either be derived anaerobically through glycolysis, or aerobically through the citric acid cycle and electron transport system. The aerobic transfer is more efficient, but the anaerobic substrate level production of adenosine triphosphate (ATP) can be effective in promoting substrate infusion into the cell. These substrates—glucose, amino acids, fatty acids, lactic acid, and glycerol—can be either metabolized to produce ATP or stored in the liver and muscle as glycogen via gluconeogenesis.

79

In hypovolemic shock states, adequate perfusion of the cellular capillary bed is crucial. The cells of the peripheral tissues—skin, connective tissue, muscle, and gastrointestinal tract—react to the inadequate perfusion of decreased circulating volume by shifting to anaerobiosis. Immediately, the following deleterious series of events occur at the cellular level:

1. Substrate transport is impaired.
2. There is a decrease in ATP and adenosine diphosphate (ADP) production with subsequent derangement of the energy-dependent ATPase molecule.
3. Membrane dysfunction occurs.
4. Sodium and water enter and potassium exudes through the membrane and cellular swelling ensues.[36]
5. The glycolytic cycle is blocked at the mitochondrial entranceway (pyruvate-acetyl coenzyme A [CoA] step).
6. Finally, only 2 moles of ATP are produced from 1 mole of glucose.

An adequately functioning citric cycle produces 38 moles of ATP; thus anaerobic circulatory collapse reduces energy production by 95 percent. Since the peripheral cellular mass is 75 percent of the total body mass, any energy deficit in this area affects the entire organism.

A review of the changes occurring on specific peripheral tissues during hypovolemic shock will be of value in the elucidation of cellular metabolic dysfunction in shock.

Nonvital Organ Energy Metabolism

SKELETAL MUSCLE CELL

Skeletal muscle adapts itself to anaerobiosis by rapidly increasing its energy output via various ATP-producing anaerobic mechanisms. These are phosphocreatine decomposition, myokinase reaction, and utilization of glycogen stores. However, during severe anaerobiosis these mechanisms are rapidly utilized, and lactic acid formation, the blind alley of anaerobic glycolysis, accelerates. Muscle mass is one of the largest producers of lactic acid in hypovolemic shock states. During severe circulatory deficiency, muscle protein is consumed as one of the main sources of stored energy, and acute catabolism of muscle mass occurs and alanine is released. Muscle branched-chain amino acids and ketones are utilized for substrate when the muscle becomes glucose-deficient. The muscle oxidizes leucine to carbon dioxide and converts the carbon skeletons of aspartate, arginine, glutamine, isoleucine, and valine into Krebs cycle intermediates. During hypovolemic shock of any cause, muscle increasingly releases branched-chain amino acids and increases their serum concentration 10-fold. Large concentrations of alanine and lactate are released and transported to the liver for conversion into glucose via gluconeogenesis, and glucose is then returned to the muscle. These cycles are called glucose–alanine and Cori (lactate) cycles.

GASTROINTESTINAL CELL

Curtailment of ATP production during hypovolemic shock profoundly affects gastrointestinal tract absorption of glucose and amino acids. The lack of perfusion through the gastrointestinal tract impairs mobilization of glucose, fatty acids, and also monoacylglycerol because of decreased lymphatic flow. Active transport is the mechanism for glucose and amino acid absorption, and the transport defect is probably due to the energy deficit. Active glucose transport is ATP-dependent and is associated with an ATPase enzyme. This is evidenced by the fact that ouabain, an ATPase inhibitor, and phlorhizin, a competitive inhibitor, interfere with glucose absorption. Amino acid absorption is also ATP-dependent, as demonstrated by the fact that 2,4-dinitrophenol, an electron transport inhibitor, impedes the concentration of L-amino acids in the gastrointestinal mucosal cells.

Recently, Barzilai et al.[2] showed that in hemorrhagic hypovolemic shock, specific gastrointestinal tract metabolic functions are impaired because of membrane energy dysfunction. Proton fluxes were measured in rabbit antral pouches with a sensitive microelectrode inserted into the mucosa. Barzilai et al. found

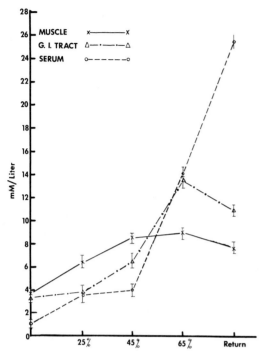

FIG. 4-1 "Wash out" phenomenon. Intracellular lactate levels in muscle and gastrointestinal tract tissue, and serum concentrations at specific increments of hemorrhage. Note increase in serum concentration and decrease in intracellular values when volume is returned ("wash out" phenomenon).

studies in our laboratory[32] showed that of all the peripheral tissues, the gastrointestinal tract is the largest producer of lactate (Fig. 4-1).

SKIN AND CONNECTIVE TISSUE CELL

Skin and connective tissue, forming 14 percent of the total body cell mass, may produce marked anaerobiosis when inadequately perfused. Since connective tissue is the transitional area of inflammatory reaction, energy deficiency severely impairs its immune response to injury and wound healing by the following mechanisms:

> Polymorphonuclear cells and other macrophages involved in the energy-requiring function of phagocytosis and opsonization are unable to clear the wound of foreign bodies. ATP-deficient collagen synthesis is inhibited in the messenger ribonucleic acid (mRNA) and transfer RNA (tRNA) processes. Ground substance cannot be produced, and fibroblasts cannot synthesize procollagen because there is interference with the translational function on the fibroblast's endoplasmic reticulum ribosomes.

Thus, low perfusion states interfere with host defense against infection and with wound healing.

Vital Organ Energy Metabolism

KIDNEY CELL

After the patient has decompensated hemodynamically, vital organs become affected with the kidney showing the first involvement. Green et al.[9] reported that in decompensated hypovolemic shocked animals there is a proportional decrease between renal pressure and flow. Sato et al.[31] documented the following renal ultrastructural alterations in human hypovolemic shock of various causes: minimal to mild changes in glomeruli; focal necrosis of

that the relative impermeability of rabbit antral mucosa to H^+ apparently protected it against acute ulceration. When the rate of H^+ back-diffusion was artifically increased to a level that was ulcerogenic in fundic mucosa by the introduction of hydrochloric acid into the pouches, ulceration also occurred in the antrum. Their findings also indicated that mucosal carbonic anhydrase had a protective function by contributing to the maintainance of normal intracellular acid–base balance in the epithelial cells, and that either acetazolamide or other potent inhibitors of anion transport that blocks chloride and bicarbonate exchange, disturbed this balance. Thus, the energy deficit of low perfusion states can produce gastric ulceration. However, the most profound effect is a markedly increased cellular anaerobiosis producing large serum lactic acid concentrations. Hemorrhagic hypovolemic shock dog tubular epithelium with an increase in the number of secondary lysosomes or residual bodies; and predominantly distal tubular casts accompanied by flattening of the tubular epithelium. The highly metabolic tubular cell function is dependent on glomerular and tubular perfusion. Energy produced by the kidney's oxidative and decarboxylating reactions is used for active reabsorption of sodium and water. It is estimated that one oxygen molecule is needed for reabsorption of 20 to 30 sodium ions. Thus, the hypoxia of depressed perfusion decreases oxygen uptake and ATP production and increases water and sodium losses.

Sodium- and potassium-activated ATPase is localized in the basolateral cell membrane of the proximal and distal nephron. The luminal brush border of proximal tubular cells is associated with a nonmitochondrial ATPase stimulated by bicarbonate and alkaline phosphatase. There is indirect evidence that ATPase is connected with either H^+ secretion or bicarbonate reabsorption. Calcium-activated ATPase is localized in the basolateral membranes of the proximal and distal nephrons. The lack of both ADP and renal cellular ATP deranges ATPase function, which interferes with sodium and hydrogen ions secretion and excretion and consequently with acid-base balance reparation.

In profound hypovolemia, anaerobic metabolism produces metabolic acidosis, negating distal tubular function. Glutaminase I, a phosphate-dependent enzyme located in the renal tubular cell's mitochondrion, increases its activity during metabolic acidosis by catalyzing ammonia formation via glutamine deamination and excreting H^+ as an ammonium salt. This oxygen-requiring enzyme is linked to the citric acid cycle because glutamine becomes glutamate so that it can ultimately enter the Krebs cycle and be converted to glucose. Recent evidence indicates that the net synthesis of glucose is not a requirement for ammonia production. However, the transport of malate and possibly oxaloacetate across the mitochondrial membrane, with subsequent conversion to phosphoenolpyruvate (PEP) by the PEP carboxykinase reaction, must be closely linked to the rate at which ammonia is being formed from glutamine within the mitochondria. The lack of substrate, the diminished ATP production, and the overwhelming metabolic acidosis impair the kidney's compensatory ability and result in intracellular edema of the proximal and distal tubules, with release of lysosomal enzymes and functional failure. If uncorrected, tubular failure and necrosis lead to persisting renal insufficiency.

LUNG CELL

Biochemically, the lung operates as a membrane exchanging oxygen for carbon dioxide, with these gases diffusing across the alveolar membrane into the red blood cells for transport to the tissues. Thus, the lung is primarily a gas exchanger passively equilibrating gases between the alveolar and red blood cells according to the ideal gas law. Minimal energy is expended in this process, and the lung functions without difficulty in hypovolemic shock states except in the presence of an alveolovascular membrane injury with accompanying edema and hyalinization.

Hemoglobin transports about 97 to 98 percent of the oxygen by a reversible molecular combination. Dissociation of hemoglobin and oxygen at tissue level is represented by the hemoglobin–oxygen dissociation curve. In hypovolemic shock, this curve moves to the right, which decreases the affinity of hemoglobin for oxygen through four mechanisms: (1) increased H^+ acidity (blood pH decrease); (2) increased carbon dioxide tension; (3) increased erythrocyte concentration of 2,3-diphosphoglycerate (2,3-DPG); and (4) increased body temperature.

The Bohr effect (increased carbon dioxide tension caused by increased hydrogen ion concentration secondary to peripheral metabolic acidosis of anaerobic metabolism) is probably due to increased carbonic acid generation and increased dissociation as expressed in the following formula:

$$H_2CO_3 \underset{\text{anhydrase}}{\overset{\text{carbonic}}{\rightleftarrows}} H^+ + HCO_3$$

2,3-DPG is a metabolic cofactor in the Embden-Meyerhof glycolytic pathway. In the erythrocyte, one 2,3-DPG molecule binds noncovalently to the α-amino group of the N-terminal valine residue of the 2 β chain of deoxyhemoglobin. Thus, 2,3-DPG pulls the equilibrium between oxyhemoglobin and deoxyhemoglobin plus oxygen to the right, favoring the deoxygenated state of hemoglobin as shown in the following formula (dissociation of oxygen from hemoglobin catalyzed by 2,3-DPG):

$$Hb\ O_2 \overset{DPG}{\rightarrow} HB \cdot DPG + O_2$$

In hypovolemic shock, erythrocytic 2,3-DPG significantly increases. According to Wilson,[45] when one is replacing volume in hypovolemic shock patients, it should be noted that the decreased 2,3-DPG content of old stored blood may yield high oxygen affinity hemoglobin that could interfere with the erythrocytic delivery of oxygen at the tissue level. Finally, elevated temperature changes in septic shock patients also move the dissociation curve to the right and increase oxygen release.

The alveolar apparatus is composed of macrophages and type I and II pneumocytes. Oxygen diffusion occurs in the membraneous type I pneumocytes, while type II pneumocytes produce surfactant, which is a lipoprotein complex containing mainly L-dipalmitoyl phosphatidylcholine.

The half-life of this saturated pulmonary lecithin is 14 hours, which suggests that active synthesis is required. Inclusion bodies in type II alveolar cells show an uptake of ^{14}C palmitate, which is indirect evidence of their synthesis in these cells. Surfactant is considered to be the substance maintaining the integrity of thin-walled alveoli by preventing the collapse and coaptation of alveolar cells. This is apparently accomplished by the dipolar effect of the fatty acid in the surfactant; the negative charges repel each other thus keeping the alveoli open as reported by Clowes.[5] According to Greenfield,[10] because of their high metabolic rate, type II cells are dependent on ATP for surfactant synthesis. In hypovolemic shock, dysfunction in type I pneumocytes may cause a membranous leak, which fills the alveoli and produces a surfactant washout, compounding the atelectasis of adult respiratory distress syndrome.

The pulmonary alveolar macrophage is a glucose- and oxygen-utilizing phagocyte. It produces hydrogen peroxide (H_2O_2) but no hydroxyl radicals, a mechanism that apparently protects the alveolar spaces where the macrophage resides. Oxygen radicals produced intracellularly or released extracellularly may be important to the macrophage in its bactericidal activity but may also expose the cell to self-destruction by oxidant injury. The soluble sulfhydryl system in erythrocytes has been shown to protect the polymorphonuclear leukocyte and macrophage cell from oxidant injury by reducing hydrogen peroxide. The hexose monophosphate pathway works to regenerate reduced nicotine adenine phosphonucleotide (NADPH) so that reduced glutathione may be replenished. Papermaster-Bender et al.[27] reported that any nascent oxygen (0^-)-releasing effect by the alveolar macrophage may damage type I pneumocytes and cause fluid to leak into the alveolus and depress type II pneumocytes surfactant production.

LIVER CELL

Schumer et al.[33] reported that hepatic cell oxygen metabolism is increased during hypovolemic shock. Mitochondrial metabolism showed uncoupling of oxidative phosphorylation. This oxygen waste without energy accumulation is a continuous process associated with changes in the character of the mitochondria. This uncoupling process produces an increase of inorganic phosphates in the liver and a decrease in the concentration of both high-energy organic phosphates, ATP and ADP.

Liver cells perform the following metabolic functions: (1) bile and cholesterol excretion, (2) gluconeogenesis, (3) detoxification, and (4) protein synthesis. Depressed perfusion secondary to all types of hypovolemic shock profoundly affects these functions.

Bile and Cholesterol Excretion. Studies on bile solubilization and excretion in hypovolemic shock states indicate a marked decrease in bile formation and excretion. It has been noted in shock patients after biliary tract surgery with external drainage that the bile secretion is suppressed. This may be attributable to the oxygen or NAD dependence of the bilirubin-solubilizing reaction of glucuronide conjugation to bilirubin. In hypovolemic shock or low-flow states a mild jaundice of 1.0 to 3.0

mg/dl is usually present. Cholesterol is either taken up or synthesized by the liver and either excreted in the bile or converted to bile acids. In hypovolemic shock, this energy-consuming process, which is ultimately needed for hormone synthesis, is markedly reduced. The biochemical effects of deranged cholesterol metabolism may be prolonged and militate against the patient's recovering from the catabolic effects of low flow states.

Detoxification.   The liver is unable to detoxify because the allosteric enzymes—glucuronidases, sulfatases, and hydroxylases—are NAD^+-dependent. This will inhibit the detoxification and solubilization of various intermediate metabolites such as serotonin, histamine, and various steroids. Oxidative reactions in the liver act to metabolize certain inert hydrocarbons. This hydroxylation occurs in the endoplasmic reticulum of the hepatic cells. Hydroxyl compounds may be further oxidized to ketones or aldehydes by the action of the enzymes' alcoholic dehydrogenases. The detoxifying function in the reticuloendothelial system of the liver may play a significant role in the neutralization of bacterial exotoxins and endotoxins.

Protein Synthesis.   Decreased urea nitrogen in the blood of hypovolemic shock patients is not surprising because the deaminating and transaminating amino acid enzymes in the liver need ATP to produce glucose or substrates to enter into the citric acid cycle. These oxidative enzymes depend on cofactors for normal functioning. Thus, severe hypovolemic shock states may produce liver failure with an attendant hyperammonemia.

HEART CELL

The heart muscle cell, with its abundant mitochondria, needs to produce high concentrations of ATP. This cell extracts lactate, glucose, and fatty acids and converts these substrates to ATP. During severe hypotension, however, anaerobic metabolism produces rather than consumes lactic acid, indicating a dependence on anaerobic glycolysis for energy. Some of the capacity of the cardiac mitochondrial citric acid cycle and electron transport system is not restored to normal function after transfusion as evidenced by persistently low levels of ATP in patients with hypovolemic shock. This translates into depressed left ventricular work, coronary flow, and ventricular oxygen consumption in posthypovolemic shock states. Rush reported that blood levels of pyruvate and lactate remain significantly elevated during this same period.[30] Lefer et al.[19] described a myocardial depressant factor that appeared to be a vasoactive peptide produced by the pancreas during hypovolemic shock. Spitzer et al.[38] demonstrated that in septic dogs the marked decrease in uptake and oxidation of free fatty acids greatly impaired myocardial energy metabolism. Concomitantly, lactate becomes a significant energy source. Thus, glycolytic metabolism may help protect the heart against anoxic injury. Furthermore, since fatty acid oxidation requires Krebs cycle intermediates when carbohydrate is oxidized, intracellular glucose is important even when oxygen is not rate limiting. Glucose transport and phosphorylation increase with anoxia, the latter because glucose-6-phosphate (G6P) inhibition of hexokinase is released as the glycolytic flux increases and G6P concentration falls. Glycolytic flux increases and phosphofructokinase (PFK) is released from inhibition by declining citrate and ATP, and PFK is activated by rising phosphate.[16] Glycogen stores are rapidly depleted during anoxia since β-phosphorylase itself is stimulated by phosphate and released from inhibition by G6P and because epinephrine induces transformation of phosphorylase β to α.

Under severely hypoxic conditions, anaerobic metabolism is unable to maintain the heart's high-energy phosphate stores. Consequently, first creatine phosphate and later ATP stores are diminished. Lactate production and glycolytic flux increase more than 20-fold. If anoxic conditions continue, acidosis produces a PFK inhibition, or rate limitation, and thus hexokinase is inhibited by the increase in G6P. If ATP falls below 2 M/g, glycoytic flux will cease because there is insufficient ATP to phosphorylate F6P. The effects of hypovolemia on heart metabolism appear to be due to the anoxic defects because the results are the same as seen in the anoxic heart.

BRAIN CELL

The average oxygen utilization by the normal human brain has been found to range from 3.3 to 3.9 ml/100 g/min and the mean oxygen consumption has been calculated to be 3.6 ml/100 g/min. Rate increases in oxygen consumption can occur during convulsions but apparently not during mental activity.

What happens metabolically in the late stages of low-flow states when the brain is poorly perfused and anoxic? The intact brain's main substrate source of energy is glucose, which is metabolized in the glycolytic and Krebs cycles and hexose monophosphate shunt. Under ordinary conditions the lactate yield is low, 6 M/g wet weight/hr, but under adverse conditions it may increase to 400 M/g wet weight/h. Normally phosphocreatine and ATP concentrations are about 3 M/g wet weight, but hypoxia causes a marked decrease of these compounds. Thus, the general requirements of brain cells for ATP production are similar to those of any other organ. The interdependence between the membrane potential and ionic concentrations is important for the nerve cell. In low-flow and anoxic states, ATP deficiency affects the sodium/potassium ATPase molecule along the membrane and, consequently, impulse propagation.

Apparently glutamic acid is the only amino acid metabolized in brain tissue. It participates in the brain's uptake of ammonia and combines with ammonia to form glutamine, which is then excreted in the plasma for liver metabolism. Glutamic acid is formed by the transamination of ketoglutarate formed in the Krebs cycle from the metabolism of glucose to produce pyruvate and then oxaloacetate. This is the brain's defense against the anoxia and ammonemia of low perfusion, and a hypoperfused liver. During hypovolemic shock the brain is the last organ to be underperfused and has the necessary enzymatic activity to support its continuing major metabolic activities. It is protected from anaerobiosis by its "autonomic cerebral metabolism;" however, because of its metabolic complexity, it will not withstand prolonged hypoperfusion. Anoxia will produce metabolic acidosis, enzyme dysfunction, cellular membrane leakage causing edema, attendant convulsion, coma, and finally death.

BIOCHEMICAL DISORDERS IN SEPSIS

Septic shock initially is an immunologic reaction characterized by a hyperdynamic phase producing increased cardiac output and decreased peripheral resistance. This reaction is secondary to endotoxin–antibody–complement complexing and leukocyte aggregation, degranulation, and lysis that results in the production of histamine, serotonin, superradicals, lysosomal enzymes, and leukotrienes. These substances induce marked capillary permeability and a third-space loss leading to hypovolemia or the hypodynamic phase of septic shock. This phase is characterized by decreased cardiac output and increased peripheral resistance. Specific and different subcellular effects occur in each of these two phases of septic shock.

Subcellular Effects in the Hyperdynamic Phase of Septic Shock

Because of increased peripheral cell perfusion, subcellular changes in the hyperdynamic phase do not result from anaerobic metabolism, but rather from alterations in the glycolytic and gluconeogenic cycles, probably via endotoxin-mediated membrane effects. Gimpel et al.[8] reported that the initial step in endotoxin-induced changes in carbohydrate metabolism is an activation of a membrane-bound enzyme, adenylate cyclase (AC). Binding of endotoxin to AC may be responsible for accelerated glycolysis, depletion of carbohydrate reserves, and hypoglycemic damage of glycolysis-dependent cells. Raymond et al.'s study in nonischemic, nonhypoxic skeletal muscle in dogs challenged by live *Escherichia coli* (*E. coli*) showed an increased lactic acid concentration due to increased glucose oxidation.[29] Similarly, we showed[14] that after 3 hours of endotoxin challenge in rats, lactic acid concentrations rose 20 to 30 percent higher than normal. Hirsch et al.[11] reported that in gram-negative sepsis in combat trauma glycolytic cycle function rose significantly above normal during the hyperdynamic phase. Studies by Vary et al.[40,41] in a chronic septic model (intraabdominal abscess of *B. fragilis* + *E. coli*) showed depression of the oxidative pyruvate dehydrogenase complex in large abscesses. This may be due to defects in energy metabolism, specifically, a decrease in acetyl-CoA precursors.

GLUCONEOGENESIS

The liver glycolytic intermediate pattern in endotoxemia has been interpreted by Williamson et al.[44] as arising from a block in an enzymatic step between fructose-1,6-diphosphate (FDP) and fructose-6-phosphate (F6P). Either fructose diphosphatase is inhibited, conserving the FDP supply, or phosphofructokinase is activated and more FDP accumulates in the metabolic pool. We showed[17] that by a regulatory "feed-forward" control loop, the elevated FDP activates pyruvate kinase, depleting phosphoenolpyruvate (PEP), and thus accounts for the lowered concentration of this substrate in perfused or intact endotoxified livers reported by Scrutton et al.[34] Williamson et al.[44] and Holtzman et al.[14] in our laboratory. A fall in glucose-6-phosphate (G6P) then results because of increased conversion into F6P and FDP. The net effect of these reactions is to route carbohydrate moieties away from gluconeogenesis. When glycogen is exhausted, the hypoglycemia of terminal sepsis and endotoxemia usually appears.

Another feature of this interpretation emphasizes the role of futile cycles in carbohydrate metabolism. These occur at the three points where glycolytic and gluconeogenic pathways do not share common enzymes. At these points substrate molecules shuttle back and forth between anabolic and catabolic enzymes. Since each turn of the cycle consumes a high-energy phosphate bond, the term "futile cycle" is aptly descriptive because no glucose is synthesized yet chemical energy is being wasted. Although futile cycling is believed to have an important control function in normal metabolism, it is capable of depleting energy stores unless it is effectively coupled to life-supporting activities. Since G6P, FDP, and PEP are generated and consumed at futile cycles, they can be considered key substrates in gluconeogenesis. Because of this functional importance, and because these three substrates give the most consistently observed changes in endotoxemia and sepsis, they deserve further attention.

Williamson et al.'s systemic explanation of the biochemical findings in endotoxified liver exposed to endotoxin is recommended by its simplicity and consistency.[44] However, Scrutton et al.[34] reported that since many details of gluconeogenic regulation have not been worked out even for normal livers, the exact site at which endotoxin exerts its direct or indirect influence on cellular metabolism remains unknown. Identification of the early metabolic changes occurring in liver in endotoxemic and septic animals could be useful in the design of therapies to arrest the catabolic debilitation of severe sepsis before it progresses to shock. Obviously, selecting animals already exhibiting the gross pathophysiology of terminal endotoxemia is not conducive to the detection of subtle metabolic changes that may be key determinants of the course and outcome of sepsis. However, Yates et al. in our laboratory found that it is also necessary to understand that assays of metabolites cannot themselves reveal the control mechanisms unless supplemented by radioactive label studies that can measure metabolic flux quantitatively.[47]

The perfused livers in Williamson et al.'s[44] studies were isolated from endotoxin-treated rats with plasma glucose of 40 mg/dl. Livers from endotoxemic rats that had not yet developed this extreme hypoglycemia were reported to show glycolytic intermediate concentrations similar to those observed in the preterminal animals, as reported by our research group.[14,17,47] This suggests that hepatic metabolism is disordered before plasma glucose reflects the full extent of the damage. Kuttner et al.[17] demonstrated that G6P underwent significant changes in concentration that preceded other metabolic responses associated with inhibited gluconeogenesis. The obvious interpretation is that endotoxin exerts its action first on hexose monophosphate-regulating enzymes and that the other changes follow from this as the pathologic condition unfolds.

Although the first enzyme or substrate to show a response to endotoxin may not have a key regulatory role, an understanding of early events could be critical in preventing the subsequent cascade of adverse changes.[20,21]

When a lethal dose of endotoxin is administered to a test animal, body defenses are overwhelmed and relentless progression of biochemical and physiologic events is triggered, culminating in death. It is necessary to know if this sequence applies to sepsis, where some host factors may insulate against the metabolic insult. This was found to be the case. In an experimental model of leakage peritonitis developing from a cecal perforation, G6P was markedly diminished within 5 hours, whereas PEP was unchanged and FDP was not significantly increased (Table 4-1). Of the three substrates previously cited as possessing regulatory roles at futile cycles, only G6P shows a response in this experimental sepsis. The liver intermediates in this model resemble the pattern reported for the 1-hour endotoxemic rat livers. Moderate sepsis and early endotoxemia both may progress to later stages only after they have induced changes in hexose mono-phosphate-regulating enzymes in the liver. This would imply that a convincing fall in G6P is a signal of other disturbances yet to come in gluconeogenesis. A minor note emerging from this observation is that if moderate sepsis acts on liver metabolism in a manner very similar to endotoxin, then it seems likely that endotoxin may be implicated as a common agent responsible for metabolic dysfunction in endotoxemia and sepsis.[12,13]

We showed that PEP was not lowered in experimental sepsis except when the rats were clearly preterminal[45] (Figs. 4-2 and 4-3). Strengthening this observation is Sharma et al.'s report that pyruvate kinase, a PEP-utilizing enzyme, is unaffected in livers from endotoxin-treated dogs, whereas levels of glucokinase and phosphofructokinase are sharply decreased.[35] Thus, of the three glycolytic intermediates believed to reflect futile cycle control of gluconeogenesis, only G6P seems to be consistently altered in early and late phases of endotoxemia and sepsis. This suggests that the other changes occurring later are secondary homeostatic readjustments of metabolic pool constituents.

TABLE 4-1. Changes in Glycolytic Intermediates in Rat Liver After Peritonitis and Fecal Implant Sepsis

Metabolite	(nmoles/g wet tissue $\pm$ SD)		
	Control (Sham-operated)	Peritonitis (Cecal Incision)	Sepsis (Fecal Implant)
Glucose-6-phosphate	234 ± 36 (N = 11)	117 ± 78^a (N = 8)	177 ± 120 (N = 15)
Fructose-6-phosphate	63 ± 18 (N = 11)	37 ± 20^a (N = 8)	58 ± 28 (N = 15)
Fructose-1,6-diphosphate	11 ± 6 (N = 11)	24 ± 8 (N = 8)	8 ± 7 (N = 15)
Dihydroxyacetone phosphate	33 ± 18 (N = 15)	55 ± 32 (N = 12)	33 ± 15 (N = 15)
2-Phosphoglyceric acid	508 ± 153 (N = 15)	578 ± 259 (N = 12)	698 ± 238^b (N = 15)
Phosphoenolpyruvate	219 ± 94 (N = 15)	235 ± 87 (N = 12)	191 ± 112 (N = 15)
Lactic acid	907 ± 305 (N = 15)	$2,158 \pm 552^a$ (N = 12)	$2,302 \pm 521^a$ (N = 15)

Fasted adult albino rats (160–200 g) were biopsied by freeze-clamp 5 hr after cecal incision peritonitis and 18 hrs after human stool capsule implant sepsis.

N = number of rats sampled.

[a] Significant to $P < 0.001$ compared to controls.

[b] Significant to $P < 0.025$ compared to controls.

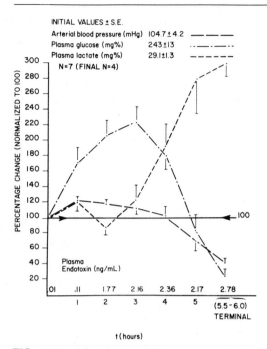

FIG. 4-2 Metabolic and hemodynamic response to plasma endotoxin in rat peritonitis after cecal incision.

An endotoxin-mediated action on glucokinase or glucose-6-phosphatase, the two enzymes that control G6P levels, would have the potential to influence glucose anabolism and catabolism in many competing pathways. Glucose-6-phosphate is the central substrate leading to glycogen formation, the pentose shunt, toward glycolysis via F6P, and back to glucose itself. The concentration of this substrate is therefore a key determinant of metabolic function as shown by Katz et al.[15] If endotoxin directly or indirectly imposes a biochemical lesion on G6P-regulating enzymes, carbohydrate metabolism could be deranged at many remote sites in many important metabolic pathways. The corollary of this fact would be that any therapy for sepsis that corrects or prevents the G6P changes ought to be highly effective. Nagler et al.[26] reported preliminary evidence that G6P injection is even more beneficial than glucose itself in some shock states.

Citric acid cycling and electron transport flux, with their attendant adenosine triphosphate (ATP) production, apparently are not inhibited in the hyperdynamic phase. However,

oxygen extraction decreases as shown by arterial venous differences and oxygen extraction ratios. Chaudry et al.[4] using cecal ligation and cecal puncture peritonitis in rats, and Balis et al.[1] in live *E. coli*-treated rats, observed no changes in adenine nucleotides in early sepsis (high-flow septic rats). In contrast Mela et al.[23] using both hemorrhagic and endotoxin shock, and Tanaka et al.[39] in *E. coli* bacteremia, reported strong inhibition of rat liver mitochondrial energy-producing reactions in the early stage of both hemorrhagic and endotoxin shock. Despite good perfusion, hepatic energy charges decreased and the mitochondrial oxidoreduction state increased, suggesting that the primary derangement in hepatic high-energy metabolism is nonanaerobic. The exact cause of this decreased oxygen utilization is still unknown. Tanaka et al.[39] reported in their study on *E. coli* bacteremia in rat liver mitochondria, that at 3 hours (hypodynamic phase), respiratory control, state III respiration, PO ratios, and phosphorylation ratios (nmols of ATP formed per milligram mitochondrial protein per minute) were all increased. Thus mitochondrial enzyme systems such as the citric acid cycle and the electron transport system are initially overstimulated and extract more oxygen. Why does this occur in the hyperdynamic phase? Hypoxia in oligemic shock decreases the substrate and oxygen supply to the cell. However, mitochondria increase their rate of oxygen extraction as measured by the arterial venous oxygen difference. Mela et al.[22,23,24] reported that liver mitochondria isolated during lethal endotoxemia in rats and dogs also showed disturbed energy production, paralleling such pathologic ultrastructural findings as swelling and morphologic membrane defects. These functional alterations indicated defective oxidative phosphorylative reactions rather than a direct inhibition of the electron transport chain.

Other energy-linked reactions such as ion transport across the membrane also show inhibition in endotoxin shock. Ion transport studies show that in the early stages of endotoxemia there is significant inhibition of energy-linked Ca^{++} accumulation by liver mitochondria. This inhibition corresponds to increased permeability of the mitochondrial inner membrane to K^+. These effects on energy-dependent ion trans-

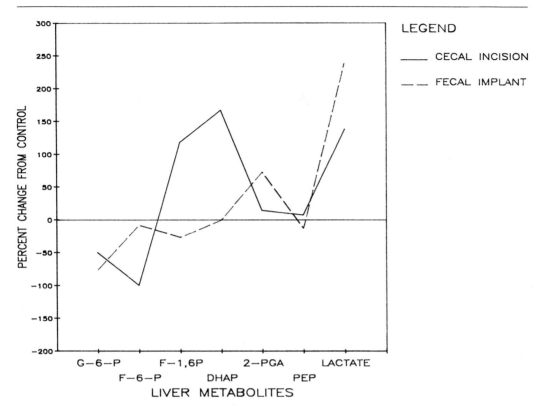

FIG. 4-3 Metabolic response of glycolytic intermediates to cecal incision and fecal implant sepsis.

port are evident in the early stages of circulatory shock when energy production is still adequate. Changes identical to those found in the liver were also monitored in the kidney; the time course of these alterations suggests that kidney mitochondria are damaged at an earlier stage of shock than liver mitochondria. Thus the inhibition of gluconeogenesis in both the liver and kidney compounds the energy deficit in these tissues and contributes to the decline in their vital functions. Heart and skeletal muscle do not experience the same degree of mitochondrial damage in early oligemic shock. Skeletal muscle cells are more resistant to high lactate concentrations and low PO_2 and pH levels than those of other tissues, so overall energy changes are minimal. Experimental studies of the hypodynamic phase of septic shock with its increased glycolysis, lactic acid production, and acidosis have shown that when these occur ATP production is reduced to 10 percent of normal.

Kuttner et al.[17] in a study of hepatic glycolytic intermediates in early endotoxemia and sepsis in rats and mice, showed gluconeogenic inhibition (Table 4-1). The glucose metabolite of glycogenolysis and gluconeogenesis, glucose-6-phosphate (G6P) significantly decreases, and lactic acid production increases indicating a decrease in gluconeogenic lactate uptake. One probable cause for these changes in septic shock is the unavailability of glycolytic flux substrates for gluconeogenesis (Fig. 4-4).

Lactic acidosis is first buffered, therefore producing an early respiratory alkalosis that is the attempt of the respiratory system to excrete water and carbon dioxide. This water contains the proton H^+ produced by the dissociation of lactic acid.

The periphery takes up plasma free fatty acids as well as very low density lipoproteins fatty acids at an increased rate if oxygen is present as in the hyperdynamic state of sepsis,

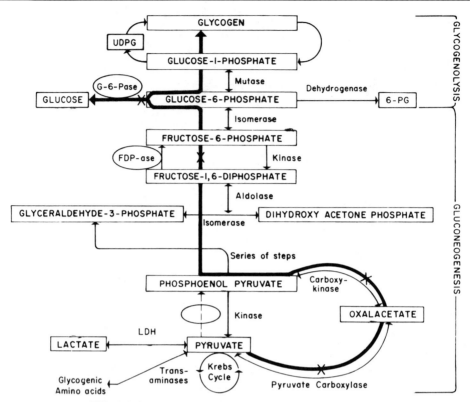

FIG. 4-4 Scheme of Glyconeogenesis and gluconeogenesis.

thus permitting free fatty acid (FFA) utilization for energy production. If oxygen delivery to the muscle cell is limited, FFA remain in the serum and cannot be used for energy generation.

Subcellular Effects in the Hypodynamic Phase of Septic Shock

Table 4-2 shows an outline of metabolic changes occurring in the hypodynamic phase of septic shock. With the loss of plasma volume, the circulatory response is similar to that of hypovolemic shock. There is release of epinephrine and norepinephrine, producing increased peripheral resistance and cardiac rate. Cardiac output is depressed because of the decreased blood volume and venous return. This is known as the hypodynamic phase of septic shock. Depressed perfusion to nonvital tissues produces deranged cellular metabolism. The lack of oxygen results in the anaerobic metabolism of glucose with increased production of lactic acid, the main cause of metabolic acidosis in the hypodynamic phase of septic shock. Impaired function of the Krebs cycle depresses ATP, or energy production. This energy deficit decreases membrane ATPase function, allowing further loss of fluid through the endothelial cells and resulting in the intracellular edema of shock. The net result of these hemodynamic changes is decreased cellular perfusion of substrate and oxygen to nonvital tissues, skin, connective tissue, muscle and gastrointestinal tract, and subsequently reduced circulation to vital tissues, the brain, lungs, heart, liver, and kidney. The lack of perfusion through the massive peripheral cellular mass produces the following hypoxic milieu: (1) anaerobic metabolism, (2) energy deficiency, (3) catabolism of

TABLE 4-2. Metabolic Changes in Hypodynamic Septic Shock

Carbohydrate metabolism
  Increased glycogenolysis
  Increased glycolysis
  Inhibited gluconeogenesis
  Lactic acidosis
  Hypoglycemia
  Increased HMP flux
  Decreased citric acid cycling

Fat metabolism
  Increased lipolysis
  Increased serum fatty acid levels
  Increased serum glycerol levels
  Increased VLDL levels

Protein metabolism
  Increased proteolysis
  Increased branched chain amino acid levels
  Increased alaninemia
  Decreased protein biosynthesis

Oxygen metabolism
  Increased oxygen extraction

Energy metabolism
  Decreased ATP levels
  Increased AMP and ADP levels

substrates including lipolysis and proteolysis, (4) membrane dysfunction. In later stages, similar metabolic alterations occur in the visceral cells leading to functional failure, inadequate metabolism for energy requirements, and finally the multisystem failure syndrome.[3]

ANAEROBIC METABOLISM

Lactate from muscle, gastrointestinal tract, and skin should become the precursor of glucose in the gluconeogenic pathway, but in the hypodynamic phase of septic shock gluconeogenesis is inhibited and lactic acid cannot be metabolized. Consequently, lactic acid remains high in the cell and in the serum, compounding the metabolic acidosis. This acidosis has a significant effect on enzyme function and inhibits gluconeogenesis and membrane function. In hypoxemia, increased flux through the glycolytic cycle is the only compensatory mechanism in the mammalian cell for increasing ATP production. Glycolysis is augmented, thus stimulating glyceraldehyde 3-phosphate dehydro-

genase (G3PD) to produce more reduced NADH. The latter then fuels the pyruvate to lactate reaction to regenerate oxidized nicotinamide adenine denucleotide (NAD), which cycles G3PD to the 1,3-biphosphoglycerate reaction. Thus 1 mole of glucose produces 2 moles of ATP rather than the 38 moles yielded by complete oxidation.

This marked ATP deficiency affects gluconeogenesis in liver and kidney because the synthetic activity of the glycolytic cycle requires energy. Additionally, glycolytic intermediates are being utilized for glycolysis.

Newer studies in our laboratory of septic shock in late peritonitis investigated the enzymes involved in the gluconeogenic inhibition at the rate-limiting steps (Apantaku et al., 1982, unpublished findings). Glucose-6-phosphatase (G6Pase), fructose diphosphatase (FDPase), phosphofructokinase (PFKase), and pyruvate kinase (PKase) in mitochondria-free supernatates from rat liver homogenates were assayed at optimal substrate levels at pH 7.4. There was a significant increase for PKase-specific activity consistent with stimulated glycolysis. Thus the metabolic lesion of septic shock is not caused by major alterations in enzyme properties, but rather by acid pH, and deficiencies in substrates and energy. This is an important finding because it negates molecular irreversibility as a concept in shock, and may permit restoration of metabolic function by hormones and substrates even in the terminal stages of sepsis.

Comparison studies[45] using both endotoxic and peritonitis septic shock models showed similar gluconeogenic inhibitions in both models, thereby suggesting a common causative agent. Since there was no profound blood pressure depression when gluconeogenic inhibition was present, this would indicate that endotoxemia is the effector of the metabolic injury in the septic and endotoxemic liver. We interpreted these similarities as an indication that endotoxemia was producing an insulin-like membrane effect on adenylcyclase increasing glycolysis and causing ATP and substrate depletion, as reported by Filkins.[7] Gluconeogenic inhibition was described by Wilmore et al.[43] in burned patients with gram-negative sepsis, and by Miller et al.[25] in preterminal patients with severe bacterial sepsis.

A new aspect in the glycolytic and gluconeogenic metabolic balance is the discovery of a new activator of rat liver phosphofructokinase, fructose-2,6-biphosphate. Addition of glucagon to hepatocytes caused a decreased in the level of this effector. Pilkis et al.[28] reported that this sugar biphosphate is more potent than fructose-1,6-biphosphate in activating liver enzyme. Since many of the effectors of phosphofructokinase also affect the activity of fructose-1,6-biphosphatase in a reciprocal manner, they tested fructose-2,6-biphosphate for its ability to modulate fructose-1,6-biphosphatase activity. They found fructose-1,6-biphosphate to be a potent inhibitor of fructose-1,6-biphosphatase. Siegel et al.[37] reported that in the hyperdynamic state of sepsis, glucagon release significantly increases, thus inducing gluconeogenesis early in the septic process. However, the insulin-like action of endotoxemia suppresses fructose-2,6-biphosphate, induces glycolysis, and probably produces the energy deficiency of sepsis.

CATABOLISM OF SUBSTRATES INCLUDING LIPOLYSIS AND PROTEOLYSIS

Peripheral cells compensate for decreases in substrates by metabolizing alternate precursors, glycerol, and fatty acids through lipolysis, amino acids such as alanine through gluconeogenesis, and branched chain amino acids for muscle metabolism.

Fat Metabolism. Spitzer et al.[38] studied metabolic and hormonal alterations in adipocytes isolated from septic shock. They found that lipolysis in septic shock is induced by the release of epinephrine, norepinephrine, adrenocorticotropin, thyrotropin, and vasopressin, all of which are released in the hypodynamic state of septic shock. These hormones function through the adenylate cyclase system. Filkins[6] reported that endotoxin alone stimulates adenylate cyclase and increases the oxidation of glucose to carbon dioxide via the hexose monophosphate shunt (HMP) shunt. Our rat liver studies by Kuttner et al.[18] showed that intravenous *E. coli* endotoxin raised glucose-6-phosphate dehydrogenase (G6PDH) activity by 49

percent. There was a significant (36 percent) acceleration in 6-phosphogluconate (6PG) consumption during endotoxemia. The cofactor, NADP, decreased significantly by 18 percent during endotoxemia. We attributed this NADP consumption to the accelerated lipogenic reaction, since lipogenesis needs more NADPH when accelerated.

This concept was further supported by Wannemacher et al.[42] who showed in rats infected with *Streptococcus pneumoniae* and live virus vaccine strain of *Francisella tularensis* that the percentage of glucose passing into the HMP shut rises from 20 to 24 percent to 46 to 49 percent at 24 hours. One function of the HMP shunt is to generate NADPH so that lipogenesis and fatty acid synthesis can be supported by the increase in NADPH. Incidentally, there is a possibility of transforming NADPH to NADH via flavin adenine dinucleotide for electron ion transport production of ATP, but again this reaction probably does not function without the oxygen acceptor.

Glycerol and fatty acids released during hypodynamic septic shock are utilized for gluconeogenesis and glycolysis, respectively. Glycerol is converted to glycerol-3-phosphate, then to 3-phosphoglycerate, and finally to glucose via the gluconeogenic pathway. Fatty acids that are oxidized are converted to acyl CoA, then to acetyl CoA, and cycled through the citric acid cycle for ATP production if oxygen is present. Again, because of absence of the oxygen receptor the aerobic oxidation of fatty acids to produce ATP is markedly limited. This yields an inhibition in the utilization of acyl glycerol and of free fatty acids, resulting in a deposition of fats in the viscera and a marked lipemia. Wolfe et al.[46] reported that some of the increased flux of FFA in the liver is incorporated in very low density lipoproteins and then released into the plasma. This elevated FFA level exerts a dampening effect on factors stimulating gluconeogenesis.

Protein Metabolism. Proteolysis in skeletal muscle occurs because there is a need for branched chain amino acids. Leucine, isoleucine, and valine, which are ketogenic, are metabolized by muscle, kidney, and liver cells. Alanine is utilized by the liver and kidney for gluconeogenesis. With inhibition of gluconeogenesis, proteolysis of the periphery becomes a futile Cori cycle. Amino acids, alanine, branched chain amino acids, fatty acids, and lactate are increased in concentration in the serum compounding the metabolic acidosis of shock.

MEMBRANE DYSFUNCTION

The metabolic changes, outlined in Table 4-2, produce derangement of membrane function. The cell membranes are composed of bipolar lipoprotein with protein receptor enzyme interspersed. These membranes, through these receptors, control the function of the cells by acting as barriers with selective permeability. The selective permeability is provided by gates and pumps as well as specific receptors for enzymes, substrates, and hormonal signals. The different techniques for transport across membranes are: (1) diffusion in which no metabolic energy is required, and (2) active transport where molecules are transported against electrochemical gradients by energy input. Thirty to forty percent of all ATP as energy is utilized by a resting patient to maintain equilibrium of water, cation, and anion electrolytes and proteins. There is an increase in energy expenditure in the septic state equal to 7 percent for each degree of temperature over normal.

In the hypodynamic state when a marked energy deficit occurs, the membranes leak fluid and sodium intracellularly, and there is a leak of potassium extracellularly because the Na/K ATPase enzyme is depleted of high-energy substrates. Shires et al.[36] proved this membrane dysfunction in studies using electrodes to measure membrane changes evolving in late hemorrhagic shock. The membrane dysfunction affects protein biosynthesis, phagocytosis, pinocytosis in absorption (digestion), and nerve impulse transmission. This depressed membrane activity is an important component of the sequential changes called multisystem failure. Study of the changes that produce membrane alterations is necessary to describe the syndrome of multisystem failure.

Sepsis or septic shock is a subcellular molecular disease. To learn what happens to the cell will contribute to treating the whole patient in a rational and effective manner.

REFERENCES

1. Balis JU, Paterson JF, Shelley SA et al: Glucorticoid and antibiotic effects on hepatic microcirculation and associated host responses in lethal gram-negative bacteremia. Lab Invest 40: 55, 1979
2. Barzilai AH, Schiessel R, Kivilaakso E, Silen W: Ulceration of rabbit antral mucosa. Surg Forum 30:9, 1979
3. Baue AE: The energy crisis in surgical patients. Arch Surg 109: 349, 1974
4. Chaudry, IH, Wichterman KA, Baue AE: Effect of sepsis on tissue adenine nucleotide levels. Surgery 85: 205, 1979
5. Clowes GHA Jr: Pulmonary abnormalities in sepsis. Surg Clin North Am 54:993, 1974
6. Filkins JP: Adrenergic blockade and glucoregulation in endotoxin shock. Circ Shock 6: 99, 1979
7. Filkins JP: Role of the RES in the pathogenesis of endotoxic hypoglycemia. Circ Shock 9: 269, 1982
8. Gimpel J, Hodgins DS, Jacobson ED: Effect of endotoxin on hepatic adenylate cyclase activity. Circ Shock 1: 31, 1974
9. Green HD, Bond RF, Rapela CE et al: Competition between intrinsic and extrinsic controls of resistance vessels of major vascular beds during hemorrhagic hypotension and shock. p. 77. In Lefer AM, Saba TM, Mela LM (eds): Advances in Shock Research, Vol 3. Alan R Liss, New York, 1980
10. Greenfield LJ: Surfactant in surgery. Surg Clin North Am 54:979, 1974
11. Hirsch EF, Fletcher JR, Lucas S: Hypotension and lacticacidemia in sepsis following combat trauma. J Trauma 12: 45, 1972
12. Holtzman SF: Metabolism in Endotoxic Shock and its Modification by Dexamethasone. University of Illinois College of Medicine, Chicago, unpublished doctoral dissertation, 1976
13. Holtzman S, Erve PR, Schuler JJ et al: Glucocorticoid effect on hepatic carbohydrate metabolism during endotoxemia. Surg Forum 25:354, 1974
14. Holtzman S, Schuler JJ, Earnest W et al: Carbohydrate metabolism in endotoxemia. Circ Shock 1:99, 1974
15. Katz J, Wals PA, Rognstad R: Glucose phosphorylation, glucose-6-phosphatase, and recycling in rat hepatocytes. J Biol Chem 4530, 1978
16. Kuttner RE, Apantaku FO, Schumer W: Glucocorticoid effect on glycolytic intermediates in septic rat heart. p. 103. In Lefer AM (ed): Advances in Shock Research, Vol. 5. Alan R Liss, New York, 1981
17. Kuttner RE, Holtzman SF, Schumer W: A time

study of hepatic glycolytic intermediates in endo-toxemic and septic rats and mice. p. 73. In Schumer W, Spitzer JJ, Marshall BE (eds): Advances in Shock Research, Vol 4. Alan R Liss, New York, 1980

18. Kuttner RE, Schumer W, Apantaku FO: Effect of endotoxin and glucocorticoid pretreatment on hexose monophosphate shunt activity in rat liver. Circ Shock 9: 37, 1982

19. Lefer AM, Barenholz Y: Pancreatic hydrolases and the formation of a myocardial depressant factor in shock. Am J Physiol 233: 1103, 1972

20. Lindbergh B, Haljamae H, Jonsson O, Pettersson S: Effect of glucagon and blood transfusion on liver metabolism in hemorrhagic shock. Ann Surg, 187:103, 1978

21. Maitra PK, Estabrook RW: A fluorimetric method for the enzymatic determination of glycolytic intermediates. Anal Biochem 7:472, 1964

22. Mela L: Mitochondrial metabolic alterations in experimental circulatory shock. p. 288. In Urbaschek B, Urbaschek R, Neter E (eds): Gram-Negative Bacterial Infections and Mode of Endotoxin Actions. Pathophysiological, Immunological, and Clinical Aspects. Springer-Verlag, New York, 1975

23. Mela L, Bacalzo LV, Jr., Miller LD: Defective oxidative metabolism of rat liver mitochondria in hemorrhagic and endotoxin shock. Am J Physiol 220: 571, 1971

24. Mela LM, Miller LD, Diaco JF, Sugerman HJ: Effect of *E. coli* endotoxin on mitochondrial energy-linked functions. Surgery 68: 541, 1970

25. Miller SI, Wallace RJ, Jr., Musher DM, et al: Hypoglycemia as a manifestation of sepsis. Am J Med 68: 649, 1980

26. Nagler AL, Seifter E, Levenson SM: Prevention of shock by glucose-phosphate therapy. Circ Shock (Abstr 51) 5:212, 1978

27. Papermaster-Bender G, Whitcomb ME, Sagone AL, Jr.: Characterization of the metabolic responses of the human pulmonary alveolar macrophage. J Reticuloendothel Soc 28:129, 1980

28. Pilkis SJ, El-Haghrabi MR, Pilkis J, et al: Fructose 2,6-biphosphate. A new activator of phosphofructokinase. J Biol Chem 256:3171, 1981

29. Raymond RM, Harkema JM, Emerson TE, Jr.: Direct effects of gram-negative endotoxin on skeletal muscle glucose uptake. J Physiol 240: H342, 1981

30. Rush BF, Jr.: Irreversibility in the post-transfusion phase of hemorrhagic shock. p. 215. In Hinshaw LB, Cox BG (eds): Advances in Experimental Medicine and Biology, Vol 23, The Fundamental Mechanisms of Shock. Plenum Press, New York, 1972

31. Sato T, Kamiyama Y, Jones RT, et al: Ultrastruc-

tural study on kidney cell injury following various types of shock in 26 immediate autopsy patients. p. 55. In Lefer AM, Saba TM, Mela LM (eds): Advances in Shock Research, Vol 1. Alan R Liss, New York, 1979

32. Schumer W: Lactate studies of the dog in oligemic shock. J Surg Res 8:491, 1968

33. Schumer W, Erve PR: Cellular metabolism in shock. Circ Shock 2: 109, 1975

34. Scrutton MC, Utter MF: The regulation of glycolysis gluconeogenesis in animal tissues. Annu Rev Biochem 37:249, 1968

35. Sharma C, Liu MS: Effect of endotoxin on the level of key rate limiting enzymes in glycolysis in the liver of normal and alloxan diabetic dogs. Circ Shock (Abstr 75) 5:227, 1978

36. Shires GT, Cunningham JN, Baker CRF, et al: Alterations in cellular membrane function during hemorrhagic shock in primates. Ann Surg 176:288, 1972

37. Siegel JH, Cerra FB, Border JR, et al: Human response to sepsis: a physiologic manifestation of disordered metabolic control. p. 235. In Cowley RA, Trump BE (eds): Pathophysiology of Shock, Anoxia, and Ischemia. Williams and Wilkins, Baltimore, 1982

38. Spitzer JA, Leach GJ, Palmer MA: Some metabolic and hormonal alterations in adipocytes isolated from septic dogs. p. 55. In Schumer W, Spitzer JJ, Marshall BE (eds): Advances in Shock Research, Vol 4. Alan R Liss, New York, 1980

39. Tanaka J, Sato T, Jones RT, et al: Aspects of high-energy metabolism in rat liver following *E. coli* bacteremia. Circ Shock 7:207, 1980

40. Vary T, Siegel JH, Nakatani T, et al: Effect of sepsis on activity of pyruvate dehydrogenase complex in skeletal muscle and liver. Am J Physiol 250: E634, 1986

41. Vary TC, Siegel JH, Nakatani T, et al: Control of pyruvate dehydrogenase complex activity in sepsis. Fed Proc (Abstr 7730) 44:1733, 1985

42. Wannemacher RW, Jr., Beall FA, Canonico PG, et al: Glucose and alanine metabolism during bacterial infections in rats and rhesus monkeys. Metabolism 29:201, 1980

43. Wilmore DW, Mason AD, Jr., Pruitt BA, Jr.: Impaired glucose flow in burned patients with gram-negative sepsis. Surg Gynecol Obst 143: 720, 1976

44. Williamson JR, Refino C, LaNoue K: Effects of *E. coli* lipopolysaccharide B treatment of rats on gluconeogenesis. p. 145. In Porter R, Knight J (eds): Energy Metabolism in Trauma. A Ciba Symposium. J. and A. Churchill, London, 1970

45. Wilson JW: The pulmonary cellular and subcellular alterations of extracorporeal circulation. Surg Clin North Am 54:1203, 1974

46. Wolfe RR, Shaw JHF, Durkot MJ: Energy metabo-

lism in trauma and sepsis: the role of fat. p. 89. In Lefer AM, Schumer W (eds): Molecular and Cellular Aspects of Shock and Trauma. Progress in Clinical and Biological Research, Vol. 111. Alan R Liss, New York, 1983

47. Yates AJP, Schumer W, Holtzman SF, Kuttner RE: Endotoxin role in peritonitis septic shock in rats. p. 63. In Schumer W, Spitzer JJ, Marshall BE (eds): Advances in Shock Research, Vol 4. Alan R Liss, New York, 1980

5

Statistical Treatment of Clinical Data

Bill Coleman
John H. Siegel

INTRODUCTION

Statistical treatment is now *de rigueur* in the health sciences. The presence of P values certifies an investigator's work as scientific, and one would no more appear in print without a P value than at a formal function without a black tie. Whether this treatment is applied wisely, or even with common sense, is an entirely different question.

As it happens, there is a theoretical rationale underlying the use of statistics. This rationale can be explained clearly, although working it out in practice takes more persistence in following mathematical derivations than many scientists are willing to use. Understanding the rationale will help the reader of a scientific paper to assess whether the data therein advanced actually support the conclusions reached and to assess the extent of the clinical situations to which the conclusions apply.

The object of this chapter is to explain the rationale of statistics, and to do this with as little mathematics and as many medical illustrations as possible. We will be explaining a system of concepts. The reader is invited to see these concepts as a system: they can be applied in combination to analyze clinical data. Various combinations can be employed according to the purpose at hand. Alternative systems are possible. (The textbook of DeGroot[9] is particularly strong in conveying the sense that the possibilities are numerous and should be selected thoughtfully.)

The general situation requiring statistical treatment is one to which we come naturally. We wish to compare the effects of treatments or of diseases by observing selected patients. Having done so we can never be entirely sure whether the effects we observe in these patients are characteristic of the treatment or disease itself or are perhaps merely due to peculiarities of the particular patients observed.

The *simplest* of these situations[3,9,11] is that in which we wish to compare a continuous measurement (say, oxygen consumption) between two groups (say, septic and nonseptic patients). This chapter will begin with an example of this kind, followed by an extended discussion of the concepts involved in analyzing this example. A variation of this situation[6,8] is when the measurement is discrete; it has a small number (perhaps only two) of possible outcomes. For example, we might want to find out if the use of a certain treatment is related to a decrease in mortality or to an increase in toxicity. *More complicated* are those situations[4,17] in which we wish to relate two variables measured in a group or even to compare such a relationship across two groups. We might want to find out if the level of circulating leucine is related to the amount of leucine administered parenterally, or if the white blood count is a certain function of time following trauma. What complicates these latter situations is that there are two levels of analysis: we have to decide on an appropriate form for the mathematical relationship between the variables before we can proceed to the purely statistical question of applying the properties observed in our sample of patients to a general population of future patients. The later parts of this chapter will be concerned with analyzing relationships.

AN EXAMPLE

A group of investigators studying the effect of lipid infusion as part of parenteral nutrition in intensive care unit (ICU) patients recently published[16] data, shown in Table 5-1, on oxygen consumption ($\dot{V}O_2$), carbon dioxide production ($\dot{V}CO_2$), and respiratory quotient (RQ).

Respiratory quotient is defined to be the ratio of $\dot{V}CO_2$ to $\dot{V}O_2$. By stoichiometry, the burning of different metabolic fuels involves different ratios of carbon dioxide produced to oxygen consumed. Therefore RQ is a function of the type of fuel utilized and its value gives information about the patient's metabolism.

The authors of this study compare septic to nonseptic patients and find that, on the average, septics had higher $\dot{V}O_2$ (144 versus 133) and lower $\dot{V}CO_2$ (126 versus 129), both of these facts tending to give lower RQ (0.87 versus 0.98). These authors then elaborately analyze their data to determine the relative contributions of $\dot{V}CO_2$ and $\dot{V}O_2$ to the difference in RQ, under conditions of lipid infusion and no lipid infusion, and finally come to speculate on the differences in metabolism likely to give rise to these data.

Table 5-1 supports an early phase of this argument. The authors conclude, on the basis of the ±'s, [a]'s, and P values with which they have decorated their table, that the difference in RQ between septic and nonseptic is genuine and is accounted for by a genuine difference in $\dot{V}O_2$, while the data do not necessarily indicate a genuine difference in $\dot{V}CO_2$. It is with the process of thought leading to these conclusions that we shall be concerned in the first part of this chapter. How and in what sense does statistical inference allow one to conclude that observed differences are genuine or, as such people importantly say, "significant?"

The answer to this question can be stated briefly, and we shall do so in the following paragraphs. Packed into the answer are many assumptions. Unpacking these assumptions will occupy us for the next section of the chapter.

Surgical ICU patients of the type studied by the authors of the lipid metabolism paper display a variety of values of $\dot{V}O_2$, $\dot{V}CO_2$, and

TABLE 5-1.   Metabolic Gas Exchange

Group	N	$\dot{V}O_2$(ml/min/m²)	$\dot{V}CO_2$(ml/min/m²)	RQ
Nonseptic	128	133 ± 27	129 ± 28	0.98 ± 0.12
		0.0001[a]	NS[a]	0.0001[a]
Septic	246	144 ± 19	126 ± 19	0.87 ± 0.10

[a] P values for Student's t-test of differences between means.
(Nanni G, Siegel JH, Coleman B et al: Increased lipid fuel dependence in the critically ill septic patient. J Trauma 24(1):14, © 1984 The Williams & Wilkins Co., Baltimore.)

RQ, as one would find on selecting several such patients at random. Indeed, the authors' notation "± ____" is an attempt to show us the range of variability that they found in their patients. Thus, although the *average* value of $\dot{V}O_2$ in the nonseptic group was 133 ml/min/m², the patients typically differed from this by 27 ml/min/m²; this typical difference is the *standard deviation*. Since there is this inherent variability in the patient population, the mean values observed by the authors in their sample are likely to be different from the mean values of the population as a whole.

The point of statistical inference is to give a quantitative evaluation of the degree to which we can believe in conclusions that are drawn from measurements having random uncertainty. There are several theories of how this can be done.[9]

The classical theory (or *sampling theory*) emphasizes the question of whether patient groups observed to be different are actually different. Is the higher $\dot{V}O_2$ observed in the septic sample a result of a difference in physiology or is it a result merely of the chance properties of that particular selection of patients? In the case of $\dot{V}O_2$, the difference in means (144 − 133 = 11) is small compared to the standard deviation (19 and 27) of either group. On the other hand, this difference appears in a large pool of cases (246 and 128 patient studies). For $\dot{V}CO_2$ the difference in means is even smaller: 126 − 129 = −3. Are either of these differences large enough to indicate more than random variability?

Is there some general way that we can assess quantitatively the strength of the evidence for an apparent difference between two groups? One way would be to determine the probability of having selected samples displaying a difference as large as (or larger than) the difference observed in our samples, computing this probability on the assumption that there really is no difference in the population at large. If the difference in our samples is very great, it will be hard to explain on the assumption that they come from a population in which there is no difference: the probability thereby assigned to samples like ours would be low. In other words, to the degree to which the observed result of the experiment (drawing the samples) is hard to explain on the basis of the theory that there is really no difference, we are compelled to abandon the theory.

In a nutshell, the *P value* is the probability assigned to reality by the theory (the *null hypothesis*) that there is no difference between groups. If this probability is low then it is hard to believe the theory. We say that the difference is *significant*.

In our example, the probabilities in question are given mathematically by *Student's t-distribution*. Using the data given in Table 5-1, the authors have calculated a number, the *t-statistic*, which they have then compared to tables of the t-distribution. On this basis they are telling us that if there really were no difference in $\dot{V}O_2$ between septic and nonseptic patients, then samples as divergent as theirs would have a probability of less than 0.0001 (1 in 10,000). This result makes it uncomfortable to believe that there is no difference. In comparison, for $\dot{V}CO_2$ they report that their result is "not significant" (NS). This means that the corresponding probability is greater than 0.05 (1 in 20) so that one does not feel especially compelled to believe that $\dot{V}CO_2$ is different between septic and nonseptic patients.

OBSERVATIONS CONCERNING THIS EXAMPLE

Randomness

Scientists (and physicians) have been making observations and drawing conclusions from them for some thousands of years. The modern science of statistics is concerned with drawing conclusions about populations on the basis of random samples. Statistical treatment is one method among many available to medical research. For it to be the method of choice in a particular problem, the laws of probability must be usable and then must be used correctly: certain conditions must be met.

THE LARGER POPULATION

There must be a larger population to which the conclusions are to be applied. A group of researchers[20] studied the effect on ICU mortality of a new teaching service organization that uses a computer-based physiologic assessment system. Part of their results are presented in Table 5-2. The authors compare mortality rates in several categories for the period 1973 to 1975 to the corresponding rates in 1976 to 1978. The data show decreased mortality in each group for the later period compared to the earlier one. The authors wish to attribute this decrease to increasing effectiveness of their computer-based ICU service. As part of their argument they perform a statistical test, called "Fisher's Exact Test,"[8] and find $P = 0.0017$ in the combined group. From this they expect us to conclude that the decreased mortality they observed would hold in general, not just in their ICU but in any ICU. We will return several times in the course of this chapter to how compelling this conclusion really is; for the moment we merely record that, validly or not, this is what the authors expect us to conclude.

As another part of their argument, these authors have to show that the decrease in mortality is not due merely to decreased severity in the cases that they see. In connection with this, one might note that the percentage of multiple trauma is slightly less: 71 of 115 (61.7 percent) in the early time period compared to 46 of 80 (57.5 percent) in the later time period. The authors offer no statistical test for this. Why? Because, it would make no sense. What larger population would be referred to? If the difference were significant, would one con-clude that any ICU using their teaching service would see fewer cases of multiple trauma?

Statistical significance does not certify that a result is important, or that it is scientific, or even that it is true; rather, it certifies that the result can be extrapolated to the larger population of which the sample is a sample. If there is no question of extrapolating to a larger population then it is ridiculous to append a P value to a result, even if that result is true.

There is a philosophical controversy concerning the meaning of probability. It is easiest to explain probability in terms of a fixed finite population. For example, in a political poll there is a fixed total population of persons eligible to vote in an election; the poll attempts to determine the number voting for each candidate, on the basis of a random sample of the whole. Medical research is usually not similarly concerned with the total population of actual cases of a certain kind, but more with the potential population of such cases. Rather than imagining that there is a fixed total population, one imagines that there is a fixed physiologic mechanism generating similar patients in response to a set of conditions. We are sampling this potential population with a view towards discovering the nature of the physiologic mechanism governing it. *In this larger sense we can take the population to be that generated by some fixed and clearly defined set of physiologic or therapeutic conditions.*

Thus in the earlier example the authors of the lipid infusion paper wish us to conclude that there is something inherent in the physiology of sepsis that makes septic patients have higher $\dot{V}O_2$, on the average, than nonseptic patients, and this assertion, whether true or not,

TABLE 5-2.   Changes in ICU Mortality

Surgery	1973–1975			1976–1978			P^a
	Total	Deaths	% Deaths	Total	Deaths	% Deaths	
No head injury							
Trauma	115	18	15.7	80	6	7.5	NS
Multiple trauma	71	12	16.9	46	4	8.7	NS
Gunshot	28	5	17.9	18	0	0	NS
All trauma	144	31	21.5	121	9	7.4	0.0017

a Fisher's Exact Test.

(Siegel JH, Cerra FB, Moody EA et al: The effect on survival of and injured patients of an ICU teaching service organized about a computer-based physiologic CARE system. 20(7):558, © 1980 The Williams & Wilkins Co., Baltimore.)

TABLE 5-3. Nutritional Support

	All Patients			Patients with Lipids		
	N	$N_2/m^2/day$	$Gcal/m^2/day$	N	$Lcal/m^2/day$	Total $cal/m^2/day$
Septic[a]	246	4.3 ± 1.9	514 ± 236	114	205 ± 93	873 ± 238
Nonseptic	128	4.6 ± 1.8	551 ± 313	34	162 ± 87	869 ± 234

[a] All differences not significant between septic and nonseptic patients.
(Nanni G. Siegel JH, Coleman B et al: Increased lipid fuel dependence in the critically ill septic patient. J Trauma 24(1):14, ©1984 The Williams & Wilkins Co., Baltimore.)

makes sense within the framework of statistical inference; it is the kind of assertion that statistical inference is designed to test.

Some uses of statistics are more puzzling. The data in Table 5-3, also extracted from the lipid infusion paper, show the differences in nutritional support between the septic and nonseptic patients. Precisely what hypothesis was it that the authors tested and are reporting that they failed to find significant? Was it the hypothesis that there is some physiologic mechanism inherent in sepsis and some pedagogic mechanism inherent in modern American medical education, mechanisms that generate patients and physicians in such a way that when a septic patient presents himself the house staff will administer a certain nutritional regimen? No. Obviously, the authors were trying to demonstrate that the results in RQ previously described were not due to some undetected difference in the quantity or quality of nutritional support. However, for this analysis the entire population was that contained within their study, so the simple description of the administered levels, without any statistical test, would have been sufficient to prove this fact. Apparently, even sophisticated authors like these feel so compelled by peer pressure to "validate" their data with statistical tests that they do not always pause to consider whether the tests mean anything.

THE SAMPLE MUST BE CHOSEN RANDOMLY

As our discussion has emphasized, the use of statistics hinges on calculating the probabilities that certain samples might be randomly drawn from populations. If the sample is drawn by any mechanism other than pure random selection, statistical inference does not apply. Although it is possible to reason validity from data not drawn randomly, it is not possible to do so using statistics. Attempts to use statistics on nonrandom data invite results of the "Dewey Defeats Truman" type.

Let us look again at the ICU mortality data shown in Table 5-2. Since there is no way of having physicians selectively not use their training, the only practical means at the authors' disposal for studying the effects of the training program is to compare the early years to the later years. But there is a general problem with the use of historical controls to assess a subsequent therapy. The selection of patients is hardly random since, by definition, all of the control patients are early and all of the treatment patients are late: the patients in each group may have numerous common characteristics that distinguish them from patients in the other group and that have nothing to do with presence or absence of treatment. Although the authors assert that these other factors are irrelevant, it is difficult to be sure what the distinguishing factor between the groups is. In the published discussion following the printed article, the discussants are free to suggest several explanations of the decrease in mortality, explanations different from that given by the authors. Even though the effect in the combined trauma group is calculated to be significant to $P < 0.0017$, the laws of probability, on which this calculation is based, may not really apply. These authors recognize the difficulty and tend to moderate the assertiveness with which they press their conclusion: "These data suggest that . . .", "These data strongly suggest that . . .", "The statistical evidence presented strongly suggests, but does not prove, since no randomized prospective study was possible, that . . ." In this way the authors closely skirt the precipice of misrepresentation, only infrequently actually falling in: "This test indicates that it was indeed . . ."

Again, these authors really had no choice. The only obvious alternative (to compare their results to those from a similar ICU) is even less satisfactory. The authors simply have to hope that their sample is approximately random and then have to present their results as honestly as possible.

In a more general form, randomness of the sample is always a problem in medical studies. Most investigators have to select patients from their own institution; only a very fortunate investigator is able to select from sufficiently many institutions to avoid the suspicion that his or her results do not generalize.

TARGET POPULATION

The target population from which the sample is drawn must be appropriate. If an investigator were to draw conclusions about oxygen consumption in sepsis on the basis of a sample drawn from an institution treating trauma patients exclusively, or cardiac surgical patients exclusively, we would be entitled to wonder how these results apply to other types of septic patients. Not only must the sample be drawn randomly, but the investigator must also take care to design the sampled population to match the population of interest.

In practice this problem is usually more subtle than the example above illustrates. Suppose an investigator is studying the survival rate of patients receiving a new chemotherapy for cancer. This chemotherapy is complex and risky. After randomly assigning 50 patients to control and 50 patients to the new treatment, the investigator finds that 10 of the new treatment patients withdraw in the middle of the study. Of these 10, 7 have died, 1 is still alive, and 2 are lost to follow-up. A first reaction might be to discard the data from the 10 withdrawals on the grounds that these patients did not complete their therapy. To discard them implies that the population studied is the group of patients who would complete therapy, and any mortality estimates are to be applied to this group. However, the clinician reading the report has a different interest. Presented with a patient who appears suitable, the clinician wishes to know what are the chances that he can pull that patient through by beginning the

new therapy. If the patient dies after withdrawing because the therapy was too complicated, it is no consolation to know that his theoretical chances would have been better if he had completed the new therapy than if he had had standard therapy.

It requires considerable thought to design a study so that the results apply to a clinically realistic population. There must be a definite protocol indicating criteria for eligibility in the study, criteria that can be objectively applied. Reading these criteria is the only way to know what population the results apply to. Given these criteria, eligible patients must be selected totally at random and not by convenience. Designing the study involves balancing the practical and ethical conduct of the study against the desirability of having the most useful possible target population. There is a special source of bias in study samples in that patients and physicians may be able to subtly influence the outcome according to their preconceptions. This must be avoided by blinding the patient and physician from knowedge of which treatment is being used, where possible, or the results must be presented at a discounted rate where it is not.

The conduct of the study must be, in every way, as close as possible to the intended clinical application.

CAUSAL RELATIONSHIPS

Causal relationships can only be inferred by prospective randomization. Our discussion of Table 5-1 has thus far stressed the obvious interpretation that sepsis results in higher $\dot{V}O_2$. Other interpretations are perfectly possible a priori: that patients with higher $\dot{V}O_2$ have a metabolic inadequacy predisposing them to sepsis, or again that there is some third condition (perhaps decreased immunocompetence) leading to sepsis and independently complicated by increased $\dot{V}O_2$. These subtleties multiply if we distinguish between the oxygen delivery and oxygen extraction components of $\dot{V}O_2$. And so on.

The application of statistics by itself does nothing to decide between the merits of these interpretations. The fact that $P < 0.0001$ only assures us that if we similarly examined a similar group of patients after the fact we would similarly observe higher $\dot{V}O_2$ in the septic group. We are not enlightened as to the mechanism bringing about this result.

If we have some causal theory, for example, that prophylactic manipulation of $\dot{V}O_2$ prevents sepsis, then the only way to establish it directly is to assign patients randomly to two groups, in one of which we prospectively intervene to produce the alleged cause and then see whether doing so also produces the alleged result. If we believed, on the contrary, that sepsis results in increased $\dot{V}O_2$, we would prove this by making one group septic, in the natural way, and seeing if $\dot{V}O_2$ becomes increased.

This last suggestion is outrageous (in a number of ways), but is meant to remind us of a hard reality of clinical research: so few interventions are ethical and feasible that opportunities for directly establishing causal relationships are limited and progress is tedious.

ETHICAL DESIGN OF STUDIES

We have just observed that the only way to establish conclusively the superiority of one treatment over another is to randomize a group of patients, some to one treatment and some to the other. Since the premise of the study is that one treatment may well be superior, an ethical conflict arises between the investigator's (and society's) need to find out the result and the study patient's right to the best treatment. There seems to be a consensus that the patient's right is inviolable and that the needs of the study are secondary. Our discussion is based on this assumption.

To protect this right of the patient the investigator is required to secure informed consent from the patient or the patient's family. It is customary to maintain that there is no reason to prefer one treatment to the other unless there is positive scientific proof to the contrary, that is, until the results of the study are in. Although customary, this attitude seems to us often to be disingenuous at best and dishonest at worst.

When a patient consults a physician in the normal course of events (whether the physician is conducting a study or not), the patient has no expectation that the physician is operating strictly on the basis of rigorous scientific *proof* and containing the range of alternatives accordingly. Rather, the patient assumes that the physician will use educated *judgment* to prescribe that treatment most likely to be beneficial, whether completely proven or not. (We are not here addressing the question of possible toxic side effects.)

In the special case where the physician is conducting a study, the investigator must be able to assure the patient that participation in the study will give him a better chance than nonparticipation, and, in fact, that the design of the study gives the patient the best possible such chance.

Although there may not be strict scientific proof of the merits of a new treatment, it is often possible to make a shrewd guess. Often a physician learns of a new treatment that appears to give greatly improved results, but in uncontrolled experiments. As a scientist, he wishes to try it at his institution, but encounters some (perhaps justified) resistance from fellow staff members (perhaps including himself) to abandoning an old method. So the staff reasonably agree on a controlled trial. Thus there is as yet nothing resembling scientific proof. Still, the likely possibilities are either that the new treatment is a chimaera or that it is substantially better. Always assigning 50 percent of the study patients to each group is not appropriate. What is needed is a flexible method that will assign the fewest possible patients to the bad treatment, if one treatment is indeed worse. Such a plan would best satisfy our conscience as attending physicians.

An example of such a flexible method is the play-the-winner rule of Zelen.[23] In its original form it applies to studies in which there are two treatments, A and B, to be compared and in which the outcome is known soon after treatment is begun. The first patient is assigned randomly to A or B, say to A. If A succeeds then the second patient is also assigned to A; if not, then B is given a turn, until it eventually fails and we return to A. This method assigns patients randomly, since each patient's assignment depends on the random outcome of the previous patient's trial and, indirectly, on those of all the preceding patients. Yet, in the long run more patients will be assigned to the preferable treatment.

This method was recently modified by Cornell and Bartlett[7] and used by them in a clinical study[2] of extracorporeal membrane oxygenation in infants. Their modification is to make each patient's assignment depend not deterministically but only probabilistically on the preceding study. This is important in a single-center study since otherwise the attending physicians know which treatment their patient will be assigned to before entering the patient in the study, a potential source of serious bias since the physician may either promote or discourage entry of the patient, depending on the treatment expected. Another important purpose of the modification is that it allows assignment to depend on however many studies happen to have a known result. Thus one does not need to know the result of the immediately preceding study. The procedure can be visualized by imagining that we start with some number, say 20, of slips of paper, half labeled "A" and half labeled "B." We put these in a hat and, drawing one at random, assign the first patient accordingly. Later, perhaps after several other patients have been similarly entered, the first patient's result becomes known. If the treatment succeeds, we replace the slip of paper in the hat; if not, we replace instead a slip designating the alternative treatment. Eventually, as the proportion of slips changes, the better treatment becomes more probable, how soon depending on the initial number of slips of paper.

This method is valid, but can have results that seem paradoxical. In Bartlett and Cornell's study only one subject was picked for the control treatment; all the rest were assigned to the experimental treatment. Nonetheless, with a sufficient number of total subjects, the random error of estimation is small enough to permit statistically valid conclusions to be drawn. At the same time, this method permitted only one patient, instead of half of the sample, to be relegated to the conventional treatment. Since the one patient on conventional treatment died while all 19 patients on the new treatment survived, the benefit of play-the-winner, compared to equal allocation, to this group of infants and their parents is obvious!

Play-the-winner is not the only such way to design a study, and even within its frame-work variations are possible. The most obvious variation is to change the number of slips of paper in the hat at the beginning; if there are more slips, then each outcome has less effect, and the allocation will be more equal. These choices do not affect the expected scientific outcome of the study, only the allocation of patients within it. One would wonder if there were not an "optimal" design. Unfortunately, it is difficult to clarify this idea of optimality, first because there are several features that one wants to optimize and that conflict with each other, and second because there is no easy way to fit these features into an unambiguous quantitative framework. For a given pair of treatments, unequal allocation will usually increase the combined sample size, putting a larger pool of subjects at risk and also delaying publication of the results and the benefit to the population at large. In some studies limitations of resources may prohibit very large samples.

Work needs to be done to clarify these issues and design intelligible ways of assessing the risks, costs, and benefits involved in the particular circumstances of each study. For the moment, we believe that for any study to be undertaken in which there is a clear risk to the patient and whose authors do not make some reasonable attempt to meet these considerations is simply unacceptable.

Significance

We now begin a second series of observations about our example. As the previous series centered around the conditions implied by the assumption of randomness, this series deals with the meaning of the term "significance."

"SIGNIFICANT" DOES NOT MEAN "IMPORTANT"

The authors of the ICU study go on to report that for all noncardiac surgical patients, they observed 211 deaths out of 1,344 cases (15.7 percent mortality) from 1973 to 1975 compared to 168 deaths out of 1,515 cases (11.1 percent) from 1976 to 1978, and that this difference was significant to $P = 0.00032$ by Fisher's

Exact Test. A reader, musing on the relation of this result to those presented above in our Table 5-2, might come to wonder how it is that this reduction from 15.7 percent mortality to 11.1 percent in all patients is so highly significant while the much greater reduction from 15.7 percent to only 7.5 percent in the trauma group without head injury is not significant at all (although it might appear to be so to the patients involved). The answer, very simply, is that this is a typical artifact of statistical testing.

It is reasonable that a larger sample will tend to have less random error—that the law of averages will cancel out aberrant data. It is, then, accordingly reasonable that the decrease in mortality in the total patient group, while modest in size, is more deserving of our belief, being observed in a larger sample (about 15 times as large as the trauma group).

There are really three distinct concepts involved:

1. The magnitude of the estimated difference in effect, which for the all patient group is
15.7 − 11.1 percent = 4.6 percent
2. The P value, 0.00032, which quantifies indirectly the believability of this estimate
3. The application of the term "significant," implying that the P value is so low that it would be foolhardy not to believe in a difference.

There is no paradox as long as we realize that the significance attaches to the believability, not to the magnitude, and even less to the clinical importance, of the estimate.

In our mania to wrap everything up in a single number we have come to emphasize the P value and to lose sight of the estimated difference, although it is the estimated difference that reflects any possible clinical significance. We thus operate a public philanthropy for the unimaginative, who can be assured that if they merely persist in studying enough cases they will be guaranteed of finding significant results and, thereby, a readership.

Rather than the P value, it would be better to report a *confidence interval* for the difference between the groups. The confidence interval is the entire range of values that can be believed consistently with the data, in just the same sense as explained above for the P value. For the P value to be less than 0.05 is equivalent to having zero (i.e., no difference in effect) con-

tained in a statistically corresponding 95 percent confidence interval. By providing readers with the whole range of believable values, we allow them to see if there are values so small as to make the difference trivial, or so large as to make the difference important, or both (indicating that no useful conclusion can be drawn without a larger sample).

IMPROBABLE EVENTS OCCUR REGULARLY

Above, we explained the P value as the probability of randomly drawing samples that would make the difference between groups appear at least as large as in the present sample, assuming that there really were no difference. Suppose our regular practice is to accept that there is a difference whenever $P < 0.05$. Out of all samples coming from populations where there really is no difference, the laws of probability assure us that 5 percent will be aberrant enough to make us think falsely that there is. Thus another way to look at the P value is that it is the probability that we will make a mistake: that we will think there is a difference when there is none.

We tend to think that each time we run a risk, if that risk is only 1 in 20 (or 0.05), then the thing risked just will not happen. On the contrary, it will happen 5 percent of the time, in fact. If we consistently test at $P < 0.05$, we should confidently expect to be wrong 5 percent of the time. Thus, we should ask, in each case, whether this level of risk is bearable. Secondly, we should resist any procedures (such as the one about to be discussed) that have the effect of raising the real significance level above the nominal significance level.

With this in mind, we can see that always setting the risk level at 0.05, regardless of what it is we are risking, is foolish, although peer pressure appears to make it impossible to do anything else.

LESS IS MORE

Doing more statistical tests is not more scientific than doing fewer tests, or, as Mies van der Rohe more tersely (and appropriately) said, "Less is more!" The structure of the data in a clinical paper can easily be quite complex. For example, the authors of the lipid infusion paper studied several other variables besides those we have excerpted in Table 5-1, including respiration, metabolism, and blood gas values. On top of this, the groups they wished to compare were not just sepsis versus no sepsis but also lipid infusion versus no lipid infusion, and all the combinations of these two pairs. Also, they were compelled to test comparisons between different modes of ventilatory support.

One can appreciate that when there are many variables to be compared or many groups among which to compare them, many tests can be done. In light of our remarks above, one appreciates as well that random chance ensures that 5 percent of these tests will show $P < 0.05$ even if there are no differences in any variables between any groups. We commonly see tables of data elaborately decorated with symbols indicating precise P values for a multitude of tests. These should be viewed with grave suspicion and not as a demonstration of their (usually well-meaning) authors' thoroughness. This is another case where our instant acquiescence to having $P < 0.05$ provides an opportunity for the industrious investigator willing to expend enough computer time to do enough statistical tests on his data.

There are two approximate methods[3] for finding the overall P value when several tests are done. Suppose, for concreteness, that we have decided ahead of time to reject the hypothesis that there is no difference if $P < 0.05$. (In this case we say that 0.05 is the α *level* or *significance level* of the test.)

First, we suppose that there are m tests to be done and that they are independent. If in the first test there is really no difference, our chance of being right as $1 - 0.05$ (or 0.95). The same is true for each of the other tests. Our chance of being right on all m of the tests is the product of these probabilities: $(0.95) \times (0.95) \times \ldots \times (0.95)$, which is $(0.95)^m$. The P value (the chance of being wrong) is then $1 - (0.95)^m$.

If the tests are not independent (for example, if we have three groups and are testing each pair of them), then this formula is inappropriate. A different approximation is obtained from Bonferroni's inequality. The chance of being wrong once is 0.05, and so the chance of being wrong m times is, at most, m times 0.05. This approximation may be extremely high, especially with a large number of tests.

We may look at this in a preventive sense. If we can forsee that we plan to do m tests at 0.05, then a (possibly very) conservative procedure is to do each test at $0.05/m$. There are other methods, such as Scheffé's or Tukey's, that are appropriate in certain specific circumstances.

How, then, can such data be analyzed? Table 5-4 continues the data of Table 5-1, subdividing each group according to the presence or absence of lipid infusion. First, we notice that three of the P values given are 0.001 or less and that it is upon these that the authors lean most heavily for subsequent interpretation. Clearly, if they take risks at a probability of, say, 0.001 (or 1 in 1,000) then they can afford to take many more than they can at 1 in 20. Second, the note at the bottom of the table indicates that the authors have used Scheffé's S method. This is a means of comparing a measurement among groups in such a way that all

TABLE 5-4. Metabolic Gas Exchange

	N	$\dot{V}O_2$ ml/min/m²	$\dot{V}CO_2$ ml/min/m²	RQ
Nonseptic (no lipid infusion)	94	136 ± 28	130 ± 29	0.97 ± 0.12
		0.09[a]	0.08[a]	0.001[a]
Nonseptic (lipid infusion)	34	124 ± 18	125 ± 22	1.01 ± 0.12
Effect of lipid in nonseptic		−12	−5	+0.04
		0.05[a] 0.0001[a]	0.05[a] NS[a]	NS[a] 0.001[a]
	132	142 ± 19	123 ± 19	0.87 ± 0.10
Septic (lipid infusion)	114	151 ± 14	134 ± 19	0.89 ± 0.09
Effect of lipid in septic		+9	+11	+0.02

[a] P values for Scheffé's method of simultaneous inference for all contrasts in the analysis of variance.

(Nanni G, Siegel JH, Coleman B et al: Increased lipid fuel dependence in the critically ill septic patient. J Trauma 24(1):14, © 1980 The Williams & Wilkins Co., Baltimore.)

possible comparisons involving that measurement have a single combined risk, instead of one risk for each pair of groups. If we were to agree ahead of time to accept any difference with $P < 0.05$, our total risk for all of Table 5-4, with its three measurements, would be three chances at 0.05, no matter how many comparisons are actually made. For this to be possible, the Scheffé procedure must be much stricter than the t-test; for example, the result labeled as $P < 0.09$ in the table (and therefore not significant at 0.05) had $P < 0.003$ by the t-test. Third, these authors regard this type of table as exploratory and use it only as a preliminary to a more probing analysis.

There is no point in using a computer package to rummage around in a set of data. The investigator should have a clear idea ahead of time what the purposes of the analysis are and should only perform those few tests that are appropriately justified, that are crucial to the interpretation, and that organize the data into an intelligible pattern.

There is similarly no point, and even a negative point, to the peer pressure and editor pressure that urges authors into these indiscriminate acts of homage to concepts that are misunderstood.

FAILURE TO FIND A REAL DIFFERENCE

The P value does not protect against the contrary error of failing to find a real difference. Let us imagine that a physician has an ICU in which the pneumonia patients have an average shunt of 40 percent with a standard deviation of 10 percent. (This approximately agrees with our measurements.) This physician wishes to investigate a new treatment that promises to reduce shunt, by randomizing 20 patients equally to control and to the new treatment and then comparing the results using the usual t-test with $P < 0.05$. In reality the new treatment *is* better; on the average, it will decrease shunt in such patients to 30 percent. How likely is he to discover this?

The physician's chances can be determined by using a chart of *operating characteristic* curves, such as the one shown in Figure 5-1 and adapted from the very thorough discussion in Gibra.[11] The actual decrease in shunt is from 40 to 30 percent, so it equals 10 percent, or 1 standard deviation. We therefore locate 1 on the horizontal axis and follow up the vertical line until it meets the n = 20 curve. This corresponds to a little more than 0.4, or about

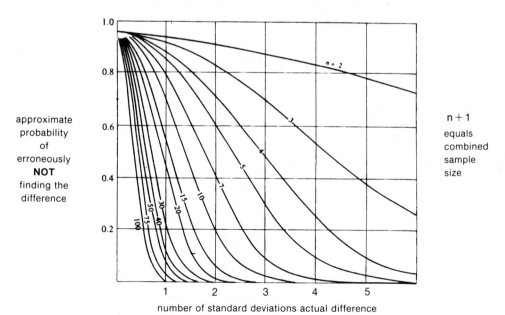

FIG. 5-1 Operating characteristic curves ($P = 0.05$). (Adapted from Gibra IN: Probability and Statistical Inference for Scientists and Engineers. Prentice Hall, Englewood Cliffs, 1973.)

42 percent, on the vertical scale. So the physician's chance of failing to discover the effectiveness of the therapy is about 42 percent. Even with a total sample size of n = 30, the chance of error would be about 20 percent.

A more practical way for the physician to read this chart, since he does not know the true amount of improvement (if any) under the new treatment, would be to follow down the n = 20 curve, corresponding to the sample size. After doing so, he would compile the information in Table 5-5 and would then have to make a judgment as to whether a reasonable chance of detecting any clinically important difference exists.

We pointed out previously that with large enough samples even clinically trivial differences become detectable. The reverse of this is that with small to moderate samples even clinically important differences are hard to detect. A low *P* value does *not* protect against failing to detect a real difference (type II error), but only against thinking there is a difference when there is none (type I error). Even worse, insisting on a low *P* value actually increases our risk of failure to detect a real difference: insisting on not being seduced by an apparent difference decreases our sensitivity to a real one.

Is it reasonable that we should treat the two types of error so asymmetrically? The inventors of the theory conceived of the situation as one in which each new result was another brick added to the edifice of science; better to turn away a good brick occasionally than to let a false one be mortared in. However we regard[13,14] this attitude of theirs, we might still feel that the physician in our example is in a different position. His object here is not eternal truth but simply to treat patients as well as possible with the materials available at this stage in history, and thereby to make progress. He must make a judgment for the particular circumstances of each study, deliberately weighing the benefits and consequences of

each type of error for his patients and for the community of patients as a whole.

If it is a question not of the benefit of a treatment but of its toxicity, then these considerations are paramount. To change our example a bit, suppose that what our physician is investigating is a vasoactive drug with a side effect of increasing shunt from 40 to 50 percent. This is again a difference of 10 percent or 1 standard deviation, although in the other direction. Our previous calculation still applies: randomizing 20 patients and then comparing them using the t-test at $P < 0.05$ gives the physician a 42 percent chance of failing to detect this toxicity. The *P* value places the burden of proof on the side of showing that there is toxicity. This is the opposite of the way it should be.

Statistics texts usually try to warn their readers that failure to reach significance does not mean that there is no difference but merely that none has been established, and this is sometimes what we read in journal articles. Yet often (as in Table 5-3 above) this is stated in such a way as to imply that there is no difference, and by the time we reach the "discussion" section we often see it explicitly concluded that there is no difference.

As in our discussion above, we recommend that the author report a confidence interval. If the confidence interval contains zero within a very narrow range of values, the reader can conclude that not only is the difference not significant but also any difference must be negligibly small in magnitude. If the interval is wide, the reader knows that no useful conclusion can be drawn without more data.

Assumptions

We have emphasized that the use of statistics involves the computation of the probabilities that certain data sets could arise in certain circumstances. To do this not only requires that probability be appropriate in the general sense we have already discussed but also that the particular probability distribution used should fit the particular circumstances of the experiment. Any statistics text will include these as-

TABLE 5-5. Chances of Detecting a Difference (in this Example)

Actual improvement in shunt (%)	5	10	15	20
Number of standard deviations	½	1	1½	2
Chance of not detecting (%)	80	42	10	2

sumptions as part of the description of each test. Here we discuss two assumptions that are commonly violated in the literature.

NORMALITY

The t-test, as well as the F-test used in analysis of variance and in regression, requires that the underlying distribution of the data be *normal,* that is, that the probabilities fit the famous bell-shaped curve centered at the mean value. There are standard *goodness of fit* tests to check this assumption, although they are not often used.

In some cases, the data are so obviously not normally distributed that no formal test is needed. Suppose, while reading an article, we are informed that cardiac index (CI) for group A is 3 ± 2 L/min/m² while for group B it is 4.5 ± 2 L/min/m² and that this difference is significant by Student's t-test to $P < 0.05$. Look again at the figures for group A. The normal distribution is symmetric about its mean and has 95 percent of its probability within 2 standard deviations. For CI to be normally distributed in this group there would have to be a 95 percent chance of finding CI between $3 - (2 \times 2) = -1$ and $3 + (2 \times 2) = 7$. There would be a 6.7 percent chance of CI less than zero and even a 2.5 percent chance of CI less than -1! These data cannot be normally distributed, the t-test cannot apply, and a P value derived from it cannot mean anything.

INDEPENDENCE OF CASES

Suppose we measure $\dot{V}O_2$ in 12 patients. If 12 turns out not to be enough, we can magically double our sample size by just remeasuring the same 12 patients. If we do this soon after the first measurements, we will get substantially the same results again, but will be much further along the road to statistical significance and fame. If we wait for a longer interval, the measurements will be a bit more independent and the result will depend a bit more on the underlying physiology than on our caprice.

Many statistical procedures depend on the assumption that the data points are sampled from independent individuals, which is often impractical in clinical and experimental work. When this assumption is not met, specific adjustments need to be made. To the degree that multiple samples in the same individual are independent and that the number of individuals sampled is larger than the number of samples per individual, these adjustments are negligible. Some of the studies discussed in this chapter are more secure from this point of view, and some are less.

RELATIONSHIPS BETWEEN VARIABLES

Linear Regression

Thus far we have discussed statistical tests of whether the average value of some measurement is different between different groups. These tests are only a preliminary method in the characterization of such differences, as we will now begin to explain.

A group of authors published a series[18,19,21,22] of papers on cardiorespiratory interactions in surgical ICU patients with cardiogenic decompensation, sepsis, or liver disease. Figure 5-2 shows the relationship they found[18] between cardiac output (CO) and total peripheral resistance (TPR) in some of these patients. The authors report that CO is predictable from TPR in these patients using the equation

$$CO = \frac{4192}{TPR} + 1.63.$$

This equation (a linear regression equation[17]) is a mathematical summary of the data, just as the average value of a variable is, except that the regression relates two variables to each other. (Incidentally, the lines plotted are not the regression line but lines of constant cardiac work. Indeed, much of the point of this figure was to show that certain of the septic

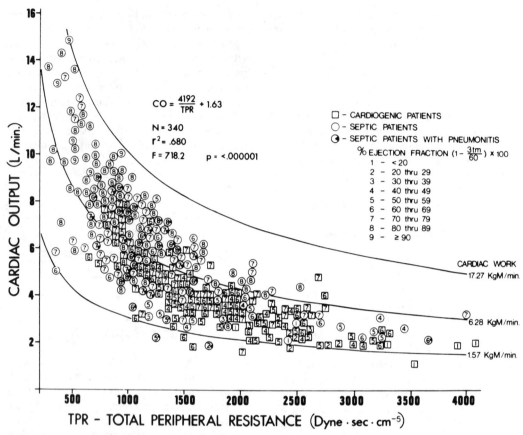

FIG. 5-2 Relation between cardiac output and total peripheral resistance in 340 studies. Individual points labeled by percent ejection fraction. Lines of constant cardiac work are shown. (Siegel JH, Giovannini I, Coleman B: Ventilation: perfusion maldistribution secondary to the hyperdynamic cardiovascular state as the major cause of increased pulmonary shunting in human sepsis. J Trauma 19: 432, © 1979 The Williams & Wilkins Co., Baltimore.)

patients are regularly doing large amounts of cardiac work.)

The equation given is derived from the sample of 340 studies that the authors chose. The statistic $r^2 = 0.680$ indicates, in a certain specific sense,[4] that the equation accounts for 68 percent of the variability in these authors' existing data. The question then remains whether this relationship would hold up in the population at large. (Just which population is that? One might well ask.) The value $P < 0.000001$ (derived from the statistic F = 718.2) gives the probability assigned to data sets as or more structured than that of these authors by the hypothesis that CO and TPR are actually unrelated in the population as a whole. Since P is so low, we feel strongly compelled to reject this hypothesis.

Meaning

Before we can go on to explain what this analysis shows that previous ones do not, we must dispose of an objection that has been made[1,15] and that has even taken in some sophisticated investigators (as we can see from the published discussion following one[22] of the present series of papers). Dealing with this objection will help us to see a fundamental feature of this type of analysis.

Without thinking too carefully, one might argue as follows. By definition, CO is related to TPR by the formula

$$CO = \frac{79.9 \, (MBP - RAP)}{TPR}$$

where MBP is mean blood pressure, RAP is right atrial pressure, and the proportionality constant 79.9 is to adjust for units of measurement. Thus we perfectly well expect CO and TPR to have the hyperbolic relationship shown in Figure 5-2, and the authors' statistical demonstration that they do so, far from being a discovery, is merely a restatement of an empty tautology.

With a bit more thought than this argument shows, one might wonder why the intercept value is found to be 1.63 rather than 0, as the equation above would predict, and wonder whether 4,192 actually equals 79.9 times the average pressure gradient. We ignore this.

Another reply is more to the point. Let us suppose a patient has MBP − RAP = 90, so as to lie on the curve shown in Figure 5-3. Further suppose that this patient has a TPR of, say, 3,000 and is thus at point 1 in the figure. The attending physician prescribes a vasodila-

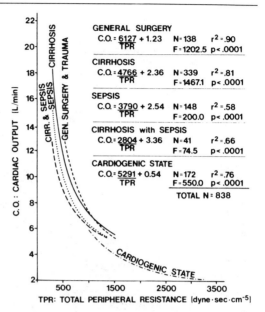

FIG. 5-4 Vascular tone relations in different clinical conditions. N, number of studies. (Siegel JH, Giovannini I, Coleman B et al: Pathologic synergistic modulation of the cardiovascular respiratory and metabolic response to injury by cirrhosis and/or sepsis: a manifestation of a common metabolic defect? Arch Surg 117: 225, © 1982 American Medical Association.)

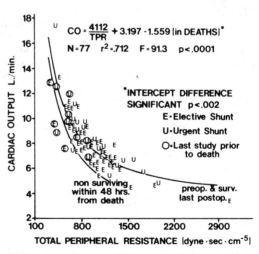

FIG. 5-5 Vascular tone abnormalities in cirrhotic patients after portal decompression. CO, cardiac output. (Siegel JH, Giovannini I. Coleman B et al: Death after portal decompressive surgery: physiologic state, metabolic adequacy, and the sequence of development of the physiologic determinants of survival. Arch Surg 116: 1130, © 1981 American Medical Association.)

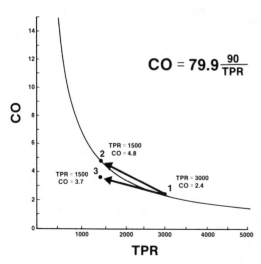

FIG. 5-3 Hypothetical alterations in vascular flow: resistance relations (vascular tone) produced by vasodilatation.

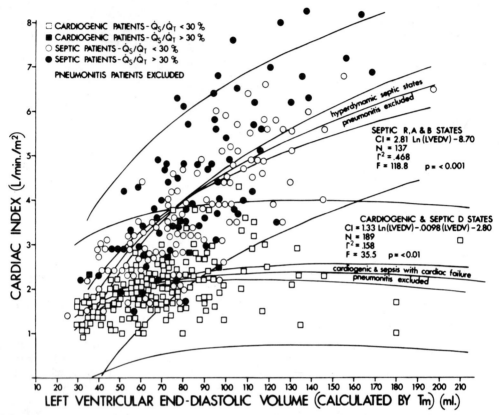

FIG. 5-6 Relation between cardiac index (CI) and left ventricular end-diastolic volume (LVEDV) for septic and cardiogenic patients. The regression and confidence limits for septic R, A, and B state patients show them to be in a different range of Starling relationships than the regression and confidence limits for cardiogenic and septic D state patients. The regression slopes of these two groups are significantly different (F ratio, 3,191; P < 0.0001). The hyperdynamic septic patients with large CI/LVEDV tend to have $\dot{Q}S/\dot{Q}T > 30$ percent. (Siegel JH, Giovannini I, Coleman B: Ventilation: perfusion maldistribution secondary to the hyperdynamic cardiovascular state as the major cause of increased pulmonary shunting in sepsis. J Trauma 19: 432, © 1979 The Williams & Wilkins Co., Baltimore.)

tor so as to bring TPR down, say to half, 1,500. Will CO thereby double, going from 2.4 to 4.8 and bringing the patient to point 2 in the figure? Not necessarily. First, there is a direct effect of the vasodilator on MBP. Next, point 2 represents more cardiac work than point 1 does. Even if the myocardium is strong enough to support this work for a sustained period, still the body is a homeostatic mechanism. If the periphery does not need a cardiac output of 4.8, then the body will adjust MBP, heart rate (HR), and ejection fraction (EFx) to give a more appropriate CO, perhaps that of point 3. The final value of CO, far from being obvious, de-pends in a complicated way on systemic needs, myocardial reserves, and the chosen balance between MBP, HR, and EFx. Each type of patient will be different, and empirically we will discover different relationships between CO and TPR depending on the type. This is illustrated in Figure 5-4, taken from a later publication[22] by these authors in which they contrast various combinations of sepsis and liver disease. In Figure 5-5 they contrast[21] the homeostasis achieved by patients surviving portacaval shunt with that of patients who die. The difference is significant to P < 0.002.

In a similar way, even basic laws of phys-

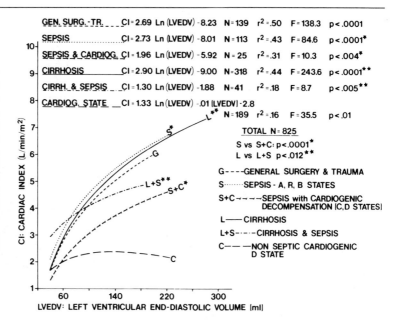

FIG. 5-7 Ventricular function relations labeled by clinical condition. N, number of studies. (Siegel JH, Giovannini I, Coleman B et al: Pathologic synergistic modulation of the cardiovascular, respiratory, and metabolic response to injury by cirrhosis and/or sepsis: a manifestation of a common metabolic defect? Arch Surg 116: 1130, © 1981 American Medical Association.)

iology apply differently in different groups of patients. Figure 5-6 is taken from one[18] of the series of papers we have been discussing. In it the authors contrast the relationship of cardiac index (CI) to left ventricular end-diastolic volume (LVEDV) as observed in a group of high-output septic patients to that observed in a group of cardiogenic patients. This relation should be given by Starling's law of the heart, but Starling's law is only asserted to be true provided other factors such as HR and MBP are constant. The point of the Starling preparation, in which Starling's law was verified, is to make these factors constant. In vivo they are not constant but adjust along with CI and LVEDV, differently in different types of patients. The two groups in Figure 5-6 are different to $P < 0.0001$. Further, in the cardiogenic group, once LVEDV is over 70 or 80 there is effectively no increase (and perhaps even a decrease) in CI with increased LVEDV. (Note how the statistics show this: $r^2 = 0.158$, implying that the relationship is weak, yet with 189 studies even this trivial relationship is significant to $P < 0.01$.)

To continue the same example, Figures 5-7 and 5-8 correspond to Figures 5-4 and 5-5 respectively. By combining such analyses, the authors of these studies were able to build up a powerful interpretation of the physiologic re-

lationships underlying the data they observed.

These examples illustrate that a knowledge of the average value of the measurements in a patient group only provides a beginning

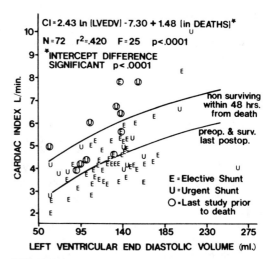

FIG. 5-8 Relation of cardiac index (CI) to left ventricular end-diastolic volume (LVEDV) in cirrhotic patients with portal hypertension. (Siegel JH, Giovannini I, Coleman B et al: Death after portal decompressive surgery: physiologic state, metabolic adequacy, and the sequence of development of the physiologic determinants of survival. Arch Surg 116: 1130, © 1981 American Medical Association.)

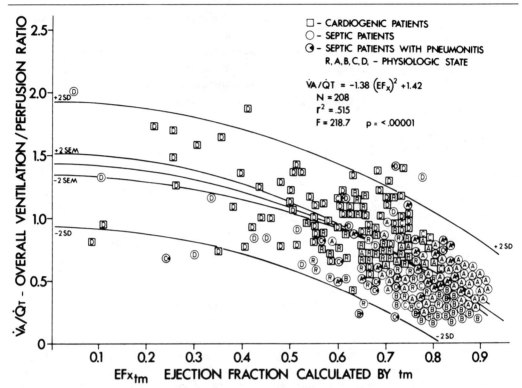

FIG. 5-9 Relation of V̇A/Q̇T to ejection fraction. Points labeled by physiologic state. Note that septic B and A state patients have the lowest V̇A/Q̇T and highest ejection fractions, and that cardiogenic and septic D state patients have a higher V̇A/Q̇T and a lower range of ejection fractions. (Siegel JH, Giovannini I, Coleman B: Ventilation: perfusion maldistribution secondary to the hyperdynamic cardiovascular state as the major cause of increased pulmonary shunting in human sepsis. J Trauma 19: 423, © 1979 The Williams & Wilkins Co., Baltimore.)

of a characterization of that group. Not only do hyperdynamic septic patients on the whole have higher CI than septic patients with cardiogenic decompensation, but they even have higher CI for any given LVEDV. As we have seen, systematically exploring the relationships between variables in a patient group gives us a picture of the physiologic adaptation typical of the group.

These examples also have a cautionary side related to our discussion of randomness. Since the relationship observed is a function of the type of patients, whenever there is a mixture of patients the overall pattern depends on which type predominates, which in turn often depends on nonrandom factors. For example, an institution seeing more high-output septics than decompensated septics will form a different picture of the physiology of sepsis than one seeing the opposite proportion. Often the effect of such mixing of types will be confusion, so that no clear pattern forms at all.

Multiple Regression

A type of physiologic adaptation can be analyzed even more closely by finding regression equations with more than one independent

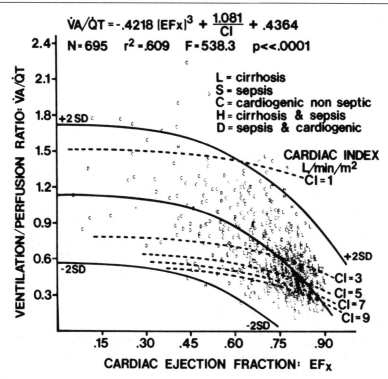

$$\dot{V}A/\dot{Q}T = -.4218 \, (EFx)^3 + \frac{1.081}{CI} + .4364$$

N = 695   r² = .609   F = 538.3   p << .0001

L = cirrhosis
S = sepsis
C = cardiogenic non septic
H = cirrhosis & sepsis
D = sepsis & cardiogenic

FIG. 5-10 Effect of cardiac ejection fraction and cardiac index (CI) on ventilation–perfusion ratio (V̇A/Q̇T). Points are labeled by clinical condition, pneumonitis excluded. All patients received mechanical ventilation at fraction of inspired oxygen of 40 percent or greater. N, number of studies. (Siegel JH, Giovannini I, Coleman B et al: Death after portal decompressive surgery: physiologic state, metabolic adequacy, and the sequence of development of the physiologic determinants of survival. Arch Surg 116: 1130, © 1981 American Medical Association.)

variable. Figure 5-9 is similar to the figures we have just been discussing. It depicts the dependence[18] of the mean pulmonary ventilation/perfusion ratio (V̇A/Q̇T) on the cardiac ejection fraction (EFx). Although this is good as far as it goes (and is intended to go), the situation is better explained (in a larger group of patients) in Figure 5-10. Here V̇A/Q̇T is predicted[22] from both CI and EFx. These two independent variables are obviously interrelated so that as EFx rises, CI also rises. According to the figure, this will place a patient to the right and down, and he or she will tend to have a low V̇A/Q̇T.

What is interesting is that these two effects are not completely dependent: even for a fixed CI, an increase in EFx is associated with a decrease in V̇A/Q̇T. To put this another way, although there are any number of means of setting CI—among them changes in EFx, MBP, TPR, and HR—these means are not equivalent in their other physiologic effects. Much of the point of the series of papers we are discussing is to show how the different cardiovascular adaptations that occur in patients with different diseases have different implications for (and are partially the result of) the need for respiratory adequacy.

More generally, we again see the point that the more we probe how relationships are set up, the more we can understand the disease process. This can be done using multiple linear regression along with an understanding of the different methods for comparing regression equations.[4]

Causality

We can sometimes be surprised by the response of actual patients to the basic laws of physiology. For example, the slightest acquaintance with respiratory physiology would make one realize that an increase in expired ventilation will empty the lung of carbon dioxide whereas a decrease will permit a buildup, as shown in Figure 5-11. Our patients are confused about this. Figure 5-12 shows them under the delusion that there is a small ($r = 0.2$) but highly significant ($F_{1,375} = 15.9$, $P < 0.0001$) positive correlation between arterial carbon dioxide tension ($PaCO_2$) and expired ventilation.

Perhaps this unscientific behavior on their part can be accounted for by examining the difference in causality between the two situations. The predictions in Figure 5-11 are appropriate when, the rate of carbon dioxide production being constant, the expired ventilation is varied and the $PaCO_2$ follows it. Our patients are under a different regimen: as their $PaCO_2$ rises, the house staff increases ventilation. The direction of causality is reversed.

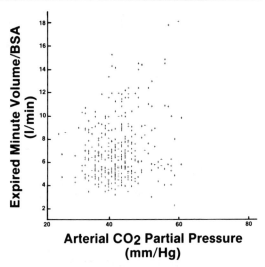

FIG. **5-12** Actual relation between $PaCO_2$ and ventilation in patients with controlled ventilation.

In different causal situations, the observed envelope of data points can be quite different.

Time

Effects become even more complicated when we consider their sequence in time. Consider a simplified metabolic model in which we assume that plasma glucose and insulin levels form a closed system.

Here again we contrast two situations by taking different variables to be the causal factor. On the left of Figure 5-13 we imagine that we administer a dose of insulin to a fasting normal subject. This gives a transient peak in plasma insulin followed slightly later by a trough in plasma glucose. On the right we administer instead a dose of glucose. The plasma glucose rise is followed by a rise in plasma insulin. Perhaps. The exact sequence depends on a number of factors. If the anabolic stimulus is too great, the glucose may overshoot and there might consequently be several cycles of "ringing" (Fig. 5-14). If we take into account the whole system of hormones and substrates

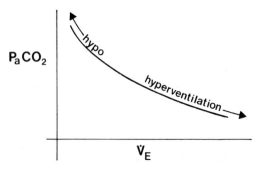

FIG. **5-11** Theoretical relation between ventilation ($\dot{V}E$) and arterial carbon dioxide tension ($PaCO_2$) in spontaneously breathing subjects.

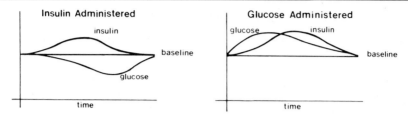

FIG. 5-13 Different causal response sequences between insulin and glucose depending on initiating factor.

with which these two actually interact, the possibilities are limitless.

The data have a structure in time. If we only take static "snapshots" of these processes, the observed correlations will depend both on the type of episode and whether we take our measurements early or late within it; we will only see part of the story. If we take measurements with a regular structure in time, we will have a better chance of uncovering a more realistic picture of the underlying physiology. We must look to see if there is a correlation of glucose measurements not just with insulin measurements taken at the same time but also with those taken at earlier or later times. This has been studied systematically.[5]

In a more positive sense, this time structure offers an opportunity. Each stage of disease response is characterized not only by the level of each physiologic measurement but also by the dynamic that restores equilibrium after any small transient disturbance. This restoration may be fast or slow, or simple or complex, and may tell us more about the patient's condition than just knowing the equilibrium level

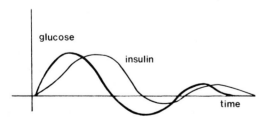

FIG. 5-14 Hypothetical metabolic "ringing" due to glucose–insulin overshoot.

does. Over long periods the patient goes through a succession of stages, each with its own equilibrium points and its own dynamics. Finding them is a basic goal of clinical research, helping us to characterize diseases and treatments.

Clustering

We have emphasized the notion that depending on the type of insult, the degree of host competence, the therapeutic regimen, and the measurement scheme, different groups of patients display different apparent physiologies. Sorting them out by using clinical criteria can become bewildering, simply because there are so many possible combinations of so many criteria. An alternative method is *cluster analysis*. For this, one would assume that all these possibilities result in only a few groups, within each of which the patients bear each other a family resemblance in their observed behavior.

An appropriate set of variables is selected, and a set of measurements for each patient is taken on these variables. Cluster analysis is a method for grouping together those patients whose measurements most nearly agree.

In one such study[12,10,19] a selection of ICU patients was classified according to their cardiovascular condition. First a reference group of general surgical ICU patients, designated as the "R state," was identified, and a set of 11 measurements for all other patients was rescaled as the number of standard deviations above or below the R state mean. Cluster

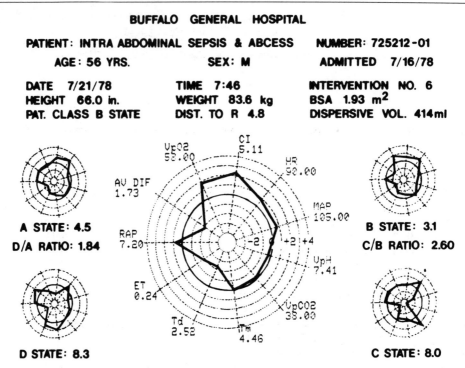

FIG. 5-15 Circle diagram of physiologic state. At corners are shown the prototype patterns for the A, B, C, and D states. In the large circle in the center is the physiologic pattern manifested by a 56-year-old man with intra-abdominal sepsis and abscess. The perfect circle in the center equals 0 standard deviations to reference control R state. Each dotted line represents 1 standard deviation from R, either increased or decreased. Adjacent to each state is the state distance in normalized units from that prototype. Patient is closest to a B state (3.1) and therefore is classified as B. The real value of each physiologic variable is given with the variable name on each ray. (Siegel JH, Cerra FB, Coleman B et al: Physiologic and metabolic correlations in human sepsis. Surgery 86: 163, 1979.)

analysis divided the remaining patients into four groups: the A state (stress response), the B state (metabolic decompensation), the C state (respiratory decompensation), and the D state (cardiogenic decompensation). Each of these groups is characterized by a clinically interpretable derangement in the 11 physiologic variables.

Subsequent patients can then be classified by the closeness with which they approximate these 5 prototypes. Figure 5-15 is redrawn from a routine computer study of a septic patient.[19] On the 11 axes of the center circle are plotted his standardized values of the 11 variables.

Thus, his cardiac index (CI) is 2 standard deviations above the R state mean, and his heart rate (HR) is 1 standard deviation above. More ominously, his arteriovenous oxygen saturation difference (AV DIF) is 2 standard deviations below R state. The four circles on the outside depict the A,B,C, and D state prototypes, and give this patient's distance from each. He is classified as B state since it is the state from which his distance is least.

As Figure 5-16 illustrates for a different patient, these patterns are seen to change in a consistent way over time, indicating the patient's progress through his disease.

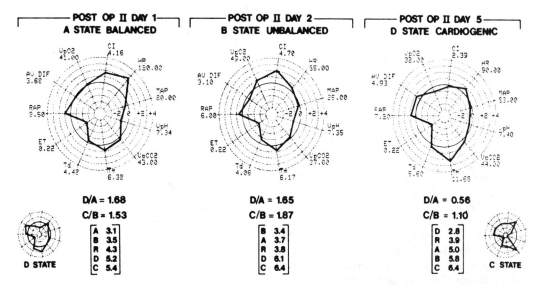

FIG. 5-16 State transitions in severe sepsis. Changing physiologic patterns together with their state distances and state distance ratios are shown for a 62-year-old man with bowel infarctions and resection who developed peritonitis and sepsis followed by wound dehiscence. Closure of dehiscence, ileostomy, colostomy, and tracheostomy were performed in a second operative procedure (op II). The state transitions following his second operation from an A-balanced physiologic state to a B state of metabolic imbalance, followed by cardiac decompensation into a D-state cardiogenic septic are shown. Small figures in the corner permit comparison of the patient's states with the prototypes of the A, B, C, and D states. (Siegel JH, Cerra FB, Coleman B et al: Physiologic and metabolic correlations in the human sepsis. Surgery 86: 163, 1979.)

CONCLUSION

Many physicians view statistical inference as inherently scientific. It is not; it is merely a tool and no more inherently scientific than any other tool. To be scientific, it must be used scientifically and, *a fortiori*, with common sense, neither of which requisites are hard to meet.

In this chapter we have tried to present a viewpoint conducive to the better use of statistics. We have not been exhaustive, but have discussed only those aspects that are part of a common theme: the meaning of probability.

In some situations, statistics are indispensible. In every experiment there is some random error, especially in the observation of the effects of treatment upon a patient. In those experiments where the outcomes can be regarded as random samples of a fixed process, statistical inference can estimate the extent to which our conclusions reflect that process.

We hope that the reader has also seen the deeper theme that lies beneath the surface of our chapter. By helping us sort out the relations and combinations of relations characteristic of groups of patients, statistics offer us an opportunity to clarify the process of disease and of treatment.

ACKNOWLEDGMENT

We are grateful to the distinguished series of research fellows who have come to us from the Department of Surgery, Centro di Studio per la Fisiopatologia dello Shock, C.N.R., Universitá Cattolica del Sacro Cuore, Rome, under Drs. Gian Carlo Castiglioni and Marco Castagneto. It was during a long visit by Dr. Ivo Giovannini that we first worked out the basics of the ideas we have here presented concerning the application of statistical techniques to physiologic research. This research has subsequently flourished in the hands of Drs. Giuseppe Nanni, Gabriele Sganga, Mauro Pittiruti, and Roberto M. Tacchino.

This work was supported in part by grants HL 29280 and HL 29281 from the National Heart, Lung and Blood Institute and NAS 9–171–86 from the National Aeronautics and Space Administration.

REFERENCES

1. Archie JD: Mathematic coupling. Ann Sur 296: 303, 1981
2. Bartlett RH, Roloff DW, Cornell RG et al: Extracorporeal circulation in neonatal respiratory failure: a prospective randomized study. Pediatrics 76(4): 479, 1985
3. Bickel PJ, Doksum KA: Mathematical Statistics: Basic Ideas and Selected Topics. Holden-Dag, San Francisco, 1977
4. Coleman B, Siegel JH: Statistical interpretation. p. 445. In Peters R, Benfield J, Peacock E (eds): Scientific Management of Surgical Patients. Little Brown, Boston, 1983
5. Coleman B, Siegel JH, Kazarinoff ND: Autocorre-
6. Coleman B, McDowell EM: Development of hamster tracheal epithelium III. Illustration of statistical methods for proportional data in biology. Anat Rec 213: 457, 1985
7. Cornell RG, Landenberger BD, Bartlett RH: Randomized play-the-winner clinical trials. Commun Stat Theory Methods 15(1): 159, 1986
8. Cox DR: The Analysis of Binary Data. Chapman and Hall, London, 1970
9. DeGroot, MH: Probability and Statistics. Addison-Wesley, Reading, 1975
10. Friedman HP, Goldwyn RM, Siegel JH: The use and interpretation of multivariable methods in the classification of stages of serious infectious disease process in the critically ill. p. 81. In Elashoff R (ed): Perspectives in Biometrics. Academic Press, New York, 1975
11. Gibra IN: Probability and Statistical Inference for Scientists and Engineers. Prentice Hall, Englewood Cliffs, 1973
12. Goldwyn, RM, Friedman HP, Siegel JH: Iteraction and interaction in computer data bank analysis—case study in physiological classification and assessment physiological classification and assessment of the critically ill. Comput Biomed Res 4: 607, 1971
13. Kuhn T: The Structure of Scientific Revolutions. Chicago University Press, Chicago, 1972
14. Lakatos I, Musgrave A (eds): Criticism and the Growth of Knowledge. Cambridge University Press, Cambridge, U.K. 1970.
15. Mrochen H, Hieronymi U, Kuckelt W: Plotting cardiac output versus total peripheral resistance. Crit Care Med 9(2): 129, 1981
16. Nanni G, Siegel JH, Coleman B et al: Increased lipid fuel dependence in the critically ill septic patient. J Trauma 24(1): 14, 1984
17. Seber GAF: Linear Regression Analysis. Wiley, New York 1977
18. Siegel JH, Giovannini I, Coleman B: Ventilation: perfusion maldistribution secondary to the hyperdynamic cardiovascular state as the major cause of increased pulmonary shunting in human sepsis. J. Trauma 19: 432, 1979
19. Siegel JH, Cerra FB, Coleman B, et al: Physiologic and metabolic correlations in human sepsis. Surgery 86: 163, 1979
20. Siegel JH, Cerra FB, Moody EA et al: The effect on survival of critically ill and injured patients of an ICU teaching service organized about a computer-based physiologic CARE system. J Trauma 20(7): 558, 1980
21. Siegel JH, Giovannini I, Coleman B et al: Death after portal decompressive surgery: physiologic

state, metabolic adequacy, and the sequence of development of the physiologic determinants of survival. Arch Surg 116: 1330, 1981

22. Siegel JH, Giovannini I, Coleman B et al: Pathologic synergistic modulation of the cardiovascular, respiratory and metabolic response to injury by cirrhosis and/or sepsis: a manifestation of a common metabolic defect? Arch Surg 117:225, 1982

23. Zelen M: Play the winner rule and the controlled clinical trial. J Am Stat Assoc 64: 131, 1969

SUGGESTED READINGS

Altman DG: Improving the quality of statistics in medical journals. p. 21. In Gore SM, Altman DG: Statistics in Practice. British Medical Association, London, 1982

Badgley RF: An assessment of research methods reported in 103 scientific articles from two Canadian medical journals. Can Med Assoc J 85: 246, 1961

Coleman B: Significance of free insulin concentrations in diabetes mellitus. J Pediatr 102(5): 800, 1983 (Letter).

Coleman B: Methodology in clinical research. In Proceedings of the 7th International Congress of Logic, Methodology and Philosophy of Science, 1983

DerSimonian R, Charette LJ, McPeek B et al: Reporting on methods in clinical trials. N Engl J Med 306: 1332, 1982

Feinstein AR, Horwitz RI: Double standards, scientific methods, and epidemiologic research. N Engl J Med 307: 1611, 1982

Glantz SA: Biostatistics; how to detect, correct, and prevent errors in the medical literature. Circulation 61: 1, 1980

Gore S, Jones IG, Rytter EC: Misuses of statistical methods: critical assessment of articles in B.M.J. from January to March, 1976. Br Med J 1: 85, 1977

Hoffman JIF: The incorrect use of chi square analysis for paired data. Clin Exp Immunol 24: 227, 1976

Lionel NDW, Herxheimer A: Assessing reports of therapeutic trials. Br Med J 3: 637, 1970

May GS, DeMets DL, Friedman LM et al: The randomized clinical trial: bias in analysis. Circulation 64(4): 669, 1981

A pillar of medicine (editorial): JAMA 195: 1145, 1966

Rosen MR, Hoffman BF: Statistics, biomedical scientists, and Circulation Research (editorial). Circ Res 42: 739, 1978

Ross OB, Jr.: Use of controls in medical research. JAMA 145: 72, 1951

Schoolman HM, Becktel JM, Best, WR, Johnson AF: Statistics in medical research: principles versus practices. J Lab Clin Med 71: 357, 1968

Schor S, Karten I: Statistical evaluation of medical journal manuscripts. JAMA 195: 1123, 1966

Schor S: Statistical reviewing program for medical manuscripts. Am Statistician 21: 28, 1967

Shott S: Statistics in veterinary research. JAMA 187(2): 138, 1985

Shuster JJ, Binion J, Moxley J, et al: Statistical review process: recommended procedures for biomedical research articles (letter) JAMA 235: 534, 1976

Statistical errors (editorial): Br Med J 1: 66, 1977

Weech AA: Statistics use and misuse. Aust Pediatr J 10: 328, 1974

White SJ: Statistical errors in papers in the British Journal of Psychiatry. Br J Psychiatry 135: 336, 1979

SECTION II

PHARMACOLOGIC CONSIDERATIONS IN THE MANAGEMENT OF SHOCK

6

Newer Pharmacologic Approaches to Shock*

Steven Sharpe

Bart Chernow

INTRODUCTION

The development of a successful therapeutic approach to septic shock remains a major problem in modern medicine. The mortality associated with septic shock is unacceptably high at 30 to 70 percent, despite the availability of modern antibiotics. Cardiogenic shock (associated with acute myocardial infarction) also has a high mortality and spinal shock remains a devastating disease. Consequently, new pharmacologic approaches for the treatment of all shock states are being developed. Areas of particular interest at present include (1) the role of prostanoids in shock states and the use

of cyclooxygenase inhibitors in shock therapy; (2) the role of the endogenous opioid systems in the pathogenesis of shock states and the use of the receptor-specific opiate antagonist naloxone, and the physiologic opiate antagonist thyrotropin-releasing hormone (TRH) as shock therapies; (3) the role of corticosteroids in the therapy of septic shock (still controversial after 20 years); and (4) the use of exogenous catecholamine therapy in the treatment of shock.

Although we discuss prostaglandins, opioid peptides, steroids, and catecholamines separately in this chapter, these agents probably have diverse, complex interactions in vivo. For example, prostaglandins inhibit endogenous norepinephrine release from the sympathetic nerve endings, possibly by decreasing calcium entry into the cell.[147] Inhibitors of prostaglandin synthesis may increase norepinephrine release, which perhaps offers one explanation for their ability to improve survival in septic shock.[70,74] In support of this concept, in experi-

* The opinions and assertions contained herein are the private ones of the authors and are not to be construed as reflecting the views of the Navy Department, the Naval Service at large, or the Department of Defense.

mental septic shock, indomethacin increases the systemic vascular resistance by stimulating the sympathetic nervous system.[258] In addition, Hughes[137] recently showed in septic patients that combination naloxone–methylprednisolone therapy improved hemodynamics in association with an augmented catecholamine response; this suggested a synergistic increase in sympathomedullary discharge in sepsis.

Much of the data presented in this chapter are from experimental shock studies. We would be negligent if we did not note the limitations of these studies:

1. Different experimental models within the same species may produce widely divergent results. Furthermore, the best animal model of human sepsis is unclear.[244] Do endotoxin boluses, live *E. coli* infusions, or "ligation and perforation" models best approximate human septic shock?

2. The dosage, timing, and route of drug administration each affect experimental results. For example, survival rates after antibiotic–steroid combination therapy are best when the drugs are given at the time of the septic insult (initiation of endotoxin or live *E. coli* infusion), rather than hours after the infusion has begun.[116,118]

3. Agents such as naloxone (opiate receptor antagonist) and nonsteroidal anti-inflammatory drugs (prostaglandin antagonists) may improve the hemodynamic parameters and survival of animal subjects having certain types of shock, but a drug's mechanism of action may be very difficult to prove *with certainty*. For example, prostaglandin antagonists improve survival in rat endotoxic shock, but these antagonists block the production of many arachidonic acid metabolites (Fig. 6-1), in addition to having nonprostaglandin-mediated effects.

4. Much of the data presented are from animal work. Experimental results differ due to interspecies variability. Final proof of efficacy in humans is only obtained with well-designed *human* studies, once animal efficacy and safety have been demonstrated.

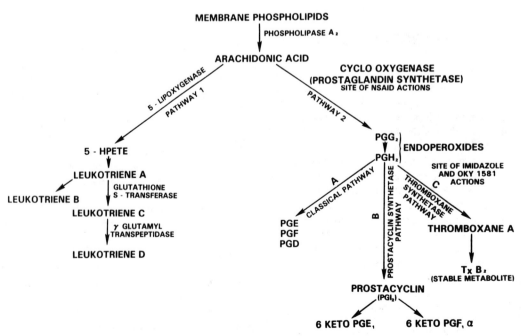

FIG. 6-1 The prostaglandin metabolic cascade. The lipoxygenase and cyclo-oxygenase pathways constitute major metabolic routes of arachidonic acid metabolism. There are three subdivisions of the cyclo-oxygenase pathway. (Fletcher JR: Prostaglandin manipulation. p. 651. In Chernow B, Lake CR (eds): The Pharmacologic Approach to the Critically Ill Patient. Williams & Wilkins, Baltimore, 1983.)

PROSTAGLANDINS AND SHOCK

History

In the 1930s, investigators[150] discovered that human semen caused uterine smooth muscle contraction or relaxation. Von Euler isolated a lipid soluble acid from this material, which he named "prostaglandins." Subsequently, it was discovered that the prostaglandins constituted a group of unique compounds. The structures of prostaglandin $F_{2\alpha}$ ($PGF_{2\alpha}$) and prostaglandin E_1 (PGE_1) were identified in 1962[15]; both have a core 20-carbon unsaturated fatty acid with a cyclopentane ring. In 1964, PGE_2 was successfully synthesized from arachidonic acid. Since then, many more prostaglandins have been discovered.

Synthesis

Although there are other prostaglandin precursors, the most important in humans is probably arachidonic acid,[79] which is either ingested or produced endogenously from its fatty acid precursor, linoleic acid. Arachidonic acid is esterified and incorporated into cellular membranes. Various stimuli activate the enzyme phospholipase A_2, which releases the arachidonic acid from the cell membranes, making it available to be metabolized via two distinct pathways to numerous important mediators with varied biologic effects (Fig. 6-1).

LIPOXYGENASE PATHWAY

Lipoxygenase catalyzes the conversion of arachidonic acid to 12-hydroperoxy arachidonic acid (HPETE) and to the hydroxy form of these acids (HETE). The leukotrienes, of which slow-reacting substance of anaphylaxis is a member,[43] are also products of the lipoxygenase pathway. The lipoxygenase pathway enzymes are found in platelets, white blood cells, and lung tissue. Lipoxygenase by-products increase vascular permeability,[51] and cause bronchoconstriction,[51,110,211] but the di-

rect role of these products in shock states remains speculative.

CYCLO-OXYGENASE PATHWAY

Cyclo-oxygenase catalyzes the conversion of arachidonic acid into the "prostanoids" (Fig. 6-1). Nonsteroidal anti-inflammatory drugs (NSAID) such as indomethacin, ibuprofen and aspirin block the activity of cyclo-oxygenase.[175] The cyclo-oxygenase enzyme catalyzes the conversion of arachidonic acid to the unstable intermediate endoperoxide prostaglandin G_2 (PGG_2), which is then converted to prostaglandin H_2 (PGH_2), which is converted in turn via one of three major subdivisions of the cyclo-oxygenase pathway to various end products. In Pathway A (Fig. 6-1), PGH_2 is converted enzymatically or nonenzymatically to the "classic" prostaglandins (PGD_2, PGE_2, PGF_2), once thought to be the prostaglandins of primary importance. In Pathway B, PGH_2 is converted via prostacyclin synthetase (concentrated in vascular endothelium) to prostacyclin (PGI_1) which relaxes vascular smooth muscle[8] and inhibits platelet aggregation.[176] Prostacyclin has a half-life of approximately 3 minutes, and is hydrolyzed nonenzymatically to a much more stable end product, 6-keto $PGF_{1\alpha}$ (often assayed as a marker of prostacyclin activity). In Pathway C, PGH_2 is converted via thromboxane synthetase (found mostly in platelets) to thromboxane A_2 (T_xA_2), also an unstable compound with a half-life of 30 seconds, which contracts vascular smooth muscle[180,222] and causes platelet[107] and leukocyte[216] aggregation. It is converted to the stable metabolite thromboxane B_2 (T_xB_2)[180,211] which is assayed as a marker of thromboxane A_2 activity. At present the balance between the opposing actions of T_xA_2 and PGI_2 is generating the most interest by investigators doing shock-related prostaglandin research.

Prostaglandin Inhibitor and Prostaglandin Shock Therapy

A number of methods are available to minimize the production of prostaglandins. It was not until 10 years after the first use of NSAIDs in the therapy of endotoxic shock[183] that these agents were discovered to inhibit prostaglandin release from tissue homogenates,[233] platelets,[212] and the spleen.[67] Aspirin decreases endoperoxidase intermediate production (PGG_2) by actually acetylating the cyclo-oxygenase enzyme.[78] Cyclo-oxygenase inhibition has numerous effects since the production of many different prostanoids is blocked. More recently, the specific thromboxane synthetase inhibitors imidazole and OKY 1581 have been utilized.[29] Prostaglandin production can also be limited by creating an essential fatty acid (arachidonic acid precursor) deficiency via nutritional depletion. This is a means of independently verifying the importance of decreased prostaglandin production using nonpharmacologic means.[39] The prostaglandins are a varied group of compounds that often have opposing effects. Certain prostaglandins, such as PGE_1,[169] PGA_1,[204] and PGI_2 have been used therapeutically in shock states, with mixed results. Lefer[154] suggests that beneficial prostaglandin effects in shock may be coronary artery vasodilatation, prevention of tachycardia, inhibition of protein degradation, lysosomal membrane stabilization, and reduced platelet aggregation. Prostacyclin, 6-keto PGE_1, and $PGF_{2\alpha}$ have some of these effects and therefore may be effective shock therapy. Prostaglandin A_1 and 6-keto $PGF_{1\alpha}$ have little of these activities, and are generally not effective agents in shock (Table 6-1).

Prostaglandins and Hypovolemic Shock

In hemorrhagic shock, using different species, investigators have demonstrated elevations in PGE_1, $PGF_{2\alpha}$, and PGA_1 levels.[73,80,81,142] These increased values indicate a rapid, shock-associated increase in prostaglandin synthesis and/or decreased clearance because prostaglandins are probably not stored to any great extent within body tissues.[154] Investigators have demonstrated that treatment with prostaglandin antagonists improves a number of hypovolemic shock-related parameters. Hypotension is reversed, probably because of increased

systemic vascular resistance.[18,156,157] Late in hypovolemic shock, Bond et al.[18] showed that PGE_2 decreases presynaptic norepinephrine release causing hypotension that is reversible with the use of prostaglandin antagonists. The balance between vasodilating and vasoconstricting prostaglandins in any given shock state may determine the vascular resistance of the patient in shock.[179] Pulmonary vascular resistance and lung water are increased in hemorrhagic shock, possibly secondary to platelet aggregation and capillary endothelial damage; both effects are minimized by aspirin therapy.[182]

Both PGE_1 and $PGF_{2\alpha}$ have been shown to decrease platelet aggregation and stabilize lysosomal membranes, as well as to improve survival in experimental hypovolemic shock.[124,243]

Prostaglandins and Endotoxic or Septic Shock

As with hemorrhagic shock, investigators have sought to understand the role of prostaglandins in the pathogenesis of septic shock. Early studies were not well controlled, but subsequently, using sensitive and specific radioimmunoassays, *endotoxin* infusions were shown to increase plasma 6-keto $PGF_{1\alpha}$ (stable metabolite of PGI_2),[19,25,106,249] T_xB_2, a stable metabolite of T_xA_2,[4,19,29,84,249,250] PGE_2[4,5,37,39] and $PGF_{2\alpha}$ levels.[5,6,37,72] Early increases in T_xA_2 were associated with increases in pulmonary artery pressures.[29] Thromboxane A_2 (vasoconstrictor and platelet aggregator) and PGI_2 (vasodilator and platelet antiaggregator) rather than the earlier discovered "classic" prostaglandins (PGEs and PGFs) may be the prostaglandins most important in the pathophysiology of endotoxin shock.[26,27,29,39,109]

Circulating T_xB_2 and 6-keto $PGF_{1\alpha}$ levels are increased following live *E. coli* infusions in baboons[230] and in rats with fecal bacterial peritonitis[28] or after intraperitoneal injections of live *E. coli* in rats.[76] In human sepsis, while moderate elevations in 6-keto $PGF_{1\alpha}$ are observed, T_xB_2 levels have only been elevated in eventual nonsurvivors.[194,196] Although cer-

TABLE 6-1. Cellular and Hemodynamic Properties of Prostaglandins

Prostaglandin	Reduces Blood Pressure	Prevents Tachycardia	Coronary Vasodilation	Prevents Platelet Aggregation	Lysosomal Membrane Stabilization	Inhibits Proteolysis
PGA_1	±	0	±	±	0	±
PGD_2	++	+	+	+++	++	++
PGE_1	++	++	++	+++	++	++
6-Keto-PGE_1	+++	+++	++	++	++	++
PGE_2	++	+	±	+	+	±
6-Keto-PGE_{1a}	0	0	0	0	0	0
PGF_{2a}	±	+	−	0	±	+
PGI_2	++++	+++	++++	++++	+++	+++

+, increase; −, decrease; 0, no effect; ±, unclear or variable effect.
(Lefer Am: Role of prostaglandins and thromboxanes in shock states. p. 366. In Altura BM, Lefer AM, Schumer W (eds): Handbook of Shock and Trauma, Vol. 1. Raven Press, New York, 1983.)

tain specific prostaglandins have been measured in shock states, Lefer[154] noted that "no one has systematically quantified the three major branches of the cyclo-oxygenase pathway, namely the prostacyclin, thromboxane, and classic prostaglandin branches in one type of shock." Such data would be extremely useful in further defining the role of prostaglandins in shock states.

What are the sources of the increased circulating prostaglandins in shock? There is evidence that (1) T_xA_2, PGI_2, and PGE prostaglandins may be produced by macrophages of the reticuloendothelial system,[38,40,149] (2) thromboxane A_2 is not produced in great quantity by circulating elements of the blood (in the rat);[42] and (3) thromboxane A_2 may be produced by cells in the lung.[140]

Earlier work in both dogs and cats showed improved hemodynamics and survival using NSAID *pretreatment;* but posttreatment NSAID use did not improve survival in these shock models.[122,186] However, NSAID posttreatment does improve survival in endotoxin shock in baboons.[75] Using live *E. coli* intraperitoneal injections in rats, Short et al.[206] demonstrated combination antibiotic–NSAID improvement in survival that was not demonstrable with either agent alone. In the rat peritonitis model, either essential fatty acid deficiency or NSAID combined with gentamicin improves survival.[28] In addition, the relatively specific thromboxane synthetase inhibitor, imidazole, improves survival[39] and hemodynamics[84] in endotoxin shock, implicat-

ing thromboxane A_2 as a cause of endotoxin-induced shock.

Which events in septic shock may be mediated by the prostaglandins? Myocardial contractility is depressed in acute endotoxemia,[92,101] and NSAIDs reverse this effect, which may be thromboxane-mediated.[52,231] Endotoxemia is associated with acute but transient increases in pulmonary artery pressures in many species,[29,105,140] which are inhibited both by NSAIDs[105,140,185] and specific thromboxane synthetase inhibitors.[29,84] Endotoxic shock in animals is often associated with disseminated intravascular coagulation (DIC). In baboons, NSAIDs had no effect, but in rats, pretreatment with thromboxane synthetase inhibitors helped prevent DIC.[4,84] Prostaglandins do not seem to alter sepsis-related histamine, serotonin, or kinin effects.

Could these effects of NSAIDs be nonspecific, nonprostaglandin-mediated effects? The following evidence supports prostaglandin mediation: (1) Fatty acid deficiency in rats minimizes the normally observed endotoxin-induced increases in circulating prostaglandins and reduces the endotoxin-associated mortality.[39] Restoration of fatty acids also restores the elevated endotoxin-associated circulating prostaglandin levels and endotoxin sensitivity.[41] (2) Even NSAIDs with very different chemical structures such as ibuprofen, indomethacin, and aspirin show similar efficacy in the treatment of endotoxemia,[71,247] and (3) the NSAID indomethacin demonstrates efficacy in the treatment of endotoxemia at doses usually associated with specific cyclo-oxyge-nase inhibition.[53,71,72]

Summary

At present, current evidence suggests that PGI_2 and T_xA_2 are more important than the "classic" prostaglandins in the pathophysiology of shock. The role of the leukotrienes in shock states remains largely unknown. Continued work with specific prostaglandin inhibitors is needed to delineate better the specific pathophysiological actions of various prostanoids. The NSAIDs are not free of adverse side effects, the most prominent being decreased renal blood flow in various shock states[69,112,113] and acute renal failure in patients with certain medical disease.[82,83,237] Costs versus benefits must be evaluated. Most important, the entire previous discussion constitutes animal, not human, studies. To determine the efficacy of prostaglandin manipulation as a therapy for shock states, well-designed, closely monitored clinical trials in humans are warranted.

OPIOID PEPTIDE SYSTEM AND SHOCK

Since the discovery of endogenous opioid peptides, investigators have studied their role in the pathophysiology of shock states because of the following clinical observations: (1) severe pain and stress (opioid related events) can induce a shock-like state;[30] (2) shock may result in pain relief (suggesting opioid release);[12] and (3) the association between hypotension and pain relief is very similar to the effects of exogenously administered opiates, such as morphine sulfate. In this section we review the history of the opiates and the present state of knowledge about opiate receptors, and different classes of opioid ligands. The use of opioid antagonists in shock states, the role of the

opioid system in the pathophysiology of shock, and the use of thyrotropin-releasing hormone (TRH) in shock are also discussed.

Historical Background and Present Knowledge

Morphine was isolated in 1803. The analgesia of opium was described in 1860. Heroin was marketed in the 1890s.[213] The existence of receptors specific for the opiates was suspected because opiates are of similar structure, minimal changes in that structure can change an antagonist to an agonist, and opiates show stereospecificity. In 1973, three different groups of investigators discovered the endogenous opiate receptor in the brain.[188,210,227] Subsequently, at least five different types of opiate receptors (μ, δ, κ, σ, and ϵ) were identified,[45,260] each receptor type probably being of different physiologic importance depending upon its specific actions. Morphine binds relatively specifically to the μ-receptor, mediating analgesia and respiratory depression. There may even be two μ-receptor subtypes, μ_1, a high-affinity site that mediates β-endorphin, opiate, and enkephalin analgesia, and a low-affinity μ_2-receptor that mediates such effects as respiratory depression. Leu-enkephalin has a high affinity for the δ-receptor, which mediates respiratory and behavioral depressant effects. Dynorphin binds somewhat specifically to the κ-receptor, which produces sedating effects.[77] Naloxone (an opiate receptor antagonist) binds selectively to the μ receptor at low doses and to the δ-receptor at higher doses. κ- and δ-receptors are probably more important in the pathogenesis of shock than μ-receptors. The μ- and δ-receptors have been the most extensively studied and best localized within the brain.[21,95] They are located in limbic areas associated with emotional control, in the hypothalamus and brain stem (areas important in autonomic function), and in periaqueductal regions important for sensing pain.

After the discovery of endogenous opiate receptors, investigators sought to find endogenous opioid ligands that bound to these receptors. In 1975, the first group of endogenous opioids, the enkephalins, was isolated.[139] Two subtypes were distinguished, leucine (leu) enkephalin, and methionine (met) enkephalin. In 1976, a second group of endogenous opioids, the endorphins, was discovered.[22,99,153] Both the endorphins and the enkephalins, as well as ACTH were found to be part of a 91-amino-acid polypeptide, β-lipotropin, (released by the pituitary) originally isolated in 1964.[22,153,164] With the discovery of dynorphin, a 17-amino-acid peptide, it is now thought that there are three general classes of opioid peptides; the endorphins, the enkephalins, and the dynorphins. These peptides may have different physiologic and/or pathophysiologic roles, associated with their distinct areas of localization. Enkephalins are found in adrenal gland, hypothalamus, nucleus tractus solitarius, nucleus ambiguous, dorsal nucleus of the vagus, spinal cord, and limbic system.[9,45,138] β-Endorphin is found in the hypothalamus and pituitary gland with axonal projections to the limbic system, midbrain, and reticular areas.[45,238] Dynorphins are located in the spinal cord, hypothalamus, and pituitary gland.[45] These areas are important in autonomic regulation and suggest an association between the opioid peptides and autonomic function.

Opiate Antagonists

NALOXONE (RECEPTOR-SPECIFIC)

Naloxone's effectiveness in reversing the hypotension of experimental shock has suggested an important role for the endogenous opioids in the pathogenesis of shock states. Naloxone has no effect on blood pressure in normotensive controls, and acts at central or peripheral cardiovascular sites to improve hemodynamics in experimental shock,[63,129,131] an effect that depends upon the integrity of the adrenal medulla.[127] In spinal shock, naloxone's effects are stereospecific and are mediated by the parasympathetic nervous system,[63,131] and by enhanced dopamine release.[62] Although termed a "pure and specific" opiate receptor antagonist, naloxone is "neither a pure antago-

nist under all conditions, nor completely selective."[58] At lower dosages, naloxone is approximately 10 to 20 times more selective for the μ rather than the δ-binding sites[34] but at higher dosages (such as those used in experimental shock) it interacts with both the μ- and δ-receptors. At these higher dosages (1 to 2 mg/kg) naloxone may alter calcium flux and lipid peroxidation, effects that opiate receptors probably do not mediate.[57] Naloxone is also able to alter the effects of some nonopiate depressants. In summary, although not a perfect opiate receptor antagonist, naloxone is an extremely useful tool, in that effective naloxone–opiate antagonism is *a necessary but not sufficient* criterion to invoke the endogenous opioids as causal in any given shock state. Sawynok et al.[199] proposed five criteria that should be met before endogenous opiates can be implicated in any given effect: (1) cross-tolerance to morphine, (2) the same effect with other opiate antagonists, (3) inactivity of stereoisomers lacking opiate antagonist activity, (4) release and increase of opioid peptides in the pathophysiologic state believed to be caused by opioid peptides, (5) potentiation of effect by agents that inhibit breakdown of endogenous opioid peptides.

A number of other opiate receptor antagonists exist that differ from naloxone in duration of action and receptor selectivity. The newer, more μ-receptor-selective, antagonists include naloxazone[187] and B funaltrexamine.[223] ICI 154129 is a more selective δ-receptor antagonist.[205] The effectiveness of these antagonists in shock states is being investigated.

THYROTROPIN-RELEASING HORMONE

Thyrotropin-releasing hormone (TRH) is a tripeptide that stimulates the release of thyroid-stimulating hormone and prolactin from the pituitary gland. It also has pharmacologic effects antagonistic to those of the opiates except that it does not reverse opiate-induced analgesia.[135] Because it does not bind to opiate receptors, TRH is termed a physiologic opiate antagonist. Thyrotropin-releasing hormone is present throughout the CNS and has a number of physiologic roles associated with its thyroid regulation.[251] Central administration of TRH can induce opiate-like withdrawal.[44] Its serum half-life is approximately 6 minutes.[177]

Opioid Systems in the Pathophysiology of Shock

ENDOTOXIC SHOCK

Based on the hypothesis that pain and shock might be connected via involvement of the endogenous opioid system, Holaday and Faden[132] demonstrated rapid naloxone reversal of the hypotension of endotoxin-induced shock in rats. With naloxone pretreatment (Fig. 6-2) an effect occurred at dosages of 0.1 mg/kg, but maximal hemodynamic effects occurred at dosages greater than 1 mg/kg/hr.[61,128] Rebolusing was sometimes required (Fig. 6-3). Survival was not improved in this model. Reynolds et al.[195] administered naloxone (2 mg/kg IV bolus and then a 2 mg/kg/hr infusion for 4 hours versus saline controls) after endotoxin-induced

hypotension in dogs. They found that naloxone improved systemic blood pressure, cardiac output, and 24-hour survival. These results have since been reconfirmed.[191] The beneficial effects of naloxone are stereospecific and dose-related[60] (prerequisites for claiming a specific opioid receptor effect). Carr et al.[32] have shown a biphasic increase in plasma β-endorphin (B-EP) levels after small doses of endotoxin in sheep, with an early 10-fold rise occurring *prior to* hypotension, suggesting a causal relationship. Naloxone administration *increased* β-endorphin release, suggesting that inhibition of release is not a factor in naloxone-induced shock reversal. Faden and Holaday[60] showed further decreases in systemic blood pressure with morphine or β-endorphin infusions following endotoxin-induced hypotension. These effects were reversed with naloxone. Rats injected with endotoxin have increased pain tolerance, an effect that is reversible with naloxone.[13]

The role of the opioid system in endotoxic shock may be at least partially mediated by the adrenal gland. The susceptibility to experimental endotoxin shock is increased (by > 60-

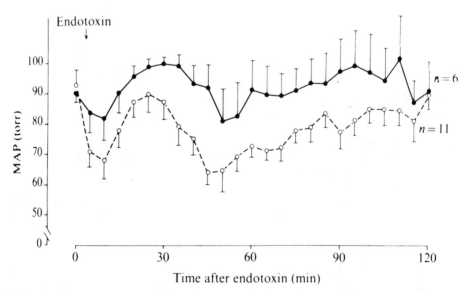

FIG. 6-2 Naloxone pretreatment. Effects on 2 hr MAP measurements after endotoxin. Pretreatment using 10 mg/kg (●) blocked the effects of 4 mg endotoxin on MAP. The groups treated with 4 mg endotoxin alone (○) had significantly lower MAP compared with preendotoxin controls. Vertical bars are ± SEM. (Holaday JW, Faden AI: Naloxone reversal of endotoxin hypotension suggests role of endorphins in shock. Nature 275:451, © 1978 by Macmillan Journals Limited.)

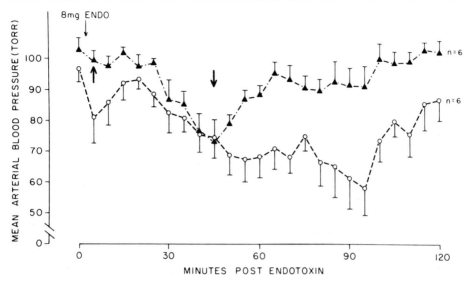

FIG. 6-3 Reversal of endotoxin shock by naloxone. After injection of 8 mg endotoxin, rats received naloxone 10 mg/kg (▲) or saline (○) after MAP reached 65 to 70 mmHg (torr). Large arrows indicate naloxone injections. Importantly, some animals required reinjection with naloxone because endotoxin effects were biphasic. Naloxone injections improved MAP. Vertical bars are ± SEM. (Holaday JW, Faden AI: Naloxone reversal of endotoxin hypotension suggests role of endorphins in shock. Nature 275:451, © 1978 by Macmillan Journals Limited.)

fold) by prior adrenalectomy in rats.[100,130,255,256] Glucocorticoid administration, which decreases circulating endogenous[127] opioid peptide levels, diminished the lethal effects of preshock adrenalectomy. Selective adrenal demedullation decreases resistance to endotoxin-induced shock in the rat and eliminates the efficacy of naloxone in shock.[127] These data suggest that endorphin release may inhibit sympathoadrenal discharge and naloxone may improve hemodynamic parameters and survival in animal models of sepsis. In addition naloxone therapy attenuates the often-observed sepsis-related decreases in platelets, polymorphonuclear leukocytes, and core temperature, and corrects sepsis-associated hypoglycemia and acidosis.[59,191]

HEMORRHAGIC SHOCK

In rats subjected to hemorrhagic shock, naloxone improves systemic blood pressure and survival compared to saline controls. In canine hypovolemia, naloxone (2 mg/kg bolus and 2 mg/kg/hr) improves inotropic function and prolongs survival[103,104,234] (Fig. 6-4). Naloxone is also effective (probably acting via a central mechanism)[133] in improving the hemodynamic parameters of hemorrhaged cats,[47] rabbits,[200] and cynomologus monkeys.

SPINAL SHOCK

Holaday and Faden[131] demonstrated decreases in body temperature, arterial blood pressure, and respirations following C7 spinal cord transections in rats. These effects were reversible with 10 mg/kg of naloxone. A small dose (48 μg) of naloxone administered peripherally had no antihypotensive effect, but the same dose given directly into the lateral cerebral ventricle reversed the spinal cord transection-induced hypotension, which suggests at least partial central mediation of naloxone's effect. Vagotomy after cord transection prevented the effectiveness of centrally administered naloxone in reversing this hypotension which suggests vagal mediation of the naloxone effect. Faden et al.[62] demonstrated (in the cat model of spinal shock) a correlation be-

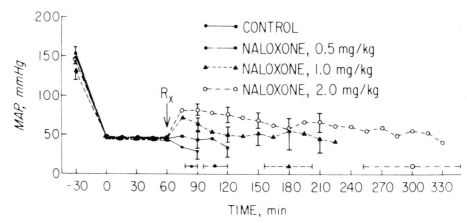

FIG. 6-4 Effect of naloxone on MAP in canine hemorrhagic shock. Values are means ± SEM for treatments shown. Naloxone produces a dose-dependent improvement in MAP when given as a bolus at + = 60 minutes followed by an infusion from + = 60 to 240 minutes intravenously. Blood reinfusion at + = 120 minutes returns MAP to baseline values in dogs that received the two higher doses of naloxone. (Gurll NJ, Vargish T, Reynolds DG, Lechner R: Opiate receptors and endorphins in the pathophysiology of hemorrhagic shock. Surgery 89:364, 1981.)

tween improved hemodynamics, centrally administered naloxone, and increased plasma dopamine levels (partially negated by the use of the dopamine antagonist, domperidone), which suggest a vagus-dopaminergic interaction. Naloxone therapy in feline spinal shock also improved neurologic recovery.[65]

Thyrotropin-Releasing Hormone: A Physiological Opiate Antagonist

Thyrotropin-releasing hormone (TRH) improves the hemodynamic variables of both hypovolemic and endotoxic shock[102,126,134] (Fig. 6-5). Blood pressure improvement and survival in rat endotoxic shock are dependent on the dose of TRH.[134] It improves neurologic recovery and survival in cats after cervical spinal trauma.[64]

The therapeutic mechanism of TRH's action in shock remains only partially defined. Most likely, TRH acts as both a physiologic opiate antagonist and as an antagonist of leukotrienes.[168] It is probably not effective via its known thyroid-stimulating properties (1) be-

cause the direct cardiovascular effects of TRH occur within minutes whereas secondary TRH-induced increases in triiodothyronine and thyroxine require several hours;[126,165] (2) because direct TRH effects remain after hypophysectomy of the rat and occur even with very low-dose direct intraventricular instillation; and (3) because TRH analogues causing much greater hemodynamic effects than TRH are only equipotent in stimulating the pituitary–thyroid axis.[135,174] If not via thyroid hormone stimulation, then how is TRH effective as shock therapy? Unlike naloxone, TRH elevates blood pressure in control rats,[102,126,134] apparently via a pressor effect[254] that remains intact in animals with spinal transections below T1, but not in the cervical region, and is not affected by autonomic (sympathetic or parasympathetic) agonists or antagonists.[11,136,254] This implies that normal autonomic pathways are not important in this pressor effect. Intravenous TRH retains its pressor effects in endotoxic shock in the rat with prior adrenal demedullation. However, it is ineffective when instilled directly into the cerebral ventricles in rat endotoxic shock in association with this same prior demedullation, which implies multiple activity pathways. Important preliminary findings[127] suggest that TRH and naloxone may be additive in the treatment of experimental shock.

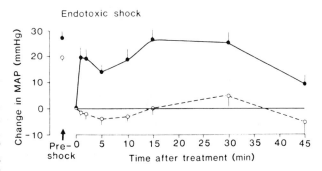

Endotoxic shock

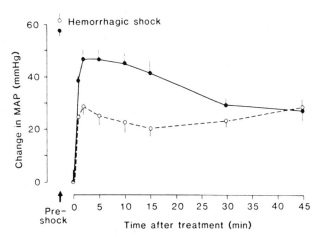

Hemorrhagic shock

FIG. 6-5 Rats received intravenous injections of either TRH (2 mg/kg; solid lines) or an equal volume of saline (dashed lines) after they were subjected to endotoxic (top) or hemorrhagic (bottom) shock hypotension. The data are expressed as changes in MAP prior to shock (preshock) and at various times after drug treatment at time 0. Vertical bars indicate the standard error of the mean; populations of rats and absolute MAP values are defined in the text. A significant increase in MAP was observed when comparing time-integrated area responses from TRH-treated rats with saline controls. (Holaday JW, D'Amato RJ, Faden AI: Thyrotropin-releasing hormone improves cardiovascular function in experimental endotoxic and hemorrhagic shock. Science 213:217, © 1981 by Macmillan Journals Limited.)

Summary

There are numerous opiate receptors, but κ and δ seem to be most important in mediating shock states. There are presently three classes of endogenous opiates, all of which are probably important in mediating various shock states. With the use of the relatively specific opiate receptor antagonist, naloxone, and the physiologic opiate antagonist, TRH, good *animal* data show that the opioid system is important in the pathophysiology of hemorrhagic, endotoxic, and spinal shock. At present, neither naloxone nor TRH is approved by the Food and Drug Administration for use in any form of human shock; they are at present only experimental. We await well-designed clinical trials in humans to demonstrate the efficacy (or lack of efficacy) of these agents in shock states.

STEROIDS AND SHOCK

Corticosteroids have been used in the therapy of shock for more than twenty years. Steroid therapy is *not* useful in hemorrhagic shock[16,190] and may be deleterious in cardiogenic shock;[197] however, steroid use in septic shock may be beneficial but remains controversial.

Several studies have demonstrated that steroids improve survival in experimental septic shock models. Hinshaw et al.[14,116-118] demonstrated in successive experiments (using live *E. coli* infusions) that (1) antibiotics and steroids in combination result in better 7-day survival (100 percent) than antibiotic therapy alone (0 percent survival); (2) early combination treatment (begun within 30 minutes of the initiation of the *E. coli* infusion) improves survival (100 percent) more than late institution of combination therapy. If steroid therapy was begun after the total dose of *E. coli* was infused, the survival was 85 percent at 7 days. If steroid therapy was begun after hypotension had persisted for 4 hours, the survival rate was 65 percent. In canine endotoxin shock, White et al.[241] showed 0 percent 7-day survival, if steroid therapy was initiated within 15 minutes of the onset of an endotoxin *bolus;* there was 83 percent 7-day survival if the steroid infusion was initiated within 15 minutes after the intitation of a 5-hour endotoxin *infusion.* Using the canine *E. coli* infusion model, Hinshaw et al.[119] demonstrated 0 percent 7-day survival if a steroid bolus was given within 15 minutes of the start of the *E. coli* infusion, 20 percent 7-day survival after antibiotic therapy alone, and 100 percent 7-day survival when giving combination antibiotic–steroid therapy within 15 minutes of the start of the *E. coli* infusion. Beller et al.,[14] using the same canine live *E. coli* model of sepsis, demonstrated that early (within 15 minutes) initiation of bolus steroids combined with bolus gentamicin therapy produced 57 percent 7-day survival, whereas therapy begun at the same time using a prolonged steroid infusion combined with bolus gentamicin produced 100 percent 7-day survival. With a slightly less toxic dose of bolus endotoxin in the dog, Hinshaw et al.[123] demonstrated a 47 percent 7-day survival using bolus steroids *alone* when therapy was started within 15 minutes of the endotoxin dose, as opposed to 20 percent 7-day survival after endotoxin injection alone. In the mouse, using a live *E. coli* intravenous infusion and intraperitoneal injections as their septic shock model, Greisman et al.[97,98] demonstrated that not only was early initiation of combination therapy important for maximum survival, but that, at least in mice, too low a dose (10 mg/kg or less) or too great a dose (60 mg/kg or greater) reduced the steroids' protective effect. In the *E. coli* infusion and cecal ligation–puncture models of septic shock in *rats* [10,56,189,224] as well, the early institution of combination antibiotic–steroid therapy produced optimal results. Steroids alone increased survival very little. Therefore, there is evidence that in the dog, mouse, rat, and baboon, and whether using endotoxin, live *E. coli,* or cecal ligation as models of septic shock, *early* combination antibiotic–steroid therapy maximizes survival. The dose and duration of infusion of steroid may also be important.

Why might steroids be effective in reducing mortality in septic shock?

1. Septic shock, particularly in its later stages in humans, is often characterized by decreased cardiac output and increased peripheral vascular resistance, as well as decreased regional blood flow. Steroids increase cardiac output[248] inotropy,[148,225] and perfusion to the brain, kidney, liver, and heart.[55,123] There is also steroid-induced local vasodilation.[3,49,55,123,148]

2. Microcirculatory damage in septic shock may be caused by complement–polymorphonuclear-leukocyte interactions that lead to endothelial damage[31,108,111] and subsequent release of white cell products. These leukocyte products may create the capillary leakage, such as in the pulmonary circulation, that is commonly associated with septic shock.[184] Steroids may protect the endothelium from white-cell-mediated damage,[7,24,207] stabilize lysosomal membranes, [155,217] prevent platelet aggregation and DIC, and prevent the initiation of the complement–white-cell interaction.[108,184]

3. In animal models of septic shock, hepatic damage, and concomitant hypoglycemia (blood glucose levels less than 50 mg/dl) are common and often associated with death.[68,116-118,120,121] Steroid administration stimulates glucose production in endotoxin-induced primate sepsis. As an associated metabolic finding in septic shock in animals, insulin levels are often reduced. Steroid–antibiotic therapy normalizes insulin levels, and prevents hypoglycemia and death.[117,119,241]

4. Mitochondrial oxidative function is disrupted in canine (live *E. coli*-induced) and rat (endotoxin-induced) septic shock. Early steroid therapy prevents this disruption of cellular function.[171,172]

5. β-endorphin, as well as ACTH, is released from the pituitary in stress[130,255] and it is believed that endorphins may cause or exacerbate the hypotension of septic shock. Exogenous steroids, via feedback inhibition, decrease not only ACTH but also pituitary β-endorphin release. However, it is not clear

that the pituitary is the source of β-endorphin.

These are proposed mechanisms of action for steroid efficacy in experimental septic shock. Are there complications associated with short-term, pharmacologic doses of steroids? A National Institutes of Health conference in 1976[66] concluded that proposed steroid-induced defects in phagocytic function are probably exaggerated. Hinshaw et al.[115] found no deleterious effects of short-term steroid on phagocytic function. Schumer,[201] in the only large recent series of steroid use in human septic shock, found an associated complication rate of 5 percent and little to justify concern that short-term boluses of corticosteroids cause complications similar to those that arise with long-term steroid therapy. However, Sprung et al.[218] found an increased rate of superinfection, at least with the use of dexamethasone in septic shock.

Having outlined convincing work that (1) demonstrates improved survival in experimental septic shock using early combination steroid–antibiotic therapy, (2) explores the multiple proposed mechanisms of steroid efficacy in septic shock, and (3) emphasizes the relative safety of short-term pharmacologic dose steroids, why is steroid usage in septic shock still controversial? In 1974, Weitzman and Berger[240] reviewed 32 previous studies of the efficacy of steroids as therapy for bacterial infections and sepsis. They wrote[240] that

only 44 percent used a concurrent control, 41 percent were prospective experimental trials, 84 percent did not use a double blind technique, and 75 percent did not allocate treatment in a random manner. Only 59 percent of the studies adequately described criteria for diagnosis of the illness treated. . . . The reports on steroid therapy for septic shock adhered less to methodologic standards than did other studies.

The authors suggested that only well-designed clinical trials could help dispel the controversy surrounding the use of steroids in septic shock. In 1976, Schumer[201] published an 8-year prospective (n = 172) and retrospective (n = 328) evaluation of the use of steroids in human septic shock. He attempted to correct for previous inadequacies of study design.[201]

The prospective study was controlled, double blind, and randomized. Both studies make specific reference to diagnostic criteria, severity of shock, presence of underlying condition, complications and statistical methodology and . . . [the study was] concerned very strictly with only two criteria, mortality rate and complication rate.

In the retrospective analysis, mortality for patients treated with steroid–antibiotic "supportive measures" was 14 percent. Without steroids, the mortality was 42.5 percent. In the prospective study, the mortality of patients treated with antibiotic-steroid-"supportive measures" was 10.4 percent, and 38.4 percent without steroids. But Young[252] criticized the study for (1) using two different steroid preparations; (2) lacking a specific discussion of "supportive measures," such as hemodynamic monitoring, used to treat the patients; (3) using differing antibiotic regimens; (4) associating deaths with septic shock that occurred up to 4 weeks after the acute episodes; and (5) having an unusually low mortality in the steroid-treated group of patients. In an editorial in 1981, Sheagren[203] wrote, "the use of a massive dose of a glucocorticoid in the patient with septic shock remains controversial. It is clear that a prospective, randomized study is needed." In 1984, Sprung et al.[218] published a smaller 3-year prospective study of 59 patients with septic shock. All patients had received antibiotic therapy and were then randomized to receive either no steroids, 30 mg/kg methylprednisolone, or 6 mg/kg dexamethasone. They found no difference in outcome and a possible increase in the incidence of superinfections with the use of dexamethasone.

If useful at all, the efficacy of steroids as adjunctive therapy to antibiotics in the treatment of septic shock seems to depend upon early administration, but how early? In the laboratory, the initiation of the septic insult is well-defined but at the bedside it is not. Do animal models of sepsis (endotoxin, live *E. coli,* or cecal ligation) really duplicate human sepsis? Do mice, rats, dogs, or primates react the same way as humans to septic shock?

Schumer,[201] despite criticisms of his study, did demonstrate considerable benefit in the use of the steroid–antibiotic combination as therapy for human sepsis. However, Spring et al.[218] did not. We hope that other well-designed human studies will further clarify the value of steroids in septic shock. At present, the controversy continues.

EXOGENOUS CATECHOLAMINES AND SHOCK

Unlike prostaglandins and opiate antagonists, which for the present at least, remain experimental as shock therapies, exogenous catecholamines are important therapeutic agents for patients in shock. In this section we review catecholamine biochemical structure, adrenergic receptor physiology (see references 125, 158, 159, and 178 for more extensive discussions), the most commonly used catecholamines, and their role in the treatment of specific types of shock.

Biochemical Structure

The core "catechol" contains a benzene ring hydroxylated at the 3 and 4 carbon positions (Fig. 6-6). Adding an amine in the form of an ethyl-amine side-chain produces a "catecholamine." Subsequent substitutions at the terminal amine group alter the compound's affinity for specific adrenergic receptors.[239,256] Sympathomimetics have catecholamine-like activity but do not have the same biochemical structure (Fig. 6-6).

Receptor Binding

Before discussing the catecholamines themselves, it is important to outline basic adrenergic receptor physiology, because these re-

ceptors mediate the known catecholamine effects. Adrenergic receptors are cell surface membrane bound glycoproteins. The original concept of a specific adrenergic receptor was introduced in 1905.[152] Adrenergic receptors were subdivided into α and β subtypes by Ahlquist in 1948,[2] based on their relative tissue responsiveness to various catecholamines. β-Receptors have since been subdivided into β_2 and β_2,[151] α-receptors into α_1 and α_2,[125] and most recently described are the dopamine$_1$ (D_1) receptors.[91]

β-RECEPTORS

β_1-Adrenergic receptors are located on the myocardial cells at the postsynaptic myoneural junction and predominantly mediate cardiac sympathomimetic effects.[220] Activation of the β_1-receptor increases both inotropy and chronotropy. Because they are also found on the surface of adipose cells, β_1-adrenergic receptor stimulation increases lipolysis.[178]

β_2-Receptors are located on vascular and bronchial smooth muscle cells and stimulation of these receptors produces vasodilatation of the pulmonary, mesenteric, and skeletal vascular beds as well as bronchodilatation.[90,173,245] These same receptors are also located on hepatocytes, pancreatic islet cells, neutrophils, and lymphocytes. β_2-Receptor stimulation causes increased hepatic glucose production, increased insulin release, and decreased granulocyte lysosomal release. Both β_1- and β_2-receptors increase cellular metabolic activity, probably by increasing the intracellular production of cyclic AMP, which in turn stimulates increased cellular enzymatic activity.[159]

α-RECEPTORS

α_1-Receptors are located on the postsynaptic membrane of the myoneural junction of vascular and genitourinary smooth muscle. Stimulation in the periphery produces vasoconstriction,[90,159] which is calcium-dependent.[219]

α_2-Receptors are located predominantly in the presynaptic regions of vascular beds where stimulation produces decreased norepineph-

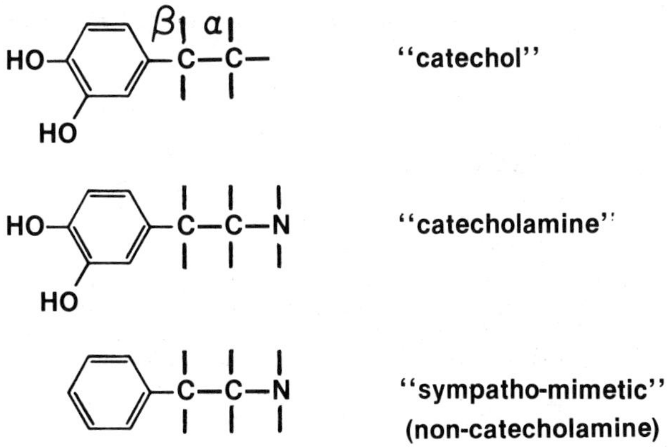

β_1 α_1

"catechol"

"catecholamine"

"sympatho-mimetic"
(non-catecholamine)

FIG. 6-6 The structure of catechols, catecholamines, and sympathomimetics. (Legan E, Chernow B: The catecholamine response to critical illness. Semin Respir Med 7(1): 88, 1985, with permission.)

rine release and vasodilatation. α_2-Receptors on pancreatic islet cells and adopocytes also inhibit both insulin release and lipolysis; α_2-receptors on vascular smooth muscle mediate vasoconstriction.[125]

DOPAMINE RECEPTORS

Dopamine$_1$ (D$_1$) receptors are found on the postsynaptic membranes of the cerebral, coronary, mesenteric, and renal vascular beds,[87,90] and stimulation produces vasodilation. Dopamine$_2$ (D$_2$) receptors are presynaptic and their stimulation inhibits norepinephrine release across the synaptic cleft.[91]

ADRENERGIC RECEPTOR REGULATION

The extent and length of exposure to catecholamines, whether exogenous, or endogenous, regulate the number and function of adrenergic receptors. Catecholamine depletion, or the use of catecholamine antagonists,[1] may result in increased sensitivity to catecholamines, due to increased receptor density on the cell surface, termed "up-regulation."[20,202] This may explain the increased risk of myocardial infarction or exacerbation of clinical unstable angina after abrupt withdrawal or β-adrenergic receptor antagonists.[202]

In contrast, prolonged, or even short-term exposure (1 to 6 hours), to catecholamines[228] may produce "down-regulation" of adrenergic receptors or catecholamine "desensitization."

Catecholamines Used in Shock Therapy

NOREPINEPHRINE

Norepinephrine (NE) stimulates α-adrenergic receptors and β_1-receptors but has little β_2-receptor activity (Table 6-2). In pharmacologic dosages it causes α_1 stimulation and consequent vasoconstriction. Norepinephrine constricts both veins and arteries. Therefore norepinephrine increases preload (by increasing venous return of blood to the heart), afterload (by increasing systemic vascular resistance), and myocardial contractility (by its β_1 stimulation), resulting in increased cardiac oxygen demand and work load. Despite these NE-induced changes, cardiac output usually remains unchanged or slightly decreased. Norepinephrine also increases coronary artery blood flow because of the increased gradient between mean arterial pressure (MAP) and left ventricular end-diastolic pressure (LVEDP) and because of NE-induced myocardial stimulation.[141] Norepinephrine constricts the renal arterial bed (cortex greater than medulla) and this may be angiotensin-II-mediated.[17] Glomerular filtration (GFR) remains unchanged, because of an increased filtration fraction, until vasoconstriction becomes intense, producing markedly diminished renal blood flow and a falling GFR. Norepinephrine causes hepatic and splanchnic vasoconstriction[96] as well as decreased intestinal motility and muscle tone.[85] It produces carotid and aortic-body-induced respiratory stimulation, and in-

TABLE 6-2. Catecholamine Effects on Adrenergic Receptors

Catecholamine	Receptor				
	Alpha$_1$	Alpha$_2$	Beta$_1$	Beta$_2$	DA
Epinephrine	+++	+++	+++	+++	0
Norepinephrine	+++	+++	+++	+	0
Isoproterenol	0	0	+++	+++	0
Dopamine[a]	0 to +++	+	++ to +++	++	+++
Dobutamine	0 to +	0	+++	+	0

+, relative degree of stimulation; 0, no stimulation.

[a] Variable, dose-dependent effects. High doses produce predominant α-adrenergic effects.

(Zaritsky A: Catecholamines and sympathomimetics. p. 483. In Chernow B, Lake CR (eds): The Pharmacologic Approach to the Critically Ill Patient. Williams & Wilkins, Baltimore, 1983.)

creases pulmonary vascular resistance. It does not constrict cerebral blood vessels, and in animals, even increases cerebral blood flow.[170] With NE infusions associated with high blood NE levels (greater than 1800 pg/ml),[209] elevations of plasma glucose, acetoacetate, B-hydroxy butyrate, and glycerol have been observed. The half-life of NE is approximately 2.5 minutes[209] and it is cleared via re-uptake in specific neuronal and extraneuronal sites,[46] and by hepatic and renal enzymatic degradation. Through intense vasoconstriction, NE can produce renal, mesenteric, and peripheral ischemia. Boluses of NE may cause severe hypertension secondary to arterial vasoconstriction, causing myocardial ischemia, myocardial infarction, or cerebral hemorrhage.[239] The primary indication for NE is the need for vasoconstriction to elevate blood pressure when other vasoconstrictors, such as high-dose dopamine, are not effective. The side effects of NE are also the direct result of vasoconstriction, but when indicated, may be helpful in the treatment of shock.

EPINEPHRINE

Epinephrine stimulates both α- and β-adrenergic receptors, with lower-dose epinephrine enhancing β- and higher dose-increasing α-adrenergic receptor activity. Via its β_1-stimulating effects, epinephrine augments cardiac inotropy, chronotropy, and cardiac output. It increases conduction velocity through the Sinoatrial (SA) and arterioventricular (A-V) node, accelerates the firing of ectopic foci, and decreases the refractory period of the myocardium in general. With predominant β-adrenergic receptor stimulation (dosages of 0.1 to 0.4 mg/kg/min), epinephrine increases *systolic* blood pressure without changing, and possibly decreasing diastolic blood pressure, the result of peripheral, β-receptor-mediated arterial vasodilatation. The epinephrine-induced increases in inotropy and heart rate result in an increase in myocardial oxygen consumption, although coronary blood flow may be increased.[239] At lower doses, because of epinephrine's predominant β-mediated arterial vasodilatation, there is less of an increase in myocardial wall tension than with NE. However, as with NE, the balance usually favors decreased cardiac efficiency (work/oxygen consumption), which may predispose to ischemia and arrhythmias.[141,226] With infusion rates greater than 20 μg/min, there is usually predominant α activity, causing intense, diffuse vasoconstriction with associated increases in preload and afterload. There are simultaneous decreases in renal, mucocutaneous, and skeletal blood flow, predisposing to ischemia in these areas. At infusion rates as low as 2 μg/min, epinephrine decreases renal blood flow (by about 10 percent) while infusion rates of 9 μg/min decrease plasma flow[94] through the kidney by approximately 25 percent. Until there is intense catecholamine-induced vasoconstriction, GFR may be maintained by catecholamine-mediated increases in the filtration fraction. Epinephrine also causes renin and angiotensin release via β stimulation of the juxtaglomerular apparatus, which may mediate further increases in blood pressure.[232] Epinephrine relaxes the bronchial smooth muscles via β_2-receptor stimulation, an effect that makes it the drug of choice for treatment of acute asthma and anaphylaxis. It decreases GI tract smooth muscle tone (β-effect) and decreases gut motility (α effect),[85] and also decreases perfusion to the stomach and small bowel.[259] It does not cause any direct cerebral vasoconstriction (epinephrine has poor CNS penetration) and in fact, probably increases cerebral blood flow by increasing the systemic blood pressure without altering cerebral vascular resistance, making it useful in cardiopulmonary resuscitation (CPR). In hepatocytes, epinephrine causes increased glucose production both by glycogenolysis and gluconeogenesis, as well as increased glycogen degradation in skeletal muscle. Epinephrine decreases insulin secretion via α-receptor stimulation and increases insulin secretion via β-stimulation, with the former effect predominating. Muscle protein catabolism is decreased[253] and, through stimulation of β-adrenergic adipocyte receptors, epinephrine enhances free fatty acid production. It is used as an in vitro stimulant to platelet aggregation, enhancing the effect of other platelet aggregating agents.[208] Epinephrine causes demargination of polymorphonuclear leukocytes and decreases leukocyte adherence.

As with NE, epinephrine is cleared within minutes, primarily by catechol-O-methyl transferase, which is concentrated in various organs, as well as by postganglionic sympathetic nerve re-uptake.[46] The major side effects of epinephrine infusions are the direct result, at lower doses, of its potent cardiac stimulation (β-mediated) and at higher doses from its vasoconstiction (α-mediated). β-Effects include ectopy, tachycardia, hypertension, and myocardial ischemia. α-Effects include hypertension, myocardial ischemia, as well as diffuse intense vasoconstriction of the mucocutaneous, splanchnic, and renal vasculature. As with NE, the desired effects of epinephrine may also precipitate the undesired side effects. Epinephrine's primary indication is for potent inotropy without the intense vasoconstriction of NE (at lower doses), for asthmatic associated bronchodilatation, and for anaphylaxis.

ISOPROTERENOL

Isoproterenol is a β-adrenergic agonist (both β_1 and β_2) with minimal α-adrenergic activity. Because of its generalized β-adrenergic effects, it is a potent cardiac stimulant and peripheral (particularly skeletal muscle) vasodilator.

Isoproterenol, via β_1-stimulation, is both a potent inotrope and chronotrope increasing myocardial oxygen consumption. Isoproterenol decreases LVEDP (preload), a β_2-mediated effect. Isoproterenol may cause some secondary increase in coronary artery blood flow[162] but generally the increase in cardiac work is greater than the increase in oxygen delivery, decreasing myocardial efficiency. Although isoproterenol increases MAP, blood flow may be shunted preferentially to skeletal muscle rather than to the splanchnic or renal arterial bed. The β_2-adrenergic-stimulated vasodilatation of isoproterenol may cause a decrease in arterial blood pressure further compromising vital organ perfusion.

Isoproterenol causes bronchial smooth muscle relaxation,[245] decreases pulmonary vascular resistance,[173] and may increase intrapulmonary shunt. Like epinephrine, isoproterenol stimulates adipocyte β-adrenergic receptors, increasing lipolysis,[239] however, because of its relatively pure β activity, isoproterenol increases insulin release (islet cell β-receptor-mediated), thereby minimizing any hyperglycemic effect. Isoproterenol is indicated for hypotension associated with bradycardia, status asthmaticus (particularly in children), and as a second-line agent to increase cardiac contractility.

DOPAMINE

Dopamine (the endogenous precursor of NE; Fig. 6-7) has its pharmacologic actions mediated by three adrenergic receptors, depending upon the rate of IV infusion. At infusion rates of 0.5 to 2 μg/kg/min, dopamine increases

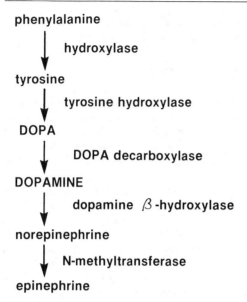

phenylalanine

→ hydroxylase

tyrosine

→ tyrosine hydroxylase

DOPA

→ DOPA decarboxylase

DOPAMINE

→ dopamine β-hydroxylase

norepinephrine

→ N-methyltransferase

epinephrine

FIG. 6-7 The endogenous catecholamine synthetic pathway. (Legan E, Chernow B: The catecholamine response to critical illness. Semin Respir Med 7(1): 88, 1985, with permission.)

renal blood flow, and GFR.[87] Urine sodium excretion is enhanced by a possible direct dopamine–renal tubular cell interaction[88,114] or by dopamine-induced *decreases* in aldosterone secretion.[91,242] Usually dopamine infusion rates between 2 and 5 μg/kg/min cause continued dopaminergic receptor stimulation associated with β-adrenergic-mediated increases in inotropy without important increases in heart rate, MAP, or peripheral resistance.[88,89] Infusion rates greater than 5 μg/kg/min cause a predominantly β-mediated effect, with probably a small residual of dopaminergic-mediated effects, as well as causing some endogenous release of NE.[146] At rates above 10 μg/kg/min, infusions of dopamine begin to produce α-adrenergic vasoconstriction with renal vascular constriction.[87,89] At infusion rates above 20 μg/kg/min, dopamine is almost entirely a potent vasoconstrictor via α-adrenergic stimulation. Dopamine-induced venoconstriction increases preload, myocardial wall tension, and therefore the tendency towards transudative pulmonary edema.[166] Increased inotropy may worsen intrapulmonary shunt by increasing blood flow to poorly ventilated areas of the lung,[144] and one investigator demonstrated an exacerbation

of hypoxic vasoconstriction associated with dopamine use.[173] Less often recognized dopamine effects include D_2-receptor stimulated inhibition of TSH and prolactin release from the anterior pituitary gland, and pancreatic islet cell inhibition of insulin release.[257]

Dopamine-induced side effects include hypertension, myocardial or peripheral ischemia, severe tachycardia, and arrhythmias. Because of its unique selective renal vasodilating effects at low doses, dopamine is indicated to improve renal blood flow and urine output, and at higher doses to increase inotropy, and at still higher doses to produce and increase blood pressure by causing vasoconstriction of peripheral arteries.

DOBUTAMINE

Dobutamine (Fig. 6-8) is almost exclusively a β_1-agonist, whose predominant effect is to increase cardiac contractility. It has very little β_2-adrenergic or α-adrenergic effect (Table 6-2).[89,215,229,235] It is less chronotropic than isoproterenol (an effect that is at least partially mediated by β_2-adrenergic cardiac receptors).[246] Dobutamine augments S-A node automaticity and increases A-V node and ventricular rates of conduction.[167] These are apparently direct dobutamine-stimulated β_1-adrenergic receptor effects without secondary dopaminergic activation or NE release.[215,229,235] Dobutamine may produce dose-dependent improvement in myocardial contractility without changes in either blood pressure or heart rate,[86,89,160,161,214] although limited β_2-stimulated vasodilatation[198,229] and heart rate-increases[50,160] can occur. At approximately 10 μg/kg/min, dobutamine usually improves cardiac output (CO), LVEDP, and LVSWI in patients with failing left ventricles. Dobutamine tends to decrease myocardial oxygen consumption. In septic shock, dobutamine increases LVSWI, MAP, and cardiac index (CI).[145] Dobutamine, unlike dopamine, has no specific effects on the renal vasculature. In the canine model, using dobutamine in dosages greater than 8 μg/kg/min, investigators demonstrated that the percentage of cardiac output provided to the kidney decreased relative to other vascular beds including the skeletal muscle vasculature.[198,235.] In human shock, dobuta-

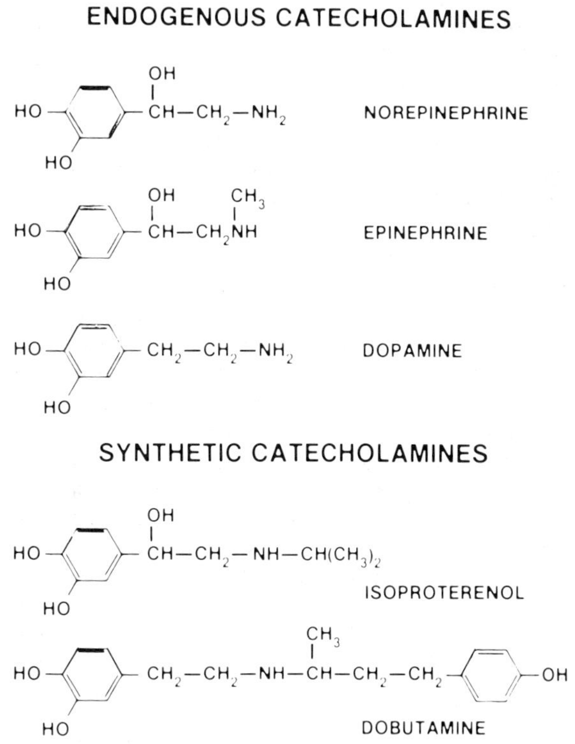

ENDOGENOUS CATECHOLAMINES

FIG. 6-8 The structure of endogenous and synthetic catecholamines. (Legan E, Chernow B: The catecholamine response to critical illness. Semin Respir Med 7(1): 88, 1985, with permission.)

SYNTHETIC CATECHOLAMINES

mine causes both urine output and cardiac output to increase.[161] As a result of alterations in blood flow relative to poorly ventilated areas, dobutamine, like epinephrine and isproterenol, can cause an increase in intrapulmonary shunt.

Dobutamine's major side effects include arrhythmias, hypertension, myocardial ischemia, and sometimes tachycardia. Dobutamine is a positive inotrope. As such it is indicated as therapy for septic shock (when cardiac output is insufficient), in congestive heart failure (CHF), and in cardiogenic shock.

Catecholamine Therapy in Specific Shock States

CARDIOGENIC SHOCK

Cardiogenic shock, particularly as the result of an acute myocardial infarction, excluding mechanical lesions such as papillary muscle rupture, has a mortality rate greater than 90 percent. Less often, primary myocardial failure can occur secondary to viral cardiac infections, sepsis, hypovolemia, or postcardiopulmonary bypass. Cardiogenic shock is the most severe form of acute congestive heart failure.

Plasma NE and epinephrine levels are increased in patients with congestive heart failure, and markedly elevated plasma NE levels may reflect more severe disease.[35,93,163] However, patients with severe CHF may have decreases in myocardial NE stores and possibly increased urinary catecholamine clearance.[35] In addition, in those patients with severe CHF (New York Heart Association Class IV) who require heart transplantation, the density of cardiac β-adrenergic receptors is decreased.[23]

Generally the combination of inotropic support (catecholamines) and mechanical or chemical vasodilator therapy is most effective in treating cardiogenic shock. Dopamine, dobutamine, and epinephrine are the most useful inotropes in this type of shock. Dopamine, in β-agonist dosages, can increase the cardiac output in cardiogenic shock but it also increases the oxygen consumption. Vasoconstriction (seen with high dosages of dopamine) should be avoided. Low-dosage dopamine (selective "renal" effect) may be helpful, particularly in conjunction with another inotrope. Dobutamine is a useful agent in this setting because it is primarily an inotrope, producing some mild vasodilatation and little tachycardia, all of which are desirable effects. Epinephrine is a potent inotrope at lower dosages (β-effect). It will increase oxygen consumption, may cause marked tachycardia, and is arrhythmogenic; however, epinephrine used carefully, in spite of its risks, may be useful when dobutamine is not effective. High-dosage epinephrine (above 20 μg/min) has potent vasoconstricting effects that are disadvantageous in cardiogenic shock. Isoproterenol is not indicated except when the cardiogenic shock is associated with bradycardia. Norepinephrine is usually not useful because its strong vasoconstrictor effects are not usually desirable in cardiogenic shock.

HYPOVOLEMIC SHOCK

As the result of significant volume or blood loss, there is a reflex increase in sympathetic outflow in hypovolemic shock which increases peripheral vasoconstriction and heart rate, in an attempt to compensate for decreased preload, declining oxygen delivery, and decreased stroke volume. Initially systemic blood pressure is maintained, at the expense of local vasoconstriction, but ultimately hypotension and shock occur. Hemorrhagic shock increases both plasma epinephrine and norepinephrine levels.[34a] These increases may be caused both by hypotension-stimulated receptor activity and secondary acidosis.[36] Biocarbonate therapy causes partial reversal of the epinephrine response.[48]

The therapy of choice for this form of shock is volume replacement. Catecholamine therapy is useful only in the acute setting as a temporizing measure until volume replacement can be initiated. Dopamine therapy in hypovolemia does not improve oliguria[182] and can result in necrosis of peripheral extremities. If secondary myocardial dysfunction persists after adequate volume resuscitation, catecholamine inotropic support may transiently be useful.

SEPTIC SHOCK

Septic shock causes increases in both plasma norepinephrine and epinephrine levels[33,54,221] that do not seem to correlate well with systemic blood pressure. The cornerstone of therapy for septic shock is antibiotic administration, in conjunction with circulatory support. The hemodynamic parameters to be maximized are preload (PCW), afterload (SVR), HR, and contractility. Early in septic shock, judicious fluid therapy may be helpful to raise filling pressures and increase the blood pressure. Low-dosage dopamine (0.5 to 2 μg/kg/min) may be helpful to increase urine output.

The vasodilatation seen in sepsis is often refractory to NE therapy. When inotropic support is indicated, dopamine[192] (β doses), dobutamine,[145,193] epinephrine, and isoproterenol[236] are all effective. For reasons cited above (see discussion of isoproterenol above), dopamine, dobutamine, or a combination of the two, using low-dosage dopamine, may be helpful. Late in septic shock, combination vasodilator–catecholamine therapy may produce short-term improvement, but probably does not affect outcome. We have now developed an improved understanding of α-adrenergic receptor function, which should lead to newer pharmacologic approaches to shock reversal in septic subjects.[34b]

CONCLUSIONS

We have examined the possible role of prostaglandins and opioid peptides in various shock states, and the possible use of prostaglandin antagonists, opiate antagonists, steroids, and catecholamines. We have seen that animal and human results do not always correlate. Most of all, it should be clear that the pathophysiology of shock states is extremely complex and, at present, only partially defined. Therapies for cardiogenic, spinal, and septic shock remain unsatisfactory and better therapies remain to be developed.

ACKNOWLEDGMENTS

This work was supported by Research Task Number M0095001.1032.

REFERENCES

1. Aarons RD, Molinoff PB: Changes in density of beta adrenergic receptors in rat lymphocytes, heart, and lung after chronic treatment with propranolol. J Pharmacol Exp Ther 221: 439, 1982
2. Ahlquist RP: A study of the adrenotropic receptors. Am J Physiol 153: 586, 1948
3. Altura BM, Altura BT, Hershey SG: Pharmacodynamic actions of corticosteroids on the microcirculation and vascular smooth muscle. p. 67. In Glenn TM (ed): Steroids and Shock, University Park Press, Baltimore, 1974
4. Anderegg K, Anzeveno P. Cook JA et al: Effects of a pyridine derivative thromboxane synthetase inhibitor and its inactive isomer in endotoxic shock in the rat. Br J Pharmacol 78: 725, 1983
5. Anderson FL, Jubiz W, Tsagaris TJ, Kuida H: Endotoxin-induced prostaglandin E and F release in dogs. Am J Physiol 228: 410, 1975
6. Anderson FL, Tsagaris TJ, Jubiz W, Kuida H: Prostaglandin F and E levels during endotoxin-induced pulmonary hypertension in calves. Am J Physiol 228: 1479, 1975
7. Anderson RR, Holliday RL, Driedger AA et al: Documentation of pulmonary capillary permeability in the adult respiratory distress syndrome accompanying human sepsis. Am Rev Respir Dis 119: 869, 1979
8. Armstrong JM, Lattimer N, Moncada S, Vane JR: Comparison of the vasodepressor effects of prostacyclin and 6-oxo-prostaglandin $F_{1\alpha}$ with those of prostaglandin E_2 in rats and rabbits. Br J Pharmacol 62: 125, 1978
9. Atweh SF, Kuhar MJ: Autoradiographic localization of opiate receptors in rat brain, spinal cord, and lower medulla. Brain Res 124: 53, 1977
10. Balis JU, Paterson JF, Shelley SA et al: Glucocorticoid and antibiotic effects on hepatic microcirculation and associated host responses in lethal gram-negative bacteremia. Lab Invest 40: 55, 1979
11. Beale JS, White RP, Huang SP: EEG and blood pressure effects of TRH in rabbits. Neuropharmacology 16: 499, 1977
12. Beecher HK: Pain in wounded men in battle. Ann Surg 123: 96, 1946
13. Belenky GL, Ruvio BA, Holaday JW: Endotoxin shock is accompanied by a naloxone sensitive increase in nociceptive latencies. Abstr Soc Neurosci 7: 798, 1982
14. Beller BK, Archer LT, Passey RB et al: Effectiveness of modified steroid-antibiotic therapies for lethal sepsis in the dog. Arch Surg 118: 1293, 1983
15. Bergstrom S, Samuelsson B: The prostaglandins. Endeavour 27: 109, 1968
16. Bihari DJ, Tinker J: Steroids in intensive care. Intensive Crit Care Digest 2: 14, 1983
17. Bomzon L, Rosendorff C: Renovascular resistance and noradrenaline. Am J Physiol 229: 1649, 1975
18. Bond RF, Bond CH, Peissner LC et al: Prostaglandin modulation of adrenergic vascular control during hemorrhagic shock. Am J Physiol 241: H85, 1981
19. Bottoms GD, Johnson MA, Roessel OF: Endotoxin-induced hemodynamic changes in dogs: role of thromboxane and prostaglandin I_2. Am J Vet Res 44: 1497, 1983
20. Boudoulas H, Louis RP, Kates RE, Dalamangas G: Hypersensitivity to adrenergic stimulation after propranolol withdrawal in normal subjects. Ann Intern Med 87: 433, 1977
21. Bowen WD, Gentleman S, Herkenham M, Pert C: Interconverting mu and delta forms of the opiate receptor in rat striatal patches. Proc Natl Acad Sci USA 78: 4818, 1981
22. Bradbury AF, Smyth DG, Snell CR et al: C fragment of lipotropin has a high affinity for brain opiate receptors. Nature 260: 793, 1976
23. Bristow MR, Ginsburg R, Manobe W et al: Decreased catecholamine sensitivity and B-adrenergic receptor density in failing human hearts. N Engl J Med 307: 205, 1982
24. Brigham K, Bowers R, Haynes J: Increased sheep lung vascular permeability caused by *E. coli* endotoxin. Circ Res 45: 292, 1979
25. Bult H, Beetens J, Herman AG: Blood levels of 6-oxo-prostaglandin F_{1a} during endotoxin-induced hypotension in rabbits. Eur J Pharmacol 63: 47, 1980
26. Bult H, Beetens J, Vercruysse P, Herman AG: Blood levels in 6-keto-PGF1$_a$, the stable metabolite of prostacyclin during endotoxin-induced hypotension. Arch Int Pharmacodyn 236: 285, 1978
27. Butler RR, Wise WC, Halushka PV, Cook JA: Elevated plasma levels of thromboxane and

prostacyclin in septic shock. Circ Shock 8: 213, 1981

28. Butler RR, Wise WC, Halushka PV, Cook JA: Gentamicin and indomethacin in the treatment of septic shock: effects on prostacyclin and thromboxane A_2 production. J Pharmacol Exp Ther 225: 94, 1983

29. Casey LC, Fletcher JR, Zmudka MI, Ramwell PW: Prevention of endotoxin-induced pulmonary hypertension in primates by the use of a selective thromboxane synthetase inhibitor, OKY 1581. J Pharmacol Exp Ther 222: 441, 1982

30. Cannon WB: A consideration of the nature of wound shock. JAMA 70: 611, 1918

31. Coalson JJ, Hinshaw LB, Guenter CA: The pulmonary ultrastructure in septic shock. Exp Mol Pathol 12: 84, 1970

32. Carr DB, Bergland R, Hamilton A et al: Endotoxin-stimulated opioid peptide secretion: two secretory pools and feedback control in vivo. Science 217: 845, 1982

33. Cavanaugh D, Rao RS, Sutton DMC et al: Pathophysiology of endotoxin shock in the primate. Am J Obstet Gynecol 108: 705, 1976

34. Chang KJ, Cuatrecasas P: Multiple opiate receptors. Enkephalins and morphine binds to receptors of different specificity. J Biol Chem 254: 2610, 1979

34a. Chernow B, Lake CR, Barton M et al: Sympathetic nervous system sensitivity to hemorrhagic hypotension in the subhuman primate. J Trauma 24: 229, 1984

34b. Chernow B, Roth BL: Pharmacologic manipulation of the peripheral vasculature in shock: Clinical and experimental approaches. Circ Shock 18: 141, 1986

35. Chidsey CA, Braunwald E, Morrow AG: Catecholamine excretion and cardiac stores of norepinephrine in congestive heart failure. Am J Med 39: 442, 1965

36. Chien, Shu: Role of the sympathetic nervous system in hemorrhage. Physiol Rev 47: 214, 1967

37. Coker SJ, Hughes B, Parratt JR et al: The release of prostanoids during the acute pulmonary response to *E. coli* endotoxin in anesthetized cats. Br J Pharmacol 78: 561, 1983

38. Cook JA, Halushka PV, Wise WC: Modulation of macrophage arachadonic acid metabolism: potential role in the susceptibility of rats to endotoxic shock. Circ Shock 9: 605, 1982

39. Cook JA, Wise WC, Halushka PV: Elevated thromboxane levels in the rat during endotoxic shock: protective effects of imidazole, 13-azaprostanoic acid, or essential fatty acid deficiency. J Clin Invest 65: 227, 1980

40. Cook JA, Wise WC, Halushka PV: Thromboxane A_2 and prostacyclin production by lipopolysaccharide stimulated peritoneal macrophages. J Reticuloendothel Soc 30: 445, 1981

41. Cook JA, Wise WC, Knapp DR, Halushka PV: Sensitization of essential fatty acid deficient rats to endotoxin by arachidonate pretreatment: role of thromboxane A_2. Circ Shock 8: 69, 1981

42. Cook JA, Wise WC, Temple GE, Halushka PV: Exchange transfusion in rats with Fluosol (FL-43), an artificial blood substitute: Effect of endotoxin (LPS) on early thromboxane (Tx) A_2 synthesis. Circ Shock 10: 230, 1983

43. Corey EJ, Clark DA, Goto G et al: Stereospecific total synthesis of a slow reacting substance of anaphylaxsis, leukotriene. J Am Chem Soc 102: 1436, 1980

44. Cowan A: Quasi-morphine withdrawal syndrome: recent developments. Fed Proc 40: 1489, 1981

45. Cox BM: Endogenous opioid peptides: a guide to structures and terminology. Life Sci 31: 1645, 1982

46. Cryer PE, Rizza RA, Haymond MW et al: Epinephrine and norepinephrine are cleared through beta-adrenergic but not alpha-adrenergic mechanisms in man. Metabolism 29 (Suppl I): 1114, 1980

47. Curtis MT, Lefer AM: Protective actions of naloxone in hemorragic shock. Am J Physiol 239: H416, 1980

48. Darby TD, Watts DT: Acidosis and blood epinephrine levels in hemorrhagic hypotension. Am J Physiol 206: 1281, 1964

49. Dietzman RH, Castaneda AR, Lillehei CW et al: Corticosteroids as effective vasodilators in the treatment of low output syndrome. Chest 57: 440, 1970

50. DiSesa VJ, Brown E, Mudge GH et al: Hemodynamic comparison of dopamine and dobutamine in the postoperative volume-loaded, pressure-loaded and normal ventricle. J Thorac Cardiovasc Surg 83: 256, 1982

51. Drazen JM, Austen KF, Lewis RA et al: Comparative airway and vascular activities of leukotrienes C-1 and D *in-vivo* and *in-vitro*. Proc Natl Acad Sci USA 77: 4354, 1980

52. Dunham BM, Grindlinger GA, Utsunomiya T et al: Role of prostaglandins in positive end-expiratory pressure-induced negative inotropism. Am J Physiol 241: H783, 1981

53. Dunn MJ, Zambraski EJ: Renal effects of drugs that inhibit prostaglandin synthesis. Kidney Int 18: 609, 1980

54. Emerson TE, Jr.: Participation of endogenous vasoactive agents in the pathogenesis of endotoxin shock. Adv Exp Med Biol 23: 34, 1971

55. Emerson TE, Jr., Bryan WJ: Regional cerebral blood flows in endotoxin shock with methyl-

prednisolone treatment. Proc Soc Exp Biol Med 156: 378, 1977

56. Fabian TC, Patterson R: Steroid therapy in septic shock. Am Surg 48: 614, 1982
57. Faden AI: Neuropeptides in shock and neural injury. p. 636. In Chernow B, Lake CR (eds): The Pharmacologic Approach to the Critically Ill Patient. Baltimore, Williams and Wilkins, 1983
58. Faden AI: Opiate antagonists and thyrotropin-releasing hormone. JAMA 252: 1177, 1984
59. Faden AI, Holaday JW: Opiate antagonists: a role in the treatment of hypovolemic shock. Science 205: 317, 1979
60. Faden AI, Holaday JW: Naloxone treatment of endotoxin shock: stereospecificity of physiologic and pharmacologic effects in the rat. J Pharmacol Exp Ther 212: 441, 1980
61. Faden AI, Holaday JW: Experimental endotoxin shock: the pathophysiologic function of endorphins and treatment with opiate antagonists. J Infect Dis 142: 229, 1980
62. Faden AI, Jacobs TP, Feuerstein G, Holaday JW: Dopamine partially mediates the cardiovascular effects of naloxone after spinal injury. Brain Res 213: 415, 1981
63. Faden AI, Jacobs TP, Holaday JW: Endorphin-parasympathetic interaction in spinal shock. J Autonom Nerv Syst 2: 295, 1980
64. Faden AI, Jacobs TP, Holaday JW: Thyrotropin-releasing hormone improves neurologic recovery after spinal trauma in the cat. N Engl J Med 305: 1063, 1981
65. Faden AI, Jacobs TP, Holaday JW: Opiate antagonist improves neurologic recovery after spinal injury. Science 211: 493, 1981
66. Fauci AS, Dale DC, Balow JE: Glucocorticosteroid therapy: mechanisms of action and clinical considerations. Ann Intern Med 84: 304, 1976
67. Ferreira SH, Moncada S, Vane JR: Indomethacin and aspirin abolish prostaglandin production release from the spleen. Nature (New Biol) 231: 237, 1971
68. Filkins JP, Cornell RP: Depression of hepatic gluconeogenesis and the hypoglycemia of endotoxin shock. Am J Physiol 227: 778, 1974
69. Fink MP, MacVittie TJ, Casey LC: Effects of nonsteroidal anti-inflammatory drugs on renal function in septic dogs. J Surg Res 36: 516, 1984
70. Fletcher JR, Herman CM, Ramwell PW: Improved survival in endotoxemia with aspirin and indomethacin pretreatment. Surg Forum 27: 11, 1976
71. Fletcher JR, Ramwell PW: Modification by aspirin and indomethacin of the haemodynamic and prostaglandin releasing effects of *E. coli* endotoxin in the dog. Br J Pharmacol 61: 175, 1977
72. Fletcher JR, Ramwell PW: Lidocaine or indo-

methacin improves survival in baboon endotoxin shock. J Surg Res 24: 154, 1978
73. Fletcher JR, Ramwell PW: Modulation of prostaglandins E and F by the lung in baboon hemorrhagic shock. J Surg Res 26: 465, 1979
74. Fletcher JR, Ramwell PW: Indomethacin treatment following baboon endotoxin shock improves survival. Adv Shock Res 4: 103, 1980
75. Fletcher JR, Ramwell PW: Indomethacin improves survival after endotoxin in baboons. Adv Prostaglandin Thromboxane Res 7: 821, 1980
76. Fletcher JR, Short BL, Casey LC et al: Thromboxane inhibition in gram-negative sepsis fails to improve survival. Adv Prostaglandin Thromboxane Leukotriene Res 12: 117, 1983
77. Florez J, Hurle MA, Mediavilla A: Respiratory responses to opiates applied to the medullary ventral surface. Life Sci 31: 2189, 1982
78. Flower RJ: Drugs which inhibit prostaglandin biosynthesis. Pharmacol Rev 26: 33, 1974
79. Flower RJ: Prostaglandins and related compounds. p. 374. In Vane JR, Ferriera SH (eds): Handbook of Experimental Pharmacology, Vol. 50. Springer-Verlag, New York, 1978
80. Flynn JT, Appert HE, Howard JM: Arterial prostaglandin A_1, E_1, F_{2a} concentrations during hemorrhagic shock in the dog. Circ Shock 2: 155, 1975
81. Flynn JT, Bridenbaugh GA, Leter AM: Clearance of PGF_{2a} during circulatory shock. Life Sci 17: 1699, 1975
82. Fong HJ, Cohen AH: Ibuprofen-induced acute renal failure with acute tubular necrosis. Am J Nephrol 2: 28, 1982
83. Friedman WF, Hirschklau MJ, Printz MP et al: Pharmacologic closure of patent ductus arteriosus in the premature infant. N Engl J Med 295: 526, 1976
84. Fukumoto S, Tanaka K: Protective effects of thromboxane A_2 synthetase inhibitors on endotoxic shock. Prostaglandins Leukotrienes Med 11: 179, 1983
85. Furness JB, Burnstock G: Role of circulating catecholamines in the gastrointestinal tract. p. 515. In Handbook of Physiology Endocrinology VI. American Physiology Society, Washington, DC, 1975
86. Gillespie TA, Ambos HD, Sobel BE et al: Effects of dobutamine in patients with acute myocardial infarction. Am J Cardiol 39: 588, 1977
87. Goldberg LI: Cardiovascular and renal actions of dopamine: potential clinical applications. Pharmacol Rev 24: 1, 1972
88. Goldberg LI: Dopamine—clinical uses of an endogenous catecholamine. N Engl J Med 291: 707, 1974
89. Goldberg LI, Hsieh Y, Resnekov L: Newer cate-

cholamines for treatment of heart failure and shock: an update on dopamine and a first look at dobutamine. Prog Cardiovasc Dis 19: 327, 1977

90. Goldberg LI, Rajfer SI: Sympathomimetic amines: potential clinical applications in ischemic heart disease. Am Heart J 103: 724, 1982

91. Goldberg LI, Volkman PH, Kohli JD: A comparison of the vascular dopamine receptor with other dopamine receptors. Annu Rev Pharmacol Toxicol 18: 57, 1978

92. Goldfarb RD, Tambolini W, Wiener SM, Weber PB: Canine left ventricular performance during LD_{50} endotoxemia. Am J Physiol 244: H370, 1983

93. Goldstein DS: Plasma norepinephrine as an indicator of sympathetic neural activity in clinical cardiology. Am J Cardiol 48: 1147, 1981

94. Gombos EA, Hulet WH, Bopp P et al: Reactivity of renal and systemic circulations to vasoconstrictor agents in normotensive and hypertensive subjects. J Clin Invest 41: 203, 1962

95. Goodman RR, Snyder SH, Kuhar MJ, Young WS: Differentiation of the delta and mu opiate receptor localizations by light microscopic autoradiography. Proc Natl Acad Sci USA 77: 6239, 1980

96. Greenway CV, Stark RD: Hepatic vascular bed. Physiol Rev 51: 23, 1971

97. Greisman SE: Experimental gram-negative bacterial sepsis: optimal methylprednisolone requirements for prevention of mortality not preventable by antibiotics alone. Proc Soc Exp Biol Med 170: 436, 1982

98. Greisman SE, DuBuy JB, Woodward CL: Experimental gram-negative bacterial sepsis: prevention of mortality not preventable by antibiotics alone. Infect Immun 25: 538, 1979

99. Guillemin R: Peptides in the brain: the new endocrinology of the neuron. Science 202: 390, 1978

100. Guillemin R, Vargo T, Rossier J et al: Beta-endorphin and adrenocorticotropin are secreted concomitantly by the pituitary gland. Science 197:1367, 1977

101. Guntheroth WG, Jacky JP, Kawabori I et al: Left ventricular performance in endotoxin shock in dogs. Am J Physiol 242: H172, 1982

102. Gurll NJ, Reynolds DG, Holaday JW, Ganes E: Improved cardiovascular function and survival using thyrotropin-releasing hormone (TRH) in primate hemorrhagic shock. Physiologist 25: 342, 1982

103. Gurll NJ, Reynolds DG, Vargish T, Lechner R: Naloxone without transfusion prolongs survival and enhances cardiovascular function in hypovolemic shock. J Pharmacol Exp Ther 220: 621, 1982

104. Gurll NJ, Vargish T, Reynolds DG, Lechner R: Opiate receptors and endorphins in the patho-physiology of hemorragic shock. Surgery 89: 364, 1981

105. Hales CA, Sonne L, Peterson M et al: Role of thromboxane and prostacyclin in pulmonary vasomotor changes after endotoxin in dogs. J Clin Invest 68: 497, 1981

106. Halushka PV, Wise WC, Cook JA: Protective effect of aspirin in endotoxic shock. J Pharmacol Exp Ther 218: 464, 1981

107. Hamberg M, Svensson J, Samuelsson B: Thromboxanes: a new group of biologically active compounds derived from prostaglandin endoperoxides. Proc Natl Acad Sci USA 72: 2994, 1975

108. Hammerschmidt DE, White JG, Craddock PR, Jacob HS: Corticosteroids inhibit complement-induced granulocyte aggregation: a possible mechanism for their efficacy in shock states. J Clin Invest 63: 789, 1979

109. Harris RH, Zmudka M, Maddox Y et al: Relationships of TxB_2 and 6-keto-PGF_a to the hemodynamic changes during baboon endotoxin shock. Adv Prostaglandin Thromboxane Res 7: 843, 1980

110. Hedqvist P, Dahlen SE, Gustaffson L et al: Biological profile of leukotrienes C_4 and D_4. Acta Physiol Scand 110: 331, 1980

111. Heflin AC, Jr., Brigham KL: Prevention by granulocyte depletion of increased vascular permeability of sheep lung following endotoxemia. J Clin Invest 68: 1253, 1981

112. Henrich WL, Anderson RJ, Berns AS et al: The role of renal nerves and prostaglandins in control of renal hemo-dynamics and plasma renin activity during hypotensive hemorrhage in the dog. J Clin Invest 61: 744, 1978

113. Henrich WL, Hamasaki Y, Said SI et al: Dissociation of systemic and renal effects of endotoxemia: prostaglandin inhibition uncovers an important role of renal nerves. J Clin Invest 69: 691, 1982

114. Hilberman M: Renal protection. In Shoemaker WC, Thompson WL (eds): Critical Care State of the Art, Vol III. Society of Critical Care Medicine, Fullerton, CA, 1982

115. Hinshaw LB: Effects of glucocorticoids in septic shock on phagocytic cells including the granular leukocytes, monocytes, and tissue macrophages. Monograph, The Upjohn Co., 1979

116. Hinshaw LB, Archer LT, Beller-Todd BK et al: Survival of primates in lethal septic shock following delayed treatment with steroid. Circ Shock 8: 291, 1981

117. Hinshaw LB, Archer LT, Beller-Todd BK et al: Survival of primates in LD_{100} septic shock following steroid/antibiotic therapy. J Surg Res 28: 151, 1980

118. Hinshaw LB, Beller-Todd BK, Archer LT et al: Effectiveness of steroid/antibiotic treatment in primates administered LD_{100} E. coli. Ann Surg 194: 51, 1981

119. Hinshaw LB, Beller BK, Archer LT, Flournoy DJ, White GL, Phillips RW: Recovery from lethal *E. coli* shock in dogs. Surg Gynecol Obstet 149: 545, 1979

120. Hinshaw LB, Benjamin B, Coalson JJ et al: Hypoglycemia in lethal septic shock in subhuman primates. Circ Shock 2: 197, 1975

121. Hinshaw LB, Peyton MD, Archer LT et al: Prevention of death in endotoxin shock by glucose administration. Surg Gynecol Obstet 139: 851, 1974

122. Hinshaw LB, Solomon LA, Erdos EG et al: Effects of acetylsalicylic acid on the canine response to endotoxin. J Pharmacol Exp Ther 157: 665, 1967

123. Hinshaw LB, Solomon LA, Freeny PC, Reins DA: Hemodynamic and survival effects of methylprednisolone in endotoxin shock. Arch Surg 94: 61, 1967

124. Hissen W, Fleming JS, Bierwagen ME, Pindell MH: Effect of prostaglandin E_1 on platelet aggregation in vitro and in hemorrhagic shock. Microvass Res 1: 374, 1969

125. Hoffman BB, Lefkowitz RJ: α-Adrenergic receptor subtypes. N Engl J Med 302: 1390, 1980

126. Holaday JW, D'Amato RJ, Faden AI: Thyrotropin-releasing hormone improves cardiovascular function in experimental endotoxic and hemorragic shock. Science 213: 216, 1981

127. Holaday JW, D'Amato RJ, Ruvio BA, Faden AI: Action of naloxone and TRH on the autonomic regulation of circulation. Adv Biochem Psychopharmacol 33: 353, 1982

128. Holaday JW, Faden AI: Naloxone reversal of endotoxin hypotension suggests a role of endorphins in shock Nature 275: 450, 1978

129. Holaday JW, Faden AI: Hypophysectomy inhibits the therapeutic effects of naloxone in endotoxic and hypovolemic shock. Physiologist 22: 57, 1979

130. Holaday JW, Faden AI: Adrenalectomy elevates beta-endorphin levels and potentiates shock susceptability which is naloxone reversible. Circ Shock 7: 222, 1980

131. Holaday JW, Faden AI: Naloxone acts at central opiate receptors to reverse hypotension, hypothermia, and hypoventilation in spinal shock. Brain Res 189: 295, 1980

132. Holaday, JW, Faden AI: Naloxone reverses the pathophysiology of shock through an antagonism of endorphin systems. p. 421. In Martin JB, Reichlin S (eds): Neurosecretion and Brain Peptides: Implications for Brain Function and Neurological Disease. Raven Press, New York, 1981

133. Holaday JW, O'Hara M, Faden AI: Hypophysectomy alters cardiorespiratory variables: central effects of pituitary endorphins in shock. Am J Physiol 241: H479, 1981

134. Holaday JW, Ruvio BA, Faden AI: Thyrotropin-releasing hormone improves blood pressure and survival in endotoxic shock. Eur J Pharm 74: 101, 1981

135. Holaday JW, Tseng LF, Loh HH, Li CH: Thyrotropin releasing hormone antagonizes beta endorphin hypothermia and catalepsy. Life Sci 22: 1537, 1978

136. Horita A, Carino MA: Centrally administered TRH produces a vasopressor response in rabbits. Proc West Pharm Soc 20: 303, 1977

137. Hughes GS: Naloxone and methylprednisolone sodium succinate enhance sympathomedullary discharge in patients with septic shock. Life Sci 35(23): 2319, 1984

138. Hughes J, Kosterlitz HW, Smith TW: The distribution of methionine enkephalin and leucine encephalin in the brain and peripheral tissues. Brit J Pharmacol 61: 639, 1977

139. Hughes J, Smith TW, Kosterlitz HW et al: Identification of two related pentapeptides from the brain with potent opiate agonist activity. Nature 258: 577, 1975

140. Huttemeier PC, Watkins WD, Peterson MB, Zapol WM: Acute pulmonary hypertension and lung thromboxane release after endotoxin infusion in normal and leukopenic sheep. Circ Res 50: 688, 1982

141. Iimura O, Wakabayashi C, Kobayashi T et al: Studies on experimental coronary insufficiency. Recent Adv Stud Cardiac Struct Metab 12: 537, 1978

142. Jakshick BA, Marshall GR, Kourik JL et al: Profile of circulating vasoactive substances in hemorrhagic shock and their pharmacologic manipulation. J Clin Invest 54: 842, 1974

143. Janssen HF, Lutherer LO: Ventriculocisternal administration of naloxone protects against severe hypotension during endotoxin shock. Brain Res 194: 608, 1980

144. Jardin F, Eveleigh MC, Gurdjian F et al: Venous admixture in human septic shock. Circulation 60: 155, 1979

145. Jardin F, Sportiche M, Bazil M et al: Dobutamine: a hemodynamic evaluation in septic shock. Crit Care Med 9: 329, 1981

146. Jarnberg PO, Bengtsson L, Ekstrand J et al: Dopamine infusion in man: plasma catecholamine levels and pharmacokinetics. Acta Anaesthesiol Scand 25: 328, 1981

147. Johnson DG, Thoa NB, Weinshilboum R et al:

Enhanced release of dopamine B-hydroxylase from sympathetic nerves by calcium and phenoxybenzamine and its reversal by prostaglandins. Proc Natl Acad Sci 68: 2227, 1971

148. Kadowitz PJ, Yard AC: Circulatory effects of hydrocortisone and protection against endotoxin shock in cats. Eur J Pharmacol 9: 311, 1970

149. Kurland JI, Bockman R: Prostaglandin E production by human blood monocytes and mouse peritoneal macrophages. J Exp Med 147: 952, 1978

150. Kurzrok R, Lieb CC: Biochemical studies of human semen. II. The action of semen on the human uterus. Proc Soc Exp Biol Med 28: 268, 1930

151. Lands AM, Arnold A, McAuliffe JP et al: Differentiation of receptor systems activated by sympathomimetic amines. Nature (London) 214: 597, 1967

152. Langley JN, Magnus R: Some observation of the movements of the intestine before and after degenerative section of the mesenteric nerves. J Physiol 33: 34, 1905

153. Lazurus LH, Ling N, Guillemin R: Beta-lipotropin as a prohormone for the morphinomimetic peptides endorphins and enkephalins. Proc Natl Acad Sci USA 73: 2156, 1976

154. Lefer AM: Role of prostaglandins and thromboxanes in shock states. p. 55. In Altura BM, et al (eds). Handbook of Shock and Trauma. Vol I. Raven Press, New York, 1983

155. Lefer AM, Martin J: Mechanism of the protective effect of corticosteroids in hemorrhagic shock. Am J Physiol 216: 314, 1969

156. Leffler CW, Passmore JC: Effects of indomethacin on hemodynamics of dogs in refractory hemorrhagic shock. J Surg Res 23: 392, 1977

157. Leffler CW, Tyler TL, Cassin S: Effects of indomethacin on cardiovascular hemodynamics of goats in hemorrhagic shock. Circ Shock 5: 299, 1978

158. Lefkowitz RJ: Direct binding studies of adrenergic receptors: Biochemical, physiologic, and clinical implications. Ann Intern Med 91: 450, 1979

159. Lefkowitz RJ: Clinical physiology of adrenergic receptor regulation. Am J Physiol 243: 1243, 1982

160. Leier CV, Hebran PT, Huss P et al: Comparative systemic and regional hemodynamic effects of dopamine and dobutamine in patients with cardiomyopathic heart failure. Circulation 58: 466, 1978

161. Leier CV, Weber J, Bush CA: The cardiovascular effects of the continuous infusion of dobutamine in patients with severe cardiac failure. Circulation 56: 468, 1977

162. Lekven J, Kjekahus JK, Mjos OD: Cardiac effects of isoproterenol during graded myocardial ischemia. Scand J Clin Invest 33: 161–171, 1974

163. Levine TB, Francis GS, Goldsmith SR et al: Activity of the sympathetic nervous system and renin angiotensin system assessed by plasma hormone levels and their relation to hemodynamic abnormalities in congestive heart failure. Am J Cardiol 49: 1659, 1982

164. Li CH: Lipotropin, a new active peptide from pituitary glands. Nature 201: 924, 1964

165. Lifschitz BM, Defesi CR, Surks MI: Thyrotropin response to thyrotropin-releasing hormone in the euthyroid rat: dose-response, time course, and demonstration of partial refractoriness to a second dose of thyrotropin-releasing hormone. Endocrinology 102: 1775, 1978

166. Loeb HS, Bredakis J, Gunner RM: Superiority of dobutamine over dopamine for augmentation of cardiac output in patients with chronic low output cardiac failure. Circulation 55: 375, 1977

167. Loeb HS, Sinno MZ, Saudye A et al: Electrophysiologic properties of dobutamine. Circ Shock 1: 217, 1974

168. Lux WE, Feuerstein G, Faden AI: Alteration of leukotriene D_4 hypotension by thyrotropin-releasing hormone. Nature 302: 822, 1983

169. Machiedo GW, Brown CS, Lavigne JE, Rush BF Jr: Beneficial effect of prostaglandin E_1 in experimental hemorrhagic shock. Surg Gynecol Obstet 143: 433, 1976

170. McCalden TA, Mendelow AD, Coull A et al: Role of catecholamines degradable enzymes and the adrenergic innervation in determining the cerebrovascular response to infused norepinephrine. Stroke 10: 319, 1979

171. Mela L: Reversibility of mitochondrial metabolic response to circulatory shock and tissue ischemia. Circ Shock (Suppl 1) 61, 1979

172. Mela L, Miller LD: Efficacy of glucocorticoids in preventing mitochondrial metabolic failure in endotoxemia. Circ Shock 10: 371, 1983

173. Mentzer RM Jr, Alegre CA, Nolan SP: The effects of dopamine and isoproterenol on the pulmonary circulation. J Thorac Cardiovasc Surg 71: 807, 1976

174. Metcalf G: Regulatory peptides as a source of new drugs. The clinical prospects for analogues of TRH which are resistant to metabolic degradation. Brain Res 257: 389, 1982

175. Moncada S, Flower RJ, Vane JR: Prostaglandins, prostacyclin, and thromboxane A_2. p. 668. In Gilman AG, Goodman LS, Gilman A (eds): The Pharmacological Basis of Therapeutics, Sixth Edition. MacMillan, New York, 1980

176. Moncada S, Gryglewski R, Bunting S, Vane JR: An enzyme isolated from arteries transforms prostaglandin endoperoxides to an unstable

substance that inhibits platelet aggregation. Nature (London) 263: 663, 1976

177. Morley JE, Garvin TJ, Pekary AE et al: Plasma clearance and plasma half disappearance time of exogenous thyrotropin-releasing hormone and pyroglutamyl-N^{31M}-methyl-histidyl prolineamide. J Clin Endocrinol Metab 48: 377, 1979

178. Motulsky HJ, Insel PA: Adrenergic receptors in man. N Engl J Med 307: 18, 1982

179. Nasjletti A, Malik KU: Interrelations between prostaglandins and vasoconstrictor hormones: contribution to blood pressure regulation. Fed Proc 41: 2394, 1982

180. Needleman P, Minkes M, Raz A: Thromboxanes: selective biosynthesis and distinct biological properties. Science 193: 163, 1976

181. Neiberger RE, Levine JI, Passmore JC: Renal effects of dopamine during prolonged hemorrhagic hypotension in the dog. Circ Shock 7: 129, 1980

182. Noble WH, Famewo CE, Garvey MB: Pulmonary vascular effects of acetylsalicylic acid, chloroquine, dextran and methylprednisolone given after hemorrhagic shock in dogs. Can Anaesth Soc J 24: 661, 1977

183. Northover BJ, Subramanian G: Anagelsic–antipyretic drugs as antagonists of endotoxin shock in dogs. J Pathol Bacteriol 83: 463, 1962

184. O'Flaherty JT, Craddock PR, Jacob HS: Mechanism of anti-complementary activity of corticosteroids *in vivo*: Possible relevance in endotoxin shock. Proc Soc Exp Biol Med 154: 206, 1977

185. Parratt JR, Sturgess RM: The effect of indomethacin on the cardiovascular and metabolic responses to *E. coli* endotoxin in the cat. Br J Pharmacol 50: 177, 1974

186. Parratt JR, Sturgess RM: E. coli endotoxin shock in the cat, treatment with indomethacin. Br J Pharmacol 53: 485, 1975

187. Pasternak GW, Childers SR, Snyder SH: Naloxazone, a long-acting opiate antagonist: effects on analgesia in intact animals and on opiate receptor binding in vitro. J Pharmacol Exp Ther 214: 455, 1980

188. Pert CB, Pasternak G, Snyder SH: Opiate agonists and antagonists discriminated by receptor binding in brain. Science 182: 1359, 1973

189. Pitcairn M, Schuler J, Erve PR et al: Glucocorticoid and antibiotic effect on experimental gram-negative bacteremic shock. Arch Surg 110: 1012, 1975

190. Raflo GT, Jones RC, Jr, Wangensteen SL: Inadequacy of steroids in the treatment of severe haemorrhagic shock. Am J Surg 130: 321, 1975

191. Raymond RM, Harkema JM, Stoffs WV, Emerson TE: Effects of naloxone therapy on hemodynamics and metabolism following superlethal dosage of E. coli endotoxin in dogs. Surg Gynecol Obstet 152: 159, 1981

192. Regnier B, Rapin M, Gory G, et al: Hemodynamic effects of dopamine in septic shock. Intensive Care Med 3: 47, 1977

193. Regnier B, Safran D, Carlet J, et al: Comparative hemodynamic effects of dopamine and dobutamine in septic shock. Intensive Care Med 5: 115, 1979

194. Reines HD, Halushka PV, Cook JA et al: Plasma thromboxane concentrations are raised in patients dying with septic shock. Lancet 2: 174, 1982

195. Reynolds DG, Gurll NJ, Vargish T et al: Blockade of opiate receptors with naloxone improves survival and cardiac performance in canine endotoxic shock. Circ Shock 7: 39, 1980

196. Rie M, Peterson D, Kong D et al: Plasma prostacyclin increases during acute human sepsis. Circ Shock 10: 232, 1983

197. Roberts R, Demello V, Sobel BE: Deleterious effects of methylprednisolone in patients with myocardial infarction. Circulation 53(3 Suppl 1): 204, 1976

198. Robie NW, Goldberg LI: Comparative systemic and regional hemodynamic effects of dopamine and dobutamine. Am Heart J 90: 340, 1975

199. Sawynok J, Pinsky C, LaBella FS: Mini review on the specificity of naloxone as an opiate antagonist. Life Sci 25: 1621, 1979

200. Schadt JC, York DH: The reversal of hemorrhagic hypotension by naloxone in conscious rabbits. Can J Physiol Pharmacol 59: 1208, 1981

201. Schumer W: Steroids in the treatment of clinical septic shock. Ann Surg 184: 333, 1976

202. Shand DG, Wood AJ: Propranolol withdrawl syndrome—why? Circulation 58: 202, 1978

203. Sheagren JN: Septic shock and corticosteroids (Editorial). N Engl J Med 305: 456, 1981

204. Shatney CH, Lillehei RC: Effects of prostaglandins in canine endotoxin shock. Acta Biol Med Ger 35: 1141, 1976

205. Shaw JS, Miller L, Turnbull MJ et al: Selective antagonists at the opiate delta receptor. Life Sci 31: 1259, 1982

206. Short BL, Gardiner M, Walker RI et al: Indomethacin improves survival in gram-negative sepsis. Adv Shock Res 6: 27, 1981

207. Sibbald WJ, Anderson RR, Reid B et al: Alveolocapillary permeability in human septic adult respiratory distress syndrome: effect of high-dose corticosteroid therapy. Chest 79: 133, 1981

208. Siess W, Lorenz R, Roth P et al: Plasma catecholamines, platelet aggregation and associated thromboxane formation after physical exercise, smoking, or norepinephrine infusion. Circulation 66: 44, 1982

209. Silverberg AB, Shah SD, Haymond MW et al: Norepinephrine: Hormone and neurotransmitter in man. Am J Physiol 234: E252, 1978
210. Simon EJ, Hiller JM, Edelman I: Stereospecific binding of the potent narcotic analgesic ^{3}H-etorphine to rat brain homogenate. Proc Natl Acad Sci USA 70: 1947, 1973
211. Smedegard G, Hedqvist P, Dahlen SE et al: Leukotriene C$_4$ affects pulmonary and cardiovascular dynamics in monkey. Nature 295: 327, 1982
212. Smith JB, Willis AL: Aspirin selectively inhibits prostaglandin production in human platelets. Nature (New Biol) 231: 235, 1971
213. Snyder SH: Opiate receptors and internal opiates. Sci Am 236: 44, 1977
214. Salomon NW, Plachetka JR, Copeland JG: Comparison of dopamine and dobutamine following coronary artery bypass grafting. Ann Thorac Surg 33: 48, 1982
215. Sonnenblick EH, Frishman WH, LeJemtel TH: Dobutamine. A new synthetic cardioactive sympathetic amine. N Engl J Med 300: 17, 1979
216. Spagnuolo PJ, Ellner JJ, Hassid A, Dunn MJ: Thromboxane A$_2$ mediates augmented polymorphonuclear leukocyte adhesiveness. J Clin Invest 66: 406, 1980
217. Spath JA, Gorczynski RJ, Lefer AM: Possible mechanisms of the beneficial action of glucocorticoids in circulatory shock. Surg Gynecol Obstet 137: 597, 1973
218. Sprung CL, Caralis PV, Marcial EH et al: The effects of high-dose corticosteroids in patients with septic shock: A prospective, controlled study. N Engl J Med 311: 1137, 1984
219. Steer ML, Atlas D, Levitzki A: Interrelations between B-adrenergic receptors adenylate cyclase and calcium. N Engl J Med 292: 409, 1975
220. Stiles GL, Strasser RH, Lavin TN et al: The cardiac beta-adrenergic receptor: structural similarities of beta$_1$ and beta$_2$ receptor subtypes demonstrated by photoaffinity labeling. J Biol Chem 258: 8443, 1983
221. Sugarman HJ, Newsome HHm Greenfield LJ: Hemodynamics, oxygen consumption and serum catecholamine changes in progressive lethal peritonitis in the dog. Surg Gynecol Obstet 154: 8, 1982
222. Svensson J, Hamberg M, Samuelsson B: Prostaglandin endoperoxides. IX. Characterization of rabbit aorta contracting substance (RCS) from guinea pig lung and human platelets. Acta Physiol Scand 94: 222, 1975
223. Takemori AE, Larson DL, Portoghese PS: The irreversible narcotic antagonistic and reversible agonistic properties of the fumaramate methyl ester derivative of Naltrexone. Eur J Pharmacol 70: 445, 1981
224. Tanaka J, Sato T, Nakatani T et al: Effects of gentamicin (GM) and methylprednisolone (MP) on survival and cardiac output in a lethal *E. coli* bacteremic rat model. Fed Proc 42: 1250, 1983
225. Tanz RD, Kerby CF: The inotropic action of certain steroids upon isolated cardiac tissue; with comments on steroidal cardiotonic structure-activity relationships. J Pharmacol Exp Ther 131: 56, 1961
226. Tarazi RC: Sympathomimetic agents in the treatment of shock. Ann Intern Med 81: 364, 1974
227. Terenius L: Characteristics of the "receptor" for narcotic analgesics in synaptic plasma membrane fraction from rat brain. Acta Pharmacol Toxicol 33: 377, 1973
228. Tohmeh JF, Cryer PE: Biophasic adrenergic modulation of B-adrenergic receptors in man. J Clin Invest 65: 836, 1980
229. Tuttle RR, Mills J: Development of a new catecholamine to selectively increase cardiac contractility. Circ Res 36: 185, 1975
230. Urist MM, Casey LC, Ramwell PW et al: Prostacyclin and thromboxane metabolism in endotoxemia or sepsis in the baboon (abstr). Association for Academic Surgery, 1981
231. Utsunomiya T, Krausz MM, Dunham B et al: Depression of myocardial ATPase activity by plasma obtained during positive end-expiratory pressure. Surgery 91: 322, 1982
232. Vander AJ: Effect of catecholamines and the renal nerves on renin secretion in anesthetized dogs. Am J Physiol 209: 659, 1965
233. Vane JR: Inhibition of prostaglandin synthesis as a mechanism of action for aspirin-like drugs. Nature (New Biol) 231: 232, 1971
234. Vargish T, Reynolds DG, Gurll NJ et al: Naloxone reversal of hypovolemic shock in dogs. Circ Shock 7: 31, 1980
235. Vatner SF, McRitchie RJ, Braunwald E: Effects of dobutamine on left ventricular performance, coronary dynamics and distribution of cardiac output in conscious dogs. J Clin Invest 53: 1265, 1974
236. Vaughn DL, Peterson E: Pathophysiology of endotoxin shock in primates and the effects of various therapeutic agents. Obstet Gynecol 134: 271, 1969
237. Walshe JJ, Venuto RC: Acute oliguric renal failure induced by indomethacin: possible mechanism. Ann Intern Med 91: 47, 1979
238. Watson SJ, Akil H, Richard CW, Barchas JD: Evidence for two separate opiate peptide neuronal systems. Nature (London) 275: 226, 1978
239. Weiner N: Norepinephrine, epinephrine, and the sympathomimetic amines. In Goodman LS, Gil-

man A (eds): The Pharmacologic Basis of Therapeutics, MacMillan, New York, 1980

240. Weitzman S, Berger S: Clinical trial design in studies of corticosteroids for bacterial infections. Ann Intern Med 81: 36, 1974

241. White GL, Archer LT, Beller BK, Hinshaw LB: Increased survival with methylprednisolone treatment in canine endotoxin shock. J Surg Res 25: 357, 1978

242. Whitfield L, Sowers JR, Tuck ML et al: Dopaminergic control of plasma catecholamines and aldosterone responses to acute stimuli in normal man. J Clin Endocrinol Metab 51: 724, 1980

243. Whitten RH, Ryan NT, Egdahl RH: PGE_2 in treatment of "irreversible" hemorrhagic shock. Surg Forum 30: 473, 1979

244. Wichterman KA, Baue AE, Chaudry IH: Sepsis and septic shock—a review of laboratory models and a proposal. J Surg Res 29: 189, 1980

245. Widdicombe JG: Action of CA on broncial smooth muscle. In Handbook of Physiology and Endocrinology VI. American Physiology Society, Washington, DC, 1975

246. Williams RS, Bishop T: Selectivity of dobutamine for adrenergic receptor subtypes. J Clin Invest 67: 1703, 1981

247. Wilson FJ, Hiller FC: Ibuprofen in canine endotoxin shock. J Clin Invest 70: 536, 1982

248. Wilson RF, Fisher RR: The hemodynamic effects of massive steroids in clinical shock. Surg Gynecol Obstet 127: 769, 1968

249. Wise WC, Cook JA, Halushka PV: Ibuprofen improves survival from endotoxic shock in the rat. J Pharmacol Exp Ther 215: 160, 1980

250. Wise WC, Cook JA, Halushka PV, Knapp DR: Protective effects of thromboxane synthetase inhibitors in rats in endotoxic shock. Circ Res 46: 854, 1980

251. Yarbrough GG: On the neuropharmacology of thyrotropin-releasing hormone (TRH). Prog Neurobiol 12: 291, 1979

252. Young JB, Landsberg L: Catecholamines in intermediary metabolism. Clin Endocrinol Metab 6: 599, 1977

253. Young LS: Pathogenesis of septic shock approaches to management. In: Aspects of the management of shock (Shine KI, moderator). Ann Intern Med 93: 728, 1980

254. Zaloga GP, Chernow B, Zajtchuk R et al: Diagnostic dosages of protirelin (TRH) elevate B.P. by non-catecholamine mechanisms. Arch Intern Med 144: 1149, 1984

255. Zaloga GP, Hostinsky C, Chernow B: Endogenous opioid peptides: Critical care implications. Heart Lung 13: 421, 1984

256. Zaritsky AL, Chernow B: Catecholamines, sympathomimetics. p. 481. In Chernow B, Lake CR, (eds): The Pharmacologic Approach to the Critically Ill Patient. Williams and Wilkins, Baltimore, 1983

257. Zern RT, Foster LB, Blalock JA et al: Characteristics of the dopaminergic and noradrenergic systems of the pancreatic islets. Diabetes 28: 185, 1979

258. Zimmerman BG, Ryan MJ, Gomer S, Kraft E: Effect of prostaglandin synthesis inhibitors indomethacin and eicosa-5,8,11,14 tetranoic acid on adrenergic responses in dog cutaneous vasculature. J Pharmacol Exp Ther 187: 315, 1973

259. Zinner MJ, Kerr JK, Reynolds DG: Distribution and arteriovenous shunting of gastric blood flow in the baboon: effect of epinephrine and vasopressin infusions. Gastroenterology 71: 299, 1976

260. Zukin RS, Zukin SR: Multiple opiate receptors: emerging concepts. Life Sci 29: 2681, 1981

SECTION III

HYPOVOLEMIC SHOCK

7

Fluid Resuscitation and Oxygen Exchange in Hypovolemia

Richard M. Peters

INTRODUCTION

The cells of the body depend on the transport of oxygen from the atmosphere to the organelles of the cells. The waste product of catabolism, carbon dioxide, then must be transported back to the atmosphere in a regulated manner to preserve the optimal pH for the metabolic process.

The gas transport system requires the coordination function of the circulation, the lungs, and the ventilatory pump (Fig. 7-1). The skillful administration of intravenous fluids can be critical in restoring and/or preserving this coordinate function.

Intravenous fluids are the most common drug given to hospitalized patients, and for intensive care unit (ICU) patients, the universal drug. They need to be considered a drug because the different fluids available have different physiologic effects and require different doses, or they have different pharmacokinetics.

The first diagram (Fig. 7-2) from the brilliant teaching syllabus of Dr. James Gamble of Harvard[5] depicts a fundamental principle of fluid therapy: the distribution of fluids between the body compartments, the internal exchange, determines whether fluid therapy wreaks havoc or enhances function. The composition and quantity of the administered fluid are critical determinants of how fluid is distributed between compartments. Without adequate amounts of fluid, the functional integrity of the circulation is compromised and fluid and other substrates do not reach the cells, nor can carbon dioxide and other wastes be removed. Since the heart and the ventilatory pump require an effective circulation to supply them with an adequate supply of oxygen and substrate for the removal of the carbon dioxide produced by the contracting muscle, the two pumps can be the victims of their own dysfunction.

157

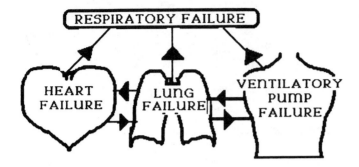

FIG. 7-1 Three systems that must have coordinated function to provide gas exchange.

AVAILABLE OXYGEN

Volume deficits are the major cause of inadequate circulation in surgical patients, and fluid overload the cause of failure of gas exchange. Precise fluid therapy is an essential of good care of the surgical patient. Optimization of gas exchange for the tissues must be the primary goal of fluid therapy. The strategy of this therapy depends on the goal, which has measurable dimensions. The most useful goal is amount of oxygen delivered to the tissues, the product of cardiac output and oxygen content of arterial blood.

Available oxygen
    = cardiac output × arterial oxygen content

Cardiac output is a function of heart rate × stroke volume. The three determinants of stroke volume are (1) the preload, end-diastolic volume of the ventricles, often erroneously equated to filling pressure; (2) the contractile strength of the myocardium; and (3) the ventricular afterload, the resistance of the systemic and pulmonary vascular beds. Preload, afterload, and contractility can all be altered by fluid exchange. Contractility of the ventricle is profoundly affected if the oxygen supply is inadequate to its needs. Hypovolemia is a major cause of inadequate coronary blood flow.

The amount of oxygen in arterial blood, the oxygen content, is controlled by (1) the hematocrit and, more precisely, the concentration of hemoglobin; (2) the efficiency of the lungs; and (3) the efficiency of the ventilatory pump (Fig. 7-1). Disorders of fluid exchange are the principal cause of deficiencies in the transfer

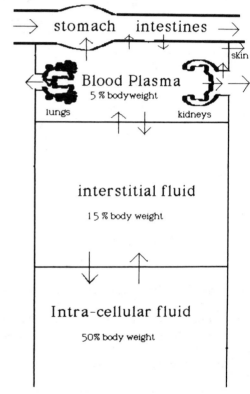

FIG. 7-2 Fluid compartments and major fluid exchange sites: gastrointestinal tract, skin, kidneys, and lungs. (Adapted from Gamble JL: Clinical Anatomy, Physiology and Pathology of Extracellular Fluid. A Lecture Syllabus. Harvard University Press, Cambridge, 1947.)

of oxygen between alveolar air and pulmonary capillary blood. Disorders of fluid exchange also change the mechanical properties of the lungs and thus increase the work required of the muscles of the chest cage. Like the heart, the effectiveness of the respiratory muscles is controlled by preload, afterload, and contractility. Also, like the heart, the preload and afterload of these muscles are profoundly altered by disorders in fluid exchange in the lungs, and the muscle contractility by the adequacy of oxygen delivery.

Thus, oxygen delivery requires two pumps, the heart and the respiratory muscles, which in turn depend on gas exchange, the delivery of oxygen and removal of carbon dioxide. We must have criteria for adequate quantity of intravenous fluids. The "physiologic criteria" accepted at this time are to maintain left heart filling pressure and cardiac output at preinjury or preoperative level. This type of control requires insertion of a Swan-Ganz catheter to measure pulmonary wedge pressure and cardiac output. In young patients with healthy hearts, central venous pressure is a reliable and may be a superior criterion of adequate cardiac filling pressure. Filling pressure is only an indirect measure of preload. If ventricular compliance is decreased, the same filling pressure will result in shorter myocardial fiber length and so a lower preload. Likewise, if afterload is increased, the cardiac output for a given preload will be less. Excessive right ventricular preload and afterload with shift of the intraventricular system can compromise left ventricular preload. Cardiac output is controlled not only by preload and afterload and contractility of the heart but also by effects of fluid therapy on the lungs and the ventilatory pump.

Unfortunately, in some studies of volume replacement comparing fluids of different composition, some investigators have not used even the presently accepted but imperfect physiologic criteria for adequacy of volume replacement. Instead, the studies have compared either equal volume of fluids of different composition or arbitrary amounts of two different fluids. As pointed out in the introduction, intravenous fluids are a form of drug and so have different potencies. The reason for the different required doses for any given volume is determined by the internal exchange of fluid. The internal exchange is controlled by the composition of the fluid.

FLUID EXCHANGE

External–Internal

The criteria for administering intravenous fluids of appropriate composition would appear to be relatively simple. Maintain the normal composition and volume of body fluids. There are circumstances where "normal" does not seem to be essential and may be less than optimal. The reason is that like all drugs, intravenous fluids have toxicity that is related principally to imperfections of substitutes for normal components of body fluids and difficulties arising from too rapid changes of colloidal osmotic pressure and/or electrolyte concentration during replacement of deficits.

Fluid exchange can be external; in clinical parlance, intake and output—or internal, the exchange between body compartments. Since Moyer[11] convinced the surgical community that often more fluid than was lost was required to restore circulatory function, an unfortunate, confusing term, "the third space" has been coined to define the location and dimensions of this excess volume (Fig. 7-3). There is no "third space." Explaining fluid requirements by stating a patient is "third spacing" becomes a substitute for understanding present knowledge of internal fluid exchange. Perhaps worse, such a quasiexplanation is uncritically accepted by many as a substitute for the knowledge about internal fluid exchange that still evades us. This chapter intends to demonstrate that the "third space" concept is a source of confusion and sloppy thinking, since the type of fluid administered can alter the size and the location of third-space fluids.

The control of internal fluid exchange provides the critical factor that limits amount and dictates composition of administered fluids. Infusion of fluids of inappropriate fluid composition or in inappropriate amounts results in excessive fluid filtration in the capillaries of the lungs and the other body tissues.

Exchange of water and solutes between the three major compartments—intravascular, interstitial, and intracellular—is determined by

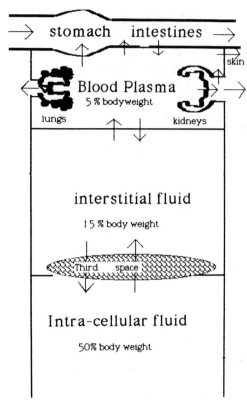

where Q_f is fluid filtered per minute, K_f is capillary membrane filtration coefficient, P_c is capillary hydrostatic pressure, P_t is interstitial fluid pressure, σ is protein reflection coefficient, Π_c is capillary oncotic pressure, and Π_t is interstitial-fluid oncotic pressure.

Figure 7-4 shows the interaction of the factors of the Starling equation. I have taken a liberty in this and Figures 7-6, 7-8, 7-9, 7-11, 7-13, and 7-14 to normalize values from different investigators from our and other laboratories. These values are made comparable to normal serum colloidal osmotic pressure values from our laboratories. All the Starling forces cannot be measured, so any discussion in-

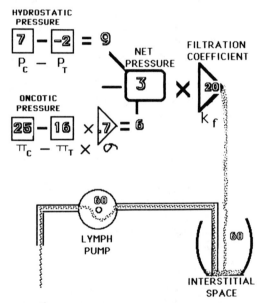

FIG. 7-3 Same as Figure 7-2, with the elusive and nonexistent "third space" shown, partly in the intracellular, partly in the extracellular space. The "third space" is of indefinite size and location. There is no general agreement as to whether it is all interstitial or partly intracellular.

the solutes in the administered fluid, the solutes in the compartment, and the permeability of the membrane separating the three compartments. Water moves freely across all membranes. Water moves into compartments with elevated osmolality and out of those with low osmolality.

The intravascular compartment is separated from the extravascular by the capillary membrane. The capillaries are freely permeable to electrolytes and water but only partially permeable to protein. The distribution of fluid across the capillary membrane has been defined by the Starling equation:

$$Q_f = K_f \left[(P_c - P_t) - \sigma(\Pi_c - \Pi_t) \right]$$

FIG. 7-4 Description of the Starling equation. Top left, the net hydrostatic pressures with normal values for the lung; the hydrostatic pressure in the capillaries, P_c, minus the hydrostatic pressure in the tissue, P_t. Bottom left, the oncotic pressure in the serum, Π_c, minus tissue oncotic pressure, Π_t, is multiplied by the reflectance coefficient (σ) (the discount for permeability of protein through the capillary membrane). The net filtration pressure is the difference between these two. The filtration coefficient ml/mmHg/min, K_f, is multiplied by the net filtration force to give the amount filtered from the capillary into the interstitium. This filtered fluid is returned to the circulation by the lymphatic pump.

volves some assumptions. The liberties inherent in such assumptions are clearly defined by a major contributor to our knowledge about lung fluid exchange, Dr. Normal Staub[3] of San Francisco, who said:

> It is easy enough to guess at suitable numbers to fit our misconceptions, but how to measure the forces in a convincing manner is a formidable problem.

The importance of this statement is that precise values are in many instances impossible to measure. However, relative values can be deduced; in particular, the sum of the forces are reasonable figures.

Starting at the top, on the left is the capillary hydrostatic pressure, P_c—the blood pressure in the capillary, a force of 7 mmHg pushing fluid out of the capillary. In the normal person, this force is enhanced by the negative interstitial pressure, -2 mmHg, which also pulls fluid from the capillary to give a net hydrostatic force of 9 mmHg pushing fluid from the capillary.

This hydrostatic force is opposed by the colloidal osmotic pressure, Π_c, or oncotic pressure of the serum, 25 mmHg in the normal patient. The tissue oncotic pressure in the lung is high, 16 mmHg, pulling fluid from the capillary for a net oncotic force of 9 mmHg. However, this force is modified by σ, the protein reflectance, a number between 0 and 1 that signifies the ability of the membrane to contain protein molecules. The capillary membrane is not completely impermeable to protein (a protein reflectance of 1) and even in disease is not totally permeable (protein reflectance of 0). The value defines the discount of the net oncotic force. The smaller σ is the greater, the discount of $(\Pi_t - \Pi_c)$. The precise value of σ is not known but is estimated to be 0.7 or 0.8 in normal lungs. As a result, the difference between $(\Pi_c - \Pi_t)$ of 9 is discounted to 6, and there is a net filtration force of 3 mmHg.

K_f is the filtration fraction, the milliliters of fluid filtered per millimeters of mercury per hour. It is shown as an equilateral triangle, the electronic engineer's symbol for an amplifier. K_f is the amplifier of the balance of factors within the brackets. When K_f rises, the gain of the amplifiers increases the ml of fluid filtered per hour for each millimeter of mercury of net filtration pressure. The normal value for K_f is estimated at 20 ml/hr/mmHg.

Q_f is the amount of fluid filtered per minute, shown as the open flask at the lower right. With a K_f value of 20 and a net filtration force of 3 mmHg, the fluid filtered, Q_f, is 60 ml/hr, all of which is pumped back into the circulation by the lymph system.

Colloid vs. Crystalloid

A good start for discussion of fluid exchange that illustrates the importance of solute composition of fluid therapy is a comparison of colloid versus crystalloid for volume replacement.[16] In collaboration with Virgilio at the San Diego Naval Regional Medical Center, we did a study in which a series of patients undergoing aortic reconstruction was randomized to receive for volume replacement either red blood cells and protein-free electrolytes or red blood cells and 5 percent albumin in electrolyte solution equivalent to serum with normal oncotic pressure. Fluids were administered to keep pulmonary wedge pressure within 3 mmHg of preoperative and cardiac output within 0.5 L of preoperative levels. We found that the electrolyte group required fluids equivalent to four times blood loss, the protein group two times blood loss. Figure 7-5 is a plot of the mean pulmonary wedge pressure and mean serum colloidal osmotic pressure through the perioperative period. In patients resuscitated with 5 percent albumin solution, serum colloidal osmotic pressure was essentially unchanged. During the immediate postoperative period, pulmonary wedge pressure was moderately elevated despite its use as a control criterion for fluid infusion. Two patients in the colloid group developed pulmonary edema. Both had some elevation in pulmonary wedge pressures but a smaller change in colloidal osmotic pressure–pulmonary wedge pressure gradient than in the crystalloid group.

For the patients resuscitated with crystal-

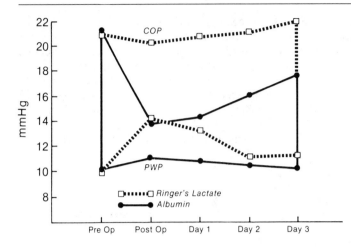

FIG. 7-5 Comparison of colloid (...) versus crystalloid (—) for volume replacement in patients undergoing abdominal aortic surgery. COP, colloidal osmotic pressure (..., —, top). PWP, pulmonary wedge pressure (..., —, bottom). The colloid-treated patients had no fall in COP but showed some rise in PWP. The crystalloid-treated patients showed a marked fall in COP and no change in PWP. Neither group had significant change in shunt fraction.

loid, note the marked fall in serum colloidal osmotic pressure and consequent fall in difference between serum colloidal osmotic pressure and pulmonary capillary wedge pressure. There is no significant rise in wedge pressure. None of these patients had pulmonary problems.

Postoperative measures of lung function showed no difference between the groups. Shires et al.[14] reported a similar study in which lung water was also measured by the double dilution method. These investigators found no increase in lung water or difference between the two groups. Clearly, simply lowering the gradient between colloidal osmotic pressure and wedge pressure does not result in increased lung water. However, significant peripheral edema developed in the patients in both studies.

The paradox of peripheral edema without pulmonary edema during hemodilution was studied by Zarins in our laboratory.[18] Zarins et al. did a study on baboons which we call isobaric plasmapheresis. The right thoracic duct was cannulated to collect lung lymph. This permitted measurements of the changes in pulmonary lymph flow rate and colloidal osmotic pressure. The animals were bled and Ringer's lactate infused to keep wedge pressure and cardiac output at control levels. The red cells and plasma were separated, and the red cells returned to the circulation. The process was repeated three times. Ringer's lactate equivalent to approximately 5 percent of body weight was required to keep the wedge pressure and car-

diac output at control level. Lung lymph increased but the wet weight of the lungs did not, signifying no increase in lung water.

Figure 7-6 shows the changes in fluid filtration in the lungs with hemodilution. With hemodilution, capillary pressure was maintained constant. No direct measures of lung interstitial fluid pressure have been made except for a few recent measurements in the lung periphery by Staub.[3] We have assumed that the lung acts like other tissues and interstitial pressure rises

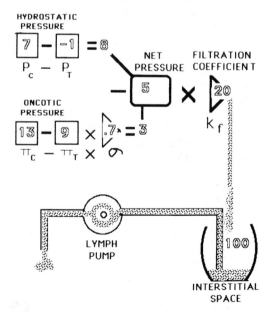

FIG. 7-6 Similar to Figure 7-4, showing results of hemodilution on normal lung fluid exchange (see text).

with increased fluid filtration. As a result, net hydrostatic pressure is reduced from 9 to 8.

Serum oncotic pressure dropped 12 mmHg, from 25 to 13. However, 7 mm of this drop was neutralized because interstitial oncotic pressure fell from 16 to 9. The fall in interstitial fluid oncotic pressure is a result of dilution and lymph removal of protein. The net oncotic force is decreased by 5 mmHg instead of 12. With the usual discount by σ, the force is reduced to 3 for a net increase in filtration force of only 2. If these compensatory forces, fall in Π_t and rise in P_t, had not occurred, the increase would be 12 mmHg. The parallel fall in Π_t as Π_c falls results in an increase in filtered volume, Q_f, from 60 to 100 ml/hr filtered well within the capacity of the lymphatic pump, so no pulmonary edema results. If the intravascular oncotic pressure remained at 16, the tissue oncotic pressure would exceed that of plasma and 240 ml/hr of fluid would be filtered.

The explanation for this protection of the lungs if best expressed by Aubrey Taylor's concept of lung edema safety factor.[15] He calculates this safety factor as equal to 20 cm of pressure. This safety factor has two major components (Fig. 7-7):

1. High interstitial protein concentration: Lowering serum oncotic pressure or raising capillary pressure results in dilution of this protein and neutralization of some of the fall in oncotic pressure.
2. Increase in lymph flow, which may be as much as 10-fold, as shown in Zarins'[18] studies: A minor component is elevation of interstitial hydrostatic pressure, P_t. Since the edema safety factor in the lung is in the region of 20 mmHg, simple hemodilution, the lowering of serum oncotic pressure, will not exceed this safety factor and so will not result in pulmonary edema.

Figure 7-8 shows the effects on net fluid filtration force of elevation of capillary pressure. The same amount of protection is provided when capillary pressure is increased to 30 mmHg. The extravascular protein, Π_t, is diluted from 16 to 9 mmHg and the net protein force, $\Pi_c - \Pi_t$, is raised to 16 but σ lowers it to 11. The tissue hydrostatic pressure, P_t, rises from -2 to -1, so the net hydrostatic force,

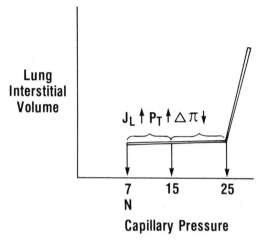

FIG. 7-7 The edema safety factor as depicted by Aubrey Taylor. Eighteen to 20 mmHg rise in net capillary pressure does not cause an increase in lung water. Increased lymphatic removal, J_L, rise in interstitial hydrostatic pressure, P_T, and fall in interstitial oncotic pressure neutralize the rise in capillary or fall in oncotic pressure. (Taylor AE, Grimbert F, Rutili G et al: Pulmonary edema: changes in Starling forces and lymph flow. p. 135. In Hargens AR (ed): Tissue Fluid Pressure and Composition. © 1981 The Williams & Wilkins Co., Baltimore.)

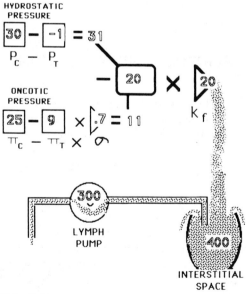

FIG. 7-8 Similar to Figure 7-4, showing the effect of rise in normal lung capillary pressure filtration exceeds the capacity of the lymphatic pump and interstitial edema results (see text).

$P_c - P_t$, is 31. To give a net force favoring filtration of 20 and with K_f of 20, 400 ml/hr (which exceeds to 200 to 300 ml/hr capacity of the lymphatic pump), edema results. Because P_c can be raised more than the edema safety factor, elevation of capillary pressure, P_c, can cause edema. Serum oncotic pressure, Π_c, cannot be changed enough to exceed the edema safety factor.

Figure 7-9 shows the effects of combination of elevation of capillary pressure and hemodilution. The edema safety factor has been spent to neutralize the high P_c. Π_t cannot be lowered significantly more nor tissue pressure increased, so a drop in serum oncotic pressure Π_c from 25 to 13 results in corresponding increase in net filtration force from 19 to 28 and filtered fluid from 400 to 560 ml. Hemodilution and elevation in P_c are additive. A drop in oncotic pressure at all levels of P_c increases fluid filtration.[8] If a patient has a drop in serum oncotic pressure due to hemodilution or other causes, he will be less protected from a rise in capillary pressure. Where serum proteins are low, control of pulmonary wedge pressure must be more precise.

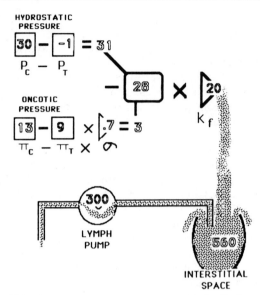

FIG. 7-9 Similar to Figure 7-4, showing the effects of normal lung hemodilution and high capillary pressure are additive (see text).

PERIPHERY HEMODILUTION

In the systemic vascular capillaries, the drop in Π_c associated with hemodilution results in interstitial edema. All the patients resuscitated from blood loss with Ringer's lactate, as did the baboons reported in Zarins' study,[18] developed systemic edema. We can measure in the periphery the tissue pressure and tissue oncotic pressure using the Scholander-Hargens wick catheter (Fig. 7-10). The catheter is polyethylene tubing with a wick of Tevdek suture tethered with polyproplene to hold it in place. The wick acts to prevent occlusion of the catheter.

Figure 7-11 shows muscle hemodilution. There is no equivalent to the lung edema safety factor in the periphery. The normal capillary

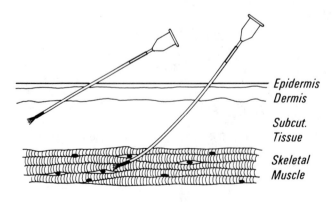

Epidermis
Dermis

Subcut.
Tissue

Skeletal
Muscle

FIG. 7-10 The Scholander-Hargens wick catheter permits measurement of interstitial hydrostatic pressure and sampling of interstitial fluid for measurement of interstitial oncotic pressure. The catheter is a small polyvinyl tube with a tethered wick.

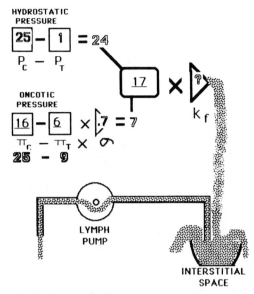

FIG. 7-11 Similar to Figure 7-4, hemodilution in the muscle and also in subcutaneous tissue causes increased interstitial fluid as shown. Because capillary pressure is higher and tissue oncotic pressure lower, the edema safety factor is less.

pressure is higher, 20 to 25 mmHg. The muscle tissue pressure is positive. Oncotic pressure of interstitial tissue is normally 8, lower than the Π_t of 16 in the lung. Therefore, the normal net filtration force is nearer 9 mmHg, as compared

with 3 mmHg in the lung. With hemodilution, the net pressure rises to 17, resulting in systemic edema.

In patients undergoing cardiopulmonary bypass using electrolyte solution as the pump prime, or when Ringer's lactate is used in aortic resection patients, filtration in the systemic beds exceeds lymphatic pump capacity. However, Kramer et al.[9] showed, as have we, that the same compensatory mechanism lowering interstitial protein concentration by lymphatic transfer to the blood raises serum protein and restores the oncotic gradient (Fig. 7-12). This homeostatic mechanism is not adequately appreciated. The interstitium stores a pool of extravascular protein. When there is acute drop in the intravascular protein due to hemorrhage, the lymphatics transfer the interstitial protein to the vascular space to restore the oncotic gradient and preserve intravascular volume. This process takes 24 to 48 hours.

Effects of Capillary Injury

The control of internal fluid exchange would be relatively simple if the only problems were to control the capillary pressure and the oncotic pressure. Unfortunately, the surgeon

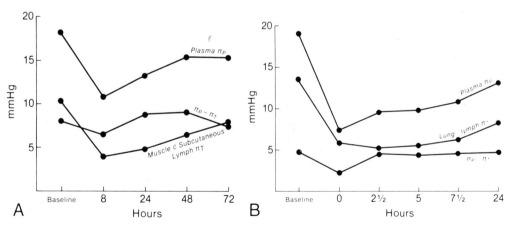

FIG. 7-12 **(A, B)** Plasmapheresis effect on plasma and lung lymph oncotic pressure. A drop in plasma oncotic pressure, Π_p, is associated with a drop in tissue oncotic pressure (Π_t). $\Pi_p - \Pi_t$ exhibits only a small fall in muscle (A) and virtually no change in the lung (B). (Modified from Kramer GC, Harms BA, Gunther RA, et al: The effects of hypoproteinemia on blood-to-lymph fluid transport in sheep lung. Circ Res 49:1173, 1981. By permission of the American Heart Association, Inc.)

faces the serious problem of edema due to injury of the capillary; in the lungs, the shock-lung or acute respiratory distress syndrome (ARDS); in the systemic circulation, burns, trauma, or sepsis.

Recent investigations show that capillary damage in the lung results from activation of the complement system and coagulation cascade. Any substances which might activate the immune or coagulation systems such as foreign protein, starch particles, or oxygenator materials, have the potential to damage lung capillaries.

What are the consequences of capillary injury? They are magnification of changes in the net Starling forces. The capillary injury increases filtration coefficient and decreases protein reflectance.

Fig. 7-13 shows: the capillary pressure, P_c, unchanged at 7, but the fluid that leaks from the capillary raises tissue pressure, P_t, to 0 from -2. $P_c - P_t$ is lowered from 9 to 7. Serum oncotic pressure, Π_c, remains at 25 but the ability of the capillary to reflect protein, σ, falls to 0.5 or less and results in a rise in tissue protein,

Π_t. As a result, $\Pi_c - \Pi_t$ falls to 3 and the drop in σ to 5 discounts the 3 to 1.5. The net filtration force rises from 3 to 5.5, a small rise that alone would be of no consequence.

However, the filtration coefficient, K_f, has risen from 20 ml/hr/mmHg to 60, so rather than 110 ml/hr, 330 ml/hr of fluid is filtered, exceeding the 200 to 200 ml/hr capacity of the lymph pump.

Hemodilution has little effect when the filtration coefficient, K_f, is increased and protein reflectance, σ, decreased. Both intra- and extravascular proteins are diluted, and the difference is about the same as if serum proteins, Π_c, were normal.

The effect of increase in pulmonary capillary pressure with an elevated filtration coefficient and depressed protein reflectance is a different matter (Fig. 7-14). A rise in pulmonary capillary pressure, P_c, emphasizes the danger of the magnifying effect of capillary injury, which causes a rise in filtration coefficient, K_f, and fall in protein reflectance, σ. There now is no safety factor of fall in tissue oncotic pressure, Π_t; rather, interstitial protein rises. The

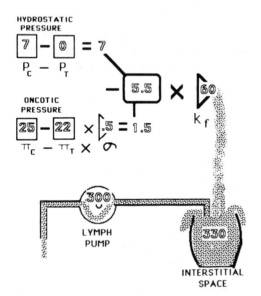

FIG. 7-13 Similar to Figure 7-4, showing the effect of capillary leak. The rise in K_f magnifies the net filtration force, exceeding the capacity of the lymphatic pump. The lung filtration coefficient is high while the protein reflectance is low.

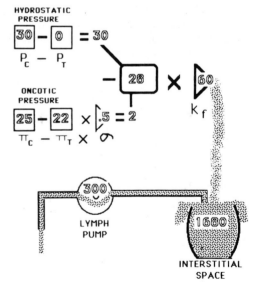

FIG. 7-14 With the addition of high lung capillary pressure to leaky capillary fluid filtration, along with high filtration coefficient and low protein reflectance, the effect of K_f amplification results in massive flooding of the lungs.

injured capillary allows protein to leak from the capillary and $\Pi_c - \Pi_t$ is only 3, while $P_c - P_t$ is 30, leaving a net filtration force of 28 to 29. Each millimeter of mercury of this force results in 60 ml fluid filtration per hour of 1,680 ml, quickly flooding the lungs.

The addition of hemodilution to high capillary pressure has little added effect if filtration coefficient is increased and protein reflectance decreased. If protein leaks across the membrane, nothing will be gained by the administration of protein. Increasing intravascular protein concentration will cause a parallel increase in extravascular protein concentration. If the capillary leak is sealed, until the excess extravascular protein is removed by the lymphatics, the extravascular protein will continue to pull fluid from the capillaries.

In both a normal pulmonary capillary bed and a damaged pulmonary capillary bed, the colloidal osmotic pressure of serum has less effect on lung fluid filtration than the pulmonary capillary pressure because changes in $\Pi_c - \Pi_t$ cannot be as great as those in $P_c - P_t$.

Artificial Colloids

The recent appearance of hetastarch (Hespan) has provided the physician with another alternative for treatment of hypovolemia. Hespan is an amylopectin that has hydroxethyl ether groups introduced into the glucose molecules and hydrolyzed so that the molecules weigh an average of 450,000 with 90 percent 10,000 to 1,000,000. The molecules less than 50,000 are rapidly excreted in the urine, resulting in excretion of 40 percent of the infused starch within 24 hours. Hetastarch is more than 99 percent excreted at the end of 2 weeks.

The artificial colloid widely used for volume replacement in Europe is dextran −70.[1] Both hetastarch and dextran can cause increased bleeding in part by dilution, but they also seem to have some direct effects that may be dose related. Doses over 1,500 ml of the standard solutions are usually not advised. Acute resuscitation with these two artificial colloids requires only two times the volume lost rather than four times the blood lost required when crystalloids are used.

We need to know what happens to the artificial colloids in the interim between infusion and excretion. We know that hemodilution with crystalloid causes an increase in lung fluid filtration in sheep[3] and baboons[18] as measured by a rise in lung lymph flow. The available studies show no increase in lung water in animals or humans when crystalloid is used for resuscitation. In the sheep studies, the oncotic pressure difference between lung lymph (thought to represent lung interstitial fluid) and plasma is maintained by washout of proteins in the lung interstitium. We need to know how much of the starch or dextrose gets into the interstitial space in the interim between administration and excretion.

Pulmonary edema, the nemesis of fluid resuscitation, does not usually occur during the period of acute resuscitation. Pulmonary edema becomes apparent 48 to 72 hours later. In a burn shock model in sheep, when dextran is infused for resuscitation during the acute stage, lung lymph flow is less than with crystalloid. However, lymph flow from the lungs is greater at 48 hours when dextran is given.[7] In the burn patient, pulmonary edema is a late phenomenon just at the time that the increase in fluid filtration with dextran is seen. Before the role in volume replacement of these artificial colloids can be clarified, it will be necessary to do studies of early and late effects on muscle and subcutaneous interstitial protein and artificial colloid compared to that of plasma to see if the presence of the artificial colloid delays the plasma protein refill or increases fluid filtration. In other words, we need to know the true useful physiologic half-life of these substances. What are the negative effects as they are excreted from the body? Just to show that a smaller volume needs to be given or that the plasma oncotic pressure is higher is not enough to tell us whether the purported advantages are real.

The controversy regarding the appropriate fluid for resuscitation from hypovolemic shock will not be resolved by stating that studies show one is better than the other or by comparing the cost of one with another. The problem centers on learning more about the effects of composition on the dynamics of internal fluid exchange.

CRITERIA FOR VOLUME INFUSED

The controversy about composition is further complicated by uncertainties that are now surfacing about the "physiologic end points" criteria for resuscitation. A worldwide epidemic of postpneumonectomy pulmonary edema serves to illustrate at least two points: (1) the type of operation or injury profoundly affects the criteria for resuscitation; (2) pulmonary edema from fluid overload is still a real clinical problem.

Postpneumonectomy pulmonary edema is almost always fatal and occurs in patients who are good risks for pneumonectomy and have an uneventful operation and early postoperative course. Twenty-four to 48 hours after the operation they develop progressive dyspnea, hyperventilation, and fall in PO_2. Unless treated immediately by intubation, ventilatory support, diuretics, and sedation, they die very quickly of hypoxemia. When consulted in Rotterdam about this problem, I wondered whether it could be similar to a problem found in a study done in 1969 by one of my colleagues, Dr. Peter Hutchin.[6] He was interested in finding out whether intraoperative infusions of large volumes of crystalloid solutions in patients undergoing pulmonary resection could block the antidiuretic effect of operation and improve the circulatory dynamics. Patients had blood loss replaced with whole blood. One group received 1,700 to 2,200 ml/m² balanced salt solution during operation and immediately postoperatively 750 ml of 5 percent glucose.

None of these patients had a CVP greater than 15. In three of 12 patients in whom wedge pressure was measured, it was below 15 cm of water. There was evidence of rales and congestion in all patients. The twelfth patient in the study developed pulmonary edema following pneumonectomy and died. The study was terminated, and Hutchin et al.[6] reached the following conclusions:

> This study demonstrates that administration of large volumes of fluids to patients undergoing pulmonary resections may lead to undesirable effects and potentially lethal consequences, particularly in patients requiring pneumonectomy. Where circulatory dynamics and urine flow may be improved to a certain extent by such treatment, the beneficial effect on the kidneys occurs at the risk of pulmonary congestion.

The recall of this study stimulated two studies: A review to compare the fluid balance for uncomplicated pneumonectomies at the University of California Medical Center, San Diego to that of patients who developed edema (Table 7-1), and a study of dog model of postpneumonectomy pulmonary edema.[19] Ta-

TABLE 7-1.   Pulmonary Edema After Right Pneumonectomy[a]

	Intake		Urine			Net Intake	
	ml	ml/kg	ml	ml/kg	EBL	ml	ml/kg
PE (N = 4)							
Mean	4,912[b]	67[c]	1,480[b]	21[b]	550	2,777	37
SD	±1,169	±14	±472	±9	±311	±1,454	±17
NP (N = 6)							
Mean	3,483[b]	46[c]	827[b]	11[b]	579	2,041	27
SD	±984	±17	±190	±4	±458	±800	±13

[a] Comparison of four patients who had PE after operation with six patients who did not. EBL, Estimated blood loss.
[b] $P < 0.10$.
[c] $P < 0.05$.
(Zeldin RA, Normandin D, Landtwing D, Peters RM: Postpneumonectomy pulmonary edema. J Thorac Cardiovasc Surg 87:359, 1984.)

ble 7-1 compares the fluid intake, blood loss, and urine output in patients undergoing right pneumonectomy who developed pulmonary edema with a like group that did not. The blood loss is similar, but the pulmonary edema patients received significantly more fluid infused and had higher urine outputs during the first 24 hours. We have complete studies on only one of the patients who developed pulmonary edema, one studied by Gibbons and the Naval Medical Center, San Diego (personal communication). To our knowledge, this is the only patient who has survived this complication. The wedge pressure was not elevated and the cardiac output was increased, as was the pulmonary artery pressure. In two other patients for whom we have data, the wedge pressure was not elevated. This, therefore, does not fit the classical definition of high pressure pulmonary edema. Review of the fluid data, however, led us to conclude, as did Hutchin,[6] that excessive fluid infusion was the initiating agent. This impression was confirmed by the study in dogs.[19]

For the conclusion that fluid overload was the cause of postpneumonectomy pulmonary edema to be accepted, we must deal with some paradoxes. The patients undergoing aortic reconstruction in both Shires[14] and Virgilio's[16] series received far more fluid than did the pneumonectomy patients who developed pulmonary edema (Fig. 7-15). It should also be noted that the variance in the amount of fluid infused in the postpneumonectomy pulmonary edema patients was large (Table 7-2). This variance was also apparent in Zeldin's study in dogs.[19] The effect of excessive volume is not uniform across patient groups. Some patients are more susceptible to pulmonary edema than others.

How can the vulnerability of patients following pneumonectomy be greater than that of patients with aortic disease, particularly since the patients who get pulmonary edema have almost all been in the good risk category? The cardiac output when measured in Gibbons' patient was elevated, but it is more important to look at the blood flow rate through the remaining left lung. The right lung is 55 percent of the total lung volume and normally receives 55 percent of the flow. (Only one patient has been reported to us as developing pulmonary edema when the smaller left lung was removed.) The flow to the left lung was increased

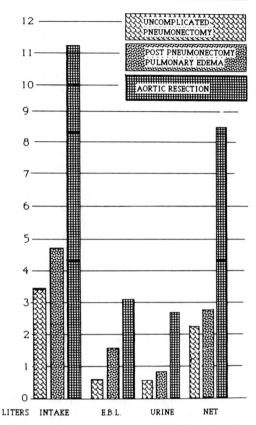

FIG. 7-15 Intake, blood loss, and urine output compared in three groups of patients listed at top right on the day of operation. Note that aortic resection patients received the most fluid but did not get pulmonary edema.

in Gibbons' patient as compared to the aortic patients (Table 7-2). The pulmonary artery pressure was also elevated in the pneumonec-

TABLE 7-2. Comparison of Pulmonary Blood Flow in a Postpneumonectomy and an Aortic Resection Patient

	Pneumonectomy	Aortic Resection
Cardiac index	4.9	2.9
Left lung	4.9	1.3
Pulmonary artery	52.0	—
Pulmonary wedge	6.0	10.0

(J Gibbons: personal communication 1981, and Virgilio RW, Rice CL, Smith DE, et al: Crystalloid versus colloid resuscitation: Is one better? A randomized clinical study. Surgery 85:129, 1979.)

tomy patients. The capillary pressure is not the same as the wedge pressure, particularly in high flow states. The pressure is between mean pulmonary artery pressure and wedge pressure. It can only be estimated at this time. Taylor et al.[15] suggested that it could be measured in patients by analyzing wedge waveform.

Figure 7-16 shows the effect of high flow in raising of capillary pressure, particularly if the mean pulmonary artery pressure is also raised. The wedge pressure may stay normal but the capillary pressure goes up because the pattern of pressure drop along the capillary is changed. The mean capillary pressure moves downstream, resulting in a higher capillary pressure without change in wedge pressure.

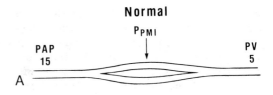

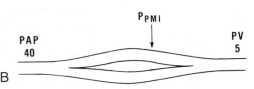

FIG. 7-16 (A) Normal relationship between pulmonary artery pressure (PAP) and pulmonary venous pressure (PV), with the mean pulmonary microvascular pressure (P_{PMI}) occurring about halfway down the stream. **(B)** When the pulmonary artery pressure rises and the vessels open, there can still be the same pulmonary venous pressure with a higher mean pulmonary microvascular pressure because the midpoint moves toward the pulmonary venous end of the circulation. (Peters RM: Postoperative respiratory failure. p. 141. In de Guia T, Lardizabal A (eds): Respiratory Failure. Proceedings of the First Boehringer Ingelheim Chest Symposium, Manila. Asia Pacific Congress Series No. 27. Excerpta Medica, Amsterdam, 1983.)

CONTROLLERS OF CARDIAC OUTPUT

There can be no question that the recognition by Moyer[11] and others of the need to give electrolyte fluid in excess of the actual amount lost was an important landmark in appropriate resuscitation. He did not, nor did his disciples, conclude that precision in the amount infused was not critical. Unfortunately, many have accepted the "third space" concept uncritically and cite it as a reason for unreasonable amount of fluid.

Much of the excessive fluid is given during the induction of anesthesia. When there is some decrease in blood pressure, the patient is considered to be "dry" and needs fluid to fill the "third space" or rehydrate it. This is not given after review of urine output or other measures of adequacy of hydration but just reflexively. The conclusion that the administration of excessive fluid is safer than not enough is correct, but this does not mean that one should be satisfied with second best. If some is good, more is not necessarily better. One can only increase the precision of fluid therapy by knowing more about the criteria for adequacy. The principal reason for giving intravenous electrolyte solutions is to provide adequate filling pressure so that the heart can pump effectively. The controllers of cardiac output are stroke volume and rate. Stroke volume is determined by the preload (length of the myocardial fibers in diastole), the afterload, and the myocardial contractility.

The level of pulmonary wedge pressure is the clinical measurement of the left ventricular preload. However, the pulmonary wedge pressure is only one of the controllers of preload. The preload—the end-diastolic volume—required depends on the stiffness or compliance of the ventricle and the transventricular pressure.

Preload = end-diastolic volume
       = ventricular compliance
           × transventricular pressure

If the ventricle is stiff, a high pressure is necessary to get the same preload. Ischemia of ventricular muscle, interstitial edema, and hypertrophy all make the ventricle stiffer.

Since the clinician estimates pulmonary capillary pressure and left heart filling pressure from the pulmonary wedge pressure, the pulmonary wedge pressure is the critical measure of competition between the heart and the lungs. Too high a pressure means increased fluid filtration; too low a wedge pressure, a fall in cardiac output. An excessive capillary pressure or capillary injury will result in flooding of the alveoli with fluid and collapse of unstable alveoli. Perfusion of unventilated alveoli causes an intrapulmonary shunt which in turn results in arterial oxygen desaturation.

The treatment of a young man who was spurned by his girlfriend and who ignited gasoline he had poured on himself provides an example of how pulmonary edema can result from the use of excessive amounts of fluid for resuscitation. He suffered 42 percent deep third-degree burns. The criteria used for resuscitation of this young man were urine output and wedge pressures with intermittent determination of cardiac output. To replace fluid loss into the burn due to capillary injury, he was given 26 L Ringer's lactate and plasma, two times the amount prescribed by the formula used for predicting fluid requirements. His admission chest roentgonogram was clear and he had no evidence of respiratory burns. As a result of this large amount of fluid, severe pulmonary edema developed on the third day.

During review of the case at morbidity and mortality conference, it was apparent that his cardiac output and urine output were both marginal to low. His physicians considered the patient to be hypovolemic with expected vasoconstriction and increased peripheral resistance. His measured wedge pressure was not excessive. Those responsible for the resuscitation defended the volume of fluid administered as essential to maintain cardiac output, without which the patient would not survive. The

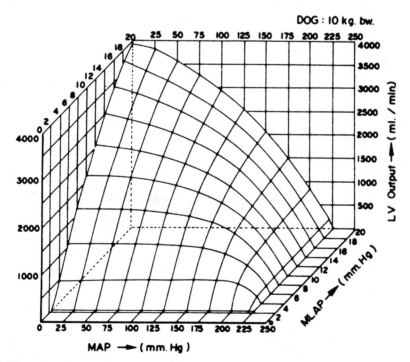

FIG. 7-17 Three-dimensional diagram of the integrated effect of changes in mean left atrial pressure (MLAP) and mean aortic pressure (mean MAP) on left ventricular outflow per minute (LV output). (Sagawa K: Analysis of the ventricular pumping capacity as a function of input and output pressure loads. p. 489. In Reeve EB, Guyton AC (eds): Physical Bases of Circulatory Transport: Regulation and Exchange. WB Saunders, Philadelphia, 1967.)

Monday morning quarterbacks did not disagree about the goal, but they criticized the strategy. Why did this young man require fluids in excess of the usual burn replacement calculations, an amount of fluid that ultimately led to pulmonary edema? Was it due to poor contractility?

The ventricular contractility is an indicator of the inherent strength of the cardiac muscle and may be affected by both the amount of interstitial fluid and cell swelling. Contractility is clearly dependent on adequate oxygen supply and can be markedly enhanced by physical conditioning and decreased by inactivity. While this young man was not an Olympic athlete, he was vigorous and was promptly resuscitated so that decreased contractility was unlikely. This conclusion is further supported by the fact that his cardiac output was over 12 L at the height of his pulmonary edema, and despite the stress of this severe burn and pulmonary edema, he has recovered from his injury.

Blood pressure was elevated to 160 systolic. The patient showed evidence of severe apprehension, shivering, and hyperactivity, all pointing to excessive afterload. A diagram by Sagawa discussed by Braunwald et al.[4] illustrates the importance of the relationship between preload and afterload (Fig. 7-17). As afterload goes up, the cardiac output for any given filling pressure goes down. The experience of cardiac surgeons in the use of afterload-reducing agents to prevent perioperative infarctions due to hypertension during induction and to increase cardiac output and reduce oxygen needs of the myocardium during the postoperative period has clearly shown the importance of Braunwald's[4] concepts in surgical patients.

These concepts are not only important to the cardiac patient; they are equally applicable to the young injured patient. With the excretion of catecholamines that are part of the response to injury, the contractility of the myocardium goes up and stroke volume will be larger for any given filling pressure. The catecholamine response to injury that increases myocardial contractility also results in vasoconstriction and an increase in afterload. The accepted criterion for fluid administration is to maintain cardiac index at least 3.0 L/min and the prein-

jury or preoperative level of wedge pressure. Since keeping the capillary pressure at the lowest level that will provide an adequate cardiac output minimizes fluid filtration, we must also ask whether it would be a better strategy to lower afterload to capitalize on the increased contractility resulting from high catecholamines. The critical question is, what is the optimal cardiac output?

Optimum Cardiac Output

There is no single value for the optimum cardiac index or filling pressure. If the myocardial contractility is increased, the preoperative filling pressure may not be the ideal one; it may be higher than is necessary. Optimum cardiac output is the cardiac output that transports to the tissues adequate amounts of oxygen to meet the metabolic demands. The oxygen consumption is increased by fever, shivering, apprehension, food intake, and decreased by sedation, starvation, and ventilator support. The amount of oxygen in each liter of blood, arterial oxygen content, is determined by the hematocrit level and the oxygen saturation—the percentage of hemoglobin carrying oxygen. The oxygen saturation is independently important because a low oxygen saturation, even if polycythemia is present to preserve oxygen content, means the PO_2 of tissues is lower and so the oxygen gradient from capillary to consuming cells is smaller. This gradient may be of critical importance if edema is present since edema lengthens the diffusion path.

The course of cellulitis in the arm of an expedition member at 5,400 m in the Himalayas gives a picture of the problem of the long perfusion path from capillary associated with a low tissue PO_2. The cellulitis would not clear despite adequate antibiotics until the individual went to a lower altitude and higher PO_2 diminished the price of long diffusion distance. Edema compromises tissue oxygenation more in the patient who has disease, causing a low arterial PO_2. Does increased interstitial fluid in skeletal muscle, heart muscle, and smooth muscle of the GI tract decrease the efficiency of muscle contraction?

Raising hematocrit does not necessarily increase available oxygen. Lowering hematocrit alters flow dynamics so that a greater cardiac output may be possible with less ventricular work, as shown in Figure 7-18.[10,13] This figure compares hematocrit on the horizontal axis, cardiac output on the vertical axis on the left, and available oxygen—cardiac output times arterial oxygen content—on the right. As hematocrit rises, arterial oxygen content increases but altered flow pressure relationships result in increased afterload and decrease in cardiac output. The curve with open circle, cardiac output vs. hematocrit, falls as hematocrit rises. The available oxygen curve is U shaped; its maximum is at hematocrit of 30. There is suggestive evidence that in resting man, a hematocrit of 30 results in greater oxygen delivery than one of 40. The afterload is less; therefore, cardiac output increase more than compensates for the lowered oxygen content. Recent studies on Everest[17] show no advantage to the polycythemia of altitude. West and associates suggest that this polycythemia is an example of maladaptation.

The physician responsible for resuscitation of the patient must understand the interaction of the factors controlling (1) oxygen needs, (2) oxygen content of arterial blood, and (3) cardiac output. The immediate task must be to deal with major blood loss but when the acute crisis of hypovolemia is coming under control, consideration of these factors in the order listed will result in the desired level of precision in volume of fluids infused:

1. Lower oxygen demands by controlling pain and apprehension.
2. Minimize muscular effort by providing ventilatory assistance if indicated.
3. Control fever.
4. Assure that gas transfer in the lungs is optimal.
5. Assure that hematocrit is in the range of 30 to 35.
6. Tune the preload and afterload to achieve the cardiac output required to meet the patient's oxygen needs.

The best index that oxygen needs are being met is the arteriovenous oxygen difference ($a\text{-}vDO_2$). A resting arteriovenous oxygen difference of 4 to 5 vol percent (ml of oxygen per dl of blood) indicates that tissue oxygen supplies are adequate and not excessive. Unless all factors are considered, inappropriate amounts and types of fluids are likely to be used. Since resuscitation requires larger quantities of fluid than were lost, the patient must excrete these fluids. Delayed onset of pulmo-

FIG. 7-18 Relationship between cardiac index and available oxygen when hematocrit is varied from 10 to 70. Cardiac index falls as hematocrit rises but available oxygen is optimal at hematocrit of 30. (Modified from Leveen et al[10] (Peters RM: Fluid exchange and oxygen delivery. p. 141. In de Guia T, Lardizabal A (eds): Respiratory Failure. Proceedings of the First Boehringer Ingelheim Chest Symposium, Manila. Asia Pacific Congress Series No. 27. Excerpta Medica, Amsterdam, 1983.

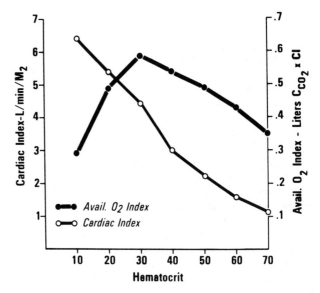

nary edema is the worst consequence of failure to excrete the excess fluids. The effects of the systemic edema on the vulnerability of tissues to infection, the rate of wound healing and the general discomfort of the patient, also may be of significant importance. At this time we do not have means of assessing their importance. However, observant surgeons are aware that a sign that the patient is on the way to recovery is the excretion of these fluids. Failure to do so is ominous. Clinical observation suggests advantages in limiting the amount of excess fluid required. The steps just discussed were addressed to limiting volume by altering the oxygen demands and the cardiac preload. Another approach is to limit volume by changing composition. The advocates of colloid solutions use this as the principal argument for use of colloids instead of crystalloids. As pointed out above, there is little evidence that this form of volume limitation is effective, and it does have the disadvantage of use of either foreign protein or starches. Another approach is to alter the electrolyte composition of the fluid administered and borrow some of the needed excess fluid from the intracellular water.

HYPERTONIC SALT SOLUTION

During exercise, man can lose many liters of water through the lungs and water in excess of salt through sweat. Man preserves extracellular and vascular fluid volume and thus cardiac output and oxygen delivery because this water loss without electrolyte increases the serum and extracellular fluid osmolality (Fig. 7-19A). To preserve intra- and extracellular osmolar balance, water moves from the intracellular to the extracellular space. This is a self-regulatory system of sharing fluid losses over the entire body water. Without this system, much smaller water losses would decrease circulatory volume to the level that would cause a fall in cardiac output. (When fluid is lost from the gastrointestinal tract, this protection of extracellular and vascular volume does not exist because the gastrointestinal

secretions are ismolar with serum. Losses from the gastrointestinal tract are not shared with the intracellular compartment.)

The shift of fluid from intracellular to extracellular space with water loss suggests an alternative to giving four times blood loss as Ringer's lactate, the use of hypertonic salt solutions. Just as exercising man raises extravascular osmolality to pull water from the cells to share extravascular losses in proportion to the relative amounts of intra- and extravascular water, hypertonic resuscitative fluids draw water from the intravascular compartment to maintain osmolar balance.

Figure 7-19B shows the results of resuscitation of a series of patients undergoing aortic surgery with Ringer's lactate solution or with an electrolyte solution of twice the osmolality of Ringer's. On the left is depicted the normal distribution of fluid and osmoles between the intracellular and extracellular spaces. Volume in liters is on the horizontal scale; millimoles per liter on the vertical scale. The areas represent the millimoles in each compartment. The calculations assume that there is no change in the total number of intracellular millimoles. With Ringer's lactate resuscitation, extracellular fluid volume increases by 8 L, intracellular by 1 L. With hypertonic salt, extracellular volume increases by only 6 liters and intracellular falls by 2 L. We have found that the movement of water from intracellular to extracellular space permits resuscitation with a volume of electrolyte solution equal to twice rather than four times the volume lost. Hypertonic fluid lowers muscular interstitial pressure and patients appear subjectively more comfortable.[12] Does it lower the oxygen diffusing path in tissues and thereby improve the delivery of oxygen to the cells?

FLUIDS AND THE VENTILATORY PUMP

Hypovolemia and pulmonary edema due to fluid overload or increased capillary permeability affect the ventilatory pump as well as

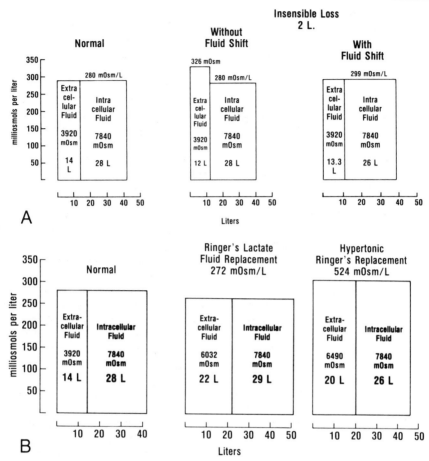

FIG. 7-19 (**A**) Effect of loss of water without electrolyte from perspiration or hyperventilation. (Left) Distribution of fluid between extra- and intracellular spaces. (Center) Loss of 2 L water with exercise from only the extracellular compartment. The extravascular milliosmoles rise from 280 to 326 and extracellular volume falls by 2 L. (Right) Because there is equilibrium between intracellular and extracellular osmolarity, fluid moves out of the cells to balance the osmolar concentration. A water loss of 2 L results in only a 700-ml reduction in extracellular fluid. (**B**) Effect of resuscitation from blood loss with hypertonic saline (right) compared with Ringer's lactate (center). The use of hypertonic fluid decreases the amount of water infused. (Peters RM: Fluid exchange and oxygen delivery. p. 141. In de Guia T, Lardizabal A (eds): Respiratory Failure. Proceedings of the First Boehringer Ingelheim Chest Symposium, Manila. Asia Pacific Congress Series No. 27. Excerpta Medica, Amsterdam, 1983.

the lungs and heart. The ventilatory pump is an injection pump rather than an ejection pump. Its preload is determined by the end expiratory volume. The afterload is determined by the stiffness of the lungs, the airway resistance (Fig. 7-20) and any restrictions to chest wall motion, such as obesity, ascites, muscle spasm due to pain.

As stroke volume of this pump—tidal volume—increases, there is greater respiratory muscle contraction and injection fraction in-

creases. For example, metabolic acidosis due to hypovolemia, fever, hyperalimentation, which increase minute ventilation, increases work and thus oxygen needs of respiratory muscles. Edematous lungs are stiff and so the respiratory muscle afterload is increased. The work of breathing per liter of ventilation is increased.

Figure 7-21 shows that when high-permeability edema, ARDS, makes the lungs stiff, the increased stiffness of lungs pulls the chest wall

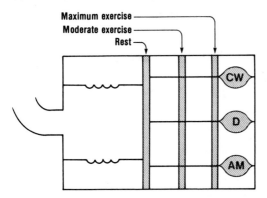

FIG. 7-20 The ventilatory pump is an injection pump. Air is pulled into the chest. The stroke volume (tidal volume) increases with exercise. End systolic volume is functional residual capacity plus tidal volume.

in, resulting in lower functional residual volume and greater preload. However, the lungs are harder to expand. After load is also markedly increased. Tidal volume and injection fraction both fall despite greater preload and lower functional residual volume. The mean pleural pressure is also lower than if the lungs were normal. To stretch stiff lungs requires more subatmospheric pressure, pleural pressure. Since the heart is in the chest and subject to the greater negative pleural pressure, the transventricular pressures are altered.

Figure 7-22 demonstrates that in the normal person, the mean pleural pressure is subatmospheric. When intraventricular pressures

are measured, their value is compared to ambient atmospheric pressure. Since the heart is in the chest, the pressure across its walls is not the difference between the chamber pressure and ambient pressure but that between chamber pressure and pleural pressure. Mean pleural pressure in the normal is about 5 mmHg subatmospheric. Preload (left atrial filling pressure) equals pulmonary pressure minus pleural pressure, 7 − (−5), or 12. For the same reason, afterload pressures shown for systole are 5 mmHg higher than the systolic extrathoracic arterial pressure.

When pulmonary edema makes lungs stiff, mean pleural pressure can fall to −15 mmHg and preload is 7 − (−15), or 22, while afterload is increased by a similar amount if the same systolic pressure is maintained.

The lower pleural pressure means that the central venous pressure minus pleural pressure (CVP-Ppl) and pulmonary wedge pressure minus pleural pressure (PWP-Ppl), the ventricular filling pressures, are increased. Cardiac afterload is increased because to maintain systemic arterial pressure at the same level, the force generated mean arterial pressure minus pleural pressure (MAP-Ppl) must be increased. The effect of a decrease in pleural pressure on transcapillary pressure in the lungs, and thus fluid filtration, is less clear.

The addition of CPAP as well as helping to expand the lungs also increases pleural pressure back towards or above normal. The increased pleural pressure lowers preload but

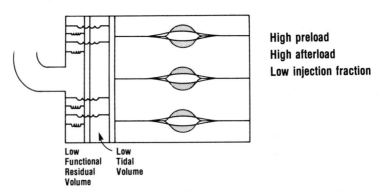

High preload
High afterload
Low injection fraction

Low Functional Residual Volume   Low Tidal Volume

FIG. 7-21 With all types of pulmonary edema, the stiff lung reduces the functional residual volume, increasing preload. The afterload is markedly increased because the lungs are hard to expand.

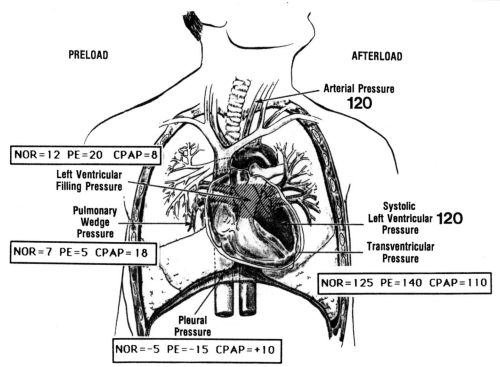

PRELOAD   AFTERLOAD

Arterial Pressure
120

NOR = 12 PE = 20 CPAP = 8

Left Ventricular
Filling Pressure

Pulmonary
Wedge
Pressure

Systolic
Left Ventricular **120**
Pressure

NOR = 7 PE = 5 CPAP = 18

Transventricular
Pressure

NOR = 125 PE = 140 CPAP = 110

Pleural
Pressure

NOR = -5 PE = -15 CPAP = +10

FIG. 7-22 Effect of changes in pleural pressure on left ventricular preload and afterload. Pulmonary edema makes the lungs stiffer so greater negative pleural pressure is necessary to inflate them. Since the heart is in the chest, a lower than normal wedge pressure, 5 vs. 7, results in high left ventricular filling pressure, 20 vs. 12. The transventricular pressure is increased from 125 to 140. CPAP raises pleural pressure, decreasing preload and afterload. CPAP, continuous positive pressure; NOR, normal; PE, pulmonary edema.

also decreases afterload, thus assisting ventricular emptying.

The ability of respiratory and cardiac muscles to maintain the required level of minute ventilation and cardiac output depends on muscle strength. Respiratory muscle strength is determined by physical conditioning and the amount of substrate and oxygen delivered to these muscles. Fatigue is the state in which energy use exceeds supply.

Macklem has emphasized the importance of the study by Aubier,[2] who showed in animals with cardiogenic shock that inadequate oxygen supply to the respiratory muscles leads to fatigue and cessation of respiration before cardiac arrest.

During spontaneous breathing with low cardiac output, anemia, or hypoxemia, the respiratory muscles deprive the rest of the body of oxygen. Figure 7-23 illustrates the failure of

delivery of adequate oxygen to prevent respiratory muscle fatigue. Hypovolemic shock results in low cardiac output, anerobic metabolism and metabolic acidosis. The acidosis results in central stimulus to ventilation. However, despite normal preload, poor oxygen supply to the respiratory muscles limits the work capacity of the respiratory muscles and minute ventilation is inadequate.

The patient with low cardiac output and/or stiff lungs due to pulmonary edema must have respirator support to remove the oxygen demands of the respiratory muscles and to increase the pleural pressure, which will decrease ventricular afterload. Ventilator support can decrease the respiratory oxygen need from 20 percent of cardiac output to only 3 percent. When cardiac output is marginal or inadequate for any reason, consideration must be given to ventilatory support and muscle paralysis to

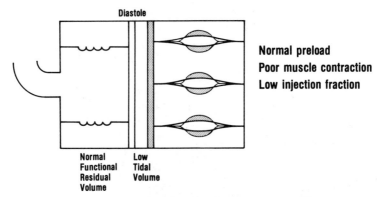

FIG. 7-23 In hypovolemic shock the lungs are normal but metabolic acidosis increases demands for ventilation to protect pH by lowering PCO_2. Low perfusion leads to low blood flow to ventilatory pump muscles. Energy use exceeds supply and ventilatory arrest can occur.

lower body oxygen consumption. Ventilator support should not be discontinued until cardiac output is restored.

better criteria for adequacy of gas exchange and the effects of fluid infused on the function of the heart, lungs, and ventilatory pump. The microvasculature and the lymphatic circulation seem most likely to hold the answers.

SUMMARY

This chapter describes the present state of knowledge regarding the appropriate fluids for resuscitation by interrelating the present knowledge of fluid dynamics with the function of the lungs and the two gas exchange pumps, the heart and the ventilatory muscles. If the reader is convinced that we have much to learn, I will be satisfied that the effort has been worthwhile. Intelligent fluid therapy demands that the physician understand the pathophysiology that is known and accept the fact that all the answers are not yet available. The use of the concept of "third space" to account for ignorance is dangerous to patients and destructive of clear thinking. Its worst effect has been to numb the minds of bright young surgeons who might help us define what kind and how much fluid is optimum in the injured patient. To determine what kind, we must know more about the distribution of various fluids immediately on infusion and as they are redistributed and excreted. To know how much, we need

REFERENCES

1. Arturson G, Thoren L: Fluid therapy in shock. World J Surg 7:573, 1983
2. Aubier M, Trippenbach T, Roussos C: Respiratory muscle fatigue during cardiogenic shock. J Appl Physiol 51:499, 1981
3. Bhattacharya J, Nanjo, Staub NC: Factors affecting lung microvascular pressure. In Malik AB, Staub NC (eds): Mechanisms of Lung Microvascular Injury. New York: Ann NY Acad Sci 384:107–114, 1982
4. Braunwald E, Ross J Jr, Sonneblick EH: Mechanisms of Contraction of the Normal and Failing Heart. 2nd ed. Little, Brown, Boston, 1976
5. Gamble JL: Clinical Anatomy, Physiology and Pathology of Extracellular Fluid. A Lecture Syllabus. Harvard University Press, Cambridge, 1947
6. Hutchin P, Terzi RG, Hollandsworth LC, et al: The influence of intravenous fluid administration on postoperative urinary water and electrolyte excretion in thoracic surgical patients. Ann Surg 170:813, 1969

7. Kramer GC, Gunther RA, Nerlich ML, et al: Effect of dextran-70 on increased microvascular fluid and protein flux after thermal injury. Circ Shock 9:529, 1982

8. Kramer GC, Harms BA, Bodai B, et al: Effects of hypoproteinemia and increased vascular pressure on lung fluid balance in sheep. J Appl Physiol 55:1514, 1983

9. Kramer GC, Harms BA, Gunther RA, et al: The effects of hypoproteinemia on blood-to-lymph fluid transport in sheep lung. Circ Res 49:1173, 1981

10. LeVeen HH, Ip M, Ahmed N, et al: Lowering blood viscosity to overcome vascular resistance. Surg Gynecol Obstet 150:139, 1980

11. Moyer CA: Fluid Balance. Year Book, Chicago, 1954

12. Shackford SR, Sise MJ, Fridlund PH, et al: Hypertonic sodium lactate versus lactated Ringer's solution for intravenous fluid therapy in operations on the abdominal aorta. Surgery 94:41, 1983

13. Shah DM, Gottlieb ME, Rahm RL, et al: Failure of red blood cell transfusion to increase oxygen transport or mixed venous PO_2 in injured patients. J Trauma 22:741, 1982

14. Shires GT III, Peitzman AB, Albert SA, et al: Response of extravascular lung water to intraoperative fluids. Ann Surg 197:515, 1983

15. Taylor AE, Grimbert F, Rutili G, et al: Pulmonary edema: Changes in Starling forces and lymph flow. p. 135. In Hargens AR (ed): Tissue Fluid Pressure and Composition. Williams & Wilkins, Baltimore, 1981

16. Virgilio RW, Rice CL, Smith DE, et al: Crystalloid versus colloid resuscitation: Is one better? A randomized clinical study. Surgery 85:129, 1979

17. Winslow RM, Samaja M, West JB: Red cell function at extreme altitude on Mount Everest. J Appl Physiol 56:109, 1984

18. Zarins CK, Rice CL, Peters RM, Virgilio RW: Lymph and pulmonary response to isobaric reduction in plasma oncotic pressure in baboons. Circ Res 43:925, 1978

19. Zeldin RA, Normandin D, Landtwing D, Peters RM: Postpneumonectomy pulmonary edema. J Thorac Cardiovasc Surg 87:359, 1984

8

Crystalloids, Colloids, and Artificial Blood Substitutes in Hypovolemia

Gerald S. Moss

Steven A. Gould

Charles L. Rice

Fluid resuscitation following shock can be divided into three phases: volume expansion, red blood cell (RBC) replacement, and correction of clotting deficiencies.

Each of these phases represents unresolved questions. Volume expansion can be accomplished with either crystalloid or colloid solutions. RBC replacement appears, at first glance, to be straightforward. What is not clear, however, are the proper physiologic "triggers" for transfusion. Finally, the diagnosis and treatment of postresuscitation bleeding remains somewhat mysterious.

This chapter reviews the issues surrounding the three phases of resuscitation.

FIRST PHASE: VOLUME EXPANSION

There has been considerable controversy over the role of resuscitation with crystalloid or colloid solutions in the subsequent development of deranged pulmonary function after major nonthoracic trauma. Colloid proponents point out that resuscitation with crystalloid alone dilutes the plasma proteins, thereby reducing plasma oncotic pressure. Reduced oncotic pressure favors fluid filtration from the intravascular to the interstitial compartment and thus sets the stage for the development of interstitial pulmonary edema.[26] It is argued that resuscitation with colloid solutions will prevent the development of interstitial pulmonary edema.[47] Crystalloid proponents point out that albumin molecules normally enter the pulmonary interstitial compartment relatively freely and are washed out via the lymphatic system and returned to the circulation.[4,59] They argue that the addition of albumin to the resuscitation fluid merely increases the albumin pool in the pulmonary interstitial compartment that must be cleared by the lymphatics.[45]

181

Studies in Rats

In 1972, Schloerb et al.[41] compared the lung water content of rats hemorrhaged and resuscitated with either Ringer's lactated solution (hereafter called Ringer's lactate) or plasmanate. Lung water was measured gravimetrically. Animals were bled 50 percent of their blood volume and 2.3 percent of body weight and then resuscitated with fluid in volumes up to six times the blood lost. The regression equations for lung water, measured gravimetrically versus infusion volume of the two test fluids, were as follows[41]:

Ringer's lactate: Lung water = 0.067 × +4.15

Albumin: Lung water = 0.236 × +3.87

The slope for Ringer's lactate-treated animals was one-fourth the value for animals treated with albumin—that is, volume for volume, lung water increased four times as much during plasmanate infusion as during Ringer's lactate infusion. Yet total protein levels in the plasmanate-treated animals were normal but were reduced as much as 50 percent of control in the Ringer's lactate-treated group.

Another way of interpreting these data is to compare the lung water value following different infusion volumes of the two test fluids. Most shock studies have shown that animals treated with plasmanate may require infusion volumes of up to twice the shed volume, whereas those treated with Ringer's lactate may need as much as five times the blood lost in order to achieve resuscitation.[46] When the respective regression equations for the two test fluids are solved using these infusion volumes, the results are similar: lung water values of 5.3 ml/g dry lung weight for Ringer's-treated animals and 5.4 for albumin-treated animals.

Schloerb and co-workers[41] also plotted lung sodium values against infusion volume for the two test fluids. Lung sodium was measured after injection of radiolabeled sodium. The regression equations for these relationships are as follows:

Ringer's lactate: Lung sodium = 10.5 × +364

Albumin: Lung sodium = 49.8 × +330

The slope of lung sodium in Ringer's lactate-treated animals is again only one-fourth the value calculated for the albumin-treated group. Electron histochemical evaluation of baboons reported from our laboratory[32] demonstrated an increase in pulmonary interstitial sodium concentration in albumin-treated animals. By contrast, baboons resuscitated from hemorrhage shock with Ringer's lactate showed no increase in pulmonary interstitial sodium concentration.

In rat studies, no data are available concerning pulmonary capillary hydrostatic pressure. Nevertheless, it is clear that for rats, withholding albumin during resuscitation does not lead to greater accumulation of pulmonary interstitial water or sodium. Similar results have been reported in rats by Collins et al.[7]

Experiments in Larger Animals

In a series of hemorrhage and resuscitation studies in baboons, we followed 2 hours of severe hemorrhage and resuscitation with either Ringer's lactated or albumin solutions.[28] Animals resuscitated with saline required five times the shed volume, whereas those treated with albumin received twice the shed volume to restore prehemorrhage vital signs. Saline-treated animals gained 10 percent of their original weight, whereas albumin-treated animals showed no change in weight. The concentration of total protein in plasma fell by approximately 40 percent in the saline-treated animals and was unchanged in the albumin-treated group. Cardiac output and acid–base status returned to normal levels in both groups. Left atrial pressures tended to be several millimeters of mercury higher in the albumin-treated animals. This setting in the saline-treated animals might be expected to be associated with increased pulmonary interstitial water. Such was not the case, however. Gravimetric measurements of lung water[29] following resuscitation as well as a battery of pulmonary function tests showed no differences between Ringer's lactate- and albumin-treated animals. Thus, it appeared that both test fluids were equally effective and equally safe.

At this point we considered the possibility that subtle degrees of pulmonary edema might not be recognized by the above-mentioned techniques. For this reason, we repeated the studies and examined the lungs by electron microscopy.[30,32] The lungs were fixed in vivo. The ultrastructural appearance of the lungs of animals treated with Ringer's lactate was not different from that of control lungs, whereas the lungs of animals treated with albumin demonstrated distortion of the interstitial space characterized by separation of individual collagen fibers and frequent empty spaces, suggesting interstitial edema. The results of examination of lung tissue at the end of the shock period also showed evidence of marked interstitial pulmonary edema.

Further studies employing electron histochemical sodium-labeling techniques showed that the lungs of animals subjected to hemorrhage shock contained large concentrations of interstitial sodium and water. These changes were reversed by resuscitation with Ringer's lactate but persisted after resuscitation with albumin. These findings are shown in Figure 8-1. This increase in pulmonary interstitial sodium concentration could increase local electrolyte osmotic pressure, thereby inducing the movement of water passively across the pulmonary capillary barrier into the interstitium.

In a similar study of hemorrhage and resuscitation, performed in monkeys, Gainsford et al.[12] found no differences in pulmonary function in animals treated with Ringer's lactate or albumin. In contrast to the results we had found in baboons,[28] Gaisford and co-workers[12] noted interstitial pulmonary edema in animals treated with Ringer's lactate, but not in those treated with albumin, as detected by electron microscopic techniques.

This difference in results between Gaisford's study and ours regarding interstitial pulmonary edema after Ringer's lactate resuscitation has two possible explanations. First, Gaisford's data suggest that the monkeys were inadvertently underresuscitated with Ringer's lactate. The infusion volume was only 65 ml/kg. Most primate studies report that at least 140 ml/kg of Ringer's lactate is necessary for adequate resuscitation over a 4-hour period. Another bit of evidence in favor of underresuscitation in the Ringer's lactate-treated group is the observation that the group had a significant base deficit at the end of resuscitation, whereas the monkeys treated with albumin did not. Since hemorrhagic shock is known to be associated with an increase in pulmonary interstitial water and sodium, it is likely that the lung changes seen in the Ringer's lactate-treated monkeys are a result of inadequate resuscitation rather than of Ringer's lactate infusion. Second, the lung tissue used for electron microscopic evaluation in the monkeys consisted of specimens taken after the animals were killed and immersion fixed. Specimens fixed in vivo, as in our baboon studies, may be more accurate because of more complete fixation and a smaller risk of postfixation artifacts.

In another hemorrhage and resuscitation study in baboons, Holcroft and Trunkey[18] measured extravascular lung water and pulmonary albumin extravasation after treatment with either Ringer's lactate or albumin. Extravascular lung water was measured using the thermal-dye technique. This method generates simultaneous indicator dilution curves by both a thermistor and a densitometer following injection of ice-cold dye. Theoretically, the thermal curve measures intravascular and total lung water, while the dye curve measures intravascular volume. The difference between the two volumes is the extravascular volume of lung water. Pulmonary extravasation of albumin was calculated by examining the ratio of pulmonary "albumin volume" to the pulmonary "blood volume" using radiolabeled albumin.

One hour after resuscitation, the extravascular lung water in the Ringer's lactate-treated animals had declined from baseline, whereas the albumin-treated animals showed a substantial increase. These changes in extravascular lung water in the albumin-treated animals are remarkably similar to the results we had reported using gravimetric measurement. In

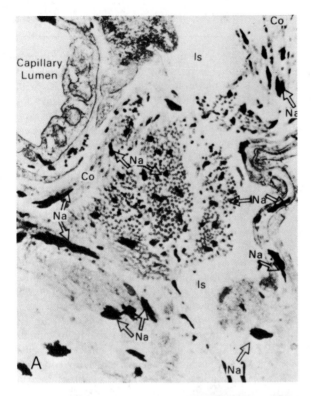

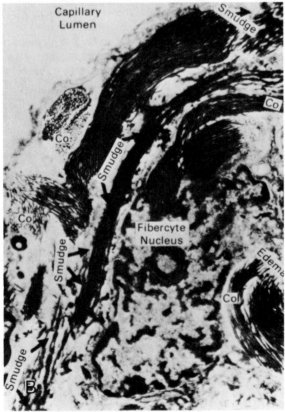

FIG. 8-1 (A) High-power view of normal lung. The precise localization of the sodium pyroantimony (Na) in and around the collagen (Co) fibers within the interstitium (Is) can be seen. Note the distribution in two planes: in transverse section, sodium can be found along the outer rims of the individual collagen fibers; in longitudinal sections, the sodium pyroantimony deposits have aggregated in geometric precision along the silhouette of the fibers. (×29,500) **(B)** High-power view of a baboon lung following hemorrhagic shock, showing distribution of sodium pyroantimony. Note the characteristic interstitial edema with smudging of sodium pyroantimony along the collagen fibers. It appears the collagen has a spongelike property for the sodium-rich edema fluid. (×20,000). (*Figure continues.*)

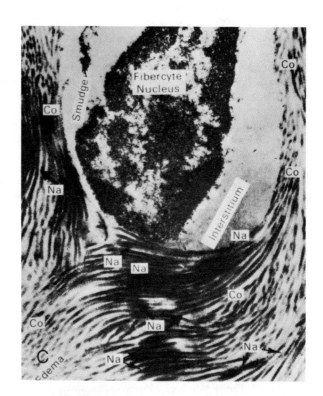

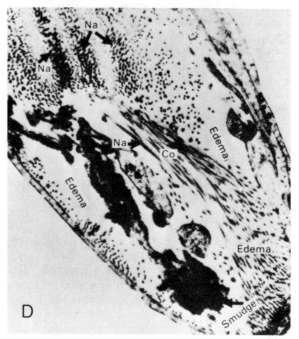

FIG. 8-1 (C) (*Continued*). Baboon lung resuscitated with Ringer's lactated solution. The interstitial space is relatively normal. Collagen fibers do not appear disrupted. Small areas of edema-rich smudges are still seen. (×27,000) Note that the distribution of sodium appears similar to that in (D) Baboon lung after resuscitation with human serum albumin. Note the marked interstitial edema, dispersal of collagen fibers and patchy areas of smudging of sodium pyroantimony. (×28,500). (Moss GS: Shock and resuscitation. p. 571. In Staub NC, Aubrey E (eds): Edema. © 1984, Raven Press, New York)

both studies, lung water is increased after resuscitation with albumin. A larger variance was seen about the mean, as compared with Ringer's-treated baboons, suggesting that the population of albumin-treated animals is different from the group treated with Ringer's lactate. These observations suggest that treatment with albumin increases the net force at the pulmonary capillary barrier in favor of transvascular fluid movement into the interstitium.

The relationship between acute hypoproteinemia and changes in lung water was studied in baboons by Zarins et al.,[60] who rapidly reduced serum albumin levels to as low as 0.8 g/dl by plasmapheresis. The plasma was exchanged for Ringer's lactate. Pulmonary wedge pressures were held constant at baseline levels. These investigators found no increase in intrapulmonary shunt or gravimetrically measured lung water. The study demonstrates that hypoproteinemia per se does not necessarily lead to pulmonary edema as long as hydrostatic pressure remains unaltered.

The effect of changes in hydrostatic pressure on lung water in the presence of hyproproteinemia was investigated by Guyton and Lindsey.[16] These workers altered hydrostatic pressure by changing the volume in a left atrial balloon in dogs rendered acutely hypoproteinemic by plasmapheresis. The pressure necessary to produce pulmonary edema fell from 23 to 13 mmHg. Thus, the principal effect of hypoproteinemia is not to produce pulmonary edema but rather to lower the threshold hydrostatic pressure that will lead to pulmonary edema.

Randomized Trials in Human Subjects

CRYSTALLOID VERSUS COLLOID

By the early 1970s, randomized trials of crystalloid versus colloid began to appear in the literature. These studies in human subjects were permissible because sufficient animal data were available, indicating that neither test fluid was more effective nor more harmful than the other. The results of some of these studies are confusing because of the differing strategies employed. In order to generate clear-cut results, several points concerning the design of these studies should be emphasized.

Blood Replacement. It is generally agreed that adequate RBC replacement is essential for successful resuscitation. If whole blood is used, however, both treatment groups receive large amounts of albumin contained in the plasma, making it difficult to interpret the results noted in the two treatment groups. Therefore, packed cells are preferable in these studies.

Physiologic End Points. The volume of albumin or Ringer's lactate given to patients should be based on physiologic end points such as right or left atrial pressures, arterial pressure, cardiac output, and urine output. The test fluids should not be given by an arbitrary formula that ignores the physiologic state of the patient.

CLINICAL STUDIES

One of the first trials in human subjects was reported in 1975 by Skillman et al.[47] They studied 16 patients undergoing elective abdominal aortic surgery. In random sequence, eight patients received a bolus of 25 percent albumin (1 g/kg) plus 1 L of 5 percent albumin, while in the operating room. The other eight patients received approximately 500 ml Ringer's lactate per hour. Lost blood was replaced with whole blood; these patients received approximately 3 L whole blood during the operation.

Patients in the colloid-treated group received 113 g albumin during the operation, 141 g on the day of surgery and 70 g on the first postoperative day. Patients in the Ringer's lactate-treated group received 31 g albumin postoperatively on the day of operation and 69 g on the first postoperative day. During the operation, both groups received the 50 g albumin present in 3 L of whole blood. No postoperative deaths were reported.

Skillman and co-workers noted a significant difference during the immediate postoperative period in plasma colloid oncotic pressure between the Ringer's lactate-treated group and the colloid-treated group (22 vs. 27 mmHg) but no difference in A-aDO$_2$. They also reported a significant correlation (P $<$ 0.05, r = 0.74) between the amount of infused sodium and A-aDO$_2$ in the Ringer's lactate-treated group, but not in the albumin-treated group. It was concluded that albumin-rich fluid was preferable because it reduced the amount of sodium-containing fluid required for adequate resuscitation.

This study does not represent a strong argument for albumin-rich fluids, since both groups received albumin, and the test fluid was given by formula. The positive correlation between infused sodium and pulmonary function was not confirmed in several subsequent studies by other investigators.

Another study involving patients undergoing elective vascular operations was published in 1979 by Virgilio et al.[54] During the operation, patients received either Ringer's lactate (N = 14) or 5 percent albumin in Ringer's lactate (N = 15) in order to maintain preoperative filling pressures, cardiac output (CO), and urine output. Blood loss was replaced by packed cells. Patients assigned to the Ringer's lactate-treated group received approximately 11 L of test fluid on the day of surgery, whereas those in the albumin-treated group received 6 L. Both groups required approximately 6.5 units of packed RBCs. Patients receiving Ringer's lactate gained 10 percent of their original body weight and developed a 40 percent reduction in plasma colloid oncotic pressure, reminiscent of the changes reported in Ringer's lactate-resuscitated baboons.[28]

During the study, no deaths occurred in either group. Virgilio and associates noted no differences between groups in intrapulmonary shunt on any day of the study. Mean ventilator time postoperatively was 23 hours in both groups. Pulmonary edema developed in two patients receiving albumin. This occurrence illustrates the central role of hydrostatic pressure in determining the volume of pulmonary interstitial water. In these patients, pulmonary edema developed after only 100 ml 5 percent albumin was infused in order to normalize a low wedge pressure. The wedge pressure abruptly rose to greater than 25 cmH$_2$O because of poor left ventricular function and was associated with frothy sputum and infiltrates

on chest radiographs. Both patients had normal plasma colloid oncotic pressure levels. No patient treated with Ringer's lactate showed the development of pulmonary edema despite reduced colloid oncotic pressure levels.

Another intriguing aspect of this study was the investigation of the relationship between pulmonary function and the gradient between plasma colloid oncotic pressure and microvascular pressure. Normally, a substantial gradient favors intravascular retention of water, since plasma colloid oncotic pressure is approximately 20 mmHg and hydrostatic pressure is 5 mmHg. As the gradient is reduced, either by a fall in plasma colloid oncotic pressure (Ringer's resuscitation) or by an elevation in microvascular pressure (albumin resuscitation), pulmonary interstitial water should increase, leading to pulmonary dysfunction, as measured by an increase in intrapulmonary shunt. No correlation was found between intrapulmonary shunt and the plasma colloid oncotic pressure–hydrostatic pressure gradient. In fact, three patients with zero or negative gradients had intrapulmonary shunt values of less than 15 percent. Conversely, six patients with normal gradients had shunt values exceeding 20 percent. Thus, Virgilio and colleagues concluded that safe resuscitation without albumin could be achieved in patients undergoing elective vascular surgery.

Lowe et al.,[21] in 1977, reported a clinical trial in 141 trauma victims from Cook County Hospital, Chicago. Thirty-six of these patients were in shock on admission. Patients received, in random sequence, either Ringer's lactate (N = 84) or 4 percent albumin solution (N = 55) in volume sufficient to restore normal vital signs and urine output. This was the first report in the literature of a group of human subjects resuscitated without any albumin at all. RBC losses were replaced with washed RBCs. These patients received an average of 5.5 L test fluid and 2 units of RBCs before surgery.

Three deaths occurred in each group. Eight patients (14 percent) in the albumin-treated group required ventilatory support after surgery, whereas three (3.6 percent) assigned to the Ringer's lactate-treated group required ventilatory support. There were no changes in a battery of pulmonary function tests, including intrapulmonary shunt and A-aDO$_2$. In addition, no correlation was found between the amount of sodium infused and any pulmonary function test in either test group. Lowe and co-workers concluded that the addition of albumin to Ringer's lactate was unnecessary to achieve successful resuscitation in this group of patients.

A criticism of this study was that too few patients were in shock on admission, so that the failure to find differences in mortality or pulmonary function with either test fluid was not surprising.[44]

In 1981, further findings in the 36 patients at Cook County Hospital, Chicago, who were in shock on admission, were published by Moss and Lowe and associates.[33] Twenty patients were assigned to the Ringer's lactate-treated group, and 16 received albumin. These patients received an average of 8 units of packed RBCs and 9 L test fluid, indicating severe injury and blood loss. Only one death occurred in this group. Two patients in each group required ventilatory support, and no differences were noted in any pulmonary function tests. Once again, no evidence could be found that albumin added to Ringer's lactate was necessary to prevent adult respiratory distress syndrome (ARDS).

Whereas Skillman and co-workers favored albumin-rich infusion fluid on the grounds that it decreased the amount of sodium infused during resuscitation, and neither Lowe nor Virgilio and their associates could find any evidence that albumin was necessary, the results of another study suggest that the infusion of albumin during resuscitation is positively harmful.

Weaver et al.[55] studied 52 patients admitted in shock from trauma. Patients were resuscitated with Ringer's lactate plus whole blood. In random sequence, selected patients also received approximately 150 g albumin during the operation and sufficient quantities of albumin postoperatively to maintain normal serum albumin levels. By the end of the operation, all patients had received approximately 10 L Ringer's lactate and 15 units of whole blood. A dramatic deterioration in pulmonary and cardiac function was noted. The ratio of inspired oxygen fraction to arterial blood oxygen tension (FIO_2/PaO_2) necessary to maintain PaO_2 above 60 mmHg was used as a measure of lung function, rather than intrapulmonary shunt measurements, in order to avoid raising the FIO_2 to 100 percent. (An elevated ratio implies deteriorating pulmonary function.) During the early postoperative period, the ratio was significantly lower in the Ringer's lactate-treated group (Ringer's lactate, 0.35; albumin, 0.67; $P < 0.05$). Later in the study, this difference was increased (Ringer's lactate, 0.26; albumin, 0.75; $P < 0.05$). Also, patients receiving albumin required ventilatory support for an average of 8 days as compared with 3 days in the group receiving Ringer's lactate.

Cardiac problems were reflected by the requirement for digitalis therapy in 16 of 27 patients assigned to the albumin-treated group, whereas only 7 of 25 in the Ringer's lactate-treated group were digitalized. Most importantly, 7 of 27 patients assigned to the albumin-treated group died, whereas none of the 25 given only Ringer's lactate died. It was concluded that albumin should not be used during initial resuscitation from trauma because of its harmful effects on the lung and heart.

This study has evoked a good deal of controversy. The strong point of this investigation is that it provides information in a group of massively injured patients requiring large amounts of resuscitative fluids. Criticism includes the following:

1. Use of whole blood in both groups during resuscitation
2. Arbitrary use of extra albumin by formula
3. Use of FIO_2/PaO_2 ratios as a measure of pulmonary function (a ratio that may not be sufficiently sensitive)
4. Increased pulmonary and cardiac complications in the albumin-treated group, raising the question of excessive resuscitation in patients assigned to the albumin group

Nonetheless, this study again suggests that resuscitation with Ringer's lactate does not lead to an increase in pulmonary interstitial water and also raises concern regarding albumin therapy.

SUMMARY OF EXPERIMENTAL AND CLINICAL STUDIES

1. There is no good evidence that Ringer's lactate resuscitation in the treatment of hemorrhagic shock produces increased pulmonary interstitial water.

2. There is some evidence that albumin resuscitation may result in albumin accumulation in lung interstitium. The clinical significance of this observation is not clear.

3. A major increase in pulmonary microvascular pressure is the most important determinant of transvascular movement of water into the pulmonary interstitium. The clinical implication of this observation is that careful monitoring of pulmonary hydrostatic pressure is crucial during resuscitation.

4. Most clinical and experimental studies suggest that there is no advantage to the administration of colloid solution rather than crystalloid in the treatment of hemorrhagic shock.

Sepsis, Resuscitation, and Pulmonary Edema

PERMEABILITY CHANGES

The question of pulmonary edema occurring as a consequence of resuscitation in septic shock is complicated by the notion that sepsis is itself associated with increased pulmonary interstitial water and increased pulmonary capillary permeability.

Increased permeability may be defined as a change in the filtration coefficient of the Starling equation. The effect of sepsis on the filtration coefficient has been studied in two different ways. The first method involves exerting a known hydrostatic pressure change in the pulmonary circuit and observing a change in lung weight. The change in weight, after correlation for intravascular fluid shifts, is regarded as the net change in interstitial volume. Dividing the change in pressure by the change in volume yields the filtration coefficient:

$$ml/(mmHg \cdot g \text{ lung tissue})$$

Gabel et al.[11] studied the effect of endotoxin on the filtration coefficient in dogs. The intact left lower lung lobe was weighed, while the pulmonary hydrostatic pressure was regulated by manipulating the balloon of a Swan-Ganz catheter threaded into the right lower lobar artery. In animals given alloxan, the filtra-

tion coefficient increased 10-fold, whereas those given endotoxin showed no change. Gabel and associates concluded that endotoxemia does not alter capillary permeability.

This study has several problems. First, no change in lung water content was observed in the dogs given endotoxin. There was no reason to expect a change in permeability if there is no change in lung water. Another problem is the interpretation of the changes in lung weight when hydrostatic pressure was increased. As Gabel et al. pointed out, this change is related not only to increased pulmonary interstitial water but to increased vascular filling as well. The slope of the weight curve was measured at various times after vascular filling was complete and was then plotted the slope against time on semilog paper. Extrapolation to time zero yielded transvascular flow; and division by changes in hydrostatic pressure then yielded the filtration coefficient. It is not clear how accurately this maneuver corrects for vascular filling.

A different method of calculating the filtration coefficient during sepsis was reported by Sturm et al.[48] The filtration coefficient was calculated by solving the Starling equation in baboons given live *E. coli*. No change was found in the filtration coefficient during the septic period. Their calculations required several assumptions. First, the reflection coefficient was assumed to be 0.8 and to remain constant during the septic period. Second, the interstitial hydrostatic pressure was assumed to be zero and to remain constant during the study. Both assumptions can be challenged. The reflection coefficient might decline during sepsis, since increased protein clearance has been reported in this setting. It is also unlikely that interstitial hydrostatic pressure remains constant.

Salt versus Colloid Resuscitation in Sepsis

The optimum fluid in which to use volume expansion in sepsis has not been well worked out. Described below are two experimental studies and two clinical trials that examine this issue.

ANIMAL STUDIES

Sturm et al.[48] infused live *E. coli* into sheep for 30 minutes. Ringer's lactate or albumin was given over a 2-hour period and titrated to elevate left atrial pressure to 12 cmH$_2$O. Both groups required approximately 15 ml/kg test fluid. At the end of resuscitation, extravascular lung water, measured by the thermal dye technique, was significantly higher in the colloid-treated group than in the Ringer's-treated group ($P < 0.05$), as shown in Table 8-1. Lung tissue analysis revealed a significantly higher concentration of albumin in the colloid-treated group.

Sturm and co-workers concluded that the higher extravascular lung water in the colloid-treated animals could be explained on the basis of increased pulmonary hydrostatic pressure and pulmonary albumin extravasation.

In a similar study, Nylander et al.[36] infused *E. coli* endotoxin into sheep. The animals were then given 20 ml/kg of either saline or homologous plasma. The Starling forces were calculated by solving the Starling equation. The interstitial pressure was assumed to be 1 mmHg and constant during the septic period; the reflection coefficient was assumed to be 0.9 and also unchanged during sepsis.

Both groups showed an approximately threefold increase in the Starling forces after infusion of test fluid. The hydrostatic pressure was slightly higher in the homologous plasma group, whereas the protein osmotic pressure was slightly lower in the saline-treated group. The authors concluded that either test fluid can worsen pulmonary edema during sepsis and that neither has a definite advantage.

CLINICAL TRIALS

In 1983 Rackow et al.[38] described 26 patients who were in shock on admission to the intensive care unit (ICU). Most of the patients were suffering from sepsis. The resuscitation protocol was designed to maintain a wedge pressure of 15 mmHg during the study period of 24 hours. Test solutions included 5 percent albumin, 6 percent hetastarch, and 0.9 percent saline. Rackow and co-workers noted that greater volumes of fluid were required to achieve adequate resuscitation in the group ad-

TABLE 8-1. Effect of Resuscitation Fluid Used on Extravascular Lung Water Following *E. coli* Septicemia

Conditions	EVLW[a] (ml/kg)
Baseline	
Control	8.8 ± 2.6
Ringer's lactate	9.2 ± 2.1
Colloid	8.0 ± 0.9
Shock	
Control	8.4 ± 2.4
Ringer's lactate	10.2 ± 2.4
Colloid	9.6 ± 2.1
Resuscitation	
Control	7.9 ± 2.5
Ringer's lactate	9.2 ± 1.7
Colloid	10.8 ± 1.9

[a] Extravascular lung water measured by the thermal dye dilution method.

ministered saline than in the groups treated with the other two fluids. Pulmonary gas exchange was not grossly different in the three groups, although COP–PCWP values were lower in the saline-treated group. Early and late mortality rates were not significantly different in the three groups.

In 1984 Metildi et al.[23] reported observations in 46 consecutive patients in the ICU with severe pulmonary insufficiency, mostly on the basis of sepsis. Fluid was administered to maintain normal acid–base balance, mixed venous PO$_2$, and PCWP. The study period was 48 hours. Test fluids were Ringer's lactate or 5 percent albumin in Ringer's lactate. No significant differences were noted in cardiac index, COP, or COP–PCWP. Improved gas exchange was noted in both treatment groups, although it was slightly better in the 5 percent albumin group. No clinical advantage was found for either fluid.

Summary

1. The increase in lung water seen in sepsis remains to be explained. Whether it results from changes in capillary permeability, changes in hydrostatic pressure, or some other process is unknown. The type of fluid used for resuscitation—crystalloid or col-

loid—does not appear to be an important factor, however.

2. Although more studies need to be done, there appears to be no advantage to infusing colloid rather than crystalloid solutions for resuscitation in septic shock.

SECOND PHASE: INCREASED OXYGEN-CARRYING CAPACITY

The indication for transfusion of blood is to restore or maintain the blood's oxygen-carrying capacity. Friedman et al.[10] attempted to look at the epidemiologic aspects of blood usage, coining the term "transfusion trigger" to identify the actual threshold used by clinicians for a blood transfusion. Their data suggest that the actual indication for blood administration may often be based on a single laboratory value, hemoglobin (Hb), rather than the individual patient's need. In order to understand the appropriate indications for a blood transfusion, the basic principles of oxygen transport should be briefly reviewed. Finch and Lenfant[9] described the oxygen transport system as "a corporate process involving several organs, each with its own regulatory system." The traditional determinants of oxygen transport are pulmonary gas exchange, blood flow, Hb mass, and Hb–O_2 affinity. The system is precisely regulated such that an alteration in one component may be balanced by compensatory changes in the remainder of the oxygen transport system to maintain oxygen equilibrium. The normal oxygen transport process will be discussed first.

Normal Oxygen Transport

Oxygen delivery is defined as the product of blood flow (cardiac output) and arterial oxygen content:

O_2 delivery
$$= \text{cardiac output} \times \text{arterial } O_2 \text{ content} \quad (1)$$

The actual utilization of oxygen by the tissues is the oxygen consumption, calculated from the CO and arteriovenous oxygen content difference using the Fick relationship:

O_2 consumption $= \text{cardiac output}$
$$\times (\text{arterial} - \text{mixed venous } O_2 \text{ content}) \quad (2)$$

The oxygen content of blood depends on the hemoglobin concentration ([Hb]), the binding coefficient of hemoglobin ($\beta = 1.39$ ml O_2/g Hb), the saturation of the hemoglobin (Sat), and the physically dissolved oxygen. The oxygen content is calculated as follows:

O_2 content
$$= (\text{Hb} \times \beta \times \text{Sat}) + (0.0031 \times PO_2) \quad (3)$$

Because the dissolved oxygen is minimal at ambient PO_2 levels, it is usually omitted. Since β is constant, the oxygen content is primarily dependent on [Hb] and saturation.

The saturation of the Hb molecule depends on the PO_2 and the Hb–O_2 affinity state, described by the sigmoidal Hb–O_2 dissociation curve (Fig. 8-2). The y axis indicates the saturation of the Hb molecule at each oxygen tension, shown on the x axis. The affinity state is characterized by the P_{50} of the dissociation curve, which is the oxygen tension at which the Hb is 50 percent saturated. The normal P_{50} value for human blood is 27 mmHg. As oxygen affin-

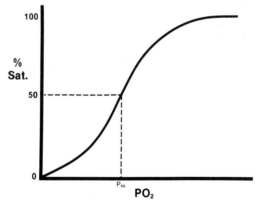

FIG. 8-2 Hemoglobin–oxygen (Hb–O_2) dissociation curve for whole blood. (Gould SA, Rice CL, Moss GS: The physiologic basis of the use of blood and blood products. p. 13. In Nyhus LM (ed): Surgery Annual. V. 16., Appleton-Century-Crofts, Norwalk, Connecticut, 1984.)

ity increases (more tightly bound), the dissociation curve shifts to the left, and the P_{50} falls. The saturation is independent of Hb concentration and at any PO_2 is affected only by left or right changes in the oxygen affinity state. Because oxygen content reflects [Hb] and saturation, the oxygen content curve will have the same sigmoidal shape as the oxygen dissociation curve (Fig. 8-3). Changes in [Hb] will determine the height of the curve, while P_{50} shifts move the curve to the left or the right.

The oxygen content curve provides a simple means of illustrating the unloading of oxygen, or the arteriovenous oxygen content difference (Fig. 8-4). The arterial PO_2 (PaO_2) is the oxygen tension at which oxygen is loaded onto the Hb molecule in the lung. The arterial content can then be read from the content curve for a known [Hb]. Oxygen is consumed during the circulation throughout the body, and the mixed venous PO_2 ($P\bar{v}O_2$) is the oxygen tension of pulmonary arterial blood at the completion of the oxygen unloading. Using the $P\bar{v}O_2$ value, the venous oxygen content can simply be read from the curve. The arteriovenous oxygen content difference (a-$\bar{v}DO_2$) can then be calculated using Equation (3) or merely read from the curve (Fig. 8-4). The a-$\bar{v}DO_2$ and CO are then multiplied, as shown in Equation (2), to obtain oxygen consumption.

The mathematics of these relationships indicate the enormous reserve that normally exists:

$$
\begin{aligned}
\text{Normal } O_2 \text{ Consumption} &= CO \times \text{a-}\bar{v}DO_2 \\
&= 5 \text{ L/min} \times 5 \text{ vol \%} \\
&= 5 \text{ L/min} \times 50 \text{ cc/L} \\
&= 250 \text{ cc/min} \\
\text{Normal } O_2 \text{ delivery} &= CO \times CaO_2 \\
&= 5 \text{ L/min} \times 20 \text{ vol \%} \\
&= 5 \text{ L/min} \times 200 \text{ cc/L} \\
&= 1{,}000 \text{ cc/min}
\end{aligned}
$$

The extraction ratio (O_2 consumed)/(O_2 delivered) is 0.25; in other words, the available oxygen is four times the normally consumed oxygen.

We have had considerable interest in evaluating the physiologic response to situations wherein the usual relationship between oxygen delivery and oxygen utilization has been al-

tered. It is in these situations that a decision must be made concerning the merits of a blood transfusion.

Disorders of Oxygen Transport

The most common indication for a blood transfusion is a low [Hb], the so-called transfusion trigger described by Friedman et al.[10] However, the oxygen transport process involves a balance between oxygen supply and demand, with a large reserve. Equation (1) demonstrates that a reduction in [Hb] in a healthy normovolemic individual might be adequately compensated by increased CO in order to maintain oxygen delivery. This increased CO provides the theoretical support for the advocates of purposeful hemodilution. We have observed this response during normovolemic hemodilution in baboons.[31] Carey,[5] Geha,[13] and Gump[15] have also documented this ability of the cardiovascular system to maintain oxygen equilibrium during hemodilution. Messmer et al.[22] showed that tissue oxygenation is easily maintained at hematocrit readings as low as 25 percent, as long as blood volume remains normal. Such results indicate that Hb concentration alone is an inadequate criterion with which to assess the need for a blood transfusion. It is common to see patients with chronic renal failure with a [Hb] of 6 to 7 g percent and persons with chronic obstructive pulmonary disease (COPD) with polycythemia and a [Hb] of 16 to 17 g percent. It is clear that there is no single magic Hb concentration for all patients.

We currently believe it more appropriate to assess the need for RBC therapy in terms of disorders of oxygen transport. These situations may be categorized as abnormalities of (1) Oxygen loading, (2) blood flow, (3) Hb mass, (4) Hb–O_2 affinity, and (5) tissue demands. Each category may change alone or in concert with one or more of the other situations. The interrelationships between the determinants of oxygen transport and the reserve mechanisms were described by Woodson.[58] The important principle is that isolated changes are rare—a

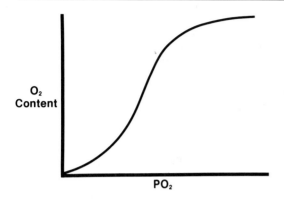

FIG. 8-3 Oxygen content curve for whole blood. (Gould SA, Rice CL, Moss GS: The physiologic basis of the use of blood and blood products. p. 13. In Nyhus LM (ed): Surgery Annual. V. 16., Appleton-Century-Crofts, Norwalk, Connecticut, 1984.)

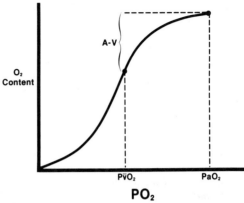

FIG. 8-4 Oxygen content curve for whole blood illustrating a-vDO$_2$ and P$\bar{v}$O$_2$. (Gould SA, Rice CL, Moss GS: The physiologic basis of the use of blood and blood products. p. 13. In Nyhus LM (ed): Surgery Annual. V. 16., Appleton-Century-Crofts, Norwalk, Connecticut, 1984.)

change in one factor is often balanced by one or more changes in the remainder to maintain oxygen equilibrium. It is unnecessary to treat every clinical disorder in the oxygen transport system—the system itself has a large reserve capacity. It is only when the reserve becomes inadequate that therapeutic interventions must be performed.

Adequacy of Oxygen Transport

The critical issue becomes the adequacy of oxygen supply. Finch and Lenfant[9] described the tissue oxygen tension as the appropriate monitor of oxygen supply. Since the P$\bar{v}$O$_2$ is the best indication of mean tissue oxygen tension, it becomes a key measurement in assessing the overall adequacy of oxygen transport in the critically ill patient. The advent of the Swan-Ganz catheter has made measurement of P$\bar{v}$O$_2$ a routine matter in the modern ICU setting.

The normal value for P$\bar{v}$O$_2$ in resting persons is 40 mmHg. As the measurement of P$\bar{v}$O$_2$ has become more frequent, the clinical importance of an abnormal value has become less clear.[2,20] Although a traditional teaching concept has stated that a reduced P$\bar{v}$O$_2$ indicates

a low CO the issue is more complex. Low P$\bar{v}$O$_2$ and high CO may occur simultaneously, confirming that there are other determinants of P$\bar{v}$O$_2$.[31,57] It is more appropriate to consider a drop in P$\bar{v}$O$_2$ as indicating either a decrease in oxygen supply (delivery) or an increase in oxygen demand. It is a nonspecific response, serving only as an important monitor of the oxygen transport system. The P$\bar{v}$O$_2$ thus becomes an indication of oxygen reserve, much like the HCO$^-_3$ level in the acid–base system.

We have used Equations (2) and (3) and the oxygen content curve to identify five etiologies of a decreased P$\bar{v}$O$_2$ (see ref. 14):

1. ↓ Arterial saturation (Sat)
2. ↓ Cardiac output (CO)
3. ↓ Hemoglobin concentration [Hb]
4. ↓ P$_{50}$
5. ↑ Oxygen consumption ($\dot{V}$O$_2$)

The first four measurements constitute oxygen delivery, and the fifth oxygen demand. These five criteria assume that each change occurs as an isolated event and that the body responds only by a decrease in the P$\bar{v}$O$_2$ in order to maintain $\dot{V}$O$_2$. In effect, as the supply (delivery) is decreased, oxygen consumption is maintained, and the reserve is depleted because of an increase in the oxygen extraction ratio (O$_2$

consumed)/(O_2 delivered). The actual utilization of oxygen remains constant (except for the situation of an increased oxygen requirement, and thus consumption).

Clinical Implications

Patients with a low $P\bar{v}O_2$ can be categorized as being in a stable or an unstable condition based on the adequacy of their hemodynamics, ventilation, urine output, and acid–base status. If a patient's condition is stable with a low $P\bar{v}O_2$, no therapy is indicated unless a true critical value is reached ($\leq$ 25 mmHg). If a patient is unstable with a low $P\bar{v}O_2$, therapeutic intervention is indicated. The appropriate therapy depends on an analysis of the five criteria and the ability to manipulate the offending variable. This will not always be feasible.

In practical terms, we consider a patient with a changing $P\bar{v}O_2$ value to be undergoing significant alterations of the oxygen transport system, which may be explained by many different conditions, only a few of which may actually be manipulated. A patient with normal lungs will have a normal saturation, and a patient with significant pulmonary disease may be quite refractory to attempts to improve his or her hypoxia. Disorders of P_{50} are actually quite rare. Oxygen consumption is a measurement that is not ordinarily manipulated; [Hb] and CO are the remaining variables. A healthy person can easily compensate for a fall in [Hb] by an increase in CO. It is the cardiac patient with a CO that cannot be augmented who might benefit from a blood transfusion when $P\bar{v}O_2$ is reduced and [Hb] is not abnormally low. In effect, a "life-threatening" anemia might exist despite only a modest reduction in Hb mass. This is a new concept, and our quantitative analysis may be helpful in confirming such an impression. To borrow a phrase from Friedman et al.[10] we believe that the $P\bar{v}O_2$ and the stability of the patient might well become the appropriate "transfusion trigger."

Transfusion

Once a decision is made that a blood transfusion is indicated to restore the RBC mass, the next issue is to identify the optimum method of transfusion. A number of choices are available (Table 8-2). In addition to merely choosing the most appropriate RBC preparation, the physician must decide whether the patient is best suited for an autologous or for a homologous transfusion.

AUTOLOGOUS BLOOD

The patient is undoubtedly the safest source of a RBC replacement. The problems of blood compatibility, immunogenicity, and hepatitis transmission become essentially nonexistent. The use of autologous blood seems to be quite limited and may be related to an inadequate educational program by its proponents. Three methods are available for the use of autologous blood: (1) preoperative collection and storage, (2) immediate preoperative collection and hemodilution, and (3) intraoperative autotransfusion.

Preoperative Collection and Storage. This technique was developed as a means of obtaining blood for patients with rare antibodies that were difficult to cross-match. The method was used most frequently during the 1960s, and certain groups have been able to satisfy most of their elective surgical blood requirements in this manner.[25]

The first descriptions involved timed withdrawal of 1 unit of blood roughly every 2 weeks, with transfusion of outdated units on day 21. This approach continued until 4 or 5 units were available at once for an elective operation. The ability of the bone marrow to maintain a normal Hb level despite continued withdrawal has been carefully demonstrated by Hamstra and Block.[17] The current availability of frozen blood storage methods has simplified the entire approach. A unit of blood can be withdrawn and frozen every 3 weeks until an adequate reserve has been obtained, obviating the issue of timed reinfusion.

The technique is thus a safe and reliable method of ensuring availability of blood for patients with unusual blood groups or prior sensitization. The two potential problems are the advance planning required and the inadvisability for patients with chronic illnesses or nutritional deficiencies. Nonetheless, we believe it is an excellent method for elective operations that could considerably reduce the need and risks of homologous blood transfusion.

Immediate Preoperative Collection and Hemodilution.   This technique is based on the cardiovascular changes that occur during the induction of normovolemic anemia. Blood is withdrawn to reduce acutely the hematocrit reading to 30 percent, and blood volume is maintained with Ringer's lactate, Dextran, or other volume expanders. A healthy individual will maintain oxygen delivery during this period of normovolemic anemia with an increase in CO. Messmer et al.[22] showed that tissue oxygenation remains normal, and advocates of purposeful hemodilution actually believe that a hematocrit reading of 30 percent is optimal.

This method can provide approximately 3 units of whole blood for intraoperative use. Although the technique has been used widely in Europe, in the United States it has been primarily limited to patients undergoing open heart operations. Since open heart operations are responsible for a large proportion of our homologous blood demand,[40] wider use of this method could have a substantial influence on the availability of blood.

Intraoperative Autotransfusion.   Autotransfusion represents a means of conserving blood during a major ongoing blood loss until the source of the hemorrhage has been controlled. The method has been extensively reviewed,[35,51] hence is not discussed in detail in this chapter.

Although the potential of autotransfusion is appealing, there are certain practical limitations to its use. The theoretical problem of contamination (infection or malignant tumor) limits its use in a variety of settings in which it might be most helpful, such as major trauma. A second concern is the required logistic support. Although several types of instruments are available, they are expensive and require the availability of trained personnel. The most serious problem, however, is the coagulopathy that occurs as a result of exposure of blood to air, peritoneal surfaces, and ex vivo mechanical devices. Several solutions have been proposed, such as systemic heparinization, collection in acid citrate dextrose (ACD), and washing before retransfusion,[37] but the problem still remains.

Although we believe that autotransfusion may have an integral role in blood replacement in the future, certain practical issues still limit its widespread application.

HOMOLOGOUS BLOOD

Most of the blood transfused in the United States is homolgous blood. Table 8-2 lists a number of products that will be discussed individually.

Whole Blood.   Approximately 28 percent of the blood administered in the United States today is in the form of whole blood.[19] With the evolution of blood component therapy (Table 8-3), there has been a steady decline in the number of transfusions given in the form of whole blood. We consider this appropriate. Since we have already stated that most transfusions are given to restore the oxygen-carrying capacity, the optimum form of replacement is packed RBCs to fulfill that indication only. While no data exist to suggest any physiologic disadvantage following whole blood transfusion, there are several theoretical advantages to the use of packed cells.

Component therapy consists of fractionation of whole blood at the time of collection into RBCs, platelets, and plasma. The use of packed cells rather than whole blood to restore oxygen carrying capacity is specific treatment, allows more efficient use of the other limited

TABLE 8-3. Blood Components

Component	Replacement	Component	Replacement
Red blood cells	O_2-carrying capacity	Fresh-frozen plasma	Clotting factors
White blood cells	Immunocompetence	Factor VIII concentrate	Factor VIII
Platelets	Platelet function	Factor IX concentrate	Factor IX

(Gould SA, Rice CL, Moss GS: The physiologic basis of the use of blood and blood products. p. 13. In Nyhus LM (ed): Surgery Annual. V. 16, Appleton-Century-Crofts, Norwalk, Connecticut, 1984.)

commodities (platelets and plasma), and avoids the undesirable effects often seen after the administration of platelet and white blood cell (WBC) debris.[6] The argument that a patient bleeding whole blood must undergo blood replacement with whole blood is no longer acceptable.

Red Blood Cells. Many physicians are still concerned that packed RBC therapy is inferior to whole blood transfusion. Criticisms have been based on two notions: (1) the plasma is usually given anyway at a later time, and (2) bleeding is more common, since the clotting factors are removed. The available data disprove both arguments.

The first argument suggests that fractionation is "make-work," since the plasma is too often given as a supplement to RBC transfusions,[42] and whole blood administration would be simpler. In examining this issue, however, Kahn et al.[19] found that plasma products are given less often with packed RBCs than with whole blood (14 percent v. 24 percent). Thus, the concurrent administration of RBCs and plasma is infrequent and is not an argument in favor of whole blood therapy.

The concern with bleeding problems has also been evaluated. Rice et al.[39] evaluated the prothrombin time (PT), partial thromboplastin time (PTT), fibrinogen, and platelet count in patients undergoing elective aortic operations for aneurysm or occlusive disease. No differences were found in these clotting measurements between patients undergoing transfusion with whole blood or with packed cells. No patient showed the development of bleeding disorders or required fresh-frozen plasma (FFP). Furthermore, there was no difference in the adequacy of volume replacement or CO between the two groups. It can be concluded that replacement of up to 1 blood volume with packed RBCs is safe and efficacious. A more

recent study by Shackford et al.[43] continued these observations in patients undergoing aortic operations. Once again, there were no significant differences in laboratory values or physiologic measurements between patients receiving whole blood and those receiving packed RBCs.

A more recent issue is the lower opsonic activity reported by Beiting et al.[3] in animals in which blood loss was replaced with packed RBCs rather than with whole blood. The clinical relevance of this laboratory finding is still unclear and will undoubtedly be the subject of future investigative work. It does not appear to be a clinically important issue.

The choice of RBCs over whole blood is still only a preliminary decision, as there are three separate RBC products. Although we consider each superior to whole blood, a number of differences deserve mention.

Packed Red Blood Cells. A concentrated suspension of RBCs is obtained by moving the supernatant plasma from the whole blood after settling or centrifugation. The RBC mass is the same as in 1 unit of whole blood. The plasma citrate level and volume of plasma are substantially reduced.

Washed Red Blood Cells. After the RBCs have been obtained by settling or centrifugation, they are washed with sterile isotonic saline colution. This process will result in a still lower plasma citrate level than will a unit of nonwashed cells. The only disadvantage is the additional time and possibility of bacterial contamination.

Frozen Red Blood Cells. The use of frozen RBCs has been an important addition to blood component therapy. A major concern with the use of liquid preserved blood has been the outdating of blood because of the limited shelf life (21 to 28 days). Despite progress in the development of better preservatives, 28 days is still a relatively brief period. Frozen RBCs can be stored indefinitely, with no apparent loss of safety or efficacy after thawing and administration. Although frozen blood is still not in widespread use, the potential impact on blood bank services is substantial. In addition to providing an indefinite shelf life, frozen blood facilitates the application of autologous blood usage, permits stockpiling of all blood groups, particularly those that are difficult to obtain, maintains normal levels of 2,3-diphosphoglycerate (2,3-DPG) and P_{50}, and may be associated with a lower risk of hepatitis transmission,[52] although the latter issue remains unsettled.

The various methods of freezing will all use glycerol to prevent crystal formation and cell membrane destruction during freezing. The blood is stored in polyvinyl bags at $-80°C$. When the cells are called for, the units are thawed and washed in order to remove the glycerol. The process of preparation for resuspension and administration is less than 1 hour. Valeri[52] documented that the survival and function of frozen RBCs is equivalent to liquid-preserved cells stored at $4°C$ for 1 week.

A frozen blood program also permits efficient use of outdated blood. Valeri and Zaroulis[53] developed a method of rejuvenating outdated RBCs by incubating them with pyruvate, inosine, glucose, phosphate, and adenine. Cells treated in this manner that have been frozen, thawed, and transfused have functioned and survived satisfactorily. This approach holds great potential for improving the resources and capabilities of the modern blood bank.

The safety and efficacy of frozen blood programs have been demonstrated by Moss et al.[27] in a wartime setting and by Szymanski and Carrington[49] and Telischi et al.[50] in civilian programs. Although a theoretical criticism of this method has been that the RBCs should be used within 24 hours or discarded, this has not proved a practical disadvantage, since most units are actually used. There are also reports suggesting that the cells can be used up to 96 hours postthaw or refrozen and still used safely.[56]

In summary, it seems clear that a frozen red cell program is safe and efficacious. Although financial and logistic issues may limit the establishment of such programs, the utilization of such a technique could have a considerable effect on chronic blood shortages in the United States.

THIRD PHASE: COMPLEMENT THERAPY IN THE TREATMENT OF HEMOSTATIC DEFECTS

The components most frequently used by surgeons are platelets and fresh-frozen plasma (FFP). This section reviews the indications for the use of these two components in massive transfusion.

Fresh-Frozen Plasma

In most patients with acute reduction in circulating volume, treatment with crystalloid solutions followed by compatible RBC transfusions, when indicated, will achieve successful resuscitation. In the case of massive transfusion, defined as blood volume replacement greater than 1.5 times the recipient volume, abnormal bleeding may occur. This hemostatic defect is characterized by oozing from the operative wound, mucous membranes, and intravenous puncture sites. The probability of developing a hemostatic defect is roughly related to the volume of infused blood and fluids.

Investigations of massively transfused patients with a hemostatic defect usually demonstrate the following changes in the coagulation profile:

1. Reduced platelet count
2. Increased bleeding time
3. Increased PT
4. Increased activated PTT
5. Decreased fibrinogen levels

In addition, studies of the coagulation profile following a 3-L plasma exchange in normal apheresis donors demonstrate similar changes.

For these reasons, the traditional explanation for the hemostatic defect following massive transfusion has been dilution of the various clotting elements. Recommendations for coagulopathy prophylaxis include administration of platelet concentrates and FFP during resuscitation and before the onset of oozing. An established coagulopathy is treated with either platelet concentrates or FFP, or both, depending on the coagulation profile. This approach is logical but should be reexamined for several reasons.

First, both platelets and FFP may transmit non-A–non-B hepatitis. Exposure to more than 2 units carries an estimated 10 percent risk of hepatitis.[1] It is important to emphasize that this often takes the form of chronic liver imflammation. The risk is likely to be the same as for whole blood. These components should therefore be used with the same precautions used for any other blood component.

Second, in the case of FFP, the observation that PT and activated PTT is abnormal in the presence of a coagulopathy is not, in itself, evidence that administration of FFP will correct the hemostatic defect. It is well known that normal clotting can still occur when the various clotting protein concentrations are substantially reduced. Furthermore, the infusion of FFP in patients who are oozing after massive transfusion and who have abnormal PT and PTT frequently fails to stop the bleeding despite normalized[24] PT and PTT. Also, prophylactic use of FFP (and platelets) has failed to reduce the incidence of coagulopathy after massive transfusion.[8]

Third, regarding platelets, there is no doubt that after the loss of more than 1 blood volume, platelet counts of 100,000 or less may be seen. In addition, the bleeding time will be abnormal in almost all massively transfused patients. However, the bleeding time and platelet count in such patients without coagulopathy are also grossly abnormal and not different from those in patients who do bleed. Furthermore, spontaneous bleeding from thrombocytopenia rarely occurs with a platelet count above 20,000, a level infrequently seen in massive transfusion.

On the basis of these observations, we recommend the following approach to component use in the third phase of resuscitation:

1. Platelet count, PT, and PTT should be measured frequently during massive resuscitation.
2. Bleeding times may not be useful.
3. Administration of components prophylactically during resuscitation is not helpful and exposes the patient unnecessarily to the risk of hepatitis.
4. If a coagulopathy develops during massive resuscitation, platelet infusions will be helpful if the platelet count is less than 100,000.
5. FFP will not be helpful in most cases of a coagulopathy. If the PT and PTT are substantially prolonged (greater than 1.5 times control), FFP infusion may be helpful.

The clinical value of FFP has been summarized in a National Institutes of Health consensus statement as follows:[34]

1. Approximately 90 percent of current FFP use is inappropriate.
2. The risk of hepatitis with FFP is similar to that associated with any other blood component.
3. The use of FFP has risen 10-fold during the last decade for no apparent reason.
4. Unacceptable indications for FFP use include the following:
   a. Volume expander
   b. Source of immunoglobin except in rare instances
   c. Source of nutrition
   d. Source of fibronectin
5. Acceptable indications include the following:
   a. Treatment of a postresuscitation clotting defect when a major decrease in clotting problems can be demonstrated
   b. Treatment of life-threatening coumadin intoxication

REFERENCES

1. Alter HJ: The dominant role of non-A, non-B in the pathogenesis of post-transfusion hepatitis: A clinical assessment. Clin Gastroenterol 9:155, 1980

2. Armstong RF, St Andrew D, Cohen SL et al: Continuous monitoring of mixed venous oxygen tension in cardio respiratory disorders. Lancet 1:632, 1978

3. Beiting CV, Kozak KJ, Dreffer RL: Whole blood vs. packed red cells for resuscitation of hemorrhagic shock: An examination of host defense parameters in dogs. Surgery 84:194, 1978

4. Brigham KL, Woolverton WC, Blake LH: Increased sheep lung vascular permeability caused by pseudomonas bacteremia. J Clin Invest 54:792, 1974

5. Carey JS: Determinants of cardiac output during experimental therapeutic hemodilution. Ann Surg 181:196, 1975

6. Chaplin H: Current concepts: Packed red blood cells. N Engl J Med 281:364, 1969

7. Collins JA, Braitberg A, Butcher HR: Changes in lung and body weight and lung water content in rats treated for hemorrhage with various fluids. Surgery 73:401, 1973

8. Counts RB, Haisch C, Simon TL et al: Hemostasis in massively transfused patients. Ann Surg 190:91, 1979

9. Finch CA, Lenfant C: Oxygen transport in man. N Engl J Med 286:407, 1972

10. Friedman BA, Burns TL, Schork MA: An analysis of blood transfusion of surgical patients by sex: A quest for the transfusion trigger. Transfusion 20:179, 1980

11. Gabel JC, Adair T, Drake RE, Traber D: Nonpulmonary contamination in the chronic sheep lung lymph preparation. Fed Proc 40:472, 1981

12. Gaisford WD, Pandey N, Jensen CG: Pulmonary changes in treated hemorrhagic shock. II. Ringer's lactate solution versus colloid infusion. Am J Surg 124:738, 1972

13. Geha AS: Coronary and cardiovascular dynamics and oxygen availability during acute normovolemic anemia. Surgery 80:47, 1976

14. Gould SA, Rosen AL, Sehgal LR et al: Is cardiac output the principal determinant of $P\bar{v}O_2$? Crit Care Med 9:273, 1981

15. Gump TE: Anemia in surgical patients. p. 105. In Collins JA, Lundsgaard-Hansen P (eds): Surgical Hemotherapy. S Karger, New York, 1980

16. Guyton AC, Lindsey AW: Effect of elevated left atrial pressure and decreased plasma protein concentration in the development of pulmonary edema. Circ Res 7:649, 1959

17. Hamstra RD, Block MH: Erythropoiesis in response to blood loss in man. J Appl Physiol 27:503, 1969

18. Holcroft JW, Trunkey DD: Extravascular lung water following hemorrhagic shock in baboon: Comparison between resuscitation with Ringer's lactate and plasmanate. Ann Surg 180:408, 1974

19. Kahn RA, Staggs SD, Miller WV, Ellis FR: Use of plasma products with whole blood and packed RBC's. JAMA 242:2087, 1979

20. Kasnitz P, Druger GL, Yorra F, Simmons DH: Mixed venous tension and hyperlactatemia. JAMA 236:570, 1976

21. Lowe RJ, Moss GS, Jilek J, Levine HA: Crystalloid vs. colloid in the etiology of pulmonary failure after trauma: A randomized trial in man. Surgery 81:676, 1977

22. Messmer K, Sunder-Plassman L, Jesch F: Oxygen supply to the tissues during limited normovolemic hemodilution. Res Exp Med 159:152, 1973

23. Metildi LA, Shackford SR, Virgilio RW, Peters RM: Crystalloid versus colloid in fluid resuscitation of patients with severe pulmonary insufficiency. Surg Gynecol Obstet 158:207, 1984

24. Miller RD, Robbins TO, Tong MJ, Barton SL: Coagulation defects associated with massive blood transfusions. Ann Surg 174:794, 1971

25. Milles G, Langston H, Dellasandro W: Autologous Transfusion. Charles C Thomas, Springfield, IL, 1971

26. Moore FD, Lyons JH, Peirce EC: Post traumatic Pulmonary Insufficiency. WB Saunders, Philadelphia, 1969

27. Moss GS, Valeri CR, Brodine CE: Clinical experience with the use of frozen blood in combat casualties. N Engl J Med 278:748, 1968

28. Moss GS, Proctor HJ, Homer LD et al: A comparison of asanguineous fluids and whole blood in the treatment of hemorrhagic shock. Surg Gynecol Obstet 129:1247, 1969

29. Moss GS, Siegel DC, Cochin A, Fresquez V: Effects of saline and colloid solutions on pulmonary function in hemorrhagic shock. Surg Gynecol Obstet 133:53, 1971

30. Moss GS, Das Gupta TK, Newson BS, Nyhus LM: The effect of saline solution resuscitation on pulmonary sodium and water distribution. Surg Gynecol Obstet 136:934, 1973

31. Moss GS, DeWoskin R, Rosen AL et al: Transport of oxygen and carbon dioxide by hemoglobin-saline solution in the red cell-free primate. Surg Gynecol Obstet 142:357, 1976

32. Moss GS, Das Gupta TK, Brinkman R et al: Changes in lung ultrastructure following heterologous and homologous serum infusion in the treatment of hemorrhagic shock. Ann Surg 189:236, 1979

33. Moss GS, Lowe RJ, Jilek J, Levine HD: Colloid or crystalloid in the resuscitation of hemorrhagic shock: A controlled clinical trial. Surgery 89:434, 1981

34. National Institutes of Health, Consensus Conference: Fresh-frozen plasma: Indications and risks. JAMA 253:551, 1985

35. Noon GP: Intraoperative autotransfusion. Surgery 84:719, 1978
36. Nylander WA, Hammon JW, Roselli RJ et al: Comparison of the effects of saline and homologous plasma infusion on lung fluid balance during endotoxemia in the unanesthetized sheep. Surgery, 90:221, 1981
37. Oller DW, Rice CL, Herman CM: Heparin versus citrate anti-coagulation in autotransfusion. J Surg Res 20:333, 1976
38. Rackow EC, Falk JL, Fein IA et al: Fluid resuscitation in circulatory shock: A comparison of the cardiorespiratory effects of albumin, hetastarch, and saline solutions in patients with hypovolemic and septic shock. Crit Care Med 11:839, 1983
39. Rice CL, John DA, Smith DE; Coagulation changes with packed cell versus whole blood transfusion. Crit Care Med 6:118, 1978
40. Roche JK, Stengle JM: Open-heart surgery and the demand for blood. JAMA 225:1516, 1973
41. Schloerb PR, Hunt PT, Plummer HA, Cage GK: Pulmonary edema after replacement of blood loss by electrolyte solutions. Surg Gynecol Obstet 135:893, 1972
42. Schmidt PJ: Red cells for transfusion. N Engl J Med 299:1411, 1978
43. Shackford SR, Virgilio RW, Peters RM: Whole blood versus packed-cell transfusions. Ann Surg 193:337, 1981
44. Shoemaker WC, Hauser CJ: Critique of crystalloid versus colloid therapy in shock and shock lung. Crit Care Med 7:117, 1979
45. Siegel DC, Moss GS, Cochin A: Pulmonary changes following treatment for hemorrhagic shock: Saline versus colloid infusion. Surg Forum 21:17, 1970
46. Siegel DC, Cochin A, Moss GS: The ventilatory response to hemorrhagic shock and resuscitation. Surgery 72:451, 1972
47. Skillman JJ, Restall DS, Salzman EW: Randomized trial of albumin vs. electrolyte solutions during abdominal aortic operations. Surgery 78:291, 1975
48. Sturm JA, Carpenter MA, Lewis FR et al: Water and protein movement in the sheep lung after septic shock: Effect of colloid versus crystalloid resuscitation. J Surg Res 26:233, 1979
49. Szymanski IO, Carrington EJ: Evaluation of large-scale frozen blood program. Transfusion 17:431, 1977
50. Telischi M, Hoiberg R, Rao KRP, Patel AR: The use of frozen, thawed erythrocytes in blood banking. Am J Clin Pathol 68:250, 1977
51. Thurer RL, Hauer JM: Autotransfusion and blood conservation. Current Prob Surg 19, 1982
52. Valeri CR: Viability and function of preserved red cells. N Engl J Med 284:81, 1971
53. Valeri CR, Zaroulis CG: Rejuvenation and freezing of outdated stored human red cells. N Engl J Med 287:1307, 1972
54. Virgilio RW, Rice, CL, Smith DE, et al: Crystalloid vs. colloid resuscitation: Is one better? Surgery, 85:129, 1979
55. Weaver DW, Ledgerwood AM, Lucas CE et al: Pulmonary effects of albumin resuscitation for severe hypovolemic shock. Arch Surg 113:387, 1978
56. Wintch R, James PM: Viability of cryopreserved red blood cells studied over 96 hours post-thaw. J Surg Res 23:88, 1977
57. Woodson RD, Wills RE, Lenfant C: effect of acute and established anemia on O_2 transport at rest, submaximal and maximal work. J Appl Physiol 44:36, 1978
58. Woodson RD: Physiological significance of oxygen dissociation curve shifts. Crit Care Med 7:374, 1979
59. Zarins CK, Rice CL, Smith DE: Role of lymphatics in preventing hypooncotic pulmonary edema. Surg Forum 27:257, 1976
60. Zarins CK, Rice CL, Peters RM, Virgilio RW: Lymph and pulmonary response in isobaric reduction in plasma oncotic pressure in baboons. Circ Res 43:925, 1978

9

Therapy of Low-Flow Shock States

John H. Siegel
Steven E. Linberg
Charles E. Wiles III

THE NATURE OF THE HYPOPERFUSION SHOCK PROCESS

Shock, as clinically encountered, is the hemodynamic manifestation of cellular metabolic insufficiency, resulting from either inadequate cellular perfusion (hypovolemic and cardiogenic), or a biochemical inability to oxidize substrates provided by an otherwise adequate perfusion (septic). In low-flow shock syndromes, the basic clinical presentation is therefore both a cause and an effect of this demodynamic disturbance, forming a vicious circle. The ability to treat victims of hypoperfusion shock properly is dependent on further knowledge of the pathogenesis of these disease processes.

Historically, studies of hemorrhagic or hy-

povolemic shock can be divided into two categories—those that have explored the actual cellular shock processes at the subcellular level, and those that have investigated the subsequent integrated compensatory and decompensatory responses in animals and human subjects. With respect to the first category of research, a considerable amount of work has been presented by Trump and colleagues.[180,183-185] These workers described the cellular and subcellular characteristics of shock in a variety of tissues from both animals and humans (Chapter 2). These microscopically visible changes appear to be progressive, and have been depicted as identifiable stages of cellular injury (Fig. 9-1). As the stage of injury progresses unmodified by treatment, a point is reached at which cell viability is no longer possible. When a critical number of cells are thus compromised, the survival of the involved organ is in danger and, depending on the organ or organs injured, the survival of the whole animal may eventually be at stake. These stages of cell injury are thought to be initiated and subsequently modified by the re-

The work reported in the chapter was supported in part by Grants HL 29280 and HL 29281 from the National Heart, Blood and Lung Institute, and by the Shock Trauma Research Fund.

201

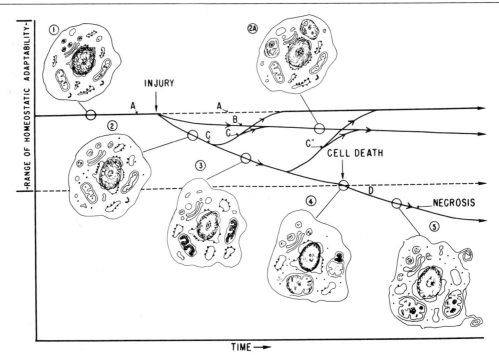

FIG. 9-1 Diagram of the stages of cellular disorganization as a result of injury. The reversible field includes those stages from which the cell can recover to normal after removal of the insult. The irreversible field includes stages after cell death when removal of the insult no longer permits recovery. (Trump BF, Valigorsky JM, Dees JH et al: Cellular change in human disease. A new method of pathological analysis. Human Path 4(1):89, 1973.)

distribution of cellular ions, calcium in particular.[181,182] This specific role of calcium in mediating cellular damage and cell death has been extensively investigated and is also reviewed in Chapter 2.

The second category of hypovolemic shock research has explored the overall integrated physiologic responses to shock that lead to hemodynamic compensation in whole animal models[24-27,29,195] and human studies.[81,87,102,131–139,143,152] These studies have shown that after hemorrhage with significant blood loss, the body uses a variety of mechanisms to maintain the blood flow to critical vital organs until volume restitution can occur through redistribution of extracellular fluid volume into the intravascular space.[47,101,102] At the organ level, maintenance of perfusion during periods of mild to moderate hypotension occurs through the autoregulation of blood flow by local control of vasoconstriction to ensure tissue oxygen delivery,[126] a mechanism en-

joyed primarily by the brain, heart, and kidneys. At the integrated level, the central nervous system (CNS) response is organized by the pattern of medullary vasomotor sympathetic discharge carried over the cardiac sympathetic efferent nerves and the efferents to the peripheral arterioles and the adrenals.[67] These are mediated by the hypotensive reduction in the level of carotid and aortic baroreceptor afferent discharges that normally inhibit the vasomotor center and through the activation of carotid body chemoreceptors by changes in pH and $PaCO_2$ that stimulate the medullary vasomotor center.[34] At the cardiac level, this increase in sympathetic efferent activity results in enhanced pumping activity by the heart[118,119] and at the peripheral vascular level in a general vasoconstrictor-mediated increase in arteriolar resistance and venous constriction with a consequent redistribution of blood volume away from the periphery into the central circulation.[60,67,190] The improved heart function results from direct catecholamine release at cardiac sympathetic nerve endings in proximity to myocardial β-adrenergic receptors[20,49,149] and by vasomotor center inhibition of vagal parasympathetic efferent outflow.[67] The result of this altered sympathetic/parasympathetic balance is (1) to increase atrial pacemaker activity and reduce atrioventricular conduction time and (2) to increase myocardial contractility directly.[119] The central redistribution of blood volume is caused by a selective vasoconstriction of peripheral arterioles and capacitance vessels at the expense of skin and skeletal muscle,[60,96] followed late in the hypovolemia or low perfusion process by vasoconstriction in the abdominal organs.[162] However, adrenergic stimuli cause coronary vasodilatation,[117,119] and increased peripheral hypercapnia and acidosis produce cerebral vasodilation (see Chapter 31), thereby protecting these two critical organs until the very last.

The immediate mechanism whereby circulating volume is restored over the immediate short term involves the movement of fluid from the extravascular to the intravascular space[101,102] as a direct result of the decreased intracapillary hydrostatic pressure associated with blood loss. At the renal level, the efferent arteriolar vasoconstriction and low flow activates the juxtaglomerular apparatus with release of renin and the subsequent angiotensin-mediated aldosterone secretion by the adrenal cortex tends to result in fluid rentention.[47,161] All these mechanisms result in an increase in circulating blood volume from its hypovolemic low point toward normal levels.[101]

In addition, at the metabolic response level, the adrenal-mediated acute increase in hepatic gluconeogenesis and the production of other osmotically active metabolic products assist in the restitution of extracellular and intravascular blood volumes at the expense of intracellular volume, through both catecholamine- and glucocorticoid secretion-controlled processes.[47] These interrelated and integrated mechanisms behind compensation can be thought of as the homeostatic attempt to ensure short-term survival. The Darwinian value of this overall response is obvious when considering the need of injured animals to escape from likely injury, to remove themselves from the cause of injury, and to recover effective cellular perfusion during the postinjury period. Without this physiologic advantage, animals would die during the hypovolemia period or would fail to reperfuse critical organ beds after trauma. There is evidence that prolonged denial of adequate perfusion of the liver and the gut may alter the metabolic and protein synthetic aspects of the normal postinjury host-defense mechanisms by which the animal or human being defends against bacterial sepsis, a severe consequence of hypovolemic shock, which may take hours or days to develop fully (see Chapters 3, 14, and 15).

A number of investigators[87,134-138,143,152] have assembled data on patients in hypovolemic shock demonstrating the now-familiar pattern of decreased cardiac index, lowered mean arterial and central venous blood pressures, increased heart rate, and increased systemic vascular resistance, underlying the redistribution of a reduced blood volume to those areas apparently in most urgent need. While these clinical data are useful in alerting the physician to the problem and undoubtedly assist in the treatment of the patient, they do not necessarily reflect either the true severity or the fundamental cellular metabolic nature of the injury. It is the cells of the body that are in trouble; with monitoring, the clinical mind set should be alerted to recognize the nature and magnitude of the primary problem, which is the reduction of oxygen delivery to the body's cells. With the development of better sensors to detect tissue and organ hypoxemia, undoubtedly less importance will be given in the future to the more traditional, but secondary, intravascular pressure and flow data now used for clinical evaluation.

Pathophysiology of Ischemic Shock

CELLULAR PATHOPHYSIOLOGY

The cells of the body undergo a known series of changes in response to ischemic or anoxic injury.[180,183-185] The earliest manifestations of ischemia appear to be attributable to alterations in cellular membrane integrity with decreases in cellular membrane potential due to ion shifts and modifications of the control of substrate oxidation.[130,181] These changes occur before any ultrastructural changes are noted.[180,182-184] Among the first morphologic changes detected by electron micrography is contraction of the inner mitochondrial compartment, which may be related to the hypoxic decrease in oxidative phosphorylation, followed by clumping of nuclear chromatin associated with the fall in intracellular pH (Fig. 9-1). The fall in oxidative phosphorylation results in a decrease in adenosine triphosphate (ATP) and other high-energy phosphates, which are required for all active cellular processes, setting the stage for the rest of the cellular morphologic response to injury. An early redistribution of cellular ions and water occurs, evidenced by swelling of the cisternae of the endoplasmic reticulum. Blebs are seen on the cell surface, perhaps indicating severe ultrastructural damage. The mitochondria soon begin to shrink and become dense, indicating the degree of biochemical change occurring in these cellular energy factories. As the point-of-no-return approaches, the mitochondria exhibit large-scale swelling and many show tiny dense aggregates. Eventually, large flocculent densities appear in the mitochondria; this event signals the death of that organelle. Nuclear chromatin soon dissolves, and the now swollen lysosomes are suspected of leaking hydrolases, which further destroy the cellular contents. Further changes occur, but in hypoperfusion shock syndromes it seems clear that the original insult is related to the reduced oxygen delivery, which results in a loss of oxidative phosphorylation, with all the other changes occurring as a direct result of this primary event. A fall in oxygen consumption ($\dot{V}O_2$) is therefore an early and definite clinical physiologic indicator of trouble, often identifying a critical level of organ perfusion and the prodromal shock syndrome before it is clinically evident.

OXYGEN CONSUMPTION

Oxygen consumption per square meter body surface area ($\dot{V}O_2/m^2$) has been shown to average 140 ml/min/m² (also calculated as 3.5 ml/kg/min, or 250 ml/min in the 70-kg "textbook" man) not only in the normal healthy individual, but also in the afebrile, resting hospitalized patient.[143,147] This value remains constant, unless altered by hypo- or hyperthermic conditions (approximately 13 percent for each degree centigrade change in body temperature,[37] or sepsis occurs, producing a hypermetabolic response.[73,84,144,155] The normal stress response to trauma, surgery, or well-controlled sepsis is associated with an increase in oxygen consumption of 15 to 35 percent.[28,73,84] In 654 observations in 165 posttrauma patients, the mean $\dot{V}O_2/m^2$ was found to be 155 ml/min/m², or 3.96 ml/kg/min, for a population with a mean age of 39.5 years.[179] When age was considered, however, the $\dot{V}O_2/m^2$ ranged from 173 ml/min/m² in the 13- to 30-year-old group, to 129 ml/min/m² in those older than 65 years (Table 9-1).

In the metabolically imbalanced state of septic multiple-organ failure syndrome, cellular failures of oxidative metabolism may occur even at high body perfusion and oxygen delivery levels.[144,155] However, in the absence of such septic toxic metabolic failure, a decrease in oxygen consumption ($\dot{V}O_2$) below the current demand for oxygen, caused by the reduced oxygen delivery occurring in low body perfusion syndromes, is compensated for by an in-

TABLE 9-1.   Oxygen Consumption in Posttrauma Patients[a]

Age Range (years)	N	$\dot{V}O_2$ ml/min/m²	$\dot{V}O_2$ ml/kg/min	Estimated $\dot{V}O_2$/min (70 kg, 1.73 BSA male)
13–30	283	173	4.28	299
31–49	166	152	3.76	263
50–65	98	136	3.36	235
>65	98	129	3.19	223

[a] Based on 645 observations in 165 patients. (Data from Tacchino RM, Siegel JH, Emanuele T et al: Circ Shock 18:360, 1986 abst.)

crease in anaerobic glycolytic metabolism, with a concomitant rise in serum lactate and in the lactate/pyruvate ratio. Such a condition is encountered throughout the body during hypovolemic or cardiogenic shock or in a localized tissue bed during periods of inflow ischemia. With the loss of perfusion volume and pressure peripherally and the consequent reduction in oxygen delivery, the $\dot{V}O_2$ is seen to fall (Fig. 9-2).

As an indicator, $\dot{V}O_2$ is potentially more useful for continuous monitoring than any one of the standard vital signs, as has been shown by Neuhof and associates[107-109] and by Siegel et al.[143,155] These workers were able to show that the true condition of the unstable patient is most accurately reflected by the $\dot{V}O_2$, and not quite so well by the heart rate and blood pressure, since these latter measurements are modified more by the compensatory response to injury than by the ischemic insult itself. Basing therapeutic decisions on the standard hemodynamic data can often lead the clinician to a false sense of security, or doom, as the case may be. For instance, the normal mechanisms of compensation may camouflage a slow but persistent intraabdominal or retroperitoneal hemorrhage, and the bedside cardiovascular alarms may not sound until the patient decompensates, just before cardiovascular arrest.

Indirect cellular metabolic monitoring by means of the $\dot{V}O_2$ can be of therapeutic value much earlier in the shock process by alerting the medical staff to reevaluate the patient before the circulatory collapse and thereby to avoid a cardiorespiratory arrest. Siegel and associates[144,150-155] demonstrated the clinical value of $\dot{V}O_2$ data when used in conjunction with other conventionally monitored as well as more advanced nonstandard clinical data. In this instance, $\dot{V}O_2$-related data become an integral component of a pattern-recognition process, permitting classification of critically ill patients into one of four abnormal conditions or "states" for qualitative and quantitative evaluation of severity.

The difference over time between the oxygen demand (assumed to equal the "stable" $\dot{V}O_2$ at the steady-state consumption for a given state of metabolic compensation), and the actual $\dot{V}O_2$, is referred to as the oxygen deficit. This oxygen deficit is therefore the integral of the decrease in $\dot{V}O_2$ below the demand, for a given period of time (graphically depicted in Fig. 9-2), together with the corresponding fall in $\dot{V}O_2$. Another way of viewing this same process is depicted in Figure 9-3, which shows the rapidly rising oxygen deficit that accumulates under actual experimental conditions, when a dog is subjected to hemorrhagic shock, even

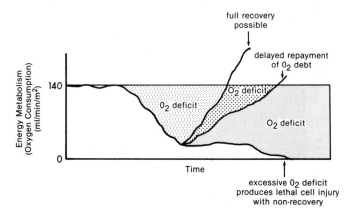

FIG. 9-2 Graphic representation of the fall in oxygen consumption that occurs following loss of perfusion to metabolizing tissues of the body, and the resulting development of an oxygen deficit. This oxygen deficit is defined as the accumulating difference over time between the oxygen demand (equal to the "stable" $\dot{V}O_2$, assumed to equal demand for the given conditions), and the actual $\dot{V}O_2$. This deficit is, therefore, the integral of the decrease in $\dot{V}O_2$ below the demand, for a given period of time.

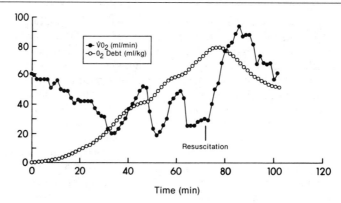

FIG. 9-3 Actual data depicting the accumulating oxygen deficit that accompanies a fall in oxygen consumption, seen during experimental hemorrhagic shock in the dog. Note spontaneous increases in $\dot{V}O_2$ as vasoconstriction and reperfusion occur with reduction in O_2 debt as volume resuscitation is instituted.

though the actual $\dot{V}O_2$ rate undergoes considerable fluctuation as attempts at homeostatic vascular compensation occur.

Although the principle of oxygen deficit has long been known, it was not until the classic experimental studies conducted by Crowell and Smith[24,26] that the importance of this variable in determing the outcome of hemorrhagic shock was demonstrated. These investigators were able to show that the oxygen deficit is very closely tied to eventual survival in an experimental hemorrhagic model (Fig. 9-4) and is a more important determinant of survival than is blood pressure. Although the latter as expected, has a strong positive correlation, it is really oxygen consumption, or a lack thereof, that reflects the metabolic bottom line.

Historically, experimental hypovolemic shock models based on the Wiggers[195] method of approach have involved controlling the preparation at a prescribed target blood pressure, for a given period of time, or until a predetermined amount of volume has to be reinfused to maintain the blood pressure at a particular depth. Survival in these models is variable[25] and even though the reduction in blood pressure is strongly related to outcome, it is not necessarily the best variable to follow, as it is largely modified by both baroreceptor and chemoreceptor reflexes[67,96] and therefore often serves as an indicator of the degree of compensation achieved rather than of cellular hypoperfusion. Crowell and Smith's work[26] has given studies of hemorrhagic shock a new and

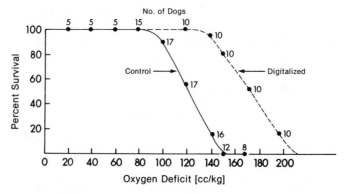

FIG. 9-4 The total oxygen deficit has been shown to be an excellent quantitative predictor of survival following hemorrhagic shock in the dog model. (Crowell JW, Smith EE: Oxygen deficit and irreversible hemorrhagic shock. Am J Physiol 206(2):313, 1964.)

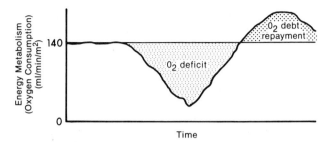

FIG. 9-5 Graphic representation of the repayment of the oxygen debt, when the oxygen consumption following resuscitation exceeds the baseline requirements for oxygen.

more meaningful marker of the true extent of metabolic injury, more closely related to cellular and organ injury and possibly a direct cause of the late multiple-organ failure frequently associated with severe shock and multiple trauma.

Oxygen Debt Repayment

After initiation of fluid resuscitation in hypovolemic survivors, there is a recovery of $\dot{V}O_2$, which exceeds the preinjury baseline for a period of time (Fig. 9-5). The "excessive" amount of oxygen consumed is referred to as repaying the oxygen debt and is quantitatively related to the preceding oxygen deficit. The actual metabolic relationship between the two is not well understood, although in another situation in which oxygen demand temporarily exceeds consumption (severe exercise), the oxygen debt repaid is approximately twice the size of the calculated oxygen deficit.[5] In shock, this quantitative relationship is generally not found in animals and humans, which may be a direct result of a wide variety of factors including the resuscitation therapy. Typically with fluid resuscitation incorporating room temperature fluids, a gradual fall in body temperature occurs that lowers the baseline $\dot{V}O_2$ during this period (Fig. 9-6). The true extent of the fall in baseline measurements compounds the efforts to quantify the actual oxygen debt and thus to estimate the extent of the metabolic injury accurately.

Cellular Pathology and Oxygen Deficit Relationships

While Crowell and Smith[26] demonstrated the relationship between survival and oxygen deficit, perhaps a finer relationship can be

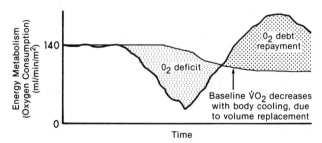

FIG. 9-6 With hemorrhage and fluid volume resuscitation there is a significant hypothermia with a fall in the baseline requirements for oxygen. Consequently, the increase in oxygen consumption required to exceed baseline needs is reduced, and repayment of the oxygen debt is achieved more quickly with an oxygen consumption that may not be that different from the preshock value.

drawn between oxygen deficit and morphologic injury to cells that relates to the previously noted work by Trump's group.[82,180,181] In a control canine hepatocyte obtained by needle biopsy prior to shock,[82] all cellular organelles appear normal (Fig. 9-7A). At a moderate oxygen deficit of 60 ml/kg, autophagic vacuoles are present, indicating definite but reversible cellular injury (Fig. 9-7B). At a severe oxygen deficit of 105 ml/kg, the mitochondria are found to be swollen, and blebbing of the cytoplasmic vesicles occurs (Fig. 9-7C). Although the injury is significant, the shock is still potentially reversible at this point, at least for the short term. This is in good agreement with the global short-term survival data presented by Crowell and Smith,[26] who showed an LD_{50} of 120 ml/kg of oxygen deficit in a similar dog model (Fig. 9-4). Whether this type of cell injury leads to multiple-organ failure after a few days remains unanswered, but preliminary studies suggest that patients who die or who have complicated posttrauma clinical courses frequently show evidence of having had a substantial period of low $\dot{V}O_2$, compatible with the accumulation of a significant oxygen deficit.

PHYSIOLOGIC PRINCIPLES UNDERLYING CARDIOVASCULAR RESPONSES IN HYPOVOLEMIC AND CARDIOGENIC SHOCK STATES

Cardiovascular and Oxygen Consumption Responses to Hypovolemia: Relationship to the Human Shock Process

Despite extensive investigation of hemorrhagic shock[24-27,29,47,130,195] and a number of excellent studies that have carefully evaluated the course of hemodynamic recovery from hypovolemia,[87,101,131-139,143,152] it has been difficult to gain much information about the evolution of the shock process in human subjects because of obvious practical and ethical considerations. Moore and colleagues conducted an extensive series of observations in young volunteers subjected to small atraumatic hemorrhage without volume replacement.[102,161] This group showed a generally small fall in cardiac output (CO), with little metabolic change seen initially. A rise in adrenocortical hormones and catecholamines was noted and the volume loss was found to have been endogenously replaced over a period of time by the movement of interstitial fluid into the intravascular space, restoring blood volume to the prehemorrhage level within 36 to 40 hours.[101]

The original human hemodynamic observations by Cornand[22] showed that hypovolemic shock patients manifested a decrease in CO with evidence of significant vasoconstriction. His studies also showed that oxygen consumption was maintained by an increased extraction of the arterial oxygen content from the arterial blood with a widening of the arteriovenous–oxygen content difference (a-$\bar{v}DO_2$, Ca-$\bar{v}O_2$), so that there was a tendency for total oxygen consumption to be maintained. However, this group of patients was not in very severe shock. Studies conducted by Weil et al.[193] and Shoemaker and colleagues[131-139] in posthemorrhagic and traumatic shock patients also demonstrated a marked reduction in CO and a rise in systemic vascular resistance. These workers, as well as MacLean[87] and Siegel,[155] observed a reduction in oxygen consumption as a key feature in human shock. All these studies show evidence of the metabolic consequences of this fall in aerobic metabolism, with increased levels of circulating plasma lactate and a rise in the lactate/pyruvate ratio. However, severe hypovolemic shock processes have also been demonstrated to be associated with a fall in body temperature and it has been speculated that this may in part be related to the reduction in oxygen consumption.

The only circumstance in which it has been possible to study the adaptive mechanisms involved in the evolution of human hypovolemic shock has been in prospective physiologic evaluations of high-risk patients undergoing major surgical procedures, in which the possibility

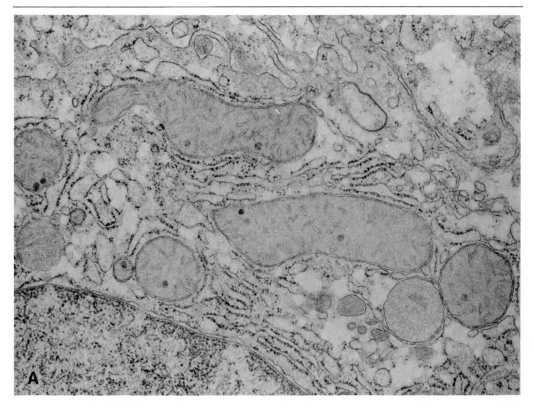

FIG. 9-7 (A) This high magnification micrograph illustrates the normal ultrastructural appearances of the nucleus and cytoplasmic organelles in the dog hepatocyte (magnification: 37,500×). (*Figure continues.*)

of extensive intraoperative blood loss has justified continuous invasive physiologic monitoring beginning before the hypovolemic period.[143,152] In some of these patients undergoing major surgery, hemorrhagic blood loss produced hypotension. Under these circumstances, two patterns of adaptation to the hypovolemic episode have been demonstrated. These are shown in Figures 9-8A–D, and represent, respectively, compensated (I) and decompensated (II) patterns of response to major intraoperative hemorrhage. These differences in the nature of the pattern of vascular compensation to hemorrhage; as discussed later, may be in part a function of age and the age-related capacity for vasomotor regulation.[179]

The compensated (I) pattern is demonstrated by patient JT (#198514) a 72-year-old man who underwent esophagogastrectomy for carcinoma of the cardiac of the stomach (Fig. 9-8A–D). He had an intraoperative blood loss in excess of 2,000 ml, requiring 2,000 ml blood products, 500 ml of colloid, and 2,000 ml Ringer's lactated solution as replacement during surgery. It can be seen that the initial period of intraoperative blood loss was associated with a fall in cardiac index (Fig. 9-8A,B). This was also associated with an initial fall in mean blood pressure (MBP) from the immediate postanesthesia induction level followed by a period of vasoconstriction which returned the MBP toward the original level and reached its peak peripheral vascular resistance (TPR) level of 3,061 dyn·sec·cm^{-5} at the nadir of the CI (1.55 L/min/m^2). Accelerated volume replacement after the lowest point of the CI was associated with a reduction in the degree of vasoconstriction, although the (MBP) rose in response to the increase in flow.

The oxygen consumption per squre meter BSA ($\dot{V}O_2/m^2$) (Fig. 9C) in this individual with a compensated (I) response was one of an ini-

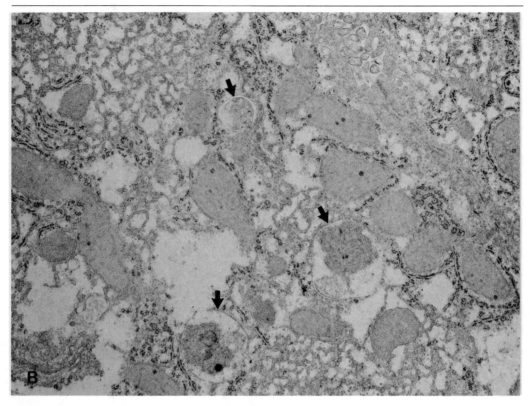

FIG. 9-7 (*Continued*) **(B)** At the end of 1 hour of moderately severe hypovolemia with an O_2 deficit of 60 ml/kg after a 20 min reinfusion, the only evidence of cell injury is an increase in the number of autophagic vacuoles (arrows). All other structures are normal (magnification: 25,000×). (*Figure continues.*)

tial decline below the preinduction level (from 120 to 60 ml/min/m²). However, the oxygen consumption began to rise back toward control levels before the lowest CI level was reached, while the vascular resistance was rising, suggesting a redistribution of blood flow to vital metabolizing organ beds. As blood volume was replaced and the CI rose toward control preanesthesia levels, the $\dot{V}O_2/m^2$ increased to acceptable levels. The return of CI to preanesthetic levels was associated with an overshoot in oxygen consumption (154 ml/min/m²), which may represent the repayment of the oxygen deficit accumulated during the preceding low-perfusion vasoconstriction period. This would also be suggested by the observation that the mixed venous pH (Fig. 9D) was seen to rise as the CI fell below 2.0 L/min/m² BSA, suggesting that the metabolic acids produced because of inadequate peripheral flow were not

being released into the circulation because of lack of perfusion of the hypoxic beds. However, as the CI rose above 2.0 L/min/m², there was a rapid fall in the venous pH to 7.32, as the body flow and oxygen consumption increased, suggesting that the reduction in vasoconstriction had permitted a reperfusion peripheral washout of metabolic acids from the formerly ischemic beds. This reduction in pH, however, was rapidly returned to acceptable levels, above pH 7.35. Except for a very brief period at the end of surgery when the rise in MBP was associated with a fall in $\dot{V}O_2/m^2$ (Fig. 9-8C), this patient demonstrated an appropriate vasoconstrictor response which allowed the patient to continue to perfuse, albeit at a reduced level, so that the oxygen deficit and its rate of accumulation were controlled to physiologically tolerable levels.

By contrast (Fig. 9-8A and B), patient EB

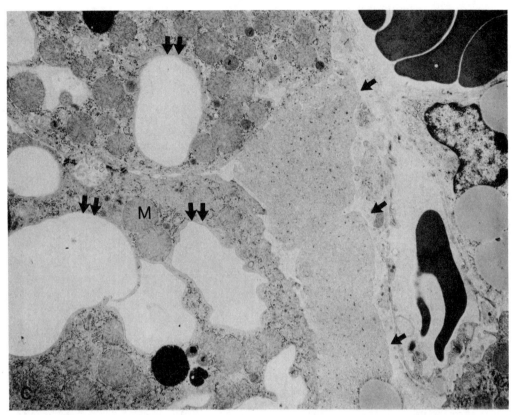

FIG. 9-7 *(Continued)* **(C)** Effects of severe hypovolemia on hepatocyte ultrastructure. This animal was subjected to a 105 ml/kg oxygen deficit. This micrograph illustrates the severe, although reversible, cellular injury. The mitochondria (M) are swollen, and there is blebbing of cytoplasmic vesicles into the space of Disse (single arrow). Several large toxic vacuoles are also seen in the hepatocytes (double arrow) (magnification: 15,000×).

(#336856) who demonstrated a decompensated (II) pattern, was an obese 39-year-old woman who underwent an abdominoperineal resection of the rectum for adenocarcinoma and who also had major blood loss. During the operative period, this patient received 3,500 ml blood products, 500 ml colloid, and 1,000 ml Ringer's lactate. In contrast to the first patient, this woman demonstrated an inappropriate maintenance of MBP (Fig. 9-8B) in the face of an almost identical reduction in CI (Fig. 9-8A). In spite of the fall of CI to below 2.0 L/min/m² BSA, the MBP was maintained, with only slight deviation, around a relatively high mean pressure, reflecting a progressive compensatory rise in TPR.

Oxygen consumption (Fig. 9-8C), which was reduced even during the immediate preoperative period, dropped to extremely low levels ($\dot{V}O_2/m^2 = 52$ ml/min/m²) as surgery was begun. At the low point of the CI response (Fig. 9-8A) (1.70 L/min/m²), the patient then manifested a sudden vasodilatory response that produced a marked hypotensive episode (Fig. 9-8B). The MBP fell from 106 mmHg to 36 mmHg. The CI was seen to rise momentarily by more than 1 L/min/m² (from 1.68 to 2.83 L/min/m²). At the same time, there was a marked increase in oxygen consumption ($\dot{V}O_2/m^2$) from 58 ml/min/m² to 187 ml/min/m² (Fig. 9-8C), suggesting that the profound peripheral vasoconstriction had produced an enormous

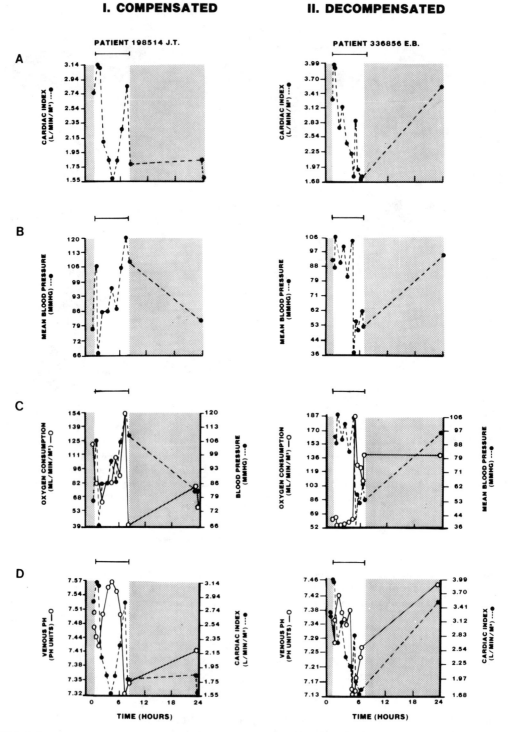

FIG. 9-8 Response patterns to hypovolemia: Compensated and Decompensated. **(A)** cardiac index; **(B)** mean blood pressure; **(C)** oxygen consumption; **(D)** mixed venous pH. In all figures, the black bar and time period designated by no shading show the intraoperative period. (Data redrawn from Siegel JH: Pattern and process in the evolution of and recovery from shock. p. 381. In Siegel JH, Chodoff PD (eds): The Aged and High Risk Surgical Patient. Grune & Stratton, New York, 1976 by permission.)

net oxygen debt that was now being repaid, after its ablation due to hypoxemic vasodilation, by increased perfusion to the previously ischemically hypoxemic tissues. This was also confirmed by the studies of venous pH (Fig. 9-8D) which demonstrated a relatively normal maintained pH during the vasoconstriction period, with a marked fall in mixed venous pH from 7.38 to 7.13 during the period of acute hypoxemic vasodilatation. This was followed by a return of mixed venous pH to 7.27 and then to 7.45, during the subsequent period of volume replacement. It is extremely interesting that even though the CI did not return to preoperative levels until 18 hours after shock, increased tissue perfusion was maintained due to the persistent vasodilatation in this patient. The oxygen consumption remained at adequate levels ($\dot{V}O_2/m^2 = 140$ ml/min/m²) in spite of persistent hypotension during the immediate postshock period, and the $\dot{V}O_2/m^2$ was actually higher than during the preceding vasoconstrictor period, with virtually no change in CI (Fig. 9-8D).

Comparison of the decompensated (II) with the compensated (I) pattern demonstrates a number of important points:

1. In the face of marked hypovolemia, the maintenance of MBP is not necessarily a beneficial response, if it occurs at the expense of deprivation of flow to peripheral tissues to the degree that oxygen consumption is impaired below a critical level.

2. Flow, as gauged by peripheral extraction of oxygen, is more important than the maintenance of perfusion pressure, provided only that a level of inflow pressure is maintained that is greater than the critical opening pressure of the vital organ vascular beds. The overall adequacy of flow can be evaluated at the bedside by the oxygen consumption response and the partition of flow by evaluation of critical organ function such as the renals by urine output, the myocardium by the absence of electrocardiographic (ECG) evidence of ischemia and the cerebral by the level of consciousness or the nature of the electroencephalogram (EEG)-evoked potentials response in the absence of a head injury.

3. Regardless of blood pressure, the degree of vasoconstriction in the presence of a reduced blood volume may be inappropriate given the level of myocardial contractile function and may produce an increase in resistance that cannot be overcome by the hypoperfusion-compromised myocardium working under unfavorable conditions of increased afterload. (This is discussed in greater detail later in this chapter).

4. Excessive peripheral vasoconstriction, by permitting metabolic acids and anaerobic by-products to build up above critical levels in the hypoxemic tissues, may have deleterious consequences when reperfusion occurs, by releasing significant quantities of metabolic acids, potassium, and other vasoactive substances into the general circulation.[2,41,47,80,91,187,194,195] There is evidence that some of these substances may in themselves produce additive myocardial depressant effects that may further impair the myocardial ability to operate against a vasoconstrictor-imposed afterload.[187] These effects may be particularly deleterious if the patient already has intrinsic cardiac disease or under circumstances in which general anesthetic agents that depress myocardial contractility are used. In addition (as discussed in Chapters 3 and 14), reperfusion of previously ischemic tissues may release substances that alter vascular permeability and that interfere with a variety of humoral reticuloendothelial and immunologic host-defense mechanisms.

This concept of low-flow-related modulation of sympathetically mediated vasoconstrictor responses, via local tissue hypoxemia, acidosis, hyperkalemia, and prostaglandin release has been extensively investigated.[74,75,80,91,120–123,163,187,188,194] These appear to be local protective mechanisms for assuring that in hypovolemia compensatory vasoregulation does not produce an excessive level of ischemia, which may result in irreversible damage. Patients who have an inappropriate balance between local or sympathetic compensatory responses are at great risk with regard to suffering the secondary injuries produced by humoral factors released by the shock process. These are also discussed at length in Chapters 3, 14, and 18.

Clinical Use of Oxygen Consumption in Acute Resuscitation

Using the $\dot{V}O_2$ data as a guide to resuscitation, it is possible to determine whether the patient is responding appropriately to volume replacement and inotropic therapy. Under actual resuscitation conditions, patients arriving in an emergency room or trauma-admitting area who are hypotensive, tachycardiac, and tachypneic, with evidence of severe blood loss have been found to fall into one of three groups. The first group is composed of those patients who, in spite of unstable cardiorespiratory status and low arterial blood pressure, are vasodilated; thus, organ perfusion persists and in reality they are metabolically stable. Although hypotension is frequently present, true circulatory shock may have existed for only a very short period; in that amount of time, they may not have experienced any significant reduction in aerobic metabolic function and have not accumulated a substantial oxygen deficit. This condition (hypotensive normoperfusor with no oxygen debt) is exemplified in Figure 9-9 (the same patient represented in Fig. 9-10, patient A). When resuscitated with volume, these patients generally recover rapidly, except for limitations imposed by special considerations centered on their anatomic injuries, such as a fatal head injury or an unstable pseudoaneurysm secondary to a thoracic aortic rupture.

A second type of patient who arrives in shock shows a severe oxidative ($\dot{V}O_2$) metabolic depression (Fig. 9-10, patient B) and is still accumulating an oxygen deficit at an alarming rate (Fig. 9-11, patient C). The emergency resuscitative needs of these patients (potentially fatal oxygen debt rate) are truly critical in that the oxygen deficit is accumulating so rapidly that the interval between reversible and irreversible cellular injury is short. On admission to the resuscitation area of the trauma center, the nonsurviving patient (B), whose data are depicted in Figures 9-10 and 9-11, was found to be accumulating an oxygen deficit at a rate greater than 2 ml/kg/min. At this rate of $\dot{V}O_2$ deficit, it would take less than 60 minutes for a lethal metabolic injury to develop, using the experimentally derived[26] criterion of 120 ml/kg debt as the LD_{50} limit. Those who regularly treat this type of patient are aware that the prehospital phase of accident extrication and transport may easily consume all or most of this critical period, leaving little time to treat the patient effectively, when time is truly critical. In spite of heroic attempts, the patient depicted here was not successfully resuscitated, and sustained a cardiac arrest shortly after the last study point shown.

A third type of patient who arrives in shock initially appears in a clinical condition

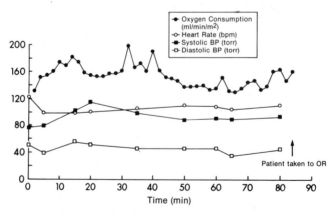

FIG. 9-9 Hypotension following posttraumatic hypovolemia due to the lack of vasoconstriction about reduced blood volume. Data obtained during the resuscitation of Patient A (see text). Although the patient was admitted tachycardic and hypotensive following traumatic injury, with obvious signs of significant blood loss, serial measurements of oxygen consumption indicated minimal detectable metabolic compromise. However, there was indication of a slight trend for an increase in oxygen consumption during the early resuscitation period as volume loss was replaced.

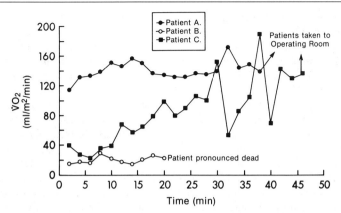

FIG. 9-10 The data presented are from 3 patients, and represent an example of each of 3 different classes of individuals who are seen in hemorrhagic shock. Those who demonstrate no metabolic deficit (Patient A), those who are metabolically unresponsive to therapy (Patient B), and those who show severe metabolic depression on admission, but quickly recover with appropriate volume resuscitation and related therapy (Patient C).

similar to that of the previous group but responds quickly to volume with an increase in $\dot{V}O_2$ (potentially reversible oxygen debt rate) (Fig. 9-10, patient C). This particular patient (C) had an initial rate of oxygen deficit accumulation that was not distinguishable from the previous patient (Fig. 9-11, patients B and C). The unknown period during which the oxygen deficit was accumulating was apparently shorter, however. Therefore, the size of the deficit was probably less than in the nonsurviving patient (B) depicted in Figure 9-10; this latter patient responded quickly to the volume infusion with an increase in $\dot{V}O_2$ to a level exceeding the expected baseline. It is worth mentioning that the improving metabolic status of the surviving patients, reflected by the increasing

$\dot{V}O_2$, was evident in the reduced rate of oxygen debt (Fig. 9-11, patient C) before the standard clinical data (blood pressure and heart rate) showed consistent improvement.

Vascular Tone as a Measure of Peripheral Vascular Functional Adequacy

Extensive experimental and clinical observations of blood pressure:flow relationships in shock and various forms of critical illness have pointed to a different degree of vascular regula-

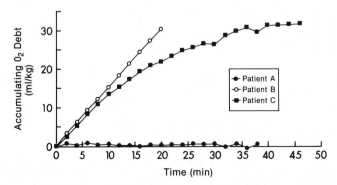

FIG. 9-11 The data presented in Figure 9–10, are redrawn to demonstrate the varying rates of oxygen deficit accumulation (O₂ debt). Patient A was admitted accumulating essentially no oxygen debt. Patients B and C were initially observed to be accumulating similar rates of oxygen debt, with the difference that with volume resuscitation, the rate of accumulation for Patient C leveled off to limit the total debt.

tion seen in patients with hypovolemic or post-traumatic nonseptic shock responses compared with that seen in patients with systemic sepsis or in patients with chronic hepatocellular disease associated with various forms of cirrhotic liver disease.[143,153,154,155] As is shown in Figure 9-12, for a given level of CI, patients with nonseptic conditions maintain a higher TPR for a given level of flow. This concept, which has been designated "vascular tone," is a useful way of characterizing the relationship between mean arterial blood pressure (MBP) and the total peripheral flow (using the CI to normalize patients for body surface area). As indicated by Green et al.,[60] vascular tone may be defined as a state of active contraction of the muscular walls of small vessels. It is generally considered subject to alteration by vasomotor nerves, hormonal or toxic substances, and metabolic by-products. In attempting to provide a method for expressing change of vasomotor activity, Green and colleagues concluded that "the most satisfactory practical expression for change of vascular tonus due to vasomotor nerve activity, and for the appearance of constrictor or dilator substances in the blood stream, is the ratio of the peripheral resistance in the experimental period to the peripheral resistance measured in the control period *at the same rate of flow.*"

While it is virtually impossible to define the entire range of vascular tone relationships in man, extensive studies by Siegel et al.[144,150,154,155] suggest a general range of "normal" vascular tone relationships. Patients in nonseptic shock not only have a higher resistance for a given level of flow than is displayed in patients with sepsis or septic shock states, but these two types of vascular tone relationships are also on opposite sides of the normal vascular tone relationship operating in control patients (who are neither septic, cirrhotic, hypertensive, nor in hypovolemic shock),[155] as demonstrated in Figure 9-12.

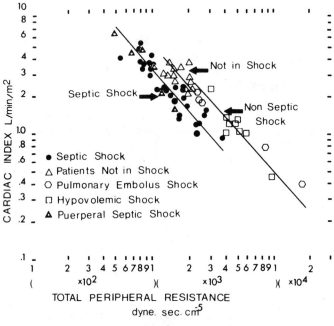

FIG. 9-12 Vascular tone relations in shock; net vascular tone. Log-log plot of the cardiac index on the *ordinate* versus the total peripheral resistance on the *abcissa.* (Siegel JH, Greenspan M, DelGuercio LRM: Abnormal vascular tone, defective oxygen transport and myocardial failure in human septic shock. Ann Surg 165:504, 1967.)

Vascular Regulation–Oxygen Consumption Relationships in Low Flow versus Septic Shock

That vascular regulation in hypovolemic shock is considerably different from that seen in sepsis is also suggested by the relationship of oxygen consumption to blood flow in hypovolemic or nonseptic shock syndromes compared with patients in hyperdynamic septic shock.[150,155] This is shown in Figure 9-13, in which the relationship of oxygen consumption ($\dot{V}O_2/m^2$) to total body flow (cardiac index) is shown. It can be seen that in patients in cardiogenic shock (as well as pulmonary embolus shock), pure hypovolemic shock, or nonseptic posttraumatic shock, *an increase in CI results in an increase in oxygen consumption until a critical level of flow is reached at which an increase in body perfusion produces no further rise in oxygen consumption.* While there

are different slopes for the flow: $\dot{V}O_2$ relationship in pure cardiogenic shock compared with trauma, in which an inflammatory response may also be present, or in sepsis, with its hypermetabolic state, these data suggest that for any given shock recovery state there is an intrinsic level of metabolic oxygen consumption which cannot be further increased by increasing perfusion alone. This $\dot{V}O_2$ level therefore represents the optimization point for maintenance of total body perfusion; the physician caring for a critically ill patient should attempt to achieve this level by adjusting volume support, vasodilatation, and cardiac inotropic support, if necessary.

In this regard, it is important to note that compared with nonseptic trauma, in patients with hyperdynamic sepsis, or with liver disease, the relationship between CI and oxygen consumption is shifted, so that a higher flow is necessary to obtain the same $\dot{V}O_2/m^2$.[150,155] Indeed, concomitant with severe sepsis involv-

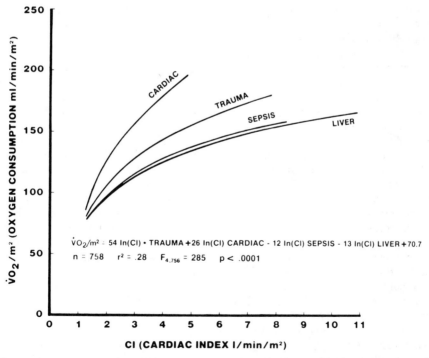

FIG. 9-13 Oxygen consumption: flow relationships in the critically ill. Regression lines derived from 758 studies from patients with cardiogenic shock, posttrauma and those with major chronic sepsis, or cirrhotic hyperdynamic liver disease. (From data of Tacchino RM, Siegel JH, Emanuele T et al: Incidence and therapy of myocardial depression in critically ill posttrauma patients. Circ Shock 18:360, 1986 (abst.))

ing a component of hepatic dysfunction (unbalanced septic B state) there are circumstances wherein marked increases in CI, rather than increasing $\dot{V}O_2/m^2$, are associated with normal or actually reduced levels of oxygen consumption.[144,150,155] Furthermore, in this septic B state, the reductions in oxygen consumption cannot be increased by further body flow increments. These data and those[144,150] discussed in Chapter 15 suggest that this type of sepsis may in fact represent not a failure of delivery of oxygen to the tissues, but rather an intrinsic cellular defect in oxidative metabolism.

Myocardial Function in Low-Flow Shock Syndromes

In patients with low-flow nonseptic shock syndromes resulting from hypovolemia, central cardiac failure syndromes (such as acute myocardial infarction), or obstructive pulmonary embolization with right heart failure, there appears to be a failure of microvascular autoregulation. The ability of the tissues to extract oxygen becomes increasingly more dependent on the level of oxygen delivery over a critical range of flow, so that the oxygen consumption ($\dot{V}O_2/m^2$) to perfusion (cardiac index) slope is steeper and shifted to the left (Fig. 9-13), perhaps representing both present $\dot{V}O_2$ needs and repayment of previous oxygen debt. The ability to maintain an oxygen consumption proportionate to the peripheral metabolic needs is a critical determinant of survival. The CO, which delivers the oxygen content of the arterial blood to the peripheral tissues and vital organs, is a function of the stroke volume that the contractile pumping action of the heart can eject times the number of beats per minute that the heart contracts.

These contractile functions are governed by determinants of myocardial mechanics. The myocardial contraction itself operates under a physiologic principle known as the force–velocity relationship.[1,8,164-171] This was originally derived from observations of contraction in skeletal muscle made by A. V. Hill,[69] who showed that when the resting length of the muscle fiber was increased, the subsequent ac-

tivation produced an increase in the developed force of contraction. In contrast to skeletal muscle, in which there is only a single mechanism for increasing the strength of contraction, cardiac muscle has two mechanisms by which myocardial force may be increased. The first of these is the classic Frank–Starling mechanism,[45,116,175] which is similar to that seen in skeletal muscle, in that increments in the resting length of the cardiac muscle fiber before contraction increase the developed force when myocardial contraction in initiated. The second mechanism, which is not seen in skeletal muscle but which is operative in cardiac muscle, is the inotropic mechanism,[1,115,116,158-160,164-168] by which alteration in the rate of activation (heart rate), or in the hormonal, or ionic biochemical environment of the cardiac muscle fiber, can increase the subsequent developed force from a constant resting fiber length.

Myocardial Mechanics and their Implications for Cardiac Function

With these two mechanisms in mind, it is important to understand that the heart muscle, and therefore the heart itself, can function in two different modes. First, the heart is a tension-generating machine under those circumstances in which the heart muscle is not permitted to shorten (Fig. 9-14B), such as during the initial period of the contraction before the heart has developed enough force to overcome the aortic diastolic pressure. This is known as the isometric contraction. Second, when the isometric tension generated by the myocardium exceeds the forces preventing any shortening, such as when the left heart intraventricular tension rises above that of the aortic diastolic pressure, the heart muscle manifests an isotonic contraction, during which it shortens externally (Fig. 9-14A). In the whole heart, this results in the ejection of blood from the ventricle.

In the in situ heart, the initial resting length of the heart muscle fiber is set by the volume of the diastolic filling, the left ventricular end-diastolic volume (LVEDV); this is known as the preload. The force of contraction after activa-

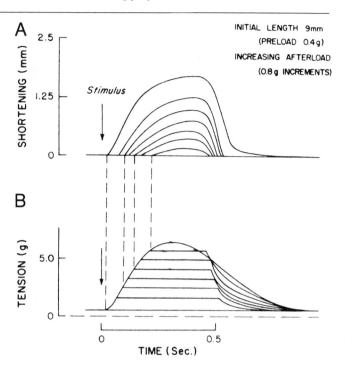

FIG. 9-14 Isometric (tension producing) versus isotonic (shortening) contractions in isolated papillary muscle. Serial isometric *tension* producing contractions at increasing afterloads (horizontal lines) shown at bottom. Upper (**A**) tracing shows successive isotonic *shortening* corresponding to the increasing *afterloads* in the lower (**B**) tracing (dotted lines). (Siegel JH, Sonnenblick EH, Judge RD, Wilson WS: The quantification of myocardial contractility in dog and man. Cardiologia 45: 189, 1964.)

tion is determined by this initial fiber length (Frank–Starling mechanism) and by the chemical–mechanical characteristics of the contractile element (inotropic mechanism). The energy imparted by this mechanicochemical transformation occurs at a rate of activation set by the inotropic level, which in turn determines the maximum velocity of shortening of the contractile element (Vmax). This Vmax is then dissipated against the intrinsic elastic components of the heart muscle itself to generate the isometric force or, having exceeded the isometric load, produces an isotonic contraction that leads to shortening against an afterload. In the in situ heart the afterload is represented by the product of the volume of blood ejected times the integral of the systolic pressure against which this ejection occurs.

As shown in Figure 9-15, at any given contractile state (Vmax) and preload (end-diastolic volume), the actual velocity of shortening (rate of volume ejection) and the magnitude of the shortening, or percentage of the diastolic volume ejected (ejection fraction) are all functions of the afterload experienced by the heart during its period of contraction. As the afterload is increased to a level greater than that which can be overcome by the heart muscle, at a given preload and contractile state, the velocity of shortening (A) and the shortening (B) decrease until the isometric point is achieved. However, myocardial (cardiac external) work is a hyperbolic function in which the work is zero at the theoretical point (Vmax) at which no load is placed on the contractile elements of the muscle; it is also zero at the point of isometricity, where no shortening occurs, since work is force generated times the degree of shortening achieved, or volume of blood ejected.[157,171] Myocardial power is developed force times the velocity of shortening; therefore, a similar relationship exists for this function.

Changing the fiber length (or the LVEDV) does not change the qualitative nature of the contractile element, nor does it alter the Vmax (Fig. 9-16). Therefore, the force–velocity relationship over the entire range of afterload describes only a single level of contractility, independent of fiber length.[164,166,174] Consequently, it is obvious that in the presence of a changing afterload, beat work or beat power cannot be used as an absolute index of contractility. Therefore, the much-used Starling–Sarnoff ven-

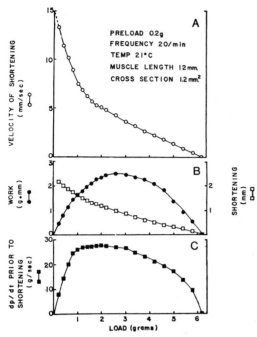

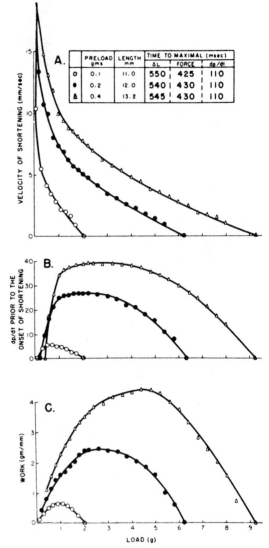

	PRELOAD gms	LENGTH mm	TIME TO MAXIMAL (msec)		
			ΔL	FORCE	dp/dt
o	0.1	11.0	550	425	110
●	0.2	12.0	540	430	110
Δ	0.4	13.2	545	430	110

FIG. 9-15 Myocardial force-velocity relations in papillary muscle. (**A**) velocity of isotonic shortening (force-velocity curve); (**B**) myocardial work and shortening; (**C**) the level of dp/dt immediately before onset of isotonic shortening. All plotted as functions of increasing *afterload* on the abcissa. The muscle was held at a single state of contractility (i.e., at constant length, constant stimulation frequency, constant temperature, and at uniform chemical inotropic background). (Siegel JH, Sonnenblick EH, Judge RD, Wilson WS: The quantification of myocardial contractility in dog and man. Cardiologia 45: 189, 1964.)

FIG. 9-16 Force-velocity and work relations with changing fiber length. (**A**), force-velocity curves; (**B**), course of dp/dt development; (**C**), myocardial work. All as functions of increasing *afterload*. (Siegel JH, Sonnenblick EH, Judge RD, Wilson WS: The quantification of myocardial contractility in dog and man. Cardiologia 45: 189, 1964.)

tricular function curves,[115,116] which relate stroke work to ventricular filling pressure or end-diastolic volume, provide only a relative, but not a unique or absolute, index of myocardial contractility (see Fig. 9-19).[23,157,164-168]

The intrinsic mechanicochemical transformation rate (Vmax) of heart muscle does not appear to be changed by increasing the resting fiber length (Fig. 9-16).[8,157,164-168,174] At a given contractile state characterized by a single Vmax, the family of myocardial force–velocity relationships produced by increasing resting fiber length, or end-diastolic volume, shows increases in the peak isometric force (load at zero velocity of shortening) that can be generated, as more of these contractile elements are

brought into aposition by stretching the myocardial fiber (Fig. 9-16A). But, since the basic elements themselves are unchanged, the maximum velocity of shortening (Vmax) remains constant; this operation at a single contractility

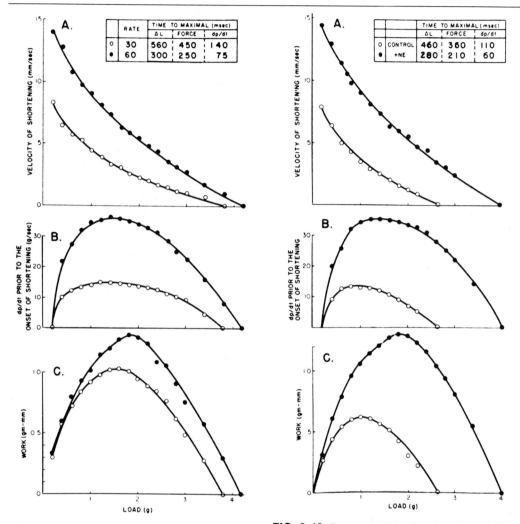

FIG. 9-17 Force-velocity and work relations with changing heart rate. **(A)**, force-velocity curves; **(B)**, course of dp/dt development; **(C)**, myocardial work. All as functions of increasing *afterload*. (Siegel JH, Sonnenblick EH, Judge RD, Wilson WS: The quantification of myocardial contractility in dog and man. Cardiologia 45: 189, 1964.)

FIG. 9-18 Force-velocity and work relations with increasing inotropic support (norepinephrine). **(A)**, force-velocity curves; **(B)**, course of dp/dt development; **(C)**; myocardial work. All as functions of increasing *afterload*. (Siegel JH, Sonnenblick EH, Judge RD, Wilson WS: The quantification of myocardial contractility in dog and man. Cardiologia 45: 189, 1964.)

has been theorized to represent the fundamental aspect of the Frank–Starling relationship.[166]

However, inotropic factors that alter the rate of activation of the contractile element, that is, increasing heart rate (Fig. 9-17), or those that alter the force and rate of force development by the mechanicochemical transformation, that is, chemical inotropic agents (Fig. 9-18), shift the force–velocity relationship to a higher (positive inotropic), or lower (negative inotropic), Vmax at the same fiber length. Increasing Vmax results in a greater shortening (increased ejection fraction) and rate of shortening (velocity of ejection) at a given afterload. From a given fiber length, increasing the Vmax also causes an increase in the maximum work that can be achieved at a given afterload (Fig. 9-18).

Finally, myocardial contraction is a time-dependent process. The activation of the contractile element, which is theorized to be both in series and in parallel with elastic elements in the myocardial fiber, occurs before and is dissipated earlier than the observed peak pressure (or tension) curve of the heart muscle.[35,157,167] The duration of the development of contractile element tension is known as the active state and it is reflected in the rate of development of the intraventricular pressure (dp/dt), provided that the valve opening occurs at no less than 30 percent of the theoretical peak isometric tension (Figs. 9-15 through 9-18).[157,159] At a constant contractile state (Vmax), the actual levels of peak tension and dp/dt increase with increasing fiber length (see Fig. 9-19). However, the durational aspects of this contractile activation, the Δt dp/dt (Fig.

9-16), and the rate of development of pressure (or tension) per unit pressure (or tension) developed, (dp/dt)/IIT, the Isometric Time–Tension index,[157-159] are constant for a given level of contractility (see Fig. 9-19). Stimuli that change the basic myocardial contractile state (Vmax) and that shift the myocardial force–velocity relationship also change Δt dp/dt and the (dp/dt)/IIT relationship to a new constant level independent of the fiber length (Fig. 9-20), end-diastolic volume, end-diastolic or pulmonary wedge pressure, or stroke work achieved (Fig. 9-20). Thus, it is possible to estimate the contractility of the intact heart either from the characteristics of intraventricular pressure development, (dp/dt)/IIT,[8,164] from the durational aspects of isometric contraction (Δt dp/dt),[157-159] or by extrapolating the velocity of shortening–afterload characteristics (V$_{CE}$)

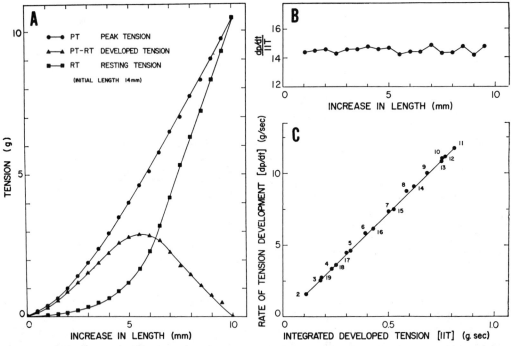

FIG. 9-19 Symmetry of length tension relations on ascending and descending portions of fiber length: tension relationship. Isometric papillary muscle held at constant temperature, chemical background, and stimulation rate. **(A)** tension versus fiber length; **(B)** dp/dt/IIT versus length; **(C)** dp/dt versus IIT. In (C) points 2–11 represent values from ascending limb and points 12–19 represent values from the descending limb of the length:tension curve shown in (A). (Siegel JH, Sonnenblick EH: Isometric time-tension relationship as an index of myocardial contractility. Circ Res 12: 597, 1963.)

that characterize the myocardial force–velocity relationship from dynamic changes in ventricular dimensions.[8,52,164,170]

As shown in Table 9-2, noninotropic agents operating on the Frank–Starling mechanism do not change the maximum velocity of contraction (Vmax), nor do they alter the duration of active state. Positive inotropic agents increase the force that can be generated from a given fiber length by changing the mechanicochemical characteristics of the contractile element, thus altering the maximum velocity of contraction (Vmax). They also increase the velocity of shortening and the degree of fiber shortening at any given afterload and shorten the duration of active state. As a result, positive inotropic agents with β-adrenergic activity, which activate adenyl cyclase and produce cAMP,[40,56,65] such as norepinephrine, dopamine, dobutamine, and isoproterenol, as well as drugs that increase Ca^{++} ion entry into the myocardium,[77,125] such as digitalis preparations and Ca^{++}, tend to increase aortic systolic pressure by increasing the velocity of aortic flow and increasing the cardiac ejection fraction from any end-diastolic volume. In general, these agents will increase CO unless there is also an afterload increase due to associated

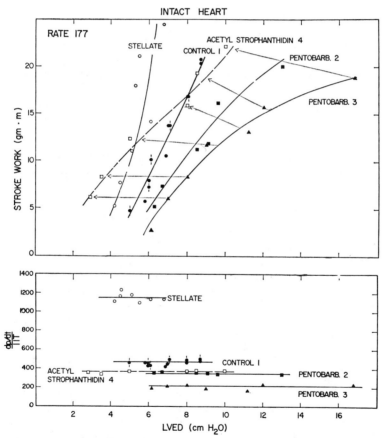

FIG. 9-20 Ventricular function curve shifts and isometric time tension relationships [(dp/dt)/IIT] with regard to effects of pentobarbital induced myocardial depression, subsequent inotropic support with a digitalis-like agent (acetyl strophanthidin) or cardiac sympathetic nerve stimulation (stellate). Canine right heart bypass. Heart paced at 177 beats per minute. Cardiac output increased in equal steps from 870 ml/min to 1790 ml/min. Note shift to the right in VF curves with pentobarbital reduction in contractility [fall in (dp/dt)/IIT], and shift to the left with inotropic agents as (dp/dt)/IIT increases. (Siegel JH, Sonnenblick EH: Isometric time-tension relationships as an index of myocardial contractility. Circ Res 12: 597, 1963.)

TABLE 9-2. Characteristics of Inotropic and Noninotropic Agents on the Parameters of Myocardial Contractility

Aspects of Contractility Intervention	Velocity Vmax	Force (P_0)	Magnitude of Active State (dp/dt)	Duration of Active State (Δt dp/dt
A. Noninotropic agents Frank-Starling mechanism; increasing fiber length (ΔL) volume infusion	Constant 0	Increase proportional to ΔL +	Increase proportional to ΔL +	Constant 0
B. Weak inotropic agents Increasing myocardial activation rate (ΔR) heart rate	Small increase +	No change or small increase 0 or +	Small increase +	Small decrease −
C. Strong inotropic agents 1. Positive inotropic agents (norepinephrine, Isuprel, digitalis, Ca^{++} glucagon, dopamine, dobutamine, amrinone)	Large increase ++ to +++	Large increase ++ to +++	Large increase ++ to +++	Large decrease − to −−
2. Negative inotropic agents (barbiturates, endotoxin, anoxia, propranolol, halothane, diethyl ether)	−−	−−	−−	++

(Siegel JH: Physiologic assessment of cardiac function in the aged and high-risk surgical patient. p. 23. In Siegel JH, Chodoff PD (eds): The Aged and High Risk Surgical Patient. Grune & Stratton, New York, 1976, by permission).

vasoconstriction with baroreceptor reflex sympathetic tone withdrawal. Finally, the reduction in the duration of active state tends to increase the diastolic filling period,[35,157,159,167] thus allowing time for increased coronary perfusion to compensate for the increased myocardial oxygen consumption produced by the inotropically mediated increased Vmax.[172]

Negative inotropic agents such as some anesthetic agents,[6,7,54,55,127,128,158,160] β-blockers,[20] ischemia,[117] toxic factors,[2,187] K^+ and Ca^{++} channel blockers,[77,125] decrease the force that can be generated from a given fiber length and reduce the maximum velocity of contraction, myocardial fiber shortening, and the velocity of shortening at any given afterload (Fig. 9-21). They also tend to increase the duration of the active state. These features result in reduced pressure generation, a lower aortic flow velocity, and a smaller ejection fraction from a given end-diastolic volume (preload) at a given afterload. They usually cause a decrease in CO and generally tend to slow the rate of myocardial contraction as well as the rate of relaxation, producing a reduced period for diastolic filling of the coronary vessels (Fig. 9-22).

The Role of Ventricular Compliance

The last major element in the basic physiologic modifiers of cardiac function is explained within the concept of ventricular compliance. The myocardial contract elements reside within the individual myocardial fibers and in a heart muscle that also contains noncontractile structural elements. These act as either in-series or in-parallel elastic factors that influence the dissipation of the energy developed by contraction.[165] They also influence the resting length–tension relationship of the non-contractile cardiac muscle. Thus, the relationship between the end-diastolic volume within the heart and the end-diastolic tension, or pressure, is changed.[79] The pressure–volume relationship of the ventricle is altered in the direction of a decreased compliance (increased pressure for a given diastolic volume) by factors that increase the degree of myocardial interstitial edema, such as myocardial contusion, acute myocarditis, and right heart failure, with increased coronary venous back pres-

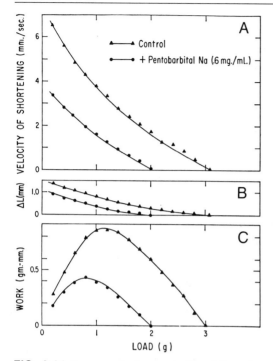

FIG. 9-21 Decrease in force-velocity relationships with negative inotropic action of pentobarbital. Isolated papillary muscle at constant initial fiber length, temperature, and stimulation rate. **(A)** velocity of shortening, **(B)** shortening (ΔL), **(C)** work. (Siegel JH, Sonnenblick EH: Quantification and prediction of myocardial failure. Arch Surg 89: 1026, 1984.)

sure.[15,16,50,140] Also, coronary vasodilator drugs or revascularization surgery, which increase coronary perfusion, may alter the actual volume of blood contained within the myocardium itself, and cardiomyopathies produce chronic fibrotic changes, both of which will reduce ventricular compliance.[30,39,140] Similar fibrotic changes occurring after repeated small infarcts may also alter the ventricular pressure–volume relationship in the direction of a reduced compliance.[140] Finally, an effective reduction in ventricular compliance occurs at very high heart rates when there is an inadequate reduction in the duration of myocardial active state, so that full myocardial relaxation fails to occur before the next cardiac activation.[173] This can occur in rapid supraventricular or ventricular tachyarrhythmias.

The ventricular compliance will be increased under circumstances that decrease the volume of blood contained in the myocardial wall. This will occur under circumstances of hypovolemic shock or following initiation of an increased ejection fraction after a previous volume overload and after relief of right heart failure that has produced high coronary venous pressures. It will also occur after acute myocardial infarction where a passive distention of the nonfunctional myocardium allows for a ballooning of the ventricular wall.[30] Under some circumstances, drugs that tend to increase right ventricular cardiac ejection, thus lowering right ventricular end-diastolic and coronary venous pressure, will also selectively increase left ventricular compliance. It has also been speculated that this occurs in some cases of right ventricular overload produced by increased pulmonary vascular resistance, where a septal shift into the left ventricle has decreased the left-sided pressure–volume relationships.[15,16,78,140] Relief of this acute septal shift by reduction of the pulmonary vasoconstriction will selectively affect the left ventricle, producing an apparent compliance increase on the left side of the heart.[140,141]

As a result of these compliance shifts, the frequently used measures of intraventricular or pulmonary capillary wedge pressure (PWP) may be in error in interpreting the cardiac work-filling pressure relationship, described by the classic Starling–Sarnoff curves.[15,39] Because of the frequency of compliance changes in various types of critical illness, measures of the LVEDV are preferable to measures of PWP or right atrial pressures (RAP) in delineating the cardiac response in hypovolemic, posttraumatic, or cardiogenic shock states. Also, cardiac physiologic measurements, which more directly characterize those functions of the myocardium that are more closely related to the durational aspects of contractile element activity, (dp/dt)/IIT or Δt dp/dt, or to the myocardial force–velocity relationships, that is, cardiac ejection fraction, or the ejection velocity–afterload relations, are more accurate guides to the effectiveness of cardiac inotropic support therapy than are indices that depend on PWP or RAP values.[15,39,113,140,142,159]

A further source of error in using any measure of contractile adequacy (Starling–Sarnoff relations) that depends on the use of PWP or RAP to estimate the relative effect of diastolic ventricular volume is the fact that if the

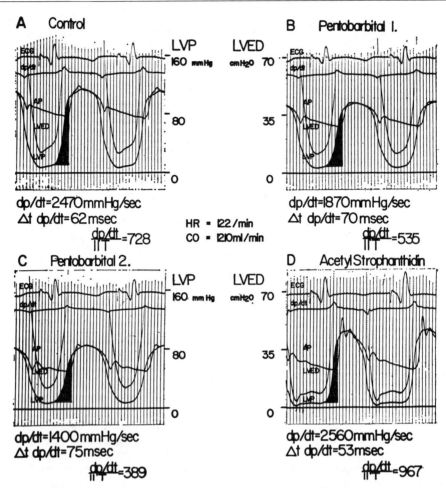

FIG. 9-22 Systolic ejection time, diastolic filling time, and Isometric Time Tension relationships in the intact canine heart in response to negative inotropic depression of myocardial force-velocity relations with pentobarbital and with recovery after use of inotropic agent (acetyl strophanthidin). Intact canine preparation on right heart bypass at constant cardiac output and heart rate. Between (**A**) and (**B**), 120 mg of sodium pentobarbital administered intravenously. Between (B) and (**C**), 120 mg of sodium pentobarbital administered intravenously. Between (C) and (**D**), 0.5 mg of acetyl strophanthidin administered intravenously. Shaded area indicates fractional integrated isometric tension (IIT), dp/dt equals maximum rate of development of isometric tension. Δt dp/dt = time from R wave to maximum dp/dt; AP = aortic pressure; LVP = left ventricular pressure; LVED = expanded left ventricular end-diastolic pressure. Time lines 0.02 seconds. Note that reduced diastolic filling time and pressure gradient between AP and LVP occurs with a prolongation in Δt dp/dt and with fall in (dp/dt)/IIT. All of these are reversed by inotropic drug therapy. (Siegel JH, Sonnenblick EH: Quantification and prediction of myocardial failure. Arch Surg 89: 1026, 1964.)

patient is maintained on mechanical ventilation, the actual value of PWP will be influenced by both the transmitted mean airway and the actual end-expiratory respiratory pressures.[11,16,78,113,140] Also, since the alveolar pressure acts as a Starling resistance to the ejection of the right heart, a high mean alveolar pressure

may in effect force the right heart to operate at a higher end-diastolic volume (RVEDV) point than is optimal for right ventricular function, so that RAP is also disproportionately increased relative to total blood volume. Consequently, both cardiac contractile status and the adequacy of fluid volume replacement can be misinterpreted, if only the cardiac work-filling pressure relationships (Starling–Sarnoff ventricular function curves) are used as a guide to the need for volume or inotropic support.

PHYSIOLOGIC GOALS OF THERAPY IN LOW-FLOW SHOCK STATES

The ultimate goal of therapy in low-flow shock states is to restore a high enough level of tissue perfusion to vital organs so that oxygen delivery will be sufficient to permit oxygen consumption to rise above critical ischemic levels. This degree of oxygen delivery will also permit repayment of any peripheral oxygen debts that have resulted in a buildup of nonoxidized metabolic substrates (lactate and other metabolic acids), so that oxidative energy metabolism can resume. Thus flow becomes more important than pressure, provided only that there is an effective driving pressure greater than the critical opening pressure of the various vascular beds. Perfusion pressure may be of particular importance in coronary, cerebral, and renal perfusion, wherein preexisting arteriosclerotic disease may substantially alter the effective critical opening pressure. However, as a general rule, if CO can be brought to a level at which maximum oxygen consumption is then achieved (Fig. 9-13), the cardiovascular component of shock therapy is probably adequate.

There is considerable urgency to the process of restoring an adequate body and organ perfusion, and immediate resuscitative efforts must be made with the fact in mind that the oxygen deficit accumulation must be halted and debt repayment begun as soon as possible. The size of the deficit is directly related to survival and most likely as well to the extent of multiple organ failure that often occurs. In hypovolemic patients, it is not uncommon to find significant rates of oxygen deficit accumulation that are rapidly developing into a lethal metabolic injury. The key to reversing this deadly trend is through the rapid use of volume and

inotropic support to restore the circulation and oxygen consumption to the hypoxic tissues (Figs. 9-10 and 9-11). The major problem in this process of resuscitation concerns the judicious use of volume. The question is often asked, "When do I stop infusing volume?," and the answer is still one that can not be given with complete authority. Experimental formulas relate the reinfused volume to the hemorrhaged volume, although the true magnitude of the volume loss is rarely, if ever, known in situations presenting in the emergency room or trauma center. Knowing the $\dot{V}O_2$ can aid the clinician in this situation, as it can be used to gauge the effectiveness of the resuscitation effort.[82,107-109,124,141,143,152-155,179] Although there is no magic number, efforts should be made to optimize $\dot{V}O_2$. If there is a rapid increase in $\dot{V}O_2$ with resuscitation, it indicates that the volume given is continuing to increase effective perfusion. When $\dot{V}O_2$ begins to level off at or near the expected posttrauma levels (Table 9-1), this suggests that the volume is approaching the volume shed; if the source of bleeding is controlled, the infusion rate may need to be decreased in order to prevent fluid overload. A slow rise from a low $\dot{V}O_2$ in response to the resuscitation efforts must be treated much more aggressively in order to save the patient. In these cases, there should be less concern about fluid overload, since a poor responder is either past the point of no return or still has a low circulating volume, whether the source of bleeding is controlled or not.

The question of the type of fluid to administer is also one of the most controversial problems in fluid resuscitation (Chapters 6 and 7). There is no statistically significant evidence that any difference exists between the final outcome of young patients (or healthy animals) resuscitated with colloid versus crystalloid.[104,129,139,141] Nevertheless, there are data that deserve mention showing that $\dot{V}O_2$ may recover more quickly with colloid than with crystalloid.[66] While much has been written about the value of hemodilution to increasing perfusion after hypovolemia,[29] in many situations the reduction in circulating red blood cell (RBC) mass and hemoglobin (Hb) concentration may have a limiting effect on oxygen delivery.[90,93] Since time is critical in a patient with a large rate of oxygen deficit accumulation, the slower the $\dot{V}O_2$ recovery the greater may be the degree of cellular and vascular permeability injury,[76,181] and this may influence the chances for a successful recovery, especially in the multiply injured or older trauma patient. However, careful quantitative prospective randomized studies that specifically address this point have yet to be performed.

The other side of the coin is that the organ responsible for maintaining an effective oxygen delivery, the heart, must also be permitted to function at an optimum level that maximizes its function under the myocardial force–velocity relationships. This means that a preload to afterload relationship should be established at which the highest level of ejection fraction is achieved that does not unduly increase intrinsic myocardial oxygen consumption. The myocardial $\dot{V}O_2$ ($M\dot{V}O_2$) is directly related to the rate of development of tension (or pressure) times the tension (or pressure) developed, times the number of contractions per minute.[172] It can be quantified approximately from an index obtained by computing the stroke power, i.e. systolic blood pressure (SBP) times stroke vol-

ume (SV) divided by ejection time (ET), [(SBP · SV)/ET], times the heart rate per minute (Fig. 9-23). As a very crude approximation, the systolic arterial blood pressure (SBP) times the heart rate can be used. However, under hyperdynamic septic or cirrhotic conditions in which vascular resistance may be reduced but the velocity of ejection is increased, this may lead to erroneous conclusions. Conditions should also be sought that permit a short ejection time to allow the longest practical period of coronary artery diastolic filling per heartbeat (Fig. 9-22). This will permit increased coronary arterial oxygen delivery to compensate for the increased myocardial oxygen consumption, provided that CO is also maintained by an adequate systemic venous volume return.

As a general rule, this means that volume infusion (preload) must be coupled with vasodilator therapy to reduce excessive systemic vascular resistance, peak and mean arterial pressure, and abnormal increases in afterload. Cardiac inotropic support also should be employed to shift the myocardial force–velocity

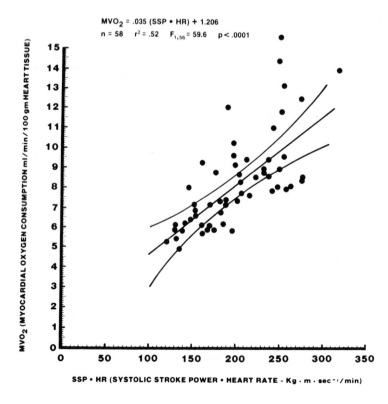

FIG. 9-23 Relationship between myocardial oxygen consumption and cardiac stroke power per minute. (Recomputed from canine data reported by Sonnenblick EH, Ross J Jr, Covell JW et al: Velocity of contraction as a determinant of myocardial oxygen consumption. Am J Physiol 209: 919, 1965.)

relationship to a higher ejection point for a given afterload, while at the same time reducing the duration of active state and thereby permitting a longer period for coronary diastolic filling at any given heart rate. This combination of agents will tend to result in increased CO and oxygen delivery and reduced ventricular end-diastolic volume and pressure, which also will tend to increase ventricular compliance by lowering coronary venous pressure.

BEDSIDE QUANTIFICATION OF CARDIOVASCULAR FUNCTION IN THE CRITICALLY ILL AND INJURED PATIENT

To achieve these goals it is necessary to use bedside techniques that permit the quantification of cardiovascular function. A number of methodologies have been proposed for the measure of cardiac output, including the use of the Fick, or thermodilution, methods for the determination of flow. These methods do not permit easy characterization of left ventricular myocardial contractile function. The CO measurements are either nonspecific with regard to helping delineate contractile dynamics, as with the Fick method, which measures only flow, or are dominated by the right ventricular contractile function, as in the case of the Swan–Ganz thermodilution curve, where the sensor lies in the pulmonary artery.[178] Studies have also been carried out using radionuclide[13,89] or radiocontrast ventriculography[33] where the left ventricular cardiac ejection fraction can be estimated and the CO determined by multiplying the stroke volume times the heart rate. Although accurate, these methods require either the intravenous introduction of radioisotopes or high osomolality iodinated dye mixtures and the application of cumbersome specialized equipment, so that they are not easy to repeat at the bedside. More recently, the improvement of dynamic methods involving noninvasive technology, such as impedance cardiography[146] or Doppler echocardiography,[92] hold promise

of being able to estimate either the velocity or durational aspects of left ventricular contractility as well as the CO. However, these methods have not been systematically tested in critically ill and injured patients over the full range of CO encountered (less than 1 L/min to greater than 20 L/min). It is expected that their value will increase as the specific instrumentation and appropriate correlation between these measures and invasive techniques is elucidated.

Specific quantification of myocardial contractile function is possible using intraventricular pressure measurements,[159] whereby the $(dp/dt)/IIT$, alone or modified as $(dp/dt)/P$, or the durational aspects of contraction, $\Delta t \, dp/dt$, can be used. A determination of contractile element velocity, VCE, using both dp/dt and the change in length, dl/dt, derived from the change in angiographic ventricular dimensions has also been used to quantify Vmax.[52,65] However, these techniques involve the introduction of a left ventricular catheter, which may be impractical for use in most critically ill patients.

Over the past 18 years, a method of simultaneously determining cardiac output and myocardial contractile function has been developed using the cardiogreen indicator dilution technique.[142,147] This approach has been effectively applied in the bedside evaluation of more than 5,000 critically ill patients over the full range of disease states and all levels of CO. It is based on a mathematical model analysis of the shape of the indicator dilution curve as well as its mass dilution characteristics, from which the CO is determined.

The principles behind this method are shown in Figure 9-24, which demonstrates cardiogreen indicator dilution curves from two patients with acute myocardial infarction shock. The CO is essentially identical, but it is obvious that there are marked differences in shape. Since the cardiogreen dye curve is obtained by injecting a bolus of indocyanine green dye into the right atrium (or pulmonary artery) with sampling of the resultant indicator dilution curve from a peripheral artery, the curve contains within its shape information concerning the dispersion characteristic of the pulmonary vascular bed and the dynamic ejection function of the left heart. These have been analyzed

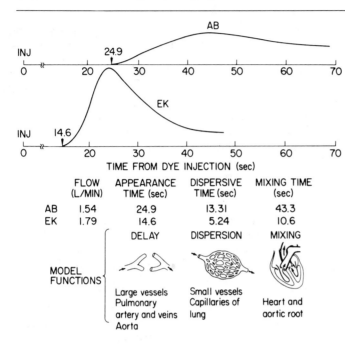

	FLOW (L/MIN)	APPEARANCE TIME (sec)	DISPERSIVE TIME (sec)	MIXING TIME (sec)
AB	1.54	24.9	13.31	43.3
EK	1.79	14.6	5.24	10.6

FIG. 9-24 Indicator dilution curves and model parameters from two patients with myocardial infarction shock, before intraaortic balloon counter-pulsation. Note that marked differences in shape of the curves are reflected in the differences in the appearance time (ta), dispersive time (td) and mixing time (tm) parameters of the model. (Siegel JH, Farrell EJ, Goldwyn RM, Friedman HP: The surgical implications of physiologic patterns in myocardial infarction shock. Surgery 72: 126, 1972.)

using a functional model of indicator dilution (Fig. 9-24) into three functions: First, an appearance time delay function, t_a, describes the passive volume transfer of the dye containing blood by the large vessels of the pulmonary artery and veins and the aorta. Second, a dispersive time function, t_d, is mainly related to the fact that the input bolus of dye is dispersed through a large volume component consisting mainly of the sum of the volumes of many branching and recombining vessels in the pulmonary small vessel and capillary bed. Weibel[192] showed that these vessels have a wide range of lengths and diameters with a nearly gaussian distribution. As a result of this structure, the flow through the pulmonary vascular bed determines the dispersive function that transforms the dye from a bolus to a distribution spread as it passes through the lung. The mean transit time for this dispersive function, t_d, has been shown to be equivalent to the mean transit time of passage of the pulmonary blood volume from pulmonary artery to left atrium.[142] As a result, when the dispersive time constant (t_d, in sec) is multiplied by the CO (in liters per second), the time factors cancel out and a computation of central dispersive blood volume (DV) is produced, which has been shown experimentally to be within 10 percent of the direct measurement of pulmonary blood volume.[142] This indicates that under ordinary circumstances the dispersive characteristics of the pulmonary vascular bed dominate the dye dilution curve spreading. The DV thus provides a means of measuring the pulmonary reservoir blood volume, which is the accommodation blood volume permitting adjustments between the right and left hearts under conditions of changing posture or stress.[191] This was confirmed in studies of critically ill patients who received sequential dye injections into the pulmonary artery and the right atrium. These patients showed no significant differences between the dispersive mean transit times, t_d, to the femoral artery measured from the two different injection sites. This finding suggests that the right heart ordinarily contributes little to the dispersive function.[142] However, in some clinical circumstances, patients with massive right heart dilatation caused by a usually fatal pulmonary embolus, or preterminal cor pulmonale, were noted to have significant right heart dispersive volumes. In addition, some patients with known ventricular or large proximal aortic aneurysms also have been shown to have significant dispersive volumes associated with these dilated vascular structures, and this has been confirmed by clinical studies before and after excision of ventricular aneurysms and in experimental preparations.[142] However, these circumstances are easily identified and indeed have diagnostic importance, since these patients invariably had pulmonary dispersive mean transit times, t_d, in excess of 7.5 seconds. The importance of recognizing an excessively long t_d was confirmed in patients in whom a massive akinetic myocardial segment following myocardial infarction shock was identified by the excessive duration of the dispersive function and confirmed by angiogram. Both abnormalities were then reduced in response to intraaortic balloon counter pulsation. As ventricular function returned, the massive dispersive component was reduced to within normal limits.[143,147] The clinical value of this measurement is that the size of the pulmonary reservoir blood volume, DV, can be established. In normal control circumstances, the pulmonary reservoir blood volume per square meter of body surface area (BSA), the DV/m^2, has been demonstrated to be approximately 200 ml/m^2 BSA. In sequential studies of patients with known hypovolemia, a low CO in the presence of a dispersive volume of less than 200 ml/m^2 BSA could be shown to be improved by additional volume transfusion. However, patients with low-flow syndromes in whom the pulmonary dispersive volume was greatly in excess of 200 ml/m^2 BSA generally did not respond well to volume infusion. Rather, they required inotropic support in order to increase CO, suggesting that in these patients a central venous overload already existed that was not improved by volume transfusion.

Third, a mixing time function, t_m, is derived from the analysis of the exponential washout downslope of the dye curve taken across the central circulation (including both right and left hearts). The t_m has been demonstrated to be dominated by the left heart, except under circumstances of massive cor pulmonale or pulmonary embolization with right heart dilatation. This washout from the heart of dye containing blood is a function of the dilution of the dye-containing left heart blood with a volume of fresh blood from the pulmonary blood volume reservoir, to replace the fraction of end-diastolic volume ejected by the dynamic action of the left ventricle. The t_m function determines the rate of disappearance of the dye curve concentration in the ventricular output stream. The t_m function has been demonstrated to be a reflection of the ejection fraction of the heart. A good heart having a large ejection fraction has a rapid exponential washout function (short t_m), and a poor heart with a low ejection fraction has a slow washout function (long t_m). The 95 percent washout point, which is equal to three washout time constants (3 t_m), can be used to compute an average minute ejection fraction[142]:

$$EFx = 1 - (3\ t_m/60)$$

This function has been shown to correlate experimentally with the durational aspects of the left ventricular contractility ($\Delta t\ dp/dt$) and therefore to be directly related to the force–velocity relationships discussed earlier.[142]

Cardiovascular Relations in Cardiogenic and Hyperdynamic Critical Illness

A simple means of estimating these time functions (t_d and t_m) from the cardiogreen dye dilution curve is shown in Figure 9-25. Thus, the dye-dilution curve can help establish three parameters—cardiac output (CO), pulmonary dispersive blood volume (DV), and cardiac ejection fraction (EFx)—which between them define the relative position of the patients cardiac function with regard to the Frank–Starling and inotropic mechanisms.[144] The effect on the cardiac index (CO/BSA) of changes in the pulmonary blood volume (the reservoir filling volume of the left heart) and the cardiac ejection fraction is shown in Figure 9-26. Unstressed control elective general surgical patients have a CI of 3 to 3.5 L/min/m^2, a pulmonary dispersive blood volume (DV/m^2) of approximately 200 ml/m^2, and cardiac ejection fraction (EFx) of 78 percent. For a given EFx, the CI is seen to increase as the DV/m^2 value is increased. Since raising the DV/m^2 in effect produces an increase in cardiac filling, this describes the Frank–Starling mechanism. At a given pulmonary reservoir volume (DV/m^2), the CI also increases as EFx rises. This describes the inotropic mechanism.

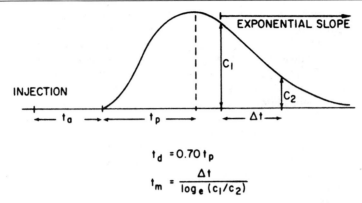

$$t_d = 0.70\, t_p$$

$$t_m = \frac{\Delta t}{\log_e (c_1/c_2)}$$

FIG. 9-25 Bedside computation of dispersive time (td) and mixing time (tm) from cardiogreen indicator dilution curve. ta = appearance time; tp = time to peak; C_1 and C_2 = two points on exponential downslope of dye curve separated by Δt. (As described by Siegel JH: Physiologic assessment of cardiac function in the aged and high-risk surgical patient. p. 23. In Siegel JH, Chodoff PD (eds): The Aged and High Risk Surgical Patient. Grune & Stratton, Inc. New York, 1976, by permission.)

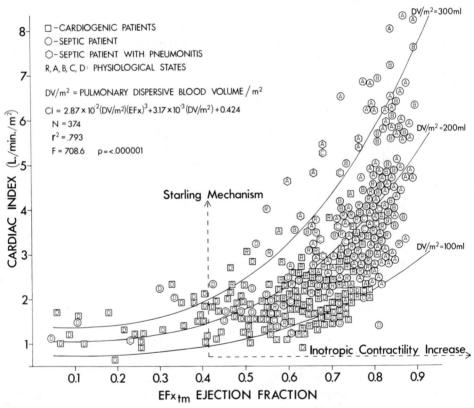

FIG. 9-26 Role of ejection fraction, computed from cardiac mixing time (tm), and pulmonary dispersive blood volume (DV/m²) on cardiac index. Effect of increases in cardiac index by the Starling mechanism versus those produced by an inotropic contractility increase are shown. Patients are labeled by type of disease condition and by physiologic state. (Siegel JH, Cerra FB, Coleman B et al: Physiological and metabolic correlations in human sepsis. Surgery 86: 163, 1979.)

Patients with cardiogenic decompensation secondary to myocardial infarction or septic myocardial depression have a reduced cardiac ejection fraction with a relatively normal or increased pulmonary blood volume (Fig. 9-26). This is in contrast to patients with hyperdynamic sepsis, who have a normal or increased pulmonary dispersive blood volume (>220 ml/m²) associated with a high ejection fraction and consequently manifest an increased CI. Patients without myocardial depression who have hypovolemic volume loss (or hypovolemic septic conditions) have a lower than normal pulmonary dispersive blood volume (<180 ml/m²). They also have a reduced LVEDV, but frequently these patients also have a compensatory increased cardiac ejection fraction in response to the sympathetic stress response, so

that the stroke volume does not fall as much as it might with a normal EFx. Identification of this circumstance permits one to increase the cardiac index by increasing the pulmonary reservoir volume (DV/m²) through intravenous infusion. Since all these data are available by virtue of a single cardiogreen indicator dilution curve, it is possible to characterize the patient fairly accurately with regard to the relative influence of preload (pulmonary dispersive blood volume or LVEDV), contractile state (cardiac ejection fraction), and relative afterload (vascular tone) effects in order to quantify more precisely the relative needs for volume infusion, vasodilation therapy, and inotropic support.

The influence of afterload is shown in Figure 9-27, which demonstrates the relation-

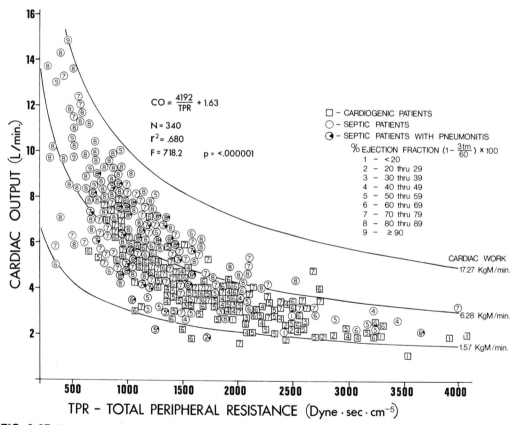

FIG. 9-27 Effect of cardiac output and total peripheral resistance on cardiac work in patients with nonseptic and septic conditions. Individual patient studies are labeled by percent ejection fraction. (Siegel JH, Giovannini I, Coleman B: Ventilation: perfusion maldistribution secondary to the hyperdynamic cardiovascular state as the major cause of increased shunting in human sepsis. Trauma 19: 432, 1979.)

ship of the CO to TPR. The normal CO is 5 to 6 L/min, and the normal TPR is 1,200 to 1,400 dyn/sec/cm^{-5}. Also shown are lines of constant cardiac work. Patients with nonseptic cardiogenic or hypovolemic conditions (squares) who have an increased total peripheral resistance also tend to have low cardiac ejection fractions (Fig. 9-27). While the cardiac work may be normal (6.28 kg M/min) or decreased, the work done is almost entirely resistive work. As a result, in this type of patient, even though cardiac work may be reduced, the myocardial oxygen consumption index (M$\dot{V}O_2$) as estimated by stroke power times heart rate (Fig. 9-23) may be normal, slightly reduced, or increased, at a time when coronary perfusion is reduced because of low CO. To increase the CO in this case, it is useful to produce a reduction in peripheral resistance by using a vasodilator agent (nitroprusside, nitroglycerine, or nitroglycerine paste).[4,19,100] Not infrequently, the accompanying use of a cardiac β-adrenergic inotropic drug at very low levels (dopamine 3 to 5 μg/kg/min, or isoproterenol 0.25 to 0.5 μg/min total dose),[18,61,94,95,141] so as to increase contractility and increase diastolic filling per contraction and only minimally increase myocardial oxygen consumption, will act synergistically with the afterload reduction to improve CO with a resulting increase in coronary perfusion.

In hyperdynamic septic patients (circles) in whom the CO is markedly increased, there is a high ejection fraction (>70 percent), but vascular resistance is reduced below control levels.[144,155] Surprisingly, although they have a lower resistance, these patients also may have an increased afterload effect, which is the product of stroke volume times the mean blood pressure during systole. As a consequence, cardiac work in sepsis may be increased, even though most of it is of a flow type. These patients also may have a markedly increased myocardial oxygen consumption, but because of the high CO and shortened systolic ejection period generally have increased coronary perfusion. Nevertheless, if there is intrinsic coronary artery disease, the demands of the hyperdynamic circulation, which appears in sepsis, or after trauma, or surgical injury may result in a relative coronary insufficiency. Under these circumstances high output failure syndromes are not uncommon in the coronary compromised patient. Septic patients may also have a metabolically induced myocardial depression,[144,155] as discussed in Chapter 15.

Cardiovascular Relations after Major Trauma

Systematic studies of the regulation of body flow (CI) in resuscitated critically ill posttraumatic patients have shown that there is a major interaction between the myocardial contractile factors (as expressed by EFx), the afterload factors (as expressed by TPR), and age.[179] This relationship is shown in Figure 9-28, in which the CI is seen to be positively correlated with increasing EFx, whereas increasing peripheral resistance (TPR) and increasing age are both negatively correlated with CI and all factors are simultaneously significant. That there are also other important regulators of CI is demonstrated by the fact that the regression intercept value is large and that the entire equation, although highly significant in 658 observations, only explains 60 percent of the variability ($r^2 = 0.596$) in flow.

The influence of these factors on total body oxygen consumption ($\dot{V}O_2$/m^2) is shown in Figure 9-29. The TPR, which is of great significance in influencing the level of CI, was not found to be significant in limiting $\dot{V}O_2$, provided there was an adequate central blood volume (DV/m^2), since with increasing TPR body oxygen extraction (Ca-$\bar{v}O_2$) increases to compensate for the low flow until shock conditions occur. As can be seen in this equation, in which all factors are simultaneously significant, the EFx and the level of the pulmonary reservoir filling volume (DV/m^2), which in turn reflects the adequacy of total body volume, were positive factors increasing oxygen consumption, whereas age was a negative factor. This is shown in further detail in Figure 9-30, in which trauma patients were divided into four age ranges (age I: 13–30; age II: 31–49; age III: 50–65, and age IV: >65). The older the age range, the lower the mean level of oxygen consumption, perhaps reflecting the reduction in metabolizing lean body mass with age, as demonstrated by Moore et al.[103] The relative effect of DV/m^2

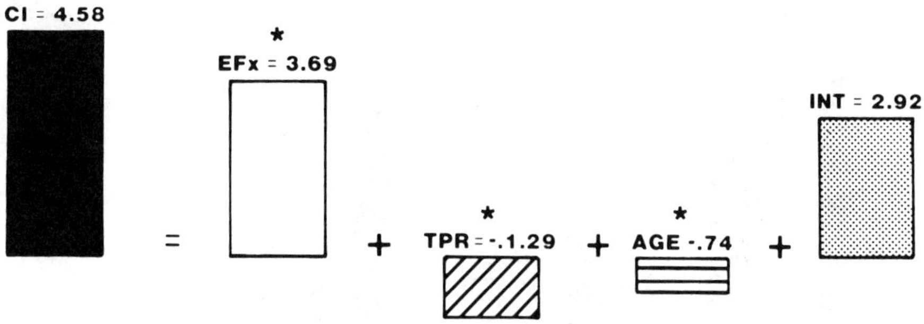

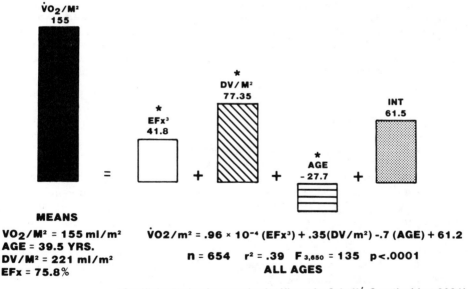

$$CI = .04876 \, (EFx) - 13.68 \bullet 10^{-5} \, (TPR) - .01881 \, (AGE) + 2.92$$

(4.58)   (75.8%)   (944 dyne/sec/cm⁻⁵) (39.9 yrs.)

(l/min/m²)

$$n = 658 \quad r^2 = .596 \quad F_{3,654} = 322 \quad p < .0001$$

*Coefficients simultaneously significant by Scheffé S method (p<.0001)

FIG. 9-28 Block diagram showing relative influence (in units of CI) of ejection fraction (EFx), total peripheral resistance (TPR), and age on cardiac index (CI). As developed from regression equation of 658 studies from posttraumatic patients. Mean values are shown in parentheses. (Tacchino RM, Siegel JH, Emanuele T et al: Incidence and therapy of myocardial depression in critically ill post-trauma patients. Circ Shock 18:360, 1986, abst.)

MEANS

$\dot{V}O_2/M^2 = 155 \, ml/m^2$
AGE = 39.5 YRS.
$DV/M^2 = 221 \, ml/m^2$
EFx = 75.8%

$$\dot{V}O_2/m^2 = .96 \times 10^{-4} \, (EFx^3) + .35(DV/m^2) - .7 \, (AGE) + 61.2$$

$$n = 654 \quad r^2 = .39 \quad F_{3,650} = 135 \quad p < .0001$$
ALL AGES

*Coefficients simultaneously significant by Scheffé S method (p<.0001)

FIG. 9-29 Block diagram showing relative effect (in units of $\dot{V}O_2/m^2$) of ejection fraction (EFx), pulmonary dispersive blood volume (DV/m²) and age on oxygen consumption per square meter BSA ($\dot{V}O_2/m^2$). Derived from regression equation of 654 studies from posttraumatic patients. (Tacchino RM, Siegel JH, Emanuele T et al: Incidence and therapy of myocardial depression in critically ill post-trauma patients. Circ Shock 18:360, 1986, abst.)

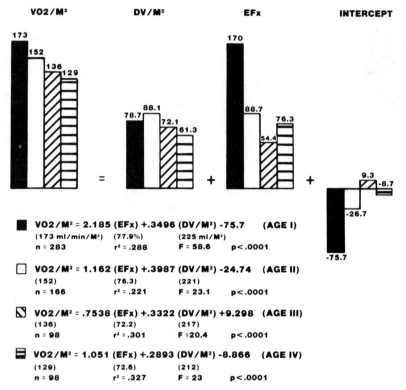

FIG. 9-30 Block diagram showing relative effects of pulmonary blood volume (DV/m²) and ejection fraction (EFx) on oxygen consumption ($\dot{V}O_2/m^2$) at four different age ranges. Age I = 13–30; age II = 31–49; age III = 50–65; age IV > 65 years. Mean values shown in parentheses. Note general decrease in mean level of oxygen consumption ($\dot{V}O_2/m^2$) with increasing age and relatively greater importance of the effect of ejection fraction in the youngest age range group. (Tacchino RM, Siegel JH, Emanuele T et al: Incidence and therapy of myocardial depression in critically ill post-trauma patients. Circ Shock 18:360, 1986, abst.)

and EFx for each age group is also shown. In this graphic display of the multivariable regression of EFx, DV/m², and age on $\dot{V}C_2/m^2$, the influence of each factor is demonstrated by multiplying its mean value times the coefficient of the regression for that variable; that is, in age I, the regression coefficient for the EFx (2.185) is multiplied by the mean EFx percentage (77.9 percent), which gives a relative value in oxygen consumption units of 170 for the EFx. This figure demonstrates that in the young trauma patient, the cardiac factor (EFx) is a major determinant of oxygen consumption. Thus, the ability of the normally responding young patient to overcome other factors that might tend to reduce CO, such as a relative reduction in blood volume, is mediated by a significant response in contractile dynamics.

This occurs even in the face of an increased afterload produced by an increased vascular tone, which raises TPR at a given cardiac index.

However, when myocardial depression supervenes, the ability to maintain an adequate cardiac output is markedly reduced in the post-trauma patient, who ordinarily maintains a higher than normal CO.[179] This is also a function of the age-related cardiac reserve, shown in Figure 9-31, demonstrating the relationship of CO to LVEDV in a series of Starling–Sarnoff ventricular function (VF) curves.[116] These VF curves have been constructed using the regression equation shown in Figure 9-31. This equation contains one term that reflects the effect of the Frank–Starling relationship (ln LVEDV) and a second term (EFx) that delineates the

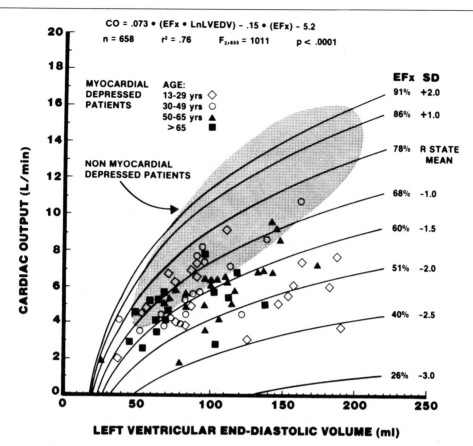

$$CO = .073 \cdot (EFx \cdot LnLVEDV) - .15 \cdot (EFx) - 5.2$$

$n = 658 \qquad r^2 = .76 \qquad F_{2,655} = 1011 \qquad p < .0001$

FIG. 9-31 Ventricular function relationships in posttraumatic patients. Cardiac output (CO) is a function of left ventricular end-diastolic volume with lines of constant ejection fraction (EFx) shown as percentages, as well as standard deviations (SD), from the mean of nonstressed R state general surgical patients. Area of nonmyocardial depressed, posttraumatic patients shown by shading. Symbols show patients with myocardial depression identified by various age ranges. There are slight differences between the actual symbol values and the mean ejection fraction line developed from the regression equation above, since one is the exact patient value and the other is based on the mean regression line for the group. Patients with myocardial depression operate on a lower ejection fraction curve and require a higher left ventricular end-diastolic volume to achieve the same level of cardiac output. (Tacchino RM, Siegel JH, Emanuele T et al: Incidence and therapy of myocardial depression in critically ill post-trauma patients. Circ Shock 18:360, 1986, abst.)

additional influence of the inotropic effect. Together these factors explain 76 percent of the variability of the CO.

Regardless of age, trauma patients who do not have myocardial depression tend to maintain a higher than normal CO for any given LVEDV (see Fig. 9-31). Using the cradiogreen dye dilution method, the mean value for the ejection fraction for the reference control (R) group of nonstressed preoperative general surgical patients studied previously was 78 percent.[143,147] Compared with this control value for EFx, patients who do not have myocardial depression following injury have a ventricular function curve that is generally shifted to the left, with a higher CO per unit LVEDV. In patients with myocardial depression, who have ejection fractions more than 1 SD below that of the R group mean (EFx ≤68 percent), the Starling–Sarnoff curves are shifted to the right with a lower CO per unit LVEDV.[179]

With regard to the effects of age as a contributing factor in myocardial depression, it is of interest to note that older trauma patients with reduced EFx generally are forced to operate at the lower end-diastolic volume range because of their higher propensity for overt cardiac failure and/or pulmonary edema, as LVEDV and left atrial pressures rise acutely with rapid volume infusion. By contrast, younger patients with comparable or more severe reductions in EFx are frequently able to maintain a near-normal CO, because the patient is able to tolerate operation at a higher LVEDV. This in part may reflect the fact that the patient with age- or disease-related chronic myocardial fibrosis may already have a less compliant ventricle, so that a smaller rise in LVEDV produces a greater increase in ventricular end-diastolic pressure than normal. This in turn raises the pulmonary venous and right atrial pressures, potentiating any tendency for pulmonary capillary transudation or venous stasis induced by contusion, shock, or sepsis. In other words, the young patient is able to operate at a higher point on a given Starling–Sarnoff curve and thereby compensates for poor contractile function due to a negative inotropic effect by being able to handle a greater ventricular fiber length preload. This in turn permits the young patient to compensate for the increased afterload produced by the product of a larger cardiac stroke volume times the increased peripheral resistance.

Another factor influencing afterload in patients with myocardial depression is also related to age; it appears to be the tendency for younger patients to maintain a somewhat higher vascular tone relationship in response to posttraumatic stress. The CI is shown as a function of the TPR for 165 posttrauma patients in Figure 9-32.[179] The region of distribution of patients without myocardial depression is shown by the shaded area. The regression equation for posttrauma patients with myocardial depression demonstrates that the cardiac index:TPR relationship is shifted to a significantly lower vascular tone in the older patient, perhaps reflecting a general loss of vascular reactivity to sympathetically mediated vasoconstrictor stimuli. Younger posttrauma patients, however, tend to be shifted to a higher resistance level per unit flow, although older patients with hypertension are also categorized in this functional region. This sympathetically induced increase in vascular tone and relative afterload, if excessive, can be of great clinical importance in reducing flow by shifting the patient to a lower cardiac ejection velocity and ejection fraction point on the myocardial force–velocity relationship. The poorer the contractility state (i.e., the lower the Vmax and the more reduced the velocity of shortening–afterload relationship), the more prominent the effect of increased TPR in reducing EFx and cardiac stroke volume and thus lowering the CI.[70,160,171] This will be discussed in considerable detail with regard to the management of specific cases in the Therapeutic Decision Making section of this chapter.

Physiologic State Classification in Heterogeneous Shock and Critical Illness Processes

The physiologic data, presented earlier from patients in various types of shock and critical illness conditions, suggest that no single variable is likely to provide an adequate description of the entire process. No one variable will enable the physician to discriminate completely among the different types of shock or to determine the degree of severity of critical illness manifested by a specific patient. To use an analogy, to attempt to delineate qualitatively and quantitatively the nature of a specific shock state from one or two measurements, such as blood pressure or heart rate, is like asking each one of the blind men of Aesop's fable to describe the elephant by using only his tactile observation of a single part of the beast. In order to define an unseen process solely on the basis of its visible parameters, one must use some technique of pattern recognition applied to multiple aspects of many individual specimens of the same class. However, when as in shock states, there are not only different kinds of shock, but a given patient may pass through several stages of a given type of shock, a comprehensive technique of multidimensional statistical analysis must be used to define the patient's physiologic state at a moment in time.[46,147] Only in this way can we study the changing pattern of physiologic compensation in response to various types of stress and the nature of recovery or decompensation in each group of patients.

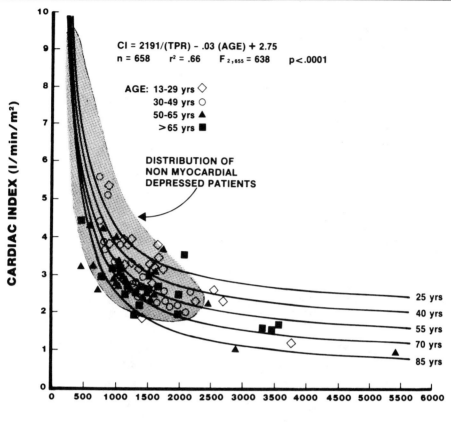

FIG. 9-32 Effect of age on peripheral resistance in 165 trauma patients. Note tendency for increased vascular tone over the entire range of flow resistance relations for younger age patients. Also, note CI and TPR distribution of nonmyocardial depressed patients, and myocardial depressed patients. (Tacchino RM, Siegel JH, Emanuele T et al: Incidence and therapy of myocardial depression in critically ill post-trauma patients. Circ Shock 18:360, 1986, abst.)

The basic statistical methodology behind this technique of multivariable physiologic analysis was developed by defining a physiologic frame of reference for the delineation of a control reference state of resting normal compensation (R state) for surgical high-risk but nonstressed patients, as well as a metric by which one may measure the magnitude and direction of a specific new patient's change in status from the reference control state (R state).[46,145,147] In defining the control population from whom to develop a concept of physiologic stability,[46] we purposely chose a group of older preoperative general surgical patients with a wide range of intercurrent diseases, but who did not have any major physiologic abnormality that would produce acute cardiovascular or cardiorespiratory decompensation. We specifically excluded from the control group patients whose acute physiologic or clinical state involved sepsis, shock, acute myocardial infarction, heart failure, cirrhotic liver disease or acute hepatic decompensation, acute pulmonary dysfunction, or trauma.[46]

After some preliminary screening, we selected a simultaneously obtained multivariable set of 11 physiologic variables (Fig. 9-33) that reflected different aspects of cardiovascular and cardiopulmonary compensation. These were the cardiac index (CI), heart rate (HR),

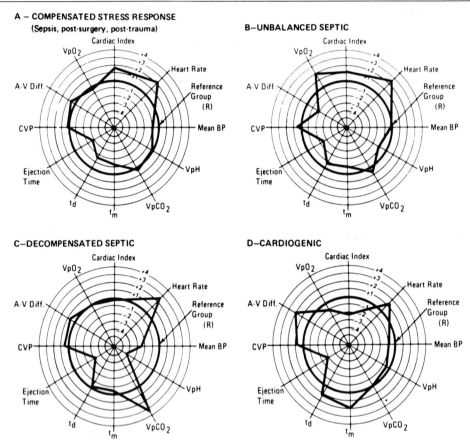

FIG. 9-33 Circle diagrams representing prototypic patterns of physiologic adaptation in various pathophysiologic states. Individual parameter values of cardiac index, heart rate, mean BP, mixed venous pH (VpH), mixed venous PCO_2 (VpCO$_2$), mixing time (tm), dispersive time (td), systolic ejection time (ET), right atrial pressure (CVP), arterio-venous oxygen difference (AV-Diff) and mixed venous O_2 tension (VpO$_2$) are normalized by the mean and the standard deviation of these values in the reference group (R state) of nonstressed general surgical patients. Individual prototypes of A-, B-, C-, and D-state patients are derived from clustering the multivariable data sets of all patients in shock in the frame of reference of the R-state group. (Siegel JH, Farrell EJ, Goldwynn RM, Friedman HP: The surgical implications of physiologic patterns in myocardial infarction shock. Surgery 72: 126, 1972.)

mean blood pressure (MBP), arteriovenous oxygen difference (Ca-$\bar{v}O_2$), systolic ejection time (ET), right atrial mean pressure (CVP), mixed venous pH ($\bar{V}$pH), mixed venous PO_2 ($\bar{V}PO_2$), and two parameters derived from the analysis of the shape characteristics of the central indicator dilution curve—the cardiac mixing time (t_m), and the dispersive time (t_d).[142,144,147] The cardiac mixing time (t_m) is directly related to the durational aspects of left ventricular contractility, and the dispersive time (t_d) under ordinary circumstances reflects the mean transit time through the pulmonary vascular bed.[142]

We used this physiologic set for the control population to establish a frame of reference. The metric by which to evaluate change from control in various forms of acute illness was created by the technique of normalizing all the individual multivariable data sets from all types of patients by the mean and standard deviation of that variable in the control reference state (R) group. This statistical device enables us to scale all variables, such as MBP, $\bar{V}$pH, and CI in standard deviations from control, rather than in individual units such as millimeters of mercury, negative logs of the hydrogen ion concentration, or liters per minute per square meter body surface area. We then subjected all the individual normalized multivariable data sets to a cluster analysis procedure previously described,[46,147] in which data-inferred groupings of patient data sets were selected by a criterion that partitions the physiologic space of the 11 variables into relatively homogenous regions. The patient samples grouped within a region were most like the 11-dimensional mean of that region and most different from the multivariate means of the other groups.

Previous studies of this classification technique showed that compared with the reference control group (R state) the entire spectrum of clinical severity in patients with trauma, sepsis, or cardiogenic shock could be viewed in terms of four pathophysiologic states (A, B, C, and D).[144,147] We can describe the prototypical patient of each of these abnormal states by the physiologic pattern of the multivariable means (see Fig. 9-33). Each pattern (dark line) is compared with the perfect circle (heavy circle) of the normalized control mean. One can evaluate the specific individual variable abnormalities manifested by the prototypical patient of each state by their difference from the R state mean in standard deviations, increased or decreased (light circles). Table 9-3 shows the actual mean values for each variable, and the standard deviations from the R state prototype are shown for each state.

Observing these prototypical patterns (Fig. 9-33), we can see that the A state patient represents a compensated stress response characteristic of an adequate reaction to sepsis, surgery, or trauma. In the A state pattern, there is a statistically significant increase in CI and HR and a decrease in ejection time. There is an increase in myocardial contractility reflected by the decrease in cardiac mixing time (t_m), which reflects a larger cardiac ejection fraction (EFx).[142] Also, a more rapid pulmonary dispersive transit time (t_d) occurs that, taken together with the increased CI, usually results in no change or an increase in the pulmonary reservoir filling volume (DV/m²). However, there are no changes in any of the parameters of oxygen extraction (Ca-$\bar{v}O_2$, P$\bar{v}O_2$) or peripheral metabolism (P$\bar{v}CO_2$ or pH$\bar{v}$). In summary, the A state represents a sympathetically mediated normal stress response in which the Ca-

$\bar{v}O_2$ remains normal while flow increases; as a result, net oxygen consumption rises to adequately meet all body demands.[46,144,147] It is of critical importance to emphasize that the A state is the normal response to stress; therefore, an injured, postsurgical, or septic patient who fails to demonstrate an A state response is manifesting an abnormal stress adaptation that usually requires urgent therapy if further pathophysiologic deterioration is to be prevented.

The B and C states (Fig. 9-33) are physiologic patterns of increasing severity characteristic of deteriorating stages in the septic process.[46,144,150] In the B state, which is also seen in nonseptic patients with hepatocellular decompensation,[151,153] a hyperdynamic cardiovascular pattern fails to supply peripheral needs adequately and, in spite of an increased CI, which characteristically occurs due to a marked reduction in TPR and vascular tone, the Ca-$\bar{v}O_2$ (A-V Diff) narrows, oxygen consumption fails to rise and indeed often falls, and a metabolic acidosis with a decrease in venous pH ensues. The C state (Fig. 9-33) occurs when a respiratory decompensation is superimposed on the septic processes of the A or B states (see Chapter 15).[144] There is a profound septic shock with a fall in MBP, in spite of a normal or increased level of CI with a further fall in the vascular tone. A combined metabolic and respiratory acidosis occurs that is matched by the corresponding impairment in oxygen exchange.[143,144,147,155]

By contrast, in the cardiogenic or D state patient (Fig. 9-33), a primary myocardial rather than a primary peripheral failure pattern occurs.[147] There is a fall in cardiac contractility and ejection fraction, (EFx) reflected by the lengthening of the cardiac mixing time. (t_m) The pulmonary dispersive mean transit time (t_d) also increases, as the CI decreases. Frequently due to left heart failure, the rise in pulmonary mean transit is disproportionately greater than the fall in CI, and the pulmonary reservoir blood volume (DV/m²) rises above control levels, reflecting pulmonary congestion. A marked widening of the Ca-$\bar{v}O_2$ occurs, which is generally proportionate to the fall in cardiac flow, reflecting the severity of the decrease in perfusion. Hypotension and acidosis may occur as well but are not characteristic statistical features of this pattern of physiologic abnormality.

TABLE 9-3. Cardiovascular Patterns in Shock

	No. of Studies	CI[a] (L/min/m²)	MBP[a] (mmHg)	Ca-v̄O₂ (AV Diff[a]) (vol %)	HR[a] (beats/min)	ET[a] (sec)	CVP[a] (mmHg)	pHv̄ (pH units)	PvO₂ (mmHg)	PvCO₂ (mmHg)	t_m[a] (sec)	t_d[a] (sec)
±1 SD from R		0.127[b]	0.0986[b]	0.159[b]	0.0730[b]	0.0565[b]	0.486[b]	0.0762	10.38	9.34	0.179[b]	0.126[b]
R	185	2.54 (0.0)	88 (0.0)	3.7 (0.0)	78 (0.0)	0.30 (0.0)	2.7 (0.0)	7.43 (0.0)	39 (0.0)	39 (0.0)	4.3 (0.0)	4.8 (0.0)
A	252	3.91 (1.48)	73 (−0.80)	4.2 (0.36)	115 (2.33)	0.21 (−2.77)	2.8 (0.05)	7.42 (−0.12)	35 (−0.36)	39 (0.01)	2.6 (−1.23)	3.0 (−1.58)
B	118	3.58 (1.18)	81 (−0.36)	1.7 (−2.03)	114 (2.29)	0.21 (−2.52)	4.9 (0.53)	7.35 (−1.00)	60 (1.98)	44 (0.57)	3.0 (−0.88)	3.6 (−1.01)
C	37	2.45 (−0.11)	51 (−2.36)	4.5 (0.56)	115 (2.32)	0.19 (−3.52)	5.5 (0.63)	7.10 (−4.27)	40 (0.13)	70 (3.31)	3.7 (−0.36)	4.4 (−0.33)
D	103	1.32 (−2.21)	72 (−0.87)	7.3 (1.88)	99 (1.42)	0.20 (−2.89)	6.5 (0.79)	7.39 (−0.52)	26 (−1.25)	40 (0.12)	10.5 (2.15)	7.0 (1.28)
Total	695											

Abbreviations: CI, cardiac index; MBP, mean blood pressure; Ca-v̄O₂ (AV-Diff), arteriovenous oxygen difference; HR, heart rate; ET, ejection time; CVP, central venous pressure; t_m, mixing mean transit time; t_d, dispersive mean transit time.

[a] Mean values represent antilog of the mean of the log values.

[b] Normalizing factor for ± SD applied to log value of corresponding R mean.

[c] Numbers in parentheses below mean values are the number of standard deviations of the normalized variable from the corresponding mean of the R group. A level of ± 1.0 SD is used as the minimum level for consideration as a physiologically important difference between means.

(Siegel JH: Pattern and process in the evolution of and recovery from shock. p. 381. In Siegel JH, Chodoff PD (eds): The Aged and High Risk Surgical Patient. Grune & Stratton, New York, 1976, by permission.)

In the case of pure hypovolemic shock, the CI falls, while the Ca-$\bar{v}O_2$ and the level of peripheral acidosis increase but, in contrast to the cardiogenic D state prototype, the cardiac ejection fraction remains normal or is increased while the pulmonary reservoir volume (DV/m^2) is reduced. The original states were derived from analysis of 695 multivariable patient data sets from 148 patients,[147] but to date we have studied more than 5,000 different patients (>15,000 studies) with a wide range of critical illnesses from seven different institutions without bringing the basic concept or the nature of the prototype states into question. However, our continuing studies suggest that the precision of classification can be increased and prognostic significance can be enhanced by adding selected respiratory and metabolic variables to this original 11 variable state classification set[143,147] (Table 9-4).

Physiologic Trajectory of Recovery

The main value of physiologic state classification is that it permits quantification of change in the patient's condition. A critical determinant of whether the patient survives after trauma is often the ability of the physician to recognize early in the patient's clinical course that a transition has occurred from a normal well-compensated A state stress response to a D state of myocardial depression, or if sepsis develops, that a state of hepatocellular decompensation has occurred, producing a change from a metabolically adequate septic A state to a B state of metabolic insufficiency (Chapter 15).

Using the quantitative measure of physiologic state, one can establish a physiologic grid in which each of the prototype state patterns (R, A, B, C, D) represents a reference point in a physiologic accommodation space.[144,145] Since every patient has some degree of similarity with each of the mean physiologic prototypes described, it is possible to classify each patient by the degree of similarity to the normal reference control R state as well as to the A, B, C, or D states. In addition, since the normalizing factors convert the individual physiologic measurements into the standard deviation of that measurement from the R state control mean, all variables have the same scale. Thus, by determining a value that is the square root of the sum of the squares of the differences between the patient's variables and the variable levels for each of these five states (R, A, B, C, D), a physiologic "distance" can be estab-

TABLE 9-4. Respiratory and Metabolic Patterns in Shock

	No. of Studies	$\frac{\text{A-aDO}_2}{\text{PaO}_2}$	PaCO$_2$ (mmHg)	pHa (pH units)	aHCO$_3$ (mm/L)	$\dot{V}O_2$ (ml/min/m^2)
±1 SD from R[a]		0.87	8.75	0.07	5.67	45.61
R	89	0.93 (0.0)[b]	34 (0.0)	7.46 (0.0)	24 (0.0)	102 (0.0)
A	149	2.3 (1.54)	33 (−0.01)	7.43 (−0.43)	23 (−0.10)	223 (2.66)
B	44	1.5 (0.70)	36 (0.33)	7.39 (−1.00)	22 (−0.21)	73 (−0.64)
C	6	9.2 (9.55)	45 (1.37)	7.17 (−4.14)	20 (−0.59)	141 (0.84)
D	81	2.7 (2.03)	30 (−0.33)	7.46 (0.0)	21 (−0.40)	87 (−0.31)
Total	369					

[a] Normalizing factor for ± SD applied to value of corresponding R mean. (Patients not on TPN support).

[b] Numbers in parentheses below mean values are the number of standard deviations (SD) of the normalized variable from the corresponding mean of the R group. A level of ±1.0 SD is used as a minimum level for consideration as a physiologically important difference between means.

(Modified from Siegel JH: Pattern and process in the evolution of and recovery from shock. p. 381. In Siegel JH, Chodoff PD (eds): The Aged and High Risk Surgical Patient. Grune & Stratton, New York, 1976, by permission.)

lished representing that patient's specific degree of similarity compared to the compensated or decompensated patterns of accommodation demonstrated in the five prototype states.[145] By virtue of this quantitative measure of physiologic state distances and state distance ratios (e.g., D/A, C/B) (Fig. 9-34), one obtains a grid that can be used to locate a given patient's position in this physiologic space from one time period to the next. This technique is similar in principle to one that might be used to define the position of a satellite in interplanatary space; it permits delineation of a physiologic trajectory, facilitating quantification of changing physiologic relationships and comparison of a given patient's time course to known patient courses in different types of disease conditions.[145]

Figure 9-35A shows three sequential circle diagrams of a patient with post traumatic myo-cardial contusion immediately after injury and during stages of resuscitative therapy. Figure 9-35B shows this patient's physiologic trajectory time course. The y axis in Figure 9-35B demonstrates that for each point in the patient's time course the quantitative "distance" similarity of the patient's data pattern to the cardiogenic decompensation of the D state is compared with that patient's similarity to a normal A state stress response. In this way, the D/A ratio axis represents the adequacy of the cardiovascular system. A patient who is very close to the cardiogenic D state decompensation is far away from a normal A state stress response and will have a low D/A ratio. A normal D/A ratio is 1; this patient's initial D/A ratio was 0.30.

On the x axis, for the same time points one can compare the patient's similarity to a state of respiratory decompensation (C state)

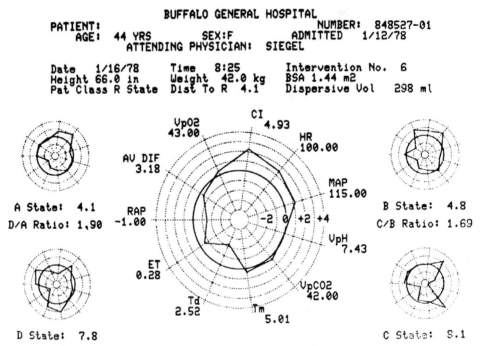

FIG. 9-34 Circle diagram of specific patient demonstrating similarities of his deviation pattern from R (dark circle) to the prototype A-, B-, C-, and D-state patterns. The allover physiologic "distance" from each prototypic pattern is seen in the A-, B-, C-, and D-state distances, presented below each small circle diagram, as well as the ratios between the various distances (D/A and C/B ratios). This permits staging of each patient's physiologic pattern at a given moment in time. (Siegel JH, Giovannini I, Coleman B: Ventilation: perfusion maldistribution secondary to the hyperdynamic cardiovascular state as the major cause of increased shunting in human sepsis. J Trauma 19: 432, 1979.)

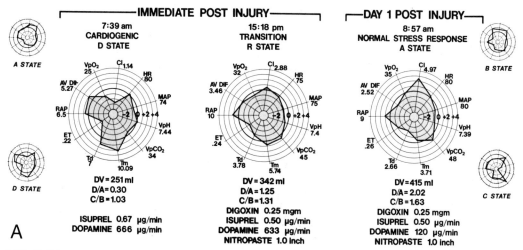

FIG. 9-35 (A) Serial circle diagrams from patient following posttraumatic myocardial contusion with acute cardiogenic failure treated with inotropic support and increase of pulmonary blood volume (DV). Conversion from D-state cardiogenic failure to normal A-state stress response by this therapy. (*Figure continues.*)

with respect to the distance to a state of metabolic insufficiency (B state), that is, the C to B state ratio. A normal C/B ratio is 1.2, this patient had an initial C/B ratio of 1.03. Patients with the severe B state metabolic insufficiency of sepsis, or nonseptic hepatocellular decompensation, will have an increased C/B ratio, whereas there is an decreased C/B ratio in patients with C state respiratory insufficiency. Within this D/A versus C/B framework, there are certain regions that have been delineated by the study of previous patient's trajectories.[145,186]

Uncomplicated preoperative patients prior to coronary artery bypass grafting (CABG) are grouped in the region defined as CABG-P. CABG patients who do well after coronary bypass surgery move immediately postsurgery into the CABG-I-O box, where there is no myocardial depression, but a mild postsurgical respiratory insufficiency. They quickly recover to the CABG-P region. However, CABG patients with severe postbypass cardiogenic decompensation, or patients with primary, or postoperative, myocardial infarction have a fall both in D/A and in C/B ratios; they fall

into the region defined as CABG-II-O, characterized by severe myocardial depression and decompensation as well as a respiratory insufficiency related to pulmonary congestion or pulmonary edema.

Preoperative general surgical elective (GSEL) patients who have no overt myocardial disease fall into the region marked GSEL-P. It can be seen that preoperative GSEL patients have some physiologic overlap with patients who are to be operated on for coronary artery surgery, as most CABG patients do not have ventricular dysfunction at rest despite coronary artery disease. However, in contrast to the CABG patients, during the first 3 days after a surgical insult, the trajectory of GSEL patients without cardiac disease is to move in the direction of an increased D/A ratio (GSEL-1-3), reflecting the normal A state stress response. They also have a mild metabolic insufficiency denoted by a small increase in C/B ratio. Within this physiologic trajectory framework we can now begin to look at the responses of severely traumatized patients.[144,186]

Figure 9-36 shows the trajectories of 16 posttraumatic patients.[186] Thirteen recovered

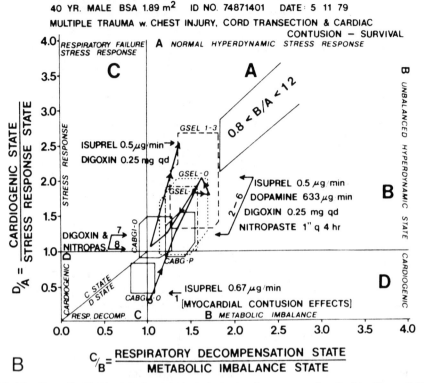

FIG. 9-35 *(Continued)* **(B)** Physiologic state trajectory showing course of patient in Figure 9-35(A). This figure compares patient's movement through recovery space to previously described envelopes of recovery trajectories. It shows the effect of various levels of inotropic support in moving patient from cardiogenic decompensation state (CABG II–0) to normal general surgical recovery envelope (GSEL 1–3). (Figs. A and B from Trunkey DD, Siegel JH, Baker SP, Gennarelli TA: Panel: Current status of trauma indices. J Trauma 23: 185, 1983.)

sufficiently after their episode of major multiple trauma to leave the ICU within the first 4 days, and three died within the first 3 days. The 13 rapidly recovering survivors all had a stress response trajectory, which moved them in the GSEL 1–3 region. They had a normal A state stress response ($\uparrow$D/A) and a very mild degree of metabolic insufficiency ($\uparrow$C/B). Thus, the GSEL envelope of normal postsurgical recoveries also defines a trajectory of injury recovery from multiple trauma.

On the other hand, the three critically ill multiple-trauma patients who succumbed within the first 3 days had their trajectories primarily located in the CABG-II-O region. All showed evidence of severe and refractory myo-

cardial injury or depression. Recognition of this fact is important—while there are many reasons why patients with serious trauma die, it indicates that patients with serious multiple trauma who have a component of myocardial depression are very likely to succumb unless treated aggressively and early. Thus the physiologic trajectory response also provides us with an index of disease severity, since the recoveries of these two groups form almost totally separate clusters of trajectories.

The prime value of the physiologic pattern and physiologic trajectory is to permit delineation of the relative importance of the various pathophysiologic factors in producing a state of critical imbalance or shock in an injured

CARE — PHYSIOLOGIC STATE TRAJECTORY PLOT

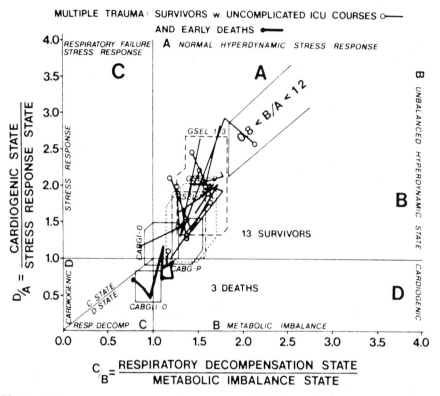

FIG. 9-36 Physiologic recovery trajectories of 16 posttraumatic patients; comparison of 13 patients with uncomplicated ICU courses, with 3 early deaths manifesting myocardial depression. (Trunkey DD, Siegel JH, Baker SP, Gennarelli TA: Panel: Current status of trauma indices. J Trauma 23: 185, 1983.)

patient. Figure 9-35A shows a series of physiologic patterns from a 40-year-old man who had been in a severe automobile accident. He had a severe chest injury with contusion and was also quadriplegic because of a cervical spine injury; he had no other injuries. Since spinal shock was considered the major factor in this patient's circulatory instability, on observing his physiologic pattern it was surprising to find that it demonstrated the D (or cardiogenic) state. Even though persistent hypotension was not present, state classification demonstrated that the magnitude of his myocardial injury was serious enough to produce a physiologic decompensation at least as severe as that seen in previously studied patients after a major myocardial infarction, following cardiac sur-

gery, or with septic or toxic myocardial depression.

By following the serial response patterns in Figure 9-35A it can be seen that in order to assist this patient to achieve a normal A state compensation, a combination of several cardiac inotropic agents and peripheral vasodilatation were required to enable him to achieve a satisfactory CO, since his intrinsic postmyocardial contusion cardiac function was insufficient to allow it to overcome the afterload, even with spinal cord transection. This therapy also helped the patient to accept a transfusion-mediated increase in pulmonary blood volume (DV) from an inadequate level of 251 ml (133 ml/m²), gradually to 342 ml (180 ml/m²), and finally to 415 ml (220 ml/m²). As a result of this therapy with vasodilatation, volume, and inotropic support, the patient returned to a classic A state and thus was able to achieve the desired normal stress response.

Figure 9-35B shows this patient's computer-generated trajectory plot, which provides an indication of how his recovery trajectory was similar or dissimilar to the recovery plots of other types of patients. His initial myocardial depression (point 1) is seen to be as severe (CABG-II-O) as that seen in primary cardiogenic failure patients or in fatal trauma cases with acute myocardial depression (Fig. 9-36). However, with volume, inotropic support consisting of isoproterenol (Isuprel), dopamine, and digoxin, and vasodilatation (nitroglycerine paste), he was moved to normal posttraumatic hyperdynamic response trajectory (points 2–6).

In this case, dependence on continued inotropic support was seen. When inotropic support with Isuprel was transiently stopped (points 7 and 8), there was a significant fall in the D/A ratio; the isoproterenol was begun again (final point) in a very low dose (0.5 μg/min) to achieve the desired stress response and return him to a normal stress-response trajectory region (GSEL 1–3).

Another type of problem that this type of physiologic index allows us to define is shown in Figure 9-37. A 52-year-old man who had a severe bowel injury developed myocardial depression secondary to a septic abscess complication of his intra-abdominal injury. He initially showed a good stress response (point 1). After bowel resection (point 2), his sepsis became severe, and a myocardial depression oc-

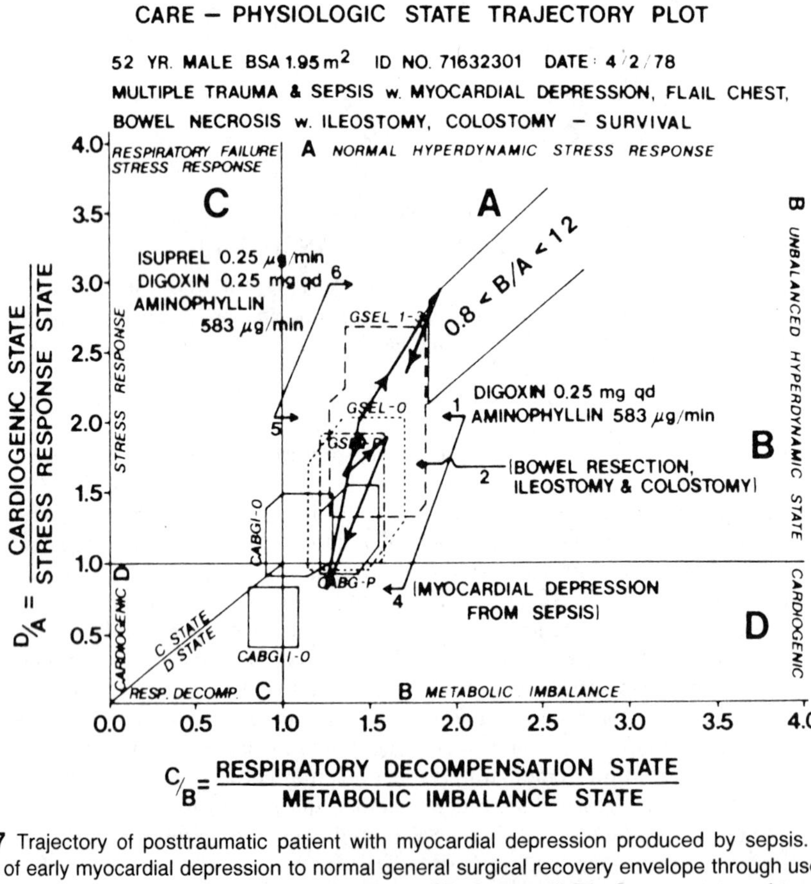

FIG. 9-37 Trajectory of posttraumatic patient with myocardial depression produced by sepsis. Conversion from state of early myocardial depression to normal general surgical recovery envelope through use of multiple inotropic agent support. (Trunkey DD, Siegel JH, Baker SP, Gennarelli TA: Current status of trauma indices. J Trauma 23: 185, 1983.)

curred (although not as severe as that following the direct myocardial contusion injury shown in Fig. 9-35). This appeared late in the clinical course (point 4) related secondary to the septic process (see Chapter 15). However, as also shown in this trajectory plot, there was a salutory physiologic response to the use of isoproterenol, digoxin, and aminophylline in returning the recovery trajectory to a normal stress response (points 5 and 6).

THERAPEUTIC PRINCIPLES IN THE MANAGEMENT OF HYPOVOLEMIC AND LOW-FLOW SHOCK STATES

Any therapeutic approach to low-flow shock must take into account the management of the abnormal cardiovascular interactions underlying the clinical presentations. Such therapy must specifically address the previously described principles of the myocardial force–velocity relationship as they effect the evolution of, and recovery from, the specific kind of low-flow shock state.

Increasing Preload

Perhaps the most important aspect of any therapeutic program designed to increase CO in the low-flow shock patient is the assurance of an adequate level of venous return so that the cardiac diastolic filling volume is maintained and the heart muscle achieves a normal or somewhat increased fiber length (preload) from which to generate tension and stroke volume. The maintenance of an adequate preload is particularly critical in the patient whose shock process is secondary to a period of hypovolemia due to extracorporeal volume loss, or to third-space sequestration of intravascular volume into a poorly exchanging region of interstitial space due to sepsis trauma or inflamma-

tion. Before failure of the contractile mechanism can be evaluated, it is necessary to attempt to achieve intravascular volume compensation by a trial of volume loading. Failure to increase CO by volume infusion without excessively increasing the pulmonary reservoir filling volume (DV) and the LVEDV establishes the presence of a depressed Starling–Sarnoff ventricular function relationship and suggests an underlying dysfunction of myocardial contractility. A rise in PWP, or RAP with a low DV and LVEDV strongly suggests that a decrease in ventricular compliance is also a factor in the poor ventricular function relation. Unfortunately, in patients with associated adult respiratory distress syndrome (ARDS) or extensive pneumonitis who require increased positive end-expiratory pressure (PEEP) and mean airway pressures for effective ventilation, PWP and thus RAP may be falsely elevated by the transmitted intra-alveolar pressures, thus making these two variables unreliable to assess either ventricular filling volumes or compliance relationships.[15,113]

Several important points need emphasizing with respect to estimating the nature and magnitude of the volume replacement required (see also the extensive discussion of volume replacement in shock presented in Chapters 7 and 8). The first of these is that the mechanism of the hypovolemia has profound implications as to the volume and type of fluid replacement, which may in turn mandate the need for inotropic support or afterload reduction to permit volume resuscitation to be made. This concept is shown in Figure 9-38, which presents a computer-generated estimate of the acute shifts in body compartment volumes in a 60-year-old 80-kg man who had a previous history of chronic cardiac disease. Using Moore's[103] estimates of body compartment volumes (Table 9-5) modified by factors for chronic disease (Fig. 9-38B),[148] two different scenarios are generated for comparison, assuming nearly complete plasma volume refill (Tables 9-6 and 9-7). In the one instance (Fig. 9-38A), an estimate was developed for the patient, assuming partial compensation for an acute gastrointestinal hemorrhage of 12 hours duration after initial volume replacement of packed RBCs, whole blood, and crystalloid (using the formula shown in Table 9-6). In spite of this therapy

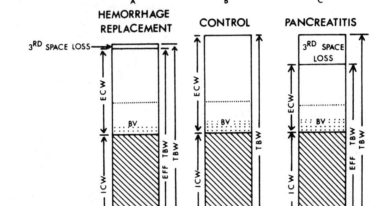

60 YEAR OLD MALE
BODY WEIGHT 80 KG
CHRONIC CARDIAC DISEASE

    A) ACUTE PROBLEM – GI BLEEDING FROM DUODENAL ULCER FOR 12 HRS
      ADMISSION HCT = 28 REPLACEMENT PACKED CELLS 500 ML
                                    WHOLE BLOOD 500 ML
                                    CRYSTALOID 500 ML

    B) EXPECTED COMPARTMENT VALUES FOR THIS CHRONICALLY ILL PATIENT
      ADMISSION HCT = 38

    C) ACUTE PROBLEM – ACUTE PANCREATITIS 12 HRS. AFTER ONSET
      ADMISSION HCT = 48   NO REPLACEMENT THERAPY

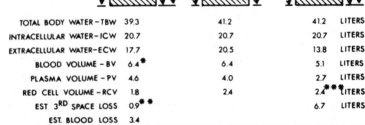

	A	B	C	
TOTAL BODY WATER – TBW	39.3	41.2	41.2	LITERS
INTRACELLULAR WATER – ICW	20.7	20.7	20.7	LITERS
EXTRACELLULAR WATER – ECW	17.7	20.5	13.8	LITERS
BLOOD VOLUME – BV	6.4*	6.4	5.1	LITERS
PLASMA VOLUME – PV	4.6	4.0	2.7	LITERS
RED CELL VOLUME – RCV	1.8	2.4	2.4***	LITERS
EST 3ᴿᴰ SPACE LOSS	0.9**		6.7	LITERS
EST. BLOOD LOSS	3.4			

        * ASSUMED TO BE CONSTANT THROUGH REPLACEMENT FLUIDS AND PLASMA REFILL
        ** AS SUGGESTED BY SHIRES (PARTIALLY INTRACELLULAR)
        *** ASSUMED TO BE CONSTANT (IE. NO DESTRUCTION OF RED CELL MASS)

FIG. 9-38 Computer model of body compartment shifts in response to hemorrhage compared to shifts produced by a third-space loss due to an inflammatory disease such as pancreatitis. Control is a 60-year-old male with chronic cardiac disease. (Siegel JH, Fickthorn J: Computer-based CARE of the aged or high-risk patient. Automated assistance in fluid management, metabolic balance, and cardiopulmonary regulation. p. 547. In Siegel JH, Chodhoff PD (eds): The Aged and High Risk Surgical Patient, Grune & Stratton, Inc., 1976 by permission.)

(Fig. 9-38A), the hematocrit (HCT) had fallen from the expected 38 to 28 percent. As shown in the bar diagram, the computation of blood loss is estimated at 3.4 L with a known replacement of only 1,500 ml RBCs and crystalloid. The remaining compensation for the intravascular deficit has been supplied by the shift of extracellular volume into the intravascular space. The implication of these data is that a cautious additional volume of at least 1,900 ml packed cells and colloid (or nearly four times that amount if crystalloid only were to be given according to Shires' estimates[129]) would have to be replaced if total body compartment compensation is to be achieved. Depending on the present level of CO and $\dot{V}O_2$ as an indication of the acute need, on the adequacy of the myocardial contractile mechanism, and on the magnitude of the afterload, a decision can be made concerning which option (colloid vs. crystal-

TABLE 9-5.   Equations Summarizing Body Composition in Humans

Body Compartment	Formula	Reference
Body surface area	$BSA = 0.007184\ BWT^{0.435}\ HT^{0.725}$	[a]
Total body water		
Male	$TBW = (0.795 - 0.0024\ BWT - 0.0015\ AGE)\ BWT$	Moore, Olesen, McMurrey, et al.[103]
Female	$TBW = (0.698 - 0.0026\ BWT - 0.0012\ AGE)\ BWT$	Moore, Olesen, McMurrey, et al.[103]
Intracellular water		
Male	$ICW = (0.623 - 0.0016\ AGE)\ TBW$	Moore, Olesen, McMurrey, et al.[103]
Female	$ICW = (0.553 - 0.0007\ AGE)\ TBW$	Moore, Olesen, McMurrey, et al.[103]
Blood volume	$BV = 0.647 + 0.112\ TBW$	Moore, Olesen, McMurrey, et al.[103]

BWT, body weight, in kg; HT, height, in cm; TBW, ICW, and BV in liters.

[a] Data from Dubois D, Dubois EF: A height–weight formula to estimate the surface area of man. Proc Soc Exp Biol, 13:77, 1916.

[b] Data from Moore FW, Olesen KH, McMurrey JD, et al: The Body Cell Mass and Its Supporting Environment. WB Saunders, Philadelphia, 1963.

TABLE 9-6.   Blood Loss Determination

Major trauma, GI bleeding, postop, blood loss GT 500 ml.

$$\text{Average HCT during hermorrhage} = \left[\left(13 - \frac{\text{Duration}}{\text{of Hemorrhage}}\right) \times \frac{\text{expected}}{\text{HCT}} + \frac{\text{present}}{\text{HCT}}\right] / \left[\left(13 - \frac{\text{Duration}}{\text{of hemorrhage}}\right) + 1\right]$$

Duration of Hemorrhage $\leq$ 12 hours

$$\text{Blood loss} = \left[\begin{array}{c}\text{Expected} \\ \text{red cell mass}\end{array} + \begin{array}{c}\text{Red cell mass} \\ \text{administered}\end{array} - \begin{array}{c}\text{Present} \\ \text{red cell mass}\end{array}\right] \Big/ \begin{array}{c}\text{Average HCT} \\ \text{during hemorrhage}\end{array}$$

$$BL_{loss} = [(BV_{exp} \cdot HCT_{exp}) + 0.32\ BL_{given} + 0.67\ PC_{given} - (BV_{pres} \cdot HCT_{pres})]/HCT_{av}$$

TABLE 9-7.   Extracellular Water Deficit

Nonhemorrhagic Conditions

$$\begin{array}{c}\text{Present} \\ \text{blood vol.}\end{array} = \left[\begin{array}{c}\text{Expected} \\ \text{red cell mass}\end{array} + \begin{array}{c}\text{Red cell mass} \\ \text{administered}\end{array} - \begin{array}{c}\text{Red cell mass} \\ \text{loss}\end{array}\right] \Big/ \text{Present HCT}$$

(1) $BV_{pres} = [(BV_{exp} \cdot HCT_{exp}) + 0.32\ BL_{given} + 0.67\ PC_{given} - (BL_{loss} \cdot HCT_{exp})]/HCT_{pres}$

$$\begin{array}{c}\text{Present} \\ \text{plasma vol.}\end{array} = \left[\begin{array}{c}\text{present} \\ \text{plasmacrit}\end{array} \times \begin{array}{c}\text{present} \\ \text{blood vol.}\end{array}\right]$$

(2) $PV_{pres} = (1.0 - HCT_{pres})\ BV_{pres}$

$$\begin{array}{c}\text{Present} \\ \text{ECW}\end{array} = \left[\begin{array}{c}\text{present} \\ \text{plasma vol.}\end{array} \times \begin{array}{c}\text{expected} \\ \text{ECW}\end{array}\right] \Big/ \begin{array}{c}\text{expected} \\ \text{plasma volume}\end{array}$$

(3) $ECW\ deficit = ECW_{exp} - ECW_{pres}$

(Siegel JH, Fichthorn J: Computer-based CARE of the aged or high-risk patient: Automated assistance in fluid management, metabolic balance, and cardiopulmonary regulations. p. 547. In Siegel JH, Chodoff PD (eds): The Aged and High Risk Surgical Patient. Grune & Stratton, New York, 1976, by permission.)

loid) might be the safest choice for preload replacement. In this regard, it is important to consider that maintenance of a sufficiently high Hb concentration in the perfusing blood reduces the need for an increased CO to supply a given level of $\dot{V}O_2$ requirement (Table 9-8); this may be a critical factor in meeting the peripheral O_2 deficit needs in a patient with limited myocardial contractile capability.[90,93]

In the second example shown in Figure 9-38C, the volume deficit effects of an acute inflammatory "third space" loss of extracellu-

TABLE 9-8. Effect of Hemoglobin Reduction on Circulatory Oxygen Delivery

At a hemoglobin of 10 g %
  Arterial: 10 g Hb $\times$ 90% sat $\times$ 1.39* = 12.5 vol% O_2
  Venous: 10 g Hb $\times$ 40% sat $\times$ 1.39 = 5.6 vol% O_2
                    Ca-$\bar{v}O_2$ Diff = 6.9 vol% O_2

For a cardiac output of 4.00 L/min:
  6.9 vol% O_2 $\times$ 4.00 L/min = 276 ml/O_2/min

At a hemoglobin of 7 g%
  Arterial: 7 g Hb $\times$ 90% sat $\times$ 1.39 = 8.8 vol% O_2
  Venous: 7 g Hb $\times$ 40% sat $\times$ 1.39 = 3.9 vol% O_2
                    Ca-$\bar{v}O_2$ diff = 4.9 vol% O_2

For a cardiac output of 4.00 L/min:
  4.9 vol% O_2 $\times$ 4.00 L/min = 196 ml O_2/min

To achieve the same oxygen consumption as with 10g Hb, cardiac output must increase:
  4.9 vol% O_2 $\times$ 5.63 L/min = 276 ml O_2/min

* 1.39 = volumes percent O_2 carried per gram hemoglobin (Hb) at 100 percent saturation. Dissolved PO_2 omitted.
  (Siegel JH: Pattern and process in the evolution of and recovery from Shock. p. 381. In Siegel JH, Chodoff PD (eds): The Aged and High Risk Surgical Patient. Grune & Stratton, New York, 1976, by permission.)

lar fluid, in this case resulting from acute pancreatitis, has been estimated for patient of the same age, body weight and with the same background of intercurrent chronic cardiac disease. In this case (estimated by formulae in Table 9-7), the extracellular fluid (ECF) shift of 6.7 L into the poorly exhanging third space has produced a rise in HCT from 38 to 48 percent by a parallel reduction in plasma volume to 2.7 L without reduction in red cell mass (2.4 L). While the implications for therapy in this type of patient (or one with a simple bowel obstruction, chemical or inflammatory peritonitis, etc.) are considerably different from that in the patient with blood loss hypovolemia, in terms of both the magnitude and type of fluid needed for replacement (lactate or bicarbonate Ringer's solution with variable amounts of potassium added in the pancreatitis case vs. packed RBCs, and colloid or balanced salt solution in the posthemorrhage case), the requirement that the cardiac function be able to accept such a large volume remains the same. Therefore, the operation of the myocardium and the peripheral vascular tone mechanisms interacting together within a family or force–velocity relationships becomes the critical determinant of survival during the volume replacement phase of therapy.[143,179]

Contractility Increasing Agents

The choice of cardiac inotropic and vasodilator agents in low-flow shock syndromes is determined by the relative degree of contractility (Vmax) increase versus the magnitude of afterload reduction required by the individual patient to raise CO and peripheral perfusion sufficiently to increase the $\dot{V}O_2$ to its optimum stable level. This is the flow and oxygen delivery rate at which no oxygen deficit accumulates and at which the body's utilization of oxidizable metabolic acids (e.g., lactate, free fatty acids, amino acids) can proceed at a level of substrate fuel clearance at which no metabolic base deficit, or mixed venous acidosis persists.

Patients with low-flow shock states due to hypovolemia also require restitution of volume loss to a level that can permit adequate cardiac filling (preload). Consequently, with myocardial depression or acute myocardial failure where Vmax is reduced by vasoconstriction has increased afterload, the combined use of both inotropic and vasodilator agents may be necessary to allow the patient to shift from a high afterload point on a decreased force–velocity curve to a reduced afterload point on a more normal or increased ($\uparrow$Vmax) force–velocity relationship (Fig. 9-21).

Several options (Table 9-2) exist with regard to the choice of cardiac inotropic agents that can increase Vmax. The β-adrenergic sympathomimetic amines act by increasing the rate of adenyl cyclase activity, which synthesizes 3',5'-cyclic adenosine monophosphate (cAMP) in the myocardial cell.[40] This in turn increases the rate of Ca^{++} transport after membrane depolarization from the specialized sarcolemmal organelles into the cytosolic locations, where actin and myosin fiber contraction occurs.[125] The force of the myofibrillar contraction is increased by the availability of Ca^{++}, so that Vmax increases.[8,77,125,167] Since the rate of conduction along the specialized Purkinje fiber system, as well as the activation rate of the pacemaker cells, is also increased by sympathomimetic amines, these agents generally tend to increase both chronotropic as well as inotropic activity. However, some agents have a relatively greater inotropic:chronotropic ratio and are generally preferred in most circumstances.

It must be remembered that all cardiac inotropic agents increase myocardial oxygen consumption ($M\dot{V}O_2$) as a function of the rate of development of tension generated and the peak fiber tension achieved.[172] Therefore, in using any inotropic drug one must achieve a sufficient increase in coronary perfusion and myocardial oxygen delivery to meet the increased myocardial oxidative requirement produced by the resultant increase in stroke power (Fig. 9-23). In general, if total CO can be increased while reducing afterload, as well as cardiac work and power, and if the aortic diastolic to LVED pressure gradient can be increased, the net increase in coronary flow relative to $M\dot{V}O_2$ produces a favorable balance.

Inotropic agents with β-adrenergic activity also act to relax vascular smooth muscle and therefore have vasodilator activity whereas those with α-adrenergic activity (norepinephrine, methoxamine) cause vascular smooth muscle contraction and vasoconstriction.[56,189] The natural sympathetic transmitter norepinephrine (NE), which is released from stores at sympathetic nerve endings in the periphery and in the heart,[49,190] exhibits both α- and β-adrenergic activity. Thus, a baroreceptor- and chemoreceptor-induced mass sympathetic response such as occurs in most low-flow shock states results in central cardiac inotropic and chronotropic activity[34,36,119] and peripheral arterial and venous vasoconstriction.[67,190] These effects raise blood pressure by increasing vascular tone, increase venous return from the venous capacitance beds and also increase the force of myocardial contraction by the Frank–Starling mechanism.[118]

Fortunately, there are no α-adrenergic receptors in the coronary vascular bed, so that NE release produces coronary vasodilatation.[20,149] Unfortunately, in hypovolemic shock states, or where intrinsic myocardial contractile depression has occurred due to direct myocardial trauma,[43,92] after sepsis[144,155] or a period of shock-induced low-flow myocardial ischemia,[117,147] the vascular capacitance beds also may be depleted of reserve volume. As a result, at a time when the myocardium may be able to respond only poorly to the levels of β-adrenergic activity provided by norepinephrine, venous return is not increased, and only the peripheral vasoconstrictor response remains effective. Under these circumstances, the relative increase in afterload is the dominant effect, further reducing cardiac ejection, which is already low by virtue of diminished preload and Vmax effects.[70,171] Consequently, there is virtually no role for the use of NE or methoxamine in low-flow, especially hypovolemic, shock states.[158,160] In this setting, one chooses a sympathomimetic agent with pure or primarily β-adrenergic effects that also has a predominance of inotropic over chronotropic activity and attempts to optimize the ability to accept an increase in intravascular volume.

DOPAMINE

The most frequently used inotropic agent is naturally occurring dopamine, which at very low doses (0.5 to 2 μg/kg/min) also appears to have a selective "dopaminagenic" effect in dilating the renal arterioles, thereby increasing renal blood flow.[111] However, this agent also has both β- and α-adrenergic activity at higher doses, so that its net effect on the circulation is very much a function of the dosage rate utilized.[56,83,86,141] At low doses of 1 to 5 μg/kg/

min, there is a weak cardiac inotropic effect with a selective increase in renal and mesenteric blood flow due to a specific regional vasodilatation of these beds. At intermediate dosage rates 6 to 15 μg/kg/min, the β-adrenergic effects become dominant (although some α-adrenergic activity is noted above 10 μg/kg/min), and there is cardiac inotropic activity and an absence of, or minimal, vasoconstrictor action. At dosage rates of greater than 15 μg/kg/min, however, the α-adrenergic action of this agent becomes dominant, and vasoconstriction with an increase in vascular tone and afterload occurs. There is a claim in the literature that sepsis specifically impairs both the α- and β-adrenergic actions of dopamine so that very large doses ($\geq$50 μg/kg/min) are necessary to achieve comparable effects.[105] However, we consider these to be inappropriate dose levels even in sepsis; we believe that other agents either alone, or in combination with lower doses of dopamine should be used instead. In those circumstances in which a critical level of arterial pressure must be maintained by vasoconstriction, for instance, in the oliguric septic shock patient on hemodialysis or hemofiltration, we have had better results using the naturally occurring catecholamine epinephrine (0.02 to 0.10 μg/kg/min), which exhibits strong β-adrenergic activity as well as α-adrenergic effects.

DOBUTAMINE

This agent is a synthetic analogue of dopamine. It has a more prominent β_1-adrenergic activity, which results in a stronger inotropic than chronotropic action. There is a mild to moderate vasodilator effect and no α-adrenergic vasoconstrictor activity.[58,114,141] As a result, this agent given in doses of 2 to 10 μg/kg/min increases Vmax, causes systemic vasodilatation, and thereby reduces afterload relative to the increase in myocardial force–velocity relationships. Alone, there does not appear to be an increase in vascular tone—indeed, there may be a decrease. Any blood pressure rise seen with this agent is due to the increase in CO, which may increase effective pressure

by shifting the patient's position on the vascular flow:resistance curve.

ISOPROTERENOL

Isoproterenol (Isuprel) is a pure β-adrenergic agent, which is undoubtedly the most powerful agent of its class on a microgram-to-microgram comparison basis. It has inotropic, chronotropic, and active peripheral vasodilatory activity.[32,56,62,65,98,143] Although an excellent agent in many situations, it is generally not used because the dosage spread between its primarily inotropic action and its chronotropic effect is small; as a result, its proper level of dosing is not well understood by most critical care specialists. When correctly used at the optimal level for cardiac inotropic activity, 0.25 to 1.0 μg/min total body dose,[18,143] there is a profound increase in CO and generally no change, or even a slight decrease, in heart rate as the increased stroke volume, flow, and dynamic pressure increases reduce the patient's endogenous baroreceptor and chemoreceptor stimulation of the vasomotor center. There is also an active peripheral vasodilator function, which may help overcome the vasoconstriction of selective beds with an increase in $\dot{V}O_2$. Finally, even at low dose there is a marked reduction in the duration of systolic pressure development with an increased period for coronary diastolic filling, which together with the increased CO appears to compensate for the $M\dot{V}O_2$ increase produced by this agent. Often when the proper low-dose therapy is used, ECG evidence of ischemia due to low-flow states is reduced. In patients with mild degrees of atrioventricular block, or sick sinus syndrome producing bradycardia secondary to low-flow states, use of this agent at slightly higher dose rates (0.5 to 4 μg/min total dose) can increase the heart rate to more effective levels.

Isoproterenol has also been claimed to attenuate pulmonary edema after acid lung injury by reducing pulmonary outflow vasoconstriction, thus preventing excess fluid flux into the interstitial space of the lung.[98] This action on the hemodynamics of pulmonary perfusion in septic hyperdynamic stress states, where selective pulmonary vasoconstriction appears to cause increased venoarterial admixture, may account for its action in reducing pulmonary shunt. At doses comparable to those used with dopamine or dobutamine (and in some individuals with atrial or ventricular ectopic activation foci), however, the level of tachycardia achieved relative to the inotropic effect is unacceptable. At high doses (0.2 to 11 μg/kg/min), the use of isoproterenol has been associated with accelerated myocardial necrosis in animals and in patients with acute myocardial infarction or chronic ischemic myocardial disease.

GLUCAGON

This naturally occurring pancreatic islet cell hormone also increases myocardial adenyl cyclase activity as well as the level of cAMP. At doses of 3 to 5 mg/hr, it has been shown to have cardiac inotropic activity in animals and in human subjects in hypovolemic and septic shock states, with very little chronotropic and no α-adrenergic activity.[31,51,59,85,112,156] However, since this agent is also a powerful stimulator of hepatic gluconeogenesis and skeletal muscle proteolysis, its use in critically ill patients is generally confined to those individuals in low-flow shock states who have previously been on agents which deplete cardiac NE stores (reserpine), or β-adrenergic blocking agents (propanolol or its derivative drugs) for chronic control of angina pectoris or hypertension.[51] In these circumstances, agents that rely for their effect or the release of endogenous cardiac NE stores or on competitive activation of β-adrenergic receptors may be ineffective in increasing myocardial contractility and cardiac output. Glucagon is an effective though weak inotropic agent under these conditions.

DIGOXIN

Digoxin, like other preparations similar to digitalis, exerts its inotropic effect by inhibiting the Na^+/K^+ exchange mechanism, maintaining membrane electrical potential.[77] This causes reversal of the slower Na^+/Ca^{++} exchange channel and results in an increase in cytosolic Ca^{++}, which acts to increase the force of contraction thus increasing Vmax.[125] This cardiac glycoside also slows atrioventricular conduction, which is of value in reducing the rate of ventricular activation in cases of rapid atrial flutter or atrial fibrillation.[99] At toxic levels, or when serum K^+ is reduced, digitalis agents alter the threshold for ventricular deplorization and can produce ectopic foci of ventricular activation, which predispose to ventricular premature contraction, bigeminy, and other ventricular dysrhythmias, including ventricular fibrillation. With rapid digitalizing doses, digoxin can induce transient peripheral vasoconstriction and microvascular mesenteric vasoconstriction with ischemia and necrosis of bowel has been reported in patients with chronic congestive heart failure. The primary route of excretion of digoxin is renal, therefore with impaired renal clearance the dose must be adjusted according to the level of creatinine clearance.[71]

Nevertheless, acute digitalization to achieve an inotropic effect is of value in selected patients after low-flow shock states.[21,58,141,143,155,159] This is especially true if primary cardiac failure or anesthetic toxicity is a cause of the inability to achieve a normal or hyperdynamic stress-response CO.[54,141,143,155,158-160] This may be seen in patients with acute myocardial infarction with acute pulmonary edema and after massive pulmonary embolization with acute right heart failure. A similar localized heart failure that can be improved by digoxin may occur with direct myocardial contusion.[43,186] However, it is important to recognize that in cardiac failure complicating acute hypovolemia, the usual signs of pulmonary congestion, rales or pulmonary edema, or hepatic congestion may be absent due to the low central blood volume. What may be seen instead is an inability to raise the CO in spite of a large rise in central venous, or pulmonary wedge, pressure as volume is reinfused. Of equal importance in utilizing acute digitalization for inotropic support in posttrauma patients is the fact that, unlike the conduction slowing effect required to control supraventricular dysrhythmias, the ventricular inotropic effect can be achieved by less than a full digitalizing dose; usually only 75 percent of the full dose is necessary. As a result, when rapid digoxin infusion is chosen for inotropic support, a total dose of only 0.75 mg is usually required.[143] This should be administered intravenously, after checking to assure a normal or slightly increased serum K^+ level, in three divided doses of 0.25 mg, 4 to 6 hours apart. If there is great urgency due to pulmonary edema, digoxin may be given intravenously as a 0.5-mg dose followed by 0.25 mg, 2 to 4 hours later. Then a low intravenous maintenance level of 0.125 to 0.250 mg can be given on a daily basis. Plasma K^+ and digoxin levels should be monitored daily in acutely ill patients receiving digoxin, especially when there also is a reduced creatinine clearance.[71]

GLUCOSE–POTASSIUM–INSULIN

On the basis of work in postcardiac bypass patients with refractory contractile depression and some shock studies, the use of glucose–potassium–insulin (GKI) has been advocated as an acute inotropic resuscitation therapy.[97] This is administered as an IV bolus of 50 ml of 50 percent glucose containing 20 mEq K^+ and 10 units of insulin. It can be effective in restoring effective contraction after cardiac arrest or during low-flow hypovolemic resuscitation. In our experience, however, this effect is generally limited in magnitude and is not particularly effective as a mode of continuous therapy. With serious or persistent contractile reductions, one of the previously discussed intravenous agents should be employed.

CALCIUM

The use of a bolus of 0.5 to 1.0 g Ca^{++} usually as calcium gluconate has also been advocated as a means of improving myocardial contractility. This may be of value in the hypovolemic patient who has rapidly received large quantities of blood anticoagulated with Ca^{++} binding agents, for whom 14.5 mEq of Ca^{++} is advocated for each 5 units of packed RBCs. Its use has also been advocated after cardiac arrest to assist the ischemia-depressed heart in order to resume a normal contractile action. However, some studies suggest a pathologic

role for Ca^{++} in the myocardial ischemia reperfusion syndrome, which should be considered when this agent is used.[182]

AMRINONE

This drug represents the first clinical use of a new class of nonglycoside, noncatecholamine cardiac inotropic and vasodilatory agents. It acts by inhibition of phosphodiesterase (PDE) III, which inactivates cAMP and at high doses may also potentiate inward Ca^{++}/Na^+ exchange.[88] It is not affected by either β-adrenergic blockade or depletion of cardiac norepinephrine by reserpine.[53,88] As a result of its PDE III-inhibiting action, amrinone has been reported to potentiate the inotropic effects of β-adrenergic agents such as isoproterenol or dobutamine. Its use at a dose range of 10 to 40 $\mu g/kg/min$ has been advocated in low-flow situations in which congestive heart failure is a prominent feature, such as after acute myocardial infarction[88] or in the low CO syndrome following cardiopulmonary bypass surgery,[53] wherein downregulation of β-adrenergic receptors may occur. In these circumstances, its vasodilator and β-adrenergic catecholamine potentiating actions make it an attractive complementary inotropic that may increase total flow while also increasing nutrient organ flow rather than cutaneous vasodilatation.[88] It also tends to increase CO with little increase in myocardial oxygen consumption because of the concomitant reduction in afterload and ventricular wall tension.[88] However, there is little present clinical work regarding its value in hypovolemic shock or in the pathologic hyperdynamic high-output cardiac failure associated with sepsis. Nevertheless, a place for this agent in combined therapy seems likely, if the preliminary good reports in cardiogenic low-flow syndromes can be substantiated in human hypovolemic and septic shock studies.

COMBINATION THERAPY USING MULTIPLE INOTROPIC AGENTS

It is frequently advantageous to use simultaneous continuous infusions of fractional doses of several of the above inotropic drugs rather than a single agent alone to achieve the desired inotropic effect in critically ill patients.[141,143] The rationale for this approach is related to the goal of reducing the specific toxicity of a given agent while maximizing the net cardiac inotropic level. For example, by combining dopamine infusion at dopaminogenic (renal vasodilator) doses of 2 to 5 μg/min/kg with low-dose isoproterenol 0.25 μg/min total dose, or dobutamine, 3 to 10 μg/min/kg, it is possible to increase cardiac ejection fraction, CO, and renal blood flow, without inducing the degree of vasoconstriction and afterload increase that would occur if dopamine alone were used at doses high enough to increase contractility in the severely depressed posttrauma or septic myocardium. Similarly, acute digitalization with low-dose daily maintenance can be supported by the addition of a low-dose continuous infusion of dopamine (3 to 5 μg/kg/min) or dobutamine (2 to 10 μg/kg/min) if the required increase in CO and $\dot{V}O_2$ does not occur. Obviously, in any given patient, the dose and mix of these agents may need to be adjusted upward to get the desired effect.

Afterload-Reducing Agents

The third major aspect of cardiovascular therapy used to increased CO and oxygen consumption in low-flow states is the administration of vasodilatory drugs to reduce an excessive afterload effect. These agents fall into several types, but in all instances it is essential that they not be used until an effort has been made to provide for adequate vascular filling (preload) proportionate to the level of contractility. Failure to ensure an effective cardiac filling volume may produce profound and unacceptable hypotension, below the level of vascular opening pressure to critical perfusion beds, when sudden vasodilatation is achieved. However, with adequate preload, the combined use of cardiac inotropic agents and vasodilators may permit optimization of force–velocity relations, so that a maximum cardiac ejection can be achieved without excessively increasing the afterload and myocardial oxygen consumption.[18,94,95,141,143,179] These agents fall into several classes.

NARCOTICS AND TRANQUILIZERS

It is often forgotten that pain and apprehension can produce intense sympathetic discharge with marked vasoconstriction and hypertension. In many instances, the simple administration of therapeutic doses of morphine or demerol will alleviate pain and anxiety and result in a reduction in vascular tone and blood pressure and an increase in CO. In a similar fashion, the use of thorazine (25 to 50 mg) or valium (5 to 10 mg) given slowly intravenously will result in a reduction in acute systemic vasoconstriction. In all these instances, and especially with the use of morphine, respiration must be monitored; in the critically ill patient, frequent blood gases must be examined to guard against hypercapnia and/or hypoxemia when these drugs are used, unless the patient is on controlled or mandatory assisted ventilatory support with a predetermined adequate lower limit. Specific vasodilators that have been of value in reducing afterload are as follows.

NITROGLYCERINE

The use of nitroglycerine either by transcutaneous administration (Nitropaste from 1 inch to 2 inches applied to the chest wall) in less severe cases, or by intravenous infusion (6 μg/min to 25 μg/min) titrated to reduce mean blood pressure 5 to 10 mmHg from preinfusion levels, is efficacious in those instances in which mild to moderate vasoconstriction occurs.[4,140] It is important to remember that the main action of nitroglycerine is to dilate the venous capacitance vessels and by lowering the venous component of peripheral vascular resistance to reduce the net impedance to flow. Consequently, the right atrial and pulmonary wedge pressures, or LVEDV, should be monitored during its use to prevent an excessive reduction in preload. However, there is a direct effect on the arterial vascular tone, most notable in the coronary circulation, where it produces vasodilatation. This makes it a valuable afterload-reducing agent in older patients who have known or suspected coronary artery disease. This agent, as Nitropaste, has been shown also to be effective in increasing CO and $\dot{V}O_2$ in patients with low-flow states secondary to septic myocardial depression.[18]

NITROPRUSSIDE

The arteriolar dilating agent nitroprusside, which also has some effect in dilating venous capacitance vessels is the most widely used intravenous agent for severe acute hypertension or major vasoconstrictor episodes.[141] It is generally administered starting at a low dose of 0.5 μg/kg/min and is gradually increased by 0.2 μg/kg/min up to a maximum level of 8 μg/kg/min in refractory hypertensive crises, or where aortic pressure must be reduced at all cost as with dissecting aneurysms, or during the preparations for surgery in patients with a thoracic aortic rupture who have an unstable pseudoaneurysm.[4,19,100,140] In some applications, this agent has been used with a computer-based Servo-controlled infusion pump set to adjust the rate of nitroprusside infusion automatically to keep the arterial blood pressure within preset limits. As with nitroglycerine, preload may also be reduced with this agent and filling pressures and CO must be monitored frequently.[140] As a guide to the adequacy of peripheral perfusion the $\dot{V}O_2$, lactate and base deficit should be determined at regular intervals during the infusion period. Because of the tendency for this agent to liberate nitrites with the formation of cyanohemoglobin, cyanosis must be clinically evaluated and quantitative co-oximetry of oxygen: hemoglobin saturation must be done and the agent may need to be discontinued.

PHENTOLAMINE

In cases in which severe hypertension must be controlled and nitroprusside is not indicated, or has not been effective, phentolamine has been useful.[13,68] This α-adrenergic blocking agent produces a profound reduction in arteriolar vasoconstriction. It is usually ad-

ministered as a continuous infusion beginning at 0.1 mg/min, increasing up to 2 mg/min at 10 to 15-minute intervals until blood pressure is controlled. In general, as the reduction in blood pressure is achieved, PWP, CO, $\dot{V}O_2$, and lactate levels should be followed to ensure that the fall in resistance is indeed productive of increased peripheral perfusion. Excessive tachycardias have been reported with the use of this agent.[141] Other antihypertension drugs are discussed in Chapter 12.

As a final comment on the use of vasodilator therapy, with the exception of the active β-adrenergic dilatation of isoproterenol, all the arteriolar vasodilator agents have been reported to reduce the hypoxic vasoconstriction in the pulmonary arterioles.[141] This may cause an increase in pulmonary shunt with a fall in PaO_2 and saturation as CO rises. Also, the use of PEEP for ventilatory support may have a greater effect in reducing venous return to the right heart in those patients receiving vasodilators that also act to dilate the venous capacitance vessels. For these reasons, both oxygen delivery, CO, percentage shunt, and $\dot{V}O_2$ must be carefully followed in any patient receiving vasodilator therapy for the treatment of low-flow shock states.

Noninotropic Mechanical Unloading

A valuable adjunctive therapy for use in low-flow cardiogenic shock is the use of the intra-aortic balloon counterpulsation (IABP) device[38,43,48,147,179] (see Chapter 11). This mechanical therapeutic measure has two main effects. The first is related to providing an increased aortic diastolic perfusion of the coronary and cerebral circulation during the period of diastolic balloon inflation. The second is related to the reduction in the subsequent systolic afterload, which impedes cardiac ejection, during the period of systolic balloon deflation by virtue of having already reduced the proximal aortic volume and pressure during the previous diastolic inflation period. This allows for a greater stroke volume and also reduced myocardial oxygen consumption (M$\dot{V}O_2$). A third effect that has been noted is an increased renal perfusion and a rise in urine output. This is thought to be due to the increased traffic over the carotid baroreceptor afferents, which inhibits the vasomotor center, thereby reducing the sympathetic efferent vasoconstrictor activity. An example of this modality of therapy is shown in Figure 9-39 for

two patients with acute myocardial infarction shock.[147] Both patients had severe D state cardiogenic myocardial depression with a reduction in cardiac ejection fraction ($\uparrow t_m$), a fall in CI, and a rise in the Ca-$\bar{v}O_2$ (A-V Diff) in an attempt to maintain $\dot{V}O_2$. The use of IABP caused a marked decrease in systolic ejection time (ET) indicating the systolic afterload re-

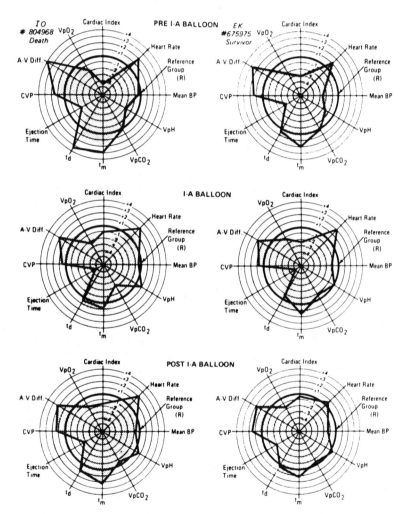

FIG. 9-39 Multivariable physiologic patterns during clinical course of recovery from acute myocardial infarction shock in two patients treated by intra-aortic balloon counter pulsation. Pre-, intra-, and post-IA balloon studies are shown. Shaded area shows D-state cardiogenic decompensation prototype mean for comparison with actual patient study (solid dark line). Note similarity of pattern during IA-balloon support with return to D-state pattern in patient IO who succumbed, versus movement toward R-state pattern in patient EK who survived after discontinuance of IA-balloon, indicating return of intrinsic myocardial contractile function. (Siegel JH, Farrell EJ, Goldwyn RM, Friedman HP: The surgical implications of physiologic patterns in myocardial infarction shock. Surgery 72: 126, 1972.)

duction permitting a higher velocity of ejection. The cardiac ejection fraction rose ($\downarrow$ t_m), and CI and $\dot{V}O_2$ increased as well. When IABP was discontinued, the surviving patient (EK#675975) was able to sustain an R state by maintaining the improved cardiac ejection fraction; thus CI was increased, even though the afterload was now increased over IABP levels. By contrast, the nonsurviving patient (IO#804968) was unable to withstand the increased afterload and the loss of the IABP supplemented coronary perfusion. As a result, the patient returned to a D state, where death occurred.

IABP has also been used successfully in acute postsurgical or posttraumatic myocardial infarction,[38,147] after cardiac contusion with refractory shock,[43,48] and in selected cases of severe septic myocardial depression,[179] although in the latter instance the mortality associated with the sepsis itself has generally been the limiting factor in survival.

STEROIDS AND ANTI-INFLAMMATORY AGENTS

The role of steroids in hypovolemic and low-flow shock states remains controversial after more than 30 years of cycles of sporadic enthusiasm and disgruntlement. Some evidence exists that the use of pharmacologic doses of methylprednisolone, or dexamethasone, may be of use in the acute endotoxin-induced phase of septic shock;[9,81,91,120–122] certain uses of these agents have been advocated in incomplete spinal cord lesions and early in head injury patients with associated circulatory instability (see Chapters 31 and 32). However, no statistically significant clinically validated study has verified any beneft in human hypovolemic shock. A variety of claims have also been made for the use of other types of anti-inflammatory agents, including prostacyclins, superoxide inhibiting agents, and antihistamine drugs in experimental studies.[74,75,141,163,188] These must await a clinically relevant and statistically significant experience before they can be advocated for use in patients.

ANTIBIOTICS

The use of prophylactic antibiotic therapy is also a topic of much disagreement. The experimental studies conducted by Fine[41,42] suggested that a major cause of refractory shock after acute hypovolemia could come from the absorption of bacterial endotoxins. Overload of the hepatic, splenic, and pulmonary RE system has been implicated in posttraumatic or hypovolemic shock deterioration (Chapters 3 and 14). This factor has been cited as a justification for antibiotic use in major hypovolemic hypotension.[12] Conversely, much literature can be cited (see Chapter 16), indicating that the use of prophylactic antibiotics merely selects out more severe pathogens with a greater incidence of serious or fatal infections. We do not advocate prophylactic antibiotics for general use, although there are situations of clear contamination, bowel injury, open fractures wtih devitalized tissues, in which antibiotic therapy for likely pathogens should be combined with volume resuscitation and cardiodynamic measures in the treatment of posttraumatic hypovolemic shock patients.

THERAPEUTIC DECISION MAKING IN POSTTRAUMATIC HYPOVOLEMIA: USE OF PHYSIOLOGIC PATTERN RECOGNITION AND RECOVERY TRAJECTORIES

Determination of the patient's physiologic state classification by the cardiogreen indicator dilution cardiac output has been used as a means of physiologic consultation in treating critically ill and injured patients. It has been useful in determining the magnitude of the hypovolemic insult and in delineating severe myocardial depression in the absence of hypotension. This type of physiologic pattern recognition has also been of great value in detecting the onset of a normal stress-response septic hyperdynamic state and its deterioration into a state of uncontrolled septic metabolic decompensation (see Chapter 15).

Hypovolemia and Myocardial Contusion (Decreased Preload and Depressed Vmax)

An example of the use of this computer-based methodology to identify and guide treatment for a serious state of myocardial depression complicating post traumatic hypovolemic shock in the absence of hypotension is shown in Figure 9-40. This patient (AS#016907) was a 24-year-old man injured in an automobile accident. He sustained a fractured pelvis with laceration of the superior gluteal artery, a ruptured spleen and a chest contusion. When resuscitated after angiographic embolization of the bleeding pelvic artery and after splenectomy and stabilization of the severe pelvic fracture, he was noted to be doing poorly with a decrease in urine output and clinical evidence of severe peripheral vasoconstriction without significant hypotension. His blood pressure was 107/85 with a mean of 93 mmHg, although he had a tachycardia of 120 bpm. However, the patient's physiologic pattern, shown in Figure 9-40A, demonstrates the absence of a normal A state stress response and the presence of a severe D state cardiogenic decompensation, equal to or greater than that commonly seen in patients sustaining an acute myocardial infarction, or due to postcoronary bypass myocardial depression. The CI was nearly 3 SD decreased below the R state mean at 1.09 L/min/m². The pulmonary blood volume (DV) was also reduced from an expected value of 358 ml (200 ml/m²) to 223 ml (125 ml/m²), indicating a marked central hypovolemia related to the major hemorrhage; myocardial function was shown to be markedly depressed with an ejection fraction (EFx) of only 44 percent, with t_m more than 2 SD below the R state mean. Indeed, in the absence of this type of computer-based physiologic assessment and pattern recognition, the nature and severity of his physio-

logic response to injury would likely have been obscured if only conventional modalities of evaluation such as blood pressure, heart rate, and urine output had been used.

The result of this use of pattern recognition technique to identify the nature of critical illness and to delineate the appropriate response to therapy is shown in Figure 9-40B. This figure demonstrates the cardiovascular and metabolic response of the patient seen previously in Figure 9-40A to the combined use of cardiac inotropic agents and additional volume replacement. In response to this therapy, the patient was enabled to achieve a normal A state stress response with an increase in CI to 4.91 L/min/m², the pulmonary blood volume rose in response to volume infusion to a more normal value of 409 ml (229 ml/m²); the cardiac ejection fraction (EFx) increased to 82 percent in response to cardiac inotropic therapy with dopamine (13 µg/kg/min) and dobutamine (11 µg/kg/min), producing a pattern nearly identical with the prototype A state stress response normally expected in this type of case.

It is of interest to note that in the A state stress response (Figure 9-40B) the patient's mean blood pressure of 69 mmHg was actually lower than that seen in the combined hypovolemic and cardiogenic shock D state shown earlier, indicating that a pathologic degree of vasoconstriction was merely masking the severe combined cardiogenic and hypovolemia induced reduction in CI. It is also worth noting that in this patient, who required a combination of increased PEEP and elevated peak airway pressures for ventilation of posttraumatic ARDS syndrome, both the pulmonary artery wedge pressure (PWP) and right atrial pressures (RAP) were elevated during both the hypovolemic cardiogenic D state and in the normal A state stress response state after therapy, even though the LVEDV values (LVV) were markedly different (Fig. 9-40A,B). This would have made it extremely difficult to arrive at an appropriate therapeutic end point merely by using the RAP or the Swan–Ganz MPA or (PWP) pressures as a guide.

The systemic oxygen debt and estimated myocardial oxygen consumption consequences of the severe flow reduction produced by a combination of hypovolemia, increased vascu-

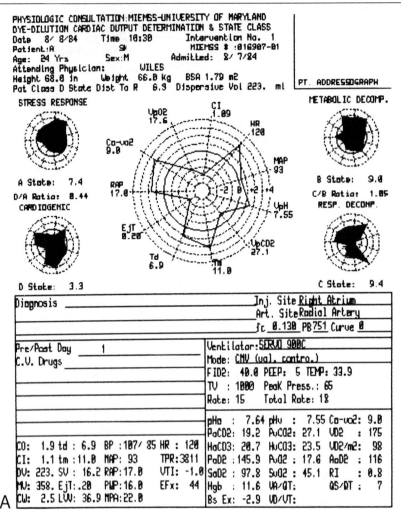

PHYSIOLOGIC CONSULTATION:MIEMSS-UNIVERSITY OF MARYLAND
DYE-DILUTION CARDIAC OUTPUT DETERMINATION & STATE CLASS
Date   8/ 8/84   Time 10:30   Intervention No.   1
Patient:A   S   MIEMSS # :016907-01
Age: 24 Yrs   Sex:M   Admitted: 8/ 7/84
Attending Physician: WILES
Height 68.0 in   Weight 66.0 kg   BSA 1.79 m2
Pat Class D State Dist To R   6.9 Dispersive Vol 223. ml

PT. ADDRESSOGRAPH

STRESS RESPONSE   METABOLIC DECOMP.

VbO2 17.6   CI 1.09
Ca-vo2 9.0   HR 120

A State: 7.4   RAP 17.0   MAP 93   B State: 9.0
D/A Ratio: 0.44   VpH 7.55   C/B Ratio: 1.05
CARDIOGENIC   RESP. DECOMP.

EjT 0.20
                     Td 6.9   VpCO2 27.1
                             TM 11.0

D State: 3.3   C State: 9.4

Diagnosis	Inj. Site Right Atrium
	Art. Site Radial Artery
	fc 0.130 PB 751 Curve 0

Pre/Post Day 1	Ventilator: SERVO 900C
C.V. Drugs	Mode: CMV (vol. contro.)
	FID2: 40.0 PEEP: 5 TEMP: 33.9
	TV : 1000 Peak Press.: 65
	Rate: 15 Total Rate: 18
	pHa : 7.64 pHv : 7.55 Ca-vo2: 9.0
	PaCO2: 19.2 PvCO2: 27.1 VO2 : 175
CO: 1.9 td : 6.9 BP :107/ 85 HR : 120	HaCO3: 20.7 HvCO3: 23.5 VO2/m2: 98
CI: 1.1 tm :11.0 MAP: 93 TPR:3811	PaO2 :145.9 PvO2 : 17.6 AaD2 : 116
DV: 223. SV : 16.2 RAP:17.0 VTI: -1.0	SaO2 : 97.8 SvO2 : 45.1 RI : 0.8
MV: 358. EjT:.20 PWP:16.0 EFx: 44	Hgb : 11.6 VA/QT: QS/QT : 7
CW: 2.5 LW: 36.9 MPA:22.0	Bs Ex: -2.9 VD/VT:

A

FIG. 9-40 (A) Physiologic consultation from 24-year-old male who sustained motor vehicle accident with ruptured spleen, fractured pelvis, hypovolemia, chest contusion, and myocardial depression (D state). Study carried out prior to initiation of cardiac inotropic support. (*Figure continues.*)

lar tone and myocardial depression can be seen in this patient. At the time of the initial study (Fig. 9-40A) when the CI was reduced to 1.09 L/min/m², the total body oxygen consumption ($\dot{V}O_2/m^2$) was only 98 ml/min/m² (2.65 ml/kg/min), producing an increased body extraction of the reduced oxygen delivery, so that the Ca-$\bar{v}O_2$ was increased to 9.0 vol percent. This is equivalent to a rate of accumulation of oxygen deficit equivalent to 1.63 ml/kg/min, assuming a normal expected mean age-dependent A state posttrauma $\dot{V}O_2$ of 4.28 ml/kg/min (Table 9-1). This is supported by

the observation that in spite of a marked reduction in $PaCO_2$ to 19.1 mmHg, produced by hyperventilation and causing respiratory alkalosis, there was a significant base deficit of -2.9 mEq/L. However, the patient may have been somewhat protected from the consequences of this rapidly accumulating oxygen deficit by the markedly reduced body temperature of 33.9°C produced by the massive infusion of intravenous fluids and bank blood.

The extremely high vascular resistance (TPR = 3,811) constituted a significant afterload affect that could not be overcome by the

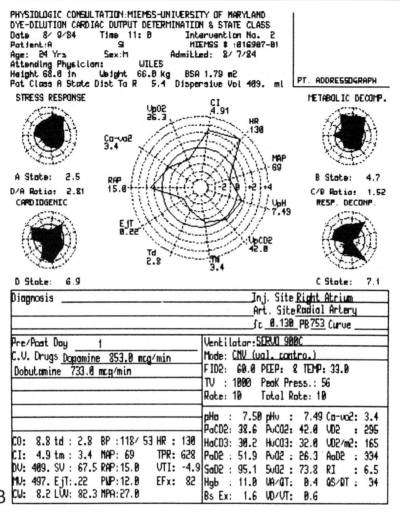

PHYSIOLOGIC CONSULTATION:MIEMSS-UNIVERSITY OF MARYLAND
DYE-DILUTION CARDIAC OUTPUT DETERMINATION & STATE CLASS
Date 8/ 9/84   Time 11: 8   Intervention No. 2
Patient:A   9   MIEMSS # :016907-01
Age: 24 Yrs   Sex:M   Admitted: 8/ 7/84
Attending Physician: WILES
Height 68.0 in   Weight 66.0 kg   BSA 1.79 m2
Pat Class A State Dist To R   5.4 Dispersive Vol 409. ml

PT. ADDRESSOGRAPH

STRESS RESPONSE   METABOLIC DECOMP.

A State: 2.5   B State: 4.7
D/A Ratio: 2.81   C/B Ratio: 1.52
CARDIOGENIC   RESP. DECONP.

D State: 6.9   C State: 7.1

Diagnosis _____   Inj. Site Right Atrium
                                   Art. Site Radial Artery
                                   Jc 0.130 PB 753 Curve _____

Pre/Post Day 1	Ventilator: SERVO 900C
C.V. Drugs Dopamine 853.0 mcg/min	Mode: CMV (vol. contro.)
Dobutamine 733.0 mcg/min	FID2: 60.0 PEEP: 8 TEMP: 33.0
	TV : 1000 Peak Press.: 56
	Rate: 10 Total Rate: 10

		pHa : 7.50 pHv : 7.49	Ca-vo2: 3.4
		PaCO2: 38.6 PvCO2: 42.0	VO2 : 295
		HaCO3: 30.2 HvCO3: 32.0	VO2/m2: 165
CO: 8.8 td : 2.8	BP :118/ 53	PaO2: 51.9 PvO2: 26.3	AaDO2 : 334
CI: 4.9 tm : 3.4	MAP: 69 TPR: 628	SaO2: 95.1 SvO2: 73.8	RI : 6.5
DV: 409. SV : 67.5	RAP:15.0 VTI: -4.9	Hgb : 11.0 VA/QT: 0.4	QS/QT: 34
MV: 497. EjT:.22	PLP:12.0 EFx: 82	Bs Ex: 1.6 VD/VT: 0.6	
CW: 8.2 LVW: 82.3	NPA:27.0		

B

FIG. 9-40 (*Continued*) **(B)** Follow-up study on patient shown previously in Figure 9-40(A) after the initiation of cardiac inotropic support with dopamine 13 mcg/kg/min and dobutamine 11 mcg/kg/min, as well as volume (A state). See text for details.

depressed myocardium (EFx = 44 percent) operating from a hypovolemia reduced LVEDV (LVV = 36.9 ml) so that only a small stroke volume (SV = 16.2 ml) could be ejected producing a low CI. Nevertheless, the external cardiac work (CW) was only slightly reduced at 2.5 kg/M/min and the index of myocardial oxygen consumption (estimated as the product of stroke power times heart rate, as in Figure 9-23) remained at nearly normal values (142 kg/M · sec⁻¹/min) compared with the mean of 156 kg/M · sec⁻¹/min seen in unstressed reference control R state patients.

The use of cardiac inotropic therapy using dopamine and dobutamine (Fig. 9-40B) enabled this patient to achieve an increased EFx (82 percent) and thereby to accommodate to the larger LVEDV of 82.3 ml induced by transfusion, thus producing a higher stroke volume (67.5 ml) and CI (4.91 L/min). The latter resulted in a marked increase of peripheral perfusion, so that oxygen consumption rose to 165 ml/min/m² as the peripheral resistance fell to 628 dyn/sec/cm⁻⁵. As body flow increased, Ca-v̄O₂ was reduced to 3.4 vol percent, the rate of oxygen uptake increased to 4.47 ml/kg/min, which appeared to be sufficient to repay the prior oxygen debt, and the metabolic acidosis and base deficit disappeared indicating adequacy of perfusion. Cardiac work rose from 2.5 kg/M/min in the D state to 8.2 kg/M/min, in the A state and the index of myocardial oxygen consumption ($M\dot{V}O_2$), which was at R state levels in spite of the low-flow cardiogenic D state, also rose fourfold ($M\dot{V}O_2 = 640$ kg/ M · sec^{-1}/min) as the patient achieved the A state compensatory response. However, since CI rose more than 4.6 times the D state value (5 SD of R above the previous D state level), as ejection fraction increased to 82 percent and ejection time decreased, it is reasonable to assume that there was adequate coronary flow to meet the myocardial oxygen demands. These demands would be expected to increase because of the increases in central blood volume and flow (which increased both myocardial preload and afterload), as well because of the increase in the Vmax of the myocardial force–velocity relationship induced by the β-adrenergic cardiac inotropic support.

Thus, in summarizing the therapeutic response in this case, not only did the use of inotropic support result in an increase in myocardial contractile dynamics, but the increase in stroke volume and flow resulted in a relative reduction in vascular tone, apparently by lowering the sympathetic reflex induced relative increase in vasoconstriction to a more appropriate stress-induced vasodilatory response. This is demonstrated by the reduction in vascular tone index (VTI), which summarizes the vascular pressure–flow relationship, from −1.0 in the hypovolemic–cardiogenic D state (Fig. 9-40A) to −4.9 in the normal–volemic hyperdynamic A state stress response (Fig. 9-40B).

Hypovolemia and Excessive Vasoconstriction (Decreased Preload and Increased Afterload)

An excessive vasoconstriction response often seen in the young trauma patient, as in the previous case, may induce an inappropriate degree of afterload. This may force the patient to operate at a disadvantagous point, on the myocardial Starling–Sarnoff relationship. As a result, even though the patient may be hypovo-lemic, the combination of a slightly reduced myocardial contractile function (Vmax) and a markedly increased afterload point on the force–velocity relationship will also result in a decreased EFx and a dilated ventricle with a very large LVEDV (LVV).

This is shown in Figure 9-41A, which demonstrates an inappropriate vasoconstrictive response in a 15-year-old patient (GO#013308) who sustained major multiple trauma with an aortic rupture, also including a pelvic fracture, a splenic laceration, an open humeral fracture, and a spinal cord contusion with a partial central cord lesion at T12–L1. As can be seen in Figure 9-41A, showing the study done after repair of the aorta, splenectomy, and external fixation of the fractures, the vascular resistance was 2185 dyn/sec/cm^{-5} at a CO of 4.7 L/min (CI = 2.5 L/min/m^2) representing a large absolute increase in vascular tone index to +4.7. This produced a marked elevation of systolic and diastolic arterial pressure (208/96) with mean pressure of 128 mmHg, nearly 2 SD higher than the R state control. The combination of a greatly increased afterload and the reflex bradycardia (HR = 50) induced by the resulting hypertension resulted in an EFx reduction to 70 percent, producing a large LVEDV of 133 ml in spite of the fact that the pulmonary reservoir blood volume (DV) was reduced to 273 ml (147 ml/m^2) from an expected level of 372 ml. This combination of unfavorable force-velocity relationship factors forced the patient to function at a less than optimal position near the flat portion of a depressed Starling–Sarnoff relationship. In spite of the low CO, the cardiac work was also increased to 8.1 kg/M/min and the index of myocardial oxygen consumption was also elevated to nearly three times control ($M\dot{V}O_2 = 414$ kg/M · sec^{-1}/min).

Simply achieving vasodilatation through the use of thorazine (Fig. 9-41B), permitted a fall in the vascular resistance to 493 dyn/sec/ cm^{-5} and a reduction in the BP to 108/56 with a mean of 72 mmHg. The heart rate rose to 100 and the EFx increased to an expected A state level of 85 percent without the use of cardiac inotropic agents. Vasodilatation with afterload reduction allowed the patient to accept the necessary volume infusion with an increase in the cardiac output to 11.7 L/min (CI = 6.25 L/min/m^2) and while the $M\dot{V}O_2$ also rose to 616 kg/M · sec^{-1}/min, this 150 percent increase

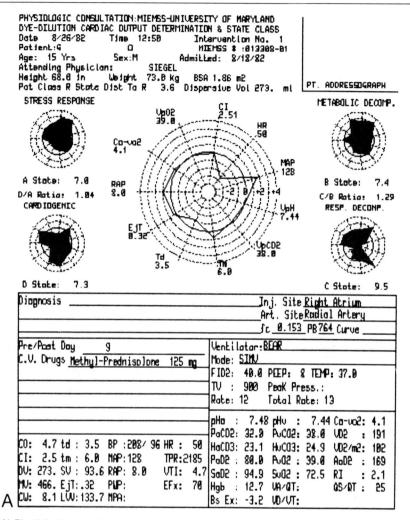

```
PHYSIOLOGIC CONSULTATION:MIEMSS-UNIVERSITY OF MARYLAND
DYE-DILUTION CARDIAC OUTPUT DETERMINATION & STATE CLASS
Date  8/26/82    Time 12:58    Intervention No.  1
Patient:G            Q         MIEMSS # :013308-01
Age:  15 Yrs     Sex:M         Admitted: 8/18/82
Attending Physician:       SIEGEL
Height 68.0 in    Weight  73.0 kg   BSA 1.86 m2
Pat Class R State Dist To R  3.6  Dispersive Vol 273. ml
                                                          PT. ADDRESSOGRAPH
     STRESS RESPONSE              CI            METABOLIC DECOMP.
                      VpO2       2.51
                      39.0            HR
                                      50
              Co-vo2                          MAP
              4.1                             128

  A State:  7.0      RAP               VpH         B State:  7.4
  D/A Ratio: 1.04    8.0               7.44        C/B Ratio: 1.29
     CARDIOGENIC                                    RESP. DECOMP.
                     EJT                 VpCO2
                     0.32                38.0
                  Td          TW
                  3.5         6.0
  D State:  7.3                                    C State:  9.5
```

Diagnosis _____	Inj. Site _Right Atrium_
	Art. Site _Radial Artery_
	_fc_ _0.153_ PB _764_ Curve _____

Pre/Post Day 9	Ventilator:_BEAR_
C.V. Drugs _Methyl-Prednisolone 125 mg_	Mode: SIMV
	FIO2: 40.0 PEEP: 8 TEMP: 37.0
	TV : 900 Peak Press.:
	Rate: 12 Total Rate: 13

	pHa : 7.48 pHv : 7.44 Co-vo2: 4.1
	PaCO2: 32.0 PvCO2: 38.0 VO2 : 191
	HaCO3: 23.1 HvCO3: 24.9 VO2/m2: 102
CO: 4.7 td : 3.5 BP :208/ 96 HR : 50	PaO2: 80.0 PvO2 : 39.0 AoO2 : 169
CI: 2.5 tm : 6.0 MAP:128 TPR:2185	SaO2: 94.9 SvO2 : 72.5 RI : 2.1
DV: 273. SV : 93.6 RAP: 8.0 VTI: 4.7	Hgb : 12.7 VA/QT: QS/QT: 25
MV: 466. EjT:.32 PLP: EFx: 70	Bs Ex: -3.2 VD/VT:
CW: 8.1 LW:133.7 MPA:	

A

FIG. 9-41 (A) Physiologic consultation on 15-year-old male admitted with a fractured pelvis, ruptured spleen, ruptured aorta, fractured humerus, and spinal cord contusion. Study performed after repair of the aorta, splenectomy, and external fixation of fractures, but prior to the administration of a vasodilator agent. (*Figure continues.*)

was much less than the 250 percent rise in CI.

The net result of this increased body flow response was to allow oxygen consumption ($\dot{V}O_2/m^2$) to rise from its previous low value of 102 ml/min/m² during vasoconstriction (Fig. 9-41A) to a more normal value for age of 179 ml/min/m² under the stress circumstances (Fig. 9-41B). The reduced $\dot{V}O_2$ of 102 ml/min/m² represents an estimated rate of oxygen deficit of 1.66 ml/kg/min and is reflected by the base deficit of −3.2 mEq/L. When $\dot{V}O_2$ rose to a more normal level of 4.58 ml/kg/min, which may still be less than required by this specific patient, the base deficit was reduced to −1.9 mEq/L.

As the outflow resistance was lowered, the patient was able to accommodate a larger pulmonary reservoir blood volume (DV = 353 ml or 190 ml/m²) at lower right atrial and pulmonary wedge pressures with essentially no increase in LVEDV because the afterload reduction permitted an increased EFx 85 percent (Fig. 9-41B). This clearly demonstrates the role of simple vasodilatation alone in the patient with high afterload, without myocardial depression (patient #013308), compared with the additional need for nonvasoconstrictor β-adrenergic inotropic support in the patient with intrinsic myocardial depression (patient #016907).

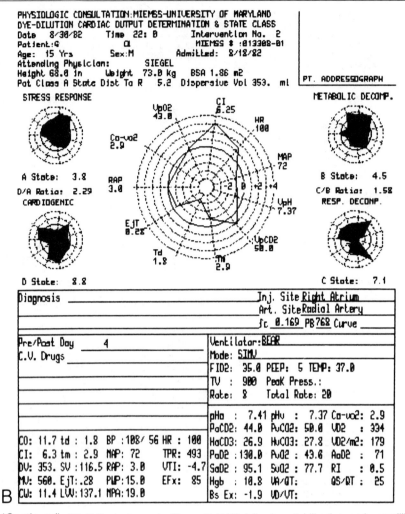

PHYSIOLOGIC CONSULTATION:MIEMSS-UNIVERSITY OF MARYLAND
DYE-DILUTION CARDIAC OUTPUT DETERMINATION & STATE CLASS
Date   8/30/82   Time 22: 0   Intervention No. 2
Patient:G   G   MIEMSS # :013308-01
Age: 15 Yrs   Sex:M   Admitted: 8/12/82
Attending Physician: SIEGEL
Height 68.0 in   Weight 73.0 kg   BSA 1.86 m2
Pat Class A State Dist To R   5.2 Dispersive Vol 353. ml   PT. ADDRESSOGRAPH

STRESS RESPONSE   METABOLIC DECOMP.

A State: 3.8   RAP   B State: 4.5
D/A Ratio: 2.29   3.0   C/B Ratio: 1.58
CARDIOGENIC   RESP. DECOMP.

D State: 8.8   C State: 7.1

Diagnosis	Inj. Site Right Atrium
	Art. Site Radial Artery
	ƒc 0.169 PB 768 Curve

Pre/Post Day 4	Ventilator:BEAR
C.V. Drugs	Mode: SIMV
	FIO2: 35.0 PEEP: 5 TEMP: 37.0
	TV : 900 Peak Press.:
	Rate: 8 Total Rate: 20

	pHa : 7.41	pHv : 7.37	Ca-vo2: 2.9
	PaCO2: 44.0	PvCO2: 50.0	VO2 : 334
CO: 11.7 td : 1.8 BP :108/ 56 HR : 100	HaCO3: 26.9	HvCO3: 27.8	VO2/m2: 179
CI: 6.3 tm : 2.9 MAP: 72 TPR: 493	PaO2 :130.0	PvO2 : 43.6	AaO2 : 71
DV: 353. SV :116.5 RAP: 3.0 VTI: -4.7	SaO2 : 95.1	SvO2 : 77.7	RI : 0.5
MV: 560. EjT:.28 PUP:15.0 EFx: 85	Hgb : 10.8	VA/QT:	QS/QT : 25
CW: 11.4 LVW:137.1 MPA:19.0	Bs Ex: -1.9	VD/VT:	

FIG. 9-41 (*Continued*) (**B**) Patient shown in Figure 9-41(A) following stabilization and vasodilitation with thorazine and administration of appropriate intravascular volume. See text for details.

Hypovolemia with Preexisting Myocardial Disease and Excessive Vasoconstriction (Decreased Preload, Reduced Vmax and Increased Afterload)

The use of these two types of agents (vasodilators and β-adrenergic inotropic drugs) in combination is often necessary when direct myocardial contusion and excessive vasoconstriction are both features of the patient's clinical course. However, the use of continuous vasodilatation and inotropic therapy is also indicated in the older patient, in whom there may be preexisting intrinsic myocardial disease prior to the acute traumatic insult, or other acute myocardial depressant factor. This use is shown in a patient (RJ#014016), a 53-year-old man with a previous history of myocardial infarction with clinically important myocardial dysfunction requiring chronic digitalization. This patient sustained an industrial accident with a severe crushing injury to the pelvis and left lower extremity. A major branch of the internal iliac artery was torn and required an-

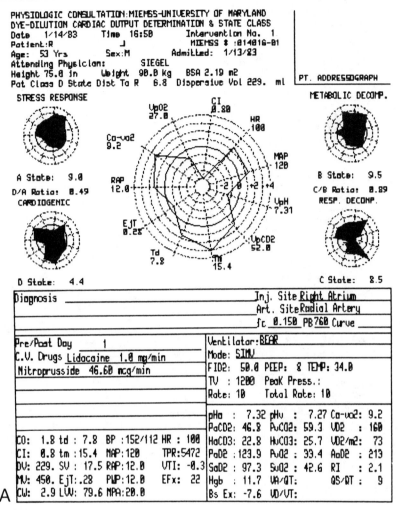

FIG. 9-42 (A) Physiologic consultation in 53-year-old male with previous history of myocardial infarction following major crushing injury of the pelvis and left lower extremity. Patient had ventricular arrhythmias and inappropriate hypertension due to excessive vasoconstriction and was maintained on low-dose nitroprusside, 0.5 mcg/kg/min and lidocaine 1.0 mg/min. (*Figure continues.*)

giographic embolization. However, there was extensive retroperitoneal and pelvic hemorrhage before arterial control. There was no chest trauma of any sort and no evidence that the patient had sustained a second acute myocardial infarction during the immediate postinjury period, based on CPK-MB studies and continuing ECG study. While no previous cardiovascular study during the preinjury period exists, this patient's immediate postresuscitation and post arterial embolization pattern of response is shown in Figure 9-42A. This demonstrates a marked hypovolemia (DV = 229 ml instead of an expected 438 ml) and an inappropriate vasoconstrictive response that enabled the patient to sustain a BP of 152/112 with a mean of 120 mmHg, in spite of a CO reduced to 1.8 L/min (CI = 0.8 L/min/m²). The excessive peripheral vascular resistance of 5,472 dyn/sec/cm⁻⁵ produced a compounding insult to the already damaged myocardium with a reduction in EFx to only 22 percent, at a relatively normal heart rate of 100 bpm. The lack of usefulness of the Swan–Ganz pulmonary wedge or right

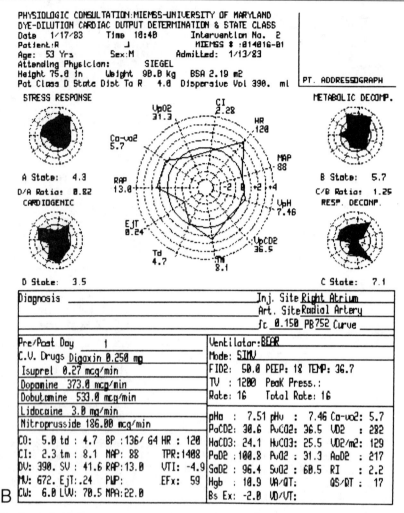

PHYSIOLOGIC CONSULTATION:MIEMSS-UNIVERSITY OF MARYLAND
DYE-DILUTION CARDIAC OUTPUT DETERMINATION & STATE CLASS
Date 1/17/83   Time 18:48   Intervention No. 2
Patient:R   J   MIEMSS # :014016-81
Age: 53 Yrs   Sex:M   Admitted: 1/13/83
Attending Physician: SIEGEL
Height 75.0 in   Weight 90.0 kg   BSA 2.19 m2
Pot Class D State Dist To R   4.0   Dispersive Vol 390. ml

PT. ADDRESSOGRAPH

STRESS RESPONSE

METABOLIC DECOMP.

A State: 4.3
D/A Ratio: 0.82
CARDIOGENIC

B State: 5.7
C/B Ratio: 1.25
RESP. DECOMP.

D State: 3.5

C State: 7.1

Diagnosis	Inj. Site Right Atrium
	Art. Site Radial Artery
	fc 0.150 PB 752 Curve

Pre/Post Day 1	Ventilator: BEAR
C.V. Drugs Digoxin 0.250 mg	Mode: SIMV
Isuprel 0.27 mcg/min	FIO2: 50.0 PEEP: 18 TEMP: 36.7
Dopamine 373.0 mcg/min	TV : 1200 Peak Press.:
Dobutamine 533.0 mcg/min	Rate: 16 Total Rate: 16
Lidocaine 3.0 mg/min	
Nitroprusside 186.00 mcg/min	pHa : 7.51 pHv : 7.46 Ca-vo2: 5.7
CO: 5.0 td : 4.7 BP :136/ 64 HR : 120	PaCO2: 30.6 PvCO2: 36.5 VO2 : 282
CI: 2.3 tm : 8.1 MAP: 88 TPR:1408	HaCO3: 24.1 HvCO3: 25.5 VO2/m2: 129
DV: 390. SV : 41.6 RAP:13.0 VTI: -4.9	PaO2 :100.8 PvO2 : 31.3 AaO2 : 217
MV: 672. EjT:.24 PWP: EFx: 59	SaO2 : 96.4 SvO2 : 60.5 RI : 2.2
CW: 6.0 LW: 70.5 MPA:22.0	Hgb : 10.9 VA/QT: QS/QT: 17
	Bs Ex: -2.0 VD/VT:

B

FIG. 9-42 *(Continued)* **(B)** Patient shown previously in Figure 9-42(A) following multiple dose inotropic support: digitalization with maintenance at 0.25 mg digoxin, isoproterenol 0.27 mcg/min, dopamine 4 mcg/kg/min, and dobutamine 6 mcg/kg/min; lidocaine has been increased to 3.0 mg/min and the nitroprusside vasodilitation to 2.0 mcg/kg/min permitting the administration of needed volume support and an increase in cardiac output. *(Figure continues.)*

atrial pressures in determining the severity of myocardial depression is shown in this patient in whom right atrial pressure and pulmonary wedge pressure were only 12 mmHg, in spite of increased blood pressure, at a time when the CI was reduced nearly 4 SD below normal because the hypovolemia had reduced ventricular filling. The magnitude of this hypodynamic response and its metabolic consequences are better seen in the marked reduction of oxygen consumption ($\dot{V}O_2/m^2$) to

73 ml/min/m² and the severe metabolic acidosis with a mixed venous pH of 7.27. This represents an estimated oxygen deficit of 1.53 ml/kg/min based on the age expected mean $\dot{V}O_2$ of 3.31 ml/kg/min (Table 9-1) for this patient. As a result of this large oxygen deficit, the base deficit was −7.6 mEq/L.

At this level of reduced preload, pulmonary reservoir volume (DV = 229 ml or 105 ml/m²), the reduced myocardial contractility was unable to overcome the excessive reflex vaso-

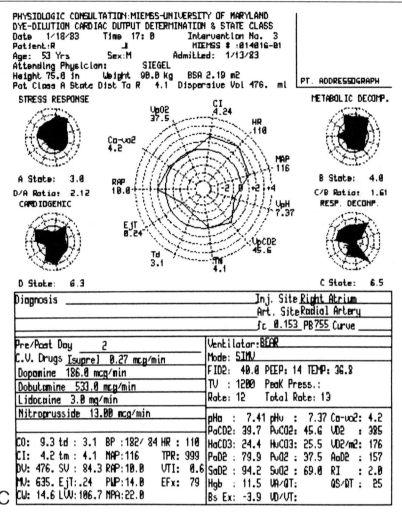

PHYSIOLOGIC CONSULTATION:MIEMSS-UNIVERSITY OF MARYLAND
DYE-DILUTION CARDIAC OUTPUT DETERMINATION & STATE CLASS
Date 1/18/83   Time 17: 0   Intervention No. 3
Patient:R   J   MIEMSS # :014016-01
Age: 53 Yrs   Sex:M   Admitted: 1/13/83
Attending Physician: SIEGEL
Height 75.0 in   Weight 98.0 Kg   BSA 2.19 m2
Pat Class A State Dist To R 4.1 Dispersive Vol 476. ml

PT. ADDRESSOGRAPH

STRESS RESPONSE

A State: 3.0
D/A Ratio: 2.12
CARDIOGENIC

D State: 6.3

VpO2 37.5
Co-vo2 4.2
RAP 10.0
CI 4.24
HR 110
MAP 116
VpH 7.37
EjT 0.24
Td 3.1
Tm 4.1
VpCO2 45.6

METABOLIC DECOMP.

B State: 4.0
C/B Ratio: 1.61
RESP. DECOMP.

C State: 6.5

Diagnosis		Inj. Site Right Atrium
		Art. Site Radial Artery
		ʃc 0.153 PB 755 Curve

Pre/Post Day 2		Ventilator: BEAR
C.V. Drugs Isuprel 0.27 mcg/min		Mode: SIMV
Dopamine 186.0 mcg/min		FIO2: 40.0 PEEP: 14 TEMP: 36.8
Dobutamine 533.0 mcg/min		TV : 1200 Peak Press.:
Lidocaine 3.0 mg/min		Rate: 12 Total Rate: 13
Nitroprusside 13.00 mcg/min		

pHa : 7.41	pHv : 7.37	Ca-vo2: 4.2
PaCO2: 39.7	PvCO2: 45.6	VO2 : 385
HaCO3: 24.4	HvCO3: 25.5	VO2/m2: 176
PaO2: 79.9	PvO2: 37.5	AaO2: 157
SaO2: 94.2	SvO2: 69.0	RI : 2.0
Hgb : 11.5	VA/QT:	QS/QT : 25
Bs Ex: -3.9	VD/VT:	

C

CO: 9.3 td : 3.1	BP :182/ 84	HR : 110
CI: 4.2 tm : 4.1	MAP:116	TPR: 999
DV: 476. SV : 84.3	RAP:10.0	VTI: 0.6
MV: 635. EjT:.24	PLP:14.0	EFx: 79
CW: 14.6 LVW:106.7	NPA:22.0	

FIG. 9-42 (*Continued*) (C) Patient shown previously in Figures 9-40(A) and (B) on continued maintenance with multiple-dose inotropic support and volume restitution now maintaining A-state response with adequate oxygen consumption ($\dot{V}O_2$/m²) increased from 73 ml/min [9-42(A)] to 176 ml/min. This has permitted reduction in the level of dopamine to 2 mcg/kg/min, without change in dobutamine, and a reduction in nitroprusside to 0.14 mcg/kg/min, as volume has been increased with sustained reduction in peripheral vascular resistance. See text for details.

constriction-induced afterload. In spite of the use of nitroprusside (46 μg/min), the EFx was only 22 percent, producing a 17.5-ml stroke volume, even though LVEDV was nearly normal (LVV = 79.6 ml). Over a several-day period of support (Fig. 9-42B) using β-adrenergic inotropic agents including isoproterenol (0.27 μg/min total body dose), dopamine (4.1 μg/kg/min), dobutamine (5.9 μg/kg/min), and digitalization, as well as an increased level of nitro-

prusside (186 μg/min) as a vosodilator agent, the vascular resistance was reduced to 1408 dyn/sec/cm⁻⁵, and the CO increased to 5.0 L/min (CI = 2.28 L/min/m²). The flow increase resulted in an initial increase of oxygen consumption to 129 ml/min/m² with a large correction of the oxygen deficit and the metabolic acidosis was reduced to a base deficit of −2.0 mEq/L (Fig. 9-42B).

As the myocardium regained its contractility over a four day period, it was possible to reduce both the rate of nitroprusside (13 μg/min) as well as that of dopamine (2.1 μg/kg/min) infusion, while still maintaining the pure β-adrenergic inotropic support with isoproterenol and dobutamine (Fig. 9-42C). This resulted in an increase in CO to 9.3 L/min (CI = 4.2 L/min/m²) at a vascular resistance of 999 dyn/sec/cm⁻⁵. The heart rate fell in spite of the potential chronatropic activity of these agents, and blood pressure rose to 182/84, which approached the patient's recorded preinjury values with a MAP of 116 mmHg. With the combination of inotropic support and vasodilation as DV was increased by volume infusion to 476 ml, the right atrial pressure actually was decreased (compared both to the initial hypo-

perfusion cardiogenic D state as well as to the studies done during recovery from cardiogenic decompensation).

Figure 9-43 shows the Starling–Sarnoff ventricular function relationships for the three patients presented above. These data show that a somewhat different therapeutic strategy was salutory in each instance, depending on the specific pathophysiologic features. In the 15-year-old trauma victim with an excessive vasoconstrictor response but only slight contractility reduction, the reflex bradycardia and low EFx together produced a dilated heart (large LVEDV) able to maintain a relatively normal, although not adequate CO. By vasodilitation alone, the afterload was reduced and the heart rate and EFx increased, so that the

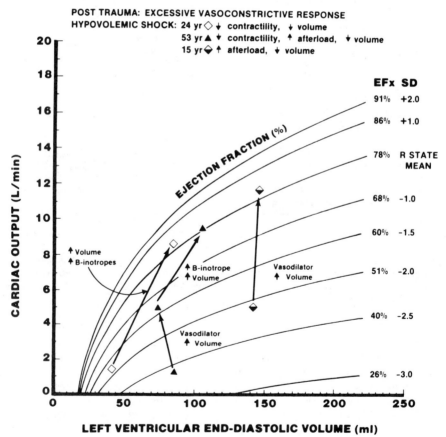

FIG. 9-43 Ventricular function relationships for 3 patients presented in Figures 9-40, 9-41, and 9-42 showing relative changes brought about by alterations in contractility and afterload in response to volume and inotropic support. See legend for Figure 9-31. See text for details.

patient was able to increase the CO at the relatively large LVEDV required by the volume infusion needed to correct the volume deficit.

In the 24-year-old with severe posttraumatic myocardial depression, major blood loss hypovolemia and increased vascular tone, the relative role of the diminished contractility with a markedly reduced EFx appeared most important. In this case, a major therapeutic thrust with nonvasoconstricting β-adrenergic inotropic agents enabled the patient to accept the required volume infusion and to increase CO by virtue of a large increase in EFx, even though LVEDV also rose to more normal levels. As flow increased, the reflex vasoconstriction decreased.

In the 53-year-old hypovolemic shock patient with previous myocardial disease, the added myocardial depression induced by a period of low flow shock made it impossible for this patient to overcome his vasoconstrictor afterload. Consequently, he required the use of a large dose of a major vasodilator agent (nitroprusside) in combination with increased doses of β-adrenergic inotropic agents just to permit him to accept volume infusion without developing acute pulmonary edema. This therapy allowed a shift to a more effective ventricular function relationship with a more normal ejection fraction. By permitting an increase in the cardiac ejection fraction to 79 percent, this in turn allowed him to accommodate to a normal pulmonary reservoir volume with only a small increase in the LVEDV. The CO then rose to a normal stress response A state level, which resulted in an acceptable body perfusion to a needed $\dot{V}O_2$ of 4.28 ml/kg/min ($\dot{V}O_2/m^2 = 176$ ml/min/m²), to repay the oxygen debt.

Refractory Myocardial Contractile Failure and Hypovolemia without Vasoconstriction (Reduced Vmax, Decreased Preload and Afterload)

The presence of a persistent low-flow syndrome due to the combination of volume deficit and myocardial failure ($\downarrow$Vmax), in spite of a reduced vascular tone response (decreased afterload), prevents the hypovolemic patient from accepting volume infusion (preload) without manifesting acute heart failure and pulmonary congestion. This is a not-uncommon consequence of a severe posttraumatic or postsurgical shock episode wherein a period of myocardial hypoxemia is complicated by subsequent acute myocardial infarction or sepsis. Often these patients have had a previous history of documented cardiac disease or are in the older age range, in which chronic occult myocardial ischemic disease is common. Not infrequently, the patient also has an associated ARDS or pulmonary congestion, which further limits oxygen delivery. Under these circumstances, the patient manifests persistent hypotension, low CI, and reduced $\dot{V}O_2$ with the maintenance of an increased PWP and RAP in spite of a low pulmonary reservoir volume (DV) and a decreased LVEDV. This pattern may be only minimally improved by β-adrenergic inotropic agents and/or digoxin; the critical level of arterial perfusion pressure and reduced venous capacitance volume makes it dangerous to use vasodilator agents, which would not be expected to have much effect anyway, since vascular resistance (afterload) is generally low.

In this setting, the addition of mechanical diastolic flow augmentation by the use of intraaortic balloon counter pulsation (IABP) can have a salutory effect, especially if combined with vasodilating β-adrenergic agents, and possibly in the future by the adjunctive use of PDE III-inhibiting agents such as amrinone. An example of the combined use of IABP with β-adrenergic support is shown in Figure 9-44.

This patient (HK#017823) was a 60-year-old man who sustained a major pelvic fracture with massive retroperitoneal hemorrhage, a splenic disruption requiring splenectomy, pulmonary contusion, and a closed head injury with facial fractures. Postinjury, his clinical course slowly worsened as his ARDS, complicated by bronchopneumonia, increased with increasing pulmonary venoarterial admixture ($\dot{Q}S/\dot{Q}T = 20\%$), A-aO₂/PaO₂ (RI = 3.6) and a rising PaCO₂ (44 mmHg) with both metabolic and respiratory acidosis (pHv = 7.25, base excess −10.4 mEq/L) (see Fig. 9-44A).

From a hemodynamic point of view, in spite

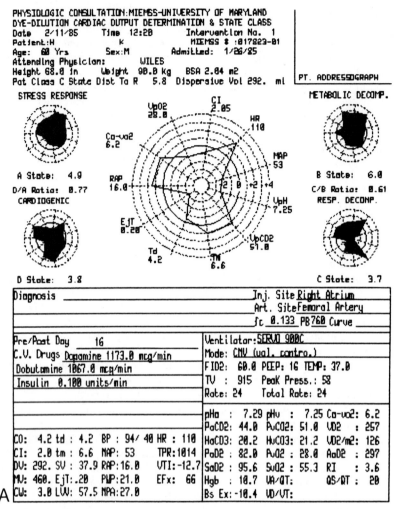

FIG. 9-44 **(A)** Physiologic consultation in 60-year-old male following major pelvic fracture with massive retroperitoneal hemorrhage, splenic disruption requiring splenectomy, pulmonary contusion, and closed head injury. Patient developed ARDS, complicated by pulmonary sepsis; patient persistently hypotensive with low cardiac output in spite of support with dopamine 13 mcg/kg/min and dobutamine 12 mcg/kg/min, with low oxygen consumption and severe myocardial depression. (*Figure continues.*)

of continuous dopamine (13 μg/kg/min) and dobutamine (12 μg/kg/min), the patient was persistently hypotensive with an arterial blood pressure of 94/40 mmHg and an MAP of 53 mmHg. The EFx was only 66 percent, indicating a severe myocardial depression with cardiogenic D state and respiratory C state decompensation. He had a persistently low CI of 2.0 L/min/m² at a high RAP and PWP (due in part to the need for 16 cm PEEP and high ventilatory pressures), even though his pulmonary reservoir blood volume was only 292 ml (reduced from an expected 408 ml) and the LVEDV was also reduced (LVV = 57.5 ml). As a result, the body oxygen consumption ($\dot{V}O_2/m^2$) was limited to 126 ml/min/m² (2.86 ml/kg/min), with an estimated age corrected oxygen deficit of 0.50 ml/kg/min. The vascular resistance (TPR = 1014) was low for the level of flow due to a reduction in vascular tone (VTI = −12.7); as a result, while total flow and cardiac minute work (CW = 3.0 Kg/M/min) were reduced, the

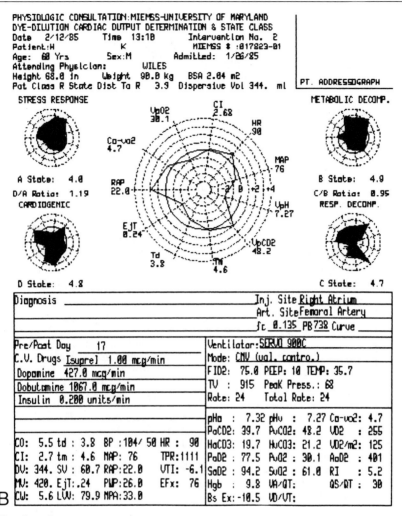

```
PHYSIOLOGIC CONSULTATION:MIEMSS-UNIVERSITY OF MARYLAND
DYE-DILUTION CARDIAC OUTPUT DETERMINATION & STATE CLASS
Date  2/12/85    Time  13:10    Intervention No.  2
Patient:H         K            MIEMSS # :017823-01
Age:  60 Yrs      Sex:M         Admitted: 1/26/85
Attending Physician:      WILES
Height 68.0 in    Weight  90.0 kg    BSA 2.04 m2
Pat Class R State Dist To R   3.9  Dispersive Vol 344. ml
```

PT. ADDRESSOGRAPH

STRESS RESPONSE

METABOLIC DECOMP.

CARDIOGENIC

RESP. DECOMP.

A State: 4.0
D/A Ratio: 1.19
D State: 4.8

B State: 4.9
C/B Ratio: 0.95
C State: 4.7

VpO2 30.1
Co-vo2 4.7
CI 2.68
HR 90
MAP 76
RAP 22.0
VpH 7.27
EJT 0.24
Td 3.8
TM 4.6
VpCO2 48.2

Diagnosis	Inj. Site Right Atrium
	Art. Site Femoral Artery
	Jc 0.135 PB 738 Curve

Pre/Post Day 17	Ventilator: SERVO 900C
C.V. Drugs Isuprel 1.00 mcg/min	Mode: CMV (vol. contro.)
Dopamine 427.0 mcg/min	FIO2: 75.0 PEEP: 10 TEMP: 35.7
Dobutamine 1067.0 mcg/min	TV : 915 PeaK Press.: 68
Insulin 0.200 units/min	Rate: 24 Total Rate: 24

	pHa : 7.32 pHv : 7.27 Co-vo2: 4.7
	PaCO2: 39.7 PvCO2: 48.2 VO2 : 255
CO: 5.5 td : 3.8 BP :104/ 50 HR : 90	HaCO3: 19.7 HvCO3: 21.2 VO2/m2: 125
CI: 2.7 tm : 4.6 MAP: 76 TPR:1111	PaO2 : 77.5 PvO2 : 30.1 AaDO2 : 401
DV: 344. SV : 60.7 RAP:22.0 VTI: -6.1	SaO2 : 94.2 SvO2 : 61.0 RI : 5.2
MV: 420. EjT:.24 PWP:26.0 EFx: 76	Hgb : 9.8 VA/QT: QS/QT : 30
B CW: 5.6 LVW: 79.9 RPA:33.0	Bs Ex: -10.5 VD/VT:

FIG. 9-44 (*Continued*) **(B)** Patient shown in Figure 9-44(A), following the introduction of intra-aortic balloon counter pulsation (IABP), low dose isoproterenol added at 1 mcg/min with a reduction of the vasoconstricting inotropic agent dopamine to 4.7 mcg/kg/min, and continuation of dobutamine at 12 mcg/kg/min. IABP followed by an increase in cardiac output and rise in mean blood pressure. (*Figure continues.*)

$M\dot{V}O_2$ index was slightly above the R state normal (196 kg/M · sec^{-1}/min) because of the increased heart rate.

The inability to support the failing circulation in this patient by inotropic agents and volume infusion resulted in the decision to add IABP (Fig. 9-44B). Within 24 hours, this modality of therapy combined with low-dose isoproterenol (1.0 μg/min total dose) enabled the CI to rise to 2.7 L/min/m² as EFx increased to 76 percent, even though the dopamine was reduced from 13.0 to 5.3 μg/kg/min. The patient

was able to accept a somewhat increased volume infusion (DV = 344 ml), and LVEDV rose (LVV = 79.9 ml), permitting a larger stroke volume (60.7 ml). However, this flow increase was not sufficient to increase $\dot{V}O_2$/m², which remained low at 125 ml/min/m² (2.83 ml/kg/min) with a persistent O_2 deficit of 0.53 ml/kg/min. The base deficit remained at −10.5 mEq/L, and respiratory insufficiency due to the septic posttraumatic ARDS also worsened as $\dot{Q}S/\dot{Q}T$ rose to 30 percent and the RI increased to 5.2.

As a result, IABP was continued and com-

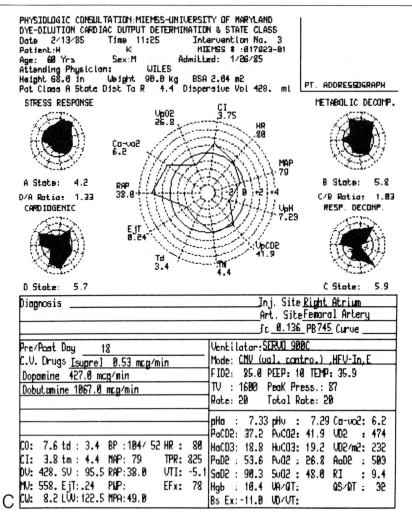

PHYSIOLOGIC CONSULTATION:MIEMSS-UNIVERSITY OF MARYLAND
DYE-DILUTION CARDIAC OUTPUT DETERMINATION & STATE CLASS
Date 2/13/85   Time 11:25   Intervention No.   3
Patient:H   K   MIEMSS # :017823-01
Age: 60 Yrs   Sex:M   Admitted: 1/26/85
Attending Physician: WILES
Height 68.0 in   Weight 98.0 kg   BSA 2.04 m2
Pat Class A State Dist To R   4.4 Dispersive Vol 428. ml

PT. ADDRESSOGRAPH

STRESS RESPONSE

A State: 4.2
D/A Ratio: 1.33

CARDIOGENIC

D State: 5.7

VpO2 26.8
Co-vo2 6.2
RAP 38.0
EJT 0.24
Td 3.4

CI 3.75
HR 80
MAP 79
VpH 7.29
VpCO2 41.9
Tm 4.4

METABOLIC DECOMP.

B State: 5.8
C/B Ratio: 1.03

RESP. DECOMP.

C State: 5.9

Diagnosis _____	Inj. Site Right Atrium
	Art. Site Femoral Artery
	fc 0.136 PB 745 Curve ___

Pre/Post Day 18	Ventilator: SERVO 900C
C.V. Drugs Isuprel 0.53 mcg/min	Mode: CNV (val. contro.) ,HFV-In,E
Dopamine 427.0 mcg/min	FIO2: 85.0 PEEP: 10 TEMP: 35.9
Dobutamine 1067.0 mcg/min	TV : 1600 Peak Press.: 87
	Rate: 20 Total Rate: 20

	pHa : 7.33 pHv : 7.29 Co-vo2: 6.2
	PaCO2: 37.2 PvCO2: 41.9 VO2 : 474
CO: 7.6 td : 3.4 BP :104/ 52 HR : 80	HaCO3: 18.8 HvCO3: 19.2 VO2/m2: 232
CI: 3.8 tm : 4.4 MAP: 79 TPR: 825	PaO2 : 53.6 PvO2 : 26.8 AaDO2 : 503
DV: 428. SV : 95.5 RAP:38.0 VTI: -5.1	SaO2 : 90.3 SvO2 : 48.0 RI : 9.4
MV: 558. EjT:.24 PLP: EFx: 78	Hgb : 10.4 VA/QT: QS/QT : 32
CW: 8.2 LW:122.5 MPA:49.0	Bs Ex:-11.0 VD/VT:

C

FIG. 9-44 (*Continued*) (**C**) Continuation of IABP support with addition of combined high-frequency ventilation (CHFV) to compensate for ARDS permitting improvement in cardiac output with rise in $\dot{V}O_2$ and use of reduced levels of inotropic support, as patient is now able to accept slightly larger volume infusion and achieve more adequate body perfusion. (*Figure continues.*)

bined high-frequency ventilation (CHFV) (see Chapter 19) was added (Fig. 9-44C) in order to lower $PaCO_2$ and to compensate for the progressive ARDS-induced respiratory failure. The continuing IABP diastolic augmentation permitted the myocardial function to compensate further in spite of the very severe respiratory and metabolic acidosis. The CI rose to 3.8 L/min/m² (CO = 7.6 L/min), EFx increased further to 78% and as a consequence of the increased inotropic response a more adequate volume balance could be achieved and DV rose to 428 ml while LVEDV increased (LVV = 122.5 ml). The resultant increase in body perfusion caused an increase in $\dot{V}O_2$/m² from 125 to 232 ml/min/m² (5.27 ml/kg/min) with an estimated oxygen deficit payback of 1.91 ml/kg/min.

Continued IABP (Fig. 9-44D) stabilized the CI at 3.4 L/min/m² (CO = 6.8 L/min) and EFx (74 percent), with an adequate $\dot{V}O_2$/m² for age of 142 ml/min/m² (3.22 ml/kg/min) at lower β-adrenergic drug support. The LVEDV remained high (LVV = 115.6 ml) and with the CHFV the better myocardial function allowed

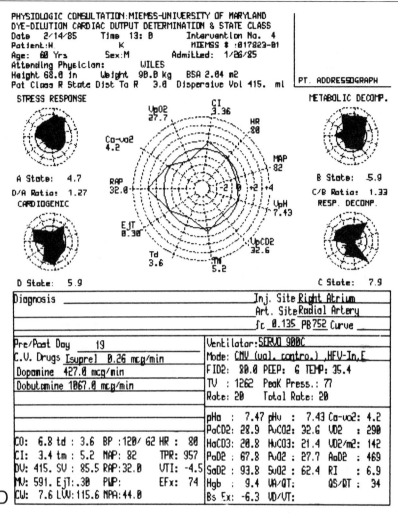

FIG. 9-44 (*Continued*) (**D**) Patient shown in 9-44 (A), (B), and (C) with continuation of IABP support and CHFV ventilation. Stability of cardiac index and $\dot{V}O_2$ at functionally acceptable levels with lessening of base deficit. See text for details.

a partial compensation for the ARDS even though the $\dot{Q}S/\dot{Q}T$ (34 percent) and RI (6.9) remained high. Arterial pH rose (pH = 7.47), and the base deficit was improved (−6.3 mEq/L) as respiratory compensation, with reduced $PaCO_2$ was produced by CHFV and the sustained high pulmonary blood flow (CO = 6.8 L/min). Stroke power per minute, the index of estimated $M\dot{V}O_2$, rose to 274 kg/M · sec^{-1}/min, but this increase was less (140 percent) than the increase in CI (164 percent). By virtue of the IABP unloading effect, it was also less than would have been expected for this level of flow

increase, if achieved by inotropic support and volume alone. Although the ultimate outcome for this patient after removal from IABP was not successful, because of the progressive septic ARDS with eventual cardiorespiratory arrest, this case does make the point that the addition of IABP to a program of nonvasoconstrictor inotropic support can achieve cardiovascular compensation at reduced inotropic drug dose levels, in order to buy time for other therapeutic maneuvers to have a chance to be successful.

A more satisfactory outcome to IABP is

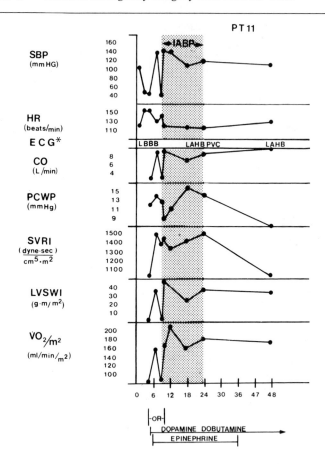

FIG. 9-45 Time course of a 43-year-old man with acute posttraumatic myocardial contusion associated with grade III hepatic laceration who developed low output syndrome during surgery. When cardiac output and hemodynamic parameters became refractory to inotropic support during surgery, IABP was begun allowing cardiovascular stability to be maintained with gradual weaning of inotropic support. SBP (systolic blood pressure), PCWP (pulmonary capillary wedge pressure), SVRI (systemic vascular resistance index), LVSWI (left ventricular stroke work index). LBBB (left bundle branch block), LAHB (left anterior hemi block), PVC (premature vent. contraction). See text for details. (Flancbaum L, Wright J, Siegel JH: Emergency surgery in patients with posttraumatic myocardial contusion. J Trauma 1986, in press.)

usually possible when a non septic refractory myocardial decompensation is the main cause of circulatory shock. This is shown in Figure 9-45 for a 43-year-old man with acute posttraumatic myocardial contusion who developed low output syndrome during surgery to control grade III hepatic lacerations.[43] After intraoperative volume infusion he became refractory to inotropic support. IABP was begun with an increase in CI and circulatory stabilization with full recovery.

CONCLUSION

The management of low-flow shock states induced by hypovolemia or primary myocardial failure requires precise bedside diagnosis of the causes and physiologic magnitude of the resultant low-flow state. The relative role of the factors that influence cardiac performance, as expressed in the myocardial force–velocity relationship, must be addressed and a therapeutic program tailored to the particular patient's quantitative set of physiologic abnormalities must be instituted. Ultimately, in nonseptic forms of circulatory instability, the test of successful shock resolution is reflected in the return of oxygen consumption to normal stress-response levels and the abolition of substantial metabolic base deficits, which indicate a mismatch between required oxygen delivery and cellular needs. It is critical to note that time is of the essence, since cellular substrate fuel–energy metabolism is in part dependent on intact membrane and ultrastructural organization and all of these can be seriously or irreversibly altered by prolonged or severe cellular hypoxemia, as indicated in Chapters 2, 3, and 4. Hypoxic injury may result in compromised host-defense mechanisms and predispose to the development of sepsis, which in itself causes an acquired disease of intermediary metabolism with profound oxidative impairment of energy engendering fuels[144,150] (Chapter 15).

Each aspect of the patient's pathophysiology must be addressed by a coordinated program of support that emphasizes flow and oxygen delivery, rather than maintenance of arterial pressure. In order to achieve these goals, the critical care surgeon or physician must be knowledgeable of, and feel comfortable with, the use of multiple therapeutic modalities. The cardiovascular therapeutic armamentarium must include preload measures (volume infusion), cardiac inotropic agents that raise Vmax without excessively increasing myocardial oxygen consumption out of proportion to the increase in coronary perfusion, and afterload-reducing drugs that reduce cardiac work and $M\dot{V}O_2$ and enhance organ perfusion through vasodilatation. When necessary, mechanical diastolic augmentation via IABP counterpulsation may be needed early during the course of shock, in support of pharmacologic

measures. The adequacy of respiratory gas exchange by appropriate choice of mechanical ventilation measures is also a key feature of low-flow shock therapy (as discussed in Chapter 19). Finally, the proper early utilization of metabolic nutritional support may be critical in enhancing cardiac and peripheral organ function during the immediate postshock recovery period, or when the hypoxemic injury leads to a secondary septic process (Chapters 15 and 17).

The net result of all these coordinated therapies is often greater than the sum of the parts. Figure 9-46) demonstrates that on a teaching ICU service knowledgeable use of the physiologic data provided by the CARE cardiorespiratory consultation methodology (CARE-CR) to guide therapy was associated with a statistically significant ($P < 0.00006$) decrease in general surgical (including posttrauma ($P < 0.0017$)) mortality in a critical care setting, comparing pre-CARE-CR and post-CARE-CR periods. While this type of sequential study of the effect of a change in therapeutic approach over time raises a certain degree of uncertainty from

FIG. 9-46 Statistical linear logistic model showing relationship between the increased percent of surgical patients studied by physiologic consultation (CARE-CR) to the reduction in actual death rate in surgical ICU patients over a 6-year-period. From a study of 2,859 patients. The proposition that increased use of CARE-CR is a predictor of a decrease in percent surgical mortality has a P > 0.00006 and enables rejection of the Null hypothesis. These data support the value of the use of the CARE-CR studies of the patients type of compensation to injury and sepsis as a means of developing and guiding appropriate surgical and pharmacologic therapy. (Siegel JH, Cerra FB, Moody EA et al: The effect on survival of critically ill and injured patients of an ICU teaching service organized about a computer-based physiologic CARE system. J Trauma. 20: 558, 1980.)

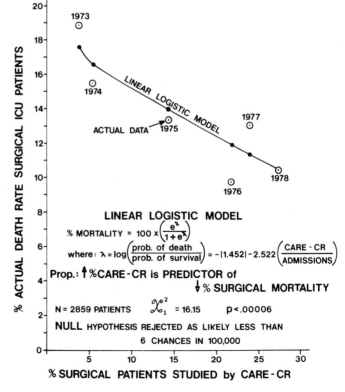

LINEAR LOGISTIC MODEL

$$\% \text{ MORTALITY} = 100 \times \left(\frac{e^{\lambda}}{1+e^{\lambda}}\right)$$

$$\text{where: } \lambda = \log\left(\frac{\text{prob. of death}}{\text{prob. of survival}}\right) = -|1.452| - 2.522\left(\frac{\text{CARE-CR}}{\text{ADMISSIONS}}\right)$$

Prop.: ↑%CARE-CR is PREDICTOR of ↓% SURGICAL MORTALITY

N = 2859 PATIENTS χ^2_1 = 16.15   p < .00006

NULL HYPOTHESIS REJECTED AS LIKELY LESS THAN 6 CHANCES IN 100,000

% ACTUAL DEATH RATE SURGICAL ICU PATIENTS

% SURGICAL PATIENTS STUDIED by CARE-CR

a statistical point of view (as discussed in Chapter 5), it nevertheless focuses attention on the likelihood that an increased availability of more precise physiologic and biochemical information, if used as the basis for therapeutic decision making, will lead to better care of the critically ill and injured surgical patient.

REFERENCES

1. Abbott BC, Mommaerts WFHM: A study of inotropic mechanisms in papillary muscle preparation. J Gen Physiol 42: 533, 1959
2. Alving BM, Hojima Y, Pisano JJ et al: Hypotension associated with prekallikrein activator (Hageman-factor fragments) in plasma protein fraction. N Engl J Med 299: 66, 1978
3. Alyono D, Ring WS, Anderson RW: The effects of hemorrhagic shock on the diastolic properties of the left ventricle in the conscious dog. Surgery 83: 691, 1978
4. Armstrong PW, Walker DC, Burton JR, Parker JO: Vasodilator therapy in acute myocardial infarction. A comparison of sodium nitroprusside and nitroglycerin. Circulation 52: 1118, 1975
5. Astrand PO, Rodahl K: Textbook of Work Physiology. McGraw-Hill, New York, 1970
6. Bendixen HH, Laver MB: Circulatory effects of thiopental sodium in dogs. Anesth Analg 41: 674, 1962
7. Bloodwell RD, Brown RC, Christenson GR et al: The effect of fluothane on myocardial contractile force in man. Anesth Analg 40: 352, 1961
8. Braunwald E, Ross J Jr, Sonnenblick EH: Mechanisms of contraction of the normal and failing heart. N Engl J Med 277: 794, 1967
9. Brigham KL, Bowers RE, McKeen CR: Methylprednisolone prevention of increased lung vascular permeability following endotoxemia in sheep. J Clin Invest 67: 1103, 1981
10. Brodie BR, Grossman W, Mann T, McLaurin LP: Effects of sodium nitroprusside on left ventricular diastolic pressure-volume relations. J Clin Invest 59: 59, 1977
11. Buda AJ, Pinsky MR, Ingels NB et al: Effect of intrathoracic pressure on left ventricular performance. N Engl J Med 301: 453, 1979
12. Burke JF: Preoperative antibiotics. Surg Clin North Am 43: 665, 1963
13. Calvin JE, Driedger AA, Sibbald WJ: The effect of phentolamine in low cardiac output syndrome as assessed by radionuclide angiography. Crit Care Med (abstr) 8: 240, 1980
14. Calvin JE, Driedger AA, Sibbald WJ: An assessment of myocardial function in human sepsis utilizing ECG gated cardiac scintigraphy. Chest 80: 579, 1981
15. Calvin JE, Driedger AA, Sibbald WJ: Does the pulmonary capillary wedge pressure predict left ventricular preload in critically ill? Crit Care Med 9: 437, 1981
16. Calvin JE, Driedger AA, Sibbald WJ: Positive end-expiratory pressure (PEEP) does not depress left ventricular function in patients with pulmonary edema. Am Rev Respir Dis 124: 121, 1981
17. Carey LC, Lowery BD, Cloutier CT: Blood sugar and insulin response of humans in shock. Ann Surg 172: 342, 1970
18. Cerra FB, Hassett J Siegel JH: Vasodilator therapy in clinical sepsis with low output syndrome. J Surg Res 25: 180, 1978
19. Chatterjee K, Parmley WW: The role of vasodilator therapy in heart failure. Prog Cardiovasc Dis 19: 301, 1977
20. Chidsey CA, Braunwald E, Morrow AG, Mason DT: Myocardial norepinephrine concentration in man: Effects of reserpine and of congestive heart failure. N Engl J Med 269: 653, 1963
21. Coleman HN III: Role of acetylstrophanthidin in augmenting myocardial oxygen consumption: Relation of increased O_2 consumption to change in velocity of contraction. Circ Res 21: 487, 1967
22. Cournand A, Riley RL, Bradley SE et al: Studies of circulation in clinical shock. Surgery 13: 964, 1943
23. Covell JW, Ross J Jr, Sonnenblick EH, Braunwald E: Comparison of the force-velocity relation and the ventricular function curve as measures of the contractile state of the intact heart. Circ Res 19: 364, 1966
24. Crowell JW: Oxygen debt as the common parameter in irreversible hemorrhagic shock. Fed Proc 20: 116, 1961.
25. Crowell JW, Ford RG, Lewis VM: Oxygen transport in hemorrhagic shock as a function of the hematocrit ratio. Am J Physiol 196: 1033, 1959
26. Crowell JW, Smith EE: Oxygen deficit and irreversible hemorrhagic shock. Am J Physiol 206(2): 313, 1964
27. Cunningham JN Jr, Shires GT, Wagner Y: Cellular transport defects in hemorrhagic shock. Surgery 70: 215, 1971
28. Cuthbertson DP: Post-shock metabolic response. Lancet 1: 433, 1942
29. Dawidson I, Haglind E, Gelin LE: Hemodilution and oxygen transport to tissue in shock. Acta Chir Scand (suppl) 489: 245, 1979

30. Diamond G, Forrester JS: Effect of coronary artery disease and acute myocardial infarction on left ventricular compliance in man. Circulation 45: 11, 1972

31. Diamond G, Forrester J, Danzig R et al: Hemodynamic effects of glucagon during acute myocardial infarction with left ventricular failure in man. Br Heart J 33: 290, 1971

32. Dodge HT, Lord JD, Sandler H: Cardiovascular effects of isoproterenol in normal subjects and subjects with congestive heart failure. Am Heart J 60: 94, 1960

33. Dodge HT, Sandler H, Ballew DW, Lord JD Jr: The use of biplane angiocardiography for the measurement of left ventricular volume in man. Am Heart J 60: 762, 1960

34. Downing SE, Siegel JH: Baroreceptor and chemoreceptor influences on sympathetic discharge to the heart. Am J Physiol 204: 471, 1963

35. Downing SE, Sonnenblick EH: Cardiac muscle mechanics and ventricular performance: Force and time parameters. Am J Physiol 207: 705, 1964

36. Downing SE, Talner NS Gardner TH: Cardiovascular responses to metabolic acidosis. Am J Physiol 208: 237, 1965

37. DuBois EF: Basal Metabolism in Health and Disease. 3rd Ed., Lea & Febiger, Philadelphia, 1936

38. Dunkman WB, Leinbach RC, Buckley MJ, et al: Clinical and hemodynamic results of intraaortic balloon pumping and surgery for cardiogenic shock. Circulation 46: 465, 1972

39. Ellis FJ, Mangano DT, VanDkye DC: Relationship of wedge pressure to end-diastolic volume in patients undergoing myocardial revascularization. J Thorac Cardiovasc Surg 78: 605, 1979

40. Epstein SE, Levey GS, Skeleton CL: Adenyl cyclase and cyclic AMP: Biochemical links in the regulation of myocardial contractility. Circulation 43: 437, 1971

41. Fine J, Frank ED, Ravin HA et al: The bacterial factor in traumatic shock. N Engl J Med 260: 214, 1959

42. Fine J: Some recent developments in the study of refractory traumatic shock. Gastroenterology, 59: 301, 1970

43. Flancbaum L, Wright J, Siegel JH: Emergency surgery in patients with posttraumatic myocardial contusion. J Trauma (in press) 1986

44. Forrester JS, Diamond GS, Parmley WW, Swann HJC: Early increase in left ventricular compliance after myocardial infarction. J Clin Invest 51: 598, 1972

45. Frank O: Zur Dynamik des Herzmuskels. Z Biol, 32: 370, 1895

46. Friedman HP, Goldwyn RM, Siegel JH: The use and interpretation of multivariate methods in the classification of stages of serious infectious disease processes in the critically ill, p 18, In Blashoff R ed: Prospectives in Biometrics. New York, Academic, 1975.

47. Gann DS, Amaral JF: Pathophysiology of trauma and shock. p. 37. In Zuidema GD, Rutherford RB, Ballinger WF (eds): The Management of Trauma. WB Saunders, Philadelphia, 1985

48. Gewetz B, O'Brien C, Kirsh, MM: Use of the intra-aortic balloon support for refractory low cardiac output in myocardial contusion. J Trauma 17: 325, 1977

49. Gilmore JP, Siegel JH: Myocardial catecholamines and ventricular performance during carotid artery occlusion. Am J Physiol 207: 672, 1964

50. Glantz SA, Parmley WW: Factors which affect the diastolic pressure-volume curve. Circ Res, 42: 171, 1978

51. Glick G, Parmley WW, Wechsler AS, Sonnenblick EH: Glucagon: Its enhancement of cardiac performance in cat and dog and persistence of its inotropic action despite beta-receptor blockade with propranolol. Circ Res, 22: 789, 1968

52. Glick G, Sonnenblick EH, Braunwald E: Myocardial force-velocity relations studied in intact unanesthetized man. J Clin Invest, 44: 978, 1965

53. Goenen M, Pedemonte O, Baele P, Col J: Amrinone in the management of low cardiac output after open heart surgery. Am J Cardiol (symp) 56: 33B, 1985

54. Goldberg AH, Maling HM, Gaffney TE: The effect of digoxin pretreatment on heart contractile force during thiopental infusions in dogs. Anesthesiology 22: 974, 1961

55. Goldberg AH, Ullrick WC: Effects of halothane on isometric contractions of isolated heart muscle. Anesthesiology 28: 838, 1967

56. Goldberg LI, Cotton M deV, Darby TD, Howell EV: Comparative heart contractile force effects of equipressor doses of several sympathomimetic amines. J Pharmacol Exp Ther 108: 177, 1953

57. Goldman S, Olajos M, Morkin E: Effects of verapamil on positive inotropic stimulation in the left atrium and ventricle of conscious dogs. J Pharm Exp Ther 222: 270, 1982

58. Goldstein RA, Passamani ER, Roberts R: A comparison of digoxin and dobutamine in patients with acute infarction and cardiac failure. N Engl J Med 303: 846, 1980

59. Goldstein RE, Skelton CL, Levey GS et al: Effects of glucagon on contractility and adenyl cyclase activity of human papillary muscle. Circulation (suppl) 42: 158, 1970

60. Green HD, Lewis RN, Nicherson ND, Heller AL: Blood flow, peripheral resistance and vascular tonus, with observations on relationship be-

tween blood flow and cutaneous temperature. Am J Physiol 141: 518, 1944

61. Gunnar RM, Cruz A, Boswell J et al: Myocardial infarction with shock: Hemodynamic studies and results of therapy. Circulation 33: 753, 1966

62. Gunnar RM, Loeb HS, Pietras RJ, Tobin JR Jr: Ineffectiveness of isoproterenol in shock due to acute myocardial infarction. JAMA 202: 1124, 1967

63. Hallermann FJ, Rastelli GC, Swan HJC: Comparison of left ventricular volumes by dye dilution and angiographic methods in the dog. Am J Physiol 204: 446, 1963

64. Harlan JM, Harker LA: Hemostasis, thrombosis and thromboembolic disorders: The role of arachidonic acid metabolites in platelet-vessel wall interactions. Med Clin North Am 65: 855, 1981

65. Harrison DC, Glick G, Goldblatt A, Braunwald E: Studies on cardiac dimensions in intact, unanesthetized man. IV. Effects of isoproterenol and methoxamine. Circulation 29: 186, 1964

66. Hauser CJ, Shoemaker WC, Turpin I, Goldberg S: Oxygen transport responses to colloids and crystalloids in critically ill surgical patients. Surg Gynecol Obstet 150: 811, 1980

67. Heymans C, Neil E: Reflexogenic Areas of the Cardiovascular System. Little Brown Co., Boston, 1958

68. Henning RJ, Shubin H, Weil MH: Afterload reduction with phentolamine in patients with acute pulmonary edema. Am J Med 63: 568, 1977

69. Hill AV: Heat of shortening and dynamic constants of muscle. Proc Roy Soc Lond Biol 126: 136, 1938

70. Imperial ES, Levy MN, Zieske H Jr: Outflow resistance as an independent determinant of cardiac performance. Circ Res 9: 1148, 1961

71. Jellife RW: Factors to consider in planning digoxin therapy. J Chronic Dis 24: 407, 1971

72. Kho LK, Shoemaker WC: Cardiorespiratory changes in acute hemorrhage. Surg Gynecol Obstet 124: 826, 1967

73. Kinney JM, Long CL, Duke JH: Carbohydrate and nitrogen metabolism after injury. p. 103. In R Porter and J Knight (eds): Energy Metabolism in Trauma. Churchill, London, 1970

74. Krausz MM, Utsunomiya T, Dunham B et al: Inhibition of permeability edema with imidazole. Surgery 92: 299, 1982

75. Krausz MM, Utsunomiya T, Feuerstein G et al: Prostacyclin reversal of lethal endotoxemia in dogs. J Clin Invest 67: 1118, 1981

76. Landis EM: Micro-injection studies of capillary permeability effects of lack of oxygen on permeability of capillary wall to fluid and to plasma proteins. Am J Physiol 83: 528, 1928

77. Langer GA: Sodium-calcium exchange in the heart. Annu Rev Physiol 44: 435, 1982

78. Lavern B, Strauss HW, Pohost GM: Right and left ventricular geometry: Adjustments during acute respiratory failure. Crit Care Med 7: 509, 1979

79. Lewis BS, Gotsman MS: Current concepts of left ventricular relaxation and compliance. Am Heart J 99: 101, 1980

80. Lewis RA, Austen KF: Mediation of local homeostasis and inflammation by leukotrienes and other mast cell-dependent compounds. Nature 293: 103, 1981

81. Lillehei RC, Longerbeam JK, Block JH, Manax WG: The nature of irreversible shock, experimental and clinical observations. Ann Surg, 160: 682, 1964

82. Linberg SE, Dunham CM, Mergner WJ, Marzella LL: The development of a clinically applicable hemorrhagic shock model. Circ Shock 13(1): 62, 1984

83. Loeb HS, Winslow EBJ, Rahimtoola SH et al: Acute hemodynamic effects of dopamine in patients with shock. Circulation 44: 163, 1971

84. Long CL, Spencer JL, Kinney JM, Geiger JW: Carbohydrate metabolism in normal man and effect of glucose infusion. J Appl Physiol 31: 102, 1971

85. Lucchesi BR: Cardiac actions of glucagon. Circ Res 22: 777, 1968

86. MacCannell KL, McNay JL, Meyer MB, Goldberg LI: Dopamine in the treatment of hypotension and shock. N Engl J Med 275: 1389, 1966

87. MacLean LD, Duff JH, Scott HM, Peretz OL: Treatment of shock in man based on hemodynamic diagnosis. Surg Gynecol Obstet 120: 1, 1965

88. Mancini D, LeJemel T, Sonnenblick EH: Intravenous use of amrinone for the treatment of the failing heart. Am J Cardiol (symp) 56: 8B, 1985

89. Marshall RC, Berger HJ, Costin JC et al: Assessment of cardiac performance with quantitative radionuclide angiocardiography. Circulation 56: 820, 1977

90. McConn R, DelGuercio LRM: Respiratory function of blood in the acutely ill patient and the effect of steroids. Ann Surg 174: 436, 1971

91. Melby JC: pathophysiology of shock. p. 115. In Schumer W, Nylus LM (eds): Corticosteroids in the Treatment of Shock. University of Illinois Press, Urbana, 1970

92. Miller FA Jr, Seward JB, Gersh BJ, et al: Two-Dimensional echocardiographic findings in cardiac trauma. Am J Cardiol 50: 1022, 1982

93. Miller LD, Oski FA, Diaco JF et al: The affinity of hemoglobin for oxygen: Its control and in vivo significance. Surgery 68: 187, 1970

94. Miller RR, Awan NA, Joye JA et al: Combined dopamine and nitroprusside therapy in congestive heart failure. Circulation 55: 881, 1977

95. Miller RR, Palomo AR, Brandon TA et al: Combined vasodilator and inotropic therapy of heart failure: Experimental and clinical concepts. Am Heart J 102: 500, 1981

96. Milnor WR: The cardiovascular control system. p 1061. In Mountcastle VB (ed): Medical Physiology. 14th Ed. CV Mosby, St. Louis, 1980

97. Mittra B: Potassium, glucose and insulin in treatment of myocardial infarction. Lancet 2: 607, 1965

98. Mizus I, Summer W, Farrukh I et al: Isoproterenol or aminophylline attenuate pulmonary edema after acid lung injury. Am Rev Respir Dis 131: 256, 1985

99. Moe GK, Mendez R: The action of several cardiac glycosides on conduction velocity and ventricular excitability in the dog heart. Circulation 4: 729, 1951

100. Mookherjee S, Keighley JFH, Warner RA et al: Hemodynamic ventilatory and blood gas changes during infusion of sodium nitroferricyanide (nitroprusside). Studies in patients with congestive heart failure. Chest 72: 273, 1977

101. Moore FD: The effects of hemorrhage on body composition. N Engl J Med 273: 567, 1965

102. Moore FD, Dagher FJ, Boyden CM et al: Hemorrhage in normal man. I. Distribution and dispersal of saline infusions following acute blood loss: Clinical kinetics of blood volume support. Ann Surg 163: 485, 1966

103. Moore FD, Olesen KH, McMurrey JD et al: The Body Cell Mass and its Supporting Environment. WB Saunders, Philadelphia-London, 1963, p 535

104. Moss GS, Siegel DC, Cochin A, Fresques V: Effects of saline and colloid solutions on pulmonary function in hemorrhagic shock. Surg Gynecol Obstet 133: 53, 1971

105. Myers ML, Jacobson A, Finley R et al: Beta receptor dysfunction in sepsis? Crit Care Med (abstr) 8: 231, 1980

106. Nachman RL, Weksler B, Feries B: Characterization of human platelet serotonin and the response to pulmonary emboli. Surgery 70: 12, 1971

107. Neuhof H, Hey D, Glaser E et al: Monitoring of shock patients by direct and continuous measurement of oxygen uptake. p. 6. In Current Topics in Critical Care Medicine. 3rd International Symposium, Rio de Janeiro 1974, Karger Basel, 1976

108. Neuhof H, Wolf H: Oxygen uptake during hemodilution. Bibl Haematologica 41: 66, 1975

109. Neuhof H, Wolf H: Method for continuously measured oxygen consumption and cardiac output for use in critically ill patients. Crit Care Med 6(3): 155, 1978

110. Ollodart R, Mansberger AR: The effect of hypovolemic shock on bacterial defense. Am J Surg 110: 302, 1965

111. Parker S, Carlon GC, Issacs M et al: Dopamine administration in oliguria and oliguric renal failure. Crit Care Med 9: 630, 1981

112. Parmley WW, Sonnenblick EH: Glucagon: A new agent in cardiac therapy. Am J Cardiol 27: 298, 1971

113. Powers SR Jr, Mannal R, Neclerio M et al: Physiologic consequences of positive end-expiratory pressure (PEEP) ventilation. Ann Surg 178: 265, 1973

114. Regnier B, Rapin MG, Gory G et al: Hemodynamic effects of dopamine in septic shock. Intensive Care Med 3: 47, 1977

115. Sarnoff SJ: Myocardial contractility as described by ventricular function curves; Observations on Starling's law of Heart. Physiol Rev 35: 107, 1955

116. Sarnoff SJ, Berglund E: Ventricular function I. Starlings's law of the heart, studied by means of simultaneous right and left ventricular function curves in the dog. Circulation 9: 706, 1954

117. Sarnoff SJ, Case RB, Waithe PE Ishacs JP: Insufficient coronary flow and myocardial failure as a complicating factor in late hemorrhagic shock. Am J Physiol 176: 439, 1954

118. Sarnoff SJ, Gilmore JP, Brockman SK et al: Regulation of ventricular contraction by the carotid sinus: Its effect on atrial and ventricular dynamics. Circ Res 8: 1123, 1960

119. Sarnoff SJ, Mithcell JH: The regulation of the performance of the heart. Am J Med 30: 747, 1961

120. Schumer W: Histamine release in endotoxin shock: Effect of dexamethasone administration. p. 235. In Hinshaw LB, Cox BG (eds): The Fundamental Mechanisms of Shock. Plenum, New York, 1972

121. Schumer W, Erve PR, Miller B et al: Steroids in the treatment of shock. p. 275. In Malinin T, Zeppa R, Drucker W, Calahan A (eds): Acute Fluid Replacement in the Therapy of Shock. Stratton Intercontinental, New York, 1974

122. Schumer W, Nyhus LM: Corticosteroid effect on biochemical parameters of human oligemic shock. Arch Surg 100: 405, 1970

123. Pitcairn M, Schuler J, Erve PR et al: Glucocorticoid and antibiotic effect on experimental gram-negative bacteremic shock. Arch Surg 110: 1012, 1975

124. Shah DM, Newell JC, Saba TM: Defects in pe-

ripheral oxygen utilization following trauma and shock. Arch Surg 116: 1277, 1981

125. Shamoo AE, Ambudkar IS: Regulation of calcium transport in cardiac cells. Can J Physiol Pharmacol 62: 9, 1984

126. Shepherd AP, Granger HJ, Smith EE Guyton AC: Local control of tissue oxygen delivery and its contribution to the regulation of cardiac output. Am J Physiol 225: 747, 1973

127. Shimosato S, Gamble C Etsten BE: Differential effects of diethyl ether anesthesia upon right and left myocardial function. Anesthesiology 28: 874, 1967

128. Shimosato S, Shanks C Etsten BE: The effects of methoxyflurane and sympathetic nerve stimulation on myocardial mechanics. Anesthesiology 29: 538, 1968

129. Shires T: The role of sodium-containing solutions on the treatment of oligemic shock. Surg Clin North Am 45: 365, 1965

130. Shires GT, Cunningham JN, Baker CRF et al: Alterations in cellular membrane function during hemorrhagic shock in primates. Ann Surg 176: 288, 1972

131. Shoemaker WC: Comparison of the relative effectiveness of whole blood transfusions and various types of fluid therapy in resuscitation. Crit Care Med 4: 71, 1976

132. Shoemaker WC: Pathophysiologic basis of therapy for shock and trauma syndromes use of sequential cardiorespiratory measurements to describe natural histories and evaluate possible mechanisms. Semin Drug Treat 3: 211, 1973

133. Shoemaker WC, Baker RJ: Evaluation and treatment of the patient in shock from trauma. Surg Clin North Am 47: 3, 1967

134. Shoemaker WC, Carey JS, Mohr PA et al: Hemodynamic measurements in various types of clinical shock. Arch Surg 93: 189, 1966

135. Shoemaker WC, Czer LS: Evaluation of the biologic importance of various hemodynamic and oxygen transport variables: Which variables should be monitored in postoperative shock? Crit Care Med 7: 424, 1979

136. Shoemaker WC, Boyd DR, Kim SF et al: Sequential oxygen transport and acid base changes after trauma to the unanesthetized patient. Surg Gynecol Obstet 132: 1033, 1971

137. Shoemaker WC, Monson DO: Effect of whole blood and plasma expanders on volume-flow relationships in critically ill patients. Surg Gynecol Obstet 144: 909, 1977

138. Shoemaker WC, Montgomery ES, Kaplan E Elwyn DH: Physiologic patterns in surviving and nonsurviving shock patients. Arch Surg 106: 630, 1973

139. Shoemaker WC, Schluchter M, Hopkins JA et al: Comparison of the relative effectiveness of colloids and crystalloids in emergency resuscitation. Am J Surg 142: 73, 1981

140. Sibbald WJ, Calvin JE, Driedger A: Right and left ventricular preload, and diastolic ventricular compliance: Implications for therapy in critically ill patients. p. 80. In Shoemaker WC, Thompson WL (eds): Critical Care Medicine. Vol. 3. Williams & Wilkins, Baltimore, 1982

141. Sibbald WJ, Calvin JE, Holliday RL, Driedger AA: Concepts in the pharmacologic and non-pharmacologic support of cardiovascular function in critically ill surgical patients. Surg Clin North Am 63: 455, 1983

142. Siegel JH: Physiologic assessment of cardiac function in the aged and high-risk surgical patient. p. 23. In Siegel JH, Chodoff PD (eds): The Aged and High Risk Surgical Patient. Grune & Stratton, Inc., New York 1976

143. Siegel JH: Pattern and process in the evolution of and recovery from shock. p. 381. In Siegel JH, Chodoff PD (eds): The Aged and High Risk Surgical Patient. Grune & Stratton, New York, 1976

144. Siegel JH, Cerra FB, Coleman B et al: Physiological and metabolic correlations in human sepsis. Surgery 86: 163, 1979

145. Siegel JH, Cerra FB, Peters D et al: The physiologic trajectory of recovery as the organizing principle for the quantification of the hormono-metabolic adaptation to surgical stress and severe sepsis. p. 177. In Schumer W, Spitzer JJ, Marshell BE (eds.) Advances in Shock Research. Liss, New York, 1979

146. Siegel JH, Fabian M, Lankau C et al: Clinical and experimental use of thoracic impedance plethysmography in quantifying myocardial contractility. Surgery 67: 907, 1970

147. Siegel JH, Farrell EF, Goldwyn RM, Friedman HP: The surgical implications of physiologic patterns in myocardial infarction shock. Surgery 72: 126, 1972

148. Siegel JH, Fichthorn J: Computer-based CARE of the aged or high-risk patient: Automated assistance in fluid management, metabolic balance, and cardiopulmonary regulation. p. 547 In Siegel JH, Chodoff PD (eds): The Aged and High Risk Surgical Patient, Grune & Stratton, Inc., 1976

149. Siegel JH, Gilmore JP, Sarnoff SJ: Myocardial extraction and production of catecholamines. Cir Res 9: 1336, 1961

150. Siegel JH, Giovannini I, Coleman B et al: Pathologic synergy in cardiovascular and respiratory compensation with cirrhosis and sepsis: A manifestation of a common metabolic defect? Arch. Surg., 117: 225, 1982

151. Siegel JH, Giovannini I, Coleman B et al: Death after portal decompressive surgery; Physiologic state, metabolic adequacy, and the sequence of development of the physiologic determinants of survival. Arch Surg 116: 1330, 1981

152. Siegel JH, Goldwyn RM, DelGuercio LRM: Hemodynamic alterations following massive fluid replacement in man. p. 10. In Fox CL, Nahas GG (eds): Body Fluid Replacement in the Surgical Patient. Grune & Stratton, New York, 1970

153. Siegel JH, Goldwyn RM, Farrell EJ et al: Hyperdynamic states and the physiologic determinants of survival in patients with cirrhosis and portal hypertension. Arch Surg 108: 282, 1974

154. Siegel JH, Greenspan M, Cohn JD, Del Guercio LRM: The prognostic implications of altered physiology in operations for portal hypertension. Surg Gynecol Obstet 126: 249, 1968

155. Siegel JH, Greenspan M, Del Guercio LRM: Abnormal vascular tone, defective oxygen transport and myocardial failure in human septic shock. Ann Surg 165: 504, 1967

156. Siegel JH, Levine MJ, McConn R, Del Guercio LRM: The effect of glucagon infusion on cardiovascular function in the critically ill. Surg Gynecol Obstet 131: 505, 1970

157. Siegel JH, Sonnenblick EH: Isometric time-tension relationships as an index of myocardial contractility. Circ Res 12: 597, 1963

158. Siegel JH, Sonnenblick EH: Quantification and prediction of myocardial failure. Arch Surg 89: 1026, 1964

159. Siegel JH, Sonnenblick EH, Judge RD, Wilson WS: The quantification of myocardial contractility in dog and man. Cardiologia 45: 189, 1964

160. Siegel JH, Sonnenblick EH, Judge RD, Wilson WS: Occult myocardial failure and vasopressors in shock. Cardiologia 47: 353, 1969

161. Skillman JJ, Lauler DP, Hickler RB et al: Hemorrhage in normal man: Effect on renin, cortisol, aldosterone, and urine composition. Ann Surg 166: 865, 1967

162. Slater GI, Vladeck BC, Bassin R et al: Sequential changes in distribution of cardiac output in hemorrhagic shock. Surgery 73: 714, 1973

163. Solomkin JS, Simmons RL: Cellular and subcellular mediators of acute inflammation. Surg Clin North Am 63: 225, 1983

164. Sonnenblick EH: Instantaneous force-velocity-length determinants in the contraction of heart muscle. Circ Res 16: 441, 1965

165. Sonnenblick EH: Series elastic and contractile elements in heart muscle: Changes in muscle length. Am J Physiol 207: 1330, 1964

166. Sonnenblick EH: Implications of muscle mechanics in the heart. Fed Proc 21: 975, 1962

167. Sonnenblick EH: Active state in heart muscle: Its delayed onset and modification by inotropic agents. J Gen Physiol 50: 661, 1967

168. Sonnenblick EH: Force-velocity relations in mammalian heart muscle. Am J Physiol 202: 931, 1962

169. Sonnenblick EH, Braunwald E, Morrow AG: The contractile properties of human heart muscle: Studies on myocardial mechanics of surgically excised papillary muscles. J Clin Invest 44: 966, 1965

170. Sonnenblick EH, Braunwald E, Williams JF Jr, Glick G: Effects of exercise on myocardial force-velocity relations in intact unanesthetized man: Relative roles of changes in heart rate, sympathetic activity, and ventricular dimensions. J Clin Invest 44: 2051, 1965

171. Sonnenblick EH, Downing SE: Afterload as a primary determinant of ventricular performance. Am J Physiol 204: 604, 1963

172. Sonnenblick EH, Ross J Jr, Covell JW et al: Velocity of contraction as a determinant of myocardial oxygen consumption. Am J Physiol 209: 919, 1965

173. Sonnenblick EH, Siegel JH, Sarnoff SJ: Ventricular distensibility and pressure-volume curve during sympathetic stimulation. Am J Physiol 204: 1, 1963

174. Sonnenblick EH, Spiro D, Spotnitz HM: The ultrastructural basis of Starling's law of the heart: The role of the sarcomeres in determining ventricular size and stroke volume. Am Heart J 68: 336, 1964

175. Starling EH: Linacre Lecture on Law of the Heart. Longmans Green, London, 1918.

176. Stern MA, Gohlke HK, Loeb HS et al: Hemodynamic effects of intravenous phentolamine in low output cardiac failure: Dose-response relationships. Circulation 58: 157, 1978

177. Sugai N, Shimosato S, Etsten BE: Effect of halothane on force-velocity relations and dynamic stiffness of isolated heart muscle. Anesthesiology 29: 267, 1968

178. Swan HJC, Ganz W, Forrester J et al: Catheterization of the heart in man with use of a flow-directed, balloon-tipped catheter. N Engl J Med 283: 447, 1970

179. Tacchino RM, Siegel JH, Emanuele T et al: Incidence and therapy of myocardial depression in critically ill post-trauma patients. Circ Shock 18: 360, 1986 (abst.)

180. Trump BF, Arstila AU: Cellular reaction to injury. p. 9. In RB Hill Jr, MF LaVia (eds): Principles of Pathobiology. 2nd Ed. Oxford University Press, New York, 1975

181. Trump BF, Berezesky IK, Cowley RA: The cellular and subcellular characteristics of acute and chronic injury with emphasis on the role of cal-

cium. p. 6. In RA Cowley, BF Trump (eds): Pathophysiology of Shock, Anoxia, and Ischemia. Williams & Wilkins, Baltimore, 1982

182. Trump BF, Berezesky IK, Laiho KU et al: The role of calcium in cell injury. A review. Scan Electron Microsc 2: 437, 1980

183. Trump BF, Ginn FL: The pathogenesis of subcellular reactions to lethal injury. p. 1. In Bajusz E, Jasmin G (eds): Methods and Achievements in Experimental Pathology. Vol 4. Karger, Basel, 1969

184. Trump BF, Laiho KA, Mergner WJ, Arstila AU: Studies on the subcellular pathophysiology of acute lethal cell injury. Beitr Pathol 152: 243, 1974

185. Trump BF, Mergner WJ: Cell Injury. p. 115. In Zweifach BW, Grant L, McClusky RT (eds): The Inflammatory Process. 2nd Ed. Vol 1. Academic Press New York, 1974

186. Trunkey DD, Siegel JH, Baker SP, Gennarelli TA: Panel: Current status of trauma severity indices. J Trauma 23: 185, 1983

187. Utsunomiya T, Krausz MM, Dunham B, et al: Circulating negative inotropic agent(s) following pulmonary embolism. Surgery 91: 402, 1982

188. Utsunomiya T, Krausz MM, Shepro D, Hechtman HB: Prostaglandin control of plasma and platelet 5-hydroxytryptamine in normal and embolized animals. Am J Physiol 241: H766, 1981

189. Walters PA Jr, Cooper TW, Denison AB Jr, Green HD: Dilator responses to isoproterenol in cutaneous and skeletal muscle vascular beds: Effects of adrenergic blocking drugs. J Pharmacol Exp Ther 115: 323, 1955

190. Walton RP, Richardson JA, Walton RP Jr Thompson WL: Sympathetic influences during hemorrhagic hypotension. Am J Physiol 197: 223, 1959

191. Wang Y, Marshall RJ, Shepherd JT: The effect of changes in posture and of graded exercise on stroke volume in man. J Clin Invest 39: 1051, 1960

192. Weibel E: Morphometry of the Human Lung. Academic Press, New York, 1963

193. Weil MH, Shubin H, Rosoff L: Fluid repletion in circulatory shock: Central venous pressure and other practical guides. JAMA 192: 608, 1965

194. Weksler BB, Ley CW, Jaffe EA: Stimulation of endothelial cell prostacyclin production by thrombin trypsin and the ionophore. J Clin Invest 62: 923, 1978

195. Wiggers CJ: Physiology of Shock. New York, Commonwealth Fund, 1950

SECTION IV

CARDIOGENIC SHOCK AND CARDIOVASCULAR CRISES

10

Acute Myocardial Infarction and Cardiogenic Shock

Robert J. Henning

INTRODUCTION

Each year, 1.3 million individuals experience an acute myocardial infarction. In the United States, the annual incidence of acute myocardial infarction among men aged 35 to 44 is 1.9/1,000 and increases rapidly for each succeeding decade to a peak incidence of 11.6/1,000 in the 65 to 74-year age group.[70] More than 50 percent of coronary deaths are sudden, usually occurring outside the hospital within 1 hour of the onset of symptoms. Sudden death is more frequently in younger than in older adults.[237] Precipitating factors[205] include strenuous physical exertion in 15 percent, modest or usual activity in 18 percent, surgical procedures in 5 percent, rest in 51 percent, and sleep in 10 percent. The elapsed time between the onset of acute symptoms and hospital admis-sion averages 8 hours and only approximately 15 percent of all patients reach the hospital within 4 hours of the onset of symptoms.[108] Indecision on the part of the patient or his family, who fail to recognize the symptoms or fail to utilize available medical facilities, are the primary reasons for delay. In more than 10 percent of the cases, physicians contribute to the delay in hospital admission.[108] Following hospitalization, 25 percent of all patients who die from acute myocardial infarction die within 24 hours, 10 percent within 30 days, 5 percent within the second month, and an additional 8 to 10 percent prior to the end of the first year.[202]

Significant reduction in the mortality of acute myocardial infarction requires public education in the symptoms and signs of acute coronary heart disease as well as training in cardiopulmonary resuscitation. Comprehensive early hospital therapy will also further improve patient survival.

CLINICAL MANIFESTATIONS

Patients with acute myocardial infarction usually have prodromal symptoms of chest pain. However, chest pain may be absent in 4 percent of patients especially if there is pre-existent atrial fibrillation or hypotension or a history of myocardial infarction, heart failure, or diabetes mellitus.[20] The chest discomfort is typically described as constricting, crushing, oppressing, compressing, squeezing, choking, or viselike. It may also be characterized as stabbing, knifelike, boring, or burning. The pain, which may persist for several hours, is typically substernal and may spread to the left and occasionally to the right side of the chest. It may radiate to the shoulders, upper extremities, neck and jaw, and the interscapular area of the back. Nausea and vomiting occur more frequently in patients with acute inferior wall myocardial infarction because of vagal stimulation and the clinical symptoms may suggest acute cholecystitis, gastritis, peptic ulcer disease, or perforation of a viscus. Conversely, pain may be overshadowed by palpitations, weakness, light-headedness, shortness of breath, or diaphoresis. Less frequently, syncope, and symptoms of a concurrent cerebral vascular episode with convulsions and paralysis are the initial manifestations of myocardial infarction.[50] Generalized weakness is usually present after the chest pain and associated discomfort of cardiac infarction have subsided.

Although the physical examination of the patient with acute myocardial infarction may be nonrevealing, the patient is usually anxious and restless. Both sympathetic overactivity and a reduction in cardiac output account for cold perspiration, pallor, and clammy, cyanotic skin. Acute dyspnea with cough producing blood-tinged sputum may indicate pulmonary edema due to acute left ventricular failure. The heart rate may vary from extremes of bradycardia to tachycardia. Arterial systolic and diastolic blood pressures are typically reduced. The pulse pressure is narrowed due to disproportional reduction in systolic blood pressure. In a minority of patients hypertension is observed due to excessive adrenergic stimulation but this usually subsides following sedation and/or analgesic medication.

Fever due to myocardial tissue necrosis may be observed within 48 hours after the initial symptoms of acute infarction. Rectal temperatures seldom exceed 38°C (102°F). The fever rarely persists beyond the seventh hospital day unless there is extension of the myocardial infarction, pericarditis, or systemic infection, typically in the lungs or urinary tract.

Twelve percent of patients admitted to the hospital with an acute cerebral vascular episode have an associated acute myocardial infarction. However, only 2 percent of patients with an acute myocardial infarction sustain a cerebral vascular accident due to embolization of mural thrombi.[50,248]

Right ventricular infarction with papillary muscle dysfunction or necrosis often produces significant jugular venous distention and tall "V" waves of tricuspid regurgitation. Infarction of more than 25 percent of the left ventricular myocardium is usually associated with congestive left heart and ultimately right heart failure with increased jugular venous pressure and jugular vein distention (Table 10-1). Reduction in ventricular ejection velocity and stroke volume account for decreased pulse pressure and peripheral arterial pulsations. A sharp, rapid carotid upstroke of brief duration is observed with acute mitral regurgitation or traumatic rupture of the interventricular septum with a left to right shunt. Moist pulmonary crackles, wheezes, diffuse coarse rhonchi, and occasional hemoptysis suggest increased pulmonary capillary pressure and pulmonary edema.

Precordial palpitation may demonstrate a

TABLE 10-1. Hemodynamic Manifestations of Left Ventricular Muscle Loss

Left Ventricular Muscle Loss (%)	Hemodynamic Manifestation
> 8	Decreased compliance
>10	Decreased ejection fraction
>15	Increased left ventricular end-diastolic pressure
>20	Increased left ventricular end-diastolic volume
>25	Clinical congestive heart failure
>40	Cardiogenic shock

(Adapted from Russell RO, Rackley CE, Pombo J et al: Effects of left ventricular filling pressure in patients with acute myocardial infarction. J Clin Invest 99:1539, 1970.)

paradoxical pulsation in the third to fifth intercostal space, or a diffuse "rippling" precordial motion reflecting dyskinesis of the anterior left ventricular wall.

The heart sounds are often decreased in intensity. The first heart sound may be indistinguishable from the second heart sound with a consequent "tic-tac" rhythm. Paradoxical splitting of the second heart sound may be due to left ventricular dysfunction with delayed closure of the aortic valve. In patients with left ventricular failure and pulmonary hypertension, the pulmonary component of the second sound (P_2) is accentuated and may be louder than the aortic closure sound. Fourth heart sounds are auscultated in more than 80 percent of patients and are due to ventricular vibrations from forceful atrial contractions into a poorly compliant ventricular chamber.[217] This hemodynamic event is often palpable at the ventricular apex when the patient is examined in the left lateral decubitus position. Third heart sounds result from vibrations originating within the damaged left ventricular wall as active rapid expansile filling is abruptly halted in early diastole by the poorly compliant left ventricle. The mortality[217] of patients with acute myocardial infarction, third heart sounds, and pulmonary edema is 20 to 40 percent.

Transient or persistent systolic murmurs due to mitral regurgitation are usually caused by papillary muscle dysfunction. These murmurs characteristically begin after the first heart sound and frequently have a crescendo–decrescendo or diamond-shaped configuration. In a minority of cases the murmur may be holosystolic in duration. The intensity and character of the murmur correlate poorly with the hemodynamic severity of the mitral regurgitation. Such murmurs may be confused with pericardial friction rubs, which occur in 20 percent of patients after the second day of hospitalization. Typical pericardial rubs however are superficial, scratching, or crunching in quality often with two or three discrete components. The first component of a pericardial friction rub occurs during early diastole, coincident with rapid ventricular filling; the second component occurs during late diastole with atrial contraction, and the third component occurs during ventricular systole.

Hepatic congestion with right upper quadrant tenderness and abnormal liver function is typically due to right heart failure caused by left ventricular failure and, less commonly, due to right ventricular infarction. A hepatojugular reflux is caused by reflux of blood into the internal jugular veins with jugular venous distention when the liver is compressed. This constitutes one sign of right ventricular failure.

Peripheral pitting edema is evidence for right ventricular failure with elevation of capillary hydrostatic pressure in excess of colloid oncotic pressure. This sign reflects subacute or chronic capillary hypertension.

LABORATORY EXAMINATION

Acute increases in the serum concentration of creatine kinase, aspartate aminotransferase (AST) (formerly glutamic oxaloacetic transaminase), and lactic dehydrogenase to more than twice the normal concentration have become standard criteria for the laboratory diagnosis of acute myocardial infarction. When the blood concentration of these enzymes is measured within the first 24 to 48 hours following sustained coronary occlusion in laboratory animals and uncomplicated myocardial infarction in humans, there is a close correlation between the total enzyme concentration in blood and the amount of myocardial necrosis.[98,218]

HEMODYNAMIC MONITORING

Although left ventricular dysfunction may be suspected at the bedside by auscultation of a decreased intensity of the first heart sound, paradoxical splitting of the second heart sound, accentuation of the pulmonary component of the second sound, third, and fourth heart (gallop) sounds, and signs of pulmonary edema, quantitation of the degree of myocardial depression on the basis of a careful physical examination alone is difficult. Considerable disparity frequently exists between the physical findings of acute myocardial infarction and actual invasive hemodynamic measurements.[83] The insertion of intra-arterial and thermistor-tipped pulmonary artery catheters is useful for quantitating alterations in cardiac output and myocardial performance and accurately guiding the clinician in the treatment of patients with complicated myocardial infarction (Table 10-2). Vascular catheters facilitate measurement of intra-arterial and pulmonary arterial pressure, pulmonary artery occlusive pressure (reflecting left ventricular end-diastolic pressure), cardiac output, arterial and venous blood gases, lactate concentration, osmolality, and colloid oncotic pressure. Intravascular catheters also facilitate the infusion of fluids or medications, the withdrawal of blood for immediate laboratory analysis and occasional phlebotomy, and provide a ready access for angiography, insertion of pacemaker catheters or the intra-aortic balloon for counterpulsation.

Hemodynamic monitoring facilitates the early recognition and diagnosis of complications of acute myocardial infarction and is useful in detecting other hemodynamic disorders.[46] Low cardiac output secondary to acute right ventricular infarction in patients with inferior-posterior wall myocardial infarction may be detected by a disproportionate elevation of right ventricular filling pressure. Acute mitral regurgitation due to papillary muscle dysfunction or dilitation of the mitral valve annulus is often characterized by a giant V wave in

the pulmonary artery wedge pressure tracing which coincides with the end of the T wave on the simultaneously recorded electrocardiogram. An increase in oxygen content in pulmonary arterial blood by ≥ 1 vol percent compared to right ventricular blood indicates the presence of a ventricular septal defect.[102] In acute pulmonary embolism, a low cardiac output is associated with increases in right atrial, pulmonary arterial systolic and diastolic pressures, but often normal pulmonary artery occlusive pressures.[43] In patients with acute cardiac tamponade and constrictive pericarditis with low cardiac output, the diastolic pressure in all four cardiac chambers is similar and diastolic filling time is shortened due to impairment of chamber filling. The diastolic pressure tracing may have a "square root" or "check" configuration in patients with pericardial constriction.

Colloid Oncotic Pressure

The diagnosis and treatment of patients with myocardial infarction complicated by acute pulmonary edema may be facilitated by the measurement of colloid oncotic pressure or "protein pressure" of the plasma.[65]

Normal human plasma has a total protein concentration of approximately 7 g/dl and a colloid oncotic pressure (COP) of 25 mmHg (range: 21 to 30 mmHg).[261] The principal oncotically active protein is albumin, which has a molecular weight of 69,000 and accounts for 67 to 75 percent of the normal colloid oncotic pressure. Globulins and fibrinogen, with molecular weights ranging from 45,000 to 1,000,000, account for most of the remaining oncotically active proteins.

The COP declines to approximately 21.5 mmHg after 4 hours in the supine position because of loss of normal gravimetric forces with reabsorption of hypo-oncotic fluid from the interstitial spaces of the lower extremities into the intravascular space. Furthermore, in critically ill patients with acute myocardial infarction there may be failure of synthesis or mobilization of albumin from the liver, and dilution of COP with the intravenous administration of large volumes of crystalloid solution. A persis-

TABLE 10-2. Indications for Right Heart Catheterization with a Balloon-Tipped Flotation Catheter

Hypovolemia with loss of >10% plasma volume
Acute right ventricular infarction with right heart failure
Ventricular septal rupture
Massive pulmonary embolism
Severe mitral regurgitation
Advanced congestive heart failure
Cardiogenic shock
Cardiac tamponade

tent reduction in COP to ≤ 14 mmHg is associated[176] with a mortality in excess of 50 percent.

In supine, healthy individuals, the pulmonary artery occlusive pressure (PAWP) ranges from 4 to 12 mmHg. Because the COP is normally between 21 and 30 mmHg, there is a net force or "COP–PAWP gradient" of 9 to 26 mmHg, which tends to retain fluid within the intravascular compartment. A persistent COP–PAWP gradient ranging between 0 and 5.9 mmHg is associated with a 50 percent incidence of acute pulmonary edema and a persistent COP–PAWP gradient of ≤ 0 mmHg is invariably associated with acute pulmonary edema regardless of the absolute value of either the COP or the PAWP.[260] Furthermore, the radiographic severity of the acute pulmonary edema is closely correlated with the COP–PAWP gradient. A COP–PAWP pressure gradient ≤ 0 mmHg is associated with ≥ 3+/4+ pulmonary edema.[260] Patients who respond to treatment invariably develop a positive gradient of ≥ 6 mmHg.

Lactate Measurements

When acute myocardial infarction reduces cardiac output and oxygen delivery to the point that aerobic metabolism is no longer maintained even under conditions of maximum oxygen extraction from capillary blood, an oxygen debt is incurred. Tissue viability is then temporarily sustained by anaerobic metabolism, which is a substantially less efficient pathway for generating adenosine triphosphate (ATP). Under anaerobic conditions, glucose does not enter the Krebs citric acid cycle via acetyl coenzyme A with the production of 38 mols of ATP, but is metabolized to lactic acid and produces only 2 mols of ATP.

Measurements of blood lactate in patients with complicated acute myocardial infarction have been compared with routine hemodynamic, respiratory, and metabolic measurements as prognostic indicators of survival or death.[118] In this investigation blood lactate consistently proved to be a more useful prognostic indicator of survival or death than the measurement of arterial pressure, pulmonary artery occlusive pressure, heart rate, mixed venous oxygen tension, or arterial pH. No patient survived in whom the arterial blood lactate was greater than 5 mmol/L for more than 12 hours, regardless of the magnitude of the stroke volume, the left ventricular filling pressure, or the cardiac work. Serial measurements of blood lactate therefore provide a useful indicator of the severity of perfusion failure and the oxygen debt in patients with acute myocardial infarction.

Peripheral Skin (Toe) Temperature Measurements

Quantitative changes in peripheral skin temperature have been demonstrated to provide a competent noninvasive indication of the presence and severity of alterations in cardiac output and tissue perfusion. The temperature gradient between the ventral surface of the first toe and the ambient room temperature (T-A gradient) has been measured and compared with established hemodynamic measurements in patients with complicated acute myocardial infarction.[119] In this investigation the T-A temperature gradient served as a more predictable indicator of survival or fatality than serial measurements of blood lactate, arterial pressure, or cardiac output. Patients who improved with treatment and ultimately survived experienced increases in the T-A gradient to more than 4°C whereas a gradient of less than 3°C over an interval of 12 hours typically was observed in patients who subsequently died.

Radionuclides: Myocardial Imaging

Rubidium, cesium, and thallium isotopes have been used by clinicians to assess myocardial perfusion. These isotopes are taken up by the same active transport mechanism responsible for potassium uptake in normally perfused myocardial cells but uptake by ischemic, infarcted, or scarred tissue is reduced or absent. In 1975, Lebowitz first reported the use of thallium 201 in assessing myocardial perfusion.[144] The energy emitted by thallium permits detection with gamma scintillation cameras and the ease of producing thallium in commercial cyclotrons and the long half-life of more than 73 hours makes it a practical isotopic marker of myocardial perfusion.

Following intravenous administration, the initial distribution of thallium 201 within the myocardium is dependent upon coronary blood flow.[11] Experimental evidence indicates a close relationship between blood flow and initial thallium 201 concentration. Accordingly, a reduction of 70 percent in normal resting blood flow may be associated with a 55 to 70 percent decrease in initial thallium 201 tissue concentrations. Regional decreases in thallium uptake may represent myocardial necrosis due to myocardial infarction, unstable angina pectoris, or coronary artery spasm. These conditions cannot be differentiated on the initial examination. However, "filling in" of defects with repeat scintigraphic examination 4 hours after the initial injection is an indication of reversible ischemia of viable myocardium. A deficit that remains unchanged for 8 hours or more is consistent with necrosis or scar tissue formation secondary to infarction. Conversely, an entirely normal study performed within the first few hours following the onset of symptoms provides reasonable evidence that acute myocardial infarction is unlikely.

Thallium images provide valuable diagnostic information as soon as regional blood flow is significantly impaired. In a study of 200 patients reported by Wackers, the diagnostic sensitivity of the procedure was 100 percent when patients were examined within 6 hours after the onset of chest pain.[255] In patients studied 6 to 24 hours after the acute event, the sensitivity was 88 percent, while only 72 percent of the patients imaged after 24 hours had a positive study. Patients with large infarctions studied within the first 24 hours had positive studies, and patients with small infarctions and nontransmural infarctions had positive studies when examined within 6 hours of the onset of chest pain. However, when the thallium test was performed between 6 and 24 hours, only 57 percent of patients with small infarctions and 70 percent of patients with nontransmural infarction had positive studies.

Myocardial Imaging with Technetium Pyrophosphate

In 1974, Bonte theorized that since hydroxyapatite $[Ca_{10}(PO_4)_6(OH)_2]$ crystals, are detected within damaged myocardial cells, the calcium-chelating agent pyrophosphate labeled with technetium 99 might become incorporated into acutely infarcted myocardial tissue.[36] Cardiac mitochondrial calcification occurs as early as 2 to 4 hours after permanent coronary occlusion and becomes marked by 12 to 24 hours. The degree of technetium 99m pyrophosphate uptake is roughly proportional to the extent of acute myocardial damage. A 20 to 40 percent reduction in normal cardiac perfusion results in maximum pyrophosphate accumulation. As blood flow is further reduced, the uptake actually decreases, and in very large myocardial infarctions accumulation of Tc pyrophosphate may occur only in the lateral zones. The total amount of technetium isotope uptake therefore is not a precise indicator of the total quantity of infarcted tissue.

Focal uptake of Tc pyrophosphate must be differentiated from diffuse uptake, as a focal uptake is more consistent with discrete myocardial necrosis. A 0 to 4+ grading system for the interpretation of Tc pyrophosphate images has been developed, which depends on the intensity of the radioactivity over the myocardium in comparison with isotope uptake in the ribs.[199] Three to 4+ focal uptake of technetium 99m pyrophosphate is compatible with acute myocardial necrosis.

The timing of the procedure with respect to the onset of clinical symptoms has a profound effect on the intensity of pyrophosphate accumulation. Imaging within the initial 8 hours of symptoms frequently fails to reveal uptake in an acutely infarcted region and maximum accumulation may not be achieved for 2 to 3 days with technetium pyrophosphate. After this time the intensity of the uptake decreases and there may be no radioactive isotope accumulation in the heart after 1 to 2 weeks.

Not all cardiac accumulations of Tc pyrophosphate, however, represent acute myocardial infarction. Patients with unstable or variant angina may demonstrate diffuse or even 2+ focal accumulations in the heart. In addition, pyrophosphate accumulaton may occur in patients with documented prior myocardial infarction, cardiomyopathy, myocardial contusion, ventricular aneurysms, calcified cardiac valves, cardiac tumors, chronic pericarditis, and occasionally adriamycin- (Doxorubicin) induced cardiopathy.[122] Extracardiac focal accumulations of Tc pyrophosphate may occur in breast tumors, rib or sternal fractures, at the site of chest electrical defibrillation, within soft tissue tumors, and at the site of skin lesions. Nevertheless, in acute myocardial infarction the sensitivity of Tc pyrophosphate in detecting acute necrosis generally exceeds 90 percent. The sensitivity is only 40 to 50 percent in nontransmural myocardial infarctions, as 3 to 4 g of tissue must be infarcted before sufficient Tc pyrophosphate uptake can be detected.[199] The incidence of false-positive tests, in which abnormal scintigrams are obtained in patients who have no confirmatory evidence of acute myocardial infarction, is 18 percent.[60,114,122,265]

Patients with persistently positive Tc pyrophosphate studies 3 or more weeks following acute infarction exhibit a higher incidence of recurrent angina and left ventricular failure than patients in whom the images revert to a normal picture within 7 to 14 days. Patients with small foci of pyrophosphate myocardial uptake have complication rates comparable to patients without infarction, whereas moderate uptake (encompassing areas of approximately 16 to 40 cm²) and high uptake (>40 cm²) may be associated with a complication rate in excess of 60 percent and a mortality rate in excess of 80 percent, respectively.[121]

Tc pyrophosphate imaging is specifically indicated for those patients in whom the electrocardiogram (ECG) or the serum enzyme levels are nondiagnostic or do not correlate with the history or the clinical findings. The technique is particularly useful in the detection of perioperative myocardial infarction following coronary revascularization surgery, estimating the extent and location of myocardial injury, and as a predictor of morbidity and mortality. Thallium 201 is useful for excluding the presence of an acute myocardial infarction within the initial 8 hours of the onset of symptoms if the myocardium perfusion scan is completely normal in appearance. If a defect is present

on initial scintigraphic examination that completely "fills in" with the repeat 4 hour examination, then reversible myocardial ischemia is present.

Within the next 10 years computer interpretation of radionucleotide scintigraphic examinations will eliminate subjective impressions, interobserver variability, and will improve the sensitivity of the radionucleotide examinations as diagnostic tests for acute myocardial infarction.

Hemodynamic Subsets

The relationship between clinical status determined by careful physical examination and hemodynamic measurements in patients with acute myocardial infarction has been recently described by Forrester and co-workers.[83,84] Patients have been classified on the basis of physical signs of tissue hypoperfusion and pulmonary congestion. Clinical "subsets" of patients with acute myocardial infarction have been defined and correlated with measurements of cardiac output and pulmonary capillary occlusive pressure in order to facilitate therapy and establish prognosis (Table 10-3).

UNCOMPLICATED ACUTE MYOCARDIAL INFARCTION

Patients with uncomplicated acute myocardial infarction generally have cardiac outputs and ventricular filling pressures (PAWP) within the normal range of 4 and 7 L/min and 2 to 12 mmHg, respectively. However, as many as 25 percent of the patients in this subset may have increases in the PAWP compatible with alterations in left ventricular compliance and "preclinical" heart failure. The left ventricular stroke work index (SWI) [SWI = (MAP–PAWP) $\times$ (S.I.) $\times$ (0.0136)] is usually between 50 and 70 g-m/m² but may be slightly de-

**TABLE 10-3.   Findings in Subsets of Patients
with Acute Myocardial Infarction**

Subset	Cardiac Index (L/min/m²)	Pulmonary Artery Occlusive Pressure (mmHg)	Mortality (%)
I: Absence of both pulmonary congestion and peripheral hypoperfusion	2.7 ± 0.5	12 ± 7	3
II: Isolated pulmonary congestion	2.3 ± 0.4	23 ± 5	10
III: Isolated peripheral hypoperfusion	1.9 ± 0.4	12 ± 5	20
IV: Pulmonary congestion and hypoperfusion	1.6 ± 0.6	27 ± 8	>60

(Adapted from Forrester JS, Diamond GA, Swan HJC: Correlative classification of clinical hemodynamic function after acute myocardial infarction. Am J Cardiol 39:137, 1977.)

creased. One-third of patients may require treatment for systemic hypertension.

These patients constitute more than 65 percent of all patients with acute myocardial infarction and require observation, bed rest, electrocardiographic monitoring for malignant cardiac arrhythmias, supplemental oxygen, and analgesic medications.

Specific Therapeutic Interventions: Narcotic Analgesics: Morphine and Meperidine

Immediate relief of pain, anxiety, and apprehension associated with acute myocardial infarction is a primary goal of therapy. Pain and anxiety may produce coronary artery spasm as well as stimulate secretion of norepinephrine, which further increases heart rate, cardiac work, and may precipitate lethal cardiac arrhythmias. The brain contains receptors for enkephalins and endorphins that diminish the response to pain. Opiates and their synthetic congeners also activate the endorphin receptors. Narcotic analgesics act upon opioid receptors in the limbic system (frontal and temporal cortex, amygdala, and hippocampus), thalamus, hypothalamus, midbrain, and substantia gelatinosa of the spinal cord.[139] Furthermore, the activity of the locus ceruleus, which plays a critical role in feelings of anxiety, fear, panic, and alarm is inhibited. The relief of pain

is relatively selective in that other sensory modalities such as touch, vibration, and hearing are not as readily obtunded. These drugs inhibit the release of acetylcholine, norepinephrine, and substance P, and alter the release of dopamine. Opiates have recently been demonstrated to inhibit neuronal activity by blocking sodium influx elicited by excitatory neurotransmitters, apparently by acting directly at the channels in the membrane of the receiving cell through which sodium passes.[235] The exact mechanism by which opioids produce tranquillity, euphoria, and other alterations of mood, however, is not precisely known.

The mechanisms responsible for the beneficial cardiac effects of narcotic analgesics is most likely vasodilatation in arterial and venous circuits by central suppression of adrenergic tone, which leads to decreased peripheral resistance and peripheral venous pooling with reduction in pulmonary congestion and myocardial oxygen consumption.[253,275] A decrease in systemic impedance facilitates forward blood flow and improves ventricular emptying unless hypotension occurs, which decreases coronary blood flow and increases myocardial ischemia.

In contrast to morphine and meperidine, pentazocine (Talwin) increases left ventricular preload and afterload, and decreases left ventricular ejection fraction and mean velocity of circumferential fiber shortening as determined by echocardiography.[145] This agent therefore may be hazardous in the treatment of patients with acute myocardial infarction.

In the presence of increased parasympathetic nervous system activity manifested by bradycardia and hypotension, morphine sulfate (a parasympathomimetic agent) should not be administered and meperidine (Demerol), a vagolytic agent, should be substituted. In the presence of sympathetic overactivity characterized by anxiety, tachycardia, and hypertension, morphine sulfate is the drug of choice for pain relief. Although morphine is generally well tolerated by patients with coronary disease when slowly administered in incremental doses of 2 to 5 mg intravenously, or 5 to 10 mg subcutaneously, larger quantities may produce systemic hypotension due primarily to expansion of the venous capacitance bed and decrease in venous return to the right side of the heart. Five milligrams of morphine is approximately equal to 40 mg meperidine.

Therapeutic doses of narcotic analgesics depress all phases of respiratory activity including rate, rhythmicity, tidal exchange, and minute volume. The responsiveness of the brain stem respiratory center is blunted to carbon dioxide accumulation but not to hypoxia. Consequently, mechanical ventilatory support should be immediately available when narcotic analgesics are used, especially in patients with obstructive airway disease.

Morphine prolongs gastrointestinal transit time, increases tone in the vesical sphincter, and therefore delays bladder emptying. It increases biliary tract pressure and may produce biliary colic. After subcutaneous administration of morphine, common bile duct pressure may increase from less than 20 cmH_2O to 200 to 300 cmH_2O for 2 hours or more.[129] Accordingly, morphine is best avoided in patients with known biliary, pancreatic, or bladder disorders and meperidine is the preferred analgesic since it does not increase bile duct pressure or cause sphincter spasm.

Morphine and the other narcotic analgesics are metabolized in the liver where they are conjugated with glucuronic acid and detoxified. These drugs must be used with caution in patients with impaired liver function. Narcotic accumulation or narcotic overdose may be manifested by alterations in mental status, marked miosis, hypotension, and respiratory depression. In this instance, naloxone 0.4 mg should be given intravenously to reverse the depressive action of the narcotic drug. If the

first injection produces only slight improvement in ventilation, a second injection of 0.4 mg is given IV after 5 minutes and a third dose may be given at 10 minutes. Naloxone has very few direct effects other than opioid antagonism. The duration of naloxone's antagonistic action is approximately 3 hours; consequently supplemental doses of naloxone will be necessary.

ARRHYTHMIA THERAPY IN ACUTE MYOCARDIAL INFARCTION

Warning Arrhythmias

Patients who experience ventricular fibrillation or life-threatening ventricular tachycardia in the setting of acute myocardial infarction were previously thought to have "warning arrhythmias," including frequent ventricular premature beats (VPBs), R on T VPBs, couplets or bigeminy, multiform premature ventricular beats, or short runs of ventricular tachycardia.[160] Although many episodes of ventricular fibrillation may be preceded by warning arrhythmias, recent investigations have demonstrated that as many as 50 percent of patients have no prior warning of potentially fatal ventricular arrhythmias.[70,152]

Arrhythmia Detection

More than 90 percent of patients who sustain an acute myocardial infarction have ventricular arrhythmias during the first 48 hours following the acute event.[113] Well-trained coronary care unit staff have detected only 45 percent of the VPBs, 15 percent of the serious ventricular arrhythmias, 13 percent of the couplets, and 7 percent of the multiform beats documented by simultaneous electrocardiographic (Holter) recordings analyzed by computer and reviewed by physicians.[220] In a separate study of arrhythmia detection in a critical care unit, only 48 percent of warning arrhythmias were detected when they occurred as a single, isolated event during a 30-minute period, and 58 percent of all episodes of ventricular tachycardia were not detected at all.[123] Vetter and Julian reported that only 36 percent of VPBs and 18 percent of the episodes of ventricular tachycardia were detected.[252] Many patients who require antiarrhythmic therapy following acute myocardial infarction therefore may not receive adequate treatment.

Pharmacologic Prevention

Lie and associates demonstrated in a randomized study that the prophylactic administration of lidocaine reduced the incidence of ventricular arrhythmias and primary ventricular fibrillation.[153] Ventricular fibrillation occurred in nine patients receiving placebo infusion and in none of the patients receiving lidocaine. Mild side effects consisting of dizziness, lightheadedness, and disorientation occurred in 15 percent of patients receiving lidocaine therapy. Wyman reported a decrease in the incidence of primary ventricular fibrillation from 6.5 percent (9 of 139) to 0.3 percent (3 of 1,026 patients) with no deaths with prophylactic administration of lidocaine following acute myocardial infarction.[274] Minor side effects occurred in 1 percent of the patients in this study. Lidocaine therapy therefore reduces the incidence of primary ventricular fibrillation, and has been recently recommended for the initial 24 to 48 hour treatment of all patients with suspected or proven acute myocardial infarction.[113]

LIDOCAINE

Lidocaine is a local anesthetic that decreases automaticity, the effective refractory period, and the action potential duration of the Purkinje fibers.[57]

Initial lidocaine administration should to-

tal 200 mg in patients without clinical evidence of heart failure or shock.[113] The drug may be administered as two 1-minute 100 mg injections, 10 minutes apart, four 50 mg injections at 5 minute intervals, or as an infusion of 20 mg/min for 10 minutes. Following the loading dose, the drug is infused in amounts of 2 to 3 mg/min. This regimen will achieve plasma concentrations averaging 2.5 μg/ml. The therapeutic concentration of lidocaine in plasma is 1.6 to 5 μg/ml. Bolus injections of lidocaine are absolutely necessary if therapeutic serum concentrations are to be promptly established, because 3 to 7 hours are required for lidocaine to reach a consistent therapeutic plasma concentration without a bolus injection. If ventricular arrhythmias persist, an additional bolus dose of 50 to 100 mg of lidocaine may be administered over a 1 to 2 minute interval and the infusion rate increased to a maximum rate of 4 mg/min.

Lidocaine is metabolized primarily by the liver and toxic concentrations may accumulate when there is hepatocellular dysfunction or decreased hepatic blood flow. In addition, propranolol and epinephrine decrease hepatic blood flow and therefore reduce the metabolic breakdown of lidocaine.

Isoniazid (INH) and chloramphenicol decrease lidocaine biotransformation and therefore prolong its duration of action, whereas phenobarbital increases it. The minimal toxic concentration of lidocaine is 6 μg/ml. Toxicity is manifested by dizziness, drowsiness, euphoria, dysarthria, blurred vision, dyspnea, muscle fasciculations convulsions, myocardial failure, and respiratory arrest. When the drug is abruptly discontinued, it decreases to subtherapeutic levels within 10 to 180 minutes.

In older patients and those with congestive heart failure, shock, and liver disease, the loading dose of lidocaine should be limited to 100 mg and the infusion dosage to 2 mg/min.[241] If symptoms and signs of toxicity occur, the infusion rate should be decreased and intermittent "stop and start" infusions should be avoided.

PROCAINAMIDE

Procainamide (Pronestyl) is useful in suppressing ventricular premature beats and recurrent ventricular tachycardia that cannot be adequately controlled with lidocaine therapy. The drug depresses cardiac muscle excitability, alters the threshold for ventricular fibrillation, and slows conduction in the atrium, the bundle of His, and through ventricular muscle.[136] The effective refractory period, the action potential duration, and the maximum velocity of fiber shortening are prolonged. The effective serum concentration is between 4 and 8 μg/L.

Rapid intravenous bolus administration and/or plasma concentrations exceeding 12 μg/ml may result in a precipitous hypotensive response, sinus arrest, widening of the QRS interval, prolongation of the QT interval, and heart block. Furthermore, in patients with acute myocardial damage, myocardial contractility may be depressed.

The major metabolite of procainamide is N-acetyl procainamide (NAPA) which has an antiarrhythmic potency 70 percent of the parent compound.[74] Therefore, serum concentrations of N-acetyl procainamide must also be monitored and maintained within a range of 3 to 8 μg/L.

If ventricular arrhythmias persist despite lidocaine therapy, which may occur in as many as 18 percent of patients with acute myocardial infarction, 100 mg procainamide may be given intravenously every 5 to 10 minutes with careful blood pressure and ECG monitoring until the arrhythmia is suppressed or a maximum dose of 1 g is administered. Following the initial loading dose of procainamide the patient should be started on a constant infusion of 2 to 5 mg/min.[141] Interruption of intravenous therapy for 3 to 4 hours is recommended before oral administration of 30 to 50 mg/kg/day of procainamide is initiated.

Procainamide is contraindicated in patients with advanced atrioventricular block and should be used with caution in the presence of intraventricular conduction disturbances. Side effects include nausea, vomiting, anorexia, fever, rash, confusion, agranulocytosis, and a lupus-like syndrome. Positive antinuclear antibodies and lupus erythematosus preparations may develop in as many as 50 percent of patients who receive more than 2 g/day for periods of several months.[120] Symptomatic fever, rash, and serositis, however, are uncommon and usually resolve once the drug is stopped.

BRETYLIUM TOSYLATE

The antiarrhythmic effect of bretylium tosylate was first described in 1965, when its protective effect in experimentally induced atrial fibrillation was reported.[151] In 1966, bretylium was shown to be more effective than lidocaine, procainamide, quinidine, dilantin, or propranolol in protecting the heart against ventricular fibrillation by raising the myocardial fibrillation threshold.[12]

Bretylium prolongs the cellular action potential duration and lengthens the effective refractory period without slowing conduction.[32] Impulse formation, spontaneous pacemaker discharge rate, and ventricular conduction velocity are not suppressed. The drug may terminate re-entrant arrhythmias by markedly prolonging cellular refractoriness without changing the propagation velocity of the cardiac impulse, or it may facilitate repolarization and increase conductivity in depolarized tissues by its catecholamine-releasing properties.

Bretylium is recommended for the treatment of life-threatening ventricular arrhythmias that fail to respond to lidocaine or procainamide therapy. Ventricular fibrillation that fails to respond to repeated direct current countershock may also respond to the combination of bretylium and countershock. Initial dosages of 5 mg/kg by rapid intravenous injection followed by a continuous infusion of 1 to 2 mg/min are recommended. Alternatively, the drug may be given intramuscularly as maintenance therapy in doses of 5 mg/kg every 4 to 6 hours. Following the injection of bretylium there may be a delay of 20 minutes to 2 hours before the onset of its antiarrhythmic action, although it may act within minutes in patients with ventricular fibrillation.

Bretylium initially causes the release of norepinephrine from adrenergic postganglionic nerve terminals; consequently, catecholamine effects on the myocardium and on peripheral arterial vessels including tachycardia, cardiac arrhythmias and hypertension are often seen shortly after administration.[164] Subsequently, bretylium blocks the release of norepinephrine in response to neuron stimulation and may produce peripheral adrenergic blockade and orthostatic hypotension. Bretylium-induced hypersensitivity to catecholamines may aggravate digitalis toxicity.

The drug should be used cautiously in patients with valvular heart disease and congestive heart failure in whom sudden alterations in arterial and pulmonary artery pressure may be dangerous. Lidocaine, procainamide, quinidine, guanethidine and dilantin may block the effect of bretylium; therefore, the dosage of these agents should be tapered and then discontinued once bretylium is instituted. The hypotensive properties of bretylium are minimized by maintaining the patient in a supine position. Should hypotension occur, volume expansion and dopamine are effective in restoring arterial pressure, although adrenergic amines such as dopamine should be administered in small concentrations because bretylium-treated patients may be extremely sensitive to catecholamines.

VERAPAMIL

Verapamil interferes with the slow inward intracellular passage of calcium ions. The drug decreases the action potential amplitude, the resting membrane potential, maximum rate of phase 0 rise (Vmax), and membrane responsiveness.[221] The spontaneous discharge rate of the sinus node is slowed by verapamil. The amplitude of the action potential in the upper and midatrioventricular nodal regions is reduced and the time-dependent recovery of excitability and the effective refractory period of AV nodal fibers are prolonged.[126]

The drug is an effective agent for the treatment of paroxysmal supraventricular tachycardia because it either converts the dysrhythmia to normal sinus rhythm or produces significant reductions in ventricular rate. In patients with atrial flutter or fibrillation, verapamil promptly decreases the ventricular rate.

When given intravenously, verapamil has a mild negative inotropic effect in patients with acute myocardial infarction, and decreases peripheral vascular resistance. The intrinsic negative inotropic effects may be offset by potent vasodilating properties with afterload reduction as demonstrated by a decrease in blood pressure and systemic vascular resistance.[75] Thus the net effect is often improved left ventricular function.

Verapamil may be administered in a dosage of 0.15 mg/kg over a period of 2 minutes intravenously. Oral verapamil, in doses of 40 to 80 mg three or four times daily, may then be administered as either a prophylactic agent or to control the ventricular rate in the presence of atrial fibrillation or flutter. The drug should not be administered to patients with sick sinus syndrome, high-degree or unstable AV block, overt congestive heart failure, or shock. Nor should it be used in the presence of β-adrenergic blockade or in conjunction with quinidine-like drugs, because shock and asystole have been reported.[21,250]

NITROGLYCERIN AND NITRATE ESTERS

Nitroglycerin and other organic nitrates have been advocated for the treatment of ischemic myocardial pain and the control of infarction size.[132,135,233] All nitrate esters produce the same pharmacologic effects as nitroglycerin. Although nitroglycerin may dilate vascular smooth muscle throughout the body, its dominant action is venodilatation leading to a reduction in venous return to the right side of the heart (preload) and therefore a decrease in cardiac work and myocardial oxygen consumption.

In the systemic arterial circulation, nitroglycerin may reduce the resistance to blood flow in large arteries and, to a lesser extent, in the small arteries and arterioles with a decline in systemic vascular resistance (afterload) unless this is overridden by reflex vasoconstriction. Significant reduction in systemic arterial pressure or stroke volume may occur in patients who have either absolute or relative hypovolemia, and may be associated with reduction in coronary blood flow and reflex tachycardia that counteracts the beneficial effects of nitroglycerin.[37,266]

Nitroglycerin causes vasodilatation of the pulmonary resistance vessels and decreases pulmonary artery pressure. Splanchnic and renal flow may also be decreased, especially in instances in which a substantial decline in arterial pressure occurs.[76]

Nitrates dilate the large epicardial coronary arteries but have little effect on the intramyocardial arteries, which are the primary coronary resistance vessels.[1] Nevertheless, collateral blood flow may be increased and retrograde flow into chronically ischemic zones of the myocardium may be enhanced. Although total coronary blood flow may decrease with nitroglycerin-induced reduction in cardiac work, myocardial perfusion is proportional to myocardial oxygen demands; endocardial perfusion and subendocardial oxygenation often improve with consequent decrease in myocardial lactate production.[269] Electrocardiographic ST segment and T wave abnormalities may therefore be reversed. At the present time, however, there is no conclusive evidence that the clinical use of nitrate preparations salvages jeopardized ischemic myocardium.

Nitrates are most useful for the relief of persistent cardiac pain not readily responsive to narcotic analgesics; they are particularly useful for treatment of coronary artery spasm.[165]

Nitrate therapy may be begun sublingually in doses of 0.3 to 0.6 mg, orally in concentrations of 10 mg, or as an intravenous infusion beginning with doses of 10 μg/min. Fluctuations in blood pressure and heart rate are most pronounced with the sublingual preparations. Slowly absorbable preparations of nitroglycerin are not customarily used for the treatment of patients with acute myocardial infarction. The dosage of nitroglycerin is progressively increased for pain control while one carefully avoids either drug-induced tachycardia or hypotension. Sublingual nitrates have significantly shorter durations of action than oral nitrates but larger amounts of oral nitrates are required for similar pharmacologic effects. A therapeutic dose of oral nitroglycerin may require 20 to 50 times the equivalent effective dose of sublingual nitroglycerin in the same patient.

β-ADRENERGIC BLOCKING AGENTS

Approximately 8 percent of all patients with acute myocardial infarction present with tachycardia, moderate fever, increased rather than decreased cardiac output, hypertension, increased left ventricular end-diastolic pressure (LVEDP), and diaphoresis.[84,256] These hemodynamic and metabolic changes may be due to a hyperadrenergic state with increased secretion of endogenous norepinephrine and epinephrine. β-adrenergic blocking agents such as propranolol (Inderal), metoprolol (Lopressor), and nadolol (Corgard), limit the inotropic and chronotropic actions of catecholamines and therefore may be used to reduce heart rate, contraction velocity, and myocardial oxygen requirements in hyperadrenergic patients.

β-Adrenergic agents have also been administered to patients with uncomplicated acute myocardial infarction in an attempt to reduce myocardial oxygen requirements, limit myocardial infarction size, and thereby reduce mortality.[183] In the United States, propranolol (Inderal) is the β-adrenergic blocking agent most frequently administered for this purpose. The drug decreases heart rate and cardiac output, prolongs and decreases the velocity of cardiac mechanical systole, and decreases blood pressure. Myocardial lactate production may be reduced and the incidence of ventricular arrhythmias is diminished. Propranolol is categorized as a class II antiarrhythmic drug. In therapeutic doses it has a depressant effect on the sinus node, prolongs atrial and AV nodal conduction times, but also shortens the effective refractory period and the action potential duration. It increases the myocardial threshold for ventricular tachycardia and fibrillation.[150]

The pharmacologic action of propranolol includes β-adrenergic receptor blockade in the tracheobronchial tree, which increases airway resistance. This may precipitate potentially fatal bronchospasm in patients with obstructive airway disease. Since β-adrenergic blocking drugs are competitive antagonists, the effects of β blockade may be overcome by β agonists such as isoproterenol.

Limitation of Infarction Size and Evidence of Reduced Mortality

Propranolol therapy has been proposed for treatment of patients with uncomplicated acute myocardial infarction.[183] For this purpose propranolol has been administered initially by slow intravenous infusion in amounts of 0.1 mg/kg in three divided doses, then orally in dosages ranging from 20 to approximately 100 mg at intervals of 4 to 6 hours. The heart rate is maintained at approximately 60 beats/min and the systolic blood pressure in excess of 90 mmHg while one is careful to avoid advanced atrioventricular block, severe bradycardia, bronchospasm, and myocardial failure.

Mueller and Ayres have reported a reduction in myocardial ischemia when patients with uncomplicated acute myocardial infarction were treated with intravenous propranolol.[182,183] The mean arterial pressure, heart rate, cardiac work, and myocardial oxygen consumption were decreased by 20 percent and the heart extracted rather than produced lactate, suggesting a favorable balance between myocardial oxygen supply and demand. Peter reported that intravenous and subsequently oral propranolol administered within 4 hours of the onset of symptoms of acute myocardial infarction reduced creatine kinase (CK) release by 30 percent in comparison with a control population but had no significant effect when administered after 4 hours of the onset of symptoms.[203]

Twenty major investigations have been reported in which patients with myocardial infarction were treated with β-adrenergic blocking agents, including propranolol, practolol, alprenolol, oxprenolol, and timolol.[3,14-17,30,51,88,130,186,187,190-192,216,232,234,245,263,264] In 11 of these studies the drugs were started within the first 48 hours following acute myocardial infarction.[14,15,16,51,88,130,187,190,191,232,234] Only the very *first* of the studies claimed a reduction in mortality,[234] but unfortunately there were scientific limitations in its randomization and placebo control studies. Subsequent randomized studies did not indicate statistically significant benefit. In one early intervention trial, only a subgroup of patients with an initial rapid heart rate had a reduced mortality with practolol therapy.[15] In a recent randomized trial involving 388 patients, comparing propranolol with atenolol and with placebo in the immediate treatment of patients with suspected myocardial infarction, there was no significant difference between the three groups with respect to mortality after 1 year.[263] In nine other studies, treatment with β-blocking drugs was started 5 days or more after the acute myocardial infarction and was continued for up to 3 years.[3,17,30,186,192,216,245,264] Seven of these trials yielded significant reductions in mortality with practolol, alprenolol, timolol, and propranolol. Practolol has subsequently been withdrawn because of problems with "occulocutaneous syndrome" and "plastic peritonitis."[186] It is not entirely clear at the present time whether the beneficial effect of β-adrenergic blockade in these studies is due to limitation of infarction size, an antiarrhythmic effect, or the prevention of subsequent infarction. These agents do decrease myocardial oxygen requirements by reducing total myocardial work; however, this occurs at the risk of a reduced myocardial inotropic state, heart failure, and bronchoconstriction.

Heterogenous patient populations, a wide variety of β-adrenergic blocking agents administered, and the frequent use of fixed dose schedules may account for the discrepancies reported in the current clinical trials.[3,14-17,30,51,88,130,186,187,190-192,216,232,234,245,263,264] At the present time, however, it appears that when β-adrenergic blockade is begun 5 days or more after the acute infarction, mortality is significantly reduced.

Calcium Channel Entry Blockers

Cardiac muscle and vascular smooth muscle are dependent on extracellular calcium and the transmembrane influx of calcium for contraction. In the presence of myocardial ischemia a cellular membrane defect permits an increased influx of calcium into the myocardial cells. Intracellular calcium concentration may then increase by as much as 50-fold in ischemic regions of the myocardium. This calcium is taken up and sequestered by the mitochondria, thus consuming adenosine triphosphate. As a result, the energy production and contractile function of the heart may be significantly impaired. Calcium channel entry blockers interfere with the amount of calcium crossing the cardiac and smooth muscle cellular membrane. Their net hemodynamic effects include (1) reduction in vascular smooth muscle tone with a decrease in coronary artery arterial and venous resistance and an increase in coronary artery blood flow, (2) a decrease in the interaction of calcium with contractile proteins thus limiting myocardial contractility, and (3) slowing of sinoatrial and atrial ventricular conduction. As a consequence, myocardial oxygen requirements are diminished. The intensity with which the various calcium channel entry blocking drugs produce these hemodynamic effects varies (Table 10-4).

In animal studies of acute myocardial infarction, some protection has been demonstrated by the calcium channel entry blockers. Infarct size has tended to be reduced, although conflicting results have been reported. Currently, the precise role of calcium channel entry blockers in the early treatment of patients with acute myocardial infarction is being investigated.[101,185]

Anticoagulant Therapy

The use of heparin or coumadin in the treatment of patients with acute myocardial infarction has been controversial since the original investigations reported in 1948.[272] Conflicting investigative reports have been largely due, over the last 25 years, to inadequate experimental design with small patient populations, suboptimal anticoagulation, a low mortality rate associated with acute thromboembolism, and significant reduction in the length of bed rest following myocardial infarction.

In the past, anticoagulation therapy has been used in the treatment of patients with acute myocardial infarction in order to[42,210,254,272]:

1. Prevent venous thrombosis and possible pulmonary embolization
2. Prevent left ventricular mural thrombus formation and systemic embolization
3. Prevent extension of myocardial necrosis
4. Reduce patient mortality

The incidence of deep venous leg thrombosis following acute myocardial infarction ranges from 32 to 37 percent as determined by the use of iodine[125] fibrinogen scanning.[210] Factors associated with an increased incidence of leg vein thrombosis include age greater than 70 years, obesity, low cardiac output, varicose veins, and prior history of myocardial infarction or thromboembolism. Anticoagulant therapy in this group is effective in preventing deep venous thrombosis in the lower extremities and reducing clinical pulmonary thromboembolic complications.[213,251,271,272] Embolization from mural wall thrombi to the brain, kidneys, or extremities may also be significantly reduced with the use of anticoagulant therapy. The British Working Party Study detected an incidence of only 1.3 percent systemic embolization in patients receiving anticoagulants.[213] In the Veterans Administration Cooperative Trial, anticoagulant therapy reduced the total number of cerebrovascular accidents from 3.8 percent in untreated patients to 0.8 percent in the group receiving anticoagulants.[251] Furthermore, there were no clinically detected embolic phenomena to the kidneys or lower extremities among treated patients, although the incidence of sys-

TABLE 10-4. Pharmokinetics of the Calcium Channel Entry Blockers

	Verapamil	Diltiazem	Nifedipine	Lidoflazine
Heart rate	↑↓	↓	↑↑	0
AV conduction	↓↓	↓	↑	0
Coronary vasodilatation	↑↑	↑↑↑	↑↑↑	↑↑↑
Contractility	↓	0	↑	0
Peripheral arterial dilatation	↑↑	↑	↑↑↑	↑↑

(Adapted from Shapiro W: Calcium channel entry blockers and ischemic heart disease. Baylor College of Medicine Cardiology Series 5(6):8, 1982.)

temic embolization was 0.6 percent in untreated patients.

There is, however, currently no secure evidence to support the use of anticoagulation with either heparin or coumadin to reduce myocardial infarction size or prevent extension of an infarct. In both the British Working Party Study and the Veterans Administration Cooperative Trial, the incidence of both in-hospital and late reinfarction was the same for both groups receiving anticoagulant and control groups.[213,251]

Full anticoagulation therapy is prescribed for patients with acute myocardial infarction who have been maintained on chronic anticoagulant therapy, or who have a history or physical findings of previous pulmonary or systemic embolization, massive cardiac enlargement, left ventricular aneurysm, refractory congestive heart failure, massive obesity, extensive varicosities or venous thrombosis of the lower extremities, or chronic inability to ambulate.[125] In such patients, the activated partial thromboplastin time (PTT) is maintained at approximately 1.5 times the control value, and is carefully monitored. Full anticoagulation is contraindicated if there is active bleeding, purpura or hemorrhagic diathesis, major hepatic or renal insufficiency, severe hypertension, open wounds, sepsis, recent surgery, or anticipated invasive vascular catheterization procedures.[105,125]

Anticoagulant Therapy Complications

In the Veterans Administration Cooperative Trial, gastrointestinal hemorrhage occurred in 0.6 percent of the patients.[251] In the British Working Party Study, major hemorrhagic complications occurred in 4.3 percent of patients receiving both heparin and phenindione.[251] Additional hemorrhagic complications reported include bleeding into the skin and muscles, especially following intramuscular injections, bleeding in the intestinal wall with resultant intestinal obstruction, addisonian crises secondary to adrenal hemorrhage, subdural hematoma formation, and retroperitoneal bleeding.[254]

Low Dose Heparin Therapy

Low dose heparin therapy, consisting of 5,000 units subcutaneously every 12 hours, has been recently popularized for prevention of deep venous thrombosis. In this instance, heparin increases the rate at which antithrombin 3 combines with and inactivates activated factor X.[33] Gallus and associates reported an incidence of deep venous thrombosis of 12.6 percent in treated patients with suspected infarctions as opposed to 22.5 percent in untreated patients.[89] Unfortunately this therapy will not prevent a thrombotic process that is in progress. Furthermore, no evidence is currently available to show whether low dose heparin therapy will reduce the incidence of pulmonary emboli or mural wall thrombus in patients with acute myocardial infarction.

Low dose heparin therapy has been recommended for patients with acute myocardial infarction unless there is evidence of active bleeding, major gastrointestinal or genitourinary disorders, or recent central nervous system or ocular surgery.[105]

Nonsurgical Coronary Artery Recanalization

Propranolol, hyaluronidase, corticosteroids, and glucose–insulin–potassium (GIK) have been used to decrease myocardial oxygen requirements, increase myocardial collateral blood flow, protect against autolytic processes, and/or increase vital substrates after acute myocardial infarction. None of these interventions has been uniformly successful. Since intracoronary thrombosis is either the cause or a consequence of acute myocardial infarction, the direct intracoronary instillation and also the intravenous administration of thrombolytic drugs has been under active study as means of increasing coronary blood flow and myocardial oxygenation in patients with acute myocardial infarction.[90-93,168] This is a potentially beneficial though as yet not fully proven option for limiting the size of the acute myocardial infarction. Streptokinase (2,000 IU/min) and streptokinase in combination with plasmino-gen (Thrombolysin, 2,000 to 4,000 IU/min) have been infused following selective coronary artery catheterization with the aid of a 0.85 mm coronary artery catheter directly into the site of thrombosis formation within 4 hours of the onset of symptoms of acute myocardial infarction. To exclude coronary spasm, nitroglycerin in doses of 0.5 mg is injected selectively into the coronary artery prior to thrombolytic therapy. Forty-seven acute myocardial infarction patients who underwent intracoronary thrombolysis have been reported by Ganz with coronary reperfusion established in 41 of 47 (87 percent) patients.[90] Left ventricular wall motion studied by contrast ventriculography, two-dimensional echocardiography, and multiple gated blood pool scintigraphy have demonstrated improvement in regional wall motion abnormalities within 12 days following reperfusion. In 18 of the 47 patients elective coronary artery bypass surgery was recommended for treatment of underlying obstructive coronary artery disease.

Mathey investigated 47 patients within 4 hours after acute myocardial infarction who underwent direct intracoronary injections of streptokinase in amounts of 3,000 IU/min for periods of 2 hours or less.[168] In 30 of the 41 patients (73 percent) recanalization of the thrombosed coronary artery occurred. Left ventricular ejection fractions increased in the majority of patients whose coronary arteries were successfully recanalized but declined in the 11 patients in whom attempts at recanalization failed. In seven patients, reperfusion was associated with ventricular fibrillation which was reversed in each instance with electrical countershock. According to both Ganz and Mathey reperfusion is usually immediately complicated by arrhythmias including ventricular premature beats, bigeminy, or isorhythmic atrioventricular dissociation. Lidocaine therapy has therefore been recommended during thrombolytic therapy. In one patient studied by Mathey, coronary artery perforation necessitated termination of the procedure. Of the 30 patients whose coronary arteries were recanalized after streptokinase infusion by Mathey, enzymatic and electrocardiographic evidence of reinfarction was observed in three patients within 10 days. Long-term anticoagulation and coro-nary artery bypass surgery were therefore recommended following recanalization.

The favorable results of intracoronary thrombolysis associated with the general goal of initiating treatment and achieving reperfusion in the shortest possible time after the onset of symptoms of acute myocardial infarction have prompted the intravenous administration of streptokinase. Eighty-one patients, reported by Ganz, received a 15 to 30 minute intravenous infusion of 750,000 to 1.5 million units of streptokinase within 3 hours of the onset of acute myocardial infarction followed by heparin anticoagulation. Reperfusion was reported in 78 of the 81 patients.[92] Major bleeding requiring transfusion of blood occurred in 10 percent of patients. Six to 22 hours after reperfusion, 6 of the 78 patients (8 percent) demonstrated signs of reocclusion as demonstrated by return of chest pain and elevation of the ST segments on the electrocardiogram. The in-hospital mortality of 6.2 percent compared favorably with the 8.6 percent hospital mortality associated with the intracoronary streptokinase study by the same investigators. Before these techniques are generally used, however, the morbidity and the mortality due to distal coronary artery embolization, coronary artery dissection and perforation, ventricular fibrillation, and major bleeding must be accurately defined.

ACUTE MYOCARDIAL INFARCTION WITH LEFT VENTRICULAR FAILURE

Patients with acute myocardial infarction may present with acute pulmonary congestion due to decreased left ventricular ejection, reduced left ventricular compliance, and increased ventricular filling pressures. The filling pressure of the left ventricle is dependent on the stiffness of the left ventricular wall, the volume of diastolic inflow into the ventricle, and the end-systolic volume.[243] In the early phase of acute myocardial infarction, ventricular compliance is increased due to noncontracting infarcted tissue that is passively stretched during systole. The infarcted tissue may subsequently become progressively more stiff (i.e., less compliant), due to the inflammatory changes and localized tissue edema quantitatively related to the mass of infarcted myocardium. These changes reduce the likelihood of systolic expansion of the infarcted segment and the hemodynamic risks of ventricular aneurysm, but at the cost of increased end-diastolic pressure. When the left ventricular end-diastolic pressure and therefore pulmonary capillary pressure exceeds plasma colloid oncotic pressure there is an increased likelihood of acute pulmonary edema. When cardiac output and left ventricular stroke work are normal (i.e., high pressure, normal flow), the acute mortality is approximately 11 percent. When the cardiac output is significantly reduced (i.e., high pressure, low flow), the mortality exceeds 40 percent.[83]

Diuretic agents such as furosemide (Lasix) or ethacrynic acid (Edecrin) and vasodilator agents such as nitroprusside (Nipride), phentolamine (Regitine), or nitroglycerin (Tridil) are useful for management of patients with acute pulmonary congestion.

Loop Diuretics: Furosemide and Ethacrynic Acid

The loop diuretics, furosemide and ethacrynic acid, redistribute renal blood flow to the cortical nephrons and primarily inhibit sodium and chloride transport and reabsorption in the ascending limb of the loop of Henle, but also in the proximal tubule of the kidney.[22] Large amounts of sodium, chloride, and water are therefore excreted into the urine, largely independent of acid–base balance. The rate of urine formation may be increased as much as 20-fold to levels that approximate one-third of the glomerular filtration rate.

The diuretic effects of furosemide are preceded by an increase in venous capacitance with a decrease in venous return and therefore a decrease in right heart and pulmonary artery pressures. Venous capacitance increases within 5 minutes of intravenous furosemide ad-

ministration, well before any diuretic effect can be documented. This effect persists for periods of approximately 20 minutes, then gradually subsides.[71,231]

Furosemide and ethacrynic acid are characterized by a prompt onset of action. Following oral administration a diuretic response occurs within 1 hour unless paralytic ileus, reductions in gastrointestinal motility, or edema of the intestine impedes absorption. Following intravenous injection a diuretic response may be observed within 10 minutes. Maximum diuresis occurs during the first 2 hours after oral administration and is usually complete within 6 hours.[230] Following intravenous administration, diuresis occurs within 30 minutes and reaches a maximum within 45 minutes. Both furosemide in doses of 40 to 100 mg and ethacrynic acid, 50 to 100 mg, may be administered orally; intravenous doses range from 20 to approximately 100 mg.

Adverse effects of furosemide and ethacrynic acid include weakness, nausea, and dizziness as well as eighth nerve damage due to drug-induced changes in electrolyte composition of the vestibular endolymph. Ethacrynic acid has also been associated with the development of skin rash and granulocytopenia. In the presence of nephrosis or chronic renal failure, the dosage of the loop diuretic must be increased. This does not significantly compromise renal function; however the incidence of undesirable side effects is increased.

Vasodilator Drugs

Vasodilator drugs are useful for the treatment of patients with heart failure, especially those with increased systemic vascular resistance who demonstrate refractoriness to diuretic agents.[116,166] Vasodilator drugs such as nitroprusside or phentolamine decrease the "afterload" or the resistance against which the left ventricle ejects blood, thereby reducing the pressure work of the left ventricle, permitting more rapid arterial runoff and increased ventricular emptying. End-diastolic volume and ventricular wall tension decrease, resulting in a decrease in myocardial oxygen consumption and an improvement in ventricular function. Venous vasodilatation may also occur with these drugs, causing pooling of blood in the venous capacitance bed and decreased ventricular "preload" or end-diastolic volume with resultant reduction in ventricular filling pressures and pulmonary congestion (Table 10-5). In these patients with complicated acute myocardial infarction, balloon-tipped flotation catheters are extremely useful for monitoring the right and left ventricular filling pressures and the cardiac output in response to vasodilating drugs.

Nitroprusside

Nitroprusside in doses of 10 to approximately 400 ug/min causes vascular smooth muscle relaxation with dilatation of both the venous capacitance bed and the arteriolar resistance bed.[44,85,175] The pharmacologically active component of nitroprusside has been postulated to be the nitroso (NO) moiety.[197] Nitroprusside decreases the venous return to the right side of the heart due to pooling of blood in the venous capacitance bed. It facilitates forward arterial blood flow by decreasing arterial vascular resistance. Accordingly, atrial and ventricular volumes and end-diastolic pressures decrease, permitting increased coronary endocardial perfusion with improvement in the oxygen supply to the myocardium. With reduction in ventricular volume there is an improvement in the alignment of the papillary muscles and reduction in mitral valvular regurgitation. In patients with congestive heart failure, nitroprusside decreases renal vascular resistance and increases renal blood flow; excretion of sodium and potassium may therefore be enhanced.[19]

In patients with mitral regurgitation, including patients with mitral insufficiency due to papillary muscle dysfunction or ruptured chordae tendinae, pharmacologic reduction with nitroprusside of the systemic vascular resistance increases the forward ejection of blood into the aorta and decreases regurgitation of blood into the left atrium.[45] Left atrial and left ventricular end-systolic and end-diastolic volumes then decrease. Reduction in the ventricular volume results in an improvement in the alignment of the papillary muscles, and an increase in the blood supply to the left ventricular free wall improves the function of these structures.

Vasodilator drugs such as nitroprusside may also reduce the magnitude of the left to right shunt across acquired intraventricular septal defects that occasionally occur with acute anteroseptal myocardial infarction.[244,246] The magnitude of the left to right shunt is largely determined by the ratio of pulmonary to systemic vascular resistance as well as the resistance offered by the defect itself. Thus in acquired ventricular septal defects with pulmonary and left ventricular volume overloads and critically lowered cardiac outputs, vasodilator-induced decreases in systemic arterial resistance increase the forward stroke volume and diminish left to right shunting and therefore pulmonary congestion. In this instance hemodynamic monitoring with the balloon-tipped flotation catheter is most useful in maximizing cardiac output without compromising systemic or coronary blood flow.

While nitroprusside may improve cardiac output in patients with acute myocardial infarction, whether or not this drug treatment re-

TABLE 10-5. Vasodilator Drugs

Drug	Dosage	Venous Tone	Arterial Resistance	Blood Pressure	Cardiac Output	PAWP	Heart Rate
Nitroprusside	8–400 μg/min	↓↓	↓↓	↔↓	↑	↓↓	↔↑
Phentolamine	0.1–2 mg/min	↓	↓↓	↔↓	↑	↓	↑
Nitroglycerin	10–200 μg/min	↓↓↓	↓	↔↓	↔↑	↓↓	↔↑
Trimethaphan	0.5–5 mg/min	↓↓	↓	↔↓	↑	↓	↔↑

(Adapted from Henning RJ, Weil MH: Treatment of Cardiogenic Shock. p. 69. In Dreifus LS, Brest AN (eds): Clinical Application of Cardiovascular Drugs. Martinus Nijhoff, The Hague, 1980.)

duces overall mortality is currently controversial.[201]

Nitroprusside-Induced Complications

In patients with increased systemic vascular resistance, stroke volume and cardiac output usually increase as systemic vascular resistance decreases and pulmonary artery occlusive pressure is decreased to 15 to 18 mmHg with nitroprusside or other vasodilator drugs. Systemic arterial pressure changes relatively little because the increase in cardiac output that follows the decline in impedance to left ventricular ejection predominates over the decrease in preload. When the pulmonary artery occlusive pressure is lowered to less than 12 mmHg, however, cardiac output and subsequently blood pressure may decrease because the reduction in preload predominates over the decline in afterload.[19,45,175,197,201,244,246] Consequently the pulmonary artery occlusive pressure should not be reduced to less than 12 to 15 mmHg when one is administering a vasodilator drug.

Direct combination of nitroprusside with sulfhydryl groups in both red blood cells and tissues liberates cyanide, which is converted in the liver to thiocyanate and subsequently excreted by the kidneys.[197] Cyanide may accumulate in the tissues in patients with significant hepatic dysfunction but clinical detection of cyanide poisoning is difficult due to lack of readily available laboratory techniques for clinical measurement. Parenteral hydroxycobolamin is currently recommended for patients with impaired hepatic function who are receiving nitroprusside to prevent cyanide accumulation.[59]

If cyanide poisoning does occur, sodium nitrite is administered to produce high concentrations of methemoglobin. Methemoglobin then competes with cytochrome oxidase for the cyanide ion forming cyanmethemoglobin and cytochrome oxidase is restored. Thiosulfate is then administered, which reacts with cyanide to form thiocyanate, which is excreted in the urine. Thiocyanate toxicity is an uncommon clinical occurrence, but problems may occur in patients with significant renal impairment when blood concentrations exceed 10 mg/100 ml.[66] The principal manifestations of thiocyanate toxicity include fatigue, nausea, anorexia, hiccupping, disorientation, psychotic behavior, and muscle spasm. Treatment consists of administration of 0.9 percent sodium chloride or dilute hydrochloric acid to hasten excretion of thiocyanate or the initiation of acute hemodialysis. Nitroprusside may also on occasion induce hypothyroidism,[193] convulsions,[81] and pulmonary arteriovenous shunting.[38]

Following abrupt discontinuation of nitroprusside, a rebound phenomenon occurs, characterized by significant increases in systemic and pulmonary artery pressure and reduction in cardiac output.[196] These changes may persist for periods of 30 minutes to 3 hours. Nitroprusside should therefore be gradually tapered over periods of 1 to 2 hours while the patient is carefully observed for signs of increasing heart failure.

Phentolamine

Phentolamine is primarily an α-adrenergic blocking agent that is chemically related to tolazoline and histamine. It antagonizes the α-adrenergic responses of norepinephrine and epinephrine.[116] The drug also has a direct vascular smooth muscle dilator effect and possibly a β-adrenergic stimulating effect.[104] In addition, phentolamine may improve myocardial metabolism by reversing insulin suppression.[162] The positive inotropic action of phentolamine may, however, be related to norepinephrine release or the unopposed β-adrenergic effects of norepinephrine, which also account for an increase in heart rate.

Phentolamine exerts greater dilator effects on the arteriolar resistance bed than nitroprusside, while nitroprusside has a greater dilating action on the venous capacitance bed than phentolamine.[174] In concentrations of 0.1 to 2 mg/min, the drug is especially useful for augmenting forward blood flow in patients with acute aortic or mitral valvular insufficiency and increased systemic vascular resistance. Because phentolamine causes less dilatation of the venous capacitance bed than nitroprusside, there is a smaller reduction in preload for a given reduction in impedance. The drug, therefore, appears to be more useful than nitroprusside in increasing cardiac output in patients in whom the left ventricular filling pressure is not markedly elevated.[174]

Gould and co-workers have administered phentolamine to patients with severe cor pulmonale[103] with resultant significant (35 percent) decline in pulmonary vascular resistance and pulmonary artery pressures. Phentolamine has also been demonstrated to have an antispasmodic effect on the lung and a prophylactic effect in subjects with allergic bronchial asthma.[134,270] At the present time however, phentolamine-induced tachycardia and the drug's high cost limit its prolonged clinical use.

Comparison of Nitroprusside with Phentolamine

The hemodynamic effects of nitroprusside have been compared with phentolamine in patients with acute myocardial infarction.[137] When directly examined in the same patients, nitroprusside was more effective in decreasing left ventricular filling pressure but phentolamine administration resulted in a more pronounced increase in stroke volume index as well as heart rate. Increases in cardiac index to mean values of nearly 4 L/min/m² with phentolamine suggested excessive myocardial stimulation. Treatment of patients with acute myocardial infarction (AMI) and mild myocardial failure with phentolamine might therefore induce extension of the ischemic zone because of the positive inotropic and chronotropic effects. However phentolamine appears to be of potential benefit in patients with AMI and severe left heart failure.[137,138]

Nitroglycerin

Nitroglycerin has been utilized in the treatment of patients with both acute and chronic low cardiac output states.[40,68,80] The actions of intravenous nitroglycerin in concentrations of 10 to approximately 200 ug/min are principally exerted on the systemic venous system with direct relaxation of smooth muscle in the venous capacitance bed and reduction in venous return to the right side of the heart. Nitroglycerin therefore may cause a rapid reduction in pulmonary vascular congestion (pulmonary edema).

Comparison of Nitroprusside with Nitroglycerin

Nitroprusside has been compared with nitroglycerin in patients with acute myocardial infarction.[137,138] In these investigations, left ventricular filling pressure declined and heart rate increased to a similar extent with both drugs when the mean arterial pressure was lowered to identical levels. In contrast to nitroprusside, nitroglycerin produced a significant decrease in stroke volume, and a slight reduction in cardiac index as a consequence of its predominant preload reducing effect. This finding was consistent with the investigations of Come[58] and also Flaherty,[79] who have shown no change or a reduction of cardiac index during intravenous administration of nitroglycerin in cases of acute myocardial infarction. In contrast, Gold,[96] Armstrong,[9] and Bussman[41] have reported that cardiac output increased with nitroglycerin therapy, especially in patients with severe left ventricular failure or increased collateral blood supply.

Chiarello reported that nitroglycerin reduced ischemic injury by increasing perfusion of ischemic areas, whereas nitroprusside *increased* ischemia due to its vasodilatory action on coronary arterioles in the nonischemic region, producing a "coronary steal" and intensifying myocardial ischemia.[48] In contrast Da Luz and Forrester reported that nitroprusside significantly improved both total coronary performance and the mechanical performance of regional ischemic myocardium.[63] This improvement was associated with an increase in regional perfusion and reduction in lactate production.[63]

At the present time either nitroprusside or nitroglycerin appears to be beneficial when administered intravenously with the aid of a Swan-Ganz catheter to patients with acute myocardial infarction and moderate to severe refractory pulmonary edema, as long as the dose is carefully titrated to avoid hypotension and tachycardia.

Digitalis Glycosides

In patients with acute myocardial failure, digitalis glycosides have been administered to enhance cardiac contractility and therefore cardiac output by increasing myocardial fiber shortening of the surviving normal and ischemic myocardium.[167,208,238] Indeed, intravenous digitalis glycosides have been demonstrated to increase the peak first derivative of left ventricular pressure in the normal myocardium and in the zones bordering ischemic tissue.[133] The direct effect on the ischemic zone of the myocardium, however, is variable. Furthermore, in myocardial infarction patients who do not have heart failure, bolus injections of rapid-acting digitalis glycosides may constrict coronary and systemic vessels.[161] Vascular resistance may then increase prior to any inotropic effect of digitalis and may augment myocardial oxygen consumption with further impairment in cardiac function and enhancement of myocardial ischemia.

The hemodynamic effects of digitalis glycosides depend, in part, on heart size.[161] In the presence of significant cardiomegaly and decreased cardiac output, digitalis decreases end-diastolic volume and pressure, resulting in a significant decline in systolic wall tension and a reduction in myocardial oxygen demand. While the augmentation in myocardial contractility produced by digitalis increases myocardial oxygen demands, concurrent reduction in myocardial wall tension counteracts the oxygen cost of augmented contractility. In patients with acute myocardial infarction without cardiomegaly, the increased metabolic cost of the positive inotropic effect of digitalis may not be entirely balanced by a reduction in end-diastolic pressure and volume and therefore myocardial wall tension. Furthermore, in these patients transient elevations of systemic arterial pressure resulting from rapidly acting glycosides may be undesirable.

Minimal increases in cardiac output and elevations of arterial pressure have been observed following administration of digitalis to patients with cardiogenic shock.[56,107,163] Since cardiogenic shock is associated with destruction of more than 40 percent of the left ventricular muscle mass it is not surprising that digitalis glycosides do not significantly improve ventricular function.

The infarcted myocardium is sensitive to digitalis glycosides and ventricular tachycardia may be provoked in patients with acute myocardial infarction who receive digitalis therapy. The threshold dosage of digitalis glycoside for inducing ventricular arrhythmias[140] is reduced 43 percent. Marked inhomogeneity of digitalis uptake in acutely infarcted myocardium, combined with localized areas of myocardial ischemia, produce different recovery times in adjacent areas of the myocardium and predispose to re-entrant cardiac arrhythmias. In addition, alterations in the renal excretion of digitalis and cardiac arrhythmias have been reported in patients with myocardial infarction and congestive heart failure. Consequently, the initial loading dose of digitalis should be reduced approximately 35 percent.

Digitalis and Cardiac Arrhythmias

Digitalis glycosides are beneficial in the treatment of cardiac dysrhythmias complicating acute myocardial infarction. Atrial fibrillation with a ventricular rate greater than 100 beats/min is an indication unless there is arrhythmia-induced hypotension with signs or symptoms of congestive heart failure, for which prompt synchronized electric shock therapy is required.[177,207,243] In less urgent situations 0.25 to 0.5 mg digoxin may be given initially intravenously and 0.25 mg given intravenously every 2 to 4 hours thereafter until the ventricular rate is controlled or a total dose of approximately 2.0 mg has been administered.

The effect of digitalis glycosides in diminishing atrioventricular (AV) conduction of atrial fibrillatory impulses is primarily due to vagal stimulation. When there is excessive sympathetic activity, adequate atrioventricular suppression may not be achieved despite large doses of digitalis.

In the setting of rapid atrial fibrillation

without hemodynamic compromise, intravenous verapamil is the drug of initial choice for prompt heart rate control. The recommended dosage is 0.07 mg/kg; administration may be repeated with 0.150 mg/kg in 30 minutes if there is no response to the initial dose. Since verapamil has negative myocardial inotropic effects, it should be used with caution in patients with congestive heart failure or in those receiving beta-adrenergic blockade therapy. Patients who do not convert to sinus rhythm with verapamil but remain in atrial fibrillation should then receive digitalis to control their ventricular rate.

Paroxysmal atrial tachycardia and atrial flutter producing hypotension should initially be treated with electrocardioversion and subsequently treated with verapamil. Verapamil is the drug of choice for treatment of paroxysmal supraventricular tachycardia without hypotension. Atrial flutter, not associated with hypotension, may be treated with either intravenous verapamil or digoxin. The effect of a single injection of verapamil lasts 30 to 60 minutes. For patients with persistent atrial flutter, digoxin therapy is indicated to control the ventricular rate.

Digitalis glycosides are of greatest benefit after acute myocardial infarction when cardiomegaly and low cardiac output states are associated with atrial fibrillation or atrial flutter. Under these circumstances the dual action of digitalis in increasing myocardial contractility and slowing heart rate serves to improve ventricular performance. Digitalis glycosides do not increase infarct size in patients who have myocardial infarction with cardiomegaly and heart failure but may increase myocardial damage when cardiac size is normal. In patients with severe pump failure (cardiogenic shock), digitalis glycosides are most useful for their antiarrhythmic effects.

Digoxin–Quinidine Interaction

In 1978 the pharmacokinetic interaction between digoxin and quinidine was recognized.[143] The use of radioimmunoassays of serum digoxin provided a simple, rapid, and reliable method for evaluating digoxin kinetics during administration of quinidine and led to the recognition of the frequent (90 percent) interaction between the two drugs. Subsequently, Leahey and colleagues as well as others found that digoxin concentrations increase from an average of 1.4 ng/ml to 3.1 ng/ml after institution of quinidine therapy.[143]

Several mechanisms for this drug interaction have been postulated. Since the concentration of digoxin in serum increases after quinidine therapy, a decrease in the distribution volume of digoxin may occur.[111] Quinidine has also been shown to reduce the renal clearance of digoxin by as much as 52 percent while the creatinine clearance remains unchanged.[72,188] The reduction in digoxin clearance appears to be dependent upon the quinidine concentration since elevations in serum digoxin correlate with serum quinidine concentration.[188] Quinidine also appears to decrease the nonrenal clearance of digoxin by altering hepatic metabolism and biliary elimination.

At the present time the digoxin dose should be reduced by 50 percent when quinidine treatment is instituted.[31] Additional adjustments of digoxin should be made after measurement of the serum digoxin concentration 4 to 5 days after the institution of quinidine.

ACUTE MYOCARDIAL INFARCTION ASSOCIATED WITH HYPOVOLEMIA

As many as 20 percent of patients with acute myocardial infarction have reductions in intravascular blood volume.[46,78,157] This may be due to the vigorous use of diuretics or high concentrations of alpha-adrenergic catecholamines, which increase capillary hydrostatic pressure and cause fluid extravasation, and may be aggravated by recurrent nausea, vomiting, diaphoresis, and failure to eat and drink. Furthermore patients with acute pulmonary edema and increased venous resistance extravasate hypo-oncotic fluid from the intravascular space into the interstitial space with consequent depletion of the circulating blood volume.[78]

Peripheral hypoperfusion due to hypovolemia may be suspected from careful physical examination. This is of major prognostic significance because the mortality rate in patients with unrecognized and therefore untreated hypoperfusion is four times greater than the mortality rate of patients with uncomplicated myocardial infarction. Intravenous fluid administration, which provides an increase in preload and an increase in end-diastolic fiber length to optimal levels, therefore serves as the cornerstone of initial therapy for patients with acute myocardial infarction and absolute or relative hypovolemia. This therapy extracts the least myocardial oxygen cost of all the available options for pharmacologic intervention.

The optimal range of left ventricular filling pressure has been stated[62,224] to be between 15 and 25 mmHg. An absolute level of left ventricular filling pressure (i.e., pulmonary artery diastolic or wedge pressure), however, may not be optimal in any given patient. Errors in zero reference, assessment of midchest position, and calibration of transducers may of themselves account for a variation of ± 7 mmHg. The pulmonary artery diastolic and wedge pressure, colloid oncotic pressure, and the cardiac output should be carefully monitored during fluid administration, and fluid challenge continued as long as cardiac output increases and colloid oncotic pressure exceeds the pulmonary artery occlusive pressure.[77,239,258,260] When measurement of colloid oncotic pressure is not available, fluid challenge may be performed utilizing the response of the pulmonary artery diastolic or wedge (occlusive) pressure as a general guideline.[117,258]

Fluid Challenge

If the pulmonary artery diastolic pressure is within 3 mmHg of the wedge pressure, the diastolic pressure may be continuously monitored during a fluid challenge. In all other patients, the wedge pressure should be monitored at 3-minute intervals. If the plasma albumin concentration is less than 3.0 g/dl or if colloid osmotic pressure, which is normally 25 mmHg (range, 22 to 28), is less than or equal to 20 mmHg, 5 percent human serum albumin, plasma protein fraction, or hydroxyethyl starch should be administered intravenously. If the plasma albumin concentration is greater than 3.0 or if colloid oncotic pressure is greater than 20 mmHg, crystalloid solutions such as 0.9 percent NaCl solution should be infused.

If the initial pulmonary artery diastolic (PADP) or wedge pressure (PAWP) is less than 12 mmHg, 200 ml fluid is administered through a peripheral intravenous line over a 10 minute interval and the pulmonary artery pressures are continuously monitored. The balloon-tipped flotation catheter is used only for pressure measurements. If the PADP or PAWP is greater than 12 but less than 16 mmHg, 100 ml fluid is administered intravenously through a peripheral intravenous line. If the PADP or PAWP is equal to or greater than 16 mmHg, 50 ml fluid is administered intravenously over 10 minutes. In less than 10 percent of patients with acute myocardial infarction, hypovolemia may be associated with an increased rather than a decreased pulmonary artery wedge pressure due to a reduction in coronary artery perfusion and myocardial failure secondary to primary hypovolemia.

If during the initial 0 to 9 minutes of fluid infusion the pulmonary artery diastolic or wedge pressure abruptly *increases* by more than 7 mmHg, the fluid challenge is discontinued; additional intravenous fluid will exceed the competence of the heart to accept fluid and cause significant reductions in cardiac output and acute pulmonary edema. If the pulmonary artery diastolic or wedge pressure increases slowly by more than 3 mmHg, but less than 7 mmHg, the infusion is completed and the patient is then observed for 10 minutes. If the pulmonary pressure remains persistently greater than 3 mmHg of the initial value, the fluid challenge is discontinued. If, however, the pulmonary pressure decreases to *within* 3 mmHg of the starting value, the fluid challenge is continued, and one should observe the response of the pulmonary artery diastolic or wedge pressure as a general guideline. Within this framework the fluid challenge is continued as long as the cardiac output increases.

The myocardial performance of the infarcted left ventricle may be assessed by serial measurement of cardiac index or left ventricular stroke work index plotted against pulmonary artery occlusive pressure, reflecting left ventricular end-diastolic pressure. The slope of the resulting line may be determined by calculating the relationship between change in cardiac index (CI) and the change in filling pressure of the ventricle (e.g., Δ CI/Δ PAWP) and correlates with measurements of angiographically determined left ventricular ejection fraction.[209] Using these techniques, serial measurements of left ventricular performance may be obtained and serve as useful prognostic indicators.

Right Ventricular Infarction

Patients who have sustained acute right ventricular infarction represent a special category: low cardiac output but normal pulmonary artery occlusive pressure.

The clinical and hemodynamic presentation of patients with right ventricular infarction depends upon the extent of right ventricular and septal involvement and the magnitude of concurrent left ventricular infarction. Transmural infarction of the posterior interventricular septum is a prerequisite for right ventricular dysfunction, since involvement of the right ventricular free wall alone is not likely to be of significant hemodynamic import.[94,128] The right ventricle contracts from apex to base rather than transversely and this is primarily impaired by septal rather than free wall infarction.

Clinically significant right ventricular infarction is characterized by distended neck veins due to right ventricular failure with increased ventricular and atrial filling pressure and, in patients with tricuspid regurgitation due to right ventricular papillary muscle dysfunction, large jugular V waves.[159] Arterial hypotension and pulsus paradoxus may be present while pulmonary congestion is usually absent.

Acute inferior and/or posterior wall myocardial infarction may be identified on the 12-lead electrocardiogram. Radionucleotide angiography and two-dimensional echocardiography provide noninvasive methods for identifying dilatation of the right ventricle with impaired wall motion and decreased ejection fraction.

The physical findings and hemodynamic profile of right ventricular infarction may simulate cardiac tamponade, constrictive pericarditis, or pulmonary embolism.[159] Cardiac tamponade may be identified by equalization of right-sided end-diastolic pressures including pulmonary artery diastolic pressure during hemodynamic studies. Absence of a pericardial effusion as demonstrated by echocardiography and radionucleotide angiography excludes cardiac tamponade. Pericardial constriction is characterized by abnormal inspiratory increase in mean right atrial pressure (Kussmaul's sign) and an early diastolic dip and plateau configuration of the ventricular pressure waveform ("square root sign"). Diastolic ventricular filling is impaired in constrictive pericarditis and systolic emptying in right ventricular infarction. When radionucleotide angiography or echocardiography demonstrates dilation and hypokinesis of the right ventricle, constrictive pericarditis is unlikely and right ventricular infarction should be suspected. Acute right ventricular failure following pulmonary embolization is characterized by a substantial increase in pulmonary artery systolic and diastolic pressure with normal pulmonary artery wedge pressure. In contrast with pulmonary embolization, right ventricular infarction does not itself account for increases in pulmonary artery pressures.

Expansion of intravascular volume utilizing fluid challenge techniques with crystalloid or colloid solutions in patients with elevated right-sided pressures and normal or near normal pulmonary artery occlusive pressures often produces significant hemodynamic improvement.[52,106] As much as 2 to 6 L may be required during an initial 24-hour period. If hypoperfusion persists following volume expansion, sodium nitroprusside, or nitroprusside in combination with dopamine, may be necessary to facilitate forward blood flow and correct hypotension. Intra-aortic balloon counterpulsation has been used to treat shock complicating right ventricular infarction and has decreased left ventricular filling pressures but has not significantly changed cardiac index or right ventricular filling pressures.[54,159] Nevertheless, the prognosis of shock complicating right ventricular infarction after appropriate therapy is significantly better than cardiogenic shock associated with left ventricular destruction.

Bradycardia and Low Cardiac Output

A less common group within the subset of patients with low cardiac output and normal or reduced ventricular filling pressures have marked bradycardia. In these patients heart rate may be accelerated and cardiac output increased to more optimal levels by the administration of atropine (0.5 to 1.0 mg IV), isoproterenol (2 mg/500 ml 5 percent dextrose/water IV), or by temporary bipolar transvenous right ventricular pacing.[64]

Myocardial Failure and Cardiogenic Shock

Approximately 40 percent of patients with acute myocardial infarction have clinically significant hemodynamic impairment.[83,84,214] In one-third of these patients, the heart is no longer able to pump an adequate supply of blood to meet the metabolic needs of the tissues of the body, with resultant anaerobic metabolism and circulatory shock.

The primary defect in this group of patients is severe impairment of left ventricular contractility due to a loss of more than 40 percent of the left ventricular muscle mass[5,112] (Table 10-1). This is most often due to a cumulative loss of muscle involving old and new myocardial infarctions.

While the syndrome of cardiogenic shock is most often caused by acute myocardial infarction it may also be due to severe valvular heart disease, cardiomyopathy, or increased ventricular work loads due to large intracardiac or systemic arteriovenous shunts.[117] Major alterations in cardiac rhythm that compromise either cardiac filling or emptying may also lead to cardiogenic shock.

The syndrome occurs more often in older patients with anterior infarction with involvement of the left anterior descending coronary artery. It appears within 6 hours following acute infarction in approximately 30 percent, and within 36 hours in approximately 85 percent of shock patients.[227] In the remaining 15 percent of patients cardiogenic shock occurs within 1 week.

In cardiogenic shock, the systolic arterial pressure is less than 90 mmHg or has declined more than 70 mmHg from a previous hypertensive level. The pulmonary artery occlusive pressure exceeds 18 mmHg while the cardiac index declines to less than 2.0 L/min/m². The increase in LVEDP is often disproportional to the increase in left ventricular end-diastolic volume because of the decrease in ventricular compliance. Cardiac work is frequently less than 1 kg/m/min. The stroke index declines from normal values of 45 to 80 to less than 25 ml/beat/m². Stroke work index[243] is less than 25 g/m/b/m². Arteriovenous oxygen difference exceeds 5.5 vol percent because of increased oxygen extraction from the smaller volumes of blood delivered to the peripheral tissues. The urine output is less than 20 ml/hour and the gradient between peripheral skin temperature (toe temperature) and ambient room temperature is within 0.5°C, reflecting sympathetic constriction of cutaneous vessels.[119] The blood lactate level characteristically exceeds 2.0 mM/L. The prognosis in patients with cardiogenic shock is extremely poor, and mortality[259] ranges from 55 to 90 percent.

Compensatory Mechanisms

In an attempt to overcome the depression of myocardial contractility, three fundamental reserve mechanisms may be called upon to support the failing heart.[115] Immediately available is the adrenergic nervous system, which stimulates heart rate and myocardial contractility and causes constriction of the peripheral vasculature. Primary pump failure may, however, be frequently accompanied by depletion of cardiac norepinephrine stores and a reduction in the inotropic response to adrenergic stimulation; therefore ventricular performance often is not increased to a completely normal level.[49]

The second compensatory mechanism is regulation of cardiac output by the Frank-Starling mechanism. Otto Frank, in 1895, demonstrated that the stroke volume of the heart may be increased, within limits, by increasing cardiac muscle fiber length.[87] Within physiological limits, an increase in myocardial diastolic fiber length is related to an increase in muscle shortening and therefore augmented capability for cardiac work. In this instance contractile tension is preserved at the expense of increased end-diastolic volume and pressure.

A third compensatory mechanism is a gradual increase in the size of myocardial contractile units with the development of left ventricular hypertrophy. Although the mass of contractile muscle may be increased by ventricular hypertrophy, the individual performance of each unit of ventricular muscle is depressed and the left ventricle functions on a lowered and depressed Frank-Starling Curve.

Strong adrenergic stimulation from both neurogenic and humoral sources maintains central aortic blood flow, increases systemic vascular resistance, and may temporarily sustain coronary and cerebral perfusion. α-Adrenergic stimulation increases venous pressure and may initially redistribute blood toward the heart and increase ventricular filling and cardiac output by the Frank-Starling mechanism. Unfortunately the increase in peripheral resistance is not precisely set at the minimal level necessary to maintain effective perfusion pressure.[53] A marked increase in peripheral vascular resistance results in a considerable increase in the work of the failing heart and precipitates further myocardial failure. Excessive vasoconstriction reduces the blood volume by increasing capillary hydrostatic pressure above colloid oncotic pressure, causing fluid extravasation. This causes hyperviscosity of blood, which further decreases tissue perfusion. A vicious cycle then occurs characterized by progressive reduction in cardiac output, reduction in systemic blood flow and blood pressure, and a progressive increase in peripheral vascular resistance.

Accumulation of lactate and hydrogen ions inhibits the breakdown of glycogen and blunts the compensatory anaerobic response to limited oxygen and high-energy phosphate availability. Cellular membrane permeability increases, and there is failure of the sodium–potassium pump with influx of calcium, sodium, and water and efflux of potassium. Cellular edema occurs with swelling of mitochondria, rupture of lysosomal membranes, and, ultimately, release of lytic enzymes. A decline in intracellular pH impairs calcium transport by the sarcolemma and sarcoplasmic reticulum and leads to a diminution and eventual cessation of myocardial contractility.[47,267]

Treatment

When the arterial systolic pressure is > 90 mmHg, mean arterial pressure is > 70 mmHg, and systemic vascular resistance is increased to > 2000 dynes/sec/cm^{-5}, vasodilator therapy with intravenous nitroprusside or phentolamine may be effective in reducing the afterload and may facilitate ventricular emptying, rapid arterial runoff, and tissue perfusion. Reducing the afterload, or the resistance against which the heart pumps blood, permits cardiac output to increase while decreasing pulmonary capillary pressure and myocardial oxygen requirements. Chatterjee and co-workers have reported a reduction in immediate cardiogenic shock mortality to 50 percent with the intravenous use of the vasodilator nitroprusside.[44]

When the systolic arterial pressure is less than 90 mmHg, mean arterial pressure is less than 70 mmHg, and/or systemic vascular resistance is not markedly increased, alternative pharmacologic interventions must be considered. Catecholamines such as dopamine and dobutamine represent immediate, short-term therapeutic alternatives[257] (Table 10-6).

DOPAMINE

Dopamine (3, 4 dihydroxyphenethylamine hydrochloride) is the natural immediate precursor of norepinephrine and is found in high con-

TABLE 10-6. Action of Catecholamines

Drug	Dosage	α_1	β_1	β_2	Blood Pressure	Cardiac Output	PAWP	Heart Rate
Dopamine	0.3–2.5 mg/min	+++	++	+	↑	↑	↔↑	↔↑
Dobutamine	0.2–1.2 mg/min	+	++++	+	↔↑	↑↑	↓	↔↑
Norepinephrine	2–20 μg/min	++++	++	0	↑↑	↔↑	↑	↔
Epinephrine	2–20 μg/min	+++	+++	++	↔↑	↑↑	↑↔↓	↑

α_1-receptors are postsynaptic activators of smooth muscle.
β_1-receptors predominate in the sino-atrial node, ventricular conduction system, and myocardium.
β_2-receptors are found in peripheral arterioles of skeletal and bronchial smooth muscles.
0 to ++++ refers to relative stimulation.
(Adapted from Henning RJ, Weil MH: Treatment of cardiogenic shock. p. 69. In Dreifus LS, Brest AN (eds): Clinical Application of Cardiovascular Drugs. Martinus Nijhoff. The Hague, 1980.)

centrations both in sympathetic nerves and the adrenal glands.[99,257] Dopamine may produce vascular smooth muscle relaxation or contraction, depending on the concentration. In doses of 0.25 to 0.5 mg/min, dopamine causes vascular smooth muscle vasodilation in the renal, mesenteric, and possibly in the coronary vascular beds.[99,169,212] This vascular effect is not antagonized by propranolol, atropine, or histamine (H_1) antagonists, but may be antagonized by phenothiazine derivatives and by apomorphine. When dopamine is administered in doses exceeding 2 mg/min, the drug acts as an α-adrenergic agonist, induces arteriolar vasoconstriction, and may increase left ventricular filling pressure and myocardial irritability.[222] The inotropic, chronotropic, and pressor responses to dopamine and other catecholamines, however, may be attenuated[247] by as much as 8 percent for each 0.1 pH unit reduction from a pH of 7.45 to 6.6. Arteriolar vasoconstriction produced by dopamine is antagonized by the α-adrenergic receptor blocking agents phentolamine (Regitine) and phenoxybenzamine (Dibenzyline).

Dopamine increases cardiac contractility and heart rate by direct action on myocardial β-adrenergic receptors and by releasing norepinephrine from myocardial catecholamine storage sites.[99] In 24 patients with cardiogenic shock treated with dopamine by Holzer and co-workers, eight patients survived.[124] Patient survival was characterized by a decrease in the left ventricular filling pressure, a slight decrease in heart rate and an increase in mean arterial pressure, and an increase in urine output compared to nonsurvivors. Loeb and co-workers compared the hemodynamic effects of dopamine with norepinephrine and isoproterenol in patients with cardiogenic shock.[158] In 13 patients, dopamine significantly increased cardiac output and stroke volume while also increasing heart rate, left ventricular end-diastolic pressure, and systemic vascular resistance. Norepinephrine did not improve cardiac output or stroke volume but did significantly increase systemic vascular resistance and mean arterial pressure. In addition, there was no significant hemodynamic difference in the measurement of mean arterial pressure, heart rate, stroke volume, systemic vascular resistance, or urine flow when these shock patients were given isoproterenol in comparison to dopamine.

The effects of dopamine on 34 patients with circulatory shock, including 19 patients with acute myocardial infarction, have been reported by Ruiz and Weil.[223] No patient with significant lactic acidosis survived, despite treatment with dopamine therapy (Table 10-7). Five patients who ultimately survived had minimal elevations of blood lactate and would have been predicted to survive independently of dopamine therapy. Accordingly, dopamine does not appear to increase survival in patients with advanced cardiogenic shock.

The effects of dopamine on myocardial oxygen requirements in patients with cardiogenic shock have been carefully investigated by Mueller and colleagues.[184] In this study, the administration of dopamine increased cardiac index, mean arterial pressure, and heart rate

TABLE 10-7. Cardiac Output and Lactate Measurements on Admission in 34 Shock Patients Treated with Dopamine

	Lactate (mm/L)	Cardiac Index (L/min/m²)
Early fatalities (N = 19)	5.4	1.8
Hospital fatalities (N = 10)	3.8	1.9
Hospital survivals (N = 5)	1.8	1.4

(Adapted from Ruiz C, Weil MH, Carlson RW: Treatment of circulatory shock with dopamine: Studies on survival. JAMA 242:165, 1979.)

while the systemic vascular resistance and the pulmonary artery occlusive pressure decreased in eight patients with established cardiogenic shock. Myocardial oxygen extraction and arterial–coronary sinus oxygen difference, however, increased. Furthermore, myocardial lactate production also increased. Consequently, the hemodynamic improvement in cardiac output and mean arterial pressure, which followed dopamine administration, occurred at the expense of increased myocardial oxygen requirements out of proportion to the available oxygen supply. Anaerobic myocardial metabolism therefore occurred with resultant myocardial lactate production rather than normal lactate extraction. These observations, like observations previously made in patients with cardiogenic shock treated with isoproterenol, pinpoint the clinical dilemma. Improvement in cardiac performance with adrenergic agonists such as dopamine is not necessarily associated with concurrent improvement in myocardial metabolism.[82,211] Dopamine may increase myocardial performance at the risk of additional myocardial ischemic injury.

DOBUTAMINE

Dobutamine, a 3-p-hydroxyphenyl-1 methyl substitution on the isoproterenol molecule, is a direct β-adrenergic receptor stimulant that causes less peripheral vasodilatation than isoproterenol.[219,249] At equivalent inotropic dosages, dobutamine produces less than 25 percent of the chronotropic effects of isoproterenol.[4] The drug was formulated and synthesized to increase cardiac performance se-

lectively without significantly altering heart rate or blood pressure.

Dobutamine has been extensively evaluated for the treatment of patients with low cardiac output states and pulmonary vascular congestion.[4,27,95,148,155,156,225] When infused at rates of 2 to 10 μg/kg/min in patients with heart failure, dobutamine increases myocardial contractility as determined by the maximum rate of change of left ventricular pressure (dp/dt) and decreases the left ventricular end-diastolic pressure. Systemic vascular resistance and pulmonary vascular resistance also decrease, reflecting an increase in cardiac output without significant changes in arterial and pulmonary arterial pressures.

DOPAMINE COMPARED WITH DOBUTAMINE

Dobutamine has been compared with dopamine in equivalent concentrations in the management of patients with primary myocardial failure.[147,154] In the investigation of Leier and co-workers, dobutamine, in concentrations of 2.5 to 10 μg/kg/min progressively increased cardiac output by increasing stroke volume, while simultaneously decreasing systemic and pulmonary vascular resistance and pulmonary capillary wedge (occlusive) pressure.[147] Heart rate did not change significantly. In comparison, dopamine increased stroke volume and cardiac output when infused in concentrations of 2 to 4 μg/kg/min. In concentrations greater than 4 μg/kg/min, dopamine produced little additional increase in stroke volume, but did increase heart rate, pulmonary artery wedge pressure, and the number of premature ventricular beats per minute. The limited capability of dopamine to augment stroke volume was related to an increase in mean arterial pressure and therefore afterload. Following discontinuation of dopamine, cardiac index and arterial pressure significantly decreased below initial measurements with a concomitant decrease in left ventricular ejection fraction, possibly due to depletion of myocardial norepinephrine.[61]

Recently Francis and co-workers have reported the use of dobutamine in the treatment of patients with cardiogenic shock.[86] Dobutamine increased arterial pressure solely by increasing cardiac output but had little or no peripheral vasoconstrictive properties. Consequently, systolic pressure increased primarily, while the mean and diastolic pressures changed slightly. Dobutamine was useful when administered early in the course of hypotension but was of no value in the treatment of advanced cardiogenic shock. Dobutamine therapy therefore appears to be most beneficial in patients who have depressed cardiac performance and elevated left ventricular filling pressure, but in whom extreme hypotension and shock have not yet occurred.

Although dobutamine administration has not been associated with myocardial necrosis as determined by cumulative serum creatine kinase release, coronary blood flow determined by radioisotopic myocardial scanning techniques has been reported to be altered.[95,171] This may, in part, be related to dobutamine's inability to increase arterial diastolic pressure and therefore coronary perfusion pressure. Consequently, the prolonged administration of dobutamine is not without some risk of ischemic myocardial injury.

NOREPINEPHRINE

Norepinephrine or levarterenol bitartrate (Levophed) is identical to the endogenous adrenal medullary hormone and also to the neurotransmitter substance released at postganglionic sympathetic nerve endings. In concentrations of 5 μg/min or less, norepinephrine has primarily β-adrenergic inotropic actions; in concentrations of 10 μg/min or greater, α-adrenergic arterial and venous vasoconstrictor activity predominates.[262] Norepinephrine has been recommended for the pharmacologic treatment of cardiogenic shock patients who are refractory to dopamine and other catecholamine therapy.[181] However, the α-adrenergic receptor stimulation associated with the use of large concentrations of norepinephrine may produce constriction of renal, mesenteric, and musculoskeletal vessels, reduction of nutritive blood flow, and increase impedance to left ventricular ejection, thereby increasing the workload on the failing heart.[2,55,109]

Intense vasoconstriction produced by norepinephrine increases capillary hydrostatic pressure above plasma colloid oncotic pressure, causing fluid extravasation into the interstitial space with resultant decrease in the circulating plasma volume. Indeed, primary hypovolemia may account for patient refractoriness to progressively larger concentrations of norepinephrine and may also explain the difficulty in weaning patients from this adrenergic agent.[229]

INDICATIONS FOR CATECHOLAMINES

Because vasopressor agents produce alterations in myocardial metabolism, their use should be restricted to brief periods and only to insure immediate patient survival. Four specific indications have been identified[117]:

1. The emergency augmentation of coronary perfusion in severely hypotensive patients with recurrent malignant cardiac arrhythmias due to myocardial ischemia, which are unresponsive to antiarrhythmic agents
2. The reversal of acute, fulminant pulmonary edema in patients in whom mean arterial pressure is not adequate for renal perfusion with consequent compromise of diuretic agents, such as furosemide and ethacrynic acid, and vasodilator drugs, such as nitroprusside
3. The emergency augmentation of cerebral perfusion in patients with significant mental obtundation secondary to severe hypotension
4. To facilitate percutaneous insertion of arterial and pulmonary arterial catheters for hemodynamic monitoring in patients with extreme hypotension

VASOPRESSOR–VASODILATOR DRUG COMBINATIONS

Vasopressor–vasodilator drug combinations, including levarterenol–phentolamine,[276] levarterenol–dibenzyline,[268] dopamine–phentolamine,[13] and dopamine–dibenzyline,[100] have been investigated for the treatment of patients with low cardiac output states. The addition of a vasodilating agent primarily emphasizes the beta effect of an α–β adrenergic catecholamine. Recently the hemodynamic effects of dopamine in combination with nitroprusside, and dobutamine and nitroprusside have been clinically examined.[172,173,240] The usefulness of dopamine is limited in the treatment of patients with low cardiac output states and severe pulmonary vascular congestion because dopamine does not uniformly reduce and may indeed increase left ventricular filling pressure. Although myocardial contractility may be improved, pulmonary venous congestion may persist due to the increase in afterload secondary to the α-adrenergic effect of dopamine. Consequently, myocardial oxygen requirements may be increased rather than decreased because of an augmentation in cardiac work produced by dopamine. This increase may be partially offset by a reduction in the left ventricular afterload and to a lesser extent preload with nitroprusside therapy. In addition arterial pressure may be maintained with dopamine in patients with extreme hypotension, permitting the use of vasodilator therapy. Recently the combination of digoxin with nitroprusside has also been shown to be more effective in augmenting left ventricular stroke work than nitroprusside alone.[206]

While such pharmacologic interventions offer attractive options, the exact myocardial oxygen cost of drug combinations is not precisely known. Consequently caution is recommended in the use of drug combinations such as dopamine and nitroprusside.

MECHANICAL CIRCULATORY ASSISTANCE

When cardiac output and tissue perfusion cannot be adequately maintained by volume loading and the pharmacologic alteration of preload, myocardial contractility, and afterload, mechanical circulatory assistance provides a potentially life-saving alternative. A wide variety of mechanical devices have been utilized in an attempt to decrease cardiac workload and maintain viable hemodynamic function. Cardiac output has been temporarily increased by devices such as the Anstadt cup,[8] cardiopulmonary bypass with either continuous or pulsatile blood flow,[26] the abdominal

left ventricular assist device (ALVAD),[189] left ventricular aortic booster pump,[29] body acceration synchronous with heart beat (BASH),[10] and intra-aortic balloon counterpulsation (IABCP).[131,178] At the present time intra-aortic balloon counterpulsation is the most widely used technique for cardiac mechanical circulatory assistance.

INTRA-AORTIC BALLOON

Insertion. In the past, a polyurethane balloon catheter was inserted under direct vision through a prosthetic Dacron cuff into the femoral artery by way of an arteriotomy and advanced from the femoral artery into the thoracic aorta and positioned immediately distal to the left subclavian artery. More recently, the percutaneous Seldinger technique has been utilized to insert the balloon catheter through a 12 Fr catheter introducer.[25,242] Balloon catheter insertions under direct vision with arteriotomies have been associated with complication rates of approximately 5 to 20 percent and mortality rates[146,195] as high as 2 percent. A percutaneous arterial insertion procedure has been associated with a 2.5 percent complication rate, including hematoma formation, false aneurysm, thrombocytopenia, lower extremity ischemia, and aortic dissection. Recently an intra-aortic balloon catheter has been developed which is inserted percutaneously over a flexible guidewire. This capability will significantly reduce the complication rate associated with percutaneous balloon catheter insertion. When the femoral site cannot be successfully cannulated because of severe atherosclerotic occlusive disease, the balloon catheter may be inserted into the aorta by way of the left axillary artery.[198] More remote alternatives include direct surgical insertion into the iliac artery or abdominal aorta.[142]

Hemodynamic Effects. Coronary and cerebral blood flow are augmented because diastolic pressure is increased in the aorta by rapid inflation of the balloon when the aortic valve is closed during ventricular diastole. Deflation of the balloon immediately prior to left ventricular systole reduces the resistance to left ventricular ejection and helps to unload the left ventricle. Balloon displacement of blood into the peripheral circulation and stimulation of aortic baroreceptors during diastolic augmentation are also important mechanisms in the unloading effect of the balloon.

With augmentation of coronary perfusion and improvement in the endocardial viability ratio,* there is more complete left ventricular emptying, a decline in end-systolic and end-diastolic volumes and pressure, and thereby a reduction in preload. Therefore IABCP is capable of reducing both preload and afterload. Consequently total myocardial work and therefore myocardial oxygen requirements are reduced.

The magnitude and duration of augmentation of the mean aortic diastolic pressure are related to three balloon-dependent variables: (1) the position of the balloon within the thoracic aorta; (2) the volume of blood displaced; (3) and the duration and timing of inflation and deflation. Premature inflation of the balloon increases the afterload, impedes blood flow, and increases intraventricular wall stress. The onset of balloon inflation should therefore be referenced against either the dicrotic notch of the arterial pressure pulse or the latter half of the T wave of the electrocardiogram. With optimal balloon counterpulsation cardiac output increases by as much as 50 percent, mean arterial pressure increases 10 to 15 mmHg, peak systolic pressure decreases 15 mmHg, and pulmonary artery occlusive pressure decreases[67,228] 5 to 10 mmHg. Coronary blood flow either remains unchanged or increases.[35] Heart rate tends to decrease while urine output increases.

Indications. Current indications for intra-aortic balloon counterpulsation include[35]:

1. Patients with acute myocardial infarction complicated by medically refractory congestive heart failure and/or cardiogenic shock
2. Patients with low cardiac output states who require cardiac catheterization or surgery
3. Patients who cannot be weaned from cardiopulmonary bypass
4. Patients with recurrent malignant cardiac arrhythmias secondary to severe hypotension

---

* $\left(\dfrac{\text{diastolic pressure time index}}{\text{tension time index}}\right)$

Contraindications. Contraindications to intra-aortic balloon counterpulsation in otherwise potentially salvageable patients include aortic valvular insufficiency, dissecting aortic or abdominal aortic aneurysm, and severe atherosclerotic occlusive disease preventing catheter passage. The presence of systemic infections is not an absolute contraindication to intra-aortic counterpulsation; patients with septic shock have been successfully treated with this method.[23] In patients with heart rates greater than 150 beats/min or grossly irregular rhythms, diastolic balloon augmentation may be inadequate due to incomplete filling and evacuation of the intra-aortic balloon. A systolic arterial blood pressure $\geq$ 60 mmHg and a pulse pressure $\geq$ 15 mmHg are necessary for balloon augmentation, while the most effective balloon pump augmentation occurs when the systolic blood pressure exceeds 80 mmHg and the diastolic blood pressure exceeds[24] 50 mmHg.

EXTERNAL COUNTERPULSATION

External counterpulsation (ECP) has been proposed as an alternative to intra-aortic balloon counterpulsation in the treatment of patients with complicated acute myocardial infarction.[236,273] With this method, uniform pressure is applied by water-filled trousers over the lower extremities during diastole, as determined from the ECG, producing diastolic pressure augmentation. The resultant positive pressure has the combined effect of increasing arterial diastolic pressure and increasing venous return to the right side of the heart. The primary limitation of the external counterpulsation device is leg discomfort and occasional leg abrasion, which prevents continuous use for longer than 3 or 4 hours.

COMPARISON OF INTERNAL AND EXTERNAL CIRCULATORY ASSISTANCE

Mueller and co-workers have compared intra-aortic balloon counterpulsation (IABCP) with external circulatory assistance in patients with cardiogenic shock.[179] Intra-aortic balloon counterpulsation effectively decreased the determinants of myocardial oxygen consumption including heart rate, left ventricular ejection resistance (afterload), and pulmonary artery wedge pressure whereas ECP moderately decreased afterload but had no effect on heart rate and left ventricular preload. Cardiac index and myocardial lactate utilization improved to a greater degree with IABCP than with ECP. Whereas IABCP decreased myocardial oxygen consumption, ECP increased myocardial oxygen consumption with only a moderate improvement of myocardial metabolism. Despite treatment with external circulatory assistance, no patient with established cardiogenic shock survived. Therefore, ECP does not appear to be hemodynamically capable of reversing cardiogenic shock, but may be of value in the treatment of patients with less complicated forms of acute myocardial infarction, especially when used with vasodilating drugs.[7,200]

CLINICAL RESULTS

Four groups of patients may be identified based on their response to intra-aortic balloon counterpulsation.[67] Group I patients demonstrate substantial improvement in cardiac output and tissue perfusion within 24 to 48 hours so that IABCP may be discontinued without marked clinical or hemodynamic deterioration (Table 10-8). Group II patients show no improvement during IABCP. Postmortem examination of these patients reveals massive myocardial infarction with severe obstructive disease of all coronary arteries. Group III patients respond to IABCP with resolution of shock but remain balloon dependent (Table 10-9). Counterpulsation for more than 72 to 96 hours in these patients does not significantly improve hospital survival. Approximately 50 percent of these patients may benefit from coronary revascularization and resection of dyskinetic segments of the left ventricle while being maintained on balloon circulatory assistance.[18,24] Patients with shock associated with

an acquired ventricular septal defect and/or severe mitral regurgitation form a fourth group in whom shock is due to a specific mechanical abnormality. In such patients intra-aortic balloon counterpulsation may increase cardiac output by as much as 35 percent, reduce pulmonary artery wedge pressure, decrease the systemic arteriovenous oxygen difference, and permit cardiac catheterization and definitive elective surgical repair.[39,97]

IABCP PLUS MEDICAL THERAPY

The results of intra-aortic balloon counterpulsation plus medical therapy for the treatment of cardiogenic shock have been summarized by Alpert and Cohn.[6] Of 253 patients with cardiogenic shock, 72 (28.5 percent) were discharged alive from the hospital. Recently Hagemeijer and co-workers have reported 13/25 (52 percent) long-term survivors, and Bolooki has reported 16/50 (40 percent) survivors with 14 patients alive more than 8 months.[35,110]

LEFT VENTRICULAR ASSIST DEVICES/ARTIFICIAL HEARTS

For patients who cannot be resuscitated or sustained by intra-aortic balloon counterpulsation in combination with pharmacologic therapy, left ventricular assist devices have recently been employed. Left ventricular assist devices are also being examined in patients with advanced heart failure due to acute myocarditis. Bernhard[28,29] has developed a mechanical pump with afferent and efferent conduits attached to the left ventricular apex and ascending thoracic aorta that is capable of pro-

TABLE 10-8. Criteria for Discontinuing the Intra-Aortic Balloon Pump

Cardiac index > 2 L/min/m²
Pulmonary artery occlusive pressure < 20 mmHg
Arterial blood pressure > 90 mmHg
Lactate < 2.5 mM/L
Dopamine requirement < 1 mg/min

TABLE 10-9. Intra-Aortic Balloon Dependence: Causes of Weaning Failures

Persistent hypotension with systolic blood pressure < 90 mmHg
Reduction in cardiac index by more than 20% or a decrease to < 2 L/min/m²
Increase in pulmonary artery wedge pressure to > 20 mmHg
Recurrent malignant cardiac arrhythmias
Recurrent severe cardiac pain and new ischemic ECG changes
Requirements for > 1.5 mg/min dopamine or large quantities of other α-adrenergic catecholamines

ducing stroke volumes as large as 85 ml and heart rates of 100 beats/min. Patients with far advanced acute left ventricular decompensation have been supported for periods of 1 to 190 hours with this device. Left ventricular improvement occurred in one-third of the patients, permitting removal of the device; patients survived 5 to 10 months. At the present time, however, insertion of the left ventricular assist device must be considered an experimental and heroic attempt to sustain life.

Surgical Management

In patients with cardiogenic shock who are unresponsive to intensive medical therapy and mechanical circulatory assistance with the intra-aortic balloon pump, acute surgical intervention must be considered. In these patients, two-dimensional echocardiography, radionucleotide angiography, and left ventricular and coronary angiography are performed to establish coronary anatomy, the location and the mass of disabled myocardium as well as the presence or absence of left ventricular aneurysm, ventricular clot, mitral valve incompetence, and/or ventricular septal defect.

In patients with high-grade proximal obstructive coronary artery disease but patent distal coronary artery vessels, aortocoronary bypass is recommended as the initial surgical procedure to determine whether improved ventricular performance may be achieved by enhancement of perfusion to ischemic areas of the myocardium. Often, however, the coronary arteries are diffusely diseased and are not amenable to bypass grafts; resection of regional dyskinetic left ventricular muscle is then the only surgical procedure possible and may be associated with mortality rates greater than 35 percent.

Mortality

The mortality rates[34,227] for patients with cardiogenic shock treated with medical therapy alone have exceeded 80 percent. The insti-

tution of intra-aortic balloon counterpulsation beginning in 1970 improved cardiac hemodynamics with resultant immediate patient survivals of 29 to 50 percent. Long-term survival rates in cardiogenic shock patients without myocardial revascularization surgery, however, averaged only 10 to 17 percent in many centers.[67,73,149,180] For this reason a more aggressive approach to the treatment of cardiogenic shock has been advocated, combining stabilization with medical therapy and intra-aortic balloon counterpulsation, cardiac catheterization, and surgical revascularization.[69,127,194,215,226] With this approach, not only have long-term survival rates of 44 to 50 percent been achieved in some centers, but substantial exercise capability has also been maintained as demonstrated by treadmill exercise tolerance.[204]

PROTOCOL FOR THE TREATMENT OF PATIENTS WITH CARDIOGENIC SHOCK[117]

Effective treatment of patients with low cardiac output states and cardiogenic shock requires a specific protocol to expedite therapy and salvage life. Our current protocol includes:

1. Insertion of intra-arterial and pulmonary arterial catheters for the direct measurement of arterial pressure, pulmonary artery pressure and occlusive pressure, cardiac output, colloid oncotic pressure, arterial blood gases, and blood lactate. Ventricular stroke work, pulmonary and systemic vascular resistance are calculated and a Frank-Starling curve is constructed.
2. Crystalloid or colloid solutions are administered intravenously by fluid challenge techniques to optimize preload, ventricular fiber stretch, and cardiac output.
3. A vasodilator drug or the combination of a vasopressor and a vasodilator drug is given to facilitate forward blood flow by reducing afterload, pulmonary vascular con-

gestion, and improving myocardial contractility.

4. Intra-aortic balloon counterpulsation is instituted for mechanical circulatory assistance in patients with persistent lactic acidosis.

5. Left ventricular angiography and coronary arteriography are performed urgently in patients who remain balloon-dependent after 48 to 72 hours of mechanical circulatory assistance, to identify coronary artery obstructive disease and mechanical abnormalities that might be corrected with emergency surgery. In patients who stabilize hemodynamically, cardiac catheterization is performed electively during their hospitalization.

6. Definitive surgical repair is performed if correctable lesions are demonstrated at cardiac catheterization.

REFERENCES

1. Abrams J: Nitroglycerin and long acting nitrates. N Engl J Med 302:1234, 1980

2. Abrams E, Forrester J, Chatterjee F et al: Variability of response to norepinephrine infusion in acute myocardial infarction. Clin Res 202, 1972

3. Ahlmark G, Saetre H, Korsgren M: Reduction of sudden deaths after myocardial infarction. Lancet 2:1563, 1974

4. Akhtar N, Mikulic E, Cohn JN, Chaudhry MH: Hemodynamic effects of dobutamine in patients with severe heart failure. Am J Cardiol 36:202, 1975

5. Alonso DR, Caulfield JB, Kastor JA: Pathophysiology of cardiogenic shock. Quantitation of myocardial necrosis: clinical, pathologic, and electrocardiographic correlations. Circulation 48:588, 1973

6. Alpert JS, Cohn LH: Medical/surgical treatment of acute myocardial infarction. p. 127. In Cohn LH (ed): The Treatment of Acute Myocardial Ischemia. Futura Publishing Company, Mt. Kisco, New York, 1979

7. Amsterdam EA, Banar J, Criley JM et al: Clinical assessment of external pressure circulatory assistance in acute myocardial infarction. Am J Cardiol 45:349, 1980

8. Anstadt GL, Schiff P, Baue AE: Prolonged circulatory support by direct mechanical ventricular assistance. Trans Am Soc Artif Intern Organ 12:72, 1966

9. Armstrong PW, Armstrong JA, Marks GS: Pharmacokinetic–hemodynamic studies of intravenous nitroglycerin in congestive heart failure. Circulation 62:160, 1980

10. Arntzenius AL, Koops S, Rodrigo FA et al: Circulatory effects of body acceleration given synchronously with the heart beat (BASH): Ballistocardiography and cardiovascular therapy. Bibl Cardiol 26:180, 1970

11. Ashburn WL, Witztum KF: Nuclear cardiology techniques. p. 239. In Karliner JS, Gregoratos G (eds): Coronary Care. Churchill Livingstone, New York, 1980

12. Bacaner MB: Bretylium tosylate for suppression of induced ventricular fibrillation. Am J Cardiol 17:528, 1966

13. Bagwell EE, Daniell HB, Freeman RF: Influence of phentolamine on cardiovascular effects of dopamine in cardiogenic shock. Arch Int Pharmacodyn Ther 208:197, 1974

14. Balcon R, Jewitt DE, Davies JPH, Oram S: A controlled trial of propranolol in acute myocardial infarction. Lancet 2:917, 1966

15. Barber JM, Boyle DM, Chaturvedi NC et al: Practolol in acute myocardial infarction. Acta Med Scand (Suppl) 587:213, 1975

16. Barber JM, Murphy FM, Merrett JD: Clinical trial of propranolol in acute myocardial infarction. Ulster Med J 36:127, 1967

17. Barber NS, Evans D, Howitt G et al: Multicenter post infarction trial of propranolol in 49 hospitals in the United Kingdom, Italy and Yugoslavia. Br Heart J 44:96, 1980

18. Bardet J, Masquet C, Kahn C et al: Clinical and hemodynamic results of intra-aortic balloon counterpulsation and surgery for cardiogenic shock. Am Heart J 93:280, 1977

19. Barstow RD, Kaloyanides GJ: Effects of sodium nitroprusside on function in the isolated intact dog kidney. J Pharmacol Exp Ther 181:244, 1972

20. Bean WB: Masquerade of myocardial infarction. Lancet 1:1044, 1977

21. Benaim ME: Asystole after verapamil. Br Med J 2:169, 1972

22. Benet LZ: Pharmacokinetics/pharmacodynamics of furosemide in man: a review. J Pharmacol Biopharmaceut 7:1, 1979

23. Berger RL, Saini VK, Long W et al: The use of diastolic augmentation with the intra-aortic balloon in human septic shock with associated coronary artery disease. Surgery 74:601, 1973

24. Bergman D: Assessment of intra-aortic balloon counterpulsation in cardiogenic shock. Crit Care Med 3:490, 1975

25. Bergman D, Nichols AB, Weiss MB et al: Percutaneous intra-aortic balloon insertion. Am J Cardiol 46:261, 1980

26. Bergman D, Parodi EN, Haubert SM et al: Counterpulsation with a new pulsatile assist device (PAD) in open heart surgery. J Assoc Adv Med Instrument 10:232, 1976

27. Berkowitz C, McKeever L, Croke RP et al: Comparative responses to dobutamine and nitroprusside in patients with chronic low output cardiac failure. Circulation 56:918, 1977

28. Bernhard WF, Berger RL, Stetz J et al: Temporary left ventricular bypass: factors affecting patient survival. Circulation 60 (Suppl 2):131, 1979

29. Bernhard WF, Lafarge CG, Bankole M et al: Biventricular bypass: physiologic studies during induced ventricular failure and fibrillation. J Thorac Cardiovasc Surg 62:859, 1971

30. Beta Blocker Heart Attack Trial Research Group: A randomized trial of propranolol in patients with acute myocardial infarction. JAMA 247(12):1707, 1982

31. Bigger JT: The quinidine-digoxin interaction. What do we know about it? N Engl J Med 301:779, 1979

32. Bigger JT, Jaffe CC: The effect of bretylium tosylate on the electrophysiologic properties of ventricular muscle and Purkinje fibers. Am J Cardiol 27:82, 1971

33. Biggs R, Denson KWE, Abmon N et al: Antithrombin III, antifactor Xa, and heparin. Br J Haematol 19:283, 1970

34. Binder MJ, Ryan JA, Marcus S et al: Evaluation of therapy in shock following acute myocardial infarction. Am J Med 18:622, 1955

35. Bolooki H: Elective and emergency use of the intra-aortic balloon pump in cardiac surgery. In Bolooki H (ed): Clinical Application of Intra-aortic Balloon Pump. Futura Publishing Company, Mt. Kisco, New York, 1984

36. Bonte FJ, Parkey RW, Graham KD: A new method for radionucleotide imaging of myocardial infarcts. Radiology 110:473, 1974

37. Borer JS, Redwood DR, Levitt B et al: Reduction in myocardial ischemia with nitroglycerin or nitroglycerin plus phenylephrine administered during acute myocardial infarction in man. N Engl J Med 293:1008, 1975

38. Brodie TS, Gray R, Swan HJC: Effects of nitroprusside on arterial oxygenation, intrapulmonic shunts and oxygen delivery. Am J Cardiol 37:123, 1976

39. Buckley MJ, Mundth ED, Daggett WM et al: Surgical management of ventricular septal defects and mitral regurgitation complicating acute myocardial infarction. Ann Thorac Surg 16:598, 1973

40. Bussman WD, Schafer H, Kaltenback M: Effects of intravenous nitroglycerin on hemodynamics and ischemic injury in patients with acute myocardial infarction. Eur J Cardiol 8:61, 1978

41. Bussmann WD, Schafer H, Kaltenback M: Wirkung von Nitroglycerin beim akuten Myocardenfarkt. IV. Intravenose Dauerinfusion von Nitroglycerin bei Patienten mit und ohne Linksinsuffizienz und ihre Auswirkungen auf die Infarktgrosse. Dtsch Med Wochenschr 101:642, 1976

42. Chambers TC, Matta RJ, Smith H, Kunzler AM: Evidence favoring the use of anticoagulants in the hospital phase of acute myocardial infarction. N Engl J Med 297:1091, 1977

43. Chatterjee K: Hemodynamic monitoring in the coronary care unit reduces mortality. p. 327 In Rapaport E (ed): Controversies in Cardiovascular Disease. WB Saunders, Philadelphia, 1980

44. Chatterjee K, Parmley WW, Ganz W et al: Hemodynamic and metabolic responses to vasodilator therapy in acute myocardial infarction. Circulation 48:1183, 1973

45. Chatterjee K, Parmley WW, Swan HHC et al: Beneficial effects of vasodilator agents in severe mitral regurgitation due to dysfunction of subvalvular apparatus. Circulation 48:684, 1973

46. Chatterjee K, Swan HJC, Ganz W et al: Use of a balloon tipped flotation electrode catheter for cardiac monitoring. Am J Cardiol 36:56, 1975

47. Chesnais JM, Coraboeuf E, Sauviat MP, Vassas MM: Sensitivity to hydrogen, lithium, and magnesium ions of the slow inward sodium current in frog atrial fibers. J Mol Cell Cardiol 7:627, 1975

48. Chiarello M, Gold HK, Leinbach RC et al: Comparison between the effects of nitroprusside and nitroglycerin on ischemic injury during acute myocardial infarction. Circulation 54:766, 1976

49. Chidsey CA, Sonnenblick EH, Morrow AG, Braunwald E: Norepinephrine stores and contractile forces of papillary muscle from the failing heart. Circulation 33:43, 1966

50. Chin PL, Kaminski J, Rout M: Myocardial infarction coincident with cerebrovascular accidents in the elderly. Age Ageing 6:29, 1977

51. Clausen J, Felsby M, Schonau J et al: Absence of prophylactic effect of propranolol in myocardial infarction. Lancet 2:920, 1966

52. Cohn J: Right ventricular infarction revisited. Am J Cardiol 43:666, 1979

53. Cohn JN: Vasodilator therapy for heart failure: the influence of impedance on left ventricular performance. Circulation 48:5, 1973

54. Cohn JN, Guiha NH, Broder MI, Limas CJ: Right ventricular infarction. Clinical and hemodynamic features. Am J Cardiol 33:209, 1974

55. Cohn JN, Luria MH: Studies on clinical shock and hypotension. II. Hemodynamic effects of norepinephrine and angiotensin. J Clin Invest 44:1494, 1965

56. Cohn JN, Tristani FE, Khatri IM: Cardiac and peripheral vascular effects of digitalis in clinical cardiogenic shock. Am Heart J 78:318, 1969

57. Collinsworth KA, Kalmon SM, Harrison DC: The clinical pharmacology of lidocaine as an antiarrhythmic drug. Circulation 50:1217, 1974

58. Come PC, Flaherty JT, Baird MD et al: Reversal by phenylephrine of the beneficial effects of intravenous nitroglycerin in patients with acute myocardial infarction. N Engl J Med 293:1003, 1975

59. Cottrell JE, Casthely P, Brodie JD: Prevention of nitroprusside induced cyanide toxicity with hydroxycobolamin. N Engl J Med 298:809, 1978

60. Cowley MJ, Mantle JA, Rogers WJ et al: Technetium 99m stannous pyrophosphate myocardial scintigraphy. Reliability and limitations in assessment of acute myocardial infarction. Circulation 56:192, 1977

61. Crexells C, Bourassa MG, Beron P: Effects of dopamine on myocardial metabolism in patients with ischemic heart disease. Cardiovasc Res 7:438, 1973

62. Crexells C, Chatterjee K, Forrester JS, Swan JHC: Optimal level of filling pressure in the left side of the heart in acute myocardial infarction. N Engl J Med 289:1263, 1973

63. DaLuz P, Forrester JS, Wyatt HL et al: Hemodynamic and metabolic effects of sodium nitroprusside on the performance and metabolism of regional ischemic myocardium. Circulation 52:400, 1975

64. DaLuz P, Forrester JS, Wyatt HL et al: Opposing efforts of increasing heart rate on global and regional ischemic myocardium function and metabolism. Circulation 52 (Suppl 2):173, 1975

65. DaLuz PL, Shubin H, Weil MH, Jacobson E, Stein L: Pulmonary edema related to changes in colloid osmotic pressure and pulmonary artery wedge pressure in patients after myocardial infarction. Circulation 51:350, 1975

66. Davies DW, Kadar D, Steward DJ et al: A sudden death associated with the use of sodium nitroprusside for induction of hypotension during anesthesia. Can Anaesth Soc J 22:547, 1975

67. Deinbman WB, Leinbach RC, Buckley MJ et al: Clinical and hemodynamic results of intra-aortic balloon pumping and surgery for cardiogenic shock. Circulation 46:465, 1972

68. Derrida JP, Sol R, Chicke P: Favorable effects of prolonged nitroglycerin infusion in patients with acute myocardial infarction. Am Heart J 96:833, 1978

69. DeWood MA, Notske RN, Hensley GR et al: Intra-aortic balloon counterpulsation with and without re-perfusion for myocardial infarction shock. Circulation 61:1105, 1980

70. Dhurandhar RW, Macmillan RL, Brown KWG: Primary ventricular fibrillation complicating acute myocardial infarction. Am J Cardiol 27:347, 1971

71. Dikshit K, Vyden JK, Forrester JS et al: Renal and extrarenal hemodynamic effects of furosemide in congestive heart failure after acute myocardial infarction. N Engl J Med 288:1087, 1973

72. Doering W: Quinidine–digoxin interaction: pharmacokinetics, underlying mechanisms and clinical implications. N Engl J Med 301:400, 1979

73. Dunkman WB, Leinbach RC, Buckley MJ et al: Clinical and hemodynamic results of intra-aortic balloon pumping and surgery for cardiogenic shock. Circulation 46:465, 1972

74. Elson J, Strong JM, Lee WK: Antiarrhythmic potency of N acetylprocainamide. Clin Pharmacol Ther 17:134, 1975

75. Ferlinz J, Easthope JL, Aronow WS: Effects of verapamil on myocardial performance in coronary disease. Circulation 59:313, 1979

76. Ferrer MI, Bradley SE, Wheeler HO et al: Some effects of nitroglycerin upon the splanchnic, pulmonary, and systemic circulation. Circulation 33:357, 1966

77. Figueras J, Weil MH: Increases in plasma oncotic pressure during acute cardiogenic pulmonary edema. Circulation 55:195, 1977

78. Figueras J, Weil MH: Hypovolemia and hypotension complicating management of acute cardiogenic pulmonary edema. Am J Cardiol 44:1349, 1979

79. Flaherty JT, Come PC, Baird MG et al: Effects of intravenous nitroglycerin on left ventricular function and ST segment changes in acute myocardial infarction. Br Heart J 38:612, 1976

80. Flaherty JT, Reid PR, Kelly DT: Intravenous nitroglycerin in acute myocardial infarction. Circulation 51:132, 1975

81. Fonzes-Dialon H, Carquet J: Sur la toxicité du nitroprusside de soude. Bull Soc Chim Biol 29:638, 1903

82. Forrester JS, DaLuz PL: Cardiac function and metabolism following dopamine in acute myocardial ischemia. In Swan HJC (ed): Use of Dopamine in Shock. III. Myocardial Infarction. Excerpta Medica, Princeton, New Jersey, 1977

83. Forrester JS, Diamond GA, Chatterjee K, Swan HJC: Medical therapy of acute myocardial in-

farction by application of hemodynamic subsets. N Engl J Med 295:1356, 1976

84. Forrester JS, Diamond GA, Swan HJC: Correlative classification of clinical hemodynamic function after acute myocardial infarction. Am J Cardiol 39:137, 1977

85. Franciosa JA, Guiha NH, Limas CJ: Improved left ventricular function during nitroprusside infusion in acute myocardial infarction. Lancet 1:650, 1972

86. Francis GS, Sharma B, Hodges M: Comparative hemodynamic effects of dopamine and dobutamine in patients with acute cardiovascular collapse. Am Heart J 103(6):995, 1982

87. Frank O: Zur dynamik des hermuskels (Z Biol 32:370, 1895; translated by Chapman CB, Wasserman E). Am Heart J 58:282, 1959

88. Fuccella LM: Report on the double blind trial with compound CIBA: 39, 089-BA (Transicor) in myocardial infarction. Quoted in Sowton E: Beta adrenergic blockage in cardiac infarction. Progr Cardiovasc Dis 10:561, 1968

89. Gallus AS, Hirsh J, Tuttle RJ et al: Small subcutaneous doses of heparin in prevention of venous thrombosis. N Engl J Med 288:545, 1973

90. Ganz W: Intracoronary thrombolysis in acute myocardial infarction. Am J Cardiol 52:92A, 1983

91. Ganz W, Buchbinder N, Marcus H et al: Intracoronary thrombolysis in evolving myocardial infarction. Am Heart J 101:4, 1981

92. Ganz W, Geft I, Shah PK et al: Intravenous streptokinase in evolving acute myocardial infarction. Am J Cardiol 53(9):1209, 1984

93. Ganz W, Ninomiya K, Hashida J et al: Intracoronary thrombolysis in acute myocardial infarction: Experimental background and clinical experience. Am Heart J 102(6):1145, 1981

94. Gewertz H, Gold HK, Fallon JT et al: Role of right ventricular infarction in cardiogenic shock with inferior myocardial infarction. Br Heart J 42:719, 1979

95. Gillespie TA, Ambos HD, Sobel BE, Roberts R: Effects of dobutamine in patients with acute myocardial infarction. Am J Cardiol 39:588, 1977

96. Gold HK, Leinbach RC, Sanders CA: Use of sublingual nitroglycerin in congestive heart failure following acute myocardial infarction. Circulation 46:839, 1972

97. Gold HK, Leinbach RC, Sanders CA et al: Intra-aortic balloon pumping for ventricular septal defect or mitral regurgitation complicating acute myocardial infarction. Circulation 47:1191, 1973

98. Goldberg DM, Windfield DA: Diagnostic accuracy of serum enzyme assays for myocardial infarction in a general hospital population. Br Heart J 34:597, 1972

99. Goldberg L: Cardiovascular and renal actions of dopamine: potential clinical applications. Pharmacol Rev 24:1, 1972

100. Goldberg LI, Talley RC, McNal JL: The potential role of dopamine in the treatment of shock. Prog Cardiovasc Dis 12:40, 1969

101. Gordon GD, Mabin TA, Isaacs S et al: Hemodynamic effects of sublingual nifedipine in acute myocardial infarction. Am J Cardiol 53(9):1228–1232, 1984

102. Gorlin R: Normal variation in venous oxygen content. In Warren JV (ed): Methods in Medical Research, Vol 7. Year Book, Chicago, 1958

103. Gould L, DeMartino A, Gomprecht RF et al: Hemodynamic effects of phentolamine in cor pulmonale. J Clin Pharmacol 12:153, 1972

104. Gould L, Fahir M, Ettinger S: Phentolamine and cardiovascular performance. Br Heart J 31:154, 1969

105. Gregoratos G, Gleeson E: Initial therapy of acute myocardial infarction. In Karliner JS, Gregoratos G (eds): Coronary Care. Churchill Livingstone, New York, 1981

106. Guiha NH, Limas CJ, Cohn JN: Predominant right ventricular dysfunction after right ventricular destruction in the dog. Am J Cardiol 33:254, 1974

107. Gunnar RM, Loeb HS, Pietras RJ: Hemodynamic measurements in a coronary care unit. Prog Cardiovasc Dis 11:29, 1968

108. Hackett TP, Cassem NH: Factors contributing to delay in responding to signs and symptoms of acute myocardial infarction. Am J Cardiol 25:651, 1969

109. Haddy FJ, Fleishman M, Emanuel DA: Effects of epinephrine, norepinephrine and seratonin upon systemic small and large vessel resistance. Circ Res 5:247, 1957

110. Hagemeijer F, Laird JD, Haalebos MMP, Hugenholtz PG: Effectiveness of intra-aortic balloon pumping without cardiac surgery for patients with severe heart failure secondary to recent myocardial infarction. Am J Cardiol 40:951, 1977

111. Hager WD, Fenster P, Mayershon M: Digoxin-quinidine interaction: pharmacokinetic evaluation. N Engl J Med 300:123, 1979

112. Harnaragan C, Bennett MA, Pentecost BL, Brewer DB: Quantitative study of infarcted myocardium in cardiogenic shock. Br Heart J 32:728, 1970

113. Harrison DC: Should lidocaine be administered routinely to all patients after acute myocardial infarction? Circulation 58:581, 1978

114. Henning H, Schelbert H, Righetti H: Dual myocardial imaging with technetium 99m pyrophosphate and thallium 201 for detecting, local-

izing, and sizing acute myocardial infarction. Am J Cardiol 40:147, 1977

115. Henning RJ: Emergency treatment of congestive heart failure. p. 43. In Weil MH, Henning RJ (eds): The Handbook of Critical Care Medicine. EM Books, New York, 1979

116. Henning RJ, Shubin H, Weil MH: Afterload reduction with phentolamine in patients with acute pulmonary edema. Am J Med 63:568, 1977

117. Henning RJ, Weil MH: Treatment of cardiogenic shock. p. 69. In Dreifus LS, Brest AN (eds): Clinical Application of Cardiovascular Drugs. Martinus Nijhoff, The Hague, 1980

118. Henning RJ, Weil MH, Wiener F: Blood lactate as a prognostic indicator of survival in patients with acute myocardial infarction. Circ Shock 9:307, 1982

119. Henning RJ, Wiener F, Valdes S, Weil MH: Measurement of toe temperature for assessing the severity of acute circulatory failure. Surg Gynec Obstet 149:1, 1979

120. Henningsen NC, Cederberg A, Hanson A, Johansson BW: Effects of long term treatment with procainamide. A prospective study with special regard to ANF and SLE in fast and slow acetylators. Acta Med Scand 198:475, 1975

121. Holman BL, Chisholm RJ, Braunwald E: The prognostic implications of acute myocardial infarction scintigraphy with technetium 99m pyrophosphate. Circulation 57:320, 1978

122. Holman L: Radionucleotide examination of the cardiovascular system. p. 363. In Braunwald E (ed): Heart Disease. WB Saunders, Philadelphia, 1980

123. Holmberg S, Ryden L, Waldenstrom A: Efficiency of arrhythmia detection by nurses in a coronary care unit using a decentralized monitoring system. Br Heart J 39:1019, 1977

124. Holzer J, Karliner JS, O'Rourke RA, et al: Effectiveness of dopamine in patients with cardiogenic shock. Am J Cardiol 32:79, 1973

125. Hurst JW, Logue RB, Walter PF: The clinical recognition and management of coronary atherosclerotic heart disease. In Hurst JW, Logue RB et al (eds): The Heart. McGraw Hill, New York, 1978

126. Husaini MH, Kvasnicka J, Ryden L et al: Action of verapamil on sinus node, atrioventricular and intraventricular conduction. Br Heart J 35:734, 1973

127. Huttler AM, Gold HK, Leinbach RC et al: Various uses of intra-aortic balloon pump. p. 169. In Cohen L (ed): Acute Myocardial Infarction—First 24 hours. New York, Verlag Gerhard Witzstrock, 1977

128. Isner JM, Roberts WC: Right ventricular infarction complicating left ventricular infarction sec-

ondary to coronary heart disease. Frequency, location, associated findings and significance from analysis of 236 necropsy patients with acute or healed myocardial infarction. Am J Cardiol 42:885, 1978

129. Jaffe JH, Martin WR: Narcotic analgesics and antagonists. p. 253. In Goodman LS, Gilman A (eds): The Pharmacological Basis of Therapeutics. Macmillan, New York, 1975

130. Kahler RL, Brill SJ, Perkins WE: The role of propranolol in management of acute myocardial infarction. p. 253. In Kattus AA, Ross G, Hall VE (eds): Cardiovascular Beta-Adrenergic Responses. University of California Press, Los Angeles, 1970

131. Kantrowitz A, Krakauer JS, Rosenbaum A et al: Phase shift balloon pumping in medically refractory shock: results in 27 patients. Arch Surg 99:739, 1969

132. Kent KM, Smith ER, Redwood DR, Epstein SE: Beneficial electrophysiologic effects of nitroglycerin during acute myocardial infarction. Am J Cardiol 33:513, 1974

133. Kerber RE, Abboud FM, Marcus ML, Eckberg TL: Effective inotropic agents on localized dyskinesis of acutely ischemic myocardium. Circulation 49:1038, 1974

134. Kerry JW: Gouendaroj M, Patel KR: Effect of alpha receptor blocking drugs and disodium cromoglycate on histamine hypersensitivity in bronchial asthma. Br Med J 2:139, 1970

135. Kim YI, Williams JF: Relief of chest pain and reduction of Q wave evolution in acute myocardial infarction by large dose sublingual nitroglycerin. Am J Cardiol 45:483, 1980

136. Koch-Wesser J: Pharmacokinetics of procainamide in man. Ann NY Acad Sci 179:370, 1971

137. Kotter V, Leitner ER, Wunderlich J, Schroder R: Comparison of hemodynamic effects of phentolamine, sodium nitroprusside and glycerol trinitrate in acute myocardial infarction. Br Heart J 39:1196, 1977

138. Kotter V, Schroder R: Nitroprusside, phentolamine and nitroglycerin in acute myocardial infarction. p. 95. In Gould L, Reddy CVR (eds): Vasodilator Therapy for Cardiac Disorders. Futura Publishing Company, Mt. Kisco, New York, 1979

139. Krieger DT, Martin JB: Brain peptides. N Engl J Med 304:876–885, 1981

140. Ku DD, Lucchesi BR: Ischemic induced alterations in cardiac sensitivity to digitalis. Eur J Pharmacol 57:135, 1979

141. Lalka D, Wyman MG, Goldreyer BN et al: Procainamide accumulation kinetics in the immediate postmyocardial infarction period. J Clin Pharmacol 18:397, 1978

142. Lambuti JJ, Cohn LH, Collins JJ: Iliac artery cannulation for intra-aortic balloon counterpulsation. J Thorac Cardiovasc Surg 67:976, 1974

143. Leahey EB, Reiffel JA, Drusin RE et al: Interaction between quinidine and digoxin. JAMA 240:533, 1978

144. Lebowitz E, Green MV, Fairchild R: 201 Thallium for medical use. J Nucl Med 16:151, 1975

145. Lee G, DeMaria AN, Amsterdam EA: Comparative effects of morphine, meperidine, and pentazocine on cardiocirculatory dynamics in patients with acute myocardial infarction. Am J Med 60:949, 1976

146. LeFemine AA, Kosowsky B, Madoff I: Results and complications of intra-aortic balloon pumping in surgical and medical patients. Am J Cardiol 40:416, 1977

147. Leier CV, Heban PT, Huss P et al: Comparative systemic and regional effects of dopamine and dobutamine in patients with cardiomyopathic heart failure. Circulation 58:466, 1978

148. Leier CV, Webel J, Bush CA: The cardiovascular effects of the continuous infusion of dobutamine in patients with severe cardiac failure. Circulation 56:468, 1977

149. Leinbach RC, Gold HK, Dinsmore RE et al: The role of angiography in cardiogenic shock. Circulation 48 (Suppl III); 95, 1973

150. Lemberg L, Castellanos A, Arcebal AG: The use of propranolol in arrhythmias complicating acute myocardial infarction. Am Heart J 80:479, 1970

151. Leueque PE: Antiarrhythmic action of bretylium. Nature 207:203, 1965

152. Lie KI, Wellens HJ, Durrer D: Characteristics and predictability of primary ventricular fibrillation. Eur J Cardiol 1:379, 1974

153. Lie KI, Wellens HJ, Von Capelle FJ, Durrer D: Lidocaine in the prevention of primary ventricular fibrillation. A double blind randomized study of 212 consecutive patients. N Engl J Med 219:1324, 1974

154. Loeb HS, Brednakis J, Gunnar RM: Superiority of dobutamine over dopamine for augmentation of cardiac output in patients with chronic low output cardiac failure. Circulation 55:375, 1977

155. Loeb HS, Khan M, Klodnycky M et al: Hemodynamic effects of dobutamine in man. Circ Shock 2:29, 1975

156. Loeb HS, Khan M, Sandye A, Gunnar RM; Acute hemodynamic effects of dobutamine and isoproterenol in patients with low cardiac output failure. Circ Shock 3:55, 1976

157. Loeb HS, Pietras RJ, Tobin JR, Gunnar RM: Hypovolemia in shock due to acute myocardial infarction. Circulation 40:653, 1969

158. Loeb H, Winslow EBJ, Rahimtoola SH et al: Acute hemodynamic effects of dopamine in patients with shock. Circulation 44:163, 1971

159. Lorell B, Leinbach RC, Pohost GM et al: Right ventricular infarction. Am J Cardiol 43:465, 1979

160. Lown B, Fakhro AM, Hood WB, Thorn GW: The coronary care unit: new perspectives and directions. JAMA 199:156, 1967

161. Lown B, Klein MD, Barr I et al: Sensitivity to digitalis drugs in acute myocardial infarction. Am J Cardiol 30:388, 1972

162. Majid PA, Saxton C, Dykes JRW et al: Automatic control of insulin secretion and the treatment of heart failure. Br Med J 4:328, 1970

163. Marcus FI: Use of digitalis in acute myocardial infarction. Circulation 62:17, 1980

164. Markis JE, Koch-Wesser J: Characteristics and mechanisms of inotropic and chronotropic actions of bretylium tosylate. J Pharmacol Exp Ther 178:94, 1971

165. Maseri A, L'Abbate A, Baroldi G et al: Coronary vasospasm as a possible cause of myocardial infarction. N Engl J Med 299:1271, 1978

166. Mason DT: Afterload reduction and cardiac performance: physiologic basis of systemic vasodilators as a new approach in the treatment of congestive heart failure. Am J Med 65:106, 1978

167. Mason DT, Awan NA, Amsterdam EA et al: New therapeutic approaches to the failing heart: recent advances in vasodilators, cardiotonics, and mechanical circulatory assistance. p. 403. In Mason DT (ed): Advances in Heart Disease. Grune and Stratton, New York, 1980

168. Mathey DG, Kuck KH, Tilsner V et al: Nonsurgical coronary artery recanalization after acute transmural myocardial infarction. Circulation 63:489, 1981

169. McDonald RH, Goldberg LI, McNay JL, Tuttle EP: Effects of dopamine in man: augmentation of sodium excretion, glomerular filtration rate and renal plasma flow. J Clin Invest 43:1116, 1964

170. McGee D, Gordon T: The Framingham study—An epidemiological investigation of cardiovascular disease. U.S. Department of Health, Education, and Welfare. HEW Publication No. (NIH) 76–1083, Washington, DC, April, 1976

171. Meyer SL, Curry GC, Dunsky MS et al: Influence of dobutamine on hemodynamic and coronary blood flow in patients with and without coronary artery disease. Am J Cardiol 38:103, 1976

172. Mikulic E, Cohn J, Franciosa JA: Comparative hemodynamic effects of intropic and vasodilator drugs in severe heart failure. Circulation 56:528, 1977

173. Miller RR, Awan NA, Joye JA: Combined dopamine and nitroprusside therapy in congestive heart failure. Circulation 55:881, 1977

174. Miller RR, Vismara LA, Williams DO et al: Pharmacological mechanisms for left ventricular unloading in clinical congestive heart failure. Differential effects of nitroprusside, phentolamine and nitroglycerin on cardiac function and peripheral circulation. Circ Res 39:127, 1976

175. Miller RR, Vismara LA, Zelis R, et al: Clinical use of sodium nitroprusside in chronic ischemic heart disease: effects on peripheral vascular resistance and venous tone and on ventricular volume, pump, and mechanical performance. Circulation 51:328, 1975

176. Morissette M, Weil MH, Shubin H: Reduction in colloid osmotic pressure associated with fatal progression of cardiopulmonary failure. Crit Care Med 3:115, 1975

177. Morrison J, Donnelly W, Killip T: Digitalis and acute myocardial infarction. Circulation 46 (suppl 2):113, 1972

178. Moulopoulous SD, Topaz S, Kolff WJ: Diastolic balloon pumping in the aorta, mechanical assistance to failing circulation. Am Heart J 63:669, 1962

179. Mueller H: Efficiency of intra-aortic balloon pumping and external counterpulsation in the treatment of cardiogenic shock. p. 191. In Ledingham I McA (ed): Recent Advances in Intensive Therapy. Churchill Livingstone, Edinburgh, 1977

180. Mueller H, Ayres SM, Conklin EF: The effects of intra-aortic balloon counterpulsation on cardiac performance and metabolism in shock associated with acute myocardial infarction. J Clin Invest 50:1885, 1971

181. Mueller H, Ayres S, Gianelli S et al: Effect of isoproterenol, L-norepinephrine, and intra-aortic counterpulsation on hemodynamics and myocardial metabolism in shock following acute myocardial infarction. Circulation 45:335, 1972

182. Mueller HS, Ayres SM: The role of propranolol in the treatment of acute myocardial infarction. Progr Cardiovasc Dis 19:405, 1977

183. Mueller HS, Ayres SM, Religa A, Evans RG: Propranolol in the treatment of acute myocardial infarction: Effect on myocardial oxygenation and hemodynamics. Circulation 49:1078, 1974

184. Mueller HS, Evans R, Ayres S: Effects of dopamine on hemodynamics and myocardial metabolism in shock following acute myocardial infarction. Circulation 57:361, 1978

185. Muller JE, Morrison J, Stone PH et al: Nifedipine therapy for patients with threatened and acute myocardial infarction: a randomized, double blind, placebo controlled comparison. Circulation 69(4):740–747, 1984

186. Multicenter International Study: Improvement in prognosis of myocardial infarction by long term betadrenoreceptor blockade using practolol. Br Med J III:735, 1975

187. Multicenter Trial: Propranolol in acute myocardial infarction. Lancet 2:1435, 1966

188. Mungall DR, Robichaux RP, Perry W et al: Effects of quinidine on serum digoxin concentration. Ann Intern Med 93:689, 1980

189. Norman JC, Mulokhea FA, Harmison LT et al: An implantable nuclear fueled circulatory support system. I. System analysis of conception, design, fabrication, and initial in vivo testing. Ann Surg 176:492, 1972

190. Norris RM, Caughey DE, Scott PJ: Trial of propranolol in acute myocardial infarction. Br Med J II:398, 1968

191. Norris RM, Clarke ED, Sammel NL et al: Protective effect of propranolol in threatened myocardial infarction. Lancet 2:907, 1978

192. Norwegian Multicenter Study Group: Timolol induced reduction in mortality and reinfarction in patients surviving acute myocardial infarction. N Engl J Med 304:801, 1981

193. Nourok DS, Glassock RJ, Solomon DH: Hypothyroidism following prolonged nitroprusside therapy. Am J Med Sci 248:129, 1964

194. O'Rourke M, Chang VP, Windsor HM et al: Acute severe cardiac failure complicating myocardial infarction. Br Heart J 37:169, 1975

195. Pace PD, Tilney NL, Lesch M, Couch NP: Peripheral arterial complications of intra-aortic counterpulsation. Surgery 82:685, 1977

196. Packer M, Meller J, Medina N et al: Rebound hemodynamic events after the abrupt withdrawal of nitroprusside in patients with severe chronic heart failure. N Engl J Med 301:1193, 1979

197. Palmer RF, Lasseter FC: Sodium nitroprusside. N Engl J Med 292:294, 1975

198. Pappas G: Intra-thoracic intra-aortic balloon insertion for pulsatile cardiopulmonary by-pass. Arch Surg 109:842, 1974

199. Parkey RW, Bonte FJ, Meyer SL: A new method for radionucleotide imaging of acute myocardial infarction in humans. Circulation 50:540, 1974

200. Parmley WW, Chatterjee K, Charuzi Y, Swan HJC: Hemodynamic effects of noninvasive systolic unloading (nitroprusside) and diastolic augmentation (external counterpulsation) in patients with acute myocardial infarction. Am J Cardiol 33:819, 1974

201. Passamani ER: Nitroprusside in myocardial infarction. N Engl J Med 306:1168, 1982

202. Pells D, Alonzo CA: Immediate mortality and five year survival of men employed with a first infarction. N Engl J Med 270:916, 1964

203. Peter CT, Norris RM, Clarke ED et al: Reduction

of enzyme levels by propranolol after acute myocardial infarction. Circulation 57:1091, 1978

204. Pierri MK, Zema M, Klingfield P et al: Exercise tolerance in late survivors of balloon pumping and surgery for cardiogenic shock. Circulation 62 (Suppl 1):138, 1980

205. Phillips C: Contributory causes of coronary thrombosis. JAMA 106:761, 1936

206. Raabe DS: Combined therapy with digoxin and nitroprusside in heart failure complicating acute myocardial infarction. Am J Cardiol 43:990, 1979

207. Rahimtoola SH, Gunnar RM: Digitalis in acute myocardial infarction. Help or hazard? Ann Intern Med 82:234, 1968

208. Rahimtoola SH, Sinno MZ, Chuquimia R et al: Effects of ouabain on impaired left ventricular function in acute myocardial infarction. N Engl J Med 287:527, 1972

209. Raphael LD, Mantle JA, Moraski RE et al: Quantitative assessment of ventricular performance in unstable heart disease by dextran function curves. Circulation 55:858, 1977

210. Rebner HS, Freshman DH: Anticoagulation in myocardial infarction. New approaches to an old problem. Cardiovasc Med 2:787, 1971

211. Reid PR, Pitt B, Kelly DT: Effects of dopamine on increasing infarct area in acute myocardial infarction. Circulation 46 (Suppl 2):210, 1972

212. Reid PR, Thompson WL: Clinical use of dopamine in the treatment of shock. Johns Hopkins Med J 137:276, 1975

213. Report of the working party on anticoagulant therapy in coronary thrombosis to the Medical Research Council: Assessment of short term anticoagulant administration after cardiac infarction. Br Med J 1:355, 1969

214. Resacknou L: Cardiogenic shock. Chest 83(6):893–898, 1983

215. Reul GJ, Morris GC, Howell JF et al: Emergency coronary artery bypass grafts in the treatment of myocardial infarction. Circulation 48 (suppl 3):177, 1973

216. Reynolds JL, Whitlock RML: Effects of a beta adrenergic receptor blocker in myocardial infarction for one year from onset. Br Heart J 34:252, 1972

217. Riley CP, Russell RO, Rackley CE: Left ventricular gallop sound and acute myocardial infarction. Am Heart J 86:598, 1973

218. Roberts R, Sobel BE: CPK isoenzymes in evaluation of myocardial ischemic injury. Hosp Prac 11:55, 1976

219. Robie N, Nutter DO, Moody C, McNay JL: In vivo analysis of adrenergic receptor activity of dobutamine. Circ Res 34:663, 1974

220. Romhilt DW, Bloomfield SS, Chow TC Fowler NO: Unreliability of conventional electrocardio-graphic monitoring for arrhythmic detection in coronary care units. Am J Cardiol 31:457, 1973

221. Rosen MR. Iluento JP, Gelkand H, et al: Effects of verapamil on electrophysiologic properties of canine cardiac Purkinje fibers. J Pharmacol Exp Ther 189:414, 1974

222. Rosenblum R: Physiologic basis for the therapeutic use of catecholamines. Am Heart J 87:527, 1974

223. Ruiz C, Weil MH, Carlson RW: Treatment of circulatory shock with dopamine: studies on survival. JAMA 242:165, 1979

224. Russell RO, Rackley CE, Pombo J et al: Effects of increasing left ventricular filling pressure in patients with acute myocardial infarction. J Clin Invest 49:1539, 1970

225. Sakamoto T, Yamada T: Hemodynamic effects of dobutamine in patients following open heart surgery. Circulation 55:525, 1977

226. Sanders CA, Buckley MJ, Leinbach RC et al: Mechanical circulatory assistance: current status and experience in combining arteriography and acute myocardial revascularization. Circulation 45:1292, 1972

227. Scheidt S, Ascheim R, Killip T: Shock after acute myocardial infarction: A clinical and hemodynamic profile. Am J Cardiol 26:556, 1970

228. Scheidt S, Wilner G, Mueller H et al: Intra-aortic balloon counterpulsation in cardiogenic shock. Report of a cooperative trial. N Engl J Med 288:979, 1973

229. Schmulzer KJ, Raschke E, Maloney JV: Intravenous L-norepinephrine as a cause of reduced plasma volume. Surgery 50:452, 1961

230. Schuster CJ, Weil MH, Besso J et al: Blood volume following diuresis induced by furosemide. Am J Med 76:585, 1984

231. Scwed JJ, Kleit SA, Hamburger JJ: Effect of furosemide and chlorthiazide on the thoracic duct lymph flow in the dog. J Lab Clin Med 79:693, 1972

232. Sloman G, Stannard M: Beta adrenergic blockade and cardiac arrhythmias. Br Med J IV:508, 1967

233. Smith ER, Redwood DR, McCarron WE, Epstein SE: Coronary artery occlusion in the conscious dog: Effects of alterations in arterial pressure produced by nitroglycerin, hemorrhage, and alpha adrenergic agonists on the degree of myocardial ischemia. Circulation 47:51, 1973

234. Snow PJD: Effect of propranolol in myocardial infarction. Lancet 2:551, 1965

235. Snyder SH: The opiate receptor and morphine like peptides in the brain. Am J Psychiatry 135:6, 1978

236. Soroff HS, Cloutier CT, Bertwell WC et al: External counterpulsation: management of cardio-

genic shock after myocardial infarction. JAMA 299:1441, 1974

237. Stamler J: Primary prevention of sudden coronary death. Circulation 52(Suppl 3):258, 1975
238. Stechel R, Zema M, Reiser P, Scherr L: Digitalis and myocardial infarction in man. Circulation 62:8, 1980
239. Stein L, Beraud JJ, Morissette M et al: Pulmonary edema during volume infusion. Circulation 57:483, 1975
240. Stemple DR, Kleiman JH, Harrison DC: Combined nitroprusside dopamine therapy in severe chronic congestive heart failure: dose related hemodynamic advantages over single drug infusion. Am J Cardiol 42:267, 1978
241. Stenson RE, Constantino RT, Harrison DC: Interrelationship of hepatic blood flow, cardiac output, and blood levels of lidocaine in man. Circulation 43:205, 1971
242. Subramanian VA, Goldstein JE, Sos TA et al: Preliminary clinical experience with percutaneous intra-aortic balloon pumping. Circulation 62(suppl):123, 1980
243. Swan HJC, Forrester JS, Diamond G et al: Hemodynamic spectrum of myocardial infarction and cardiogenic shock. Circulation 45:1097, 1972
244. Synhorst DP, Laur RM, Doty DB: Hemodynamic effects of vasodilator agents in dogs with experimental ventricular septal defects. Circulation 54:472, 1976
245. Taylor SH, Silke B, Ebbutt A et al: A long term prevention study with oxprenolol in coronary heart disease. N Engl J Med 307(21):1293, 1982
246. Tecklenberg PL, Fitzgerald J, Allaire BI et al: Afterload reduction in management of postinfarction ventricular septal defect. Am J Cardiol 38:956, 1978
247. Thompson L, Schwartz E: Cardiovascular responsiveness to catecholamines in acute metabolic and respiratory acidosis in dogs. Fed Proc 28:742, 1969
248. Thompson PL, Robinson JS: Stroke after acute myocardial infarction: Relation to infarct size. Br Med J 2:457, 1978
249. Tuttle RR, Mills J: Development of a new catecholamine to selectively increase cardiac contractility. Circ Res 36:185, 1975
250. Vaughn-Neil EF, Snell NJC, Bevan G: Hypotension after verapamil. Br Med J 2:529, 1972
251. Veterans Administration Cooperative Clinical Trial: Anticoagulants in acute myocardial infarction. JAMA 225:724, 1973
252. Vetter NJ, Julian DG: Comparison of arrhythmia computer and conventional monitoring in coronary care unit. Lancet 1:1151, 1975
253. Vismara LA, Mason DT, Amsterdam EA: Cardiocirculatory effects of morphine sulfate: mech-

anisms of action and therapeutic application. Heart Lung 3:495, 1974
254. Vreeben J: Anticoagulant therapy in myocardial infarction. In Meltzer LE, Dunning AJ (eds): Textbook of Coronary Care. Charles Press, Philadelphia, 1972
255. Wackers FJ, Buseman SE, Samson G: Value and limitation of thallium 201 scintigraphy in acute phase of myocardial infarction. N Engl J Med 295:1, 1976
256. Webb SW, Adgey AAJ, Pantridge JF: Autonomic disturbance at onset of acute myocardial infarction. Br Med J 3:89, 1972
257. Weil MH, Henning RJ: Vasopressor and vasodilator therapy of shock. p. 309. In Weil MH, Henning RJ (eds): Handbook of Critical Care Medicine. Year Book Medical Publishers, Chicago 1978
258. Weil MH, Henning RJ: New concepts in diagnosis and fluid therapy of shock. Anesth Analg 58:124, 1979
259. Weil MH, Henning RJ: Shock complicating myocardial infarction. p. 3. In Weil MH, Henning RJ (eds): The Handbook of Critical Care Medicine. EM Books, New York, 1979
260. Weil MH, Henning RJ, Morissette M, Michaels S: Relationship between colloid osmotic pressure and pulmonary artery wedge pressure in patients with acute cardiorespiratory failure. Am J Med 64:643, 1978
261. Weil MH, Morissette M, Michaels S et al: Routine plasma colloid osmotic pressure measurements. Crit Care Med 2:229, 1974
262. Weil MH, Shubin H, Carlson RW: Treatment of circulatory shock: Use of sympathomimetic and related vasoactive agents. JAMA 231:1280, 1975
263. Wilcox RG, Roland JM, Banks DC et al: Randomized trial comparing propranolol with atenolol in immediate treatment of suspected myocardial infarction. Br Med J 280:885, 1980
264. Wilhelmsson C, Vedin JA, Wilhemsen L et al: Reduction of sudden deaths after myocardial infarction by treatment with alprenolol. Lancet 2:1157, 1974
265. Willerson JT, Parkey RW, Bonte FJ: Pathophysiologic considerations and clinicopathological correlates of technetium 99m stannous pyrophosphate myocardial scintigraphy. Semin Nucl Med 10:54, 1980
266. William DO, Amsterdam EA, Mason DT: Hemodynamic effects of nitroglycerin in acute myocardial infarction. Decrease in ventricular preload at the expense of cardiac output. Circulation 51:421, 1975
267. Williamson JR, Woodrow ML, Scaipa A: Calcium binding to cardiac sarcolemma. Recent ad-

vances in the study of cardiac structure. Metabolism 5:61, 1975

268. Wilson RF, Sukhriander R, Thal AP: Combined use of norepinephrine and dibenzyline in clinical shock. Surg Forum 30:31, 1961

269. Winbury MM: Redistribution of left ventricular blood flow produced by nitroglycerin. Circ Res 1(suppl):140, 1971

270. Wisniewski JM: Prophylactic action of regitine in experimental histaminic and allergic bronchial asthma. Arch Int Pharmacodyn Ther 49:56, 1964

271. Wray R, Maurer B, Shillingford J: Prophylactic anticoagulation therapy in the prevention of calf vein thromboses after myocardial infarction. N Engl J Med 288:815, 1973

272. Wright IS, Marple CD, Beck DF: Report of the committee for the evaluation of anticoagulants in the treatment of coronary thrombosis. Am Heart J 36:801, 1948

273. Wright PW: External counterpulsation for cardiogenic shock following cardiopulmonary bypass surgery. Am Heart J 90:231, 1975

274. Wyman MG, Lalka D, Hammersmith L et al: Multiple bolus technique for lidocaine administration during the first few hours of an acute myocardial infarction. Am J Cardiol 41:313, 1978

275. Zellis R, Mansour EJ, Capone RJ: The cardiovascular effects of morphine: the peripheral capacitance and resistance vessels in human subjects. J Clin Invest 54:1247, 1974

276. Zucker G, Levine J: Pressor and diminished local vasoconstrictor effects of levarterenol-phentolamine mixtures. Arch Intern Med 104:607, 1959

11

Intra-Aortic Balloon Counterpulsation in Refractory Shock

David Bregman
Peter Kaskel

INTRODUCTION

The last 20 years have witnessed the emergence of circulatory assist devices in the treatment of hemodynamically compromised patients. Many of the early mechanical designs have become victims of technical obstacles and await further biomedical advances. One device, in particular, has seen a dramatic rise to prominence, becoming the treatment of choice for temporarily stabilizing severe hemodynamic deterioration secondary to myocardial ischemia or pump failure. The intra-aortic balloon (IAB) owes its success to the elegance and simplicity of its operating principles matched with the availability of sophisticated but reliable electronic and pneumatic technology. This combination has resulted in the use of over 700,000 intra-aortic balloons in the United States alone.

In 1962, Moulopoulos et al.[64] suggested the use of a single-chambered intra-aortic balloon positioned in the descending thoracic aorta to function as a counterpulsator. The balloon is inflated in diastole beginning with closure of the aortic valve and is held in inflation until the onset of ventricular systole, when the balloon is rapidly deflated (Fig. 11-1).

The inflation of the balloon displaces 40 cm³ of aortic blood, both towards the coronary tree, thus augmenting coronary perfusion pressure, and downward into the descending aorta (Fig. 11-2). The augmentation of the diastolic pressure and mean arterial pressure seen at the coronary ostia can increase coronary blood flow, especially across tight lesions where flow is often pressure-dependent. Deflation of the balloon occurs at the moment of left ventricular ejection, and creates a "vaccum" effect, helping the ventricle in expelling its volume. The collapsing balloon thus reduces the circulatory impedance seen by the left ventricle, and therefore reduces the mechanical work required by the myocardium to maintain a given cardiac output. A reduction in mechanical work is ac-

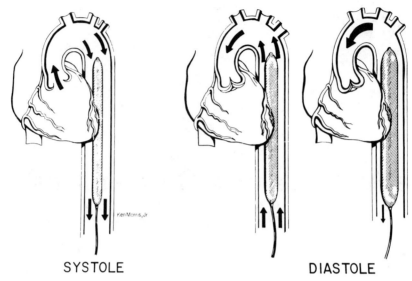

SYSTOLE   DIASTOLE

FIG. 11-1 Mechanism of action of the intra-aortic balloon. Balloon inflates during systole, increasing coronary blood flow, and deflates during diastole, causing ventricular unloading.

companied by a reduction in myocardial oxygen requirements, which is why intra-aortic balloon pumping (IABP) can often bring into balance the metabolic needs of an ischemic myocardium, with its compromised blood flow.[30]

Six years after its experimental introduction, Kantrowitz reported in 1968 the first successful clinical application of a single-chambered IABP.[47] Since that time, several qualities have emerged to make the IABP especially attractive to the clinician: (1) IABP is the only treatment that can increase mean arterial pressure while reducing circulatory impedance; (2) coronary blood flow is augmented even in the hypotensive state,[76] (3) circulatory support can be instituted within 5 minutes, utilizing the new percutaneous IABs; (4) IABP support can be maintained for an extended period of time with a minimal amount of hemolysis; (5) IABP can be instituted prophylactically during high-risk procedures; (6) IABP can produce dramatic reversals of the clinical manifestations of ischemic heart disease if initiated early. In addition, it has been demonstrated that IAB counterpulsation can limit the size of an evolving myocardial infarction if it is instituted soon after the coronary occlusion.[33,59,69,78]

For these reasons intra-aortic balloon pumping has emerged as the single most impor-

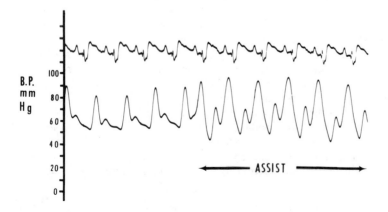

B.P.
mm
Hg

FIG. 11-2 Hemodynamic response to IABP. Note diastolic augmentation and ventricular unloading during assist in a patient with cardiogenic shock.

◄——— ASSIST ———►

tant mechanical support adjunct in the treatment of refractory left ventricular power failure.[12,13,18,19,41,80,81]

CLINICAL SYSTEM FOR IABP

Our clinical experience most recently has been with the Datascope System 90 (Datascope Corporation, Paramus, NJ) (Fig. 11-3). The System 90 has incorporated several significant improvements over its predecessors, the Datascope System 80, 82, and 83. Particular attention has now been devoted to redesigning and simplifying the operating controls, since nursing staff and other paramedical personnel are running the balloon pump console with greater frequency. As a result, the setting of two prominent slide controls is essentially all that is needed for proper operation of the balloon pump. The System 90 utilizes a nonfade

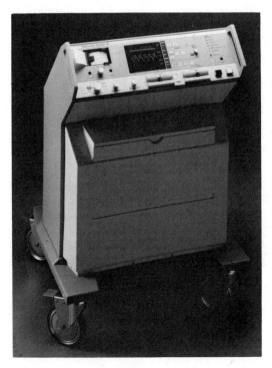

FIG. 11-3. Modern balloon-pump-driving console.

physiologic monitor, which gives excellent viewing of all pertinent data. In addition, it has the advantage of being able to freeze the tracing so that the pumping waves may be critically analyzed. In addition, the System 90 incorporates an electrosurgical interference suppression module (ESIS) that virtually eliminates interference from an electrocautery during surgery. The result is an electrocardiographic (ECG) signal essentially free of noise and a reliable triggering of the balloon pump console even during the use of an electrosurgical unit. The balloon pump console is also considerably quieter than its precedessors. System 90 has built-in battery power that allows it to be easily transported with the patient and has an automatic filling mode.

Inflation and deflation of the balloon are accomplished by alternately applying pressure and "vacuum" to a closed circuit consisting of the intra-aortic balloon and a slave balloon within a safety chamber. This circuit can be precharged with a fixed amount of either carbon dioxide or helium. Carbon dioxide is an inherently safer driving gas because it is more soluable in blood than helium. However, because helium has a lighter molecular weight it can outperform carbon dioxide at very high heart rates with smaller balloon catheters. Consequently, since the System 90 is designed to utilize either gas, optimal balloon pump operation can occur over a wide clinical spectrum.

Since the introduction of this device by Moulopolos et al.,[64] the design and construction of the intra-aortic balloon have undergone an interesting evolution. Beginning with a single-chamber, sausage-shaped device, Austen[53] at Massachusetts General Hospital developed a trisegmented balloon that inflated its midsection first, followed by the two end chambers. Any blood believed trapped between the balloon and aorta with the single chamber balloon would be expelled by this three-chamber device. Paralleling the introduction of this trisegmented model, Bregman et al. developed a unidirectional dual-chambered balloon.[15,19] By incorporating a small proximal chamber that inflated earlier than the large distal chamber, this dual-chambered balloon produced unidirectional blood flow towards the aortic root. In addition to this dual-chambered balloon, a new percutaneous single-chambered balloon has recently been introduced into clinical use.

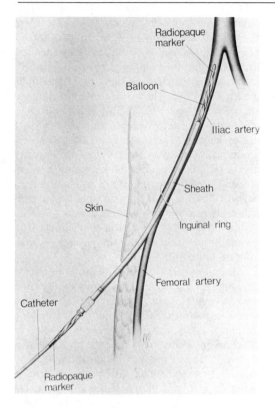

Radiopaque marker

Balloon

Iliac artery

Sheath

Skin

Inguinal ring

Femoral artery

Catheter

Radiopaque marker

FIG. 11-4 Schematic diagram showing insertion of furled 40 cc percutaneous intra-aortic balloon through a 12.5 Fr sheath in the common femoral artery.

The advantage of a percutaneous IAB is rapid balloon insertion into the femoral artery, thereby reducing the time needed for hemodynamic stabilization (Fig. 11-4).

MECHANISM OF BALLOON ACTION

The unidirectional dual-chambered intra-aortic balloon has a spherical distal chamber that inflates early in diastole and occludes the aorta.[13] This is followed sequentially by the inflation of a narrower cylindrical proximal pumping chamber, in the same diastolic interval, which displaces intra-aortic blood entirely (unidirectionally) towards the aortic root. Both chambers are completely deflated by an active vacuum just prior to ventricular ejection. Two human balloon configurations are available. For the average-sized adult patient with a normal-caliber common femoral artery, a 30 cc dual-chambered balloon is utilized with an 18-mm O.D. distal occluding balloon and a 14 mm proximal pumping balloon. For a patient with a larger vascular tree, a 35 cc dual-chambered proximal pumping balloon is available with a 20 mm occluding balloon and a 16 mm proximal pumping balloon. Both are mounted on a 12 Fr catheter.

The percutaneous intra-aortic balloon is a single chambered 40-ml sausage-shaped balloon designed to allow the balloon membrane to be wrapped around a central wire stylet.[16,17] A tightly wrapped balloon allows insertion of the balloon catheter into the femoral artery via a modified Seldinger technique. By relying on previously established percutaneous insertion (Fig. 11-4) technology, the percutaneous IAB can be inserted with great speed; an average time of 5 minutes is not uncommon. Because it requires no surgical supplies, the location of balloon pump insertions can be widened. Recent work has demonstrated that the effectiveness of the percutaneous intra-aortic balloon is comparable to the dual-chambered balloon.

IDEAL BALLOON FUNCTION

The primary goals of IABP are to implement the maximal increase in coronary blood flow during diastole and at the same time effect a decrease in left ventricular work.[32] Realization that these two beneficial effects are dependent upon one another permits maximal benefit to be otained from each factor in the following fashion. The diastolic augmentation ordinarily begins at the dicrotic notch. One can encroach upon the dicrotic notch to begin balloon inflation slightly earlier in diastole. Provided the patient does not have premature ventricular contractions from this manipulation, it can be performed in patients who appear to be responding poorly to the balloon pumping to give them an additional benefit. The right-hand side or downslope of the augmentation is the part most intimately involved with the ventricular unloading aspect of balloon pumping. If the fall in end-diastolic pressure is too great, the following sequence of events occurs. Such a fall essentially means that the balloon has collapsed too soon before the aortic valve has opened. Since blood must flow to occupy the space of the formerly expanded balloon, it will flow retrograde from all branches of the aorta, including the coronary arteries.[14] Therefore one must effect a compromise and have some fall in end-diastolic pressure, but not an excessive fall. In our experimental work, which has been substantiated in our clinical experience, this fall should not exceed 10 mmHg.

We initially place the balloon as far proximally in the aorta as possible (that is, with the tip of the balloon just distal to the left subclavian artery). Be sure to feel the pulse in the left arm so that the tip of the balloon is not in the subclavian orifice and is not occluding the left subclavian inflow.

In the clinical setting, heart rates of up to 140 beats /min can be followed when helium is used. If the rate is higher, simply assist on 1:2 (every other beat) until the rate slows, when 1:1 assist can be instituted. Weaning a patient from the IABP is undertaken by changing the assisting sequence from a 1:1 to a 1:3 ratio.

INTRA-AORTIC BALLOON INSERTION

Indications

1. Crescendo, preinfarction, or unstable angina refractory to medical therapy in preparation for coronary angiography and surgery

2. Preoperative support of patients with acute myocardial infarction complicated by a ventricular septal defect or acute mitral insufficiency
3. Support of unstable patients requiring cardiac catheterization and possible surgery
4. Support of patients during emergency cardiac catheterization, coronary angioplasty, or streptokinase infusion
5. Cardiogenic shock patients within the first 8 hours after the onset of shock
6. Support of patients with complicated myocardial infarctions with recurent chest pain and evidence of infarct extension
7. Intractable tachyarrhythmias refractory to medical therapy
8. Preoperative support of medical patients requiring cardiac transplantation
9. Support of cardiac patients for noncardiac surgery
10. Support of patients in whom balloon angioplasty has failed

The only absolute contraindications to IABP are wide-open aortic insufficiency and the presence of an acute dissecting aortic aneurysm. Minor aortic insufficiency should not contraindicate clinical use.[89] A relative contraindication is the presence of an aortic aneurysm or history of previous operation on the aorta. This must be evaluated in light of the exigency of the clinical picture.[43]

Percutaneous Method

In 1979 a single chambered 40 ml percutaneous intra-aortic balloon (Percor) was constructed around a central wire. The IAB was wrapped manually, which then allowed for percutaneous insertion into the femoral artery through a 12 Fr sheath via the modified Seldinger technique[17] (Fig. 11-4). Percutaneous balloon insertion requires approximately 5 to 10 minutes and has been successfully performed in the cardiac catheterization lab, coronary care unit, operating suite, and recovery room. Difficulties with percutaneous insertion were encountered when advancing the IAB through tortuous and atherosclerotic vessels.

In these circumstances arterial injury, dislodging of thrombus, or failure to insert the balloon often occurred. Difficulties in manually wrapping the percutaneous balloon necessitated a mechanical device to perform uniform wrapping of the balloon membrane. There have been reported instances of hand wrapped IABs failing to unfurl at the onset of balloon pumping because of initial overwrapping.

A dual-lumen intra-aortic balloon (Percor DL) was developed with a flexible inner lumen that allows the balloon to be advanced over a 0.038 inch J-tip safety guidewire that has already been positioned in the descending thoracic aorta (Fig. 11-5). To gain access to this central lumen necessitates removal of the wrapping knob with its attached support wire. When the IAB is in place, the J-tip guidewire is removed, which allows one to monitor central aortic pressure through the balloon (Fig. 11-6).

In a further balloon design advance, the wrapping knob has been incorporated at the base of the IAB catheter and is an integral part

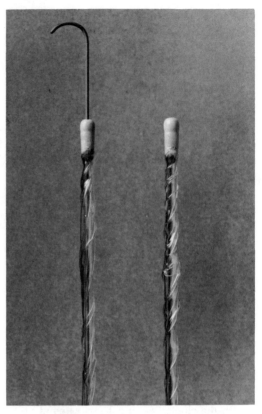

FIG. 11-6 Dual-lumen IAB can be inserted over a 0.030 inch J-tip safety guidewire to ensure passage into thoracic aorta.

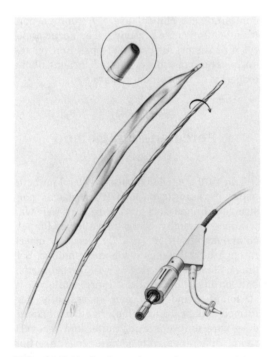

FIG. 11-5 Mechanism of wrapping percutaneous double-lumen balloon.

of the balloon. This knob rotates the inner lumen a mechanically fixed number of turns and causes the balloon membrane to wrap around the inner lumen. Access to the inner lumen now only requires removing the support wire, and not the wrapping knob. The sterile IAB package is designed to act as a passive wrapping guide for the balloon membrane when the wrapping knob is being rotated. The dual-lumen intra-aortic balloon (DL-II), which incorporates the wrapping knob, is available on either 10.5 or 12 Fr catheters. A new 8.5 Fr single-lumen IAB with a mechanical wrapper has been developed for those patients with severe peripheral vascular disease or small femoral arteries (Fig. 11-7). It is believed that the slimmer catheter will allow more blood to flow distal to the IAB and thus prevent limb ischemia. The Percor Stat, a pre-wrapped percutaneous balloon has recently been introduced.

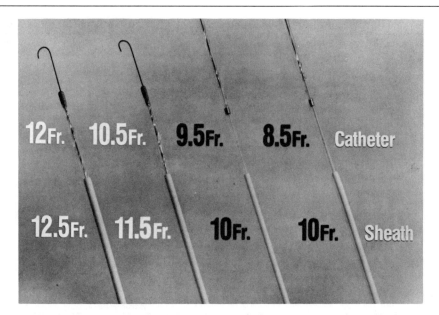

FIG. 11-7 Family of percutaneous IABs. Note that smaller balloons must use helium as the driving gas.

CLINICAL EXPERIENCE AT COLOMBIA PRESBYTERIAN MEDICAL CENTER

Our clinical experience at the Columbia Presbyterian Medical Center has been with both the dual-chambered unidirectional IAB and, more recently, with the new percutaneous intra-aortic balloon. From February, 1972, to June, 1983, a total of 274 patients have undergone intra-aortic balloon pump insertion at the Presbyterian Hospital. Of these 274 patients, 125 had unidirectional balloon insertion and the remaining 149 had percutaneous intra-aortic balloons. We will review the clinical data for percutaneous IABP.

Percutaneous Intra-Aortic Balloon

Percutaneous IAB insertion was attempted in 155 patients from February, 1979, to June, 1983, at Columbia Presbyterian Medical Center (Table 11-1). Successful insertion was accom-

plished in 149 of 155 patients (96 percent). In 10 patients the initial insertion attempt failed. However, 4 of the 10 patients eventually underwent successful IAB implantation using the long inserter technique.

Indications in these patients were broadly divided among medical and surgical groups. Of the 149 patients, 74 received the IAB for a surgical indication: intraoperative low cardiac output in 61, postoperative low output in 11, and cardiac arrest in 2. Medical indications for counterpulsation included unstable angina in 27, postinfarction angina in 19, cardiogenic shock in 10, acute ventricular septal defect complicating myocardial infarction in 4, recurrent ventricular tachycardia in 1, and 3 unsuccessful Gruntzig procedures. When homedynamic decompensation occurred in the three patients undergoing transluminal angioplasty, the IAB was inserted and emergency coronary revascularization was carried out. The patients subsequently were discharged from the hospital. Only one patient received the IAB prophylactically for unstable angina prior to a general surgical procedure. This patient survived and the balloon was removed in the immediate postoperative period.

The location of the balloon insertion varied. Sixty-one patients had the balloon im-

TABLE 11-1. Percutaneous IABP at Columbia Presbyterian Medical Center, 1979–1983

Successful Insertions	CCU	Catheterization Lab
Preoperative		
Unstable angina with general surgery	1	—
Unstable angina with cardiac surgery	13(2)[a]	10
Unstable angina—treated with medication	2(1)	1
Postinfarction angina—treated with medication	2(1)	4(1)
Postinfarction angina with surgery	10(1)	3
Cardiogenic shock—treated with medication	2	3(2)
Cardiogenic shock with surgery	1	4(1)
Recurrent ventricular tachycardia—medication	1	—
Failed Gruntzig procedure with emergency surgery	—	3
Acute VSD with surgery	1	2(1)
Acute VSD without surgery	—	1(1)
Anesthesia support for open heart surgery	2	9(1)
Perioperative		
Low output—OR	61(38)	
Postoperative		
Low output	11(6)	
Cardiac arrest	2(1)	
Total number assisted	149	
Total number discharged	92(62%)	

[a] Numbers in parentheses indicate deaths.

planted in the operating room, 13 in the open heart recovery room, 40 in the cardiac catheterization laboratoy, and 35 in the cardiac care unit.

Of the 75 patients in whom the IAB was successfully inserted for a medical indication (Fig. 11-8) 59 (79 percent) eventually underwent a cardiac procedure whereas 16 were treated medically. Only 6 of the 59 patients undergoing preoperative IAB support combined with definitive surgical procedures died. In contrast, 45 of 74 patients (61 percent) requiring intraoperative or postoperative IAB died.

The first 102 patients undergoing successful percutaneous intra-aortic balloon insertion were reviewed for vascular complications, which were noted in 15 (14.7 percent).[17] Of these 15 patients with vascular complications, 6 had limb ischemia responding to balloon removal, and 6 patients had limb ischemia requiring a thrombectomy and femoral artery repair. The remaining three patients all required surgical exploration, two for control of hemorrhage and one for repair of a large femoral false aneurysm.

Additional Percutaneous Balloon Guidelines

During our first 4 years of clinical experience with percutaneous IABP at the Columbia Presbyterian Medical Center, certain steps have been taken to reduce the "hazards" associated with this technique.[15]

1. The percutaneous IAB *must* be inserted by a physician skilled in the Seldinger technique of cardiac catheterization. Clearly, those institutions adhering to this suggestion have reduced morbidity associated with the procedure.

2. Ideally, the insertion procedure should be carried out under fluoroscopic control.

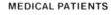
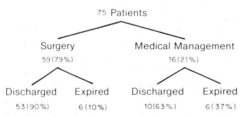

MEDICAL PATIENTS

75 Patients

Surgery 59(79%) — Medical Management 16(21%)

Discharged 53(90%) — Expired 6(10%) — Discharged 10(63%) — Expired 6(37%)

FIG. 11-8 Percutaneous IABP at the Columbia Presbyterian Medical Center, 1979 to 1983.

3. In critically ill patients undergoing cardiac catheterization, who have poor ventricular function, study of the aortoiliac system is highly desirable as a guide for subsequent balloon insertion.

4. In high-risk cardiac surgical patients undergoing open heart surgery in whom an intra-aortic balloon was not inserted prior to anesthetic induction, we recommend obtaining femoral artery access with an arterial needle and then a guidewire, which are maintained in the sterile operative field. If IABP is subsequently required for separation from cardiopulmonary bypass, arterial access is already established.

5. Finally, balloon removal should be carried out in the following manner. The balloon is deflated and pulled down to (but not into) the sheath. The femoral artery immediately distal to the balloon is tightly compressed and the balloon and sheath are then removed as a unit. Blood is allowed to spurt from the artery for a few seconds and then the compression is shifted over the puncture site for 30 minutes. Distal pulses are monitored with a Doppler apparatus and manual compression is adjusted so that an audible pulse is registered. With this technique we have occasionally retrieved specimens of thrombus that leave the femoral artery and therefore have not embolized distally.

It is clear from these remarks that attention to detail will significantly reduce the potential morbidity associated with percutaneous IABP.

CLINICAL APPLICATIONS

Myocardial Infarction with Shock

It was initially believed that the IABP would be the physician's salvation in the management of patients with acute myocardial infarction and shock. In fact, a given patient in the shock syndrome secondary to acute myocardial infarction who was placed on IABP support invariably showed some clinical improvement. However, as the major experiences with support of cardiogenic shock patients on intra-aortic balloons have evolved throughout the world, [5,7,28,37,47-49,52,67,72,86] certain basic and consistent observations have been made. Offering balloon support to patients who have been in shock for extended periods of time is not practical.[76] Although frequently there was an improvement in the patient's hemodynamics, organ function had usually reached irreversible deterioration, and the ultimate outcome of these patients has been uniformly fatal.[50] Therefore it appears more advisable to try to insert the intra-aortic balloon early during cardiogenic shock insult.[26,36,56]

A more recent report by Hagemeijer et al.[42] involved 25 class III or IV myocardial infarction shock patients who were treated with IABP during a 4-year period. Twenty of these 25 patients were successfully weaned from the IABP, and 6 died within 3 months, 5 within the first 10 days of balloon weaning. Of the 14 patients who survived for more than 34 months, 13 are still alive at the time of the report, 12 of whom were functional class II. Six have resumed full activity. This report indicates that even perhaps without surgery, with the early application of IABP a significant patient survival can be achieved.

An overall survival rate of approximately 50 percent has been reported[11] for patients in cardiogenic shock either secondary to a mechanical defect complicating acute myocardial infarction or treated with a combination of IABP and surgery. In a recent report[11] of IABP use in 728 patients, the IABP-related mortality was only 0.8 percent, and the survival of a large number of patients with acute myocardial ischemia was attributed to the use of IABP. The success of this treatment modality, coupled with its low mortality rate has encouraged many authors[2,6,28,51,57,61,74,85] to advocate the earlier institution of IABP support for cardiogenic shock. It is recommended that all cardiogenic shock patients placed on IABP support undergo complete cardiac catheterization. This is usually performed within 12 hours of the insertion of the intra-aortic balloon pump.

The unresolved question at this time is how next to proceed with the patient's care. If the patient is completely stable on the intra-aortic balloon pump, it has been suggested that the maximum benefit from the balloon will be achieved within 5 days and the patient can then be weaned. If the catheterization studies then dictate surgery, this can be performed usually during the same hospitalization. However, if the patient becomes balloon-dependent and cannot successfully be weaned from the intra-aortic balloon and associated pharmacologic adjuncts, this situation has uniformly led to 100 percent mortality even if surgical intervention is attempted. An exciting development in this regard has been the report by Reemtsma et al.[73] Noting that cardiogenic shock patients who do well on IABP support and have favorable anatomy during cardiac catheterization for revascularization, may do best with rather prompt surgical intervention that would include coronary revascularization and the avoidance of infarctectomy. The patients who may best profit from this therapeutic route seem to be those who respond most promptly to the balloon and who have major ischemic changes on their electrocardiogram that return to normal with the onset of intra-aortic balloon pumping. At present, for the cardiogenic shock patient requiring intra-aortic balloon pump support and, ultimately, coronary revascularization surgery, the overall survival as mentioned, is now being reported in excess of 50 percent.[9]

Myocardial Infarction without Shock

As evidence has accumulated supporting the use of IABP in postmyocardial infarction patients with shock, many authors[6,22,23,29,51,57,74,85] have supported the earlier institution of balloon pump therapy. Leinback et al.[57] recently studied the reversibility of myocardial ischemia through IABP use in patients with anterior myocardial infarction but without shock. Their criteria for selection were that the patients be under the age of 65 with pain and anterior ST segment elevation resistant to morphine, oxygen, and, in many cases, nitroglycerine. Continuous electrocardiographic monitoring was used and, as soon as current therapy failure was observed, IABP therapy was instituted.

Five of the eleven patients studied responded with an 84 percent fall in ST elevation in 1 hour, while maintaining precordial R waves and good ventricular function. The other six responded poorly, with a 40 percent fall in ST elevation in 1 hour, Q wave development, and poorer residual left ventricular function. Positive response correlated well with the presence or absence of complete left anterior descending coronary artery occlusion as demonstrated by coronary angiography. Thus, experimental documentation supports aggressive IABP therapy in the case of anterior infarction with residual anterior descending coronary artery patency.

High-Risk Patients Requiring Cardiac Catheterization

At present there is little doubt that a patient who has evidence of either a significant degree of left ventricular failure, ventricular tachyarrhythmia, or one of the acute mechanical complications of myocardial infarction can be safely brought through cardiac catheterization without significant risk.[19,25,39,65,83] Indeed in the author's institution 31 such intra-aortic balloon patients have been studied by the Judkins technique, and no patient with IABP support has experienced cardiac arrest or major complications in the catheterization laboratory. The advent of percutaneous IABP now makes balloon pumping readily available for all cardiac catheterization patients.[17] During the catheterization, the balloon is momentarily switched off as the guidewire passes the balloon into the thoracic aorta. As soon as this occurs, however, the balloon is returned to full function, and the catheterization proceeds uneventfully. Clearly the intra-aortic balloon pump has significantly reduced the potential complications of cardiac catheterization in these critically ill patients. Cooper et al.[31] reported on 63 high-risk myocardial revascularization patients who had preoperative IABP. Only six patients required rapid institution of cardiopulmonary bypass after anesthetic induction despite marked drop in blood pressure in 50 percent of the patients. There were two instances of postpump power failure with two deaths in this series. The author concluded from this experience that preoperative IABP is a valid method of limiting morbidity associated with coronary surgery in high-risk patients.

Preoperative IABP in High Risk Cardiac Patients

The risks of early infarction and deaths in patients with acute coronary insufficiency are generally considered greater than in patients with stable angina. The most appropriate therapy, however, and the timing of that therapy, are points of significant controversy. Scully et al.[77] have studied the effects of preoperative IABP in 42 patients with acute coronary insufficiency complicated by abnormal left ventricular hemodynamics and refractory resting pain. Aggressive medical therapy had previously failed in all cases.

The perioperative mortality rate, when compared to that for similar patients treated before the use of IABP, was lowered from 25 to 8 percent. Similar results have been achieved by Weintraub et a.[85] and McEnany et al.[61] Weintraub et al.[84] recently reported on 60 patients with medically refractory unstable angina who received both intra-aortic balloon support and myocardial revascularization. The mortality rate was less than 2 percent, similar to that of elective revascularization of patients with stable angina. In addition, inotropic support and duration of stay both in intensive care and in the hospital were decreased in the preoperative IABP group. Bolooki et al.[10] also report a shorter bypass time and Feola et al.[38] have noted an improvement in metabolic status as measured by decreased cardiac lactate production. Others have applied IABP[43,54,55,66] preoperatively in cases of decreased left ventricular function but the interpretation of the data is not as clear as in the case of acute coronary insufficiency. During a 30-month period, 2,333 patients underwent open heart surgery at the Emory University Hospital.[34] Overall use of IABP in the perioperative setting was 3.2 percent. Survival to discharge from the hospital was made possible by IABP in 40 of 62 patients (65 percent) who were in cardiogenic shock at the end of cardiopulmonary bypass.

Perioperative IABP

Myocardial failure following cardiopulmonary bypass constitutes a major complication of cardiac surgery, occurring in 4 percent of all bypass operations performed at the Massachusetts General Hospital[61] since 1971. McEnany et al.[61] report that in their review of 728 cases in which IABP therapy has been instituted, the most common indication (30.1 percent) for IABP therapy has been myocardial failure following cardiac surgery. Of these 54.2 percent survived.

Seventy-three percent of the cases of perioperative IABP use were for coronary artery disease, while 24.4 percent of patients had undergone valve replacement. Survival was achieved in 55.5 percent of the coronary artery disease group and 58.2 percent in the valve replacement group. Of note is the fact that of the combined fatalities, 79 percent occurred in the operating room while only 21 percent took place after several days of IABP therapy and removal.

McEnany and his colleagues report that the most dramatic application of IABP is in helping wean those patients from cardiopulmonary bypass in whom intraoperative ischemic damage or myocardial infarction precluded autonomous circulation. The group believes that the balloon acts as a temporizing device, supporting the patient at a lower level of myocardial work and oxygen demands, while the ischemia can be reversed by normal coronary perfusion, perhaps augmented by the increased diastolic pressure. Still, surgical correction of lesions which inhibit adequate perfusion is essential. While perioperative IABP can reduce the occurrence of myocardial ischemia during induction of anesthesia and surgery, it cannot compensate for inadequate surgical treatment.[82] The use of IABP for weaning from cardiopulmonary bypass is clearly the most established use of balloon support. Most cardiac surgeons now believe that the availability of a balloon pump in a center performing open heart surgery should be mandatory.[24,25]

Patients with Crescendo Angina Refractory to Medical Therapy

The patient with recent onset of accelerated angina refractory to medical therapy or the patient in the immediate postinfarction period who continues to have chest pain is at major risk either of incurring or extending myocardial damage.[6]

In a recent report by Levine et al.,[58] 93 patients with severe unstable angina pectoris refractory to standard medical therapy (which included β-blockade, nitrates, heparin, oxygen, and bedrest) were treated with IABP, early angiography, and myocardial revascularization surgery. Sixty patients were in the preinfarction group and 49 of these had complete relief of pain when the balloon was inserted. Forty-two of the 60 patients had typical ischemic changes, and 18 had a variant anginal pattern. Thirty-three patients were in the postinfarction angina group (less than 10 days), 25 had typical angina, and 8 had variant angina. Twenty-six of these patients had relief of pain with the IABP. Therefore, in 75 of the 93 patients (81 percent) the balloon interrupted ischemic attacks, and in the remainder of the patients the frequency of ischemic attacks was markedly reduced. In all 93 patients on balloon support, angiography was uncomplicated. Of significance is that 52 percent of the patients in this group had triple-vessel coronary artery disease. All patients underwent open heart surgery and 2 of the 60 preinfarction patients died. There were a total of five deaths (4.5 percent in this group. Two patients (one patient in each category) showed no postoperative Q waves (a 2.2 percent incidence). In a late follow-up study of this group, 74 percent of the patients were angina-free.

This experience and that of Weintraub et al.[85] and McEnany et al.[61] demonstrate that IABP provides maximal perioperative myocardial protection in the patient with acute ischemia before open heart surgery and is certainly a major advance in the care of these challenging patients. However, IABP does carry with it a certain morbidity. McEnany et al.[61] have reported that a decrease in their use of blockade therapy and calcium channel blockers, increased willingness to maintain propranolol

therapy up to the time of operation, and the skillful use of vasodilators during induction of anesthesia coupled with wedge pressure monitoring have allowed the satisfactory medical management of more patients with crescendo angina, and the safer administration of anesthesia to patients with active myocardial ischemia.

Postinfarction Angina

Patients who have sustained a recent myocardial infarction and subsequently develop anginal pain are at high risk of a second infarction in their already compromised myocardium. Bardet et al.[6] have reported a series of 21 patients with postinfarction angina (2 to 15 days after acute myocardial infarction) who did not respond to medical therapy. The IABP therapy resulted in prevention of anginal pain and ST segment changes in all patients. Of note is that in two patients Q waves that appeared during the anginal attack disappeared without a shift of the QRS axis after a few hours of IABP therapy. Transient Q waves associated with angina pectoris and with Prinzmetal's angina have been attributed to reversible ischemia. Bardet et al.[6] suggest that viable myocardium may be electrically silent and may recover normal activity when the balance between myocardial oxygen supply and demand is restored.

The great risk of death in patients with post infarction angina and impending extension of a recent myocardial infarction unresponsive to medical therapy warrants more aggressive therapy. The IABP technique stabilizes the clinical condition of such patients and thereby allows coronary arteriograms and operative intervention to be completed if the lesions are amenable to bypass surgery.

Tachyarrhythmias and Ventricular Irritability

The increase in coronary blood flow associated with IABP as well as the decrease in myocardial wall tension as a result of the acute reduction in left ventricular afterload form an ideal combination to cope with ventricular tachyarrhythmias either in the coronary care unit or for the postoperative surgical patient.[14] The treatment of tachyarrhythmias after open heart surgery with the IABP can frequently be definitive. In the setting of the coronary care unit, however, many patients can be stabilized, and their arrhythmias will decrease significantly in frequency. It is the author's policy to catheterize every medical patient on an intra-aortic balloon whose indication for insertion has been ventricular tachyarrhythmias so that the patient's anatomy can be defined and surgical intervention can proceed if indicated.

Mundth et al.[67,68] have indicated that in the medical setting, life-threatening, recurrent ventricular tachyarrhythmias in the acute postinfarct phase and in chronic coronary disease can be controlled initially with IABP as a prelude to cardiac catheterization and surgery. Ten patients with recurrent ventricular tachyarrhythmias were operated upon, and seven survived.

Williams et al.[87] have reported success with IABP therapy even when no surgically correctable lesion is present, and recommend this therapy for all patients who develop ventricular or low nodal arrhythmias refractory to standard therapy.

Culliford et al.[35] utilized IABP therapy for a patient with recurrent ventricular tachycardia. For the 72 hours before counterpulsation was begun, this patient received electrical cardioversion 120 times and high doses of antiarrhythmic agents. Counterpulsation abolished this arrhythmia dramatically. The patient was discharged home 3 weeks later and returned to full activity. Culliford et al.[35] believe IABP should be considered as a useful adjunct in the treatment of all such patients.

Septic Shock

Sepsis is usually responded to by an increase in cardiac output, the limitation of which is posed by both Starling's law and the functional cardiac reserve of the individual patient. Ultimately, the patient in septic shock will go into a low cardiac output state and, if

the appropriate medical therapy fails, will die. Berger et al.[9] reported on the fortuitous use of IABP in a septic shock patient who was initially thought to have a myocardial infarction with a low cardiac output state. The distinct improvement in this patient prompted its use in a second individual. In both of these patients cardiac output could be maintained while the appropriate pharmacologic treatment, including antibiotics and steroids, could be administered. The author's experience has also justified the concept of IABP in the low-output septic shock setting. Indeed, Berger's two initial patients ultimately were discharged from the hospital.

Pediatric Intra-Aortic Balloon Pumping

There have been very few instances of pediatric intra-aortic balloon counterpulsation in the world literature.[14] Vascular access poses a significant problem in these children. Since difficulties encountered in the placement of the intra-aortic balloon in children are usually due to the small size of femoral arteries, Mayer[60] suggests that the subclavian–innominate approach may be more feasible. With current technology, however, the only reasonable access in the infant is that directly through the ascending aorta with IABP. In older children, access can be accomplished through the peripheral route, as in two of the above cases. With pediatric IABP, the diastolic augmentation is usually, at best, equal to systole. However, systolic unloading is always achieved, as in the adult. There are presently three different sizes of pediatric balloons available to the clinician (Fig. 11-9, Table 11-2).

Management of Subendocardial Ischemia

Therapy with IABP is more physiologically sound, that the administration of inotropic drugs,[21] which increase oxygen requirements. Balloon deflation reduces afterload and lowers

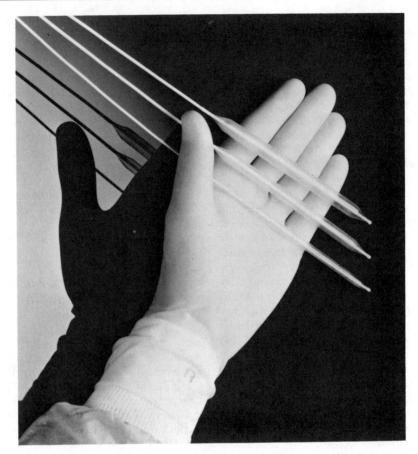

FIG. 11-9 Pediatric intra-aortic balloons.

oxygen demands while inflation simultaneously augments supply. In addition, intramural pressure is lowest at the end of diastole rather than at the beginning,[4] as in the ventricular lumen. While unassisted systemic blood pressure decreases throughout diastole as blood drains off peripherally, IABP-supported diastolic blood pressure remains much higher, thus providing pressure during the period in which the myocardium is most amenable to accepting blood flow.

The effects of IABP on transmural coronary flow distribution in nonischemic and segmentally ischemic canine myocardium were studied by Swank et al.[79] The IABP was shown to increase epicardial flow, endocardial flow, and the endocardial/epicardial flow ratio significantly in the nonischemic myocardium. In the segmental ischemic preparation, however, a 30 percent decrease in the endocardial/epicardial flow ratio was observed when IABP was employed. Cardiac edema resulting in constriction of the nutrient supply to the subendocardium was postulated as the reason for the observed preferential flow to the epicardium with IABP during ischemia.

TABLE 11-2. Pediatric Intra-Aortic Balloon Specifications

Balloon Volume (cc)	Patients' Approximate Age Range (years)	Patients' Approximate Weight Ranges (kg)
2.5	<1	3–8
5.0	1–2.5	8–13
7.0	>2.5	13–18

Cardiac Arrest

Since IABP insertion may be accomplished rapidly and efficiently, it thus appears ideal for the emergency situation. The hemodynamic effects of IABP actuation on left and right ventricular performance are immediate and cannot be duplicated by pharmacologic agents. These unique effects decrease right and left ventricular myocardial oxygen requirements (systolic unloading), increase biventricular indices of myocardial oxygen supply (diastolic augmentation), and increase right and left ventricular external performance (stroke volume) by the conversion of less efficient pressure work to more efficient volume work. Approximately one third of the patients undergoing IABP support for postinfarction cardiogenic shock without additional surgery survive. As major institutions gain experience with the technique of IABP and confidence in their own capabilities with this therapeutic modality, there is a strong call in the literature[2,6,29,30,51,57,74,77,85] for earlier initiation of IABP therapy. The realization that ischemic heart disease is a reversible process inspires us to intercede before irreversible damage is done.[70] Certainly IABP carried with it a certain morbidity and mortality,[61] but its proven effectiveness and ease of initiation have led to the use of IABP as and adjunct in resuscitative measures following cardiac arrest of any cause.[46] Time and further study will delineate the safe and effective role of IABP for this application. Percutaneous IABP will play a role in this setting.[30]

Community Hospital Use

In most instances, in the medical setting IABP use has ultimately been a prelude to cardiac catheterization and open heart surgery. It is not practical to assume that every hospital with an intra-aortic balloon pump would have these facilities. With the advent of coronary care units, many patients with acute ischemic and mechanical complications of myocardial infarction are being cared for in community hospitals. Accordingly, several community hospitals have purchased IABP equipment and have begun to insert intra-aortic balloons in selected patients in their coronary care units.[8,61] A new mobile balloon pump system, the Datascope System 84, is a portable stretcher with an integral balloon pump console whose use can facilitate interhospital transportation. Patients with early cardiogenic shock are primarily those with preinfarction angina refractory to medical therapy and patients who have incurred one of the mechanical complications of acute myocardial infarction. These hospitals have formed a liaison with a major university hospital, and the patients are then transferred to that major hospital on balloon support for additional definitive therapy when required.

McEnany et al.[61] have reported that 32 of their 747 IABPs were started at peripheral community hospitals and the patients transported to the Massachusetts General Hospital while receiving diastolic augmentation support.

Recently, Bass et al.[8] have reported on their use of IABP in a private 280 bed hospital. After thoroughly training their nursing and supporting staff, they were able to report a survival rate of 44 percent, comparable to that of major university centers.

Hines et al.[44] inserted the intra-aortic balloon in 27 patients in cardiogenic shock secondary to myocardial infarction. Four patients died within 1 hour after insertion. Of the remaining patients, 20 were weaned, 17 of these survived hospitalization, and 12 became long-term survivors. These results indicate that counterpulsation is feasible at the local hospital level and that early institution of IABP may improve long-term results.

Complications

SURGICAL INSERTION

Major complications in McEnany et al.'s report of 728 cases occurred at a rate of 8.5 percent.[61] The IABP-related mortality was only 0.8 percent. Other authors have reported higher rates of both morbidity and mortality. Some acute complications,[45,71] associated with IABP include arterial insufficiency of the catheterized limb, arterial emboli, retrograde aortic dissection, localized injury to the thoracic wall, balloon rupture with gas embolism, retroperitoneal aortoiliac hemorrhage, femoral artery false aneurysm, postischemic neuritis, pericardial tamponade secondary to anticoagulants, thrombocytopenia, and certain immunologic abnormalities. Important hazards can occur with IABP. However, these have been diminished in most series with greater experience. Novel approaches for balloon insertion have been developed by Cleveland,[27] Phillips et al.,[72] and Merrill et al.[63]

In a series of 100 patients who underwent perioperative IABP at the Columbia Presbyterian Medical Center, a 2 percent complication rate and zero incidence of IABP related deaths were achieved. Bahn et al.[3] suggest that from a series of patients undergoing cardiac catheterization, a subgroup with increased likelihood of needing IABP can be selected. These patients should receive one aortoiliac injection of contrast material at the end of their catheterization to determine the degree of vessel irregularity, stenosis, and/or tortuosity that may be present. This procedure carries little additional risk and assists greatly in the choice of site for subsequent balloon insertion, if that is necessary.

PERCUTANEOUS INSERTION

Goldman and associates[40] compared the complication rates between the patients receiving the surgically inserted IAB and the newer percutaneously inserted balloon. In 389 patients, 299 balloons were inserted surgically, while 90 were placed percutaneously. Inability to insert the balloon was recorded in 5.7 percent of the surgical procedures, while only 4.4 percent of the percutaneous balloons encountered such difficulty. Vascular complications, including aortic dissection, perforation, bleeding, and femoral occlusion occured in 14.6 percent of the surgical attempts while only 10.0 percent suffered similar results in the percutaneous series.[40]

Alcan et al.[1] reported a 90.2 percent rate of successful insertion with the percutaneous technique, whereas surgical placement was successful 90 percent of the time, Percutaneous complications included 6 thromboembolic occlusions and one hematoma, or 15.2 percent in a series of 51 patients. Surgical insertion resulted in 10 thromboembolic occlusions, 2 hematomas, 2 bacteremias, and 1 aortic dissection, or 15.6 percent in a series of 100 patients.

Clearly, percutaneous insertion offers no greater risk than the surgical technique. If careful attention is given to the details of percutaneous insertion, such as allowing only physicians skilled in catheterization techniques to insert the IABs, mandatory fluoroscopy, and utilizing the new smaller French wire-guided balloons, complications resulting from percutaneous balloons should be significantly reduced.[15]

New Balloon Designs

Because of the difficulty in inserting balloons by the peripheral route, Wolfson et al.[88] reported on a modified trisegment intra-aortic balloon with the addition of a 1 mm central lumen. This design would allow for arterial pressure measurement, contrast injection, and guidewire passage. Concurrent with this, a series of percutaneous dual-lumen intra-aortic balloon catheters were developed by Datascope Inc. (Fig. 11-7). These single-chambered percutaneous balloons utilized a flexible inner lumen that allowed the balloon membrane to be wrapped about it while it was advanced over a guidewire.[62] This would enable percutaneous balloon insertion through any arterial tortuosity that could be negotiated by a small-diameter guidewire. In addition to this a mechanical wrapping knob has been engineered into the balloon catheter to determine correct balloon membrane wrapping and unwrapping precisely. The previous technique of hand wrapping the percutaneous balloons allowed too much margin for error. But perhaps the most promising development has been the introduction of a dual-lumen 10.5 Fr percutaneous IAB and a 9.5 and 8.5 Fr single-lumen percutaneous IAB which come pre-wrapped. Because these new balloon catheters are so thin, it is hoped that their insertion will be less traumatic on atherosclerotic vessels. For the same reason the catheters will allow more blood flow distal to the insertion site, thus reducing the potential for limb ischemia, especially in small patients. Therefore we believe that we are approaching a new level of expertise, where the clinician can expect rapid institution of circulatory support with diminished associated vascular complications.

REFERENCES

1. Alcan KE, Stertzer SH, Wallsh E: Comparison of wire-guided percutaneous insertion and conventional insertion of intra-aortic balloon pump in 151 patients. Am J Med 75: 24, 1983
2. Bahn CH: Cardiac catheterization and intra-aortic balloon counterpulsation. Letters to the editor. Am J Cardiol 42: 873, 1978
3. Bahn CH, Vitikainen KJ, Anderson CL, Whitney RB: Vascular evaluation for balloon pumping. Ann Thorac Surg 27: 476, 1979
4. Baird RJ, Adiseshiah M, Okumori M: The gradient in regional myocardial tissue pressure in the left ventricle during left diastole: its relationship to regional flow distribution. J Surg Res 20: 11, 1976
5. Bardet J, Masquet C, Kahn JC et al: Clinical and hemodynamic results of intra-aortic balloon counterpulsation and surgery for cardiogenic shock. Am Heart J 93: 280, 1977
6. Bardet J, Rigaud M, Kahn JC et al: Treatment of post-myocardial infarction angina by intra-aortic balloon pumping and emergency revascularization. J Thorac Cardiovasc Surg 74(2): 299, 1977
7. Baron DW, O'Rourke MF: Long-term results of arterial counterpulsation in acute severe cardiac failure complicating myocardial infarction. Br Heart J 38: 285, 1976
8. Bass J, Jr., Katzman L, Pois AJ: Experience with intra-aortic balloon counterpulsation in a community hospital. Am Surgeon June, 44: 324, 1978
9. Berger RL, Saini VK, Long W et al: The use of diastolic augmentation with the intra-aortic balloon in human septic shock with associated coronary artery disease. Surgery 74: 601, 1973
10. Bolooki H, Williams W, Thurer RJ et al: Clinical and hemodynamic criteria for use of the intra-aortic balloon pump in patients requiring cardiac surgery. J Thorac Cardiovasc Surg 72(5): 756, 1976
11. Bourdarias JP, Gourgon R, Bardet J: Mechanical circulatory assistance by intra-aortic balloon pumping. Intensive Care Med 4: 28, 1978
12. Bregman D: Intra-aortic balloon in open heart surgery. N Engl J Med 284: 393, 1971
13. Bregman D: Clinical experience with the dual-chambered intra-aortic balloon and system 80. J Cardiovasc Surg 15: 193, 1974
14. Bregman D: Mechanical support of the failing heart. In Ravitch MM (ed): Current Problems in Surgery. Yearbook, Chicago; 1976
15. Bregman D: Percutaneous intra-aortic balloon pumping: a time for reflection. Chest 82: 397, 1982
16. Bregman D, Bolooki H, Malm JR: A simple method to facilitate difficult intra-aortic balloon insertions. Ann Thorac Surg 15: 636, 1973
17. Bregman D, Casarella WM: Percutaneous intra-aortic balloon pumping—initial clinical experience. Ann Thorac Surg 29: 153, 1980
18. Bregman D, Goetz RH: Clinical experience with a new cardiac assist device—the dual-chambered intra-aortic balloon assist. J Thorac Cardiovasc Surg 62: 577, 1971
19. Bregman D, Goetz RH: A new concept in circulatory assistance—the dual-chambered intra-aortic balloon. Mt Sinai J Med 39: 123, 1972
20. Bregman D, Kripke DC, Goetz RH: The effect of synchronous unidirectional intra-aortic balloon pumping on hemodynamics and coronary blood flow in cardiogenic shock. Trans Am Soc Artif Intern Organs 16: 439, 1970
21. Buckberg GD: Left ventricular subendocardial necrosis. Ann Thorac Surg 24(4): 379, 1977
22. Buckley MJ, Leinbach RC, Kastor JA et al: Hemodynamic evaluation of intra-aortic balloon pumping in man. Circulation (Suppl. II) 41(42): 130, 1970
23. Buckley MJ, Mundth ED, Daggett WM et al: Surgical therapy for early complications of myocardial infarction. Surgery 70: 814, 1971
24. Buckley MJ, Mundth Ed, Daggett WM et al: Surgical management of ventricular septal defects and mitral regurgitation complicating acute myocardial infarction. Ann Thorac Surg 16: 598, 1973
25. Carlson RG, Baltaxe HA, Bregman D et al: Veno-arterial perfusion with membrane lung and/or intra-aortic balloon during arteriography and surgery for coronary artery disease. In Norman JC (ed): Coronary Artery Medicine and Surgery: Concepts and Controversies. Appleton-Century-Crofts, New York; 1974
26. Carlson RG, Rees JR, Baltaxe H et al: Mechanical cardiopulmonary support during arteriography and surgical correction of coronary insufficiency producing myocardial infarction with cardiogenic shock. J Assoc Advance Med Instrument 6: 244, 1972
27. Cleveland JC: Insertion of an intra-aortic balloon through a limb of an aorto-femoral graft after

AVR, double CAB, and resection of an abdominal aortic aneurysm. Cardiovasc Dis 6: 191, 1979

28. Cohn LH: Intra-aortic balloon counterpulsation in low cardiac output states. Surg Clin North Am 55: 545, 1975

29. Cohn LH, Alpert J, Koster J et al: Changing indications for the surgical treatment of unstable angina. Arch Surg 113: 1312, 1978

30. Coletti RH, Kaskel PS, Bregman D: Measurement of coronary blood flow during open chest cardiac compression with flow augmentation by intra-aortic balloon pumping. Am Soc Artif Intern Organs 12: 1, 1983

31. Cooper GN, Jr., Singh AK, Vargas LL, Karlson KE: Preoperative intra-aortic balloon assist in high risk revascularization patients. Am J Surg 133: 463, 1977

32. Corday E, Swan HJC, Lang TW et al: Physiologic principles in the application of circulatory assist for the failing heart. Am J Cardio 26: 585, 1970

33. Cox JL, McLaughlin VW, Flowers NC, Horan LG: The ischemic zone surrounding acute myocardial infarction: its morphology as detected by dehydrogenase staining. Am Heart J 76: 650, 1968

34. Craver JM, Kaplan JA, Jones EL et al: What role should the intra-aortic balloon have in cardiac surgery. Ann Surg 189: 769, 1979

35. Culliford AT, Madden MR, Isom OW, Glassman E: IABP for refractory ventricular tachycardia. JAMA 239: 431,1978

36. Dunkman WB, Leinbach RC, Buckley MJ et al: Clinical and hemodynamic results of intra-aortic balloon pumping and surgery for cardiogenic shock. Circulation 46: 465, 1972

37. Ehrich DA, Biddle TL, Kronenberg MS, Yu PN: The hemodynamic response to intra-aortic balloon counterpulsation in patients with cardiogenic shock complicating acute myocardial infarction. Am Heart J 93: 274, 1977

38. Feola M, Wiener L, Walinsky P. 35 al: Improved survival after coronary bypass surgery in patients with poor left ventricular function: role of intra-aortic balloon counterpulsation. Am J Cardio 39: 1021, 1977

39. Gold HK, Leinbach RC, Sanders CA et al: Intra-aortic balloon pumping for control of recurrent myocardial ischemia. Circulation 47: 1197, 1973

40. Goldman BS, Hill JJ, Rosenthal GA: Complications associated with use of intra-aortic balloon pumping. Can J Surg 25: 153, 1982

41. Goetz RH, Bregman D, Esrig B, Laniado S: Unidirectional intra-aortic balloon pumping in cardiogenic shock and intractable left ventricular failure. Am J Cardiol 29: 213

42. Hagemeither F, Laird JD, Haalebos MMP, Hugenholtz PG: Effectiveness of intra-aortic balloon pumping without cardiac surgery for patients with severe heart failure secondary to a recent mycardial infarction. Am J Cardio 40: 951, 1977

43. Gunstensen J, Goldman BS, Scully HS et al: Evolving indications for preoperative intra-aortic balloon pump assistance. Ann Thorac Surg 22: 535, 1976

44. Hines GL, Delaney TB, Goodman M, Mohtashemi M: Intra-aortic balloon pumping two year experience. J Thorac Cardiovasc Surg 78: 140, 1979

45. Hyson EA, Ravin EC, Kelley MJ, Curtis AM: Intra-aortic counterpulsation balloon: radiographic considerations. Am J Roentgenol 128: 915, 1977

46. Go Sr, Hibbs, CW, Trono R et al: Intra-aortic balloon pumping: theory and practice—experience with 325 patients. Artif Organs 2(3): 249, 1978

47. Jackson G, Cullum P, Pastellopoulos A et al: Intra-aortic balloon assistance in cardiogenic shock after myocardial infarction or cardiac surgery. Br Heart J 39: 598, 1977

48. Jacobey JA, Craddock LD, Wolf PS, Beckwitt HJ: Clinical experience with counterpulsation in coronary artery disease. J Thorac Cardiovasc Surg 56: 846, 1968

49. Johnson SA, Scanlon PJ, Loeb HS et al: Treatment of cardiogenic shock in myocardial infarction by intra-aortic counterpulsation and surgery. Am J Med 62: 687, 1977

50. Kantrowitz A, Tjonneland S, Freed PS et al: Initial clinical experience with intra-aortic balloon pumping in cardiogenic shock. JAMA 203: 135, 1968

51. Kuhn LA: Management of shock following acute myocardial infarction part II. Mechanical circulatory assistance. Am Heart J 95(6): 789, 1978

52. Kveim M, Cappelen C, JR., Froysaker T, Hall KV: Intra-aortic balloon pumping in the treatment of cardiogenic shock follow-up in open heart surgery. Scand J Thorac Cardiovasc Surg 10: 231, 1976

53. Laird JD, Madras PN, Jones RT et al: Theoretical and experimental analysis of the intra-aortic balloon pump. Trans Am Soc Artif Intern Organs 14: 338, 1968

54. Lamberti JJ, Resnekov L: Cardiac assist devices. Annu Rev Med 29: 571, 1978

55. Lefemine AA, Kosowsky B, Madoff et al: Results and complications of intra-aortic balloon pumping in surgical and medical patients. Am J Cardiol 40: 416, 1977

56. Leinbach RC, Gold HK, Dinsmore RE: The role of angiography in Cardiogenic shock. Circulation (Suppl. III) 47(48): 95, 1973

57. Leinback RC, Gold HK, Harber TW et al: Early intra-aortic balloon pumping for anterior myocardial infarction without shock. Circulation 58(2): 204, 1978

58. Levine FH, Gold HK, Leinbach RC et al: Management of acute myocardial ischemia with intra-aortic balloon pumping and coronary bypass surgery. Circulation (Supply. 3) 56: 61 1977

59. Maroko PR, Bernstein EF, Libby P et al: Effects of intra-aortic balloon counterpulsation on the severity of mycardial ischemic injury following acute coronary occlusion. Circulation 45: 1150, 1972

60. Mayer JH: Subclavian artery approach for insertion of intra-aortic balloon. J Thorac Cardiovasc Surg 76: 61, 1978

61. McEnany MT, Kay HR, Buckley MJ et al: Clinical experience with intra-aortic balloon pump support in 728 patients. Circulation (Suppl. 1) 58(3): 124, 1978

62. Merav AD, Solomon N, Montefusco CM, Bregman D: A new guidable double lumen percutaneous intra-aortic balloon. Trans Am Soc Intern Organs 27: 592, 1981

63. Merrill JR, McClusky D, Logan WD: Improved technique of intra-aortic balloon insertion. Ann Thorac Surg 26: 262, 1978

64. Moulopoulos SD, Topaz S. Kolff WJ: Diastolic balloon pumping (with carbon dioxide) in the aorta—a mechanical assistance to the failing circulation. Am Heart J 63: 669, 1962

65. Mundth ED: Preoperative intra-aortic balloon pump assistance. Ann Thorac Surg 22: 603, 1976

66. Mundth ED, Buckley MJ, Daggett WM et al: Surgery for complications of acute myocardial infarction. Circulation 45: 1279, 1972

67. Mundth ED, Buckley MJ, Daggett WM et al: Intra-aortic balloon pump assistance and early surgery in cardiogenic shock. Integrated medical–surgical care in acute coronary artery disease. Adv Cardiol 15: 159, 1975

68. Mundth ED, Yurchak PM, Buckley MJ et al: Circulatory assistance and emergency direct coronary-artery surgery for shock complicating acute myocardial infarction. N Engl J Med 283: 1382, 1970

69. Nachlas MM, Sieband MP: The influence of diastolic augmentation on infarct size following coronary artery ligation. J Thorac Cardiovasc Surg 53: 698, 1967

70. Olinger GN, Bonchek LI, Keelan MH Jr, et al: Unstable angina; the case for operation. Am J Cardiol 42: 634, 1978

71. Pace PD, Tilney NL, Lesch M, Couch NP: Peripheral arterial complications of intra-aortic balloon counterpulsation. Surgery 82(5): 685, 1977

72. Phillips SJ, Gordon DF, Zeff RH et al: Cardiogenic shock treatment by augmentation with a pulsatile assist device. JAMA 240: 1376, 1978

73. Reemtsma K, Drusin, Edie R et al: Cardiac transplantation for patients requiring mechnical circulatory support. N Engl J Med 298: 670, 1978

74. Roberts AJ, Alonso DR, Combes JR et al: Role of delayed intra-aortic balloon pumping in treatment of experimental myocardial infarction. Am J Cardiol 41: 1202, 1978

75. Sanders CA, Buckley MJ, Leinbach RC et al: Mechanical circulatory assistance, emergency coronary angiography, and acute myocardial revascularization. Circulation 45: 1292, 1972

76. Scheidt S, Wilner G, Mueller H et al: Intra-aortic balloon counterpulsation in cardiogenic shock. Report of a cooperative clinical trial. N Engl J Med 288: 979, 1973

77. Scully HE, Bunstensen J, Williams WG et al: Surgical management of complicated acute coronary insufficiency. Surgery 80(4): 437, 1976

78. Sugg WL, Webb WR, Ecker RR: Reduction of extent of myocardial infarction by counterpulsation. Ann Thorac Surg 7: 311, 1969

79. Swank M, Singh HM, Flemma RJ et al: Effect of intra-aortic balloon pumping on nutrient coronary flow in normal and ischemic myocardium. J Thorac Cardiovasc Surg 76: 538, 1978

80. Talpins NL, Kripke DC, Goetz RH: Counterpulsation and intra-aortic balloon pumping in cardiogenic shock. Circulatory dynamics. Arch Surg 97: 991, 1968

81. Talpins NL, Kripke DC, Yellin E, Goetz RH: Hemodynamics and coronary blood flow during intra-aortic balloon pumping. Surg Forum 19: 122, 1968

82. Webb WR, Parker FB, Jr., Neville JF, Jr., Hanson EL: Coronary artery disease: Surgical management of acute emergencies. NY State J Med 73: 2572, 1973

83. Webb WR, Parker FB, Jr., Neville JF, Jr., Hanson EL: Acute mechanical complications of coronary arterial disease. Arch Surg 109: 251, 1974

84. Weintraub RM, Aroesty JM, Paulin S et al: Medically refractory unstable angina pectoris. Am J Cardiol 43: 877, 1979

85. Weintraub RM, Aroesty JM: The role of intra-aortic balloon pumping and surgery in the treatment of preinfarction angina. Chest 69: 707 (editorial), 1976

86. Willerson JT, Curry GC, Watson JT et al: Intra-aortic balloon counterpulsation in patients in cardiogenic shock, medically refractory left ventricular failure and/or recurrent ventricular tachycardia. Am J Med 58: 183, 1975

87. Williams EH, Tyers GFO, Carter SL, Williams DR: Ventricular arrhythmias following mitral valve replacement: control with intra-aortic balloon counterpulsation. Chest 68(5): 641, 1975

88. Wolfson S, Geha AS, Hammond GL et al: Preliminary report: modification of intra-aortic balloon for pressure measurement, contrast injection and

guidewire passage. Am J Cardiol (abstr), 39: 260 1977

89. Yellin E, Levy L, Bregman D, Frater R: Hemodynamic effects of intra-aortic balloon pumping in dogs with aortic incompetence. Trans Am Soc Artif Intern Organs 19: 389, 1973

SUGGESTED READINGS

Bregman D: Intra-aortic balloon: new developments, techniques, complications, and results. In Attar S (ed): New Development in Cardiac Assist Devices. Praeger, New York, 1985

Bregman D: Recent advances in balloon counterpulsation. p. 51. In Utley JR (ed): Perioperative Cardiac Dysfunction, Vol. III. Williams & Wilkins, Baltimore, 1985

Bregman D, Bailin MT, Kaskel P: Mechanical support of the heart and circulation. p. 291. In Bartlett R (ed): Life Support Systems in Intensive Care. Yearbook, Chicago, 1984

Bregman D, Haubert SM, Self MA: Intra-aortic balloon counterpulsation: a primer. J Cardiovasc Med 9: 607, 1984

Bregman D, Kaskel PS: Counterpulsation techniques. In Taylor (ed): Cardiopulmonary Bypass. Chapman and Hall, London (in press)

Bregman D, Kaskel PS: Clinical experience with percutaneous intra-aortic balloon pumping. p. 16. In Unger F (ed): Assisted Circulation 2 Springer-Verlag, Berlin, 1984

Bregman D, Kaskel PS: Current status of percutaneous intra-aortic balloon pumping. In Yingkai W (ed): International Practice in Cardiothoracic Surgery. Science Press, Beijing, China, 1985

Colletti RH, Kaskel PS, Bregman D: Coronary blood flow augmentation by intra-aortic balloon pumping during open chest cardiopulmonary resuscitation. Trans Am Soc Artif Intern Organs 29:93, 1983

12

Hypertensive Crises
Mark M. Applefeld

INTRODUCTION

Hypertension is a common disease that affects 30 to 40 million Americans. Despite this incidence, marked sudden and sustained elevations of systolic and/or diastolic blood pressure occur infrequently among this population. Nonetheless, such clinical events constitute true medical emergencies as they may be characterized by arteriolar spasm, necrotizing arteriolitis, and secondary end-organ damage. As a consequence, patients who experience a hypertensive crisis may develop encephalopathy, neuroretinitis, renal failure, and/or left ventricular failure. These target organ effects in a hypertensive crisis usually dictate that immediate, intensive drug therapy be instituted even before complete specific diagnostic studies can be performed. With successful drug therapy, these complications of hypertensive crises may be reversible. However, the degree to which such reversibility occurs is a function of the immediacy with which treatment is instituted as well as the baseline level of organ function upon which hyptertensive crises occur.

Inherent in this statement is the need for the physician to assess rapidly the degree of target organ damage caused by the severely elevated blood pressure. This assessment becomes important both in judging the rapidity with which treatment must be instituted and as in the selection of the appropriate drug(s) to be used. Thus, the physician must determine whether signs of encephalopathy (i.e., headache, nausea, vomiting, convulsions, muscle twitching, or coma), retinopathy (i.e., "cotton wool" exudates, striated hemorrhages, or papilledema); myocardial ischemia (i.e., angina pectoris, or ST-T wave electrocardiographic changes) or congestive failure (i.e., dyspnea, orthopnea, raised jugular venous pressure, edema, atrial or ventricular gallops); or renal insufficiency (i.e., azotemia, proteinuria, or red blood cell casts) are present.

In a severely traumatized and/or anesthetized patient the clinical assessment of a hypertensive crisis may be more difficult because

351

specific symptoms and/or signs indicating end-organ damage may not be elicited or may be overshadowed by other disease processes. Accordingly, the physician must occasionally respond to the absolute level of blood pressure alone without having a complete history or even a complete data base. A hypertensive crisis that occurs suddenly and unexpectedly in a previously normotensive individual suggests acute glomerulonephritis, pre-eclampsia, or drug ingestion (e.g., amphetamines, phencyclidine). When a hypertensive crises occurs in a previously hypertensive patient, chronic glomerulonephritis, pyelonephritis, or connective tissue disorders are likely causes. A pheochromocytoma or renovascular cause may present as a hypertensive crisis either with or without antecedent hypertension. This chapter will focus on the pathophysiology of a hypertensive crisis, specific disease entities associated with such emergencies, and the appropriate pharmacologic management of this potentially life-threatening condition.

sion to institute aggressive antihypertensive therapy is made.

Clinically, there are several circumstances in which rapid reduction (i.e., within minutes) of elevated blood pressure is required. These include hypertensive encephalopathy; severe uncontrolled hypertension from any cause (e.g., in the malignant stage of chronic hypertension or in association with a pheochromocytoma, head injury, or severe burns), rebound hypertension after cessation of antihypertensive therapy; following the ingestion of tyramine-containing foods such as ripened cheeses, red wine, or overripe fruits by patients who take monamine oxidase (MAO) inhibitors or, with the use of drugs such as phenylpropanolamine or phencyclidine. Other circumstances that call for immediate therapy include severe hypertension accompanying left ventricular failure, acute myocardial infarction, intracranial hemorrhage and/or aneurysm, or severe hypertension occurring during or soon after open heart surgery. Finally, severe hypertension in association with persistent postoperative bleeding from vascular suture sites, dissecting aortic aneurysms, or severe epistaxis also usually requires urgent therapy.

PATHOPHYSIOLOGY

Although there is no uniformity of opinion about the exact level that defines hypertensive crisis, most authorities agree that diastolic blood pressures exceeding 120 mmHg are a cause for urgent therapy. Frequently, the diastolic blood pressure in a hypertensive crisis is usually in the range of 130 to 140 mmHg. The level at which a raised systolic blood pressure presents a threat to be dealt with emergently is less clear. For example, while a 40-year-old man may not tolerate an acute rise in systolic blood pressure to 200 mmHg, such levels are frequently observed in an ambulatory elderly patient and are, in fact, well tolerated. Thus, in addition to the absolute level of blood pressure (systolic or diastolic), the time interval over which such changes have developed as well as associated end-organ damage must also be considered before a deci-

Hypertensive Encephalopathy

Hypertensive encephalopathy is characterized clinically by headache (frequently described as severe and pounding in nature), visual loss, focal neurologic deficits, seizures, confusion, somnolence, stupor, and ultimately coma. As the mean arterial pressure progressively rises, the cerebral vessels become constricted.[3,13,14] When the mean arterial pressure reaches 180 mmHg, cerebral vasodilation begins to occur. Initially vasodilation begins in areas with less muscular tone and subsequently spreads throughout the entire cerebral circulation. In turn, the latter permits a "breakthrough" of cerebral blood flow with hyperperfusion of the vascular system under exceedingly high pressure. Fluid extravasation occurs into the perivascular tissue space and causes cerebral edema and the syndrome of hypertensive encephalopathy. The degree to which these changes occur is dependent upon the preexistent level of blood pressure as well as the extent to which long-standing hypertension has caused thickening of the arteriolar wall. In turn, this latter pathophysiologic principle helps to explain the following clinical observations:[3]

Why previously *normotensive* individuals who suddenly become hypertensive may develop encephalopathy at lower levels of blood pressure than do individuals who have long-standing hypertension

Why, when blood pressure is lowered, hypertensive patients who may have thickened cerebral arterioles are not able to tolerate a sudden drastic reduction of blood pressure without experiencing symptoms of cerebral *hypoperfusion*

The raised systolic blood pressure and elevated peripheral vascular resistance that accompany a hypertensive crisis each lead to an increased afterload and cardiac work. In turn, these alterations raise the myocardial demand for oxygen at a time when such oxygen supplies are limited. These pathophysiologic events may precipitate congestive failure by causing a reduction in left ventricular ejection fraction. Further, if occlusive coronary artery disease is also present, these events may precipitate angina pectoris and/or a myocardial infarction.

The kidney is another target organ[5] of a hypertensive crisis. In the setting of long-standing hypertension, thickening of the arteriolar walls and consequent luminal narrowing of the renal blood vessels occur. When the blood pressure becomes acutely elevated under these circumstances, fibrinoid necrosis of the renal arterioles occurs and causes obliteration of the arterial lumen. These processes lead to glomerular ischemia and nephron destruction with subsequent oliguria and azotemia. The renal ischemia thus produced stimulates the release of renin, which compounds the hypertensive state further (via release of renin substrate and the potent vasoconstrictor, angiotensin). This latter sequence of events accelerates the vascular damage even further. Aldosterone levels are also raised, leading to an expansion in blood volume and an increased blood pressure. A therapeutic dilemma exists: untreated hypertension promotes these patholophysiologic and biochemical changes whereas lowering of blood pressure under these circumstances may transiently cause renal function to deteriorate even further and may also stimulate this sequence.

Laboratory abnormalities that may be observed in a hypertensive crisis include elevated blood urea nitrogen and creatinine levels, hypokalemia, evidence of intravascular coagulopathy (e.g., fragmented red blood cells, thrombocytopenia, lowered fibrinogen levels), proteinuria, microscopic hematuria, and red blood cell casts. Cardiomegaly, pulmonary vascular congestion, and/or pulmonary edema may be noted on chest x ray; ST segment depressions, T wave inversions, or ST segment elevations (if acute myocardial infarction occurs), may be seen on electrocardiography.

SPECIFIC DISEASE PROCESSES

Aortic Dissection

Aortic dissection occurs primarily in men aged 40 to 70. Over 50 percent of the patients who sustain a dissecting aortic aneurysm have a prior history of hypertension. They may have an even greater degree of hypertension after aortic dissection occurs. This is particularly true in those patients with distal (i.e., type 3) dissections. An important management principle in this disease is that the systolic pressure should be reduced to approximately 100 to 120 mmHg, *provided* that this level is compatible with adequate perfusion of vital organs (i.e., brain, heart, and kidneys).[17] This should be accomplished through the use of agents that reduce the force and velocity of left ventricular contraction so that a major stimulus to further aortic dissection may be decreased.

During Cardiac Surgery

It has been recently recognized that as many as 50 percent of patients undergoing coronary artery bypass surgery will become hypertensive before being placed on cardiopulmonary bypass, immediately after bypass is completed, or during the initial postoperative period.[7,15,18] Fewer patients (approximately 5 percent) undergoing valve replacement develop this complication. The pathogenesis of hypertension in these circumstances is unknown and there have been no consistent changes in cardiac output, heart rate, systemic vascular resistance, or blood volume. There are conflicting data on the importance of the renin–angiotensin system in this process; both decreased renin[18] activity and increased angiotensin II levels[7] have each been described. The variability in patient data and in surgical and anesthetic techniques in these series makes meaningful comparison of these data difficult.

In Quadraplegic Patients

Beginning approximately 3 months after injury, autonomic hyperreflexia may develop in many patients who have sustained high transverse spinal cord lesions.[8] Among such patients, the stimulation of muscle groups below the level of injury may elicit hypertension, sweating, flushing, and headache. Triggers for this syndrome include manipulation of the perineum and genitalia, distention of the bladder or rectum, or traction on the viscera. Hypertension occurring in this setting may be severe, prolonged, and may result in stroke or even death. In some patients with autonomic hyperreflexia, the total circulating blood volume may be "relatively" reduced, since these individuals have an inability to increase their peripheral venous tone. Thus, they may become severely hypotensive if placed in a seated or head-up position immediately after the hypertensive attack. This effect may be even more pronounced in conditions that exacerbate peripheral venous pooling (e.g., hot environments, fever, or infection) or by the use of drugs (e.g., β-blockers) that depress myocardial contractility.

In Cerebrovascular Events

Particularly in those with pre-existent hypertension, many patients who sustain cerebral injury (e.g., subarachnoid or intracerebral bleeding, lacunar strokes, thrombotic or embolic strokes, delirium tremens, or trauma) develop transient, severe elevations in blood pressure. Such patients generally should not be treated with aggressive antihypertensive therapy since the consequent abrupt reduction in blood pressure may cause further ischemia and deterioration in cerebral function. Also, patients with brain stem or thalamic lesions may exhibit severe fluctuations in blood pressure. The latter are not usually amenable to antihypertensive therapy. Thus, the management of hypertension among such patients is predicated upon consistent and sustained reduction in blood pressure as long as cerebral function does not deteriorate further as a consequence.

THERAPY

There are several general guidelines in the selection of an agent to treat a hypertensive crisis. The first is that one must assess the urgency required to lower the patient's blood pressure. Thus, the absolute level of blood pressure is only part of the problem. The physician must pay attention to the end-organ effects of hypertension: Are encephalopathy, papilloedema, or fresh hemorrhages or exudates present? Does the patient have evidence of acute pulmonary edema, myocardial ischemia, or left ventricular failure? Is azotemia or proteinuria present? The presence of any of the above symptoms and/or signs suggests the need for more urgent management (within hours) of hypertension rather than a more gradual (over 1 to 2 days) course. The age of the patient and other medical and/or surgical problems must also be considered. Thus, an abrupt decrease in blood pressure from 220/110 mmHg to 120/80 mmHg is more likely to be associated with signs of cerebral, cardiac, or renal insufficiency in a 75-year-old man than in a 35-year-old man. Stated another way, elderly patients are more dependent upon higher perfusion pressures than are younger patients. This dependence is probably the result of decreased compliance (i.e., increased stiffness) of the blood vessel wall as well as the presence of occlusive atherosclerotic vascular disease in such patients. Finally, there are relatively few agents available to lower blood pressure promptly. Each drug has specific pharmacokinetic actions and definable adverse effects. In addition, these agents frequently stimulate reflex arcs that tend to diminish their hypotensive effects. Thus, the agent(s) employed by the physician must be based upon his or her familiarity with these drugs as well as his knowledge of their potential adverse effects.

SPECIFIC AGENTS[1,2,4,6,9–12,16,19]

Diazoxide

Diazoxide is a potent, rapidly acting antihypertensive drug (Tables 12-1 and 12-2). It is structurally related to the thiazide diuretics but does not cause natriuresis as do the latter agents. Diazoxide's hypotensive action is medi-

ated via direct arteriolar vasodilation through as yet undetermined mechanisms. Thus, as the elevated peripheral vascular resistance and blood pressure decline, an increase in heart rate, stroke volume, and cardiac output usually occur. Following the administration of diazoxide, reduced glomerular filtration and renal blood flow usually cause an increased renal tubular reabsorption of sodium. In turn, this may expand the intravascular volume, precipitate congestive heart failure, and cause resistance to other hypotensive agents. Consequently, it is important to administer a potent diuretic (e.g., furosemide or ethacrynic acid) concomitantly with diazoxide.

Diazoxide is 90 percent protein bound and has a half-life of 10 to 31 hours. The duration and magnitude of the drug's hypotensive effect are dependent upon its rate of infusion and the severity of hypertension. High concentrations of unbound drug in the systemic circulation are needed if a hypotensive effect is to be achieved. Thus, for maximal effect, diazoxide (300 mg or 5 mg/kg) must be administered rapidly by an intravenous route. The onset of the initial hypotensive effect occurs within 1 to 5 minutes and peaks within 2 to 5 minutes. A second, more sustained hypotensive phase persists for 3 to 6 hours. If an adequate hypotensive response does not occur within 30 minutes, a second dose of diazoxide may be given. As much as 1,200 mg diazoxide may be administered during a 24 hour period. Following the administration of diazoxide, the patient should remain supine for at least 30 minutes and the blood pressure should be recorded every 5 min-

TABLE 12-1. Drugs Commonly Used in the Management of Hypertensive Crises

Drug	Route of Administration	Usual Adult Dosage	Onset of Effect	Duration of Action
Nitroprusside	IV drip	25–500 μg/min	Immediate	Duration of drip
Hydralazine	IV/IM	10–20 mg	± 15 min	3–6 hr
Methyldopa	IV	250–500 mg over 30 min	1–2 hr	4–8 hr
Diazoxide	IV push	300 mg bolus	1–2 min	½–6 hr
Trimethaphan	IV drip	0.5–25 mg/min	Immediate	Duration of drip
Nitroglycerin	IV drip	5–? μg/min	Immediate	Duration of drip
Propranolol	IV	1–3 mg	2–5 min	3–6 hr
Reserpine	IM or IV	0.25–5 mg	2–3 hr	2–8 hr
Clonidine	Oral	0.1–0.2 mg	30–60 min	6–8 hr
Phentolamine	IV	0.1–2.0 mg/min	Immediate	5–15 hr

TABLE 12-2. Major Adverse Effects and Precautions to Be Observed in Drugs Used to Treat Hypertensive Crises

Drug	Adverse Effects	Precautions
Nitroprusside	Nausea Vomiting Muscle twitching Thiocyanate toxicity	Light-sensitive
Hydralazine	Tachycardia Headache Flushing Drug fever	May precipitate angina pectoris and arrhythmias in patients with ischemic heart disease
Methyldopa	Sedation Drug-induced hepatitis Drug fever	
Diazoxide	Hyperglycemia Nausea Vomiting	Causes sodium retention and edema formation; use with a diuretic
Trimethaphan	Urinary retention Paralytic ileus Orthostatic hypotension	Depresses cardiac contractility
Nitroglycerin	Headache Tachycardia	Exaggerated drug sensitivity in patients with raised blood alcohol levels or normal–low pulmonary capillary wedge pressure
Propranolol	Bradycardia Depresses myocardial contractility May precipitate bronchospasm	
Reserpine	Sedation Coma	
Clonidine		Rebound hypertension after drug is stopped
Phentolamine	Tachycardia	

utes. Excessive hypotension may be treated by elevation of the lower extremities or, if needed, by infusions of either a normal saline or pressor agent.

Adverse side effects of this drug include nausea, abdominal discomfort, sodium and water retention, postural hypotension, transient myocardial or cerebral ischemia, flushing, or weight gain. Transient hyperglycemia, which is usually not excessive, may persist as long as 12 hours after diazoxide is given. However, in diabetic patients, insulin doses may need to be increased. Other side effects include hyperuricemia, skin rash, fever, leukopenia, and thrombocytopenia. A major disadvantage to the use of diazoxide is the physician's inability to titrate the dose of the drug to a desired clinical response. In an effort to overcome this disadvantage, an alternative method[10] of administering diazoxide has been used. Depending upon the response of the patient's blood pressure, as many as three 100 mg doses of diazoxide may be administered intravenously at 15 to 20 minute intervals. Following these initial increments, further 100 mg doses may be given as needed as 4 to 6 hour intervals. Using this latter method, excessive drug-induced hypotension is generally avoided.

Sodium Nitroprusside

Sodium nitroprusside is a potent, rapidly acting intravenous agent that relaxes all vascular smooth muscle independent of sympathetic tone (see Fig. 12-1). Its hypotensive action is said to reside in the nitroso group on the nitroprusside radical. As a vasodilator, the nitroso

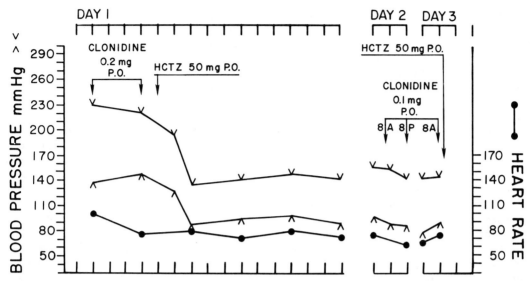

FIG. 12-1 This 53-year-old black man had a history of "borderline" untreated hypertension for 1 year. Two days prior to admission he complained of dizziness and blurred vision associated with near syncope. He was admitted because of these symptoms. Examination showed an alert man in no acute distress. Blood pressure was 230/140 mmHg; heart rate, 100/min. Fundoscopic examination showed minimal AV nicking but no hemorrhages or exudates. There were scattered bibasilar rales and a prominent atrial gallop (S4) but no evidence of congestive heart failure. No neurologic deficits were noted. Urinalysis showed trace proteinuria without hematuria or casts; electrocardiogram, left ventricular hypertrophy with repolarization changes consistent with myocardial ischemia. Because of the relative paucity of physical findings and the absence of neurologic deficits, this patient's accelerated hypertension was treated with oral doses of clonidine. He was discharged on clonidine after 2 days of hospitalization.

group is 500 to 1,000 times more potent than the nitrates. Nitroprusside's onset of action is rapid but persists only 1 to 2 minutes after its infusion is discontinued. Nitroprusside decreases both the systemic vascular resistance and the venous return. The resultant fall in arterial pressure usually causes a mild compensatory tachycardia that is mediated via the baroreceptors. Generally, renal blood flow and glomerular filtration remain constant during drug infusion. Infusion of nitroprusside should begin at 0.5 μg/kg/min and should be titrated upwards in 0.5 μg/kg/min increments until the desired reduction in blood pressure has been achieved. Infusions should be controlled by a constant-rate drug delivery pump for maximum patient safety. Nitroprusside is light-sensitive, and thus, both the bottle and infusion line must be protected by aluminum foil. This necessitates that a prepared bottle of nitroprusside be replaced every 4 hours.

Nitroprusside has been used to treat se-

vere hypertension occurring in a variety of circumstances, including that complicating pheochromocytoma, during/after cardiac surgery, or in acute myocardial infarction. However, because the maximum dP/dt increases after nitroprusside administration in dogs,[9] this drug is contraindicated in the management of dissecting aortic aneurysm.

Adverse effects of nitroprusside include nasal stuffiness, dizziness, weakness, muscle fasciculations, and nausea. Prolonged infusions, particularly in patients with renal insufficiency, may cause accumulation of thiocyanate, a product of nitroprusside metabolism. Manifestations of thiocyanate toxicity include weakness, nausea, tinnitus, psychosis, and hypothyroidism. Thus, thiocyanate levels should be monitored during nitroprusside infusions and the drug should be discontinued upon clinical signs of toxicity *or* when blood thiocyanate levels of greater than 10 to 12 mg/dl are reached.

Hydralazine

Hydralazine causes direct dilatation of smooth muscle in the peripheral arterioles. As with other antihypertensive medications, this vasodilatation stimulates a reflex increase in cardiac output, stroke volume, renal blood flow, and heart rate. Plasma levels of hydralazine are directly correlated with the drug's hypotensive effect. For the management of hypertensive emergencies, hydralazine should be administered parenterally in doses of 10 to 20 mg. When given in this manner, the drug's action begins within 10 to 30 minutes and persists for 3 to 6 hours. Once control of hypertension is achieved with a parenteral dose, oral administration may be used. Hydralazine is metabolized by the liver. Thus, to achieve the same hypotensive effect, an oral dose of the hydralazine should be three to four times greater than a parenteral dose.

Hydralazine's advantages are that its effects are noted in the supine position, that it has a predictable onset of action after administration, and that it rarely causes hypotension, sedation, or somnolence. Hydralazine may be particularly effective in a hypertensive crisis that complicates glomerulonephritis, preeclampsia, or eclampsia. Contraindications to the use of hydralazine are the presence of unstable angina pectoris, acute myocardial infarction, or dissecting aortic aneurysm.

Adverse drug effects include tachycardia, arrhythmias, headache, nausea, vomiting, drug fever, and peripheral neuropathy. The cardiac stimulation induced may provoke and/or exacerbate angina pectoris in patients who have ischemic heart disease. Thus, hydralazine should be used cautiously, if at all, in such individuals.

Methyldopa

Methyldopa reduces blood pressure by causing arteriolar vasodilatation. Renal and cerebral blood flow are usually maintained and there is generally no change in cardiac output or heart rate. Methyldopa is cleared by the kidneys, and patients who have renal insufficiency are often more sensitive to its hypotensive effects. Given intravenously, methyldopa is usually administered over 30 minutes in doses of 250 to 500 mg. After intravenous administration, the drug's hypotensive effect begins within 3 hours and persists for 4 to 8 hours. Adverse effects of methyldopa include lethargy and drowsiness, which usually decrease after several days of therapy. However, these effects may confuse the clinical picture in a patient with a stroke, intracranial hemorrhage, or neurotrauma. Thus, methyldopa is not recommended in the management of hypertensive crises in such patients. A Coombs'-positive hemolytic anemia occurs in 20 percent of patients and occasionally drug fever may be observed. Hepatic injury may also occur and ranges from mild "transaminitis" to fulminant hepatic necrosis. Since methyldopa does not affect renal blood flow, it may be particularly useful in treating the azotemic patient who has a hypertensive crisis (see above for cautionary statement). The usual oral dosage of methyldopa is 250 to 500 mg every 6 hours.

Reserpine

Reserpine depletes norepinephrine from the adrenergic nerve endings and interferes with neurotransmission at postganglionic sites. Thus, smooth muscle relaxation occurs with a consequent fall in heart rate, blood pressure, and peripheral vascular resistance. Since the onset of reserpine's action is slow (2 to 3 hours) regardless of which parenteral route is employed, it is usually given intramuscularly in 1 to 5 mg doses. Administration may be repeated after 4 hours. Caution is advised as drug accumulation, and thus excessive hypotension, may occur. Adverse drug effects include somnolence, vertigo, weakness, headache, depression, decreased gastrointestinal motility, bradycardia, and second degree AV block. The duration of reserpine's action is prolonged and is measured in days. Thus, with the availability of agents that are more potent and relatively easier to use, reserpine has now been generally relegated to a second-line drug in the management of a hypertensive crisis.

Trimethaphan Camsylate

Trimethaphan camsylate blocks acetylcholine at the postganglionic nerve terminal but has no effect on preganglionic release of acetylcholine or its metabolism. Cardiac output falls in response to this drug; however, heart rate usually does not rise. These changes, in conjunction with a decrease in renal blood flow and reflex increase in renovascular resistance, may cause a deterioration of renal function. Thus, other hypotensive agents may be preferable in hypertensive patients who also have renal disease. Trimethaphan is given intravenously by a rate-controlled infusion pump. The initial dose should be 0.5 to 1.0 mg/min with appropriate increments to control the blood pressure. Usually 3 to 5 minutes should elapse between any increases in dosage. The onset of trimethaphan's action is immediate. A limitation of trimethaphan is that its hypotensive effect is most completely expressed with the patient in the upright position. This obviously limits its use in severely ill patients who are usually recumbent. It has been suggested that elevation of the head of the bed on 4 to 6 inch blocks (which would make the lower portion of the body relatively dependent) will help promote the hypotensive effects of trimethaphan. Prolonged drug infusions may cause sodium retention, constipation, paralytic ileus, and pupillary dilatation. The latter may make accurate neurologic assessment more difficult. Trimethaphan depresses cardiac contractility and reduces maximum aortic dP/dt. Because of these effects, the drug is often used in the management of acute aortic dissection. After trimethaphan is stopped, the duration of its hypotensive action persists only a few minutes.

Phentolamine

Phentolamine competitively inhibits the binding of norepinephrine at α-adrenergic receptor sites. Its use is almost specifically limited to the management of hypertensive crises in patients who have a pheochromocytoma and

in hypertension caused by either MAO inhibitor interactions or the withdrawal of clonidine. A hypotensive effect usually may be achieved by infusions of 0.1 to 2.0 mg/min with adjustments in the amount of the drug given as needed to obtain the desired effect. The onset of hypotension is prompt but usually short lived (5 to 15 minutes) after the drug is discontinued.

Propranolol

Propranolol is the prototypical β receptor blocker and may be given either orally or intravenously. Although its use in hypertensive crises is almost exclusively restricted to those caused by dissecting aortic aneurysms, recent studies suggest a wider application. Intravenous doses of 0.1 to 0.5 mg/kg infused at 0.25 to 1.0 mg/min will result in adequate β blockade. Because of its large volume of distribution, plasma levels of propranolol after a single dose decline rapidly, with a secondary half-life from hepatic metabolism of 3 to 6 hours. Despite its hepatic metabolism, chronic renal insufficiency may also elevate blood propranolol levels as a consequence of decreased hepatic tissue binding. The most important adverse effects of propranolol are its negative inotropic and chronotropic cardiac effects as well as its bronchospastic effects. Thus, caution should be exercised when administering propranolol to patients who have known cardiovascular or pulmonary diseases. Newer β-blocking drugs[16] are without these adverse effects although their role in the management of hypertensive crises remains uncertain. Other notable adverse effects of propranolol include diarrhea, fatigue, hypoglycemia, or aggravation of myasthenia gravis or peripheral vascular disease.

Nitroglycerin

Nitroglycerin, although not generally classified as an antihypertensive drug, may be very specific when hypertension occurs as a consequence of an acute myocardial infarction, a prolonged anginal episode, or myocardial ischemia complicating cardiac surgery. The rationale for using intravenous nitroglycerin in these instances is that it produces a hypotensive effect while improving myocardial blood flow and thus reducing myocardial ischemia. Intravenous nitroglycerin should be administered by a rate-controlled drug infusion device. Dosing should begin at 5 μg/min with increments of 5 to 10 μg/min every 3 to 5 minutes until hypertension is controlled. After a dose of 20 to 25 μg/min is reached, 10 to 20 μg increments may be used. The polyvinyl chloride tubing of intravenous administration sets may absorb 40 to 80 percent of the total amount of nitroglycerin in the final concentration of the mixture. Higher rates of absorption by the tubing occur when infusion rates are low, when the concentration of nitroglycerin in solution is high, or when the tubing length is long. This is particularly true during the early stages of drug administration. However, the absorption of nitroglycerin is neither constant nor self-limiting and there are no reliable formulas to determine the extent of drug uptake by polyvinyl tubing. To alleviate this problem, manufacturers have developed nonpolyvinyl chloride tubing, which absorbs less than 5 percent of an intravenous nitroglycerin mixture. Most published reports describing the intravenous use of nitroglycerin have used polyvinyl chloride tubing. Thus, if nonpolyvinyl chloride tubing is used, excessive amounts of nitroglycerin will be administered if the doses published in these reports are administered. The onset and cessation of nitroglycerin's hypotensive effects occur within minutes.

Other than reflex tachycardia, headache, and an exaggerated hypotensive effect there are no significant adverse drug effects. Finally, there are no upper limits to the dose of nitroglycerin that may be used. Occasionally individuals will display a marked sensitivity to the effects of nitroglycerin, particularly in those patients with a normal or low pulmonary capillary wedge pressure or elevated blood alcohol levels. In such patients, extreme hypotension and cardiovascular collapse may occur. Thus, the drug should be given cautiously under these circumstances.

Clonidine

Clonidine is a centrally acting α-adrenoceptor antagonist which causes a reduction in sympathetic tone. After an initial dose, stimulation of peripheral α-adrenergic receptors may occur and produce transient vasoconstriction. This drug acts rapidly, with a decline in blood pressure beginning 30 to 60 minutes following an oral dose. The hypotensive effects peak within 2 to 4 hours and persist for 6 to 8 hours. In those instances in which the patient's blood pressure is raised but clinical symptoms are not striking, this drug may be given orally in lieu of other intravenous agents (Fig. 12-2). Recommended doses are 0.1 to 0.2 mg with total daily doses of 0.8 to 2.4 mg. If clonidine is used, it should not be abruptly discontinued because rebound hypertension may occur within 16 to 48 hours. This rebound may be treated by restarting and/or slowly tapering clonidine or by using α-adrenergic blocking agents. This potential adverse effect has generated concern about the routine use of clonidine, particularly in patients whose reliability is uncertain.

Diuretics

In addition to the above-mentioned drugs, diuretics (particularly the loop diuretics) have facilitated the management of a hypertensive crisis. As well as reducing the sodium retention many of these agents cause, the diuretics also act to decrease an expanded intravascular volume. Thus, they act synergistically with other antihypertensive agents. Its potency, ease of administration, and relative lack of adverse effects make furosemide the diuretic of choice in these circumstances. Furosemide should be rapidly administered intravenously, beginning at doses of 20 mg. Doses may be increased as needed to 100 to 200 mg. Diuresis usually begins within 30 minutes and may last for 2 to 3 hours. Patients who are elderly, who have normal renal function, or who have not previously been on diuretic therapy may have an exaggerated response to furosemide. Thus, un-

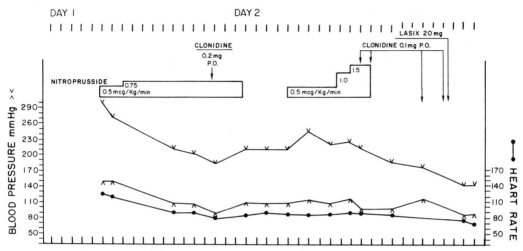

FIG. 12-2 This 47-year-old black woman had a 20 year history of hypertension. Five months earlier she stopped her antihypertensive medications and sustained an intracerebral hemorrhage with residual aphasia. On the day of admission she was found to be unresponsive, experiencing generalized tonic/clonic seizures. Examination showed an unresponsive patient with no nucchal rigidity. Blood pressure was 270/150 mmHg; pulse, 124/min. A few subretinal hemorrhages were observed bilaterally; there was neither papilloedema nor exudates. The patient did not have evidence of congestive heart failure. Blood urea nitrogen level was 18 mg/dl; creatinine, 1.0 mg/dl. There was 2+ proteinuria; an ECG was normal. This patient's hypertensive crisis was treated with increasing doses of nitroprusside. After her blood pressure was controlled, clonidine was added to her regimen and nitroprusside was ultimately discontinued. She was discharged from the hospital in an improved condition on clonidine (0.6 mg twice daily), minoxidil (2.5 mg twice daily), and hydrochlorothiazide (50 mg twice daily).

der these circumstances smaller initial doses of this drug are suggested.

CONCLUSIONS

From the above pharmacologic armamentarium, the physician who treats patients with hypertensive crises must choose the most appropriate agent (Table 12-3). It should be apparent that there are circumstances in which certain drugs may be preferable. For example, trimethaphan and propranolol are preferable for acute aortic dissection, methyldopa is preferable in the hypertensive crisis associated with moderate renal insufficiency, and nitro-

glycerin is the drug of choice in the patient with ischemic heart disease.

In managing a patient who has a hypertensive crisis, it is important to monitor vital parameters closely. Such individuals should be treated in intensive or critical care units where their level of consciousness, heart rate and rhythm, blood pressure, and urine output can be observed. There is no rule as to whether or not intra-arterial monitoring needs to be performed in these patients. With the availability of accurate, noninvasive blood pressure recording devices (i.e., Doppler), such patients may be closely evaluated without the need for invasive monitoring. However, in patients with aortic dissection, left ventricular failure or intracerebral hemorrhage, intra-arterial monitoring may be preferable since rapid changes in blood pressure may be especially detrimental. In these latter conditions, thermodilution catheters should also be used as appropriate to

TABLE 12-3.   Suggested Drugs for Hypertensive Crises

Disease	Preferred Drug	Alternatives	Use with Caution
Malignant hypertension	Nitroprusside	Diazoxide Trimethaphan Hydralazine Methyldopa Clonidine Reserpine	
Hypertensive encephalopathy	Nitroprusside	Trimethaphan Diazoxide Hydralazine	Reserpine Methyldopa
Stroke	Nitroprusside	Trimethaphan Diazoxide	Reserpine Methyldopa
Hypertension with bleeding from vascular sites, postoperative hypertension	Nitroprusside	Methyldopa Hydralazine Diazoxide Trimethaphan	
Hypertension during or after cardiac surgery	Nitroglycerin	Nitroprusside Methyldopa	Diazoxide Hydralazine
Left ventricular failure (with or without MI)	Nitroglycerin	Nitroprusside Trimethaphan	Diazoxide Hydralazine
Dissecting aortic aneurysm	Trimethaphan	Reserpine Methyldopa Propranolol	Diazoxide Hydralazine Nitroprusside
Head injuries	Nitroprusside	Trimethaphan Diazoxide	Reserpine Methyldopa
Hypertensive crises in the paraplegic	Nitroprusside	Trimethaphan Methyldopa	
Pheochromocytoma, MAO inhibitor reactions, clonidine withdrawal	Phentolamine	Nitroprusside	All others

(Adapted from Kirkendall WM: Hypertensive emergencies. In Hunt JC Cooper T, Frohlich ED et al (eds): Hypertension Update: Mechanisms, Epidemiology, Evaluation and Management. Health Learning Systems, Bloomfield, New Jersey, 1979.)

monitor right heart pressures. Following control of the hypertensive crisis and with the establishment of clinical stability, oral antihypertensive medications should be started if indicated. Long-term prognosis following a hypertensive crisis depends on its duration, reversibility, and the extent of end-organ damage.

ACKNOWLEDGMENT

The author thanks Ms. Bonnie Jane Dooley for her assistance in preparing the manuscript.

REFERENCES

1. Finnerty FA: Treatment of hypertensive emergencies. Heart Lung 10: 275, 1981
2. Hansson L, Hunyor SN, Julius S: Blood pressure crises following withdrawal of clonidine with special reference to arterial and urinary catecholamine levels and suggestions for acute management. Am Heart J 85: 605, 1973
3. Kaplan NM: Clinical Hypertension. Williams and Wilkins, Baltimore, 1978
4. Keith TA: Hypertensive crisis: recognition and management. JAMA 237: 1570, 1977
5. Kincaid-Smith P: Malignant hypertension: mechanisms and management. Pharmacol Ther 9: 245, 1980
6. Kirkendall WM: Hypertensive emergencies. In

Hunt JC, Cooper T, Frohlich ED et al (eds): Hypertension Update: Mechanisms, Epidemiology, Evaluation and Management. Health Learning Systems, Bloomfield, New Jersey, 1979.

7. Landymore RW, Murphy DA, Kinley CE: Hypertension following myocardial revascularization: its prevalence and etiology. Can J Surg 23: 468, 1980

8. Naftchi N, Demeny M, Lowman EW, Tuckman J: Hypertensive crisis in quadriplegic patients. Circulation 57: 336, 1978

9. Palmer RF, Lasseter KC: Nitroprusside and aortic dissecting aneurysm. N Engl J Med 294: 1403, 1976

10. Ram CVJ, Kaplan NM: Individual titration of diazoxide dosage in the treatment of severe hypertension. Am J Cardiol 43: 627, 1979

11. Romankiewicz JA: Pharmacology and clinical use of drugs in hypertensive emergencies. Am J Hosp Pharm 34: 185, 1977

12. Rutsaert RJ, De Broe ME: The management of hypertensive emergencies. Acta Clin Belg 35: 354, 1980

13. Skinhoj E, Strandgaard S: Pathogenesis of hypertensive encepalopathy. Lancet 1: 461, 1973

14. Strandgaard S, Olesen J, Skinhoj E, et al: Autoregulation of brain circulation in severe arterial hypertension. Br Med J 1:507, 1973

15. Taylor KM, Morton IJ, Brown JJ et al: Hypertension and the renin–angiotensin system following open heart surgery. J Thorac Cardiovasc Surg 74: 840, 1977

16. Wilson DJ, Wallin JD, Vlachakis ND et al: Intravenous labetalol in the treatment of severe hypertension and hypertensive emergencies. Am J Med 75: 95, 1983

17. Wolfe WG, Moran JF: The evolution of medical and surgical management of acute aortic dissection. Circulation et al: 56: 503, 1977

18. Wallach R, Karp RB, Reves JG et al: Pathogenesis of paroxysmal hypertension developing during and after coronary bypass surgery: a study of hemodynamic and humoral factors. Am J Cardiol 46: 559, 1980

19. Wood DE, Bogonoff MD, Finnerty FA Jr et al: The treatment of malignant hypertension and hypertensive emergencies. JAMA 228: 1673, 1974

13

Venous Thrombosis and Acute Pulmonary Embolism

Lazar J. Greenfield

INTRODUCTION

Effective management of critically ill patients is focused appropriately on their functional derangements and can be based on careful monitoring of physiologic performance. In venous thrombosis however, there is no reliable means of monitoring the disorder, and it can result in the silent propagation of a deep venous thrombus to the point that it becomes life-threatening pulmonary thromboembolism. The mortality of pulmonary thromboembolism in the critically ill patient can only be estimated, but the realistic estimate of 200,000 deaths per year in which it was the sole cause or a major contributing factor[7] underscores the need for prophylaxis, early diagnosis, and therapy.

PATHOPHYSIOLOGY

Although efforts to identify a common coagulation factor abnormality in patients with venous thrombosis have not been successful, Seeger and Marciniak[27] identified a naturally occurring inhibitor of activated Factor X in 1962, which was subsequently named antithrombin III. A congenital deficiency of this substance was found later in a small group of patients and was correlated with a strong predisposition to the development of venous thrombosis.[8] Antithrombin deficiency has also been associated with arterial thrombosis in patients following vascular surgery.[32] The classic association between venous thrombosis and malignancy as pointed out originally by Trousseau[34] has also been found to provide an early sign of an occult cancer most commonly involving lung, gastrointestinal tract, breast, and uterus.[12] Additional clinical correlations have demonstrated significantly increased risk of venous thrombosis in patients with hyperlipoproteinemia,[20] oral contraceptive use, smoking history, and obesity.[24] Less well documented evidence exists for enhanced risk in the presence of advanced age, heart disease, trauma, sepsis, and non-O blood type.[22]

In surgical patients, stasis is probably the most important factor since there is a significant reduction in lower extremity venous flow following induction of general anesthesia, which persists throughout the procedure. There is also a relationship between the duration of bed rest and the incidence of venous thrombosis, which provides the stimulus for early ambulation. Vessel wall injury also can occur in collapsed vessels when the intimal walls are in contact and some intimal injury can be demonstrated after hypoxemia. Although routine histologic examination of veins containing thrombi fails to show an inflammatory response consistent with vessel wall injury, ultrastructural study shows leukocytic attachment between endothelial intercellular junctions in areas of venous stasis after trauma at a remote site. These changes can become the nidus for the formation of a propagating thrombus. Once a nidus of thrombus begins in the presence of stasis, the substances that promote platelet aggregation, including activated Factor X, thrombin, fibrin, and catecholamines, remain at high concentration in that area. Opposing this process is the fibrinolytic system of the blood and vein walls. The endothelium of the vein wall contains an activator that converts plasminogen into plasmin, which lyses fibrin. As might be expected, however, the fibrinolytic system is inhibited after surgery and trauma, and there is also less activity in the veins of the lower extremity than in the upper extremity.

When contrast medium is injected in supine, immobilized patients, it may remain in venous valve sinuses for as long as an hour, confirming the stasis existing in the soleal veins. This is the favored location for the formation of a nidus of thrombus as described. Successive layering of platelets, fibrin, red cells, and leukocytes produces an organized white thrombus that is more adherent to the vein wall than the propagating red thrombus, which extends into the venous stream (Fig. 13-1). The latter free-floating thrombus is much less likely to cause symptoms and more likely to result in embolism. If the original thrombus becomes attached to the opposite wall, it causes interruption of flow, retrograde thrombosis, and signs of venous stasis in the extremity. Subsequent edema formation within the confines of the deep fascia produces pain and a characteristic Homans' sign elicited by forcible dorsiflexion of the foot, although the latter is by no means specific for venous thrombosis.

The site of venous obstruction determines the level at which swelling is observed clinically. Swelling at the thigh level always implies obstruction at the level of the iliofemoral system, while swelling of the calf or foot suggests obstruction at the femoropopliteal level. Autopsies suggest that it is more common for thrombi to originate in the soleus veins and then propagate proximally, but there is also evidence of primary thrombosis of femoral and iliac venous tributaries. Resolution of deep vein thrombosis (DVT) with recanalization will affect the competence of the valves within the veins and can result in the postphlebitic syndrome. Complete spontaneous lysis of large thrombi is relatively uncommon and even when patients are treated adequately with heparin to prevent further thrombosis, complete lysis occurs in less than 20 percent of cases. It seems likely that complete dissolution of small asymptomatic calf-vein thrombi is a more common occurrence, but the actual frequency is unknown.

DIAGNOSIS

Major venous thrombosis involving the deep venous system of the thigh and pelvis produces a characteristic clinical picture of pain, extensive pitting edema, and blanching that has been termed phlegmasia alba dolens or "milk leg." Association with pregnancy may

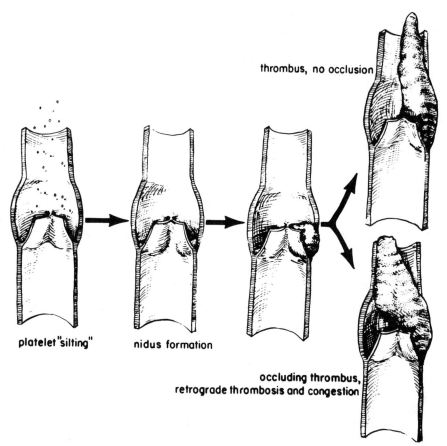

thrombus, no occlusion

platelet "silting"   nidus formation

occluding thrombus,
retrograde thrombosis and congestion

FIG. 13-1 The evolution of venous thrombosis begins with stagnant flow that permits silting of platelets, which form a nidus in the venous valvular sinus. The cycle of fibrin retraction and thrombin release aggregates more platelets as the thrombus enlarges and usually extends into the stream without occlusion, or it may occlude the vein with retrograde thrombosis. (Greenfield LJ: Acute venous thrombosis and pulmonary embolism. p. 971. In Hardy JD (ed): Hardy's Textbook of Surgery. JB Lippincott, Philadelphia, 1983.)

relate to hormonal effects on blood, relaxation of vessel walls, or mechanical compression of the left iliac vein at the pelvic brim, resulting in the term "milk leg of pregnancy." It was originally believed that the blanching was due to spasm and compromise of arterial flow, but arteriograms fail to confirm this, and efforts to achieve sympatholysis to overcome "vasospasm" are ill-advised, since usually the subcutaneous edema is responsible for the blanching. In addition to pregnancy, other mechanical factors that can affect the left iliac vein include compression from the right iliac artery or an overdistended bladder and congenital webs within the vein. These factors are responsible

for the observed 4:1 preponderance of left versus right iliac vein involvement.

With further progression of venous thrombosis to impede most of the venous return from the extremity, there is danger of limb loss from cessation of arterial flow. The clinical picture is characteristic, with sufficient congestion to produce phlegmasia cerulea dolens, or a blue leg. With the loss of sensory or motor function, the diagnosis can be made on clinical grounds and treatment started. Venous gangrene is likely unless an aggressive approach is utilized to remove the thrombus by open thrombectomy and restore blood flow. A variant of this disorder associated with malignant disease occurs peripherally in the leg and has a high mortality.

These major complications occur in less than 10 percent of the patients with venous thrombosis. In fact, only 40 percent of patients with venous thrombosis have any clinical signs of the disorder. In addition, false-positive clinical signs occur in up to 50 percent of patients studied.[21] Because of this there has been a great deal of interest in the development of screening tests that could reveal thrombi before they became evident clinically. Of course, contrast venography provides direct evidence of both occlusive and nonocclusive thrombi, but it is invasive and requires that the patient move to a radiography suite. Ideally, the screening test would be accurate, noninvasive, and performed at the bedside. Although the ideal has not been achieved, a number of tests have proved useful.

Ultrasound

The Doppler probe can be used to detect major venous thrombi with a high degree of accuracy, but is a subjective form of testing dependent on the examiner's experience. The principle is straightforward, based on the impairment of an accelerated flow signal produced by intraluminal thrombi.[31] The examination begins at the ankle, with identification of the posterior tibial vein signal adjacent to the artery. The flow signal should be altered by distal and proximal compression producing, respectively, augmentation and interruption of flow, which also can be produced by the Valsalva maneuver. The same maneuvers are repeated over the superficial and deep femoral veins and can be done over the popliteal vein. Failure to augment flow on compression below or release of interruption of flow above the probe suggests venous thrombi. The sensitivity of the test exceeds 90 percent but the specificity is 5 to 10 percent lower due to the possibility of other mechanical problems (Baker's cyst, hematoma, and others) interfering with venous flow. A negative Doppler ultrasound examination is reassuring but a positive or equivocal test should be confirmed by contrast venogra-

phy. A negative test is *not* reassuring when thromboembolism is suspected, since the thrombus may have been evacuated from the extremity. It is also less sensitive to calf vein thrombi, but can be used in patients in traction or who are wearing a plaster cast.

Impedance Plethysmography

Impedance plethysmography (IPG) measures the volume response of the extremity to temporary occlusion of the venous system. The diagnosis of venous thrombosis depends on the changes in venous capacitance and rate of emptying after release of the occlusion.[36] A proximal thigh cuff is inflated to 40 to 50 mmHg pressure for 50 to 120 seconds or until maximum filling has occurred, documented by plateau of the electrical signal. The inflation cuff is then rapidly deflated, allowing rapid outflow and reduction of volume in a normal limb. Prolongation of the outflow wave suggests major venous thrombosis with 95 percent accuracy and is much more reliable than any voluntary technique of venous occlusion (Fig. 13-2). The source of error with this technique as with all of the noninvasive methods lies in the detection of calf vein thrombosis or definition of new pathologic change in patients with old postthrombotic sequelae. The strain gauge plethysmograph can be used in a similar fashion. A positive IPG test can be used to make therapeutic decisions in the absence of clinical conditions that may produce false-positive results, such as cardiac failure, constrictive pericarditis, hypotension, arterial insufficiency, or external compression of veins.

Radio-labeled Fibrinogen

Clinical application of labeled fibrinogen has been facilitated by the development of portable scintillation counters for bedside use. After iodine blockage of the thyroid gland, the counts are obtained from marked locations on the lower extremities and expressed as a per-

PLETHYSMOGRAPHIC CALF OUTFLOWS

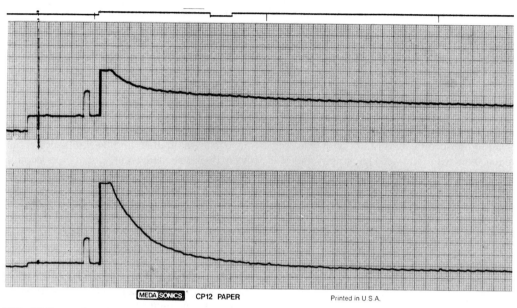

MEDASONICS   CP12 PAPER   Printed in U.S.A.

FIG. 13-2 Plethysmographic tracing shows normal response (below) to proximal thigh occlusion by pneumatic cuff. In contrast, the presence of an obstructing thrombus limits the volume increase after occlusion and prolongs the drainage downslope when the cuff is released (above). (Greenfield LJ: Complications of venous thrombosis and pulmonary embolism. p. 409. In Greenfield LJ (ed): Complications in Surgery and Trauma. JB Lippincott, Philadelphia, 1984.)

centage of the radioactivity measured by counting over the heart. An increase of 20 percent or more in one area indicates an underlying thrombus. The test permits sequential scanning of the extremities over a period of days and is most sensitive to thrombi forming in the veins of the calves shortly after an operative procedure.[9] It does not permit detection of thrombi in pelvic veins, and it cannot be used in an extremity in which there is a healing wound, fracture, cellulitis, arthritis, edema, ulceration, or superficial thrombophlebitis, because false-positive results are likely. It is also contraindicated in patients under 30 years of age and women of childbearing age. In the absence of these conditions it is quite accurate, however, showing 90 percent positive correlation with contrast venograms. A negative correlation usually is explained by cessation of active thrombosis and failure to incorporate the tagged fibrinogen, making the test useful in differentiating between old and new venous thrombi.

Venography

The injection of contrast material for direct visualization of the venous system of the extremity is the most accurate method of confirming the diagnosis of venous thrombosis and the extent of the involvement. Injection is usually made into the foot while the superficial veins are occluded by tourniquet. A supplementary injection into the femoral veins may be required to visualize the iliofemoral system. Both filling defects and nonvisualization can be found and provide an assessment of the threat of a thrombus such as one seen to be floating free and extending into the iliofemoral system

(Fig. 13-3). Potential false-positive examinations may result from external compression of a vein or washout of the contrast material from collateral veins. The procedure can also be performed with isotope injection using a gamma scintillation counter to record flow of the isotope. Delayed imaging of persistent "hot spots" may also reflect isotope retention at the sites of thrombus formation. A perfusion lung scan can also be obtained for baseline comparison and to detect silent embolism. There is less definition of deep vein thrombi with this technique than with contrast venography but it is a valuable technique for sequential study of patients and avoids the potential thrombogenesis of the injection of contrast medium.

Assay of Fibrin/Fibrinogen Products

The degradation of intravascular fibrin can be detected by measuring the plasma products of the lysis of fibrin or fibrinogen. Both fibrinopeptide A and fibrin fragment E can be detected by radioimmunoassay, but are not specific for acute venous thrombosis. A negative test could conceivably have some value in excluding the diagnosis but the tests are difficult and will require more investigation and simplification.

PROPHYLAXIS

Theoretically it should be possible to prevent formation of venous thrombi either by eliminating or reducing venous stasis or by altering blood coagulability. The belief that early ambulation prevents stasis and reduces the formation of thrombi has been the subject of controversy, and studies using tagged fibrinogen have not supported this assumption. One explanation for this is that early ambulation often consists of having the patient walk to a chair and sit, whereupon the legs are subjected to even more stasis. Other efforts, including electrical stimulation of calf muscles and passive motor-driven flexion of the foot, have not proved cost-effective or acceptable to patients.

There has been more interest in the prophylactic use of anticoagulant drugs and drugs that inhibit platelets, such as aspirin and dipyridamole. The latter drugs are under continuing evaluation for this role, but published reports have shown limited and variable protection from their use. However, good data support the use of preoperative oral anticoagulant therapy with coumarin derivatives in high-risk patients. Unfortunately, this increases the risk of hemorrhage, and with the added difficulties of laboratory control of prothrombin time, there has not been widespread acceptance of this approach. The administration of dextran 40, which produces a variety of effects on platelets and clotting factors, has been demonstrated to reduce the incidence of detectable thrombi, but it too can produce hemorrhagic problems as well as allergic reaction and, in older patients, congestive failure.

In an effort to minimize the problems associated with anticogaulant prophylaxis, there has been more acceptance of the administration of heparin, prior to and following surgery in low ("mini") doses that do not alter the laboratory clotting profile. Generally, a 5,000 unit dose is given subcutaneously 2 hours preoperatively and then every 8 or 12 hours postoperatively for 6 days. This appears to provide protection for most high-risk groups with the exception of those undergoing orthopedic procedures. The beneficial effect may be due to the enhancement of heparin cofactor (antithrombin III) as a natural inhibitor of activated Factor X. Although some studies have failed to show protection, Kakkar et al.,[23] in a randomized series of 4,121 patients, showed protection against fatal pulmonary embolism as well as deep venous thrombosis. There is a higher incidence of bleeding and wound complications associated with t.i.d. heparin prophylaxis. Since its major benefit appears to be reducing the incidence of calf vein thrombosis, which is of questionable clinical significance, the definition of optimal prophylaxis remains unresolved. For the general population of surgi-

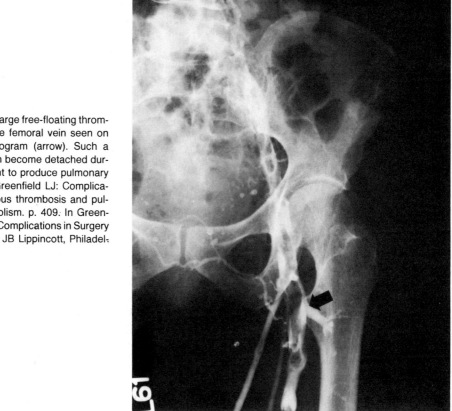

FIG. 13-3 Large free-floating thrombus within the femoral vein seen on contrast venogram (arrow). Such a thrombus can become detached during movement to produce pulmonary embolism. (Greenfield LJ: Complications of venous thrombosis and pulmonary embolism. p. 409. In Greenfield LJ (ed): Complications in Surgery and Trauma. JB Lippincott, Philadelphia, 1984.)

cal patients under age 40 years, the risk of DVT is low and prophylaxis can be limited to early ambulation with or without graduated compression stockings. For patients over age 40 who have undergone major surgical procedures, the risk is moderate and prophylaxis should be considered, such as intermittent pneumatic compression or low-dose heparin administered subcutaneously b.i.d. The patients at highest risk (age over 40, obese, and with malignant disease, history of DVT, or major trauma) need more protection, which might include low-dose heparin, intermittent pneumatic compression, oral anticoagulants, or dextran.[3] Low dose heparin should not be used in neurosurgical patients because of the consequences of any intracranial bleeding. For these patients, external pneumatic compression is the prophylaxis of choice.

NONSURGICAL TREATMENT

The approach to management of the patient with deep venous thrombosis is based on minimizing the risk of pulmonary embolism, limiting further thrombosis, and facilitating resolution of existing thrombi to avoid the postphlebitic syndrome.

Initially, the patient is placed at bed rest with the foot of the bed elevated 8 to 10 inches. Further improvement in venous return can be obtained by application of elastic bandages, which must be reapplied twice daily to avoid a tourniquet effect as they loosen. Generally, pain, swelling, and tenderness resolve over 5 to 7 days, at which time ambulation can be permitted with continued elastic support. Standing still and sitting should be prohibited to avoid the increased venous pressure and stasis.

Anticoagulation

The foundation of therapy for deep venous thrombosis is adequate anticoagulation, initially with heparin and then with coumarin derivatives for prolonged protection against recurrent thrombosis. Unless there are specific contraindications, heparin should be administered in an initial dose of 100 to 150 units/kg intravenously. Heparin is an acid mucopolysaccharide that neutralizes thrombin, inhibits thromboplastin, and reduces the platelet release reaction. It may be administered by continuous or intermittent intravenous doses regulated by whole blood clotting time. Bleeding complications can be minimized by doses of heparin that prolong the laboratory clotting times in the range of twice normal with no loss of effectiveness. Continuous intravenous infusion regulated by an infusion pump seems to minimize the total dose required for control and is associated with a lower incidence of complications.

The side effects associated with heparin treatment include bleeding, thrombocytopenia, hypersensitivity, arterial thromboembolism, and osteoporosis. Bleeding is more likely to occur in elderly women, in patients treated with aspirin, or after recent surgery or trauma. It has been well demonstrated that bleeding can occur when the results of laboratory monitoring tests are within the therapeutic range, which may be due to the effect of heparin on platelets. Some evidence suggests that the risk of bleeding is proportional to the dose administered and that the risk is lessened by continuous rather than intermittent intravenous infusion.

Arterial thromboembolism can complicate heparin administration by any route and is more common in the elderly. It tends to occur after 7 to 10 days of therapy and is associated with thrombocytopenia. This complication carries a high morbidity and mortality rate and requires immediate cessation of heparin treatment. Thrombocytopenia as a complication is due to an immune reaction but is rapidly reversed when heparin is stopped, usually within 2 days. Hypersensitivity to heparin may take the form of a skin rash or, rarely, may produce anaphylaxis. Subcutaneous injections that result in urticaria may become necrotic as an unusual form of sensitivity. Osteoporosis has been seen in patients on long-term heparin therapy for more than 6 months. It is probably due to a direct effect on bone resorption, and can be avoided by shorter periods of treatment and dosages less than 15,000 units/day.

Oral administration of anticoagulants is begun shortly after initiation of heparin therapy, since several days are usually required to bring the prothrombin time within the therapeutic range of 1.3 to 1.5 times the control value and to provide the maximal antithrombotic effect. The coumarin derivatives block the synthesis of several clotting factors, and prolongation of the prothrombin time beyond the range suggested is associated with a high incidence of bleeding complications. The nonhemorrhagic side effects are uncommon but include skin necrosis, dermatitis, and a syndrome of painful blue toes. Skin necrosis is heralded by painful erythema in areas of large amounts of subcutaneous fat and is reversible if the drug is stopped. Fortunately, the administration of vitamin K usually can rapidly restore the prothrombin time. After an episode of acute deep venous thrombosis, anticoagulation should be maintained for a minimum of 3 months; some investigators favor 6 months for thrombi in the larger veins. Many drugs interact with the coumarin derivatives, such as barbiturates, and therefore a routine for regular monitoring of prothrombin time is essential after the patient leaves the hospital. Oral anticoagulants are teratogenic and should not be used during established or planned pregnancy. In the pregnant patient, heparin is the drug of choice and, for long-term management, subcutaneous self-administration should be taught. This regimen allows a normal delivery and can be continued postpartum.

Fibrinolysis

There has been great interest in the use of fibrinolytic agents to activate the intrinsic plasmin system. Both streptokinase and urokinase have been used and found to be effective although they are associated with a high incidence of hemorrhagic complications. Streptokinase is also associated with allergic reactions in 10 percent of patients; these reactions vary from urticaria to anaphylaxis. In addition, there is no advantage over heparin in the treatment of recurrent venous thrombosis or when thrombosis has existed for over 72 hours. The lytic agents are contraindicated in the postoperative or posttraumatic patient. Fatal pulmonary embolism has also been reported following lytic therapy for a long, free-floating thrombus.[10]

SURGICAL APPROACHES

Operative Thrombectomy

A direct surgical approach to remove thrombi from the deep veins of the leg via the common femoral vein has been employed and facilitated by the use of Fogarty venous balloon catheters and an elastic wrap to milk the extremity. Although the operative results are impressive, venograms obtained prior to discharge from the hospital show rethrombosis in the majority of patients, and there does not seem to be any lesser incidence of the postphlebitic syndrome. Consequently, the procedure is now usually reserved for limb salvage in the presence of phlegmasia cerulea dolens and impending venous gangrene.

Vena Cava Interruption

Adequate anticoagulation usually is effective in managing deep venous thrombosis, but if recurrent pulmonary embolism occurs during anticoagulant therapy or if there is a contraindication to anticoagulation, a surgical approach is necessary. Mechanical protection is also indicated as prophylaxis against recurrence of embolism for the patient who has required pulmonary embolectomy and in some high-risk patients who could not tolerate recurrence (Table 13-1).

Early surgical efforts to prevent recurrence of pulmonary embolism were directed to the common femoral vein, which was ligated bilaterally. This resulted in a high incidence of sequelae due to stasis in the lower extremities and an unacceptable rate of recurrent pulmonary embolism. The next approach was ligation of the inferior vena cava below the renal veins, which added the adverse effect of a sudden reduction in cardiac output. This effect, coupled with stasis sequelae and recurrent embolism through dilated collateral veins, led to efforts to compartmentalize the vena cava by means of sutures, staples, and external clips to provide filtration without occlusion.

Since these procedures required general anesthesia and laparotomy, the next logical step was to devise a transvenous approach that could be performed under local anesthesia. The Mobin-Uddin "umbrella" unit was the first to be inserted from the jugular vein and positioned fluoroscopically below the renal veins, where it usually produced thrombosis of the vena cava (70 percent of cases).[6] It also has been associated with complications of proximal thrombus formation and lethal migration into the pulmonary artery.

The Greenfield cone-shaped filter was developed to maintain patency after trapping emboli and to permit continued flow to avoid stasis and facilitate lysis of the embolus (Fig. 13-4). It can be inserted from either the jugular vein or the femoral vein; the latter is used when the jugular vein is too small or in patients with open wounds of the neck.[14] The rate of recurrence with this device has been 2 to 4 percent and its long-term patency rate of better than

TABLE 13-1. Indications for Insertion of a Vena Caval Filter

Recurrent thromboembolism in the face of adequate anticoagulation

Documented thromboembolism in a patient who has a contraindication to anticoagulation

Complication of anticoagulation forcing therapy to be discontinued

Chronic pulmonary embolism with associated pulmonary hypertension and cor pulmonale (class V patient)

Immediately following pulmonary embolectomy

Septic pulmonary embolism

Relative indications: patient with more than 50 percent of the pulmonary vascular bed occluded (class III) who would not tolerate any additional embolism; patient with a propagating iliofemoral thrombus despite anticoagulation; patient with a large free-floating iliofemoral thrombus shown on venogram

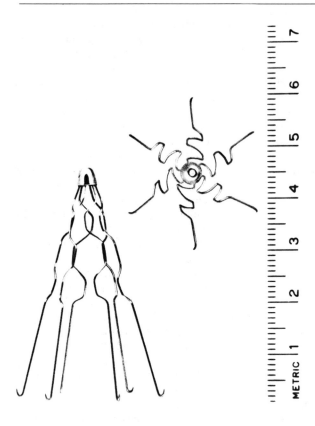

FIG. 13-4 The Greenfield filter permits trapping of emboli without loss of patency because of the geometry of the cone. If a thrombus is trapped in the filter, flow can continue around it to facilitate lysis and avoid the stasis sequelae of complete vena caval occlusion. (Greenfield LJ: Complications of venous thrombosis and pulmonary embolism. p. 412. In Greenfield LJ (ed): Complications in Surgery and Trauma. JB Lippincott, Philadelphia, 1984.)

95 percent allows it to be placed above the renal veins when necessary for embolism control, such as when there is thrombus within the renal veins or vena cava.[17] Another device, the Hunter balloon, occludes the vena cava after being positioned below the renal veins and contributes to stasis sequelae.

The complications of filter insertion range in severity from minor wound hematomas due to early resumption of anticoagulation to potentially lethal migration of the device into the pulmonary artery as documented with the Mobin-Uddin umbrella. The most common complication with the Greenfield filter has been misplacement in 7 percent of cases.[14] When misplacement occurs below the diaphragm, the patient has inadequate protection but the location (renal or iliac vein) poses no regional problem. A second filter can be placed in the appropriate location or the misplaced filter can be retrieved using a guidewire; this procedure is always advocated for misplacement into the right heart.[15] Misplacement has not occurred in our experience since the technique of routine guidewire insertion prior to filter discharge was adopted[19] (Fig. 13-5). Air embolism can occur during jugular insertion but the risk is minimized by having the patient hold his or her breath while the vein is open. In some patients the veins may be too small or fragile to permit insertion of the carrier catheter and, rarely, the patient may be too obese to permit fluoroscopy.

Recurrent embolism after filter placement has been seen in 2 to 4 percent of cases and may be due to a source of thrombus outside of the filtered flow such as the upper extremities or the right atrium. In one case a tilted filter was found to have allowed proximal thrombus formation, but this responded to treatment with urokinase and oral anticoagulation.[17]

Secondary infection of the Mobin-Uddin umbrella has been reported and required removal of the device. Secondary infection of captured thrombus within a Greenfield filter has been produced in the laboratory but the stainless steel filter and thrombus were readily sterilized by antibiotics.[25] The capture of a very

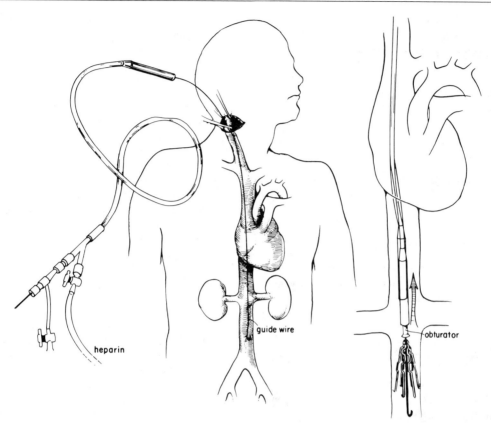

FIG. 13-5 Routine placement of a guidewire prior to passage of the carrier and discharge of the filter facilitates insertion and promotes axial orientation of the filter. (Greenfield LJ, Stewart JR, Crute S: Improved technique for Greenfield vena caval filter insertion. Surg Gynecol Obstet 156: 217, 1983.)

large embolus within a filter has the potential to occlude the vena cava suddenly with a precipitous fall in blood pressure. In a patient with known prior pulmonary embolism, this event can be mistaken for recurrent pulmonary embolism. If this diagnostic error occurs and vasopressor therapy is used, the results will be poor. The basic distinction between functional hypovolemia and right ventricular overload can be made by the measurement of central venous pressure and PaO_2. The response to volume resuscitation for the patient with sudden vena caval occlusion should be dramatic.

There is one circumstance in which migration of a Greenfield filter is possible after discharge: when there is failure to flush heparinized saline through the cylindrical carrier and a thrombus forms within it during the period of positioning under fluoroscopy. The thrombus can then tether the limbs of the filter, preventing their expansion and fixation to the wall of the vena cava. For optimal protection, a continuous drip of heparinized saline can be attached directly to the insertion catheter by intravenous tubing.

OTHER TYPES OF VENOUS THROMBOSIS

The term thrombophlebitis should be restricted to describing disorder of the superficial veins characterized by a local inflammatory process that is usually aseptic. The cause in the upper limb is usually acidic fluid infusion or prolonged cannulation. In the lower extremities it is usually associated with varicose veins and may coexist with deep vein thrombosis. The association with the injection of contrast material can be minimized by washout of the contrast material with heparinized saline.

Thrombophlebitis Migrans

The condition of recurrent episodes of superficial thrombophlebitis has been associated with visceral malignancy, systemic collagen vascular disease, and blood dyscrasias. Involvement of the deep veins and the visceral veins has also been described.

Subclavian Vein Thrombosis

This disorder is most likely to be secondary to an indwelling catheter and can occur in children. It may also occur as a primary event in a young, athletic person ("effort thrombosis") presumably as a result of injury at the thoracic inlet. There is usually a good response to elevation and anticoagulation, although some venous insufficiency and discomfort with exercise may persist.

Abdominal Vein Thrombosis

Thrombosis of the inferior vena cava can result from tumor invasion or propagating thrombus from the iliac veins. Most commonly, however, it results from ligation, plication, or insertion of partially occluding caval devices such as the Mobin-Uddin umbrella. Any caval filtration device can become totally occluded by a trapped massive thrombus, with sudden reduction in venous return and cardiac output as described previously. Thrombosis of the renal vein is most likely to occur in association

with the nephrotic syndrome. It can be a source of thromboembolism and has been treated successfully by suprarenal placement of the Greenfield filter.[30]

Portal vein thrombosis can occur in the neonate, usually secondary to propagating septic thrombophlebitis of the umbilical vein. Collateral development leads to esophageal varices. Thrombosis of the portal, hepatic, splenic, or superior mesenteric vein in the adult can occur spontaneously, but usually is associated with hepatic cirrhosis. Thrombosis of mesenteric or omental veins can simulate an acute abdomen but usually results in prolonged ileus rather than intestinal infarction.

Hepatic vein thrombosis (Budd-Chiari syndrome) usually produces massive hepatomegaly, ascites, and liver failure. It can occur in association with a congenital web, endophlebitis, or polycythemia vera. Although some success has been reported using a direct approach to the congenital webs, the usual treatment is a side-to-side portocaval shunt to allow decompression of the liver. The development of pelvic sepsis after abortion, tubal infection, or puerperal sepsis can lead to septic thrombophlebitis of the pelvic veins and septic thromboembolism. Ovarian vein and caval ligation have been the traditional operative treatment but the emphasis should be on drainage or excision of the abscesses and appropriate antibiotic therapy. We have also used the Greenfield filter in this situation since it is inert stainless steel and avoids the development of an intraluminal abscess after ligation of the vena cava.

PULMONARY THROMBOEMBOLISM

The clinical significance of major pulmonary embolism can be appreciated based on its annual mortality, estimated to be 90,000 deaths in the United States alone. It is estimated that 5 of every 1,000 adults undergoing major surgery will die from massive pulmonary embolism. Since it represents the most important complication of deep vein thrombosis, it is of particular concern to surgeons whose patients are prone to develop deep vein thrombosis in the immediate postoperative period. The full spectrum of the disorder ranges from asymptomatic minor embolism to sudden death from massive embolism.

Diagnosis

The signs and symptoms of an embolic episode obviously depend primarily on the quantity of embolus involved and, to a lesser extent, on the cardiopulmonary status of the patient. In the classic presentation, the patient suddenly develops chest pain, cough, dyspnea, tachypnea, and anxiety. Although hemoptysis has traditionally been associated with pulmonary embolism, it is actually an uncommon sign; when present it usually occurs late in the course and probably represents pulmonary infarction. Objectively, the patient with major embolism usually shows tachycardia, an increased pulmonary second sound, cyanosis, prominent jugular veins, and varying degrees of collapse. Less commonly, there may be wheezing, a pleural friction rub, splinting of the chest wall, rales, low-grade fever, ventricular gallop, and wide splitting of the pulmonic second sound. The incidence of these findings is shown in Table 13-2.

The differential diagnosis includes esophageal perforation, pneumonia, septic shock, and myocardial infarction. Since all of these entities are life-threatening, it is mandatory that an orderly approach be formulated to confirm or reject the working diagnosis. Laboratory studies in general are not very helpful in the differential diagnosis. The following determinations are particularly useful in the evaluation of suspected major embolism.

ELECTROCARDIOGRAPHY

The most common electrocardiographic change associated with pulmonary embolism is nonspecific ST and T wave changes (66 percent of patients). More specific signs of right ventricular overload such as the often quoted S_1, Q_3, T_3 pattern are seldom seen. Consequently, the primary value of the electrocardiogram is to exclude the presence of a myocardial infarction. Unfortunately, the finding of a myocardial infarction does not exclude the diagnosis of pulmonary embolism, and in some cases a lung scan or pulmonary angiogram may be required to exclude the diagnosis of embolism.

CHEST RADIOGRAPHY

Although the chest radiograph may suggest the diagnosis of pulmonary embolism because of central vascular enlargement, asymmetry of the vascular markings with segmental or lobar ischemia (Westermark's sign), or pleural effusion, these signs are nonspecific. The chest radiograph then serves to exclude other diagnostic possibilities such as pneumonia, pneumothorax, esophageal perforation, or congestive heart failure. It also is essential in the interpretation of a lung scan, since any radiographic density or evidence of chronic lung disease makes a perfusion defect in that area

TABLE 13-2. Clinical Manifestations of Major Pulmonary Embolism

Symptoms	Incidence (%)	Signs	Incidence (%)
Dyspnea	80	Tachypnea	88
Apprehension	60	Tachycardia	63
Pleural pain	60	Accentuated P_2	60
Cough	50	Rales	51
Hemoptysis	27	S_3 or S_4	47
Syncope	22	Pleural rub	17

(Adapted from Urokinase Pulmonary Embolism Trial: A national cooperative study. Circulation (suppl) 2:47, 1973.)

less likely to represent pulmonary embolism. Chronic lung disease also reduces the applicability of lung scanning to the diagnosis.

ARTERIAL BLOOD GASES

The widespread availability of blood gas and pH determinations has improved the assessment of all critically ill patients and provides important support for the diagnosis of pulmonary embolism. Hypoxemia with PaO_2 less than 60 mmHg is found in the majority of patients and thought to be due to shunting by overperfusion of nonembolized lung and widened alveolar–arterial oxygen gradient due to reduced cardiac output. The reduction in arterial PCO_2 that follows major embolism is the most discriminating finding since hypoxemia can be seen in several disorders likely to be misdiagnosed as massive embolism,[11] such as septic shock. In the absence of hypoxemia and hypocarbia, the diagnosis of major embolism in the severely ill patient can be excluded with a high level of confidence, and an alternative diagnosis should be sought.

CENTRAL VENOUS PRESSURE

In the patient with systemic hypotension, the central venous pressure can provide valuable information as well as access for administration of drugs and fluids. Low central venous pressure virtually excludes pulmonary embolism as the primary cause of the hypotension, since massive embolism almost always is accompanied by right ventricular overload and elevated right atrial pressures. Elevated right ventricular filling pressures may be transient, however, as hemodynamic accommodation occurs, and in subacute or chronic embolism the central venous pressure may be normal.

LUNG SCAN

Availability and widespread usage of lung photoscanning has led to overemphasis on this test and a tendency to overdiagnose pulmonary embolism. In the presence of a normal chest radiograph and in a nonhypotensive patient, the lung scan is a valuable screening test that has increasing validity as the size of the perfusion defect approaches lobar distribution. Smaller peripheral perfusion defects are much more difficult to interpret, since pneumonitis, atelectasis, or other ventilation abnormalities alter pulmonary perfusion. A normal lung scan, on the other hand, usually excludes the diagnosis of pulmonary embolism. Adding a ventilation scan for combined ventilation–perfusion imaging increases the accuracy of the diagnosis of thromboembolism provided that there are at least two moderate size or one large area of ventilation–perfusion mismatch. The assumption that the underperfused regions of the lung after embolism will remain normally ventilated, producing the mismatch in the scans, is clouded by the known physiological effect of bronchoconstriction produced by embolism. Adding the additional variable of wide variance in scan interpretation among observers makes the diagnosis much more reliable when based on arteriography.[2]

PULMONARY ARTERIOGRAPHY

Selective pulmonary arteriography is the most accurate method of confirming the presence, size, and distribution of pulmonary emboli. The procedure is invasive, requiring passage of a cardiac catheter into the main pulmonary artery for injection of a bolus of contrast medium. A rapid film changer produces a series of radiographs that outline areas of decreased perfusion and usually show filling defects or the rounded trailing edge of impacted emboli. Straight cutoffs of the smaller pulmonary arteries are more difficult to interpret, particularly if there is associated chronic lung disease that tends to obliterate pulmonary vessels. The procedure can be performed at low risk, although this is the most hazardous group of patients for this type of study, which usually carries[3] a 0.5 percent mortality.[2] Avoiding injection of contrast into a main pulmonary artery minimizes the complication rate. Additional useful information is obtained prior to contrast injection by measuring pulmonary arterial pressures. A normal pulmonary angiogram excludes the diagnosis of pulmonary embolism in acutely ill patients. Although the resolution rate for pulmonary emboli is unpredictable, it is unrealistic to assume that a negative arteriogram within a week of the clinical event might miss the diagnosis because of rapid fibrinolysis. In the report from the Urokinase Pulmonary Embolism Trial,[35] the earliest complete resolution was not seen before 14 days.

Pathophysiology

Although deep vein thrombosis (DVT) precedes pulmonary embolism, less than 33 percent of patients with documented pulmonary embolism show signs of venous thrombosis. Despite this, it is estimated that 85 to 90 percent of all pulmonary emboli originate from the veins of the lower extremity while the remainder arise from the right side of the heart or other veins. In fact, the lower incidence of DVT after embolism may reflect the evacuation of the thrombus from the lower extremity. In addition, the emboli tend to be multiple, fragmenting either in the right side of the heart or during impaction into the pulmonary vascular bed. Older thrombi, however, contain laminated fibrin layers that make them more solid and more difficult to lyse.

Once the embolus has lodged and interrupted pulmonary blood flow, the ratio of regional ventilation to perfusion increases, and the lung responds by bronchoconstriction to reduce wasted ventilation. This response is mediated by local reduction in CO_2 output, since it can be prevented by ventilation with increased concentration of CO_2. Some experimental studies also suggest a generalized neural reflex vasoconstriction, but even if this occurs in humans, it is not likely to be as significant a factor in survival as the mechanical effect of major vascular occlusion. Similarly, the effects of vasoactive humoral agents can be demonstrated in animals, and there is good documentation that serotonin is elaborated from platelets adherent to the embolus, which also contributes to the bronchoconstriction observed. The ability of heparin to inhibit the release of serotonin adds further weight to the early use of this drug. Other vasoactive agents such as histamine and prostaglandins may play a role in humans, but the net effect is a reduction in size of peripheral airways, reduced lung volume, and reduced static pulmonary compliance.

The hypoxemia that characterizes major embolism is thought to be due to a ventilation–perfusion imbalance secondary to the ventilation changes described above, although the findings in some patients resemble true arteriovenous shunting. The latter becomes anatomically possible if there is an unobliterated foramen ovale that opens in the presence of elevated right atrial pressures. Such an opening can also allow passage of a venous embolus into the systemic circulation, which then is termed paradoxical embolism. Although there may be some improvement in PaO_2 after supplemental oxygen is administered, the effects usually are minimal. The return of pulmonary blood flow effected by embolectomy restores respiratory gas exchange but the ischemia appears to result in some loss of capillary integrity, causing interstitial pulmonary edema, or overt pulmonary hemorrhage.

Pulmonary infarction as a consequence of embolism is relatively rare and associated clinically with problems of poor systemic perfusion such as shock or congestive heart failure. In these patients the symptoms include pleuritic chest pain, dyspnea, cough, and hemoptysis. The signs include fever, tachycardia, splinting, and occasionally friction rub. There is usually prominent leukocytosis, an elevated lactic dehydrogenase level, and bilirubinemia. A wedge-shaped density usually is seen on chest radiography.

The pulmonary vascular and cardiac effects of embolism are a direct consequence of the degree of obstruction of the pulmonary vascular bed. Occlusion of more than 30 percent of the vascular tree is required to begin to elevate mean pulmonary artery pressure, and usually more than 50 percent occlusion is required to reduce systemic pressure. The degree of pulmonary hypertension produced is proportional to the extent of angiographic vascular occlusion, but in a previously normal patient, the limit of pressure generated by the right ventricle is approximately 40 mmHg. The fate of pulmonary embolism in patients is not easy to predict although a great deal of experimental work in animals has been reported. Injection of autologous thrombi into the pulmonary circulation of dogs is followed by relatively rapid recovery of pulmonary function and objective evidence of lysis over a period of weeks. Activation of plasminogen to plasmin, which is found in high concentration in the pulmonary circulation, promotes this fibrinolytic effect. Unfortunately, the resolution of aged thrombi proceeds more slowly and is hampered further by impaction of the embolus and isolation from pulmonary blood flow. Consequently, resolution after massive embolism in patients is unpredictable and often incomplete. It is not unusual to find residual fibrin strands or webs in the pulmonary arteries at autopsy as remnants of prior embolism.

Classification and Management

The hemodynamic variables mentioned above provide a means of classifying patients that uses five grades of severity and is a useful guide to therapy and prognosis[16] (Table 13-3). The minor degrees of embolism (class I and II) usually can be managed by anticoagulants alone with a satisfactory outcome. Heparin is selected for initial treatment in a dose range designed to prolong the partial thromboplastin time to at least twice normal. At this dosage of approximately 150 units/kg, there is adequate protection against further attachment of thrombi and platelets to the embolus. Heparin should be administered intravenously by pump-regulated continuous infusion in a dose that maintains the activated partial thromboplastin time at twice normal. Many clinicians also begin oral anticoagulation therapy with coumarin derivatives shortly after starting heparin administration, to allow several days' overlap of the drugs as prothrombin time is extended into the therapeutic range.

In some patients, however, anticoagulants cannot be used because of associated problems (e.g., peptic ulcer disease), and management must involve a mechanical means of protection against recurrent embolism as outlined previously (Table 13-1). Other patients, in whom anticoagulation appears to be adequate, sustain recurrent embolism and become candidates for

surgical intervention. The third indication for a surgical procedure is to protect against recurrent embolism in a patient who has sustained massive pulmonary embolism requiring open or catheter embolectomy. In these patients, even though a satisfactory embolectomy of the pulmonary circulation has been performed, the original focus of venous thrombosis remains untreated and is very likely to promote recurrent embolism, usually of major size.

There are additional relative indications for vena caval procedures to prevent embolism. One is in the high-risk patient over 40 years of age who is obese, has a serious associated medical illness (e.g., heart disease) or malignant disease, with a history of recent DVT, and who is about to undergo major surgery. Another relative indication exists in the patient with a long, free-floating thrombus at the groin level. The final relative indication is in the patient in whom 40 to 50 percent of the vascular bed has been occluded by embolism (class III) and who would most likely not be able to tolerate an additional embolus, particularly if there is associated cardiac or pulmonary disease.

Pulmonary emboli may accumulate gradually over a prolonged period if they fail to lyse and progressively obliterate small pulmonary arteries. The clinical picture in this case is then of chronic cor pulmonale because significant pulmonary hypertension results from changes in the pulmonary vascular bed (class V). The presentation may be subtle with only dyspnea or syncope on exertion but there is a loud P_2 and right ventricular strain on the electrocardiogram. The sequence may also not be accompanied by significant respiratory symptoms and may explain the cause in some of the patients considered to have primary pulmonary hypertension. From the time that the diagnosis is made there is a very limited life expectancy and the patient may benefit from a vena caval procedure to prevent further embolism even if the disorder is primary pulmonary hypertension.[18] The rationale is that these patients develop right heart failure predisposing to DVT and pulmonary embolism, which is lethal even if small. When acute cardiopulmonary decompensation occurs in these patients after embolism, they are not good candidates for embolectomy because of fixation of the older thrombi to the pulmonary arterial wall.

TABLE 13-3. Classification of Pulmonary Thromboembolism

Class	Symptoms	Gases (mmHg)	PA Occlusion (%)	Hemodynamics
I	None	Normal	<20	Normal
II	Anxiety, hyperventilation	$PaCO_2$ <80 $PaCO_2$ <35	20–30	Tachycardia CVP[a] elevated, $\overline{PA}$[b] >20 mmHg
III	Dyspnea, collapse	$PaCO_2$ <65 $PaCO_2$ <30	30–50	CVP[a] elevated, $\overline{PA}$[b] >25 mmHg, blood pressure <100 mmHg
V	Dyspnea, syncope	$PaCO_2$ <50 $PaCO_2$ <30–40	>50	$\overline{PA}$[b] >40 mmHg, CVP[a] elevated, CO low, no shock

[a] CVP = central venous pressure.
[b] $\overline{PA}$ = mean pulmonary artery pressure.
(Greenfield LJ, Peyton MD, Brown PP, Elkins RC: Transvenous management of pulmonary embolic disease. Ann Surg 180:461, 1974.)

They should be classified separately (class V) and managed by long-term anticoagulation and filter placement.

In cases in which the emboli originate from a septic focus, usually the pelvis in a female patient, the classic treatment has been vena caval ligation with ligation of the ovarian or spermatic veins. It must be recognized, however, that large collateral veins develop as a consequence of vena caval occlusion, that may then become the avenues of recurrent embolism. For this reason, we have used the Greenfield filter at either suprarenal or infrarenal levels in conjunction with antibiotic therapy that can sterilize the stainless steel device.[25]

The methods of vena caval protection were reviewed in the preceding section on acute deep venous thrombosis. It is worth repeating that the present transvenous methods of permanent implantation of devices in the inferior vena cava will probably be greatly enhanced by further technologic improvements.

Pulmonary Embolectomy

For those patients who sustain massive embolism (class III and IV), management must be a coordinated and rapidly responsive effort, since otherwise patients may survive for only a matter of minutes. As indicated earlier, it is critical to document the presence of massive pulmonary embolism by pulmonary arteriography since the clinical diagnosis, regardless of "classic" appearance, is often in error. The initial approach to patients who have either tran-

sient collapse (class III) or persistent systemic hypotension (class IV) should include full heparinization and administration of inotropic drugs if necessary to support the circulation while the diagnosis is confirmed. Isoproterenol (4 mg in 1,000 ml 5 percent dextrose in water) is useful initially because of its bronchodilator and vasodilator effects as well as its positive inotropic cardiac effect. It may provoke arrhythmias, however, and necessitate use of dopamine. For the class II patient who responds to heparin and does not require vasopressors for systemic pressure or urine output, careful monitoring is essential to determine whether anticoagulation alone will control the disorder. Under most circumstances the spontaneous lysis of pulmonary emboli will proceed over a period of days and can be documented by serial lung scans. The rate of clearing may be prolonged for weeks, particularly after sizable embolism, and may be incomplete. The latter condition has been observed in association with persistent pulmonary hypertension even after additional lytic drugs were administered (e.g., urokinase). Lytic agents, however, may become a useful adjunct in the future.

The direct surgical approach to pulmonary embolism was used as early as 1908 by Trendelenburg,[33] who advocated a direct approach to the pulmonary artery at thoracotomy. Without circulatory support, the number of survivors of these efforts was very small, and the first successful case in the United States was not reported until 1958 by Steenberg and coworkers.[29] A modification of this technique using hypothermia to temporarily occlude the circulation was reported by Allison et al.[1] in 1960. The very high mortality rate associated with

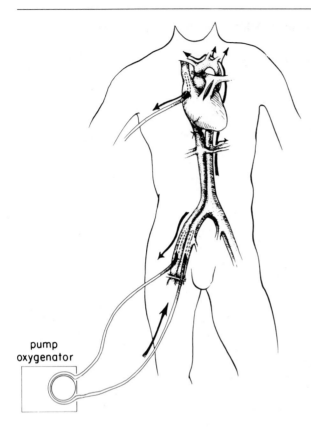

FIG. 13-6 The patient who sustains massive pulmonary embolism with shock (class IV) and fails to respond to resuscitation must be supported by partial bypass and considered for open pulmonary embolectomy. The partial bypass is accomplished by cannulation of the femoral artery and vein under local anesthesia. After general anesthesia is induced and a median sternotomy performed, insertion of a cannula into the superior vena cava and connection to the pump permit conversion to total bypass by snare of the inferior vena cava. The main pulmonary artery is opened, and the emboli are extracted by forceps and suction. (Greenfield LJ: Acute venous thrombosis and pulmonary embolism. p. 418. In Hardy JD (ed): Hardy's Textbook of Surgery. JB Lippincott, Philadelphia, 1983.)

pump
oxygenator

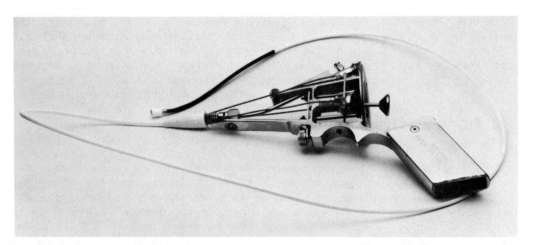

FIG. 13-7 The cup device for catheter embolectomy is attached to a steerable catheter that permits entry into branches of the pulmonary artery through either the femoral or jugular vein after insertion under local anesthesia. The catheter is positioned under fluoroscopy near the embolus identified by angiography. (Reprinted with permission from Greenfield LJ: Pulmonary embolism: Diagnosis and management. In Ravitch A (ed): Current Problems in Surgery. © 1976 by Year Book Medical Publishers, Inc., Chicago.)

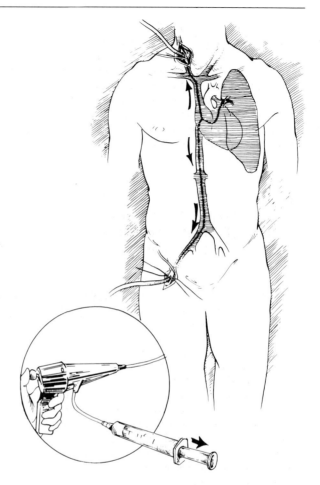

FIG. 13-8 Either the femoral or jugular veins provide access for the embolectomy catheter. The steerable cup is directed under fluoroscopy to the region of the pulmonary artery in which the embolus was identified. After injection of contrast medium to verify proximity to the embolus, the embolus is aspirated into the cup and held there by syringe vacuum while the entire catheter and embolus are withdrawn. (Greenfield LJ: Complications of venous thrombosis and pulmonary embolism. p. 419. In Greenfield LJ (ed): Complications in Surgery and Trauma. JB Lippincott, Philadelphia, 1984.)

the Trendelenburg procedure prompted the use of extracorporeal circulation to bypass the impacted pulmonary circulation. Embolectomy during cardiopulmonary bypass was reported first by Sharp[28] in 1962. Since then partial bypass support has also been utilized. Under local anesthesia, the femoral artery and vein are cannulated for venoarterial bypass. The equipment is fully portable (Fig. 13-6) and the patient can be supported during pulmonary arteriography, then transported to the operating room where general anesthesia and thoracotomy can be performed more safely with the patient on partial cardiopulmonary bypass. Once the sternotomy is performed, the partial bypass can be converted to total bypass by insertion of a superior vena caval catheter; the pulmonary emboli are then removed through a pulmonary arteriotomy.

Open pulmonary embolectomy still carries a high mortality rate, however, and the most serious complication is uncontrollable pulmonary hemorrhage that may follow restoration of pulmonary perfusion.[4] Consequently, an alternative approach utilizing local anesthesia has been suggested by Greenfield et al. for transvenous removal of pulmonary emboli.[16] A cup device attached to a steerable catheter (Fig. 13-7) is inserted in the femoral or jugular vein, and the cup is positioned adjacent to the embolus seen on arteriography. The position is verified by injection of contrast medium through the catheter. Then syringe suction is applied to aspirate the embolus into the cup where it is held by suction as the catheter and captured embolus are withdrawn (Fig. 13-8). Clinical experience[13] with the technique has been reported in 15 patients and showed that emboli could be extracted in 13 (87 percent) with an overall survival of 73 percent. Emboli could not be removed when they had been impacted for more than 72 hours, or if the patient had cardiac arrest at the time of angiography in which case open embolectomy was required. Placement of a Greenfield vena caval filter after removal of sufficient emboli to produce near normal hemodynamics protected the patients from recurrent embolism.

tory function and relief of pulmonary hypertension.[26] For the majority of patients with severe pulmonary hypertension, however, the outlook is poor unless they receive maximum protection from recurrent embolism, which, in our experience, has required both anticoagulation and placement of a vena caval filter.[18]

Chronic Pulmonary Embolism and Pulmonary Hypertension

Recurrent thromboembolism may lead to progressive obliteration of the pulmonary vascular bed if the thrombi fail to undergo lysis. The resultant pulmonary hypertension produces exertional dyspnea and signs of right heart strain with cor pulmonale. With further progression of right heart overload, tricuspid insufficiency may develop. This disorder may be difficult to distinguish from primary pulmonary hypertension although the latter is more likely to be found in women under 20 years of age without a history of deep venous thrombosis. Severe pulmonary hypertension is a serious problem, usually limiting the life expectancy to less than 2 years from diagnosis.

Open thrombectomy for chronic occlusion was first performed by Allison et al.[1] in 1958 and remains a possibility for improving pulmonary blood flow. Unfortunately, for patients to be eligible for this procedure, their occlusion must involve the proximal portion of the pulmonary arterial tree and the distal bed must be patent. The physiologic basis for continued distal patency after proximal occlusion is via bronchial arterial collateral flow. The procedure also has a significant mortality rate, reported at 38 percent by Cabrol et al.[5] in a series of 16 patients. The complications of the procedure reported by these authors include hemorrhagic pneumonitis, cardiac failure, persistent pulmonary hypertension, pulmonary edema, hemothorax, empyema, and pulmonary infarction. The long-term results in surviving patients have been favorable, with improved respira-

REFERENCES

1. Allison PR, Dunhill MS, Marshall R: Pulmonary embolism. Thorax 15: 273, 1960
2. Bell WR, Simon TL: A comparative analysis of pulmonary perfusion scans with pulmonary angiograms—from a national cooperative study. Am Heart J 92: 700, 1976
3. Bonnar J, Walsh J: Prevention of thrombosis after pelvic surgery by British dextran 70. Lancet 1: 614, 1972
4. Brown A, Muller D, Buckberg G: Massive pulmonary hemorrhagic infarction following revascularization of ischemic lungs. Arch Surg 108: 795, 1974
5. Cabrol C, Cabrol A, Acar J et al: Surgical correction of chronic postembolic obstruction of the pulmonary arteries. J Thorac Cardiovasc Surg 76: 742, 1968
6. Cimochowski GE, Evans RH, Zarius CK et al: Greenfield filter versus Mobin-Uddin umbrella: the continuing quest for the ideal method of vena caval interruption. J Thorac Cardiovasc Surg 79: 358, 1980
7. Coon WW, Willis PW III, Keller JB: Venous thromboembolism and other venous disease in the Tecumseh Community Health Study. Circulation 48: 839, 1973
8. Ekberg O: Inherited antithrombin deficiency causing thrombophilia. Thromb Diath Haemost 13: 576, 1965
9. Flanc C, Kakker VV, Clarke MB: The detection of venous thrombosis of the legs using ^{125}I-labeled fibrinogen. Surgery, 55: 742, 1968
10. Goldsmith JC, Lollar P, Hoak JC: Massive fatal pulmonary emboli with fibrinolytic therapy. Circulation 64: 1068–1069, 1982
11. Goodall RJR, Greenfield LJ: Clinical correlations in the diagnosis of pulmonary embolism. Ann Surg 191(2): 219–223, 1980

12. Gore JM, Appelbaum JS, Greene HL et al: Occult cancer in patients with acute pulmonary embolism. Ann Intern Med 96: 556, 1982

13. Greenfield LJ: Intraluminal techniques for vena caval interruption and pulmonary embolectomy. World J Surg 2: 4559, 1978

14. Greenfield LJ: Technical considerations for insertion of vena caval filters. Surg Gynecol Obstet 148: 422, 1979

15. Greenfield LJ, Crute SL: Retrieval of the Kimray-Greenfield® vena caval filter. Surgery 88(5): 719, 1980

16. Greenfield LJ, Peyton MD, Brown PP, Elkins RC: Transvenous management of pulmonary embolic disease. Ann Surg 180: 461, 1974

17. Greenfield LJ, Peyton R, Crute S, Barnes R: Greenfield vena caval filter experience: late results in 156 patients. Arch Surg 116: 1451, 1981

18. Greenfield LJ, Scher LA, Elkins RC: KMA-Greenfield® filter placement for chronic pulmonary hypertension. Ann Surg 189: 560, 1979

19. Greenfield LJ, Stewart JR, Crute S: Improved technique for Greenfield vena caval filter insertion. Surg Gynecol Obstet 156: 217, 1983

20. Hanson EC, Levine FH: Hyperlipoproteinemia as a significant risk factor for pulmonary embolism in patients undergoing coronary artery bypass grafting. Ann Thorac Surg 33: 593, 1982

21. Hirsh J, Hull R: Comparative value of tests for the diagnosis of venous thrombosis. World J Surg 2: 27, 1978

22. Jick H, Porter J: Thrombophlebitis of the lower extremities and ABO blood type. Arch Intern Med 138: 1566, 1978

23. Kakkar VV, Carrigan TP, Spindler JR et al: Efficacy of low doses of heparin in prevention of deep vein thrombosis after major surgery: a double-blind, randomized trial. Lancet 2: 101, 1972

24. Petitti DB, Wingerd J, Pellegrin F, Ramcharon S: Risk of vascular disease in women. JAMA 242: 1150, 1979

25. Peyton JWR, Hylemon MB, Greenfield LJ et al: Comparison of Greenfield filter and vena caval ligation for experimental septic thromboembolism. Surgery 93(4): 533–537, 1983

26. Sabiston DC, Jr., Wolfe WG, Oldham HN, Jr. et al: Surgical management of chronic pulmonary embolism. Ann Surg 185: 699, 1977

27. Seeger WH, Marciniak E: Inhibition of antiprothrombin C activity with plasma. Nature (London) 193: 1188, 1962

28. Sharp EH: Pulmonary embolectomy: successful removal of a massive pulmonary embolus with the support of cardiopulmonary bypass: a case report. Ann Surg 156: 1, 1962

29. Steenburg RW, Warren R, Wilson RE, Rudolf LE: A new look at pulmonary embolectomy. Surg Gynecol Obstet 107: 214, 1958

30. Stewart JR, Peyton JWR, Crute SL, Greenfield LJ: Clinical results of suprarenal placement of the Greenfield vena cava filter. Surgery 92(1): 1–4, 1982

31. Strandness DE, Schultz RD, Sumner DA, Rushmer RF: Ultrasonic flow detection. A useful technique in the evaluation of peripheral vascular disease. Am J Surg, 113: 311, 1967

32. Towne JB, Bernhard VM, Hussey C, Garancis JC: Antithrombin deficiency—a cause of unexplained thrombosis in vascular surgery. Surgery 89: 735, 1981

33. Trendelenburg F: Uber die operative behandlung der Embolie der Lungenarterie. Arch Klin Chir, 86: 686, 1908

34. Trousseau A: Phlegmatia alba dolens. p. 654. In: Clinique Medicale de l'Hotel-Dieu de Paris, Ed. 2, Vol. 3. J.B. Bailliere, Paris, 1865

35. Urokinase Pulmonary Embolism Trial: A national cooperative study. Circulation (Suppl) 2: 47, 1973

36. Wheeler HB, Mullick SC: Detection of venous obstruction in the leg by measurement of electrical impedance. Ann NY Acad Sci 170: 804, 1970

SECTION V

SEPSIS AND SEPTIC SHOCK SYNDROME

14

Immunobiologic Consequences of Trauma and Sepsis

Marc E. Lanser

INTRODUCTION

Infection is the principal cause of death following resuscitation from blunt injury.[88] In some cases, the original tissue injured is the site of infection, such as an area of soft tissue or bony injury, peritoneum following hollow viscus perforation, operative intervention following solid organ injury, or pneumonia following lung contusion. In most cases however, infections are associated with invasive monitoring devices such as intravenous and arterial catheters, urinary catheters, endotracheal tubes and tracheostomies, chest tubes, and peritoneal drainage catheters. Such infections frequently result in secondary bacteremias; however, in a small number of bacteremias, no source of infection can be identified. No study has been performed to date comparing the frequency and type of infections secondary to invasive monitoring devices in the trauma population to infections occurring in a nontraumatized population submitted to similar invasive monitoring. Such a study, though difficult to perform, would be needed in order to define the role of trauma per se in altering host-defense functions and in increasing susceptibility to infection in this monitored population. The generally accepted 20 to 30 percent incidence of infectious complications among traumatized patients appears high and is certainly in need of explanation.

The organisms responsible for these infections are of interest. Schimpff et al.[88] performed an epidemiologic study of the causative organisms responsible for 25 infections in 21 trauma patients. Six patients were admitted with infection, while 15 patients acquired these infections in hospital. These nosocomial infections were caused by organisms of ordinarily low virulence, (Table 14-1) and in most instances followed colonization of the patient from the environment as well as from attending personnel. The finding of an increased incidence of nosocomial infections following trauma due to

TABLE 14-1. Organisms Cultured in 19 Nosocomial Infections from 15 Trauma Patients

Organism	Number of Times Isolated	Percent
Pseudomonas sp	6	25
Staph. epidermidis	5	25
Staph. aureus	2	8
E. coli	3	13
Other gram-negative rods	4	17
Enterococcus	1	4
Alpha Streptococcus	1	4
Candida	1	4
Clostridia perfringens	1	4
Total	24	

(Modified from Schimpff SC, Miller RM, Polakavetz S, Hornick RB: Infection in the severely traumatized patient. Ann Surg 179:352, 1974.)

organisms of low virulence has been noted by others[2] and provides a rationale for the hypothesis that trauma may result in decreased host resistance to infection.

Although definitive proof of this hypothesis is unavailable from clinical studies, experimental studies have been performed that support its validity. Esrig et al.[33] found hemorrhagic shock to increase mortality due to intraperitoneal injection of *E. coli* from 0 to 90 percent. Conolly et al.[22] reported an increased incidence of subcutaneous infections after inoculation of bacteria in animals subjected to blunt trauma. These as well as a few other studies[1,89] are the only experimental evidence that trauma does alter susceptibility to infection. In none of these studies were the mechanisms responsible for this increased susceptibility investigated. Increased susceptibility to infection following burn injury has been somewhat better documented than that following hemorrhage or trauma.[1,55,58] These studies have consistently demonstrated increased mortality from experimental infections after thermal injury. Increased susceptibility is evident within 24 hours and lasts up to 4 days. This period is often followed by increased resistance to infection. These changes are important, as they appear to parallel the changes seen in functional activity of the reticuloendothelial system (RES) following thermal injury.[87]

These simple but important experiments form the basis of the notion that decreased resistance to infection occurs following injury. No clinical studies have been published to prove this hypothesis. Nevertheless, because of the magnitude of the problem of posttraumatic sepsis, much work has focused on the factors responsible for this phenomenon. This chapter considers alterations in lymphocyte, neutrophil, and reticuloendothelial function and their potential roles in mediating decreased resistance to infection following injury. Humoral factors as they relate to cellular function and prospects for therapeutic interventions to improve host–defense function following injury are also discussed.

LYMPHOCYTE FUNCTION FOLLOWING INJURY

Lymphocytes are important mediators of both cellular and humoral immunity. Production of immunoglobulin and its regulation are considered specific immune functions, while all other functions may be considered nonspecific in the sense that products of lymphocyte activation are not antigen specific. These lymphokines affect activity of other cells, notably other lymphocytes and macrophages (Table 14-2). Macrophages and monocytes are also capable of modulating lymphocyte activity and activity of other macrophages.[11,39,96] These cell types are considered together insofar as they effect lymphocyte function.

Immunoglobulin production requires not only intact B cells but T-cell, B-cell, and macrophage interaction. Binding of antigen to

TABLE 14-2. Soluble Lymphocyte Products (Lymphokines) Affecting Other Cell Types

Product	Cell Type(s) Affected	Reference
Interleukin 2	T cells	48, 105
Macrophage activating factor γ-interferon	Macrophages	50, 77, 107
Colony-stimulating factor	Macrophages	67

macrophages results in internalization and modification of antigen. The kind of antigen modification is not well defined. Presentation of antigen by macrophages to lymphocytes (helper-inducer cells bearing Ly1[+] surface antigen) displaying autologous HLA-DR antigens results in T-helper/inducer cell formation.[18,32] Mature helper cell formation is complex and probably occurs via interaction of helper cell precursors (Ly1) with amplifier cells (Ly123). Both are activated by interaction with macrophages bearing HLA-DR–Ag complexes; both cell types are capable of giving rise to mature helper cells.[18] Helper cells may be subdivided on the basis of surface antigen components into Ly1:Qa1[+] and Ly1:Qa1[-]. Signals from both cell types are necessary for optimal activation of B cells. Furthermore, Ly1:Qa1[+] cells are capable of inducing Ly123 cells to manifest suppressor activity, perhaps by transformation to Ly23 cells. A feedback inhibition system involving these subsets of T cells is responsible for modifying the immune response.

Macrophages may not only induce helper cells but may induce suppressor T-cell formation.[96] Data indicate that a subpopulation of macrophages with different I-region antigenic determinants are capable of suppressor cell induction. Usui et al.[96] found that the cell responsible for the induction of the first-order suppressor cell is an Ia-bearing macrophage.

Suppressor cell induction by macrophages may also depend on the functional activity of the macrophage population. Blockade of the RES, which consists of Kupffer cells and other macrophages, with colloidal carbon before intraperitoneal immunization with sheep red blood cells (SRBCs) results in a decrease in the number of SRBCs needed for suppressor cell induction.[106] The increased suppressor activity generated by RES blockade may be attributed to prolonged antigen circulation due to decreased RES clearance of antigen. This in turn results in relative antigen overload. Persistence of antigen has not been documented, although SRBC clearance is known to be depressed following RES blockade. Furthermore, since RES blockade results in a relatively minor prolongation of SRBC circulation, it is difficult to attribute suppressor cell induction to antigen persistence. It appears more reasonable that blockade of a subgroup of splenic

macrophages results in T suppressor cell induction. Regardless of the precise mechanism(s) involved, the relationship of RES blockade to T suppressor cell formation has important implications.

B-cell deficiency results in decreased immunoglobulin production and recurrent bactericidal infections. Large decreases in immunoglobulin levels have not been demonstrated following blunt injury, although IgG and IgM levels show a modest transient decrease following thermal injury.[27] The immunologic response to soluble recall antigens such as tetanus toxoid appears to be intact, although this has not been extensively studied.[4,40] By contrast, the primary antibody response, which requires not only intact B cells but antigen presentation by macrophages bearing Ia antigens and T helper/inducer cell interaction, may be defective following injury.[4,65] Miller and Claudy[66] investigated the primary antibody-forming response of spleen cells isolated from mice following burn injury. In vitro primary antibody production to sheep red blood cells was deficient from 5 to 8 days following a 20 percent third-degree burn. This decrease in antibody production was not due to a B-cell defect, as these cells were competent when isolated from the burn animal, but was due rather to the generation of suppressor T cells following burn injury.[66] The primary antibody response following blunt trauma has not been investigated. Decreased primary antibody formation to neoantigens, due to increased suppressor T-cell activity following trauma, could result in decreased resistance to nosocomial bacteria encountered in intensive care units.

In contrast to intact B-cell immunity, T-cell functions are abnormal following injury. Blunt trauma results in a decrease in the total number of circulating lymphocytes.[12,17] This decrease is due primarily to a fall in the T-lymphocyte population, although small decreases in B-cell numbers have been documented. The degree and duration of such a decrease in circulating T cells are related to the degree of injury and appear to be inversely related to cortisol levels. Bauer et al.[12] were unable to demonstrate any adverse effects of such a decrease. In an experimental model of surgical trauma in mice, Bolton et al.[17] demonstrated a transient decrease in T- and B-cell numbers lasting from

2 to 24 hours and proportional to the severity of injury. Adrenalectomy abolished this lymphopenic response. These studies would seem to implicate cortisol in the regulation of lymphocyte number (although not function) following injury. Burn injury results in a similar but greater depression of T lymphocytes than either blunt or surgical trauma.[104] This transient decrease in T-cell number following injury does not appear to be of any significant biologic consequence insofar as resistance to infection is concerned.

Greater attention has been focused on the generation of suppressor cells following burn and trauma than on the changes in absolute numbers of T and B cells. Assays of lymphocyte activity are performed using a number of stimulants of DNA formation and can be measured by uptake of ^{3}H-thymidine within the newly formed DNA. Mitogenic stimulants most often used are concanavalin A (Con A), phytohemagglutinin (PHA), or pokeweed mitogen; the first two are predominantly T-cell stimulants, while the latter is predominantly a B-cell stimulant. Antigenic stimulants include bacterial lipopolysaccharide (LPS) and SRBCs. Allogenic stimulants are HLA incompatible cells. The use of mitogens measures only proliferative responses to a stimulant and as such may not reflect biologically relevant functions such as in vivo antibody or lymphokine production. This is especially true of Con A and to a lesser extent of PHA. Both mitogens preferentially stimulate suppressor T cells, although other T-cell subsets are stimulated as well.[9] Preferential T suppressor cell stimulation is dose dependent. Low doses may result in only slight suppressor cell induction while high doses may result in substantial suppressor cell induction. Low proliferative responses to Con A may therefore be due to a small percentage of T lymphocytes, inappropriate dosing, or even low numbers of T suppressor cells capable of responding to Con A. Thus, the results of Con A or PHA stimulation assays using whole lymphocyte (and monocyte) populations must therefore be interpreted with caution.

Keeping these limitations in mind, suppression of proliferative and other cell-mediated responses have been documented following trauma. Wang et al.[98] investigated the proliferative response of spleen cells (T cells,

B cells, monocytes, and macrophages) to allogenic stimulants in a mixed lymphocyte culture (MLC). They also tested the cytolytic activity of lymphocytes to mastocytoma cells after activation in allogeneic culture. The MLC response of splenocytes from traumatized mice was significantly decreased at 2 days postinjury. The cytolytic activity of these cells after activation in culture for 5 days was also decreased. This decrease was evident from 2 hours to approximately 6 days after injury. Removal of macrophages from the coculture restored cytolytic activity to normal. Furthermore, addition of traumatized splenocytes or macrophages suppressed a normal ongoing MLC. The cells responsible for suppression of cytolytic activity belonged to a subclass of macrophages bearing Ia antigens. Prostaglandin inhibitors such as indomethacin and acetylsalicylic acid reversed this macrophage-mediated suppression, indicating that macrophage production of prostaglandins may play a role in this suppression. Prostaglandin E (PGE) is released by suppressor cells during the effector phase of lymphocyte reactivity[38] and may have a role in induction of suppressor cells themselves. Addition of prostaglandin inhibitors may work by either inhibiting macrophage or suppressor T-cell production of PGE. In either case, the role of prostaglandins, specifically PGE, in immune suppression is probably an important one. PGE has been implicated as a mediator of postburn immunosuppression by Ninnemann and Stockland.[71]

The cell responsible for suppression of lymphocyte responsiveness following burn injury may be different from that following nonburn trauma. Splenocytes from burned mice are capable of MLC suppression from 4 to 7 days after injury.[66,102] Depletion of T cells with specific antisera eliminates the suppressive effect. These results are consistent with the formation of T suppressor cells. More recently, the identity of the suppressor cell generated following burn has been confirmed using monoclonal antibody to eliminate various T-cell subsets from the MLC. The results indicate that burn generates a suppressor–inducer (Ly1), which then induces the formation of mature suppressor cells (Ly2).[51] Suppression eventually subsides due to feedback inhibition of suppressor–inducer formation. The importance of suppressor

T cells in actually reducing resistance to infection following burn has not been investigated, however.

In addition to experimental work, clinical studies have attempted to define the role of suppressor cell populations in compromising host resistance to infection following burn injury. Miller and Baker[65] correlated the clinical course of burn patients with the in vitro response of their lymphocytes to PHA and their ability to inhibit an ongoing MLR. The PHA responses were markedly depressed in patients who eventually succumbed to infection. Patients who had less severe septic episodes and who responded to antibiotics had supranormal PHA responses. The patients with no sepsis had normal PHA responses. The severity of burn was greater in those patients who had fatal infections and lowest PHA responses. Inhibition of an ongoing MLR was greatest using the most severely burned patients' cells. Although the early PHA response could not differentiate those patients who would and who would not become septic, it was reliable in predicting a fatal outcome. Removal of T cells reversed the MLR inhibition. These studies imply, but do not confirm, that the suppressor cell is a T cell. Munster et al.[69] investigated a series of antigenic stimulants as well as the mitogens Con A and PHA. Longitudinal study revealed progressive decreases in responses to all stimulants except PHA in nonsurvivors. Progressive increases in responses of survivors' cells occurred. There appeared to be no predictive value in terms of development of sepsis. These results were opposite to those of Miller et al.[65] These discrepancies may be explained by the differences in dosages of Con A employed, in view of the variable effect of Con A on suppressor cell induction. Wolfe et al.[103] were able to differentiate nonseptic from future septic patients on the basis of the PHA response before the onset of sepsis. The number of patients in each group was small (nine and four), and only group mean PHA values and not daily values were reported, making the results difficult to interpret. Large differences in depression of the PHA response were apparent between severe burns (81 percent) and less severe burns (39 percent), and the correlation between burn size and depression of the PHA response was quite good. One may conclude that burn size may be the most important independent variable determining both the PHA response and mortality following burn injury. It should be noted that decreases in the PHA mitogenic response has not been a universal finding.[69] Detailed studies investigating other clinical manifestations of T-cell suppression are needed in order to form a complete picture of the biologic significance of suppressor cell formation following burn.

In conclusion, the evidence is substantial that a suppressor cell population is induced for a variable period (usually 4 to 10 days) following burn injury. The evidence for such a phenomenon following nonburn trauma is much less complete. Although intuitively such suppressor cell formation should be related to the development of septic complications following injury, data concerning this important point are far from conclusive. Simultaneous alterations in neutrophil, reticuloendothelial and humoral defense functions (see below) make it extremely difficult to attribute the development of sepsis following injury to any one particular cellular defect.

HUMORAL FACTORS AFFECTING LYMPHOCYTE FUNCTION FOLLOWING TRAUMA

Normal feedback systems exist for the limitation of antibody and lymphokine production from activated B and T cells. The details of this negative feedback system have not been delineated, but undoubtedly they involve induction of suppressor cell activity. As antigenic stimulation proceeds in vitro, T cells bearing Ly123 antigens (suppressors) increase in number, resulting in decreased antibody production. Dysfunction of this negative feedback system may be responsible for the development of numerous autoimmune diseases. There is evidence that following injury, abnormal increases in normal negative feedback mediators as well as appearance of abnormal suppressive factors occur. These factors result in suppression of T-cell function following injury. Prostaglandins E_1 and E_2 are thought to be normal mediators of the immune response; their secretion by macrophages or suppressor T cells, or both, results in decreased T-cell cytolytic activity and decreased antibody production by B cells. Large increases in circulating PGE occur following burn injury.[41] Suppression of the MLC reaction occurs upon addition of burn serum containing elevated levels of PGE, although a direct correlation has not been established between actual percent suppression of the MLC and PGE concentration. In vitro addition of pure PGE_1 and PGE_2 to the MLC reaction also results in a dose-related suppression, which implicates elevated PGE levels following burn as a cause of the observed immunosuppression.

Interleukin 2 (IL-2), or T-cell growth factor, is an important lymphokine that mediates differentiation and proliferation of cytotoxic T lymphocytes (CTL) and enhancement of secretion of macrophage activating factor (MAF) and interferon.[48] Large amounts of IL-2 result in suppressor T-cell induction and decreased CTL activity.[95] Large quantities of IL-2 are released into the circulation after trauma, presumably by macrophages. Such increased quantities of IL-2 may be responsible for immune depression following injury, although this remains speculative, as no studies have been reported correlating IL-2 levels with in vitro lymphocyte suppression following injury.

Mannick and Schmid[61] reported the isolation of a protein subfraction from normal plasma with immunosuppressive properties. This fraction, designated immunoregulatory α-globulin (IRA), inhibits a wide range of T-cell-mediated responses. Appearance of large amounts of a polypeptide with properties resembling IRA have been reported following trauma by Constantian et al.[23] In their series of 109 patients, only 29 were trauma victims; the others were general surgical patients. Suppressive activity was assayed using PHA stimulation of normal lymphocytes. Following minor and moderate injuries, suppressive activity lasted approximately 5 days. In the sera of severely traumatized patients, suppressive activity lasted up to 4 weeks. The amount of suppressive activity correlated with the clinical course as well as with the degree of injury. Although not stated, it appeared from this report that increased suppressive activity was observed in association with sepsis rather than before its development. Others have reported burn sera suppression of the PHA response of normal lymphocytes[5,103]; this suppressive activity is present in sera of all patients regardless of clinical course.[103] Following nonburn trauma, serum suppressive activity appears to correlate somewhat better with the clinical course, being increased only during sepsis.[23]

The available data indicate that serum suppressive activity, at least as measured by suppression of lymphocyte responsiveness to PHA alone, is not an important determinant of host resistance to infection following injury. The limitations of the PHA assay must be kept in mind when evaluating the results of these types of studies.

NEUTROPHIL FUNCTION FOLLOWING TRAUMA

Intact neutrophil function is extremely important for local control of bacterial infections. Numerous syndromes characterized by severe, recurrent infections in association with decreased bactericidal activity have been identified.[10] In general, these recurrent infections have most often been due to gram-positive organisms. Isolated defects in chemotactic activity in association with recurrent infections have also been reported.[79] These chemotactic defects are far less common than either those involving bactericidal activity alone or a combination of bactericidal and chemotactic defects. The existence of these clinically important syndromes is relevant to the study of neutrophil activity following trauma, as injured patients succumb most often to uncontrolled bacterial sepsis following resuscitation. The finding of defects in neutrophil function following trauma, resembling those occurring spontaneously would, for example, be more consistent with the development of the types of infections observed following injury than would alterations in lymphocytic functions. A basic understanding of the physiology of bactericidal activity and chemotaxis is necessary in order to appreciate the alterations of these functions that occur following injury.

Overwhelming experimental evidence supports the view that bacteria are killed predominantly via oxygen-dependent mechanisms. Superoxide (O_2^-) and hydrogen peroxide (H_2O_2), essential for bactericidal activity, are generated by reduction of oxygen by the NADPH oxidase enzyme system.[10] This enzyme system catalyzes the following reaction:

$$2 O_2 + NADPH \rightarrow 2 O_2^- + NADP^+ + H^+$$
$$2 O_2^- + 2 H^+ \rightarrow O_2 + H_2O_2$$

Hexose monophosphate shunt activation regenerates NADPH by the oxidation of glucose to CO_2 and a five-carbon sugar, with $NADP^+$ serving as electron receptor. Production of H_2O_2 as well as hexose monophosphate shunt activity are secondary to the activation of the enzyme NADPH oxidase. All the oxygen consumed during the so-called respiratory burst can be accounted for by O_2^- production.[81]

The NADPH oxidase enzyme is thought to be a pyridine nucleotide-dependent flavoprotein made up of FAD, cytochrome b, and protein.[35] Electron transfer proceeds from NADPH to FAD and then from cytochrome b to O_2, to form O_2^-. Decreased bactericidal activity may result from either defective cytochrome b or flavoprotein comprising the NADPH oxidase complex.

Superoxide may be an important bactericidal species in vivo, although the role for this molecule has been difficult to demonstrate in vitro. Eighty percent of the O_2^- generated is converted to H_2O_2 via superoxide desmutase (SOD). H_2O_2 does have important in vitro bactericidal activity in conjunction with chlo-

ride ion and myeloperoxidase (MPO).[59] The complex of H_2O_2–MPO–C1 (the myeloperoxidase system) is extremely bactericidal, as first shown by Klebanoff.[49] The steps responsible for bacterial killing are halogenation of bacterial amino acids, unstable chloramine formation, and decomposition to aldehyde and free C1[94]:

$$COOH - R\text{-}CHNH_2 + H_2O_2\text{-}MPO\text{-}Cl$$
$$\rightarrow RCHNHClCOOH \rightarrow RCHO + CO_2 + NH_3 + Cl^-$$

Both aldehydes and chlorinated bacterial amino acids are capable of bacterial cell destruction, but the evidence indicates that these are not the most important mechanisms. Singlet oxygen $(^1O_2)$ formed from the reactions

$$OCl^- + H_2O_2 \rightarrow {}^1O_2 + Cl^- + H_2O \text{ and } O_2^- + H_2O_2$$
$$\rightarrow {}^1O_2 + Cl^- + H_2O$$

is thought to be the most important oxygen-derived microbicidal species. Confirmation of the importance of singlet oxygen is lacking because of the difficulty of its specific detection; however, a role for this molecule would seem to resolve some of the difficulties in attributing effective bactericidal activity exclusively to toxic aldehyde production or halogenated amino acid destruction of cell walls. Finally, hydroxyl radical $(OH\cdot)$, perhaps generated by the reaction $O_2^- + H_2O_2 \rightarrow OH\cdot + OH^- + O_2$ (see ref. 13), has been shown to be an active bactericidal species in vitro, although the actual contribution of this molecule to bactericidal activity in vivo remains controversial. A summary of the reactions involved in phagocyte destruction of bacteria is shown in Table 14-3.

TABLE 14-3. Reactions Involved in Formation of Oxygen-Derived Bactericidal Compounds

Reaction	Bactericidal Species Formed
$2 O_2 + NADPH \xrightarrow{\text{NADPH oxidase}} NADP^+ + H^+ + 2O_2^-$	O_2^-
$2 O_2^- + 2 H^+ \longrightarrow O_2 + H_2O_2$	H_2O_2
$R\text{-}CHNH_2 - COOH \xrightarrow{\text{H}_2\text{O}_2\text{-MPO-Cl}} RCHO + CO_2 + NH_3 + Cl^-$ bacterial wall	RCHO
$Cl^- + H_2O_2 \xrightarrow{\text{MPO}} ClO^- + H_2O$ $CO^- + H_2O_2 \longrightarrow {}^1O_2 + Cl^- + H_2O$ $O_2^- + H_2O_2 \longrightarrow {}^1O_2 + Cl^- + H_2O$	 $^1O_2$ $^1O_2$

Measurement of bactericidal activity may be made directly, by measuring the number of surviving bacteria following incubation with neutrophils or indirectly by measuring products of bactericidal-related metabolism. Nitro-blue tetrazolium (NBT) reduction by phagocytes is dependent on respiratory burst activity, and more specifically by O_2^- generated by NADPH oxidase. Reduction of NBT has been used as a convenient screening test for intact bactericidal metabolism. It is depressed in diseases characterized by lack of burst activity. The effect of a number of nonspecific serum factors, as well as phagocytic cell maturity on NBT reduction has resulted in severe limitations in the use of this test. Nevertheless, under strictly defined conditions, this test remains useful as an indirect measurement of bactericidal activity.

We have preferred to use chemiluminescence measurements as a means of monitoring bactericidal activity. The emission of light by stimulated neutrophils was first described by Allen et al.[7] The origin of the emitted light was originally thought to be due to relaxation to ground state of singlet oxygen ($^1O_2$); however, oxidation of other cell membrane constituents or intracellular molecules followed by secondary relaxation may also result in light emission.

Whatever the details of light production, chemiluminescence may be viewed as indirectly reflecting the production of both excited oxygen species and bactericidal activity. The amount of light generation can be amplified by the incorporation in the assay of a cyclic hydrazide, such as luminol.[6] Oxidation of luminol creates activated carbonyl groups that emit large amounts of light upon relaxation. Such light is readily measured in an adapted liquid scintillation counter or in a specially designed photometer. Under specified assay conditions, the amount of light generated correlates well with O_2^- production, hexose monophosphate shunt activity, and actual bacterial killing.[7,43] Although chemiluminescence has the advantage of rapidity and reproducibility, it is acknowledged that the amount of light detected is dependent on a number of variables, such as pH, divalent cations, glucose, and temperature.[37] Furthermore, a number of soluble stimuli such as phorbol myristate acetate (PMA), FMLP, and antigen–antibody complexes are capable of chemiluminescence generation. Phagocytosis is unnecessary,[26] as the respiratory burst and O_2^- production results from membrane "activation" before engulfment.[26,91]

ABNORMALITIES IN NEUTROPHIL BACTERICIDAL ACTIVITY FOLLOWING TRAUMA

Neutrophil bactericidal activity has not been investigated following experimental trauma. Alexander et al.[3] observed cyclic alterations in bactericidal activity of neutrophils from patients following burn. The degree of neutrophil dysfunction appeared to be related to the severity of injury. When examined on a daily basis, large decreases in bactericidal activity appeared to precede the onset of bacteremia. Bactericidal activity of the patients' neutrophils was never equal to the control population. Because the relationship of local bacterial proliferation to the development of documented bacteremia is difficult to analyze, it cannot be concluded that these decreases in neutrophil bactericidal activity resulted in decreased resistance to infection per se. Furthermore, septic processes may have profound effects on bactericidal activity, even without bacteremia. A most conservative interpretation of the data would be that decreases in bactericidal activity are related to bloodstream invasion rather than failure in local control. This difference in interpretation does not negate the potential biologic importance of the findings in this study. Unfortunately, other careful clinical studies have not been performed in a prospective way to further validate this hypothesis.

Elective surgery provokes a 25 percent decrease in bactericidal activity for approximately 1 week, with parallel decreases in intracellular myeloperoxidase.[31] Such decreases in enzyme levels have been attributed to degranulation, with the loss of this enzyme. Such degranulation could account for the decrease in killing capacity deserved. In view of the large (six- to sevenfold) variation in myeloperoxidase activity between different animal species, the significance of such small changes in enzyme levels as a cause of decreased resistance to infection is doubtful. Furthermore, no increased incidence of infection could be demonstrated following a 25 percent decrease in bacterial killing capacity in this surgical population. We recently studied a number of injured patients using chemiluminescence as an index of neutrophil bactericidal activity. We were unable to demonstrate a decreased chemiluminescence response of the patients' isolated washed neutrophils following injury[54] or any difference in response of neutrophils from nonseptic patients or from those in whom sepsis developed. These findings are in agreement with those of Ogle et al.,[76] who found increased numbers of C3b receptors on neutrophils following burn, along with normal or increased bactericidal activity. Clinical studies of bactericidal activity following burn and trauma are complicated by a number of poorly controllable

factors such as drug administration. Many drugs including antibiotics depress neutrophil bactericidal activity.[101] However, we believe that significant intrinsic neutrophil bacterial killing defects do not occur following trauma in the absence of septic complications.

In contrast to the large amount of data concerning serum-mediated effects on lymphocyte function, little has been published concerning serum-mediated effects on neutrophil activity. Using Latex particles as targets, we examined the chemiluminescence response of normal neutrophils incubated in patients' sera following trauma.[54] Patients were divided into those with an uncomplicated posttrauma course and those in whom sepsis had developed. The degree of injury as assessed by an injury severity score was similar in both patient groups. The patients who later developed sepsis had serum that markedly impaired the chemiluminescence response of normal neutrophils (Fig. 14-1). Although sepsis did not occur in any patient before the fourth day following trauma, a dif-

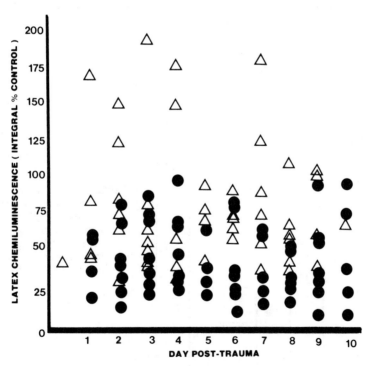

FIG. 14-1 Chemiluminescence response of normal neutrophils incubated in nonseptic or septic trauma serum. Sepsis did not supervene before posttrauma day 4 in any patient. $P < 0.05$ by ANOVA. (△) nonseptic, $N = 10$; (•) septic, $N = 9$.

ference in serum-mediated chemiluminescence was evident immediately after injury. This serum-mediated defect persisted during sepsis and reverted to normal only after the resolution of the infection (Fig. 14-2). Subsequent analysis of the patients' sera revealed the presence of an inhibitor responsible for this decrease in the chemiluminescence response.[54] Although an association was established between decreased serum-mediated chemiluminescence activity and the subsequent development of sepsis, a definite cause and effect could not be proved by this study.

Increased proteolytic activity following trauma may result in the generation of a number of protein cleavage products potentially capable of inhibiting neutrophil function. Fluid-phase C3b, thought to be generated following injury, markedly inhibits neutrophil bactericidal activity.[75] Prostaglandins generated in large amounts following burn also inhibit the chemiluminescence response in vitro. All these serum factors represent potential mediators of serum suppression of neutrophil bactericidal activity. These observations need to be ex-

tended, and the site of action of the suppressor needs to be defined.

ABNORMALITIES IN NEUTROPHIL CHEMOTAXIS FOLLOWING TRAUMA

Directed neutrophil migration (chemotaxis) is the result of a complex series of events resulting in alterations in the cell cytoskeleton.[14] Serum chemotactic factors include the complement-derived factors C3a, C5a, activated factor B, proteolytic enzymes kallikrein and plasminogen activator, and proteolytic fragments such as fibrin-split products and collagen fragments. Neutrophils retain receptor sites for these compounds. Activation involves detection of chemotactic concentration gradients across the cell body, activation

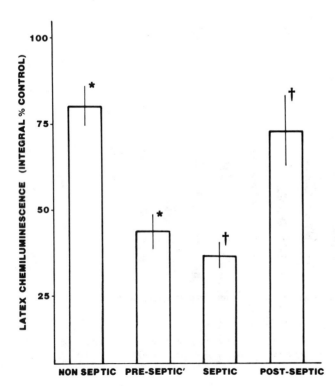

FIG. 14-2 Chemiluminescence response of normal neutrophils incubated in sera from various periods posttrauma in septic patients. Sepsis was defined as a positive blood culture or identification of abscess or gross soft tissue infection. *$P < 0.05$; †$P < 0.05$.

of membrane-bound Na-K-ATPase, and influx of K^+, Mg^{++}, and Ca^{++} with efflux of Na^+.[70] Extracellular concentrations of these ions have profound effects on in vitro chemotaxis and should be taken into account when comparing serum activity from different patients. Intracellular cyclic guanine monophosphate (GMP) and adenosine monophosphate (AMP) appear to regulate the chemotactic response in an unspecified way;[42] increased intracellular cAMP inhibits chemotaxis, while decreased concentrations augment the response. Assembly of microtubules and subsequent microfilament contraction–relaxation is dependent on local cytoplasmic Ca^{++} availability and its regulation. Orientation of the cytoskeleton in parallel with the chemoattractant gradient leads to oriented movement.

Defects in chemotaxis may be due to intrinsic cellular dysfunction. Such dysfunction may result from defective cytoskeletal formation, abnormal GMP : AMP ratios, or membrane defects. These membrane defects may be congenital, such as those associated with neonatal syndromes, or acquired such as those associated with diabetes.[79] Most intrinsic defects in chemotaxis remain uncharacterized. Chemotactic defects associated with recurrent pyogenic infections have been identified. These cellular defects are usually found in association with defects in bactericidal activity but may occur as isolated abnormalities. Infections are usually cutaneous, pulmonary, or pharyngeal. The fact that isolated defects in chemotaxis are associated with clinical disease lends credence to the concept that chemotactic defects following injury may result in increased susceptibility to bacterial infection.

Decreased chemotaxis has been documented following nonburn as well as burn injury.[28] This decrease appears within hours after injury and lasts from 1 to several weeks, depending on the injury severity. Following an experimental 60 percent burn, neutrophil migration into the peritoneum after intraperitoneal injection of bacteria is markedly depressed for at least 1 week after injury.[57] This decrease in in vivo migration correlates with an in vitro decrease in chemotaxis, which appears to be serum mediated. Following experimental hemorrhagic shock, immediate decreases in chemotaxis can be demonstrated,[29]

but this is by no means a universal finding and may depend on the animal species studied. The duration of such a defect or its effect on resistance to sepsis following hemorrhage has not been investigated.

Clinical studies have predominantly identified cellular chemotactic defects, although serum-mediated chemotactic defects have usually not been searched for in a systematic way. Factors such as the severity of burn injury may affect cellular function, while larger burns may result in the generation of serum inhibitors of chemotaxis. The degree of chemotactic depression early after burn injury does not appear to predict the relative risk of developing sepsis.

Following blunt injury, both cellular and serum-mediated abnormalities have been documented,[60] although the corresponding importance of each of these components has not been defined. Preliminary characterization of a naturally occurring 110,000-dalton chemotaxis inhibitor has been described.[21] These various factors may be quite adherent to neutrophil membranes, so that differentiation between serum and cellular components may be difficult. The duration of the chemotactic defect following blunt injury is somewhat less than that following burn injury, perhaps reflecting the lesser severity of the blunt trauma. The early chemotactic response of neutrophils from nonseptic patients has not differed from that of future septic patients, nor has the degree of severity of the chemotactic defect been shown to be related to the development of infection.

RETICULOENDOTHELIAL FUNCTION FOLLOWING TRAUMA

The RES is comprised of macrophages situated in the liver (Kupffer cells), spleen, bone marrow, and lung, as well as mobile macrophages within soft tissues. Ninety percent of the phagocytic capacity of the RES resides in liver Kupffer cells. All cells of the RES, including Kupffer cells, are derived from bone marrow precursors.[25] These cells then undergo a change in phenotype, with alterations in phagocytic, metabolic, and antigen-processing functions. This discussion is confined to Kupffer cell phagocytosis of circulating antigen.

Ninety percent of an injected bacterial load is cleared by the liver in one passage. These cells are not limited to phagocytosis of bacteria, however. Kupffer cells actively remove foreign cellular antigens, platelet aggregates, tissue fragments, viral antigens, antigen–antibody complexes, and altered proteins.[83] These cells possess Fc, C3, and fibronectin receptors.[73,82] In acquiring enhanced phagocytic capacity, Kupffer cells have lost much of their capacity as antigen-presenting cells. Their role in classic immunity remains obscure.

Modulation of Kupffer cell phagocytic activity is important to understand in order to appreciate the role of this cell in host defense following trauma. Saturation of Fc and C3 receptors following injection of IgG or complement-coated particles results in a reversible depression of receptor-mediated phagocytosis.[73] This depression lasts for 6 to 12 hours and is related to the dose of particles used. Trauma may result in the discharge into the circulation of particulate matter, including antibody–antigen complexes capable of occupying these receptors. This trauma-induced RES depression may explain the decreased clearance of bacteria, antigens, or other complement-activating particulate matter following receptor occupation.

Bacterial clearance by the RES is depressed following intravenous injection of a number of different types of particles capable of activating the alternative complement pathway,[45] implying that occupation of receptor sites does have a role in depression of such clearance. A similar depression of bacterial clearance has been demonstrated following experimental trauma.[46]

Another important factor modulating RES uptake of various particles is the concentration of opsonic fibronectin in plasma. The physiologic role of this 440,000-MW glycoprotein in RES function has been fully reviewed by Saba and Jaffe.[85] This molecule possesses binding sites for collagen, bacteria, complement components, and cell membranes.[82] Its depletion results in RES "blockade," characterized by decreased clearance of gelatinized test particles. Trauma results in depression of reticuloendothelial phagocytic function as measured by particle[8] or bacterial clearance.[46] In association with this depression, there is a corresponding fall in opsonic fibronectin levels.[84] As a result of decreased RES uptake, the number of particles trapped in the lung increases. In addition to RES depression, increased particle entrapment in the lung is partly due to neutrophil margination and phagocytosis, as neutropenic animals do not demonstrate increased lung localization of particles in spite of RES depression.[52] Traumatic depression of RES function seems to be associated with neutrophil margination within the pulmonary vascular bed. These marginated neutrophils then may act as a competitive phagocytic filter in the lung. A scheme of the possible relationship between RES depression and posttraumatic respiratory distress is shown in Figure 14-3.

Administration of purified fibronectin to rats following mild surgical trauma results in correction of RES phagocytic defects and reduction in the lung localization of particles.[84] These results have not been duplicated following either RES blockade or burn injury.[52] In these cases, fibronectin administration is only partially successful in restoring RES phagocytic activity. Administration of cryoprecipitate, rich in opsonic fibronectin, to septic trauma and surgical patients results in restoration of fibronectin levels and is associated with temporary improvement in some cardiorespiratory parameters.[90]

Clinically it is difficult to measure RES phagocytic function directly, as this involves injection of radiolabeled colloidal particles such as microaggregated albumin.[44] Because of the close correlation between fibronectin levels and RES function in experimental trauma, fibronectin concentrations have been used as a noninvasive index of RES function. This assumption may not entirely be justified, as discrepancies between these two variables following burn and infection have been noted. Factors affecting RES phagocytic function other than opsonic fibronectin levels are probably important under most conditions. Nevertheless, we have found that levels of this protein are of predictive value following trauma. Figure 14-4 shows the effect of blunt trauma on op-

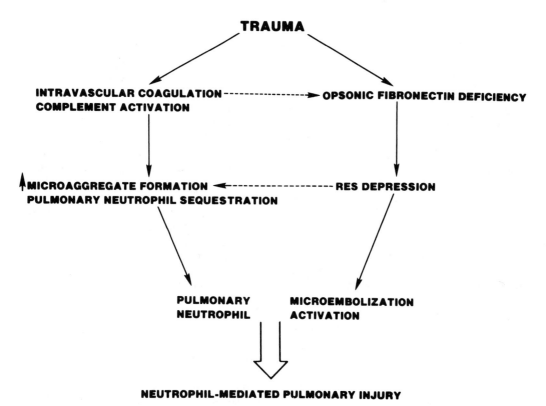

FIG. 14-3 Proposed pathophysiology of ARDS in relationship to RE phagocytic depression.

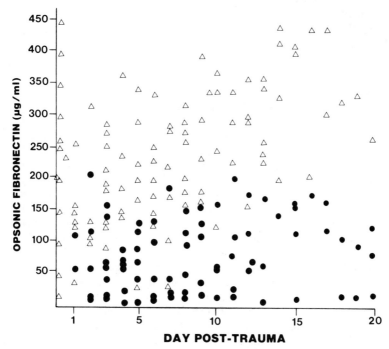

FIG. 14-4 Daily serum opsonic fibronectin levels from nonseptic and septic trauma patients. Sepsis did not supervene prior to posttrauma day 4 in any patient. $P < 0.001$ by ANOVA. ($\triangle$) nonseptic; ($\bullet$) septic.

sonic fibronectin levels. Patients in whom sepsis subsequently developed had significantly lower levels of this protein, even immediately after injury, as compared with nonseptic patients. These low levels returned to normal following the resolution of sepsis. Until actual measurements of RES phagocytic function are performed in these patients, one cannot state unequivocably that decreased RES phagocytic activity is responsible for an increased risk of the development of sepsis following injury. Fibronectin depletion itself has been found to increase susceptibility to infection in experimental animals,[53] so it is not unreasonable that trauma-induced depletion would have similar results. It must be recognized, however, that administration of this protein has not as yet been shown to reduce susceptibility to infection following trauma in either experimental animals or human subjects.

CUTANEOUS ANERGY IN RELATIONSHIP TO HOST DEFENSE FUNCTION FOLLOWING INJURY

The delayed hypersensitivity reaction (DHR) is predominantly a T-cell and macrophage-mediated inflammatory response to locally injected recall antigens. Production of IL-2, macrophage activating factor, and other lymphokines from activated T cells results in macrophage recruitment and activation. The response is modulated by suppressor T cells and possibly by neuropeptides such as substance P and somatostatin.[78]

Anergy is defined as the lack of response to skin tests to which the individual has previously been exposed. Anergy is associated with numerous medical conditions such as viral illnesses, vaccination, syphilis, malnutrition, cirrhosis, advanced age, and proliferative blood disorders. The mechanisms responsible for anergy in these conditions are not completely understood, although soluble mediators from suppressive T cells appear to be important. Macrophage dysfunction and altered neuropeptide secretion may have a role in the production of anergy as well.

Meakins et al.[64] found an association between anergy and increased mortality in a heterogeneous general surgical population. Reversal of the anergic state after operation or drainage of abscesses was associated with clinical improvement and a reduced mortality. The degree of anergy seems to be correlated with the severity of injury[63] and of infection.[62] Since patients have not, in general, been carefully stratified to control for the degree or type of illness, one cannot conclude that anergy per se is an independent variable that determines the development of sepsis. In evaluating a homogeneous group of elective surgical patients, most of whom had malignancy, a nonsignificant higher incidence of sepsis and mortality was found in the anergic subgroup. These two subgroups of reactive and anergic patients did not seem to have the same severity of illness, as a greater number of patients with advanced inoperable malignancy were in the anergic group.

Moderate injury as well as surgical trauma are associated with temporary reversible anergy.[30,92] The degree and duration of anergy are related to the severity of injury, but differences in outcome between reactive and anergic patients with the same severity of injury have not been demonstrated. Patients with more severe injuries and who are anergic have a higher incidence of sepsis and mortality than do those with less severe injuries who are reactive. Anergy persists for 4 days to 2 weeks following injury[20] but is prolonged in patients in whom sepsis develops. When delayed hypersensitivity is tested immediately after injury, there is little difference in the incidence of sepsis in anergic patients compared with reactive patients.

Following a standard, clean surgical procedure of moderate severity (nephrectomy), almost all patients exhibit anergy and decreased lymphocyte reactivity.[92] These alterations begin with induction of anesthesia and last 4 to 5 days in the case of depressed lymphocyte reactivity and 2 weeks in the case of anergy.

In general, the results of delayed hypersensitivity testing have not correlated with in vitro lymphocyte reactivity testing. This is not surprising in view of the complex cellular and humoral interactions that comprise the generation of the DTH response. The coexistence of a circulating immunosuppressive serum factor with anergy has been reported,[56] but this has not been a universal finding.

In summary, in numerous clinical conditions, delayed hypersensitivity reactivity reflects host resistance. These include malignancy, infection, and perhaps malnutrition.[93] Under these circumstances, anergy is a function of the severity of illness and may not be a truly independent variable determining host resistance to infection. Nevertheless, anergy does have predictive value in these conditions. By contrast, the appearance of anergy after surgery or trauma is a universal finding following all but the most trivial of injuries. The presence of anergy itself does not predict the development of septic complications under these circumstances; however, specific abnormalities responsible for the anergic state certainly could contribute to increased susceptibility to infec-

tion following injury. Hypersensitivity testing should be conducted within the context of investigative protocols with proper stratification of patients in an attempt to clearly define the role of anergy as a predictor of increased susceptibility to infection following injury.

ALTERATIONS IN COMPLEMENT ACTIVITY FOLLOWING INJURY

The complement system subserves many important biologic functions related to host defense. These include opsonization of bacteria and other antigens, promotion of phagocytosis of antibody–antigen complexes, direct cell lysis, neutrophil adherence and chemotaxis, and regulation of T- and B-cell activity.[100] Complement activation proceeds via the construction of enzyme complexes containing catalytic sites composed of serine proteases. The basic outline of the sequential activation of the complement pathways is shown in Figure 14-5. C3 con-

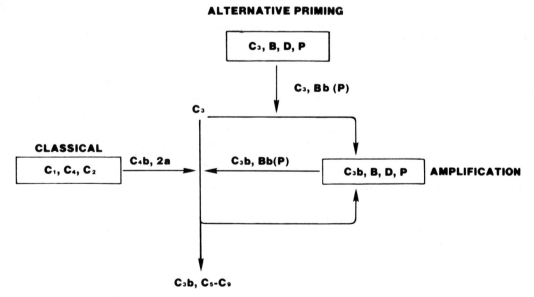

FIG. 14-5 Complement activation via classic and alternative pathways.

version represents the confluence of the classic and alternative complement pathways. The C3 convertases are C4bC2a in the classic pathway and C3bBb in the alternative pathway. In addition, an amplification loop exists, resulting in repetitive activation of C3 by membrane-bound C3b in conjunction with circulating factors B and D. Cleavage products C3a and C5a produced during complement activation have chemotactic, anaphylotoxic, and immune-modulating activity. C3a suppresses in vitro antibody production via activation of suppressor–inducer cells (Ly1), but it has no effect on the lymphocyte proliferative response.[68] C5a augments in vitro antibody production via activation of macrophages, perhaps by increasing their IL-1 production. Fluid-phase-generated C3b has been shown to be a strong inhibitor of neutrophil bactericidal activity.[75] Generation of large amounts of fluid-phase C3b following injury could therefore adversely affect neutrophil function.[100] These immunoregulatory properties of complement fragments may have important implications for the immune response following injury, when activation of the complement system occurs.

Control of the alternative pathway cascade occurs after nascent C3b formation. Competition between factors B and β-1-H (C3b inactivator–accelerator) for bound C3b determines whether alternative pathway activation occurs. This depends on the surface properties of the particle to which the C3b is attached.[34] Nonactivators of the alternate pathway favor β-1-H binding to C3b. This results in inactivation of C3b by C3bINA (C3b inactivator).

Classic pathway activation proceeds following noncovalent binding of the C1 complex (C1q $_{\text{C1s2}}^{\text{C1r2}}$) to an antibody–antigen complex.[80] It is now appreciated that many substances bind C1 in the absence of antibody.[24] These include bacterial lipid A, CRP complexes, certain gram-negative bacteria, and cellular membranes. Following C1 binding, further activation is controlled by C1 inactivator, which is capable of dissociating C1r and C1s and C1q. The exposed collagenlike part of C1q following removal of C1r and C1s may bind to fibronectin as well as to other cell membranes.[80] In this way, fibronectin may mediate clearance of various parti-

cles capable of binding C1 but incapable of activating the entire complement cascade.

Most studies of complement alterations following injury have been in the area of burns. Using a standard CH_{50} titration technique as a measure of functional classic pathway activity, only relatively minor and transient (4- to 5-day) decreases in activity have been documented.[16,36] Immunoreactive C_4 levels are decreased in a corresponding fashion. These mild changes in classic pathway activity are similar to those described following blunt and penetrating injury, and do not seem to be of major biologic significance. Alternative pathway activity is affected to a much greater degree than is classic pathway activity.[36] Measurement of immunoreactive levels of factors B and D following burn do not reveal striking abnormalities. By contrast, functional hemolytic activity of the alternative pathway is markedly depressed (approximately 90 percent) following burn. Studies comparing nonseptic and septic burn patients have not been performed using this sensitive technique. Such decreases are undoubtedly capable of reducing the host-defense response to neoantigens to which the host has no prior immunity. The decrease in such activity is probably due to activation of the alternative pathway by the burn injury. Nonburn trauma has not been adequately investigated, but indications are that similar decreases in alternative pathway activity exist. Decreased opsonic activity of sera for a number of bacteria has been demonstrated following burn injury. This decrease is found only with certain bacterial strains and does not correlate with measured immunoreactive levels of complement components.[15] This is not surprising in view of the enormous excess of most complement components in serum.

Trauma-induced activation of the alternative complement pathway may have several adverse effects. Decreased resistance to nosocomial bacteria may result if prior exposure has not occurred. Generated C3a and C5a may affect T-cell function, resulting in depression of the primary antibody response. Generation of fluid-phase C3b as well as other complement cleavage products has been shown to affect neutrophil activity adversely. Nonimmune binding of C1q to membrane fragments and damaged platelets may result in RES depression by depleting fibronectin. Microaggregates formed following trauma may be cleared by either fibronectin or C3b-mediated binding to reticuloendothelial cells. Such binding may result in decreased C3 and fibronectin–receptor availability for subsequent bacterial clearance.

THERAPEUTIC MANIPULATION OF IMMUNITY AND FUTURE PERSPECTIVES

Immunomodulation has the potential of reversing a number of the aforementioned abnormalities in various host-defense functions following injury. Difficulty arises from the fact that a clear cause-and-effect relationship between any one abnormality and decreased resistance to infection cannot be demonstrated. If decreased resistance to infection following trauma is indeed multifactorial, improvement in any one function could not be expected to modify outcome. Without a better understanding of the contribution of each of the numerous host-defense functions following injury, empirical therapy would appear to be premature. Experimental animal models may to a large extent help to clarify these problems. No detailed immunologic studies have as yet been performed using experimental models of injury. This work is critical before widespread acceptance of immunomodulating therapy in patients can be achieved.

Attempts have been made to alter lymphocyte reactivity following injury. Kupper et al.[51] restored in vitro lymphocyte reactivity in rats following burn by administration of low-dose cyclophosphamide. This drug has also been shown to improve delayed hypersensitivity reactivity; apparently, it works by destruction of suppressor-inducer cells without affecting other cell types at the dosage given. Changes in resistance to infection following such therapy have not been investigated.

Plasma exchange has been used on a limited basis in an attempt to eliminate putative serum suppressor factors generated following burn injury.[72] Such therapy has the theoretical advantage of eliminating several serum factors responsible for suppression of lymphocyte neutrophil and RES function. In one recent case of serum-mediated depression of neutrophil chemiluminescence (15 percent of normal), plasma exchange increased the chemiluminescence response to 50 percent of normal, with return to pretherapy levels within 12 hours following plasma exchange.[54] Plasma exchange has been used in a small number of patients following burn. Lymphocyte reactivity was partially restored, accompanied by "improvement" in clinical course. Within the context of a controlled clinical trial and using measurement of host-defense variables in order to monitor results, the use of this modality appears justified. In view of our current understanding of the pathophysiology of host-defense failure following injury and the apparent importance of poorly defined serum factors, plasma exchange using fresh-frozen plasma offers the potential of significant benefit.

Attempts have been made to correct RES function following injury by infusion of fibronectin-rich cryoprecipitate. Fibronectin levels can be restored in both experimental animals[84] and human subjects[86] with such therapy, and reticuloendothelial phagocytic function can be corrected in experimental animals. In a clinical report, transient improvement in cardiopulmonary function did occur[90] although the benefit was short lived. Appropriate controls have not been included in any of the clinical trials using this form of therapy, nor has resistance to infection been evaluated. Fibronectin levels can also be increased with plasma exchange (M.E. Lanser, unpublished data), though perhaps not as rapidly as with cryoprecipitate or opsonic fibronectin infusion. Until more experimental data are accumulated confirming the efficacy of fibronectin administration as immunotherapy, the use of plasma exchange for this purpose would seem to be preferable.

Other experimental, nonspecific immunomodulators, such as levamisole, FMLP, bacillus Calmette-Guérin (BCG), and glucagon, have not been applied clinically to any significant degree following injury. Investigation with these compounds is continuing, but clinical applicability remains remote.

REFERENCES

1. Alexander JW: Effect of thermal injury upon the early resistance to infection. J Surg Res 8: 238, 1969
2. Alexander JW, Hegg M, Altemeier WA: Neutrophil Function in Selected Surgical Disorders. Ann Surg 168: 447, 1968
3. Alexander JW, Meakins JL: A physiological basis for the development of opportunistic infections in man. Ann Surg 176: 273, 1972
4. Alexander JW, Moncrief JA: Alterations of the immune response following severe thermal injury. Arch Surg 93: 75, 1966
5. Alexander JW, Ogle CK, Stinnett JD, MacMillan BG: A sequential, prospective analysis of immunologic abnormalities and infection following severe thermal injury. Ann Surg 188: 809, 1978
6. Allen RC, Loose LD: Phagocytic activation of luminol-dependent chemiluminescence in rabbit alveolar and peritoneal macrophages. Biochem Biophys Res Commun 69: 245, 1976
7. Allen RC, Stjernholm RL, Steele RH: Evidence for the generation of an electronic excitation state(s) in human polymorphonuclear leukocytes and its participation in bactericidal activity. Biochem Biophys Res Commun 47: 679, 1972
8. Altura BM, Hershey SG: RES phagocytic function in trauma and adaptation to experimental shock. Am J Physiol 215: 1414, 1968
9. Armitstead JG, Ewan PW: Concanavalin A-induced suppressor cells. J Clin Lab Immunol 13: 1, 1984
10. Babior BM: Oxygen-dependent microbial killing by phagocytes. N Engl J Med 298: 721, 1978
11. Baker CC, Miller CL, Trunkey DD, Lim RC: Identity of mononuclear cells which compromise the resistance of trauma patients. J Surg Res 26: 478, 1979
12. Bauer AR, McNeil C, Trentelman E, et al: The depression of T lymphocytes after trauma. Am J Surg 136: 674, 1978
13. Beauchamp C, Fridovich I: A mechanism for the production of ethylene from methional: The generation of hydroxyl radical by xanthine oxidase. J Biol Chem 245: 4641, 1970
14. Becker EL: Stimulated neutrophil locomotion. Arch Pathol Lab Med 101: 509, 1977
15. Bjornson HB, Bjornson HS, Altemeier WA: Serum-mediated inhibition of polymorphonuclear leukocyte function following burn injury. Ann Surg 194: 568, 1981
16. Bjornson AB, Altemeier WA, Bjornson HS, et al: Host defense against opportunist microorganisms following trauma. Ann Surg 188: 93, 1978
17. Bolton PM, Kirov SM, Donald KJ: The effects of major and minor trauma on lymphocyte kinetics in mice. Aust J Exp Biol Med Sci 57: 479, 1979
18. Cantor H and Gershon RK: Immunological circuits: Cellular composition. Fed Proc 38: 2058, 1979
19. Cheung K, Archibald AC, Robinson MF: The origin of chemiluminescence produced by neutrophils stimulated by opsonized zymosan. J Immunol 130: 2324, 1983
20. Christou NV, McLean APH, Meakins JL: Host defense in blunt trauma: Interrelations of kinetics of anergy and depressed neutrophil function, neutrophil status and sepsis. J Trauma 20:833, 1980
21. Christou NV, Meakins JL: Neutrophil function in surgical patients: Two inhibitors of granulocyte chemotaxis associated with sepsis. J Surg Res 26: 355, 1979
22. Conolly WB, Hunt TK, Sonne M, Dunphy JE: Influence of distant trauma on local wound infection. Surg Gynecol Obstet 128: 713, 1969
23. Constantian MB, Menzoian JO, Numberg RB, et al: Association of a circulating immunosuppressive polypeptide with operative and accidental trauma. Ann Surg 183: 73, 1977
24. Cooper NR: Activation and regulation of the first complement component. Fed Proc 42: 134, 1983
25. Crofton RW, Desselhoff-den Dulk MM, Van-Furth R: Origin, kinetics and characteristics of kupffer cells in the normal steady state. J Exp Med 148: 1, 1978
26. Dahinden CA, Fehr J, Hugli TE: Role of cell surface contact in the kinetics of superoxide production by granulocytes. J Clin Invest 72: 113, 1983
27. Daniels JC, Larson DL, Abston S, Ritzmann SE: Serum protein profiles in thermal burns. I: Serum electrophoretic patterns, immunoglobulins and transport proteins. J Trauma 14: 137, 1974
28. Davis JM, Dineen P, Gallin JI: Neutrophil degranulation and abnormal chemotaxis after thermal injury. J Immunol 124: 1467, 1980
29. Davis JM, Stevens JM, Peitzman A, et al: Neutrophil migratory activity in severe hemorrhagic shock. Circ Shock 10: 199, 1983

30. Dawson CW, Ledgerwood AM, Rosenberg JC, Lucas CE: Anergy and altered lymphocyte function in the injured patient. Am Surg 48: 397, 1982

31. El-Maallem H, Fletcher J: Effects of surgery on neutrophil granulocyte function. Infect Immun 32: 38, 1981

32. Engleman EG, Benike CJ, Grumet FC, Evans RL: Activation of human T lymphocyte subsets: Helper and suppressor/cytotoxic T cells recognize and respond to distinct histocompatibility antigens. J Immunol 127: 212, 1981

33. Esrig BC, Frazee L, Stephenson SF, et al: The predisposition to infection following hemorrhagic shock. Surg Gynecol Obstet 144: 915, 1977

34. Fearon DT, Austen KF: Activation of the alternative complement pathway due to resistance of zymosan-bound amplification convertase to endogenous regulatory mechanisms. Proc Natl Acad Sci USA 74: 1683, 1977

35. Gabig TG: The NADPH-dependent O_2^--generating oxidase from human neutrophils. J Biol Chem 258: 6352, 1983

36. Gelfand JA, Donelan M, Burke JF: Preferential activation and depletion of the alternative complement pathway by burn injury. Ann Surg 198: 58, 1983

37. Glette J, Solberg CO, Lehmann V: Factors influencing human polymorphonuclear leukocyte chemiluminescence. Acta Pathol microbiol Immunol 90: 91, 1982

38. Goodwin JS: Modulation of concanavalin A-induced suppressor cell activation by prostaglandin E_2. Cell Immunol 49: 421, 1980

39. Gorczynski RM: Control of the immune response: Role of macrophages in regulation of antibody and cell-mediated immune responses. Scand J Immunol 5: 1031, 1976

40. Havens WP, Boch DG, Siegel L: Capacity of seriously wounded patients to produce antibody. J Clin Invest 33: 940, 1954

41. Heggers JP, Loy GL, Robson MC, et al: histological demonstration of prostaglandins and thromboxanes in burned tissue. J Surg Res 28: 110, 1980

42. Hill HR, Estenson RD, Quie PG, et al: Modulation of neutrophil chemotactic responses by cyclic 3′,5′ guanosine monophosphate and cyclic 3′, 5′ adenosine monophosphate. Metabolism 24: 447, 1975

43. Horan TD, English D, McPherson TA: Association of neutrophil chemiluminescence with microbicidal activity. Clin Immunol Immunopathol 22: 259, 1982

44. Ilo M, Wagner H: Studies of the reticuloendothelial system (RES). I: Measurement of the phagocytic capacity of the RES in man and dog. J Clin Invest 42: 417, 1963

45. Jenkin CR, Rowley D: The role of opsonins in the clearance of living and inert particles by cells of the reticuloendothelial system. J Exp Med 114: 363, 1961

46. Kaplan JE, Scovill WA, Bernard H, et al: Reticuloendothelial phagocytic response to bacterial challenge after traumatic shock. Circ Shock 4: 1, 1977

47. Kelso A, Glasebrook AL: Secretion of interleukin 2, macrophage activating factor, interferon, and colony-stimulating factor by alloreactive T lymphocyte clones. J Immunol 132: 2924, 1984

48. Kelso A, MacDonald HR, Smith KA, et al: Interleukin 2 enhancement of lymphokine secretion by T lymphocytes: Analysis of established clones and primary limiting dilution microcultures. J Immunol 132: 2932, 1984

49. Klebanoff SJ: A peroxidase-mediated antimicrobial system in leukocytes. J Clin Invest 46: 1078, 1967

50. Klein JR, Raulet DH, Pasternack MS, Bevan MJ: Cytotoxic T lymphocytes produce immune interferon in response to antigen or mitogen. J Exp Med 155: 1198, 1982

51. Kupper TS, Greene DR, Chaudry IH, et al: A cyclophosphamide-sensitive suppressor T cell circuit induced by thermal injury. Surgery 95: 699, 1984

52. Lanser ME, Saba TM: Neutrophil mediated lung localization of bacteria: A mechanism for pulmonary injury. Surgery 90: 473, 1981

53. Lanser ME, Saba TM: Opsonic fibronectin depletion and sepsis: Cause or effect? Ann Surg 195: 340, 1982

54. Lanser ME, Mao P, Brown G, et al: Serum-mediated depression of neutrophil chemiluminescence following blunt trauma. Ann Surg 202: 111, 1985

55. Liedberg CF: Antibacterial resistance in burns. II. The effect of unspecified humoral defense mechanisms, phagocytosis, and the development of bacteremia. An experimental study in the guinea pig. Acta Chir Scand 121: 351, 1961

56. McLaughlin GA, Wu AV, Saporoschetz I et al: Correlation between anergy and a circulating immunosuppressive factor following major surgical trauma. Ann Surg 190: 297, 1979

57. McManus AT: Examination of neutrophil function in a rat model of decreased host resistance following burn trauma. Rev Infect Dis 5(S5): S898, 1983

58. McRipley RJ, Garrison DW: Increased susceptibility of burned rats to pseudomones aeuru genosa. Proc Soc Exp Biol Med 115: 336, 1964

59. McRipley RJ, Sbarra AJ: Role of the phagocyte in host–parasite interactions. XII. Hydrogen peroxide-myeloperoxidase bactericidal system

in the phagocyte. J Bacteriol 94: 1425, 1967

60. Maderazo EG, Albano SD, Woronick CL, et al: Polymorphonuclear leukocyte migration abnormalities and their significance in seriously traumatized patients. Ann Surg 198: 736, 1983

61. Mannick JA, Schmid K: Prolongation of allograft survival by an alpha globulin isolated from normal blood. Transplantation 5: 1231, 1967

62. Meakins JL, Chistou NV, Shizgal HM, MacLean LD: Therapeutic approaches to anergy in surgical patients: Surgery and levamisole. Ann Surg 190: 286, 1979

63. Meakins JL, McLean APH, Kelly R, et al: Delayed hypersensitivity and neutrophil chemotaxis: Effect of trauma. Ann Surg 18: 240, 1978

64. Meakins JL, Pietsch JB, Bubenick O, et al: Delayed hypersensitivity: Indication of acquired failure of host defenses in sepsis and trauma. Ann Surg 186: 241, 1977

65. Miller CL, Baker CC: Changes in lymphocyte activity after thermal injury. J Clin Invest 63: 202, 1979

66. Miller CL, Claudy BJ: Suppressor T-cell activity induced as a result of thermal injury. Cell Immunol 44: 201, 1979

67. Moore RN, Hoffeld JT, Farrar JJ, et al: Role of colony-stimulating factors as primary regulators of macrophage functions. Lymphokines 3: 119, 1981

68. Morgan EL, Weigle WO, Hugli TE: Anaphylatoxin-mediated regulation of the immune response. I. C_3a-mediated suppression of human and murine humoral immune responses. J Exp Med 155: 1412, 1982

69. Munster AM, Winchurch RA, Burmingham WJ, Keeling P: Longitudinal assay of lymphocyte responsiveness in patients with major burns. Ann Surg 192: 772, 1980

70. Naccache P, Freer RJ, Showell HS, et al: Cation fluxes and chemotaxis in leukocytes. Fed Proc 35: 604, 1976

71. Ninnemann JL, Stockland AE: Participation of prostaglandin E in immunosuppression following thermal injury. J Trauma 24: 201, 1984

72. Ninnemann JL, Stratta RJ, Wanden GD, et al: The effect of plasma exchange on lymphocyte suppression after burn. Arch Surg 119: 33, 1984

73. Nishi T, Bhan AK, Collins AB, McCluskey RT: Effect of circulating immune complexes on Fc and C_3 receptors of Kupffer cells *in vivo*. Lab Invest 44: 442, 1981

74. Ogle CK, Ogle JD, Alexander JW: Comparison of C_3 levels in patients' sera using both anti BIC/1A and anti-C_3b. Fed Proc 39: 700, 1980

75. Ogle JD, Ogle CK, Alexander JW: Inhibition of neutrophil function by fluid phase C_3b of complement. Infect Immun 40: 967, 1983

76. Ogle JD, Ogle CK, Noel JG, Alexander JW: De-termination of C_3b receptors on normal and patient polymorphonuclear neutrophils with C_3b-coated fluorescent microspheres. Arch Surg 120: 104, 1985

77. Pace JL, Russell SW, Schreiber RD, et al: Macrophage activation: primary activity from a T-cell hybridoma is attributable to interferon-γ. Proc Natl Acad Sci USA 80: 3782, 1983

78. Payan DG, Levine J, Goetzl EJ: Modulation of immunity and hypersensitivity by sensory neuropeptides. J Immunol 132: 1601, 1984

79. Quie PG, Cates KL: Clinical conditions associated with defective polymorphonuclear leukocyte chemotaxis. Am J Pathol 88: 711, 1977

80. Reid KBM: Proteins involved in the activation and control of the two pathways of human complement. Biochem Soc Trans 11: 1, 1983

81. Root RK, Metcalf JA: H_2O_2 release from human granulocytes during phagocytosis: Relationship to superoxide anion formation and cellular catabolism of H_2O_2: Studies with normal and cytochalasin B treated cells. J Clin Invest 60: 1266, 1977

82. Ruoslahti E, Engvall E, Hayman EG: Fibronectin: Current concepts of its structure and functions. Cell Res 1: 95, 1981

83. Saba TM: Physiology and physiopathology of the reticuloendothelial system. Arch Intern Med 126: 1031, 1970

84. Saba TM, Cho E: Reticuloendothelial systemic response to operative trauma as influenced by cryoprecipitate or cold-insoluble globulin therapy. J Reticuloendothel Soc 26: 171, 1979

85. Saba TM, Jaffe E: Plasma fibronectin (opsonic glycoprotein): Its synthesis by vascular endothelial cells and role in cardiopulmonary integrity after trauma as related to reticuloendothelial function. Am J Med 68: 577, 1980

86. Saba TM, Blumenstock FA, Powers SR: Cryoprecipitate reversal of opsonic α_2 surface binding glycoprotein deficiency in septic surgical and trauma patients. Science 201: 622, 1978

87. Schildt BE: Function of the RES after thermal and mechanical trauma in mice. Acta Chir Scand 136: 359, 1970

88. Schimpff SC, Miller RM, Polakavetz S, Hornick RB: Infection in the severely traumatized patient. Ann Surg 179: 352, 1974

89. Schweinburg FB, Frank HA, and Fine J: Bacterial factor in experimental hemorrhagic shock. Am J Physiol 179: 532, 1954

90. Scovill WA, Annest SJ, Saba TM, et al: Cardiovascular hemodynamics after opsonic alpha-2-surface binding glycoprotein therapy in injured patients. Surgery 86: 284, 1979

91. Sklar LA, Jesaitis AJ, Painter RG, Cochrane CG: Ligand/receptor internalization: A spectroscopic analysis and a comparison of ligand

binding, cellular response and internalization by human neutrophils. J Cell Biochem 20: 193, 1982

92. Slade MS, Simmons RL, Yanis E, Greenberg LJ: Immunodepression after major surgery in normal patients. Surgery 78: 363, 1975

93. Spanier AH, Pietsch JB, Meakins JL, et al: The relationship between immune competence and nutrition. Surg Forum 26: 332, 1976

94. Strauss RR, Paul BB, Jacob AA, et al: Role of the phagocyte in host-parasite interactions. XXII. H_2O_2-dependent decarboxylation and deamination by myeloperoxidase and its relationship to antimicrobial activity. J Reticuloendothel Soc 7: 754, 1970

95. Ting CC, Yang SS, Hargrove ME: Induction of suppressor T cells by Interleukin 2. J Immunol 133: 261, 1984

96. Usui M, Aoki I, Sunshine GH, Dorf ME: A role for macrophages in suppressor cell induction. J Immunol 132: 1728, 1984

97. Wang BS, Heacock EH, Mannick JA: Characterization of suppressor cells generated in mice after surgical trauma. Clin Immunol Immunopathol 24: 161, 1982

98. Wang BS, Heacock EH, Wu AV, Mannick JA: Generation of suppressor cells in mice after surgical trauma. J Clin Invest 66: 200, 1980

99. Ward PA, Bergenberg JL: Defective regulation of inflammatory mediators in Hodgkins disease: Supernormal levels of chemotactic-factor inactivator. N Engl J Med 290: 76, 1974

100. Weigle WO, Morgan EL, Goodman MG, et al: Modulation of the immune response by anaphylatoxin in the microenvironment of the interacting cells. Fed Proc 41: 3099, 1982

101. Welch WP, Davis D, Thrupp LD: Effect of antimicrobial agents on human polymorphonuclear leukocyte microbicidal function. Antimicrob Agent Chemother 20: 15, 1981

102. Winchurch RA, Munster AM: Post-traumatic activation of suppressor cells. J Reticuloendothel Soc 27: 83, 1980

103. Wolfe JH, Saporoschetz I, Young AE, et al: Suppressive serum, suppressor lymphocytes and death from burns. Ann Surg 193: 513, 1981

104. Wood GW, Volenec FJ, Mani MM, Humphrey LJ: Dynamics of T-lymphocyte subpopulations and T-lymphocyte function following thermal injury. Clin Exp Immunol 31: 291, 1978

105. Yamanoto JK, Farrar WL, Johnson HM: Interleukin 2 regulation of mitogen induction of immune interferon (IFNγ) in spleen cells and lymphocytes. Cell Immunol 66: 333, 1982

106. Yoshikai Y, Miake S, Matsumoto T, et al: Effect of stimulation and blockade of the mononuclear phagocyte system on the induction of suppressor T cells of delayed footpad reaction to SRBC in mice. Immunology 6: 241, 1981

107. Zlotnik A, Roberts WK, Vasil A, et al: Coordinate production by a T cell hybridoma of α interferon and three other lymphokine activities: Multiple activities of a single lymphokine? J Immunol 131: 794, 1983

15

Sepsis, Abnormal Metabolic Control, and the Multiple Organ Failure Syndrome

John H. Siegel
Thomas C. Vary

THE HOST RESPONSE TO SEPSIS

Sepsis is a disease of host response to invasion by infectious organisms. It represents a complex interaction of primary humoral and secondary cellular immunity. The humoral response induces a primary sequence of relatively nonspecific immunologic reactions in which preformed antibodies and acute phase proteins such as C-reactive protein and opsonic fibronectin bind to antibody proteins on the cell walls of the offending organisms.[7,67,74,137] Hageman factor is activated, which initiates coagulation in areas of injury and bradykinin-mediated permeability changes.[90,137] This is followed by activation of the classic sequence of complement activation[136,137] (in some in-

stances the alternative or properdin pathway may also be activated[40]) in which C5a enhances leukocyte or macrophage aggregation and opsonization of the bacterial or fungal organism and C3a, by inducing leukocyte production of oxygen free radicals in the form of superoxides, results in damage to the micro-organism's cell membrane.[3] These two phenomena, aided by the bacterial trapping in fibrin and fibronectin binding, facilitate bacterial ingestion by defending white cells and promote changes in the invading organism's internal milieu that facilitate leukocyte bacterial killing and lysis.[67,137] Other aspects of these "septic" mechanisms induce blast transformation and proliferation of leukocytes, promote their migration and adherence to the invading organisms, and to nonviable or damaged tissue, as well as inducing the production of leukocyte proteases, which complete the work of bacterial destruction and dead tissue proteolysis, thereby facilitating their removal[67,137] (see Chapter 3). Other less well defined eicosanoid and humoral factors liberated by this process also activate the reticuloendothelial system, induce stimulation of

The work reported in this chapter was supported in part by grants HL 29280 from the National Heart Lung and Blood Institute and GM-36139 from the National Institute of General Medical Sciences and by the Shock Trauma Research Fund.

411

cellular immunity, and change the balance between suppressor, helper, and killer lymphocytes to deal with the secondary organism and tissue-specific aspects of this process[77,85,88,93,99, 137,160] (see Chapter 14). In the course of this humoral response, a number of mediators of vasoconstriction (thromboxane A_2), vasodilatation (prostacyclin), and vascular permeability changes (prostaglandins and leukotrienes) are produced that may act beneficially or deleteriously on the effectiveness of the host response and, in some instances, may cause specific aspects of the multiple organ failure syndrome[16,24,56,58,68,72,73,77,100,161,171] (see Chapters 3, 14, and 18).

Finally, to complete the host response, a metabolic mediator, interleukin I, is produced by macrophage activation and interacts with a complex neuroendocrine alteration in the hormonal balance that regulates body metabolism.[5,7,25-27,34,81,156] These mechanisms shift metabolic balance from a state of homeostasis and anabolism to one of oxidative catabolism and muscle proteolysis with an alteration in the fuel-energy balance between skeletal muscle, liver, and adipose tissue.[11,20,21,71,82-84,95,109,119,124,124,143,151,169] This altered interorgan metabolic balance results in a shift of glucose metabolism away from the peripheral tissues to the liver.[71,82,124,125,151,153,174] At the same time, the hepatocytes appear to be activated to increase production of a variety of acute phase proteins that are essential in the primary humoral aspects of host defense and damage control,[67,81,118] at the expense of other hepatic proteins that are more important for the homeostatic functions of nutritional transport.[118] In addition, there may be direct effects of bacteria or bacterial components on the metabolic control of the balance between carbohydrate and lipid metabolism that are tissue-specific and may enhance the altered interorgan substrate-energy flow.[95,98,143,152,153,158,175]

In summary, rather than being a disease process caused by infectious organisms, sepsis is an acquired disease of intermediary metabolism induced by the host response to invasion by infectious agents. The nature and magnitude of this metabolic disorder are not specific to any particular infectious agents, having been demonstrated to occur with bacterial, fungal, and viral organisms.[33,165] The metabolic dysfunction initiated by sepsis induces a fundamental shift in the pattern of physiologic abnor-

malities and dynamic metabolic interrelations involved in the regulation of energetic substrate flux between skeletal muscle, liver, and adipose tissue, thus modifying the normal balance of control by neuroendocrine mechanisms.

Specifically, sepsis alters regulation of utilization of glucose, lipids, and amino acid substrates, as well as the generation of oxidative energy. The amino acid abnormalities appear to interact with the stress-induced sympathetic response because of a defect in the hepatocyte metabolism of aromatic amino acids.[20,45,105,108,125,131,157] Evidence has accumulated that strongly suggests that this particular defect is related to the production of pathophysiologic vasoactive substances that produce a characteristic abnormality of peripheral vascular pressure flow relations (reduced vascular tone). These sepsis-induced aromatic amino acid abnormalities in vascular tone are similar to those found in patients with cirrhotic hepatocellular disease. In both sepsis and cirrhotic liver disease the reduction in vascular tone appears to be the key initiating factor in the development of the hyperdynamic cardiovascular response.[131] However, a reflex sympathetic cardiac inotropic compensation for these septic vascular tone abnormalities is necessary for the compensatory septic hyperdynamic state, which always occurs unless the myocardial contractile response is depressed by the septic episode, or by pre-existing cardiac disease.[29,123,125,131] This response, which is associated with an increase in oxygen consumption,[86,125,131,133] had been demonstrated to be critical for survival in severe sepsis.[29,133,146,162]

The hyperdynamic cardiovascular response is also accompanied by an increase in pulmonary blood flow[129,130] and this interacts with septic immunologic mediator-induced alterations in pulmonary capillary permeability[58,122,155] to produce the septic adult respiratory distress syndrome (ARDS). This pathologic phenomenon in turn reduces respiratory gas exchange in the lung and is not infrequently the fatal aspect of the septic process.[28,86,122,129,134,155] This is discussed in greater detail in Chapter 19.

However, the aspect of the septic process that influences the probability of survival most strongly is the magnitude of the fuel-energy defect produced by the sepsis-mediated abnormalities in intermediary metabolism. The initial phase of the septic metabolic response is directed at the skeletal muscle, where a reduction in muscle glucose oxidation is associated with increased proteolysis. However, when these defects become severe they induce a form of protein/calorie malnutrition that has been called the "septic autocannibalism" of skeletal muscle.[21] This phenomenon, which may be linked to the mediator-induced macrophage production of interleukin I[5,34] or its proteolysis-inducing factor (PIF),[27] changes the balance between the hepatic elaboration of normal host defense acute phase proteins and the reparative synthesis of osmotically active and nutritional transport proteins. This occurs at the same time as it enhances proteolysis of muscle proteins with release into plasma of endogenous amino acids needed for energy generation and protein synthesis in the liver.

Under circumstances where the septic process becomes uncontrolled (whether bacteria are cultured in the blood stream or not), the level of fuel-energy metabolism in the liver also becomes abnormal at the same time as skeletal muscle protein catabolism is further enhanced and urea synthesis is markedly increased. Under these circumstances, there appears to be a reprioritization of acute phase proteins with a reduced capability for the synthesis of reparative and nutritional substance transporting proteins and a shift toward the synthesis of complement-activating, superoxide scavenger, and protease-inhibiting plasma proteins.[118]

When this deteriorating phase of the septic response occurs, there frequently is evidence of a reduction in oxidative metabolism correlated to the decreased organ clearance of a number of body fuels. This alteration in oxidative energetic metabolism can be detected from physiologic studies carried out at the bedside: the patient manifests a progressive hyperdynamic high cardiac output state at the same time as a reduction in the extraction of oxygen by the periphery. In this instance the arteriovenous oxygen content gradient narrows disproportionately to the increase in total body flow, so that total oxygen consumption decreases even though oxygen delivery is increased.[125,132,133] Clinically, such patients are characterized by evidence of a progressive inflammatory response with leucocytosis, fever, tachycardia, peripheral vasodilatation with a bounding pulse pressure, and evidence of an extremely high cardiac output state. They also

demonstrate a progressive inability to metabolize intravenously administered carbohydrates, amino acids, and eventually the fats used for nutritional support and show rising plasma levels of glucose, lactate, alanine, and triglycerides. As a result, despite an iatrogenically administered high-calorie intake, they manifest marked muscle wasting and weight loss, which may be hidden at times by a tendency to interstitial fluid retention and edema.

When the final phase of septic metabolic failure is reached, there is evidence of progressive primary hepatocellular dysfunction, initially manifested by alterations in the organ clearances of a variety of substrates metabolized by the liver, later by the appearance of incompletely metabolized byproducts of hemoglobin metabolism with a rising bilirubin level, and eventually by evidence of hepatocyte damage with leakage of hepatocellular enzymes into the peripheral plasma. At the final stage of this process even the fundamental processes of urea synthesis and finally gluconeogenesis may be interfered with, so that an actual reduction in blood urea nitrogen and preterminal hypoglycemia may occur. In conjunction with this deteriorating metabolic aspect of the process, which has been called the multiple organ failure syndrome (MOFS), not only are myocardial and late pulmonary failure detected, but renal decompensation also occurs.[6,37,47,48] This is initially manifested by a high-output renal failure with a falling creatinine clearance, later by tubular failure, and finally by oliguria. The ubiquitous nature of these cellular abnormalities and the generalized nature of the failures in the metabolic process also can be seen in the development of profound skin test anergy, selective failures of acute phase protein synthesis, lymphopenia, and inadequate wound healing.[6,16,47,48] The development of this multiple organ failure, which is primarily a cellular failure, represents a serious and usually fatal transition in the septic patient.[6,16,47,124]

These are primarily failures of various aspects of the metabolic host defense mechanisms. While they are initiated by the invasion of pathologic organisms (often of high virulence), they may eventually become secondary defects, themselves permitting host invasion and tissue destruction by normally nonpathogenic organisms of little or no virulence in the noncompromised host. As a result, bacterial saprophytes, protozoic organisms, fungi, mycoplasmic, or viral organisms may appear and flourish in the deteriorating host, who becomes a defenseless culture medium.

Of greatest interest with regard to the cause of sepsis is the observation that major trauma and/or hemorrhagic shock appears to produce factors that interfere with the initial host defense response mechanisms to enhance the development of sepsis and lead to MOFS.[72,73,77,142] By observing the changes in the physiologic and metabolic aspects of this defense response over time, it becomes possible to predict the likelihood of development of severe sepsis as well as the probability of survival, based on the initial and sequential adaptive responses to traumatic or surgical injury.[146] It also may be possible, by the use of pattern recognition techniques, to identify these interactive failures and quantify the response to therapy early in the patient's course. As will be shown, this may enable the surgeon or intensive care physician to intervene at the critical time with the correct combination of physiologic, antibiotic, and nutritional therapies to support the appropriate surgical measure to drain or excise the septic process, prior to decompensation of the host response. To this end, a number of major efforts have been undertaken to provide a quantitative staging of the septic process using cardiovascular and metabolic variables that can be obtained at the bedside and reflect the adequacy of the host defense response to sepsis.[46,125,127,128,132,143]

APPLICATION OF PATTERN RECOGNITION TO THE QUANTIFICATION OF CARDIOVASCULAR AND METABOLIC ABNORMALITIES IN HUMAN SEPSIS

The nature of the metabolic and physiologic response in sepsis can be identified by the pattern of physiologic adaptation. This pattern reflects the adequacy of the organization of host defenses and arises out of the degree of intactness of the cellular and interorgan fuel-energy metabolism and the adequacy of the immunologic response mechanisms. A method for quantifying the pattern of physiologic abnormalities in patients with or without sepsis has been developed that uses the principles of statistical pattern recognition.[46,127,128,132] This method has been applied to a set of simultaneously obtained multivariable physiologic data from patients with various forms of shock or critical illness. This approach to pattern recognition is based on the use of a frame of reference and a scale of change derived from a concept of a normal adaptive stress response to injury. The importance of such a quantification method for use in clinical studies is obvious, since, unlike in experimental studies where a known type and quantity of bacterial inoculum can be introduced at a particular moment and the evolution of course of the process studied, in the clinical situation the time of the initiating insult, the magnitude of the bacterial or fungal challenge, and the nature of the specific patient's host defense are all variables whose parameters and magnitude are generally unknown. As a result, the human septic process may proceed slowly, or with great rapidity, and may induce a mild, minimal, or considerable host defense response which can be quantified by the varying patterns of organ adaptation to the septic process.

The changing temporal pattern of physiologic compensation is seen in Figure 15-1, which demonstrates the time course of the cardiac index, oxygen saturation and oxygen consumption, arterial PCO_2 and total peripheral resistance from a 62-year-old woman with severe intra-abdominal sepsis. In contrast to patients with hypovolemic shock (Chapter 9), in severe sepsis and septic shock there is an increased, rather than a decreased, cardiac index, which in this patient tended to be greater than 4 L/min/m² throughout most of her course. Oxygen consumption was normal, increased, or actually decreased at a time when cardiac index was at its highest. The decrease in oxygen consumption was not due to failure of delivery, but rather to a failure of oxygen extraction, since at the time of the lowest oxygen consumption the mixed venous oxygen saturation, and content, rose so that the arteriove-

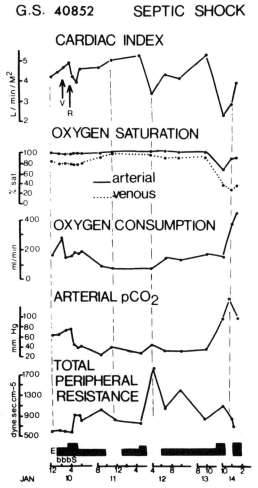

G.S. 40852   SEPTIC SHOCK

FIG. 15-1 Clinical course of patient in hyperdynamic septic shock. A 62-year-old woman with subdiaphragmatic abscess after anastomotic leak from esophagojejuneostomy following total gastrectomy for carcinoma of the stomach. E, epinephrine drip; black bar, isoproterenol infusion (2 to 4 μg/min); b, 44 mEq sodium bicarbonate; S, 1 gm solumedrol; V, 500 ml/lactated Ringers in push; R, initiation of volume cycle respirator support. (Siegel JH, Greenspan M, DelGuercio LRM: Abnormal vascular tone, defective oxygen transport and myocardial failure in human septic shock. Ann Surg 165: 504, 1967.)

nous difference narrowed. This can be seen from the time course of arterial and mixed venous oxygen saturations in Figure 15-1. At these times in this spontaneously breathing patient, there was also a tendency for hyperventi-

lation so that the arterial PCO_2 also reached its lowest point. Throughout most of the course, the peripheral pressure flow/relationships are also seen to be abnormal, with a marked reduction in total peripheral resistance at the time of high cardiac output.

To quantify these processes requires a quantitative classification methodology in order to obtain a bedside index of severity. This has practical considerations in the management of the various aspects of organ failure in the septic patient. The technique that has been developed uses multivariable physiologic data analysis from the pattern of physiologic and metabolic data obtained from control patients and those with various forms of shock and critical illness.[46,125-129] The fundamental principle behind this approach is that the frame of reference and the necessary scale to measure change can be developed from normally responding general surgical patients, based on the concept that there is a control unstressed state and a normal adaptive stress response to injury. By applying statistical clustering techniques,[46,132] it has been possible to delineate four abnormal physiologic patterns whose recognition can permit a quantitative classification of the spectrum of clinical severity in patients with various forms of trauma, sepsis, or cardiogenic illness.[125,127] This methodology has been implemented on a minicomputer so that rapid assessment of the patient's physiologic state can be obtained from bedside physiologic studies.[126]

Classification of Physiologic State

By quantitatively comparing an individual patient to the prototypical, or mean, patient variable pattern of the nonstressed control reference state (R) and each of the four pathophysiologic states (A,B,C, and D) in Figure 15-2, one can assess the nature and severity of an individual patient's physiologic compensation at a given moment in time[126,127] (see Chapter 9). As will be shown later, in sepsis each of these pathophysiologic states has a direct correlation with a specific pattern of biochemi-

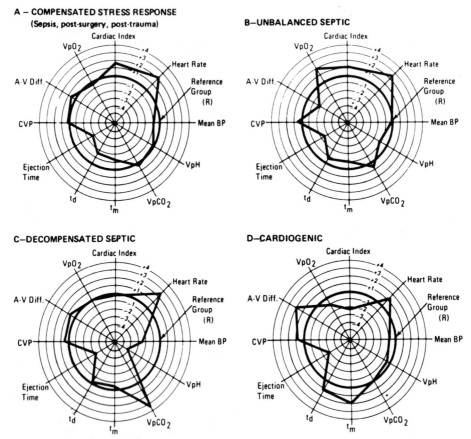

FIG. 15-2. Circle diagrams of physiologic states. Shown are the prototype mean patterns for the A, B, C, and D states. The perfect dark circle in the center of each pattern equals 0 standard deviations from the reference control (R) state. Each dotted line represents 1 standard deviation from R, either increased or decreased. The rays of the circle diagram represent respectively cardiac index, heart rate, mean blood pressure, mixed venous pH (VpH), mixed venous CO_2 tension ($VpCO_2$), cardiac washout time (t_m), pulmonary mean transit time (t_d), cardiac ejection time, right atrial pressure (CVP), arteriovenous oxygen content difference (A-V Diff) and mixed venous oxygen tension (VpO_2). (Siegel JH, Farrell EJ, Goldwyn RM, Friedman HP: The surgical implications of physiologic patterns in myocardial infarction shock. Surgery 72: 126, 1972.)

cal abnormalities that suggests a particular type of fuel-energy deficit. The A to B state transformation can be interpreted as showing the presence and the severity of the hepatic aspect of septic MOFS.[108,125,131]

In physiologic terms, the A state is a normal stress response seen in compensated sepsis and after trauma or major operative intervention. It is characterized by a sympathetic response in which heart rate (HR) and cardiac index (CI) increase, and there is an improve-

ment in contractility (a reduced cardiac washout time [tm] equals an increased ejection fraction [EFx]). The oxygen consumption index ($O_2CI = A\text{-}VO_2Diff \times CI$) increases. This sympathetic adaptation response occurs without any evidence of metabolic abnormality and minimal respiratory dysfunction. The failure to achieve an A state response in the presence of a major septic or posttraumatic stress is an abnormal physiologic response pattern.

The B state is also a hyperdynamic cardiovascular state, but it represents a more severe stage of deterioration in the septic process. The increased cardiac index and other evidences of sympathetic response (reduced tm and increased EFx, increased heart rate, decreased systolic ejection time [ET] are insufficient, or unable, to supply peripheral needs. Consequently, the consumption of oxygen is normal or reduced, when it should be increased, because of a disproportionately reduced arteriovenous oxygen extraction gradient compared to the increase in body flow (CI). A metabolic acidosis always occurs, although it may be masked by compensatory respiratory alkalosis. As will be shown later, this B-state reduction in the consumption of oxygen is a direct manifestation of reduced cellular oxidative metabolism. In the C state, respiratory decompensation is superimposed on the unbalanced septic process and on the metabolic acidosis seen in the B state, and retention of carbon dioxide with profound respiratory acidosis occurs.

In contrast to the B and C states, the D, or cardiogenic state, represents a pattern of primary myocardial rather than peripheral failure. In this state, there is a decrease in myocardial contractile function manifested by a prolonged cardiac washout time (tm) reflecting a reduced ejection fraction (EFx).[128,130,145] The cardiac index falls, and the A-VO$_2$Diff (Ca$-\bar{v}$O$_2$) widens as the body's extraction of oxygen increases to compensate for the low flow state. Thus, the D state is a delivery failure rather than an extraction failure (B state) of oxygen consumption. Unless hypovolemia is also associated with the cardiac failure, which may occur in hemorrhage or after surgery, the pulmonary blood volume (DV/m^2) rises. Hypotension and acidosis may occur. Although this pattern is characteristic of acute myocardial infarction, it also occurs in patients after cardiac surgery who show myocardial depression and after a period of profound hypovolemic shock. However, it also occurs as a result of biventricular septic myocardial depression, where it appears to be a manifestation of myocardial metabolic insufficiency occurring in association with the transition to, or after a period of, B state hyperdynamic metabolic insufficiency.[125,130,131]

CARDIOVASCULAR RESPONSE TO SEPSIS

Extensive analysis of the relationship between the metabolic abnormalities and the physiologic ones reflected in the physiologic state suggests that the septic cardiovascular response is an adaptation to the underlying fundamental metabolic abnormalities in intermediary metabolism. As a result, it is possible to interpret the cardiovascular dynamics in sepsis as reflecting the level of adequacy of the physiologic response to the underlying pathologic metabolic process that created the imbalance. For instance, the transformation from A to B state appears to indicate the development of a significant degree of hepatic insufficiency. As is shown in Figure 15-3, the cardiovascular response in patients with sepsis, compared to those without sepsis, is best demonstrated with regard to the relationship between peripheral resistance (TPR) and cardiac output.

In Figure 15-3, the patients are labeled by the closest physiologic state "distance" (see Chapter 9) to the prototypic patterns shown in Figure 15-2. This figure also demonstrates lines of constant cardiac minute work (normal nonseptic patients of similar age have a cardiac output between 5 and 6 L/min with a peripheral vascular resistance of 1200 to 1500 dyne sec cm^{-5} and a mean cardiac work of 6 kg m/min). As is shown in this figure, hyperdynamic septic patients in the A and B state of septic decompensation have increased cardiac outputs, which are generally greater than 6 L/min with a peripheral resistance level of less than 1100 dyne sec cm^{-5}.

Statistical analysis has demonstrated that this alteration in the vascular pressure/flow relationship of the body (vascular tone) is the primary physiologic vascular manifestation of the septic process.[129,131,133] As shown in Figure 15-4, and commented on earlier in Chapters 5 and 9, there are different relationships between cardiac output and total peripheral resistance in patients who manifest a hyperdynamic response to general surgical procedures, or to trauma, compared to those who have sepsis,

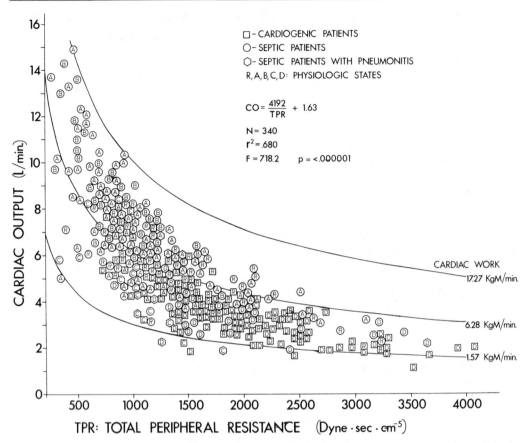

FIG. 15-3 Relation between cardiac output and total peripheral resistance labeled by classification of physiologic state (R,A,B,C,D). Lines of constant cardiac work in kg/min. (Siegel JH, Cerra FB, Coleman B et al: Physiological and metabolic correlations in human sepsis. Surgery 86: 163, 1979).

or intrinsic hepatocellular disease secondary to cirrhotic liver disease. In each of these groups, the vascular tone, which is defined as the level of peripheral vascular resistance at a given cardiac output, decreases as a function of the degree of chronic hepatocellular disease, or the acute hepatocellular dysfunction induced by sepsis. When both chronic and acute hepatocellular metabolic abnormalities are combined, such as in the patient with cirrhotic liver disease who also has sepsis, the vascular tone relationship is the lowest, as shown in Figure 15-4. These relationships are all highly significant and the differences between them have been also demonstrated to be significant.[131]

As will be discussed later, an explanation

for this reduction in vascular tone as a function of the magnitude of the interaction between chronic and acute liver disease appears to be the presence of an abnormal vascular smooth muscle vasodilator, the false neurotransmitter octopamine,[131] which has been demonstrated to be produced by a hepatic defect in the intermediary metabolism of the aromatic amino acids tyrosine and phenylalanine.[42] This metabolic defect occurs both in decompensatory cirrhotic liver disease and in severe sepsis and is a manifestation of the magnitude of the hepatocellular defect appearing in the B state of metabolic insufficiency, which is a prominent feature of both conditions.

Extensive studies by Siegel et al.[123,125,129-133] have suggested that the high cardiac output

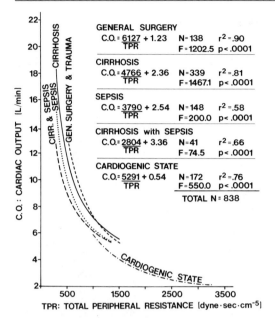

GENERAL SURGERY
$$C.O. = \frac{6127}{TPR} + 1.23 \quad N = 138 \quad r^2 = .90$$
$$F = 1202.5 \quad p < .0001$$

CIRRHOSIS
$$C.O. = \frac{4766}{TPR} + 2.36 \quad N = 339 \quad r^2 = .81$$
$$F = 1467.1 \quad p < .0001$$

SEPSIS
$$C.O. = \frac{3790}{TPR} + 2.54 \quad N = 148 \quad r^2 = .58$$
$$F = 200.0 \quad p < .0001$$

CIRRHOSIS with SEPSIS
$$C.O. = \frac{2804}{TPR} + 3.36 \quad N = 41 \quad r^2 = .66$$
$$F = 74.5 \quad p < .0001$$

CARDIOGENIC STATE
$$C.O. = \frac{5291}{TPR} + 0.54 \quad N = 172 \quad r^2 = .76$$
$$F = 550.0 \quad p < .0001$$

TOTAL N = 838

FIG. 15-4 Vascular tone relations in patient groups with various surgical conditions. (Siegel JH, Giovannini I, Coleman B et al: Pathologic synergistic modulations of the cardiovascular, respiratory, and metabolic response to injury by cirrhosis and/or sepsis: A manifestation of a common metabolic defect? Arch Surg 117: 225, 1982.)

response in patients with sepsis is a sympathetic adaptation to the abnormal vascular tone response. This hyperdynamic response to sepsis represents a critical determinant of survival as shown by Clowes and his colleagues[29] and MacLean et al.[86] It has also been demonstrated that the patient with sepsis who has overt or occult myocardial failure cannot compensate for the vascular instability produced by severe sepsis, whereas the septic hyperdynamic patient with good myocardial function has a reasonable chance of survival.[88,123,127,130,145,162] This may be due to the fact that a critical determinant of the septic patient's ability to meet the increased peripheral metabolic needs is predicated on the heart's ability to sustain a high cardiac output. This in turn means maintaining a large cardiac metabolic requirement.

As also shown in Figure 15-3, patients with hyperdynamic A and B states have an increased level of cardiac work ranging between 7 and 17 kg m/min. This is similar to the work requirements seen in moderately heavy exercise in trained athletes. However, in contrast to the cardiac response to normal exercise, which is maintained for only a few minutes, this increase in level of cardiac work is maintained for days, or even weeks, in the severely ill, hyperdynamic septic patient. The nutritional implications of such a large cardiac work requirement are obvious and reflect the fact that the fuel and energy requirements for the myocardium must be very large. Previous studies have suggested that in hyperdynamic B state septic patients, where the oxidative metabolism of other organs appears to be impaired, cardiac work accounts for nearly 50 percent of the variability in total body oxygen consumption.[125,130]

Septic Myocardial Depression and Cardiac Failure

The enormous demand of the myocardium for energy may account for the frequent occurrence of occult and overt myocardial depression and for the high output cardiac failure seen in septic states. When myocardial failure occurs, there is usually a transition from the septic A toward the septic B state of hyperdynamic cardiovascular adaptive response. This is accompanied by a myocardial metabolic decompensatory state that may produce a low-output myocardial failure of the cardiogenic D state type.

This can be seen in Figure 15-5, which shows the development of myocardial depression in sepsis in a 44-year-old woman with intra-abdominal sepsis secondary to infected pancreatic pseudocyst. This patient progressed from a hyperdynamic A state pattern (on postoperative day 5) to an early cardiogenic D state pattern (on the morning of postoperative day 6), characterized by a rise in tm and a reduction in ejection fraction and a fall in cardiac output. The use of inotropic support which corrected the myocardial depression and returned the tm and ejection fraction toward the normal stress response levels, revealed that the patient had

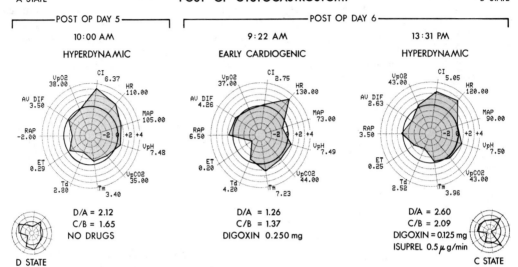

FIG. 15-5 Development of myocardial depression in sepsis. Circle diagrams of physiologic states. At the corners, are shown the prototype patterns for the A, B, C and D states. The three large circles in the center are the physiologic septic patterns manifested by a 44-year-old woman with an infected pancreatic pseudocyst. The physiologic values are given together with the name of the variable on each day. The perfect circle in the center of each pattern represents 0 standard deviations from the reference control (R state). Each dotted line represents 1 standard deviation from R, either increased or decreased. Below each patient pattern are the state distance ratios (D/A and C/B) from the state prototypes. The physiologic state of this patient was classified as A during the initial phase of the septic acute respiratory distress syndrome (10:00 am, postoperative day 5), D during early myocardial depression, (9:22 am, postoperative day 6), and B state after inotropic resuscitation (13:31 pm, postoperative day 6) showing that myocardial depression was associated with a transition from A to B state. (Siegel JH, Giovannini I, Coleman B: Ventilation: perfusion maldistribution secondary to the hyperdynamic cardiovascular state as the major cause of increased pulmonary shunting in human sepsis. J Trauma 19: 432, 1979.)

in fact moved from an A to B state with a narrow Ca-v̄ oxygen gradient (A-V Diff) and a fall in oxygen consumption index (O_2CI) from 222 ml/m² in the A state to 133 ml/m² in the hyperdynamic B state response.

The cardiogenic failure that occurs with sepsis is similar in terms of hemodynamic consequences to that seen with other forms of cardiac failure. However, patients with sepsis who go into cardiogenic failure D state and do not respond to inotropic support have an extremely high mortality. This appears to be due to the fact the myocardium is supporting the entire physiologic response to sepsis; by enabling the peripheral tissues to have access

to the maximum possible substrates and oxygen they are able to metabolize under the conditions of severe septic metabolic inhibition. When cardiac failure superimposes a low flow on a sepsis-stimulated hyperdynamic metabolism, the effects of a relative ischemia compound the metabolic insufficiency of sepsis. Understanding the septic patient's dependence on adequate myocardial function has major therapeutic implications. It will affect the requirement for early cardiac inotropic support (such as digitalis, isoproterenol, dopamine, or dobutamine) and the need for the use of vasodilator agents and volume loading to maintain the hyperdynamic cardiovascular response when there is any evidence of myocardial decompensation, but *before* a fall in cardiac output is allowed to occur.[123,129,130]

Vascular Tone and Myocardial Contractile Interrelations in Sepsis

The reason that the septic patient with a depressed myocardial contractile function usually is able to maintain a high cardiac output is related to the fundamental physiologic lesion of reduced vascular tone. As is shown in Figure 15-6, which demonstrates individual cardiac contraction force–velocity relations (see Chapter 9), the reduction in vascular tone permits the hyperdynamic septic patient with occult or overt myocardial failure to operate at a more favorable reduced afterload point on a depressed (low Vmax) force-velocity (FV) relationship. This allows the heart to maintain a higher ejection fraction (EFx) point on this FV curve than would be possible if a normal vascular tone relationship forced cardiac operation at a higher afterload point. (Figure 15-6).

These principles are shown in a series of estimated force–velocity (FV) curves obtained from analysis of the cardiac ejection fraction (EFx), the cardiac ejection time (EjT), the left ventricular volume (LVV), and the aortic systolic, mean, and diastolic pressures.[145] These

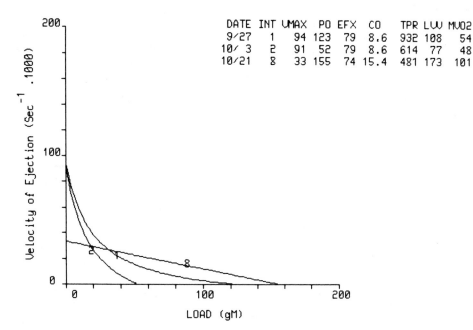

```
Pt : W           , K            ID :    381  Date of 1st Study : 9-27-85
Drugs (10/21) : Dopamine  480.0 mcg/min     , Dobutamine  333.0 mcg/min
```

DATE	INT	VMAX	PO	EFX	CO	TPR	LVV	MVO2	STATE
9/27	1	94	123	79	8.6	932	108	54	A
10/ 3	2	91	52	79	8.6	614	77	48	A
10/21	8	33	155	74	15.4	481	173	101	B

FIG. 15-6 Estimated force-velocity relations from a 22-year-old male following multiple trauma that included pelvic fracture, hepatic lacerations, and splenic fracture with development of postinjury septic complication. This figure demonstrates the reduction in force velocity relations with the fall in Vmax as the patient transitions from A to B state with pathologic hyperdynamic vascular tone reduction. Velocity intercept is estimated Vmax. Load intercept is maximum isometric load point (P_0). Location of intervention number (INT) on FV curve is velocity-load point at which ejection fraction is completed. The fall in peripheral resistance (TPR=481 dyne sec cm^{-5}) allows the patient (INT 8) to maintain a near normal ejection fraction (EFx=74 percent) even though he is operating on a depressed force-velocity relationship with a large fiber length (LVV=173 ml) that raises the afterload intercept point (P_0 = 155 g m). (Tacchino RM, Siegel JH, Goh KC et al, unpublished work, 1986.)

sequential studies are of the FV dynamics of a 22-year-old man who developed B-state sepsis following major multiple injury including a severe pelvic fracture, hepatic laceration, and splenic fracture. The FV curves show that a decrease in myocardial contractility characterized by a reduction in Vmax had occurred with the transition from A to B state. These studies also show that during the initial period of A state sepsis when Vmax was essentially constant (INT 1 and 2) the fall in TPR from 932 to 614 dyne sec cm^{-5} permitted the same EFx (79 percent) to be maintained at a lower LVV and fiber length, because the ejection fraction point (indicated by the position of the curve number on the FV relationship) could occur at a lower afterload. More important to the compensatory dynamics of the B state myocardial depression (INT 8) is the observation that the marked further reduction in vascular tone evidenced by the fall in TPR to 481 dyne sec cm^{-5} allowed compensation for the hyperdynamic increase in cardiac output (from 8.6 to 15.4 L/min), which increased LVV from 108 ml to 173 ml. It can be seen that while the ventricu-

lar fiber length and P_o increased, and the EFx point was shifted to a higher afterload on a depressed FV curve, the low resistance allowed the EFx to remain at nearly A state levels (74 percent). It is obvious from examination of the FV relationship that if the effective afterload point at which EFx was allowed to occur was forced further to the right by ill-advised vasoconstrictor therapy, without an adequate increase in Vmax, the EFx would decline even further, forcing the heart to dilate and raising the LVV to failure levels. As a final point it is important to note that even though the Vmax and EFx are higher in INT 1 and 2 than in 8, the large LVV and afterload range actually cause the estimated myocardial oxygen consumption index (MVO$_2$) to rise at a time when the myocardial contractility is most depressed. This is another reason for attempting to achieve a move favorable FV relationship that allows cardiac ejection at the lowest practical afterload. Force–velocity relationships can be increased by the use of inotropic support or by resolution of the septic process by surgical drainage and antibiotic therapy. By manipulat-

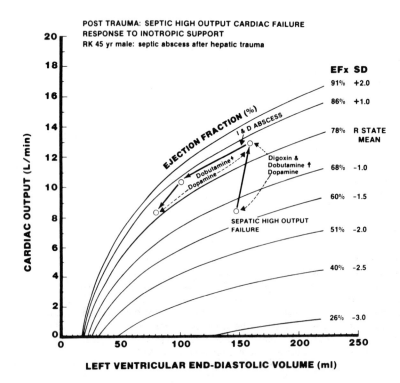

POST TRAUMA: SEPTIC HIGH OUTPUT CARDIAC FAILURE
RESPONSE TO INOTROPIC SUPPORT
RK 45 yr male: septic abscess after hepatic trauma

EJECTION FRACTION (%)

I & D ABSCESS

Dobutamine↑
Dopamine

Digoxin &
Dobutamine ↑
Dopamine

SEPATIC HIGH OUTPUT
FAILURE

EFx	SD
91%	+2.0
86%	+1.0
78%	R STATE MEAN
68%	-1.0
60%	-1.5
51%	-2.0
40%	-2.5
26%	-3.0

CARDIAC OUTPUT (L/min)

LEFT VENTRICULAR END-DIASTOLIC VOLUME (ml)

FIG. 15-7 Serial ventricular function relationships in septic high cardiac output failure showing response to inotropic support and drainage of septic abscess (I&D) in a 45-year-old male who developed sepsis secondary to hepatic abscess after trauma. Shown are mean lines of constant ejection fraction (EFx) with standard deviations, plus or minus, from the R state mean EFx. (Tacchino RM, Siegel JH, Emanuele T et al: Incidence and therapy of myocardial depression in critically ill post trauma patients. Circ Shock 18: 360, 1986.)

ing agents that increase intrinsic contractility (Vmax) and reduce afterload one can optimize the point of function on the force–velocity relationship of the posttraumatic septic patient.

Myocardial failure, as reflected in a shift to an abnormal Starling–Sarnoff ventricular function (VF) relationship, is also common in the patient with posttraumatic sepsis in whom a myocardial contractile dysfunction may be compounded by the septic and injury-mediated metabolic requirement to maintain a high car-

diac output. As a result, a septic high-output failure occurs. This is shown in Figure 15-7, which shows the physiologic time course of a 45-year-old man who developed a septic hepatic abscess after major liver trauma. In the initial study shown in this figure, the patient had a hyperdynamic cardiac output of 8.6 L/min but was forced to maintain a large left ventricular end-diastolic volume (LVV) (high-output failure) because of the reduced ejection fraction (> 1 standard deviation below the R

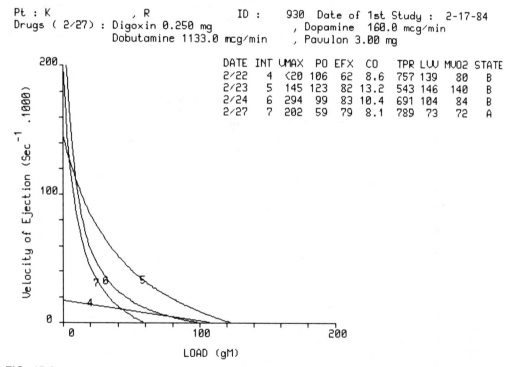

FIG. 15-8 Estimated force-velocity relationships from patient presented in Fig. 15-7 demonstrating the role of inotropic support and surgical drainage in resolving the myocardial contractile depression. Intervention 4 (INT 4) corresponds to the initial septic high output failure point shown in Fig. 15-7. The Vmax is markedly depressed, but the low peripheral vascular resistance (TPR) due to the decreased vascular tone permits a reduced ejection fraction (EFx=62 percent) to occur from a large LVV, which is, however, capable of maintaining an increased cardiac output (8.6 L/min). Inotropic support with digoxin, doubtamine and dopamine (INT 5) permits an increase in Vmax permitting an increased EFx, which allows the necessary rise in cardiac output to occur despite an increase in afterload (P_0 ↑). Incision and drainage of the hepatic abscess (between intervention 5 and 6) and an increased inotropic support level with dobutamine permits a further increase in Vmax, so that an increased cardiac output can be maintained with an increased EFx with eventual reduction in ventricular volume (LVV), as the Vmax rises to a hyperdynamic level. This allows the increased ejection fraction to be maintained at a lower afterload point as the transition from the septic B to A state occurs, with reduction in metabolic needs. Note that during the point of most increased cardiac output, the myocardial oxygen consumption index (MVO_2) is nearly twice that required by the patient when in a compensated A state response (INT 7). (Tacchino RM, Siegel JH, Goh KC et al, unpublished work, 1986.)

state mean of 78 percent). In this patient the use of inotropic support with digoxin, dobutamine, and dopamine permitted the patient to meet the demands of the hyperdynamic circulation and to increase the cardiac output to 13.2 L/min with an increase in the oxygen consumption index from 126 ml/min/m² to 202 ml/min/m², even though he remained in a B state of metabolic insufficiency. Incision and drainage of the hepatic abscess, which resolved the B state, allowed the patient to return to nearly the same level of cardiac output as previously, but with a lower left ventricular end-diastolic volume, since the ejection fraction was maintained at greater than 80 percent. This shift in the Starling–Sarnoff ventricular function re-

lationship was a direct result of the improvement in myocardial contractile function.

As shown in the estimated force–velocity relationship (Fig. 15-8) [INT 4] for the first VF point shown in Figure 15-7, this patient had a severe reduction in Vmax in spite of low-dose dopamine as a consequence of his septic B state decompensation. His low TPR facilitated a borderline effective EFx, to meet the hyperdynamic demands but at the cost of maintaining a large LVV. However, the resultant cardiac output was not adequate to meet body demands. To prepare the patient for surgery, digitalization and an increased level of dobutamine were administered. The Vmax rose (Fig. 15-8) [INT 5], allowing the cardiac output to

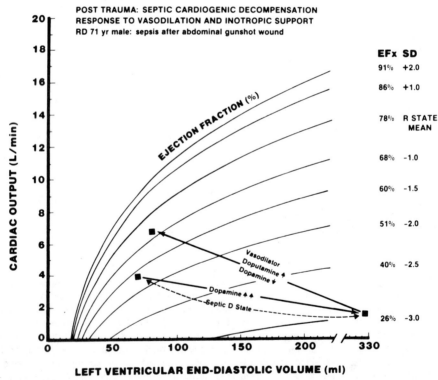

FIG. 15-9 Ventricular function relationship in aged trauma patient, with preexisting compensate heart disease, showing acute septic cardiogenic decompensation with response to combination of vasodilitation and inotropic support. The patient was a 71-year-old male who developed severe sepsis after an abdominal gunshot wound. Use of vasodilator therapy, plus nonvasoconstricting inotropic support, permits recovery from sudden low output cardiogenic failure (D state) with acute reduction in ejection fraction (EFx). Proper manipulation of force-velocity relations allows cardiac output to rise to a higher level needed for septic compensation with reversal of septic D state as EFx rises. (Tacchino RM, Siegel JH, Emanuele T et al: Incidence and therapy of myocardial depression in critically ill post trauma patients. Circ Shock 18: 360, 1986.)

increase, but afterload (the product of the increased ejection volume and the blood pressure against which it is ejected) also increased. Drainage of the septic focus (see Fig. 15-7), accompanied by an additional increase in inotropic support level (Fig. 15-8) [INT 6] allowed the Vmax to rise further and the shift in the FV curve allowed the same EFx to occur at a lower afterload level, thus reducing the LVV and shifting the VF curve (Fig. 15-7) while permitting an increased cardiac output. The combination of these factors also allows a reduction in the index of myocardial oxygen consumption (MVO_2). With stabilization and return to a hyperdynamic A state, the Vmax remained high but the body demands for perfusion were reduced and an effective cardiac output could be maintained at low afterload with a level of EFx that maintained a low LVV and MVO_2 without compromising body needs (Fig. 15-8) [INT 7].

True septic cardiogenic decompensation in the trauma patient with preexisting cardiac disease that causes a low-output failure syndrome produces a disastrous situation. In this case, the low flow results in an ischemic reduction in oxygen consumption that compounds the septic metabolic failures and frequently requires the use of both cardiac inotropic and peripheral vasodilator agents to permit recovery. This is shown in Figure 15-9, which demonstrates the ventricular function relations of a 71-year-old man with pre-existing myocardial disease who developed sepsis after an abdominal gunshot wound. The patient developed a cardiogenic septic D state with a fall in cardiac output from 4.2 L/min to 2.4 L/min, as the ejection fraction declined from 44 to 26 percent. The left ventricular end-diastolic volume rose to 330 ml, despite use of an inotropic agent with a mild vasoconstrictor properties: dopamine at 6 μg/min. In this patient the reduction of the dopamine to 4 μg/kg/min, the addition of dobutamine at 5 μg/kg/min and the use of a vasodilator agent, nitroglycerine, permitted the patient to shift the ventricular function relationships to the left by a combination of afterload reduction and inotropic support. Consequently the patient was able to maintain a higher cardiac output (6.8 L/min) at approximately the same end-diastolic volume as before the D state decompensation, because the ejection fraction was increased from 26 to 62

percent. Studies by Cerra and co-workers[18] have demonstrated the value of combined vasodilation and inotropic support therapy in D state septic patients, by increasing cardiac output and oxygen consumption to levels that prevent the addition of ischemia to the septic oxidative abnormality.

Acute Adult Respiratory Distress Syndrome in Hyperdynamic Septic States

Development of the septic process is associated with a sequence of events leading to altered permeability of the alveolar capillary membrane.[122] A variety of clinical events that have platelet and white cell activation and aggregation in the lungs as a common feature have been implicated as initiators of this phenomenon[28,58] (see Chapter 18). The induction of immune complexes by trauma or sepsis has been demonstrated to initiate the complement activation response, which also may be initiated by a variety of leukocyte chemotaxins for bacteria.[40,77,135,136] It has been speculated that opsonization and complement activation initiate a leukocyte response, which in turn results in production of superoxides and the oxides of arachidonic acid.[3,77,137] The elaboration of arachiodonic acid and the cyclo-oxygenase cascade results in the formation of thromboxane A_2.[56,58,77,171] In association with this response there is platelet and neutrophil aggregation on the capillary and endothelial membranes, with formation of microthrombi, which amplifies the effects of platelet aggregation. The net result of these microemboli in the pulmonary circulation is a diversion of blood flow from some alveolar segments to others.[28,130] In addition, the white cell superoxides, neutral proteases, and leukotrienes alter the permeability characteristics of the alveolar capillary membrane so that the fluid moves from capillary intravascular space into the pulmonary interstitial area,[52,77,122,140,147] with the formation of the ARDS of sepsis (see Chapters 18 and 19 for a full discussion of ARDS).

It is not generally appreciated that the local microcirculatory phenomena, which occur as a result of sepsis-induced platelet aggregation and permeability changes, are further influenced by the cardiovascular adaptive response to the lowered peripheral vascular tone that occurs in sepsis.[130] These phenomena together produce abnormalities in the cardiopulmonary ventilation/perfusion ($\dot{V}A/\dot{Q}T$) relationships. This is demonstrated in Figure 15-10, which shows the mean ventilation/perfusion ratio ($\dot{V}A/\dot{Q}T$) as a function of the alteration in cardiac index in a group of critically ill patients maintained on continuous ventilatory support.[125]

The patients are labeled with regard to their physiologic state (R, A, B, C, D,). The sep-

tic patients are represented by circles and the patient with nonseptic or cardiogenic syndromes are represented by squares. A normal resting ventilation/perfusion ratio has been demonstrated to be approximately 0.8 and the normal cardiac index is approximately 3 L/min/m². The hyperdynamic patients in the A or B state of sepsis are seen to have cardiac indices greater than 4 L/min/m². They also have lower ventilation/perfusion ratios than normal and indeed the patients with B state sepsis are seen to have the lowest $\dot{V}A/\dot{Q}T$ ratios, which are frequently less than 0.4. This

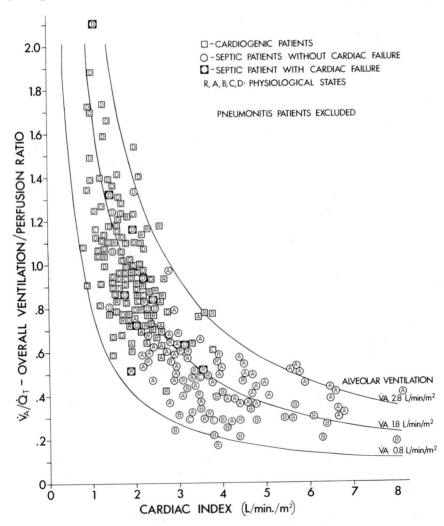

FIG. 15-10 Relationship between ventilation perfusion ratio ($\dot{V}A/\dot{Q}T$) to cardiac index, labeled by physiologic state. Also shown are lines of constant alveolar minute ventilation ($\dot{V}A$). All patients maintained on constant ventilator support a minute volumes of 9 to 24 L/min. (Siegel JH, Cerra FB, Coleman B et al: Physiological and metabolic correlations in human sepsis. Surgery 86: 163, 1979.)

group of septic patients also includes those with the lowest TPR. As a consequence of afterload reduction, they frequently have left-shifted Starling curve relationships since this permits an increase in cardiac ejection fraction. Evidence has been presented that the shift in the Starling-Sarnoff curve appears to lower the left ventricular end-diastolic volume as well as left atrial and pulmonary venous pressures, despite the maintenance of a very high pulmonary blood flow.[125,130]

The resultant alteration in pulmonary out-flow pressure appears to produce a redistribution of blood flow so that a very large portion of the increased pulmonary blood flow is diverted to the dependent lung segments with the lowest alveolar ventilation. This appears to explain the $\dot{V}A/\dot{Q}T$ abnormalities and markedly impairs the already abnormal pulmonary gas exchange, since as the CI rises, it produces a larger physiologic shunt ($\dot{Q}S/\dot{Q}T$) while also increasing the ventilatory dead space/tidal volume ratio (VD/VT) (Fig. 15-11).

Due to the permeability changes induced

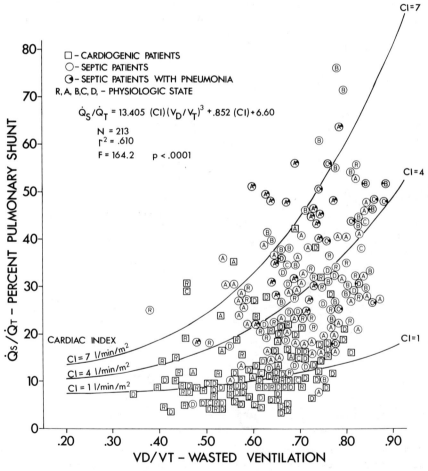

FIG. 15-11 Relation of increase in percent pulmonary shunt ($\dot{Q}S/\dot{Q}T$) to rise in physiologic dead space (VD/VT), as a function of increasing cardiac index (CI) and altered physiologic state. Note that patients with severe sepsis, without pneumonitis or septic ARDS, show an increase in shunt as a function of rise in CI with substantial increases in VD/VT, especially in B state sepsis. This indicates evidence of increasing ventilation: perfusion maldistribution with septic A to B state deterioration. (Siegel JH, Giovannini I, Coleman B: Ventilation: perfusion maldistribution secondary to the hyperdynamic cardiovascular state as the major cause of increased pulmonary shunting in human sepsis. J Trauma 19: 432, 1979.)

by complement activation with resultant thromboxane, prostanoid, and superoxide formation, this marked disparity of increasing blood flow through a diminishing fraction of the alveolar capillaries enhances the formation of interstitial and pulmonary edema in the dependent lung. Consequently, the septic patient very rapidly develops a markedly edematous lung with eventual collapse of alveolae and the formation of alveolar exudates. These in turn form a medium for the development of bronchopneumonia producing alveolar necrosis and subsequently, the late fibrosis of the lung that represents the final stage of ARDS[28,155] (see Chapter 19).

While posttraumatic ARDS can occur in the absence of sepsis, it is important to recognize that the septic pulmonary process is an integral part of the septic metabolic and physiologic response. Although its degree of severity may vary, the initial pulmonary insufficiency of sepsis is a *direct* consequence of the sympathetic cardiovascular compensation to the metabolically induced alterations in peripheral vascular tone and the immunologically induced changes in lung capillary permeability. These, in turn, are manifestations of the pathophysiologic host defense quantified by the physiologic and metabolic state classifications. Thus the state classification provides a means of staging the severity of the septic process and an organizational framework for understanding the interrelationship of the development of ARDS with that of the septic hyperdynamic state and the metabolic degeneration into what has been called the MOFS of sepsis.

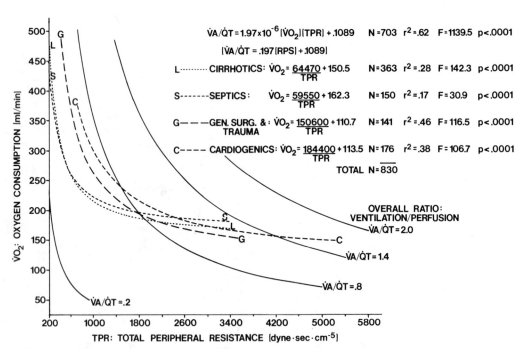

FIG. 15-12 Relation of abnormalities in ventilation:perfusion ($\dot{V}A/\dot{Q}T$) to metabolic and physiologic abnormalities in oxygen consumption ($\dot{V}O_2$) and total peripheral resistance (TPR). Regression lines and values for various groups of surgical patients. Note that patients with sepsis or cirrhotic liver disease have a lower oxygen consumption for a given level of peripheral resistance. They also tend to fall in the lowest range of $\dot{V}A/\dot{Q}T$. The fall in $\dot{V}A/\dot{Q}T$ is related both to the decrease in total peripheral resistance and $\dot{V}O_2$. (Siegel JH, Giovannini I, Coleman B et al: Pathologic synergistic modulation of the cardiovascular, respiratory, and metabolic response to injury by cirrhosis and/or sepsis: A manifestation of a common metabolic defect? Arch Surg 117: 225, 1982.)

Septic and Cirrhotic Physiologic and Metabolic Relations as a Reflection of Hepatocellular Dysfunction

The influence of either chronic (cirrhotic) or acute (septic) hepatic dysfunction and the similarity of the effects of their metabolically induced alterations in vascular tone on the pulmonary ventilation/perfusion ratio is shown in Figure 15-12. This figure demonstrates that cirrhotics or septics, who have been previously shown to have a lower vascular tone than patients with cardiogenic syndromes, following general surgical intervention, or with trauma, have a lower TPR for a given level of oxygen consumption. This figure also demonstrates that the same patients have a reduced $\dot{V}A/\dot{Q}T$ as a function of the $\dot{V}O_2$ to TPR relationship. These physiologic interrelations further emphasize the critical role of metabolic adequacy in setting the basal level for peripheral pressure/flow relations and for the distribution of ventilation and perfusion in the lung.

Both vascular tone and $\dot{V}A/\dot{Q}T$ are further reduced in either septic or cirrhotic patients who manifest the B state of metabolic insufficiency where the component of hepatic dysfunction reflected by a low $\dot{V}O_2$ is most pronounced.[125,131]

PATTERNS OF METABOLIC INSUFFICIENCY AND THEIR RELATIONSHIP TO CARDIORESPIRATORY ABNORMALITIES IN TRAUMA AND SEPSIS

The evolution of a septic process in the previously traumatized patient has provided an opportunity to study the temporal sequence of the evolution of the cardiovascular and metabolic response with an eye to delineating the pertinent interrelationships. These are shown in Figures 15-13 to 15-18, for a group of 26 patients who sustained major trauma; 10 of these became septic and 16 remained nonseptic throughout their course. There were no differences in the initial injury severity scores in the two groups of patients, nor was there any significant difference in age or pattern of illness.[108,109,118]

Time Course of the Hyperdynamic Response

In this particular group of patients, all those who became septic manifested an A-state response. As shown in Figure 15-13 patients who developed septic trauma (ST) and those who had a nonseptic trauma course (NST) were seen to have similar levels of cardiac index during the first 5 days following resuscitation and surgery for their traumatic injury. However, after 5 days the septic patients showed a gradual increase in cardiac index, whereas the cardiac index returned toward the normal levels for nontraumatized individuals in the nonseptic patients. This difference between ST and NST patients was also seen in oxygen consumption. During, the initial 7 days following injury, oxygen consumption remained high in both groups. However in those patients who became septic, there was further increase in oxygen consumption after 7 days, whereas oxygen consumption tended to fall toward normal levels in the nonseptic patients.

Parameters of the Host Defense Inflammatory Response

Figure 15-14 shows two aspects of the acute inflammatory response to injury. In the initial posttrauma period there is a rise in C-reactive protein (CRP) in both septic and nonseptic trauma patients. This acute phase protein has been demonstrated to play a critical role in facilitating opsonization of bacteria as well as in initiating complement activation that

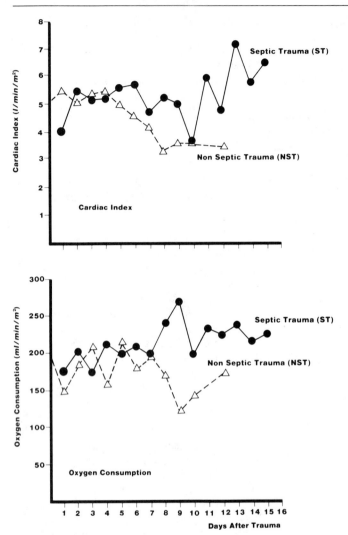

FIG. 15-13 Cardiovascular and metabolic responses after trauma and sepsis, in 10 septic and 16 nonseptic patients. Mean values over postinjury course for cardiac index (CI) and oxygen consumption ($\dot{V}O_2$) are shown for trauma patients who developed sepsis (ST) and compared to those who had nonseptic courses (NST). Note increase in CI and $\dot{V}O_2$ in ST patients as sepsis becomes established between 5 and 7 days after injury. (Sganga G, Siegel JH, Brown G et al: Reprioritization of hepatic plasma protein release in trauma and sepsis. Arch Surg 120: 187, 1985.)

potentiates bacterial cell killing.[67] The rise in CRP was statistically significant both in the early (<5 days after trauma) and late (>5 days posttrauma) period in the septic trauma patients compared to the nonseptic patients.[118] With recovery from nonseptic trauma, the CRP levels returned towards a normal level (<2 μg/ml) although they did not reach it within the period of study. Conversely, within the first 3 days after injury, the white cell count tended to be lower in those patients who eventually developed sepsis. Then, as sepsis became overt, a marked leukocytosis occurred,

whereas in the posttraumatic nonseptic patients it tended to be increased, but at an intermediate level, until recovery. This latter course undoubtedly reflects the sterile inflammatory processes associated with injury. It is of interest in this group of patients that when the white cells were studied for their ability to manifest chemiluminescence (which reflects the superoxide-producing capability of the leukocytes), there was a reduction in the capability for leukocyte superoxide formation in the injured patients who went on to sepsis.[72,73] This appears due to the presence of an inhibiting factor in

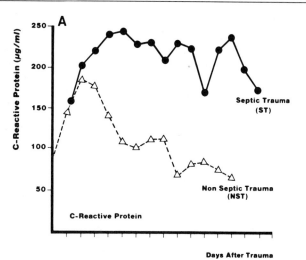

FIG. 15-14 Nature of the inflammatory response after trauma in 10 septic and 16 nonseptic patients. Comparison of rise in mean values for (A) C-reactive protein (CRP) and (B) white blood cell count in patients with sepsis following trauma (ST) compared to those who had nonseptic courses (NST). Note early rise in C-reactive protein at time of immediate posttrauma leukopenia in trauma patients who went on to have septic courses and persistance of the high CRP levels throughout the septic course. (Sganga G, Siegel JH, Brown G et al: Reprioritization of hepatic plasma protein release in trauma sepsis. Arch Surg 120: 187, 1985.)

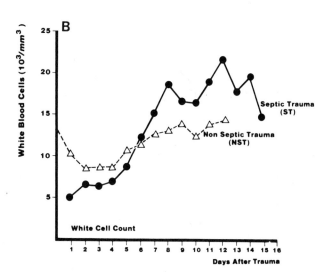

the plasma of the preseptic and septic trauma patients, since when the plasma was replaced with normal plasma, leukocytes from posttraumatic patients actually showed a increased capability for superoxide formation.[72] These same patients also demonstrated reduced opsonic fibronectin levels.[72,73] However, whether the decreased fibronectin is a cause or an effect, or is unrelated to the appearance of this leukocyte-inhibiting factor, has not been clearly identified. Nevertheless, these data suggest that defects in the host defense mechanism are manifest from the very beginning of the posttraumatic process at a time when bacterial invasion due to injury may be present, but before overt sepsis or bacteremia has occurred.

Time Course of the Metabolic Response to Injury

The metabolic response to injury has been characterized by abnormalities in the plasma levels of glucose and its gluconeogenic precursors. This is demonstrated in Figure 15-15, which shows that the evolution of the septic process is associated with an increased level of plasma glucose in preseptic trauma patients; this tends to rise toward hyperglycemic levels as the septic process becomes overt. Both NST and ST patients were receiving similar amounts of glucose administered in their total parenteral nutrition (TPN). There was no statistically significant difference between the nutritional support in the two groups. Also shown in Figure 15-15 are the increased plasma levels of alanine, which is a major gluconeogenic precursor in the preseptic and septic trauma patient.

There is a similar rise in aromatic amino acids as sepsis evolved after injury. This is shown in Figure 15-16, which demonstrates an increased plasma level of both phenylalanine and tyrosine in septic trauma patients as the septic process became manifest 5 days after the traumatic insult.

Time Course Pattern of the Hepatic Acute Phase Protein Response

Compared to levels in nonseptic patients, the hepatic acute phase (AP) protein response in those who become septic demonstrates in-

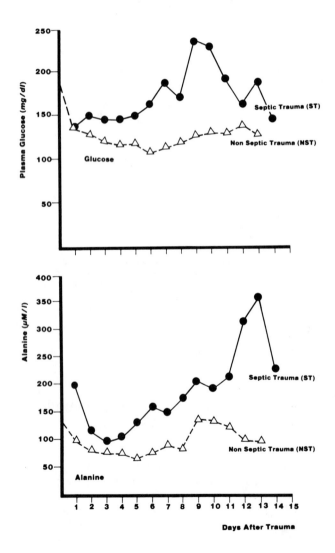

FIG. 15-15 Gluconeogenic response to trauma in 10 septic and 16 nonseptic patients, mean values for plasma glucose and alanine in patients with sepsis after trauma (ST) compared to those with nonseptic posttrauma courses (NST). Note early rise in plasma glucose associated with increase in plasma alanine in ST patients with progressive increase as to the septic course evolves. (Siegel JH, Pittiruti M, Sganga G et al, unpublished work, 1986.)

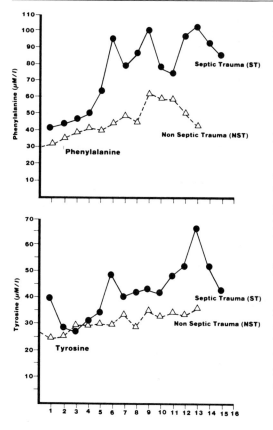

curred earlier in the time course of the septic response than did that of fibrinogen or ceruloplasmin. This differential response suggests that there may be differential rates of synthesis and or utilization of some hepatic AP proteins compared to others. However, AP proteins largely involved in carrier functions, such as transferrin and albumin, and the scavenger protein α-2 macroglobulin show no evidence of an increase in plasma levels early in the septic process compared with NST patients. They demonstrate a reprioritization as sepsis becomes overt with an actual fall (Fig. 15-18) in plasma levels of these acute phase hepatic proteins late in the septic course compared to the faster-turnover AP proteins such as CRP, α-1-antitrypsin, fibrinogen, and ceruloplasmin[118] (Fig. 15-17).

As will be discussed later in greater detail, these data suggest that there is a differential response, both with regard to time and degree of sepsis severity, in the hepatic synthesis of various acute phase host defense proteins between patients with a normal posttraumatic inflammatory response and those who go on to develop posttraumatic sepsis.

FIG. 15-16 Plasma aromatic amino acids response after trauma in 10 septic and 16 nonseptic patients. Mean values for plasma phenylalanine and tyrosine in patients with sepsis following trauma (ST) compared to those with nonseptic posttrauma courses (NST). Note increase in circulating level of phenylalanine and tyrosine as sepsis evolves after injury with maintenance of high levels of aromatic amino acids during the clinically evident septic period. (Siegel JH, Pittiruti M, Sganga G et al, unpublished work, 1986.)

THE NEUROENDOCRINE RESPONSE TO TRAUMA AND SEPSIS AND ITS PHYSIOLOGIC AND METABOLIC STATE CORRELATES

creased plasma levels (synthesis?) of the acute phase proteins involved in the inflammatory and coagulation response and in the levels of superoxide and protease scavenging AP proteins, as sepsis evolves. As seen in Figure 15-17, C-reactive protein, fibrinogen, α-1-antitrypsin and ceruloplasmin are shown to be increased in the septic trauma patient compared to the nonseptic patients.[118]

However, the increase in plasma levels of some AP proteins, CRP, and α-1-antitrypsin oc-

The increase in the circulating level of glucose and its gluconeogenic precursors, nongluconeogenic amino acids, and lipid metabolites as sepsis evolves and progresses from the A to B state, compared to nonseptic trauma, is accompanied by an alteration in the hormonal balance. This is shown in Figure 15-19, in which the various parameters of cardiovascular function used for physiologic state classification are compared to the plasma levels of metabolites and horomones in terms of standard deviations (increased or decreased) from the mean values

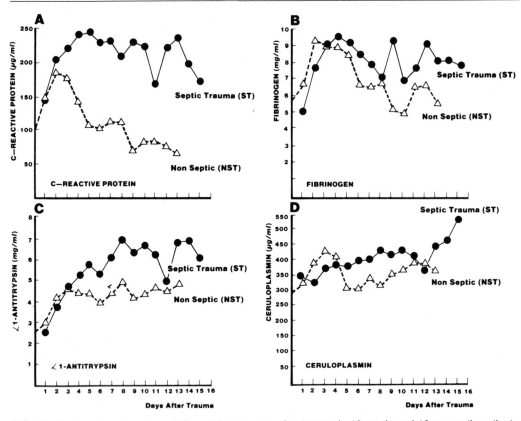

FIG. 15-17 Hepatic acute phase (AP) protein response after trauma in 10 septic and 16 nonseptic patients. Mean values for C-reactive protein **A,** fibrinogen **B,** α-1-antitrypsin **C,** and ceruloplasmin **D.** Patients with sepsis developing after trauma (ST) are compared to patients with nonseptic posttrauma courses (NST). Note early rise of CRP and α-1-antitrypsin in patients who later become clinically septic between 5 and 7 days. The fibrinogen response and ceruloplasmin response tend to be increased in sepsis, but only after the fully developed septic clinical picture is demonstrated. (Sganga G, Siegel JH, Brown G et al: Reprioritization of hepatic plasma protein release in trauma and sepsis. Arch Surg 120: 187, 1985.)

in nonseptic, reference control (R state), preoperative general surgical patients (Fig. 15-19).

Glucose-Regulatory Hormones: Insulin and Glucagon

The characteristic features of the progression from nonseptic injury to the A (compensated) and B (decompensated) states of sepsis are that sepsis (and in particular the fall in the consumption of oxygen that occurs as the B state evolves) is associated with progressive increases in the circulating blood levels of glucose and its metabolites (including lactate and pyruvate), the branched chain amino acids (leucine, isoleucine, and valine), the aromatic amino acids (phenylalanine and tyrosine), and the group of amino acids involved in synthesis of urea (proline, ornithine, argenine) and urea, as well as the plasma levels of triglycerides. As the level of triglycerides increases, the level of oxidized ketone bodies (acetoacetate) decreases and the ratio of reduced to oxidized ketone bodies (β-hydroxybutyrate/acetoacetate) rises. These changes in plasma substrate levels in sepsis occur as the plasma level of

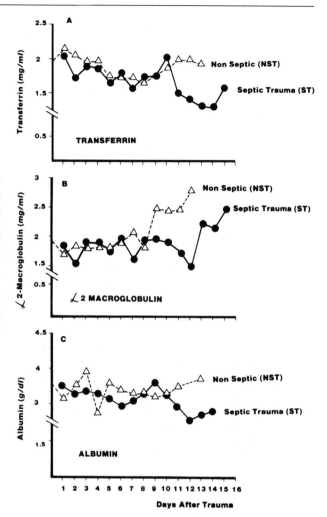

FIG. 15-18 Hepatic acute phase protein response after trauma in 10 septic and 16 nonseptic patients. Mean values from patients with sepsis developing after trauma (ST) and those with nonseptic posttrauma courses (NST). Note decrease in transferrin and albumin and relative decrease in α-2-macroglobulin in patients with well established sepsis following injury. (Sganga G, Siegel JH, Brown G et al: Reprioritization of hepatic plasma protein release in trauma and sepsis. Arch Surg 120: 187, 1985.)

circulating glucagon, which reaches a peak in the septic B state, rises enormously. Although this septic rise in glucagon is also associated with an increase in the plasma level of insulin, in sepsis the glucagon/insulin ratio remains extremely high and is reversed compared to normal.[78,84,125]

Catecholamines and False Neurotransmitters in Sepsis

In addition to the rise in glucagon seen in severe sepsis, there are also rises in epinephrine and corticosteroids early in the septic process.[31,44,78,84,125,143,156,170] However, late in the septic course when the A to B state transition occurs, there is a tendency for urinary levels of catecholamines to decrease. Furthermore, as is shown in Figure 15-20 with the development of the B state in either sepsis or cirrhotic liver disease, the fall in TPR, the narrowing of the A-$\tilde{V}O_2$ Diff, and the reduction in oxygen consumption ($\dot{V}O_2/m^2$) are asociated with a rise in the aromatic amino acids (tyrosine and phenylalanine, which are normally precursors of dopamine and the naturally occurring catecholamines) and with the appearance of the false neurotransmitter octopamine. This increase in the circulating level of octopamine, known to be an abnormal by-product of tyro-

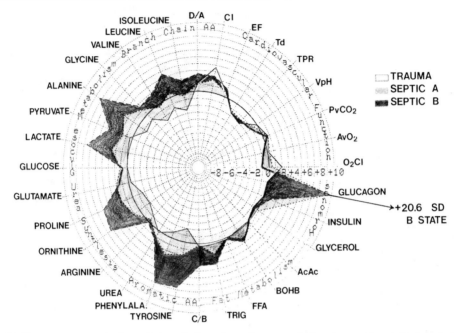

FIG. 15-19 Hormono-metabolic and physiologic patterns in nonseptic trauma and in septic A and septic B states. Dark circle in figure equals 0 standard deviations of each variable from the mean of a group of nonseptic general surgical patients in the control state (R). Each dotted line represents 1 standard deviation from R state, either increased or decreased. CI, cardiac index; EF, ejection fraction; Td, pulmonary dispersive mean transit time; TPR, total peripheral resistance; VpH, mixed venous pH; $PvCO_2$, mixed venous PCO_2; AvO_2, arteriovenous oxygen content difference; O_2CI, oxygen consumption index; AcAc, acetoacetate; BOHB, betahydroxybutyrate; FFA, free fatty acids; TRIG, triglycerides. Plasma levels of other amino acids, urea, glucose precursors, and hormones are as indicated in the figure. (Siegel JH, Cerra FB, Coleman B et al: Physiological and metabolic correlations in human sepsis. Surgery 86: 163, 1979.)

sine metabolism, also has been demonstrated to occur in patients with severe liver disease who go into hepatic coma.[42,131]

It has been postulated that this increase in octopamine represents the diversion of tyrosine away from the normal synthesis of dopamine and catecholamines to the production of false neurotransmitters.[42] Octopamine has been demonstrated to have only 1 percent of the vasoconstrictor power of the true neurotransmitter at sympathetic nerve endings (neurepinephrine) and as a result may produce a competitive vasodilator influence.[1,64] This may be the metabolic link between the alterations in hepatic function induced by sepsis and the reduced vascular tone relationship that appears to be the fundamental pathophysiologic lesion underlying the development of the septic hyperdynamic state.[131]

ALTERED FUEL: ENERGY METABOLISM IN SEPSIS

Increased Muscle Proteolysis and Enhanced Oxidation of Amino Acids: Septic Autocannibalism

Injury and the subsequent development of sepsis have been shown to initiate enhanced proteolysis. This is primarily from muscle, but breakdown of other supporting tissues may also play a contributing role. A number of recent investigative studies have suggested that

RELATION OF OCTOPAMINE AND COMA TO METABOLIC PATTERNS
IN CIRRHOTIC PATIENTS WITH PORTAL HYPERTENSION

RELATION OF OCTOPAMINE AND AMINO-ACIDS TO
METABOLIC PATTERNS IN SEPSIS

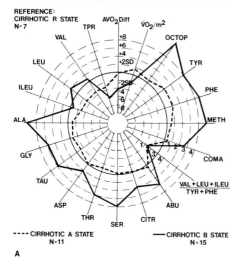
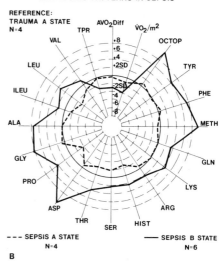

A

B

FIG. 15-20 Comparison of the relationship of plasma octopamine to plasma amino acid metabolic patterns in cirrhosis (**A**) and sepsis (**B**) with evolution of the B state of metabolic insufficiency. Dark circles in middle of the figures equals mean value for cirrhotic R state patients in cirrhotic liver disease pattern and for nonseptic trauma A state patients in septic pattern. Each dotted line represents 2 standard deviations from reference circle. AvO₂Diff, arteriovenous oxygen content difference; $\dot{V}O_2/m^2$, (oxygen consumption/m^2 body surface area; OCTOP, octopamine; TYR, tyrosine; PHE, phenylalanine; METH, methionine; GLN, glutamine; LYS, lysine; ARG, arginine; HIST, histidine; SER, serine; THR, threanine; ASP, aspartate; PRO, proline; GLY, glycine; ALA, alanine; ILEU, isoleucine; LEU, leucine; VAL, valine; TPR, total peripheral resistance. (Siegel JH, Giovannini I, Coleman B et al: Pathologic synergistic modulation of the cardiovascular, respiratory, and metabolic response to injury by cirrhosis and/or sepsis: A manifestation of a common metabolic defect? Arch Surg 117: 225, 1982.)

the enhanced proteolysis of trauma and sepsis may be initiated by the macrophage release of interleukin I, or its active fragment, PIF, which has been demonstrated in vitro to induce muscle proteolysis.[5,7,25-27,34] In the presence of trauma, and especially when sepsis develops, there appears to be an enhanced use of proteolytically derived, as well as exogenously infused, amino acids as oxidative fuels. The resultant deamination of these amino acids results in increased production of urinary urea nitrogen. Figure 15-21 demonstrates that while both the nonseptic and clinically septic trauma patients have increases both in muscle loss (estimated from 3-methylhistidine production)[167] and urinary urea production, there is an increased slope to this relationship in septic trauma, such that a larger quantity of urinary urea is produced for any given level of muscle loss.[109]

That this is primarily due to the increased muscle catabolism is seen in Figure 15-22. Here the septic trauma increase in urea production is shown to be significantly dependent on the enhanced muscle catabolism that occurs in sepsis and is only minimally influenced by the exogenously administered amino acids generally increased iatrogenically in septic patients.[109] While the reasons for this dependence of urea production on muscle catabolism are not clear, the humoral (interleukin I) and hormonal (glucagon, catecholamines, cortisol) mediators of muscle proteolysis may be linked in their time sequence with the increased liver oxidative metabolism and glucose synthesis so that the factors that stimulate muscle catabolism may also enhance gluconeogenic deamination, amino acid oxidation, and hepatic urea synthesis.

The factors that initiate muscle proteolysis are not clearly understood, but they appear to be different from the normal hormonal control

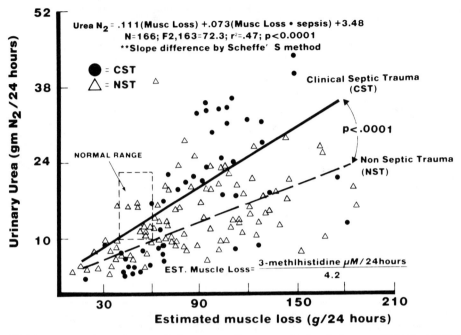

FIG. 15-21 Relation of muscle proteolysis to urea nitrogen production in trauma. Clinically septic trauma (CST) versus nonseptic trauma (NST) patients. (Pittiruti M, Siegel JH, Sganga G et al: Arch Surg, submitted for publication, 1986.)

mechanisms. An important factor may be the direct overstimulation of proteolytic mechanisms by an increase in the circulating levels of both the inflammatory humoral and stress-induced hormonal agents.[156] However, in the absence of injury and sepsis, administration of these hormones alone, or in a quantity and ratio to one another to produce levels similar to those found in sepsis does not induce the septic metabolic picture.[23,30,44,63,78,156] The second difference is that the proteolysis and the resultant amino acid gluconeogenesis of injury and especially that of sepsis cannot be substantially inhibited by administration of glucose, as can be done in starvation proteolysis.[11,21,82,119] Nor can muscle proteolysis in sepsis be prevented by infusion of insulin, as can be used to prevent the muscle proteolysis of diabetes mellitus.[41,110-112] As will be discussed, the inability of the septic skeletal muscle to inhibit its own proteolytic breakdown by oxidizing glucose as a metabolic fuel (the so-called "insulin resistance" of sepsis), ap-

pears to be due not to true insulin receptor inhibition, but to a postreceptor blockade.[8] This may be caused by a reduction in the activity level of pyruvate dehydrogenase, the critical regulating enzyme that permits pyruvate to be decarboxylated to acetyl-CoA for tricarboxycylic acid cycle (TCA) oxidation.[125,151-154]

In addition, other preferred fuel sources for muscle, which ordinarily tend to inhibit proteolysis under conditions of normal starvation or diabetes, do not rise sufficiently to compensate for the muscle's glucose oxidation limitations. Ketone bodies developed from acetyl-CoA and its precursors, which rise in circumstances of starvation,[166] or when true insulin deficiency occurs as in diabetes mellitus[98,166] do not increase proportionately to muscle needs in sepsis.[98,104,120,125,143,158,169] Thus the skeletal muscle is forced to have a greater reliance on fatty acid fuels, and may also become more dependent on the oxidation of the ketoacids of the branched chain amino acids (leucine, isoleucine, and valine) for energy

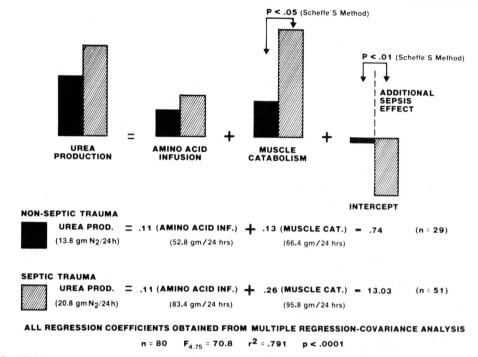

FIG. 15-22 Relative effect of amino acid infusion and muscle catabolism on urea production in septic and nonseptic trauma. The relative influence of each factor on urea production is determined from the covariance regression equation by multiplying the mean value of each variable by its β-coefficient, which converts each effect into urea production units. All differences tested by the Scheffé method of simultaneous analysis of all contrasts. (Pittiruti M, Siegel JH, Sganga G et al: Arch Surg, submitted for publication, 1986.)

metabolism.[12,19,21,45] These later ketoacids appear to be obtained through the mechanism of muscle proteolysis discussed earlier.[21,57,116]

The proteolytic mechanism liberates all of the amino acids in the sequence of actin and myocin and other structural proteins that undergo the proteolytic effect. As shown in Figure 15-23, muscle is able to utilize only the branched chain amino acids (BCAA) to any significant extent for its own Krebs TCA oxidation cycle. To carry out this oxidation, these BCAA first must be deaminated and the resultant amino acid ammonia group is transaminated via glutamate to the muscle's own pyruvate (derived from muscle glycogen or other pyruvate precursors such as glucose or lactate) to form alanine or glycine. In a similar fashion glutamine is transaminated from glutamate and these amino acids are liberated into the circulation to be carried to the liver, gut, and kidney.

The other amino acids in the protein sequence that are liberated by proteolysis generally cannot be metabolized by skeletal muscle and are released into the plasma unaltered, in a quantity that reflects the magnitude of the proteolytic process. In addition, since most septic patients receive amino acid nutritional sources by TPN or enteral feeding, the proteolytically derived amino acids add to the exogenously administered amino acids. The combination of these two effects tends to raise the plasma amino acid level.

That this is a real effect and that the liberation of amino acids into the plasma from the enhanced proteolysis of sepsis is of significance is shown in Figure 15-24, which demonstrates the plasma levels of valine as a function of the grams of exogenously administered amino acids in TPN.

It can be seen that in the nonsurviving sep-

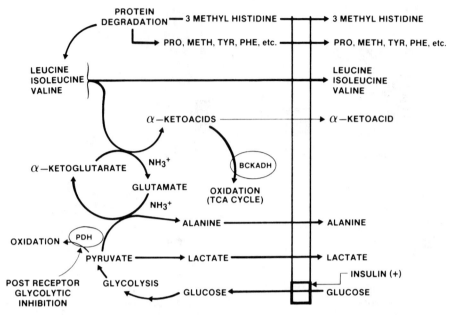

FIG. 15-23 Effect of sepsis on skeletal muscle proteolysis, pathways of branched chain amino acid, and glucose metabolism. Septic protein degradation is accelerated with increased release of 3-methylhistidine. Proteolysis liberates branched chain amino acids (leucine, isoleucine, and valine), which are either released into blood or transaminated to α-ketoacid. The BCAA α-ketoacids are either released into blood or undergo oxidation via branched chain ketoacid dehydrogenase (BCKADH). In sepsis, glucose uptake at insulin sensitive site is either normal or increased. Glycolysis appears unaffected but pyruvate oxidation is limited by postreceptor inhibition due to decreased pyruvate dehydrogenase complex activity (PDH↓). Glucose carbon (Pyruvate) is either reduced to lactate or transaminated from BCAA liberated NH_3^+ via glutamate to form alanine.

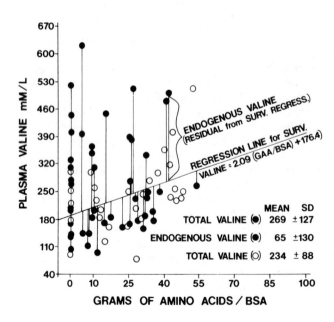

FIG. 15-24 Estimation of endogenous plasma valine release in septic deaths as residual from regression for grams of amino acid (GAA) per meter body surface area (BSA) in septic survivors. Dark circles represent data from patients who died; open circles are data from survivors. (Cerra FB, Siegel JH, Coleman B et al: Septic autocannibalism. Ann Surg 192: 570, 1980.)

tic patients who have increased clinical proteolysis, as evidenced by muscle wasting, there is a significant net increase in the levels of endogenous BCAA, in this case valine, from the regression line for the survivors. Similar effects have been shown for isoleucine and leucine.[21] These data suggest that in addition to the muscle's own deamination and oxidation of BCAA, a substantial amount of branched chain amino acids over and above muscle needs are released into the plasma. This can also be seen in Figures 15-25, which demonstrates the increasing levels of plasma alanine as a function of the circulating levels of leucine, isoleucine, and valine released by the excess proteolysis. As shown in Figure 15-25A, the higher levels of plasma alanine can be predicted by the increased levels of these three branched chain amino acids and the alanine precursor, pyruvate. Also, nonsurviving patients in septic A and B states where increased proteolysis is present have the highest levels of plasma alanine and alanine precursors in their plasma. Figure 15-25B shows that the increased release of branched chain amino acids (upon which the rise in plasma alanine level is dependent) is also accompanied by increasing plasma levels of non-muscle-metabolized amino acids, in this case tyrosine. An identical response is seen for proline and a wide variety of other actin- and myosin-derived amino acids.[17,21,125] These data and that reported by others[25,26,45,84,119,157,169,174] support the conclusion that with sepsis a generalized muscle proteolysis occurs, with muscle cell deamination of BCAA and transamination of NH_3 to pyruvate. The end result of this process liberates increased levels of the carrier amino acid alanine into the plasma. Similar results are seen for glycine and glutamine.

The amino acids released into the plasma, and those administered exogenously, are utilized either as oxidative fuels or for synthetic processes related largely to protein synthesis. Normalization of the amino acid pattern generally occurs through the regulation of oxidative catabolism, transamination, and protein synthesis of acute phase proteins in the liver, although protein synthesis during recovery in skeletal muscle and wound repair will also utilize significant quantities of amino acids.

Figure 15-26 shows the catabolic pathways

of the liberated amino acids and the glucose and lipid catabolic substrates, as well as the sequence of amino acid participation in urea synthesis. All of these pathways occur primar-

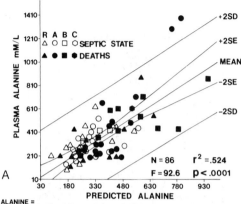

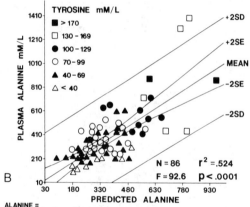

FIG. 15-25 (A) Prediction of alanine from endogenous branched chain amino acid (BCAA) levels and pyruvate. Points labeled by physiologic state (R, A, B, C) and by survival or death. ENDOILEU and ENDOVAL represent endogenous isoleucine and endogenous valine respectively, computed as shown in Fig. 15-24. Note that the highest levels of BCAA-pyruvate predictors of alanine are associated with the highest plasma alanine levels and occur in septic A, B, and C state deaths. **(B)** Prediction of alanine from endogenous BCAA and pyruvate, this figure is identical to Fig. 15-25(A), except that the points are labeled by the plasma level of tyrosine. Note that the highest plasma alanine and BCAA-pyruvate predictor levels are associated with the highest plasma tyrosine levels. (Cerra FB, Siegel JH, Coleman B et al: Septic Autocannibalism. Ann Surg 192: 570, 1980.)

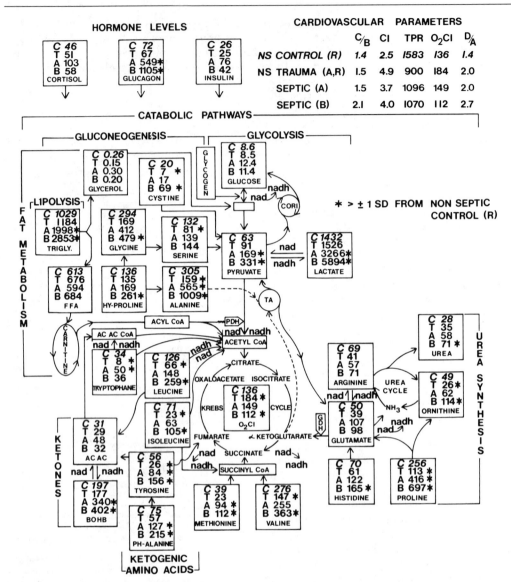

FIG. 15-26 Diagram of catabolic pathways for oxidation, gluconeogenesis and urea synthesis from amino acids in nonseptic R state controls, nonseptic trauma and septic A and B states of physiologic adaptation. Also shown are the cardiovascular parameters including cardiac index (CI), total peripheral resistance (TPR), oxygen consumption index (O_2CI), and the D/A and C/B state distance ratios as well as the plasma hormone levels of cortisol, glucagon, and insulin. The respective plasma levels of triglycerides, free fatty acids, and the ketone bodies acetoacetate (AcAc) and betahydroxybutyrate (BOHB) are also shown. This diagram demonstrates the relative sites of entry into the Krebs tricarboxylic acid cycle and shows that the plasma levels of circulating amino acids, glucose, lactate, and triglycerides tend to rise with transition from nonseptic to septic states, with the highest levels of being seen in B state sepsis where oxygen consumption is also reduced. All values given in μmole/l plasma, except glucose and glycerol, which are in mmol/l; urea, which is in mg percent; cortisol, which is in nanograms/ml; glucagon, which is in picagrams/ml; and insulin which is in μU/ml. See text for details. (Siegel JH, Cerra FB, Coleman B et al: Physiological and metabolic correlations in human sepsis. Surgery 86: 163, 1979.)

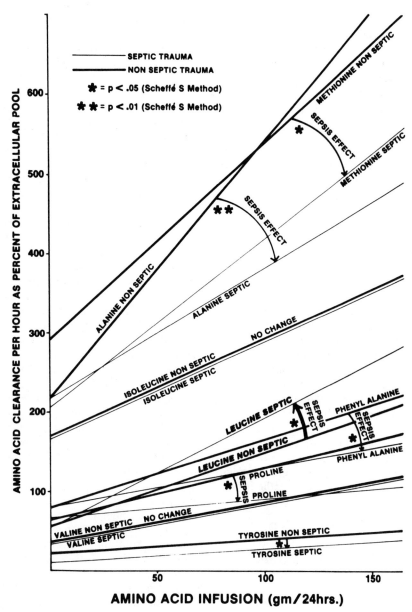

FIG. 15-27 Differential amino acid clearance in sepsis. Comparison between amino acid clearance per hour (as percent of extracellular pool) per gram of amino acid infusion, including both exogenous and endogenous sources. Note that the rate of clearance increases as a function of the amino acid infusion rate. However, the slope (rate of rise in clearance) of all amino acids is decreased by sepsis, except for that of the branched chain amino acids (leucine increases, isoleucine and valine remain unchanged). *P* values tested by the Scheffé method for the simultaneous determination of all contrasts. (Pittiruti M, Siegel JH, Sganga G et al: Increased dependence on leucine in post traumatic sepsis: leucine/tyrosine clearance ratio as indicator of hepatic impairment in septic multiple organ failure syndrome. Surgery 98: 378, 1985.)

ily in liver or kidney. This figure also shows the circulating plasma levels of the regulatory hormones, cortisol, glucagon, and insulin found in trauma and in sepsis.[125] For comparison Figure 15-26 demonstrates the respective plasma levels in nonseptic control general surgical patients in an R state, nonseptic trauma patients, and septic A or septic B state patients. The amino acid levels in each group are presented together with their respective mean cardiovascular parameters and oxygen consumption values. This figure also indicates the major catabolic pathways for the amino acids that can participate in gluconeogenesis, the ketogenic amino acids, and the primary amino acid sequence of urea synthesis. It also demonstrates where in the Krebs tricarboxycylic cycle the ketogenic, branch chain, and sulfur-containing amino acids enter for oxidation. The points of critical control at the preparatory enzymes (pyruvate dehydrogenase [PDH] and glutamate dehydrogenase [GDH]) are shown. The branched chain amino acids, leucine and isoleucine, also require a branched chain ketoacid dehydrogenase for conversion to acetyl-CoA. These processes will be discussed in greater detail in the section on regulatory control. However, the important point this diagram leads us to consider is that the maintenance of the plasma levels is a function of the input of amino acids into the plasma from proteolysis and exogenous amino acid sources and is also a function of the rate of clearance from the plasma by the various organs that utilize amino acids for oxidative catabolism or synthetic processes.

Amino Acid Clearances

As shown by Pearl and colleagues[105] and by Pittiruti et al.,[108] there are significant differences in amino acid clearance in septic versus nonseptic trauma. This is shown in Figure 15-27, which demonstrates amino acid clearances as a function of the rate of amino acid infusion from both exogenous and endogenous sources in patients with nonseptic trauma and in patients in whom sepsis has complicated the traumatic episode. The first point made by this fig-

ure is that in either condition the individual amino acid clearances increase in either condition as a function of the rate of amino acids infused. Second, at any TPN infusion rate, the amino acid clearances are decreased in septic trauma patients compared to the nonseptic trauma patients for all amino acids, except the branched chain amino acids.[108] Isoleucine and valine clearances show no change (which is a relative increase compared to a nonbranched chain amino acids) and leucine clearance undergoes an actual increase as a function of the sepsis effect.

When septic survivors are compared to those patients who go on to septic death with multiple organ failure (Fig. 15-28), a significant increase in the clearance of the branched chain amino acids occurs as sepsis worsens.[108] In contrast, there is a further significant decrease in the clearance of the aromatic amino acid tyrosine. These changes are of particular interest in view of the cardiovascular and metabolic evidence presented earlier, which suggests a negative effect on hepatic metabolic function in sepsis compared to nonsepsis. This effect becomes of increasing importance as septic deterioration from the A to the B state occurs. Using a standard amino acid TPN mixture with a constant leucine/tyrosine concentration ratio, the differential in clearance rates between the BCAA and tyrosine is of great importance in quantifying the degree of hepatic dysfunction, since tyrosine is mainly catabolized in the liver, but the branched chain amino acids can be used by peripheral tissues such as skeletal muscle at a time when glucose metabolism is impaired. Under these circumstances there may also be enhanced hepatic utilization of branched chain amino acids. Thus at a constant intravenous infusion ratio for these two amino acids, the leucine clearance divided by the tyrosine clearance is a sophisticated index of hepatic function in trauma and sepsis.[108]

The importance of amino acid clearance primarily for oxidative purposes and for gluconeogenesis in nonseptic and septic posttrauma patients is shown in Figure 15-29. This figure presents the mean group (NST, septic survivors and septic deaths) clearances of key amino acids, compared to the uptake of glucose, the level of oxygen consumption, and magnitude of urea production with regard to their stan-

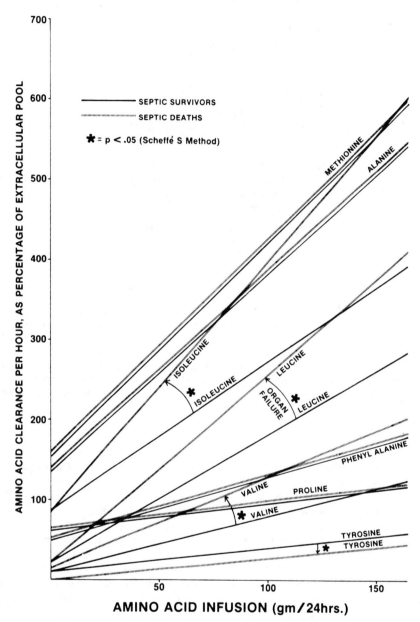

FIG. 15-28 Increased clearance of branched chain amino acids in septic nonsurvivors as multiple organ failure syndrome develops. Axes the same as in Fig. 15-27. Note that with development of septic multiple organ failure syndrome tyrosine clearance decreases, but all of the branched chain amino acids show an increase in clearance in septic nonsurvivors. (Pittiruti M, Siegel JH, Sganga G et al: Increased dependence on leucine in post traumatic sepsis: leucine/tyrosine clearance ratio as indicator of hepatic impairment in septic multiple organ failure syndrome. Surgery 98: 378, 1985.)

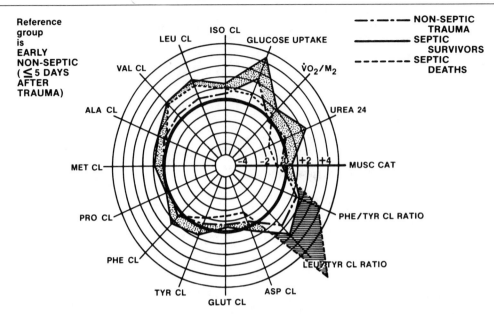

FIG. 15-29 Amino acid clearances during the late clinical course (greater than 5 days) after trauma in nonseptic trauma, septic survivors, and septic deaths. Dark circle represents the mean of patients with early nonseptic trauma studied immediately after injury. Each circle (increased or decreased) represents 1 standard deviation from the nonseptic reference group. For comparison are shown the late courses of nonseptic trauma survivors, septic survivors, and septic deaths with MOFS. Note that the prominent features of the septic MOFS deaths are the decrease in glucose uptake and the reduced oxygen consumption. There is also a decrease in urea production, marked increases in the phenylalanine/tyrosine clearance ratio and in the leucine/tyrosine clearance ratio. (Pittiruti M, Siegel JH, Sganga G et al: Increased dependence on leucine in post traumatic sepsis: leucine/tyrosine clearance ratio as indicator of hepatic impairment in septic multiple organ failure syndrome. Surgery 98: 378, 1985.)

dard deviations from patients with nonseptic syndromes seen early after trauma.[108] As this figure demonstrates, compared to NST patients at the same point in their time course, surviving posttrauma patients with sepsis evolving more than 5 days after trauma show increased oxygen consumption, increased glucose uptake, increased muscle catabolism, and increased urea production, as well as increases in the clearances of the branched chain amino acids, alanine, methionine, and the aromatic amino acids phenylalanine and tyrosine. Compared to NST, surviving septic patients also have small increases in the leucine/tyrosine clearance ratio. However, in ST patients who go on to die, with deterioration of the septic process leading to MOFS, the clearance of tyrosine is decreased while that of the branched chain amino acids remains increased. In these patients, oxygen consumption falls and urea production is reduced as the leucine/tyrosine ratio and the

phenylalanine/tyrosine clearance ratio rise disproportionately. These metabolic abnormalities of amino acid clearance and oxygen consumption reflect the development of hepatocellular failure occurring with the evolution of the B-state septic pattern.

The catabolism of the cleared amino acids for oxidative energy metabolism and gluconeogenesis that require deamination leading to urea synthesis (as opposed to their use as building blocks in protein synthesis) is seen in Figure 15-30. Here the relationship of the clearances of alanine and glutamine–glutamate (the carrier amino acids derived from muscle use of branched chain amino acids for oxidative catabolism) to the hepatic production of urea is shown. It can be seen that over the same range of glutamate–glutamine and alanine there is a significant increase in the rate of urea production in patients with septic trauma compared to nonseptic trauma.

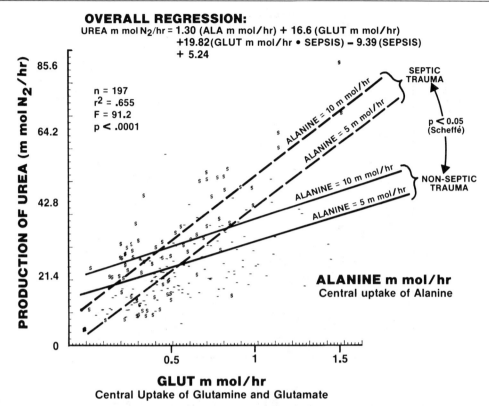

OVERALL REGRESSION:
UREA m mol N_2/hr = 1.30 (ALA m mol/hr) + 16.6 (GLUT m mol/hr)
+19.82(GLUT m mol/hr • SEPSIS) – 9.39 (SEPSIS)
+ 5.24

FIG. 15-30 Increased role of carrier amino acids, alanine, and glutamine/glutamate on the production of urea in septic and nonseptic trauma. Patients with septic trauma labeled as *s* and patients with nonseptic trauma labeled with minus sign. Note that over the same range of glutamine/glutamate clearance there is an increased slope of the alanine clearance as it relates to the production of urea. All differences evaluated by the Scheffé simultaneous method of comparison of all contrasts. The covariance regression equation is also shown. (Pittiruti M, Siegel JH, Sganga G et al: Arch Surg, submitted for publication, 1986.)

The major role of alanine in sepsis is as a substrate for gluconeogenesis, which occurs in liver and kidney (see Fig. 15-26). As is shown in Figure 15-31, which compares septic trauma to NST patients over the same range of alanine clearance, when the glucose uptake rate is decreased (reflecting decreased oxidative utilization of glucose by peripheral tissues), the glucose pool and the level of plasma glucose rise significantly. These data emphasize two points in the management of the septic patient. The first is that gluconeogenic amino acids primarily represented by alanine become a major glucose precursor in sepsis. This is similar to the circumstances found in diabetes mellitus by Felig.[41] Secondly, under circumstances where decreased glucose utilization occurs in sepsis, TPN amino acid mixtures high in alanine may unnecessarily exaggerate the already existent hyperglycemia by promoting gluconeogenesis to a greater degree than the resultant glucose can be cleared from the circulation by peripheral tissues. These two facts have profound implications for management of the septic patient with regard to nutritional support and provide insight into the disorder of metabolic control initiated by the septic process.

Lactate Acidemia

Associated with the inability to utilize glucose is a increased production of lactate, which rises in proportion to the increase in pyruvate

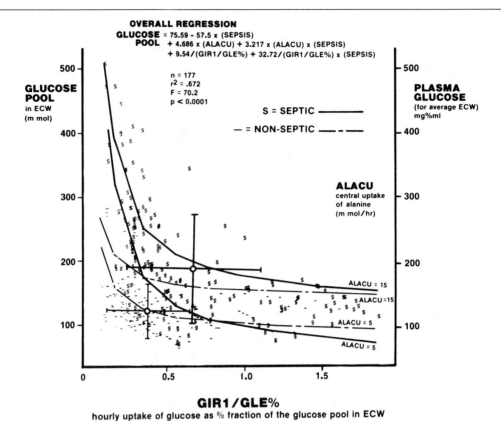

OVERALL REGRESSION
GLUCOSE = 75.59 - 57.5 x (SEPSIS)
POOL   + 4.686 x (ALACU) + 3.217 x (ALACU) x (SEPSIS)
      + 9.54/(GIR1/GLE%) + 32.72/(GIR1/GLE%) x (SEPSIS)

n = 177
r^2 = .672
F = 70.2
p < 0.0001

S = SEPTIC ————
— = NON-SEPTIC —— - ——

GLUCOSE POOL in ECW (m mol)

PLASMA GLUCOSE (for average ECW) mg%ml

ALACU central uptake of alanine (m mol/hr)

GIR1/GLE%
hourly uptake of glucose as % fraction of the glucose pool in ECW

FIG. 15-31 Gluconeogenic role of alanine clearance in increasing glucose pool and plasma glucose levels in severe septic versus nonseptic trauma patients. Note that as the glucose uptake decreases, indicating the development of severe "insulin resistance," there is a rise in plasma glucose and the glucose pool as a function of the level of central alanine uptake. This suggests that increased gluconeogenesis from alanine precursors in a major factor in the septic hyperglycemia. The covariance regression equation is also shown. (Siegel JH, Pittiruti M, Sganga G, unpublished results, 1986.)

and which is also proportionate to the increase in alanine seen in the septic patient.[125] This is shown in Figure 15-32, which demonstrates that compared to nonseptic general surgery and trauma patients, septic patients show a marked increase in plasma lactate levels, although the lactate/pyruvate ratio remains relatively constant. This increase in lactate, pyruvate, and alanine is highest in the B state or A to B state transition patients and occurs at a time when oxygen consumption is reduced. This suggests that the glucose intolerance seen in the septic patient represents an inability to oxidize lactate as well. This implies a post insulin receptor inhibition of the critical regulatory enzyme pyruvate dehydrogenase that con-

verts pyruvate to acetyl-CoA and therefore mediates the oxidation of pyruvate precursors, lactate and glucose, by controlling entry into the Krebs tricarboxycylic acid cycle. A rise in lactate has a poor prognosis if uncorrected therapeutically.[10,125,138]

Lipid Metabolism

Another aspect of the altered substrate metabolism in sepsis is in lipid metabolism. This can be seen in Figure 15-26. With progres-

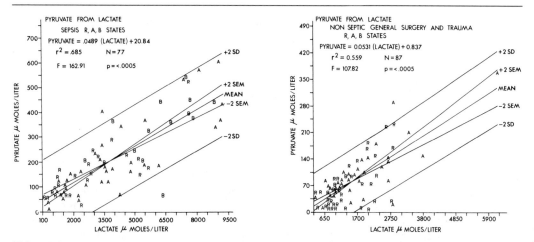

FIG. 15-32 Relationship of plasma pyruvate to plasma lactate levels. Comparison of relationship in septic states with that seen in nonseptic general surgical and trauma patients after resuscitation. Note that the relationship (β-coefficient) between lactate and pyruvate is the same in both conditions. However, septic A and B state patients tend to have higher levels of both pyruvate and lactate indicating that there is not an ischemic shift to excess lactate production, but rather a back pressure because of the reduced oxidation of pyruvate, so that the ratio between pyruvate and lactate remains constant throughout. (Siegel JH, Cerra FB, Coleman B et al: Physiological and metabolic correlations in human sepsis. Surgery 86: 163, 1979.)

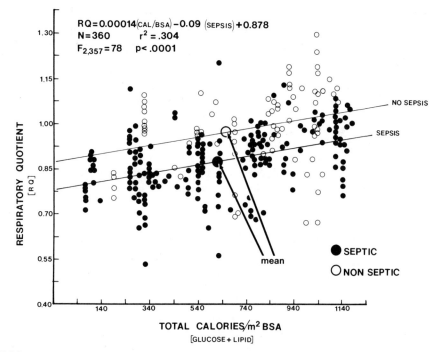

FIG. 15-33 Effect of an increase in total daily calorie input on respiratory quotient (RQ) in septic and nonseptic patients. Note that for any given calorie level the RQ is lower in the patients with sepsis. Covariance regression equation is also shown. (Nanni G, Siegel JH, Coleman B et al: Increased lipid fuel dependence in the critically ill septic patient. J Trauma 24: 14, 1984.)

TABLE 15-1. Metabolic Gas Exchange in Sepsis

Group	N	$\dot{V}O_2$ (ml/min/m²)	$\dot{V}CO_2$ (ml/min/m²)	RQ
Nonseptic	128	133 ± 27 ⌐	129 ± 29 ⌐	0.98 ± 0.12 ⌐
		0.0001[a]	NS[a]	0.0001[a]
Septic	246	144 ± 19 ⌐	126 ± 19 ⌐	0.87 ± 0.10 ⌐

[a] P-values for Student's t-test of differences between means.

(Nanni G, Siegel JH, Coleman B et al: Increased lipid dependence in the critically ill septic patient. J Trauma 24: 14, 1984.)

sion of the septic process the level of circulating triglycerides rises, even though there are only small increases in circulating levels of free fatty acids and ketone bodies. At the same time there is a marked shift in metabolism as measured by the respiratory quotient (RQ). The RQ provides information about the relative proportion of carbohydrate versus lipid fuels metabolized. A respiratory quotient of 1.0 indicates that carbohydrate or gluconeogenic amino acids alone represent the major caloric fuel utilization source. A respiratory quotient of less than 1 indicates that an alteration in the metabolic fuel utilization has occurred with a dependence on lipid sources as the primary oxidative fuel. A respiratory quotient of greater than 1.0 indicates that the input of carbohydrate and other fuel sources is in excess of metabolic needs, so that carbon fragments (via cytosolic acetyl-CoA and malonyl-CoA) are being converted to lipids and net lipogenesis is occurring. The increased utilization of lipids in sepsis is seen in Figure 15-33, which compares the respiratory quotient of nonseptic critically ill patients with septic critically ill patients. In both septic and nonseptic patients, as the total caloric input is increased there is a tendency for the respiratory quotient to rise. This indicates the ability of nutritional support both to satisfy metabolic needs and to contribute to lipogenesis.[95,176] However, the fuel set-point is different in nonseptic and septic patients for a given level of caloric input. Patients with sepsis tend to have a lower respiratory quotient for any given daily level of calories,[95,143,176] which suggests that their basic metabolic balance is shifted toward oxidation of lipid fuels over carbohydrate (Table 15-1). This is consistent with observations that glucose intolerance occurs and that lactate, glucose, and pyruvate levels rise as the septic process becomes more severe.[82,83,119,125,169]

Table 15-2 shows that the septic patient will preferentially utilize lipid sources if these are provided and that increased oxidation of lipids is the cause of the drop in the respiratory quotient, since the level of oxygen consumption increases when lipid fuels are given although the level of carbon dioxide production does not change, thus producing the fall in RQ. This preferential utilization of lipids is also shown in Figure 15-34, in which septic patients are compared with regard to their response to increasing total calories when a glucose-only TPN is utilized as the fuel source versus a glucose-plus-lipid TPN fuel mixture.[95]

TABLE 15-2. Metabolic Gas Exchange: Effect of Lipids and Sepsis

	N	$\dot{V}O_2$ (ml/min/m²)	$\dot{V}CO_2$ (ml/min/m²)	RQ
Nonseptic (no lipid infusion)	94	136 ± 28 ⌐	130 ± 29 ⌐	0.97 ± 0.12 ⌐
		0.09[a]	0.08[a]	0.001[a]
Nonseptic (lipid infusion)	34	124 ± 18 ⌐	125 ± 22 ⌐	1.01 ± 0.12 ⌐
Effect of lipid in nonseptic		⌐ −12	⌐ −5	⌐ +0.04
		0.05[a] 0.0001[a]	0.05[a] NS[a]	NS[a] 0.001[a]
Septic (no lipid infusion)	132	142 ± 19 ⌐	123 ± 19 ⌐	0.87 ± 0.10 ⌐
Septic (lipid infusion)	114	151 ± 14 ⌐	134 ± 19 ⌐	0.89 ± 0.09 ⌐
Effect of lipid in septic		⌐ +9	⌐ +11	⌐ +0.02

[a] P-values for Scheffé's method of simultaneous inference for all contrasts in the analysis of variance.

(Nanni G, Siegel JH, Coleman B et al: Increased lipid fuel dependence in the critically ill septic patient. J Trauma 24: 14, 1984.)

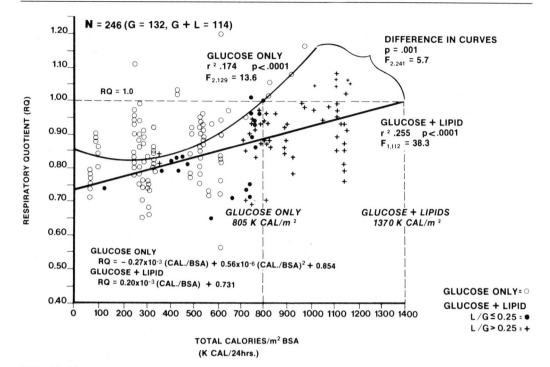

FIG. 15-34 Influence of nutritional fuel on respiratory quotient (RQ) in sepsis. Comparison of glucose-only TPN with TPN containing glucose-plus-lipid. Note that the use of glucose-only fuel rapidly raises respiratory quotient to 1.0. Thus, glucose-only calories tend to produce lipogenesis at relatively low daily intake. In contrast, glucose-plus-lipid fuel maintains an RQ of less than 1.0 up to a much higher calorie level, suggesting increased oxidation and energy production. (Nanni G, Siegel JH, Coleman B et al: Increased lipid fuel dependence in the critically ill septic patient. J Trauma 24: 14, 1984.)

When only glucose is used as the calorie source, there is a rapid increase in the respiratory quotient in septic patients. An RQ of 1.0 is reached at approximately 800 kcal/m², at which point net lipogenesis occurs. In contrast, in the same patients when oxidation is compared using a glucose-plus-lipid calorie source, the initial respiratory quotient is lower and the respiratory quotient of 1.0 is reached at a much higher total caloric level, 1400 kcal/m². This suggests that a more economical source of oxidative energy can be found in the use of lipid fuels and re-emphasizes that the control of oxidative fuel utilization is of critical importance in the septic patient. It also suggests that the increased hepatic lipid synthesis in sepsis may have a survival advantage by providing a usable fuel for peripheral oxidation when glucose oxidation is inhibited.

CELLULAR BIOCHEMISTRY OF METABOLIC CONTROL

In normal humans and animals, there is a fine balance between anabolism and catabolism. Following a meal, anabolism predominates and energy stores are sequested from the injested meal. These energy stores include glycogen, which is mainly stored in the liver and muscle; triglycerides, which are derived both from injested fats and from excess glucose consumption; and proteins, which can be considered amino acid stores. Between meals and in some pathologic conditions, these energy stores are broken down. Experimental studies show that glucose incorporated into liver or carcass glycogen is readily utilized. For example, normal rats show a loss of 99.5 percent of liver glycogen and 70.3 percent of carcass glycogen after 48 hours of starvation.[144] However, the glucose released is not sufficient to sustain the energy needs of the body for more than a short period of time. Fatty acids liberated from triglyceride pools in adipose tissue are either directly oxidized by peripheral tissues or taken up and partially oxidized in hepatic tissue with the formation of ketone bodies. Ketone bodies can serve as useful fuels for many tissues including heart, lung, skeletal muscle, and brain. The body's adaption to use alternative fuels to glucose is of fundamental importance to the survival of the organism.

Conservation of glucose carbon is also of vital importance. Certain cells, such as erythrocytes and cells of the renal medulla and central nervous system, have an absolute requirement for glucose, which translates[112] into approximately 180 g glucose/24 hr. Less than one-half of this demand for glucose can be supplied by the limited hepatic stores of glycogen. Of greater importance for the generation of glucose fuel is the ability of the liver to synthetize glucose from carbon precursors using gluconeogenesis. The liver synthesizes glucose from glycerol, lactate, and gluconeogenic amino acids (Fig. 15-35).

Glycerol is derived from adipose tissue following the breakdown of triglycerides. The remaining precursors for gluconeogenesis are derived from the recycling of glucose through lactate and pyruvate with muscle glycogen contributing significantly to the lactate pool for gluconeogenesis. As discussed earlier, the gluconeogenic amino acids are derived from the breakdown of proteins, particularly in skeletal muscle.

Hormonal Regulation of Metabolic Control

Many of these processes are under hormonal control. This serves to regulate the flow of glucose carbon to ensure adequate levels of blood glucose. These so-called metabolic hormones can be broadly categorized into two groups: anabolic and catabolic. The principal anabolic hormone is insulin. It is of major importance in fuel storage, promoting the synthesis of glycogen, triglycerides, and proteins. At basal levels, insulin has an important anticatabolic role in restraining glycogenolysis, gluconeogenesis, and lipolysis. Growth hormone is also anabolic, but only with respect to protein metabolism; growth hormone stimulates amino acid transport and protein synthesis. The major catabolic hormones are glucagon, cortisol, and catecholamines. None of these hormones itself totally opposes the anabolic actions of insulin,

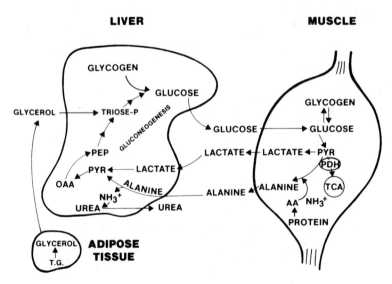

FIG. 15-35 Interorgan transfer of glucose carbon as alanine and lactate between liver and skeletal muscle. Role of glycerol from adipose tissue as glucose precursor. PYR, pyruvate; PDH, pyruvate dehydrogenase complex; TCA, tricarboxylic acid cycle; AA, amino acids; OAA, oxaloacetate; PEP, phosphoenolpyruvate; TRIOSE-P, triose phosphates; TG, triglycerides; AA, free amino acids.

but these hormones can counterbalance the actions of insulin by acting together. Glucagon has its major effects on the liver promoting gluconeogenesis, amino acid uptake, ureagenesis, and hepatic protein catabolism.[36,70] This latter effect of glucagon has been demonstrated to be secondary to a decreased intracellular glutamine level.[96] Cortisol enhances extrahepatic protein catabolism and promotes hepatic utilization of mobilized amino acids for gluconeogenesis. Catecholamines stimulate lipolysis and glycogenolysis in both hepatic and extrahepatic tissues.

Monitoring the septic patient has demonstrated that the normal balance between anabolic and catabolic processes is altered in the direction of catabolic metabolism.[78,84] This results in pathologic alterations in glucose, fatty acid, and amino acid metabolism. The pattern of alterations in the plasma level of these fuels is superimposed on changes in the plasma hormonal levels. Changes in carbohydrate metabolism after trauma and during sepsis include hyperglycemia, insulin resistance, elevated output of hepatic glucose, and increased gluconeogenesis. The metabolic alterations that occur in sepsis are numerous and all of them probably contribute to a cascade of secondary alterations that result from the initial traumatic or septic episode and collectively lead to the patterns of changes observed in plasma from critically ill patients. The most dramatic change in the catabolic hormones occur with glucagon, which rises to extraordinary high levels. Although the rise in glucagon is accompanied by a rise in immunoassayable insulin, the insulin/glucagon ratio is reversed compared to the post absorptive state. This reversal of the insulin/glucagon ratio may be responsible in part for the accelerated rate of glucose production by the liver observed in sepsis. Insulin and glucagon both have immediate and delayed effects on hepatic glucose production.[36,75] The rapid effects of glucagon are observed within seconds and may be mediated in part by changes in the concentration of cAMP[36] (Figure 15-36).

The delayed effects usually appear within hours and involve changes in the synthesis or degradation of enzymes in the metabolic pathway of glucose production.[36,75,164] Catecholamines also stimulate both glycogenolysis and gluconeogenesis. Plasma catecholamines, epinephrine and norepinephrine, have been demonstrated to rise progressively with increasing severity of injury as assessed by the Injury

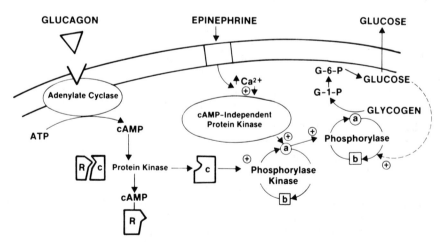

FIG. 15-36 Hormonal regulation of glycogenolysis in liver by glucagon and epinephrine. Glucagon acts through a cAMP-dependent protein kinase, while epinephrine functions through a cAMP-independent protein kinase. Both protein kinases act to increase phosphorylase kinase, which in turn activates phosphorylase b. A (+) shows sites of activation. G-6-P, glucose-6-phosphate; G-1-P, glucose-1-phosphate; cAMP, 5'-3' cyclic Adenosine Monophosphate; R, regulatory subunit cAMP-dependent protein kinase; C, catalytic subunit cAMP-dependent protein kinase; Ca^{2+}, calcium stimulation of protein kinase.

Severity Score.[31,44] Dopamine levels are also elevated, but appear to be related to norepinephrine levels. Both epinephrine and norepinephrine rise to plasma levels considered able to produce metabolic changes.[30] Regression analysis has revealed that plasma epinephrine concentrations are a more important stimulus for hyperglycemia following severe injury than is the severity of the injury itself.[44] Recent studies have demonstrated that the stimulation of hepatic glucose output by catecholamines is not necessarily mediated through changes in cAMP, as is the case with glucagon.[9,23,148] Instead it appears that catecholamines may activate glycogenolysis more effectively through a cAMP-independent mechanism involving α-adrenergic receptors, rather than through the cAMP-dependent mechanisms mediated through β-adrenergic receptors. The α-adrenergic activation of glycogenolysis is due to an increase in phosphorylase a. This effect may be mediated by alterations in Ca^{2+} influx and may be best explained by a stimulation of Ca^{2+}-sensitive phosphorylase kinase[9,148] (Fig. 15-36).

However, alterations in the plasma insulin/glucagon ratio, or catecholamine levels, are not solely responsible for enhanced glucose production. Unlike other conditions, the increased gluconeogenesis observed in sepsis is not suppressed by infusion of glucose.[82,119] This lack of response to glucose has been proposed to occur as a result of enhanced and continued delivery of gluconeogenic precursors from peripheral tissues.

Regulation of Glucose Metabolism and Control of Glucose Oxidation

In addition to alterations in hepatic glucose metabolism, glucose metabolism in peripheral tissue is also altered in sepsis. Glucose intolerance is commonly observed despite normal or accentuated insulin secretion following injury, burn shock or sepsis. Despite this insulin response, glucose intolerance and hyperglycemia persist. This suggests that certain target tissues of the injured or septic patients are relatively insensitive to the effects of circulating insulin. Glucose consumption by central and peripheral nervous systems, renal medulla, bone marrow, erythrocytes, and leukocytes is not insulin-dependent. The primary effect of insulin is to enhance the uptake of glucose in peripheral tissues, mainly skeletal muscle and fat. Since only a small proportion (1 percent) of a glucose load is taken up by adipose tissue, the major effect of insulin appears to be on muscle tissues. Hence it would appear that the skeletal muscle is where the insulin resistance occurs. This resistance to the effects of circulating insulin could be due either to changes in the sensitivity of the insulin receptor to circulating insulin or to a postreceptor defect related to alterations in intracellular metabolism. The sensitivity of the insulin receptor to circulating insulin appears to be normal. Therefore, intracellular glucose metabolism appears to be altered in sepsis, and may be responsible, in part, for the insulin resistance observed.

Most physiological control of glucose utilization occurs at the level of cell membrane glucose uptake (transport and phosphorylation), cytosolic glycogenolysis (phosphorylase), and glycolysis (phosphofructokinase) and mitochondrial oxidation (pyruvate dehydrogenase).[150] In vivo tracer studies in patients and septic animal models have shown that sepsis results in an increased glucose uptake.[8,11,71,82,119,120,168,174] In septic patients glucose utilization and lactate and alanine production are increased, which suggests that the processes of glucose uptake and glycolysis are normal or accelerated in sepsis. However, the increased glucose uptake was not accompanied by increased rate of glucose oxidation. Instead, the glucose carbon is realeased from peripheral tissues into the venous blood as lactate and alanine and returned to the liver (or kidney) to be converted into glucose by the process of gluconeogenesis (Fig. 15-37). Thus, glucose carbon is conserved. This interorgan relationship with the conservation of glucose carbon as lactate and alanine may account for the increased rate of glucose carbon turnover (recycling) in sepsis.

Glucose oxidation can be regulated either by the formation of pyruvate or by the entry of glucose carbon into the TCA cycle. Pyruvate can be formed from glycolysis (from glucose

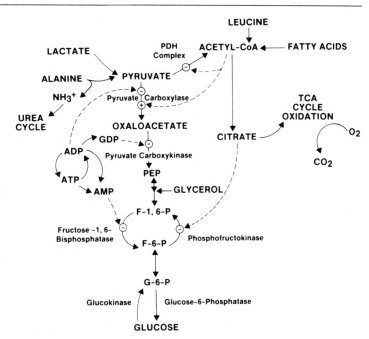

FIG. 15-37 This figure shows the regulation of hepatic gluconeogenesis by adenine nucleotides, acetyl-CoA and citrate. Dotted lines show sites of activation (+) or inhibition (−) by various metabolites. AMP, Adenine nucleotide 5′ monophosphate; ADP, Adenine nucleotide 5′ diphosphate; ATP, Adenine nucleotide 5′ triphosphate; GDP, Guanosine-5′ diphosphate; PEP, phosphoenolpyruvate; F-1,6-P, Fructose-1,6-bisphosphate; F-6-P, Fructose-6-phosphate; G-6-P, Glucose-6-phosphate.

or glycogen) and from amino acids. Estimates of glucose recycling in sepsis[8,11,71,82,119,120,168,174] suggest that the rate of pyruvate formation is probably not rate-limiting for glucose oxidation. Thus, the entry of glucose carbon into the tricarboxylic acid cycle may be the limiting step for glucose oxidation in sepsis. The mitochondrial pyruvate dehydrogenase (PDH) complex catalyzes the oxidative decarboxylation of pyruvate in the presence of the cofactors CoA and NAD to form carbon dioxide and acetyl-CoA and NADH, and allows for entry of pyruvate into the TCA cycle.[110-112] The pyruvate dehydrogenase complex (Fig. 15-38) is regulated by end-product inhibition and by reversible phosphorylation catalyzed by a pyruvate dehydrogenase kinase and phosphatase.[79] The phosphorylated form of the complex is inactive. The dephosphorylated form is active and allows for flux through the complex. The oxidative decarboxylation of pyruvate to acetyl-CoA by the pyruvate dehydrogenase complex is of special importance to glucose homeostasis because it necessarily depletes the body of glucose carbon.[110-112]

In experiments with isolated tissue preparations, it has been possible to show that a specific inhibition of the pyruvate dehydrogenase reaction is involved in the impairment of glucose oxidation during starvation, in alloxan-diabetes, sepsis, and by the oxidation of fatty acids and ketone bodies in liver, heart, and skeletal muscle.[110-112] Glucose oxidation is impaired while lactate, pyruvate, and alanine output are undiminished.[55,111] The overall contribution of inhibition of the pyruvate dehydrogenase reaction to the inhibition of glucose oxidation can be substantial. For example, in rat hearts perfused with buffer containing glucose and insulin, addition of acetate can completely inhibit glucose oxidation, whereas the rates of pyruvate, lactate, and alanine formation are inhibited[97] by only 60 to 70 percent.

In contrast to starvation, alloxan-diabetes, and high-fat diets, the regulation of the pyruvate dehydrogenase complex in liver and skeletal muscle appears to be different in sterile inflammation and sepsis[151,153] (Fig. 15-39). Sterile inflammation increases the proportion of active pyruvate dehydrogenase activity in hepatic tissue (Fig. 15-39). However, the effect of sepsis on the proportion of active pyruvate dehydrogenase complex appears to be dependent on the severity of the septic episode. In livers from animals with a small abscess, the effect of sepsis on the proportion of active pyru-

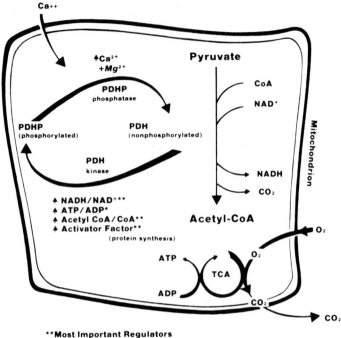

FIG. 15-38 Interconversion cycle regulating the phosphorylation/dephosphorylation of pyruvate dehydrogenase complex (PDH) in mammalian cells. CoA, Coenzyme A; PDH, Pyruvate Dehydrogenase Complex; PDHP, Phosphorylated Pyruvate Dehydrogenase Complex; NAD⁺(H), Nicotinamide Adenine Dinucleotide (Reduced); ATP, Adenosine 5'-Triphosphate; ADP, Adenosine 5'-Diphosphate; TCA, Tricarboxylic Cycle.

vate dehydrogenase complex is similar to that observed in sterile inflammation. When the abscess size is increased the proportion of active pyruvate dehydrogenase complex is reduced relative to sterile inflammation and the small septic abscess.

A different response in the proportion of active pyruvate dehydrogenase complex in skeletal muscle is observed in sterile inflammation and sepsis (Fig. 15-39). Introduction of a sterile abscess does not alter the proportion of active pyruvate dehydrogenase complex compared to control animals. The effect of sepsis, whether a small or large septic abscess, is to lower the proportion of active pyruvate dehydrogenase complex. Hence, in contrast to hepatic tissue, the effects of sepsis are independent of the severity of the septic episode. These data suggest that an early response to sepsis is a decreased proportion of active pyruvate dehydrogenase complex activity in skeletal muscle. Since decreased pyruvate dehydrogenase activity is associated with a decreased pyruvate oxidation, the decreased pyruvate dehydrogenase activity may provide a biochemical explanation for the shift in skeletal

muscle glucose metabolism in sepsis. Furthermore, this may be responsible for the sepsis-induced "insulin resistance."

A frequent complication in septic patients is lactic acidosis, which may contribute to the observed mortality.[10,102,138] From the studies described above, it is evident that the increased plasma lactate levels may occur secondary to an inhibition of the PDH complex. Although many different therapies for hyperlactatemia in sepsis have been attempted, none have proven successful when the treatment of the underlying sepsis is not effective. Recent studies demonstrate that the administration of dichloroacetate can reverse the hyperlactatemia occurring in chronic severe septic animals.[154] The decrease in circulating plasma lactate levels (Fig. 15-40A) was associated with a corresponding decrease in tissue lactate levels in both liver (Fig. 15-40B) and skeletal muscle (Fig. 15-40C). Similar results have been found in normal humans and in patients with lactic acidemia secondary to renal or hepatic disease and infection.[138,139]

Dichloroacetate reduces circulating lactate, pyruvate, and alanine in other pathologic

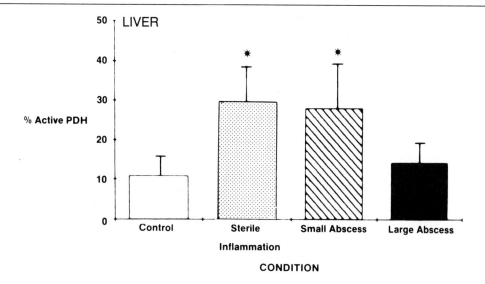

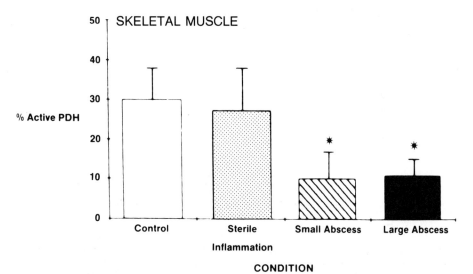

FIG. 15-39 Effect of sterile inflammation and large and small abscesses on hepatic and skeletal muscle pyruvate dehydrogenase activity levels. Studies from 250 g rat model in which a rat fecal-agar pellet was inserted into the intra-abdominal cavity. The pellet was either sterile, or contained biclonal bacterial inoculum consisting of 10^6 *E. coli* and 10^8 *Bacteroides fragilis.* Small abscess pellet (0.8 ml volume) produced a 3 to 4 ml pus containing abscess, large pellet (1.5 ml volume) produced 11 to 12 ml volume abscess. Liver and skeletal muscle samples frozen in situ 7 days after intra-abdominal introduction of pellet. Results are presented as a percentage of total PDH complex existing in active form. Note, differential effect on skeletal muscle and liver with regard to effect of small abscess and the difference between effect on PDH in skeletal muscle in septic abscess compared to sterile inflammation suggesting additional septic down-regulation. Variables shown are means ± SE for 10 to 14 animals in each group. * $P < 0.005$ vs control, Scheffé analysis of all contrasts. (Vary TC, Siegel JH, Nakatani T et al: Am J Physiol, 250:E634, 1986.)

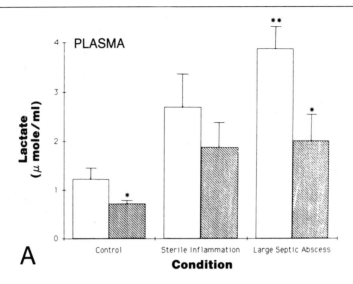

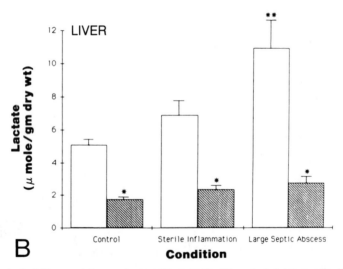

FIG. 15-40 Effect of dichloroacetate on plasma (**A**), hepatic (**B**) and skeletal muscle (**C**) lactate levels in sterile inflammation and large chronic septic abscess. Liver (**B**) and skeletal muscle (**C**) samples from control rats, or rats with sterile inflammatory, or chronic septic abscess (open bars) were frozen in situ 7 days following the intra-abdominal introduction of a rat fecal-agar pellet that was either sterile or inoculated with 10^6 *E. coli* and 10^8 *Bacteroides fragilis*. Blood samples were withdrawn from the inferior vena cava. Lactate determined in neutralized perchloric acid extracts by standard spectrophotometric techniques. Dichloroacetate (DCA) (1 mmol/kg) was injected intraperitoneally and this injection was repeated 30 and 60 minutes after the initial dosage. After the final DCA injection, the tissues were sampled and plasma was taken from the IVC (shaded bars). Values are means ± SE for 4 to 18 animals in each group. Units are nmol/g dry weight for tissues and μmol/ml for blood plasma. Plasma [$P < 0.05$ compared to animals without DCA (open bars); ** $P < 0.001$ compared to control animals]. Liver and skeletal muscle [* $P < 0.001$ compared to animals without DCA (open bars); ** $P < 0.005$ compared to control animals (open bar)]. (*Figure continues.*)

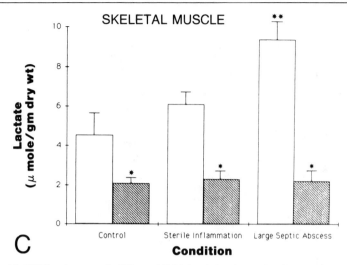

FIG. 15-40(C) *(Continued)*. Effect of DCA in skeletal muscle. (Data from ref. 154.)

conditions by activating the PDH complex[35,60] (Fig. 15-41). Dichloroacetate (DCA) noncompetitively inhibits the PDH kinase, allowing the unopposed activation of the phosphorylated PDH complex by the phosphatase.[163] An

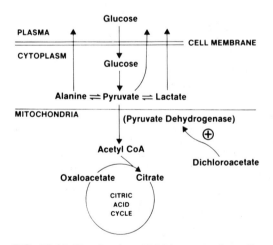

FIG. 15-41 Site of action of DCA in mammalian cells, DCA activates pyruvate dehydrogenase, thereby increasing the flux of 3-carbon compounds into the tricarboxylic acid cycle and decreasing the release of lactate, pyruvate, and alanine into the circulation. (Blackshear PJ, Fang L S-T, Alexrod L: Treatment of severe lactic acidosis with dichloroacetate. Diabetes Care 5:391, 1982.)

increased pyruvate dehydrogenase activity would lead to increased flux into the citric acid cycle. Consequently, the release of lactate, pyruvate, and alanine from peripheral tissues into circulation will be decreased and fewer three-carbon fragments would be available for gluconeogenesis.[51] The fall in plasma lactate and alanine with DCA has been documented in nonseptic diabetic humans[138,139] and in septic rats with a large chronic abscess.[154] Dichloroacetate activates PDH complex in liver (Fig. 15-42A) and skeletal muscle (Fig. 15-42B) from septic animals. Since plasma glucose levels in chronically septic rats are not decreased by dichloroacetate, the effects of dichloroacetate on plasma lactate are not due to decreased pyruvate formation via glycolysis, secondary to hypoglycemia. Thus, dichloroacetate decreases blood lactate and alanine concentrations in septic animals by activating the pyruvate dehydrogenase, and hence, pyruvate oxidation, in skeletal muscle and hepatic tissues.

A differential response in the regulation of the PDH complex in liver and skeletal muscle was observed in sterile inflammatory and septic animals with a large chronic abscess. In liver, the proportion of active PDH was increased in sterile inflammation relative to control animals. However, the proportion of active PDH complex in livers from septic animals with

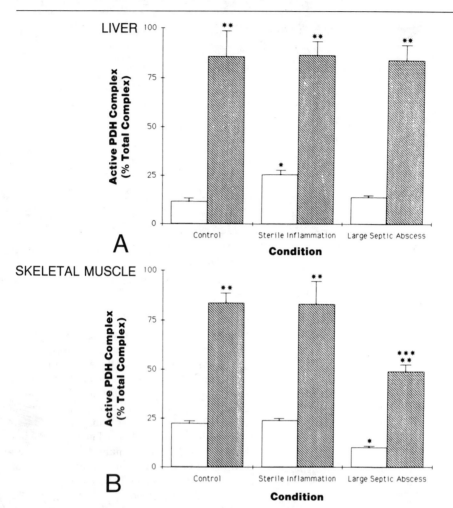

FIG. 15-42 Effects of dichloroacetate on hepatic (**A**) and skeletal muscle (**B**) percentage of active pyruvate dehydrogenase (percent PDHa) in sterile inflammation and large chronic septic abscess. Liver and skeletal muscle samples from rats were frozen in situ 7 days after the intra-abdominal introduction of a sterile or bacterial inoculated fecal-agar pellet as described in Fig. 15-40. Dichloroacetate (DCA) was administered as described in Fig. 15-40. Extracts of frozen tissues were assayed for active and total PDH complex activity . The results are expressed as the percentage of total PDH complex existing in the active form. Total complex (sum of active and inactive forms) was not different in DCA treated animals. Non-DCA, open bars; post-DCA, shaded bars. Values shown are means ± SE for 4 to 10 animals in each group. [* $P < 0.001$ compared to control without DCA (open bar); ** $P < 0.001$ DCA (shaded bars) compared to animals without DCA; *** $P < 0.005$ DCA after septic abscess (shaded bar) compared to control animals with DCA administration]. (Data from ref. 154.)

a large chronic abscess was reduced relative to sterile inflammatory animals. Despite these differences in the proportion of active PDH complex, the hepatic PDH complex was activated to the same extent following injection of dichloroacetate in each of the conditions examined (Fig. 15-42A).

In contrast to liver tissue, the proportion of active PDH complex was not affected by sterile inflammation in skeletal muscle. However, the proportion of active PDH complex was decreased relative to control and sterile inflammation in septic animals. In skeletal muscle, following injection of dichloroacetate, the activation of PDH complex in control and sterile inflammatory rats was similar. The magnitude of the dichloroacetate-induced activation of the PDH complex was similar to that observed in liver. However, dichloroacetate did not activate PDH in skeletal muscle from septic rats with a large chronic abscess to the same extent as in either control or sterile inflammation (Fig. 15-42B).

Despite this less than full activation of the PDH complex in skeletal muscle from septic animals, the activation was sufficient to lower skeletal muscle lactate levels (Fig. 15-40C). The demonstration of a differential response to sterile inflammation and sepsis in liver and skeletal muscle with dichloroacetate administration is of importance in understanding the interorgan fuel energy flux. It also suggests a specific septic factor that nonreversibly down-regulates PDH activity in muscle.

The molecular mechanisms responsbile for the reduced responsiveness of skeletal muscle PDH complex from septic animals to activation by dichloroacetate are unknown at present. Resistance to activation by injection of dichloroacetate cannot be due merely to the decreased initial proportion of active PDH complex observed in skeletal muscle from septic rats. In normal rat hearts perfused with 3-hydroxybutyrate, the proportion of active complex is low (10 percent) and addition of dichloroacetate to the perfusate fully activates the PDH complex. However, in hearts from alloxan-diabetic rats, compared to nondiabetics given DCA (92 percent), the diabetic effect lowering the proportion of active PDH complex (8 percent) persists when the concentration of active complex is changed (64 percent) by perfusion with dichloroacetate.[149] It has been suggested that this effect of alloxan-diabetes on limiting the activation of PDH by dichloroacetate is due to the activation of the pyruvate dehydrogenase kinase reaction by a factor termed kinase/activator.[65] Increasing the PDH kinase reaction results in multisite phosphorylation, which partially limits reactivation by the phosphatase. Hence, the PDH complex becomes locked in a phosphorylated, inactive state. Preliminary experimental studies by the authors suggest that the PDH kinase activity of skeletal muscle is stimulated at least twofold in sepsis, compared to sterile inflammation or

control (Vary TC, Siegel JH, unpublished results, 1986). The rate constant for inactivation of PDH kinase by ATP is similar to that observed in starvation or diabetes.[50] These data suggest that sepsis may activate existing control mechanisms in a nonphysiologic manner.

The results of the present study in septic rats with hyperlactatemia treated with dichloroacetate are noteworthy for two reasons. First, they show the drug's potential usefulness as treatment for lactic acidosis associated with sepsis. Second, they suggest that part of the underlying pathogenesis of lactic acidosis in sepsis may be a reduced pyruvate oxidation, secondary to an inhibition of the pyruvate dehydrogenase complex activity. Further investigations of the use of dichloroacetate in treating lactic acidosis associated with severe human sepsis appear warranted.

Although these studies provide information on the regulation of the proportion of active pyruvate dehydrogenase complex in sterile inflammation and sepsis, the mechanisms responsible for these changes are unknown. The proportion of active pyruvate dehydrogenase complex is determined by the relative rates of the pyruvate dehydrogenase kinase and phosphatase. The pyruvate dehydrogenase kinase is accelerated by increases in the mitochondrial $[acetyl\text{-}CoA]/[CoA]$, $[ATP]/[ADP]$, and $[NADH]/[NAD]$ concentration ratios[66] (Fig. 15-38). In skeletal muscle, the $[acetyl\text{-}CoA]/[CoA]$ concentration ratio appears to be the important regulator of the pyruvate dehydrogenase kinase activity.[2,50] The skeletal muscle $[acetyl\text{-}CoA]/[CoA]$ concentration ratio is low in control and sterile inflammatory animals, but is elevated threefold in septic animals.[151,153] These results suggest that changes in the $[acetyl\text{-}CoA]/[CoA]$ concentration ratio may be in large part responsible for the alterations in the proportion of pyruvate dehydrogenase activity observed in sepsis. The mechanisms responsible also may involve increased phosphorylating activity of pyruvate dehydrogenase kinase.

In muscle, the acetyl-CoA/CoA concentration ratio is a sensitive index of the availability of metabolic fuels to be oxidized by the tricarboxylic acid cycle.[97] The ratio is increased when noncarbohydrate fuels such as fatty acids are the major oxidative substrate (Fig. 15-43). Since the acetyl-CoA/CoA ratio is elevated

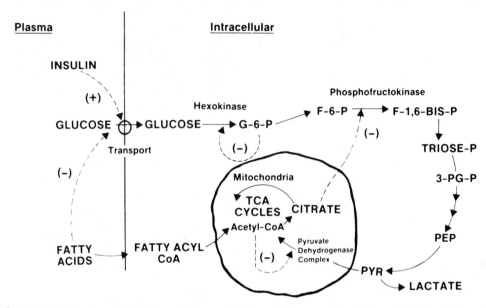

FIG. 15-43 Mechanism for regulation of glucose oxidation by increased free fatty acid (FFA) oxidation. End-product regulation by acetyl-CoA derived from fatty acyl-CoA oxidation or glucose causes inhibition of pyruvate dehydrogenase complex. Citrate derived from increased TCA cycle utilization of FFA inhibits Phosphofructokinase, buildup of G-6-P inhibits Hexokinase. Fatty acids may also inhibit glucose uptake at membrane level. Glucose transport is stimulated (+) by insulin in muscle tissue. G-6-P, Glucose-6-phosphate; F-6-P, fructose-6-phosphate; F-1,6 BISP, fructose-1,6-biphosphate; triose-P, triose phosphates; 3-PG-P, 3-phosphoglycerate phosphate; PEP, phosphoenolpyruvate; PYR, pyruvate.

in skeletal muscle from septic rats at a time when muscle PDH activity is reduced, this suggests that septic skeletal muscle is more dependent on noncarbohydrate fuels. The net effect of increased fatty acid fuel utilization would be a decreased rate of glucose oxidation and a conservation of glucose carbon. Analysis of respiratory quotients[94,95] and of indirect calorimetry[143] data in septic patients has demonstrated an increased dependence on fatty acids for oxidation, thus supporting the concept of altered fuel utilization in human sepsis.

Altered Branched Chain Amino Acid Metabolism in Normal Posttraumatic and Septic Skeletal Muscle

In the normal postabsorptive state, plasma alanine, the gluconeogenic substrate, can be derived from transamination of pyruvate with a nitrogen donor, as well as from protein stores[41] (Fig. 15-23). In the human forearm, alanine release is greater than can be accounted for by its concentration in skeletal muscle proteins.[57,113] This suggests that a significant amount of alanine released is synthesized from pyruvate derived from glucose as its carbon precursor and a nitrogen source. The potential nitrogen donors includes the branched chain amino acids (leucine, isoleucine, valine) and glutamine. Studies in postabsorptive humans have demonstrated that about 40 percent of the circulating plasma alanine can be derived from endogenous protein, whereas 60 percent is derived from de novo synthesis. In addition at least 20 percent of the nitrogen required for de novo synthesis comes from leucine.[57] Leucine (valine and isoleucine) nitrogen is presumed to be incorporated into alanine through a series of reversible transamination reactions involving the transfer of leucine nitrogen to glutamate via branched chain aminotransferase and the subsequent transamination of glutamate with pyruvate, forming alanine via glutamate or pyruvate.[69] The rate of alanine synthesis therefore will be determined by either the rate of leucine appearance, or the rate of pyruvate availability; as mentioned above, this is regulated by a number of factors.

There appears to be a differential pattern of branched chain amino acid metabolism in normal skeletal muscle and liver. In normal skeletal muscle, the aminotransferase activity is high and oxidative decarboxylation of the corresponding α-ketoacid is rate-limiting for leucine oxidation.[69] In isolated rat skeletal muscle, only about 50 percent of the leucine undergoing transamination is oxidized. The corresponding α-ketoacids are released into the blood. The α-ketoacids of branched chain amino acids are a normal constituent of human plasma and the concentration of individual keotacids is low. The normal concentration of all three α-ketoacids of branched chain amino acids in human plasma is approximately 0.1 to 0.4 mM. In liver, the α-ketoacids are readily oxidized, because the activity of the branched chain α-ketoacid dehydrogenase (BCKDH) is higher than the transaminase.[69] In the rat, the activity of the branched chain complex (milliunits/mg protein) is approximately 10 (liver), 4 to 6 (kidney), and 3 (heart or skeletal muscle).[80] The BCKDH is also regulated by a phosphorylation/dephosphorylation cycle analogous to the pyruvate dehydrogenase complex.[38,39,76] It appears that the branched chain α-ketoacid dehydrogenase (BCKDH) complex may be inactivated by phosphorylation in muscle, but protected in some way from inactivation in the liver. Recently, studies have demonstrated that the liver possesses extra amounts of the catalytic subunit of the enzyme, called activator protein, which can restore flux through phosphorylated branched chain amino acid dehydrogenase.[9] Hence, in liver it is unlikely that the activity of the branched chain dehydrogenase is rate-limiting for branched chain amino acid oxidation. It is suggested that activator protein affords a mechanism whereby branch chain ketoacids formed by transamination in extrahepatic tissues are degraded mainly in the liver with the possible formation of glucose and ketone bodies as ubiquitous fuels. Complete hepatic degradation of branched chain amino acids leads to the formation of HMG CoA (from leucine), succinyl-CoA (from valine), and acetyl-CoA and succinyl-CoA

(from isoleucine). Leucine and isoleucine are ketogenic and valine and isoleucine are glucogenic. However, the activity of the branched chain dehydrogenase complex may limit branched chain amino acid oxidation in muscle tissues. The absolute contribution of branched chain amino acids to energy metabolism is at present still debatable. In the absence of other exogenous substrates, leucine oxidation in heart muscle could only account for about 5 percent of the total oxygen consumption, even at supraphysiological plasma leucine concentrations. Furthermore, leucine, as sole substrate, could not provide sufficient energy to maintain normal cardiac function. Hence, it is doubtful that leucine represents a significant energy source in cardiac muscle tissues. The studies are less clear in the case of skeletal muscle, but a more important oxidative role in sepsis has been suggested.

It has been noted that concentrations of the branched chain amino acids are closely associated with nitrogen conservation. Thus, low circulating levels of leucine, as occur following administration of insulin, are associated with decreases in urinary urea and total nitrogen excretion. In contrast, high concentrations of plasma branched chain amino acids are associated with increased proteolysis. Protein wasting is a general feature of the trauma or septic patient. The increased proteolysis results in the release of amino acids from the protein stores, particularly skeletal muscle. The rate of release of amino acids from the leg increases two to five times in traumatized or septic patients compared to normal people following an overnight fast. When the molar percent of amino acids in muscle proteins is compared with the molar percent of amino acids released, it appears that the majority of amino acids are released in proportion to their concentration in muscle protein. However, it is well established that under conditions of negative nitrogen balance, large amounts of alanine and glutamine, in excess of their concentrations in proteins, are released from muscle to serve as a major source of carbon for glucose synthesis by liver.

In vitro studies have shown that leucine inhibits urea synthesis[89] and as noted below, may stimulate hepatic protein synthesis.[89] Addition of leucine causes an inhibition of citrulline synthesis and corresponding formation of glutamate and glutamine with either NH_3^+ or alanine as the nitrogen source.[89] The inhibition of urea synthesis by leucine was also observed when a mixture of 15 different amino acids at physiologic concentrations replaced alanine. An established effect of leucine is a marked activation of glutamate dehydrogenase in direction of glutamate synthesis, but it has no effect on the rate of glutamate deamination. If the inhibition of urea synthesis by leucine occurs in vivo, the amounts of nitrogen excreted as urea, or stored as glutamine, may be dictated in part by the intracellular leucine concentration.

Control of Muscle Proteolysis

The stimulus for enhanced muscle catabolism during sepsis is at present unknown. Studies of burn patients suggest that cortisol is a major determinant in the catabolic response.[168] Some of the proposed effects of cortisol have been confirmed in normal subjects with artificially elevated cortisol levels. However, in the postoperative state and most probably in sepsis, cortisol is of less importance, and the metabolic effects appear to be the net result of an integrated response to several hormones with the possibility of additional factors. Insulin conserves muscle protein by both stimulating protein synthesis and inhibiting protein degradation.[49,62,91] However, in sepsis and trauma, breakdown of muscle proteins, as measured by 3-methylhistidine release, is increased despite normal or increased insulin concentrations.[108,109,167] In addition, branched chain amino acids, especially leucine, have similar protein-sparing effects. Protein-sparing and possibly direct protein synthesis stimulation may be the mechanisms by which the beneficial effects of high branched chain amino acid infusions given as TPN are mediated.[14,43,116,121]

Both metabolic alterations and increased muscle proteolysis have been induced by interleukin-1,[3,25-27,34,81] which is produced by macrophages stimulated by activated complement. However, interleukin-1 has not been demonstrated in human blood, but a low-molecular-weight protein that produces similar effects has been isolated from patients with trauma and

sepsis. This low-molecular-weight substance, called PIF, has the ability to induce protein degradation and release of amino acids from muscles incubated in vitro at rates three to five times normal.[25-27]

Control of Hepatic Acute Phase Protein Synthesis

While it is clear that net proteolysis occurs in skeletal muscle during sepsis, the liver appears to increase its protein-synthesizing machinery. Important studies have demonstrated increased rates of hepatic protein synthesis following trauma or during infection.[81,159] However, it is still not entirely clear whether there is a preferential synthesis of endogenous or secretory proteins during sepsis. Most studies have simply measured whole-liver protein synthetic rates. Increased rates of synthesis of both endogenous and secreted proteins have been observed, but the quantitative relationships between the two have not been fully elucidated. The increased protein synthesis in liver coincides with enhanced uptake (or clearance) of amino acids. It has been suggested that the increased hepatic protein synthetic activity is caused by, or is dependent upon, an increased supply of amino acids from periphery. Much of the evidence for a role in amino acids in regulating protein synthesis comes from studies using isolated perfused liver.[43,106] In these systems it is possible to demonstrate enhanced rates of protein synthesis with increasing concentrations of amino acids. However, the mechanisms involved in this phenomenon do not appear to be involved with charging of the transfer RNA (tRNA), or limitation of the initiator methionyl-tRNA$_f^{MET}$, messenger RNA (mRNA) levels, or with increased amino acid oxidation.[43,106] Instead lower rates of synthesis in liver perfused with amino acid deficient medium may be a result of inhibition of peptide chain initiation, which caused polysomal disaggregation. The mechanism by which amino-acid deprivation affects the initiator complex remains unknown.

Trauma and sepsis have been shown to increase the hepatic synthesis and secretion into the plasma of a number of proteins referred to as acute phase proteins. The acute phase proteins include C-reactive protein, fibrinogen, ceruloplasmin, α_1-antitrypsin, transferrin, and α-2-macroglobulin. Many of these acute phase proteins are linked to the host's ability to resist or control infection.[67] These functions include complement activation and opsonization needed for bacterial killing (C-reactive protein), coagulation, surface structure and support lattice functions needed for leukocyte entrapment of foreign material (fibrinogen); superoxide scavenging (ceruloplasmin α-2-macroglobulin) and inactivation of excess proteases needed to prevent damage to viable cells (α_1-antitrypsin). In sepsis and trauma, interleukin-1 has been demonstrated to increase the synthesis of acute phase proteins in vitro.[81] Studies in patients have demonstrated a differential response in the plasma acute phase protein profile in trauma and sepsis. The presence of sepsis, whether clinically evident or not, modifies the posttraumatic acute phase protein response to favor plasma increase in some acute phase proteins, while affecting a decrease in the level of other proteins that may not be as critical to survival.[118] In both nonseptic and septic patients during the first 2 to 3 days after injury, there was a rise in plasma C-reactive protein, fibrinogen, α_1-antitrypsin, and ceruloplasmin levels. In nonseptic trauma patients, levels of C-reactive protein, fibrinogen, and ceruloplasmin all return toward normal values while α_1-antitrypsin levels remain elevated. In the trauma patients who go on to show clinical signs of sepsis, C-reactive protein, fibrinogen, α_1-antitrypsin, and ceruloplasmin levels all remain elevated. There was an early decrease in the transferrin level, or stability of the α_2-macroglobulin and albumin levels in patients with and without sepsis, followed by decrease in septic patients as sepsis progressed. The mechanisms for these changes are unknown. However, it is worth noting that alterations in synthesis of acute phase protein in mouse liver are associated with alterations in the mRNA for these proteins, and changes in albumin synthesis in rats rendered alloxan-diabetic are also mediated by alterations in the level of albumin mRNA.[106] These findings suggest that the differential pattern of protein synthesis between skeletal muscle and liver

may occur through transcriptional regulation of protein synthesis.

Lipid Metabolism

The metabolic course of traumatized or septic patients demonstrates that endogenous fatty acids become the primary fuel for oxidative metabolism. This conclusion is based upon analysis of respiratory quotients[95] and indirect colorimetry studies.[15,143] The same increased dependence upon fatty acid metabolism is observed in conditions such as starvation and diabetes.[110-112] In starvation, the mobilization of fatty acids from adipose tissue is coupled with an enhanced hepatic capacity for synthesizing ketone bodies. The mechanisms response for this enhanced ketogenic capacity include both increased substrate (fatty acids) and an increase in the glucagon levels leading to an increased glucagon/insulin ratio.[87] In addition, it appears that utilization of fatty acids by muscle tissue is dependent upon the delivery of fatty acids to the tissue.[103] As the plasma free fatty acid (FFA) concentrations are increased in starvation and diabetes, there is an increase in fatty acid extraction and oxidation. However, fatty metabolism is regulated differently in septic or injured patients compared to normals. In normal subjects, a close relationship exists between plasma FFA levels and FAA turnover rates over a wide variety of physiologic conditions. This normal relationship between plasma FFA concentration and turnover does not occur in injured or septic patients. In general, FFA turnover is higher than would have been predicted by the plasma FFA concentration.[119,120,175]

The release of FFA from adipose tissues in sepsis is variable; some reports show fatty acid release is increased and others show it to be decreased. Despite unaltered arterial plasma FFA acids, fatty acids are continually released into the blood and delivered to the liver. After removal of FFA from the plasma, FFA may either be oxidized or re-esterified into triglycerides. Increased hepatic triglycerides are a characteristic feature of sepsis, giving rise to the histologic observations of increased lipid droplets. Part of the increase in hepatic tri- glycerides may be due to re-esterification. The increased re-esterification of fatty acids in liver may also lead to increased rate of triglyceride secretion from the liver as very-low-density li- poprotein (VLDL-TG). Hypertriglyceridemia is also a characteristic feature of sepsis. Virtually all studies of progressive sepsis have shown increased plasma level of triglycerides as the septic process worsens. In addition to an in- crease in triglyceride synthesis, an impairment in triglyceride disposal mechanisms may also exist. Lipoprotein lipase is the enzyme is re- sponsible for the clearance of plasma triglycer- ides. Reduced lipoprotein lipase activity has been observed in muscle and adipose tissue from septic animals.[107,117] Concomitant with the

lowered lipoprotein lipase activity, triglyceride concentrations were increased.

Regulation of Ketone Body Formation

The normal response of the liver to an in- creased delivery of fatty acids is the synthesis of ketone bodies (3-L-hydroxybutyrate and acetoacetate). In conditions such as starvation and diabetes, ketogenesis is increased second- ary to increased fatty acid mobilization from adipose tissue. This increased fatty acid mobi- lization is thought to occur as a result of de-

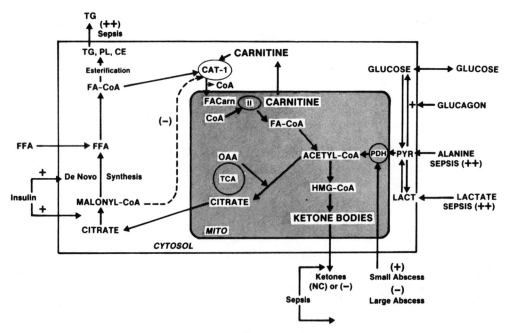

FIG. 15-44 Septic alteration of metabolic regulation of hepatic fatty acid oxidation, ketogenesis, fatty acid synthesis, and carbohydrate metabolism. Malonyl-CoA (---) derived from citrate and cytosolic acetyl-CoA inhibits carnitine:acyl CoA transferase I. [Carnitine:acyl CoA transferases (I and II) are bound to inner mitochondrial membrane in vivo, but for clarity the reactions are shown away from membrane.] The effect of hormones (insulin or glucagon) and small and large septic abscesses to increase (+), or inhibit (−) particular synthetic pathways or oxidation of specific substrates are shown. FFA, long-chain fatty acids; FA-CoA, long-chain fatty acyl-CoA; FA Carn, long-chain fatty acyl carnitine; CoA, coenzyme A; OAA, oxaloacetate; PYR, pyruvate; LACT, lactate; TCA, tricarboxylic cycle; TG, triglycerides; PL, Phospholipids; CAT-1, carnitine:acyl-CoA transferase I; II, carnitine:acyl transferase II; PDH, pyruvate dehydrogenase complex; MITO, mitochondria; HMG-CoA, β- hydroxy-β-methyl glutaryl-CoA. (Vary TC, Siegel JH, Nakatani T et al: A biochemical basis for depressed ketogen- esis in sepsis. J Trauma 26: 419, 1986.)

creasing insulin concentrations. In addition, an increase in the glucagon/insulin ratio appears to enhance the hepatic ketogenic capacity.[87] Although there is a rise in plasma glucagon levels and the glucagon/insulin ratio in sepsis, plasma insulin levels either remain constant or increase. Despite this increase in the glucagon/insulin ratio, the plasma ketone body levels in sepsis are lower than expected given the hormonal environment. Thus, sepsis appears to induce changes in hepatic fatty acid metabolism that prevent (or reverse) maximal rates of ketogenesis.

The rate of ketone body formation is a function of both the rate of influx of fatty acids from adipose tissue to liver and the extent to which the liver is capable of forming ketone bodies from fatty acids. Liver from septic animals perfused in vitro demonstrates a decreased ability to synthetize ketone bodies from long-chain fatty acids.[158] The primary regulatory event of hepatic long-chain fatty acid oxidation and ketone body synthesis is the carnitine/acyl CoA transferase I (CAT-1) reaction (Fig. 15-44). The carnitine acyl CoA transferase I is competitively inhibited by malonyl-CoA.[87] It also has been proposed that insulin stimulates formation of malonyl-CoA as a mechanism by which it inhibits ketogenesis.[13,173]

Malonyl-CoA is the first committed intermediate in the conversion of glucose into fat and its concentration is known to fluctuate in parallel with the rate of fatty acid synthesis.[87] It is believed that malonyl-CoA inhibits ketogenesis by interfering with the formation of long chain acyl carnitine. Malonyl-CoA would serve as an internal regulator to turn off ketogenesis whenever de novo fat synthesis occurs. Under conditions such as carbohydrate feeding (low glucagon/insulin), the malonyl-CoA levels are elevated, fatty acid synthesis is brisk, and the opposing pathway of fatty acid oxidation and ketone body formation is suppressed. The physiological role of malonyl-CoA appears to be as a mechanism to ensure unidirectional flow of carbon from glucose (or other precursors of pyruvate) to triglycerides, by suppressing the activity of carnitine/acyltransferase I and thereby preventing the futile reoxidation of newly synthesized fatty acids. In ketotic states, (high glucagon/insulin), malonyl-CoA levels fall, lipogenesis ceases, and the carnitine/acyl transferase I step is deregulated. The resulting activation of fatty acid oxidation and ketogenesis is further enhanced by increases in tissue carnitine content. In sepsis there is also a rise in glucagon/insulin ratio. However, the levels of both insulin and malonyl-CoA are elevated and not depressed, as in simple starvation.[152] The increase in malonyl-CoA may be responsible in part for the depressed rates of ketogenesis observed in sepsis.

Regulation of Hepatic Fatty Acid and Triglyceride Synthesis

Fatty acids are synthesized de novo in the cytosol by the addition to malonyl-CoA of two carbon units obtained from acetyl-CoA catalyzed by the multienzyme complex called fatty acid synthase. Malonyl-CoA is synthesized in the cytosol from acetyl-CoA via acetyl-CoA carboxylase. This is an irreversible step requiring acetyl-CoA, bicarbonate, and ATP, and the formation of a carboxybiotin intermediate. Acetyl-CoA generated in mitochondria cannot penetrate the inner mitochondrial membrane, therefore mitochondrial acetyl-CoA is not the direct precursor for de novo fatty acid synthesis. Acetyl-CoA condenses with oxaloacetate to form citrate, which can then be transported to the cytosol via the tricarboxylate anion carrier. In the cytosol, acetyl-CoA is reformed from citrate in a reaction catalyzed by citrate lyase.[75] The level of malonyl-CoA is elevated in livers from septic animals (Fig. 15-45). Since previous reports[54] have demonstrated a direct relationship between malonyl-CoA and rates of fatty acid synthesis, it is anticipated that lipogenesis may be stimulated in livers from septic animals at the same time as ketone body formation is inhibited or depressed (Fig. 15-46).

The overall rate of fatty acid synthesis is regulated in part by the formation of malonyl-CoA via acetyl-CoA carboxylase. Acetyl-CoA carboxylase exists as a protomer, which has low activity, and as polymer that is active.[53] Polymerization of the enzyme is dependent upon citrate.[92] Long-chain fatty acyl CoA esters favor dissociation.[101] Since fatty CoA esters are

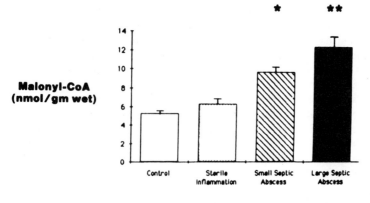

FIG. 15-45 Malonyl-CoA levels in control sterile inflammation and small and large chronic septic abscesses in rat model. Legend as in Fig. 15-39. * $P < 0.05$ compared to control; ** $P < 0.01$ compared to control. (Vary TC, Siegel JH, Nakatani T et al: A biochemical basis for depressed ketogenesis in sepsis. J Trauma 26: 419, 1986.)

known to accumulate as the exogenous fatty acid rises, fatty acids indirectly enhance their own oxidation by feedback inhibition of malonyl-CoA synthesis. In addition to activation by citrate, the *acetyl-CoA carboxylase* undergoes reversible phosphorylation.[13,59,87,172] Glucagon stimulates a cAMP-dependent protein kinase, which in turn phosphorylates the enzyme.[59,172] This phosphorylation has been associated with an inhibition of lipogenesis. Insulin also re-

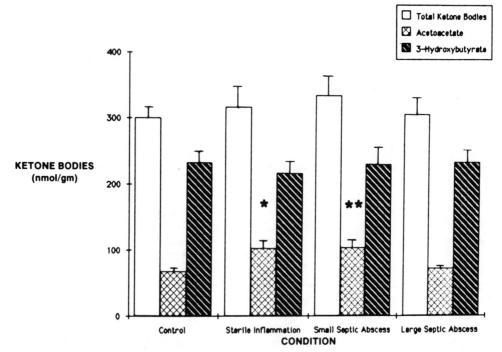

FIG. 15-46 Total ketone bodies, acetoacetate and betahydroxybutyrate levels in control, sterile inflammation and small and large septic abscesses. * $P < 0.05$ compared to control; ** $P < 0.01$ compared to control. There is a change in the oxidized to reduced ketone body ratio, but there is no significant alteration in the level of total ketone bodies in sterile inflammation or sepsis compared to control. Legend as in Fig. 15-39. (Vary TC, Siegel JH, Nakatani T et al: A biochemical basis for depressed ketogenesis in sepsis. J Trauma 26: 419, 1986.)

sults in phosphorylation of acetyl-CoA carboxylase.[13,173] In contrast to glucagon, the phosphorylation is catalyzed by a cAMP-independent protein kinase that phosphorylates a site distinct from the glucagon-induced cAMP-dependent phosphorylation. The effect of insulin is to stimulate acetyl-CoA carboxylase activity and enhance lipogenesis. At present there is no information concerning the regulation of acetyl-CoA carboxylase activity in sepsis.

MULTIPLE ORGAN FAILURE SYNDROME

As the patient's condition deteriorates in sepsis, a pattern of metabolic abnormalities develops that suggest a major pathologic abnormality in the normal interorgan regulation of substrate and fuel energy metabolism. This pattern of abnormalities finds its most abnormal picture with the development of the septic B state described earlier on the basis of hemodynamic studies. As a hypothesis for the manner in which this metabolic failure evolves, Figure 15-47, proposes that the normal muscle–liver–adipose-tissue cycle of substrate metabolism between these organs is altered by the septic insult.[123,125] A hypothesis for this is suggested from the work of Clowes,[25-27] Wannemacher et al.,[159] and others,[5,7,34] which indicates that the septic process initiates the production of interleukin I, which mediates an as yet unknown inflammatory proteolysis mechanism independent of the normal hormonally regulated proteolytic mechanisms initiated by the neuroendocrine axis.

These stress activated normal neuroendocrine mechanisms produce a heightened release of glucagon, corticosteroids, and catecholamines and potentiate the inflammatory

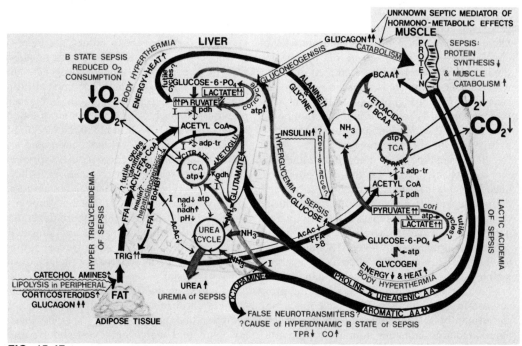

FIG. 15-47 Interorgan metabolic fuel-energy deficits and hepatic formation of false neurotransmitter pathophysiologic vasodilators in hyperdynamic B state sepsis and the multiple organ failure syndrome. See text for explanation. (Siegel JH: Relations between circulatory and metabolic changes in sepsis. Ann Rev Med 32: 175, 1981.)

proteolytic response. While other tissues participate, the net increase in muscle catabolism liberates large quantities of amino acids proportionate to the actin and myosin composition of the muscle. This is a major factor in the stress response to injury and sepsis, since the increased flux of amino acids into the circulation is used by the liver for acute phase protein synthesis, a process also stimulated by interleukin I.[81,159] Initially, the muscle can utilize a wide range of substrates for oxidative energy generation, such as glucose, fatty acids, and ketone bodies, as well as the ketoacids of the branched chain amino acids. However, as the sepsis evolves, there appears to be a specific defect in the muscle's ability to utilize glucose, due to a postreceptor blockade. As noted earlier, experimental studies have suggested that this may be secondary to a reduction in activity of muscle pyruvate dehydrogenase.[151,153,154] Under these conditions there is increased utilization of the branched chain amino acids which then enter the muscle's TCA cycle for oxidation.[45,57,69] The increased amount of branched chain amino acid ammonia nitrogen, which is detoxified by transamination with pyruvate derived from muscle glucose or glycogen, is converted to alanine, glycine, and glutamine, which are then released into the circulation and transported by the plasma to the liver.[57,119] As a result, the amount of these NH_3^+-carrier amino acids released is far in excess of that in muscle protein. In the liver, the transamination is reversed and the alanine is transaminated with α-ketoglutarate to form hepatic pyruvate and glutamate.[41,69]

In the hepatocyte, in nonseptic trauma or the compensated A state, the pyruvate produced by this transport mechanism is apparently utilized to form acetyl-CoA. Under these circumstances in early sepsis, PDH activity has been demonstrated to rise[151,153] and oxygen consumption increases.[123,125,133] This may be a mechanism to generate increased energy, which may be of value in assisting hepatic detoxification and acute phase synthetic processes. In addition, the increased glucagon elaborated by the pancreas in response to the neuroendocrine influence stimulates pyruvate carboxylase (PC), the initial step in gluconeogenesis. This increase in PC enzyme activity, which is energy-consuming, facilitates the

eventual reconversion of pyruvate to glucose-6-phosphate (G-6-P) as part of the gluconeogenic pathway.[70] As a result of G-6-P hydrolysis, there is increased formation of glucose from liver and kidney, which have similar gluconeogenic mechanisms. This accounts for the hyperglycemia of sepsis, which is further exaggerated by the fact that peripheral glucose oxidation may be diminished relative to production, as noted earlier. In skeletal muscle, PDH activity falls in sepsis[151,153] and increased equilibration of pyruvate with lactate produces an increased lactic acidemia.[125,154] The increased plasma lactic acid may also form a substrate for hepatic gluconeogenesis, as well as for oxidative metabolism in liver and heart, where PDH activity is increased.

However, as the septic process progresses in severity, there is evidence that pyruvate dehydrogenase activity in the liver may also become reduced.[151,153] In addition, a substantial proportion of the acetyl-CoA generated from glucose and other sources appears to be diverted to lipid formation, with movement of TCA cycle citrate from the intramitochondrial location to the cytosol where the formation of malonyl-CoA occurs.[87,98,101,104,152] Malonyl-CoA is the first obligatory precursor of fatty acid synthesis and appears to induce the increase in triglyceride formation that occurs in sepsis. Further experimental evidence suggests that the rise in hepatic malonyl-CoA concentration that occurs in sepsis, especially in late sepsis, may be responsible for suppression of ketone body formation.[86,152] In nondiabetic septic patients, a low ketone level has been noted and there is only a small increase as sepsis becomes more severe and changes from the A to B state[125] (Fig. 15-26). This has the net affect of denying an easily utilizable fuel source to the skeletal muscle, making it more dependent on branched chain amino acids and long chain fatty acids for oxidation, since glucose utilization appears to be suppressed (insulin resistance of sepsis).

Finally, as the B state of sepsis develops, there is an absolute reduction in oxygen consumption that may reach extremely low levels, far below that seen even at rest under normal circumstances, despite evidence of increased metabolic demands.[123,125,131,133] During this time, there also appears to be an impairment in the complete oxidation of the ureagenic amino acids that ordinarily enter the tricarboxycyclic acid cycle via glutamate.[17,108,109,125] This may reflect a depression in glutamate dehydrogenase activity as well. However, this has not been proven by any study. As a result, proline and related ureagenic precursor amino acids increase and very late in the septic process there is evidence that urea synthesis also may be impaired, reflecting the magnitude of cellular hepatic injury.[109] The impairments in amino acid and lipid metabolism generally occur earlier in sepsis than other aspects of hepatic dysfunction, such as the rise in bilirubin, the failure to detoxify a variety of drugs, or the rise in hepatic enzymes in the plasma.

In the specific case of the aromatic amino acids tyrosine and phenylalanine, the impairment of hepatic oxidative metabolism is very great. At a constant TPN infusion rate, the clearance of the aromatic amino acid tyrosine, which is metabolized almost entirely by liver, represents a very good indicator of the magnitude of the hepatic insult. As the hepatic injury of sepsis progresses with development of MOFS, there is an increasing disparity between the rising clearance of leucine, which is largely metabolized in the periphery, and the falling clearance of tyrosine which is metabolized almost entirely in the liver.[108] As a result, the increased leucine/tyrosine clearance ratio reflects the relative degree of hepatic to peripheral insufficiency occurring as MOFS progresses to a fatal outcome (Fig. 15-48A). This figure demonstrates the normal rise in leucine tyrosine clearance ratio with increased rates of standard TPN amino acid infusion occurring in survivors, compared to that occurring in patients dying of MOFS. The difference in slope is highly significant. Also shown in this figure is the time course of the surviving septic patient shown in Figure 15-7, who developed high-output cardiac failure during a period of B state decompensation. As can be seen in this figure, the evolution of the decompensatory response was marked by an increase in the leucine/tyrosine clearance ratio that responded to the surgical drainage of hepatic abscess with resolution of the drift toward the leucine/tyrosine clearance ratio characteristic of septic MOFS deaths. This occurred during the same time as the resolution from the septic B to septic A

state and the improvement in the myocardial ventricular function relationship with a fall in cardiac output toward normal hyperdynamic levels. This demonstrates the link between the cardiovascular, hepatic, and oxidative defects occurring in this group of patients. Figure 15-48B shows a similar plot of the time course of a patient dying of late multiple organ failure secondary to progressive sepsis originating in a major crushing injury of the face and frontal sinus with aspiration and gram-negative pneumonitis that eventually progressed to high-output renal failure and hepatic failure. In this nonsurviving patient the septic deterioration and final progression to MOFS were characterized by a progressive worsening of the leucine/tyrosine clearance ratio.

As noted earlier, with impairment of aromatic amino acid metabolism there is evidence that abnormal false neurotransmitter by-products of tyrosine, such as octopamine, are formed.[131] This latter substance, which has been demonstrated to produce abnormal reductions in vascular tone, also appears to cause an increase in the $\dot{V}A/\dot{Q}T$ ratio and thereby increases pulmonary shunting. Thus, as septic hepatic insufficiency occurs with impairment of amino acid metabolism, there is a parallel increase in the vascular tone abnormalities reflected by the physiologic state classification and evidence of a progression of the physiologic consequences of the septic ARDS syndrome. This linkage between abnormal hepatic function and ARDS appears to be an important component of septic MOFS.[6,16,47,48,130,131] In addition, there also appears to be evidence of myocardial depression that occurs frequently during the septic A to B state transformation.[125,130] This may reflect the fact that similar metabolic abnormalities that block the inotropic receptors sites permitting Ca^{++} entry, or limit substrate utilization may be occurring at the cardiac level.[22] However, at the present time no specific myocardial metabolic defects have been demonstrated in experimental studies.

Finally, an abnormal lipid metabolic relationship appears to be involved in the deteriorating MOFS response to sepsis, with increasing diversion of acetyl-CoA derived citrate via malonyl-CoA into the formation of increased levels of triglycerides,[152] which rise to ex-

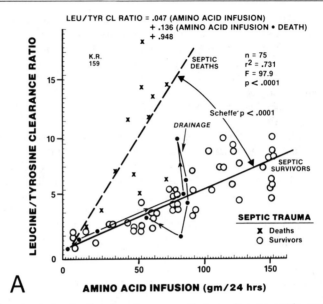

FIG. 15-48 (A) Alteration in leucine/tyrosine clearance ratio in posttrauma septic nonsurvivors compared to septic survivors. Septic MOFS deaths have significantly higher leucine/tyrosine clearance ratio per gram amino acid infusion, at constant leucine/tyrosine infusion ratio in TPN. Differences between two slopes determined by the Scheffé method for the simultaneous analysis of all contrasts. Also shown is time course of a surviving septic patient following development of hepatic abscess with MOFS and course of recovery after abscess drainage. Note alteration in the leucine/tyrosine clearance ratio as sepsis with hepatic component worsens. Improvement in course after I & D of abscess followed by reduction in the leucine/tyrosine clearance ratio to within the normal range. (*Figure continues.*)

tremely high levels during the B state transformation[125] (Fig. 15-26). Early in the septic process, lipid appears to be favored as a fuel source and patients with A state sepsis have a respiratory quotient generally < 1. This tends to drop further as sepsis progresses.[95] However, in the last stages of septic MOFS there may be impairment of the long chain fatty acid oxidation and the RQ may rise to 1. This may in part be related to the fact that septic patients show evidence of excessive carnitine loss, which may be a limiting factor after prolonged sepsis in the utilization and mitochondrial transfer of acyl-CoA esters for β-oxidation.[94] Whether carnitine loss is the critical factor is unknown, but there is clear evidence that the balance between the oxidation of fatty acids and the synthesis of triglycerides is markedly altered. This would be consistant with observations that reduced cytosolic carnitine promotes triglyceride synthesis.[150] The resulting hypertriglyceridemia of sepsis

that occurs in septic MOFS suggests that a futile cycle of fat metabolism may occur in B state sepsis.[125,175]

Reprioritization of Hepatic Protein Synthesis

The inability to oxidize a variety of metabolic fuels seen in progressive sepsis is paralleled by abnormalities in the hepatic synthesis of acute phase proteins. In nonseptic trauma or inflammation, there is evidence that the hepatic synthesis of a wide variety of acute phase proteins is enhanced.[67,81,118,159] This may be part of the inflammatory response mediated by interleukin I and similar agents.[34,81] In sterile inflammatory injury secondary to trauma, a variety of insults have been demonstrated to cause a rapid increase in synthesis of C-

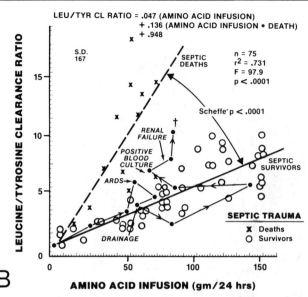

FIG. 15-48 (B) (*Continued*). Leucine tyrosine clearance ratio in posttrauma septic nonsurvivors compared to septic survivors. Legend as in Fig. 15-48(A). Shown in this figure is the time course of patient dying from progressive septic multiple organ failure syndrome. Demonstrating that progressive organ failure, including ARDS and high output renal failure, is associated with increases in the leucine/tyrosine clearance ratio. (Pittiruti M, Siegel JH, Sganga G et al: Increased dependence on leucine in post traumatic sepsis: leucine/tyrosine clearance ratio as indicator of hepatic impairment in septic multiple organ failure syndrome. Surgery 98: 378, 1985.)

reactive protein (CRP),[67,118] which plays a major role in nonspecific opsonization and complement activation that may be of importance in the control of bacterial invasion.[67,136,137] In addition, there is also increased formation of fibrinogen, which plays a major role in the coagulation process, of α-1-antitrypsin, α-2-macroglobulin, and ceruloplasm, all of which play a role in the inactivation of proteases and in superoxide scavenging.[67] Only the plasma level of albumin, which has a slower time constant for synthesis than the acute phase proteins, appears to be impaired in ordinary trauma or sterile inflammatory injury.[11]

However, in the septic patient, there is evidence of a reprioritization of hepatic acute phase proteins that becomes very marked as the septic process progresses to MOFS[118] (Fig. 15-49). The production of C-reactive protein is favored throughout all forms of sepsis and continues to be maintained at a high level, even when other synthetic processes such as urea synthesis and the formation of other acute

phase proteins are impaired. In Figure 15-50 urinary urea production and the plasma levels of C-reactive protein are compared in septic survivors and septic MOFS deaths with patients in nonseptic trauma. Both synthetic processes are seen to be impaired as the leucine/tyrosine clearance ratio increases. However, there is a statistically significant increase in both urea production and C-reactive protein levels in septic survivors compared to nonseptic trauma patients independent of the leucine/tyrosine (LT) clearance ratio. In contrast, in septic MOFS deaths the level of urea production is seen to be markedly diminished, suggesting a preterminal hepatic failure of urea synthesis, whereas C-reactive protein levels are maintained at extremely high levels both early and late in the MOFS process and appear to be independent of the LT clearance ratio. These data suggest that as the MOFS syndrome develops, certain synthetic processes become uncontrolled and favored over others. The production of C-reactive protein and α-1-antityp-

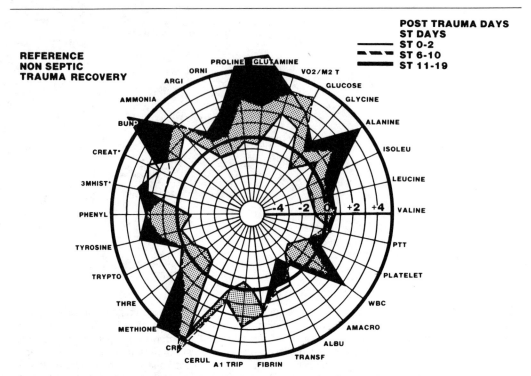

FIG. 15-49 Metabolic and acute phase protein abnormalities in septic trauma patients. The dark inner circle represents mean of nonseptic trauma patients following recovery, each circle (increased or decreased) represents 1 standard deviation from nonseptic trauma mean. Shown are the progressive alterations in oxygen consumption, glucose precursors, amino acids, urea precursors, and the acute phase proteins as sepsis progresses. Note reprioritization of acute phase proteins in late sepsis (11 to 19 days following the development of the septic course). ISOLEU, isoleucine; PTT, prothrombin time; AMACRO, α-2-macroglobulin; ALBU, albumin; TRANSF, transferrin; FIBRIN, fibrinogen; A-1-TRIP, α-1-antitrypsin; CERUL, ceruloplasmin; CRP, C-reactive protein; THRE, threanine; TRYPTO, tryptophane; PHENYL, phenylalanine; 3M HIST, 3-methylhistidine; CREAT, creatinine; BUN, blood urea nitrogen; ARGI, arginine; ORNI, ornithine; V̇O₂/m², oxygen consumption/m². (Sganga G, Siegel RH, Brown G et al: Reprioritization of hepatic plasma protein release in trauma and Arch Surg 120: 187, 1985.)

sin appears to be preserved despite the deterioration of a wide range of other synthetic and catabolic processes. The significance of this is unclear but it appears to represent a loss of regulation of the prioritized acute phase synthetic process even while other energy-engendering processes of fuel utilization and detoxifying processes are impaired.

However, as sepsis progresses in time and severity, there appears to be a reprioritization in the appearance of acute phase (AP) hepatic proteins. The increased CRP production is paralleled by increased levels of α-1-antitrypsin and to some extent an increase in fibrinogen, but there is evidence that the synthesis of ceru-

loplasm, α-2-macroglobulin, albumin, and transferrin is impaired and plasma levels of these AP proteins drop to low values (Fig. 15-49). This prioritization becomes more striking when the plasma levels of the various acute phase proteins are normalized with regard to their respective leucine/tyrosine clearance ratio (at a constant input infusion ratio of leucine and tyrosine) which puts the level of hepatic function in perspective.

Figure 15-51 shows that as the L/T ratio rises, reflecting deteriorating hepatic function, the increase in C-reactive protein in both nonseptic and septic patients is paralleled by a rise in α-1-antitrypsin. However, there are

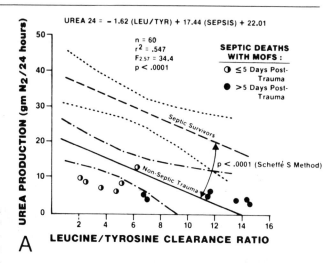

$$\text{UREA 24} = -1.62 \,(\text{LEU/TYR}) + 17.44 \,(\text{SEPSIS}) + 22.01$$

$n = 60$
$r^2 = .547$
$F_{2.57} = 34.4$
$p < .0001$

SEPTIC DEATHS
WITH MOFS :

◖ ≤5 Days Post-Trauma
● >5 Days Post-Trauma

Septic Survivors

Non-Septic Trauma

$p < .0001$ (Scheffé S Method)

FIG. 15-50 Effect of sepsis on urea production and C-reactive protein (CRP) as function of the leucine/tyrosine clearance ratio in posttraumatic survivors: (**A**) urea production and (**B**) CRP dependence covariance regressions. Note increased intercept, but similar slopes for septic effect in surviving patients. Values for septic deaths with MOFS drawn by circles for the early and late posttrauma periods after the development of sepsis. (Siegel JH, Pittiruti M, Sganga G et al, unpublished work, 1986.)

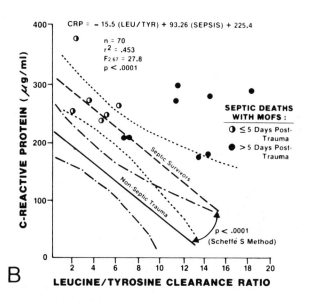

$$\text{CRP} = -15.5 \,(\text{LEU/TYR}) + 93.26 \,(\text{SEPSIS}) + 225.4$$

$n = 70$
$r^2 = .453$
$F_{2.67} = 27.8$
$p < .0001$

SEPTIC DEATHS
WITH MOFS :

◖ ≤5 Days Post-Trauma
● >5 Days Post-Trauma

Septic Survivors

Non-Septic Trauma

$p < .0001$
(Scheffé S Method)

smaller increments in the rise of fibrinogen (and in ceruloplasmin) in septic patients proportionate to that of CRP, but a large reduction in the increase in transferrin and α-macroglobulin compared to the CRP rise in the septic patients contrasted to nonseptic trauma. These data have lead to the hypothesis that as more of the muscle-released amino acids are diverted to become oxidative sources, due to the progressive septic limitations on oxidation of other fuels, there may be a inability to synthesize all acute phase proteins at the same rate.[118]

Therefore, those with the highest turnover rates may be given preference for synthesis over the others and a functional reprioritization may thus occur favoring the complement-activating CRP and the antiprotease α-1-antitrypsin at the expense of the antioxidant scavengers ceruloplasm and α-2-macroglobulin and the iron-binding AP protein transferrin. This type of reprioritization may also be occurring in a wide range of other structural and functional proteins and may account for the general failure of protein synthesis seen in late sepsis.

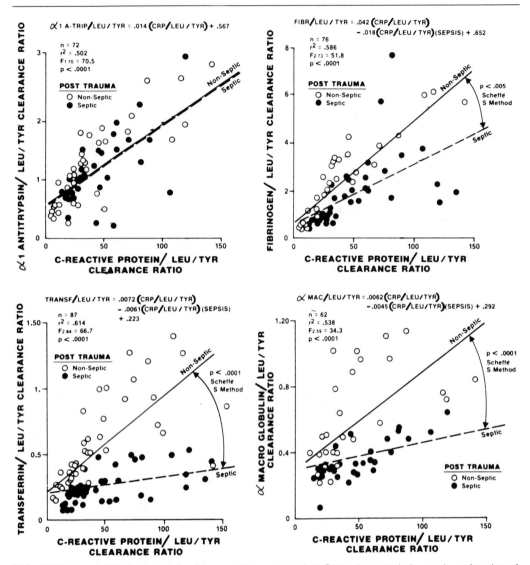

FIG. 15-51 Reprioritization of acute phase proteins compared to C-reactive protein in sepsis as function of the leucine/tyrosine clearance ratio. See text for details. Regression equations for each relationship are shown in the figure. (Siegel JH, Pittiruti M, Sganga G et al, unpublished work, 1986.)

The implications of these abnormalities in acute phase protein synthesis for the defense against bacterial invasion may be of importance. A number of studies have suggested that host defense also may be impaired in other factors related to protein synthesis. There is evidence that bacterial opsonizing fibronectin is decreased after injury and sepsis,[72,74] which may be due to increased binding or decreased production, or both. Polymorphonuclear cell superoxide formation in the septic patient appears impaired[72,73] by an abnormal circulating polypeptide. Polymorphonuclear chemotaxis has also been noted to be decreased.[135,137] Lymphocyte responsiveness may be reduced,[88,93] and skin test reactivity to test antigens decreases to the point of anergy in the severely sick septic patient.[16,24] Synthesis of albumin also appears to decrease markedly in late sepsis and clinical evidence of impairment in wound healing may reflect a defect in collagen synthesis as well. At the same time there is stimulation of fibrin deposition, immune complexes, and complement-activating processes necessary for white cell ingestion of microorganism and their killing by leukocyte-free radical elaboration. In more normal circumstances these processes promote bacterial control and the healing of the injury produced by trauma and sepsis, but in MOFS the balance between host defense and self-destruction is lost. Thus, clinical MOFS appears to reflect a runaway proteolysis of host tissues, with fundamental defects in oxidative energy metabolism and cellular immunologic responsiveness. There is also an inability to synthesize a wide range of critical proteins involved in detoxification of permeability changing substances and the prevention of excessive host cell injury from superoxide formation and proteases.

PHYSIOLOGIC STATE AND ITS BIOCHEMICAL CORRELATES AS A GUIDE TO TREATMENT

Linkage has been demonstrated between the progressive abnormalities in substrate oxidation with the appearance of abnormal vasoactive metabolic products of altered aromatic amino acid utilization and the physiologic pattern characterized as the B state of metabolic insufficiency. The relationship of this B state pattern to the presence of hepatic insufficiency in host defense protein synthesis suggests that careful bedside physiologic studies can provide a guide to the nature and urgency of therapeutic support. The physician can be guided by these in elaborating a comprehensive therapeutic approach to severe metabolic septic insufficiency. This therapeutic protocol, guided by the pattern of physiologic and metabolic defects, may require cardiac inotropic, ventilatory and nutritional support measures, with the occasional need for hemodialysis and

ultrafiltration in patients with oliguric failure. However, most important is the recognition that this pattern of defects indicates the presence of an inadequately drained, or antibiotic resistant septic process and mandates an aggressive therapeutic approach.

Therapeutic Implications of the Physiologic and Metabolic Abnormalities in Human Sepsis

Movement toward the B state indicates that the patient is not too sick to operate upon, but is too sick not to explore if there is a reasonable clinical question of an inadequately drained septic process. This is demonstrated in Figure 15-52. This 24-year-old patient sustained major multiple trauma secondary to a motor vehicle accident, with hepatic laceration, lung contusion with subsequent pulmonary sepsis and empyema, severe crushing injuries to the right lower extremity, and a closed head injury. He underwent immediate repair of his hepatic laceration and debridement of his open tibial injury with excision of necrotic muscle tissue. Subsequent to injury and emergency surgery a severe septic state developed. At the time of the first study shown (Fig. 15-52A) the empyema had already been drained. However the patient maintained a hyperdynamic state with a cardiac output of 12.2 L (CI, 5.6 L/min/m²) and a typical A state level of oxygen consumption ($\dot{V}O_2$/m², 182 ml/min) with evidence of metabolic acidosis (pH 7.37 with a base excess of -10.2 mEq/L and a hyperdynamic post septic pulmonary shunt ($\dot{Q}S/\dot{Q}T = 21$ percent, RI = 0.6).

In the 4 days following the study shown in Figure 15-52A the patient became progressively more septic (Fig. 15-52B). His cardiac output remained hyperdynamic but, there was a worsening of the metabolic acidosis. The pH decreased to 7.27 and the base excess declined to -14.1 mEq/L. Of concern was the shift from an A to a B state with an increase in mixed venous PO_2 and a decrease in the arteriovenous oxygen difference from 3.3 volume percent to 2.5 volume percent, even though cardiac

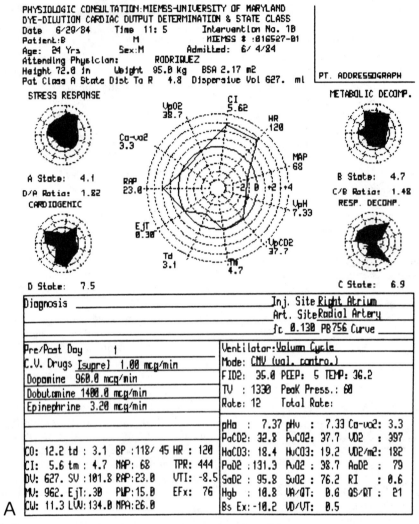

PHYSIOLOGIC CONSULTATION:MIEMSS-UNIVERSITY OF MARYLAND
DYE-DILUTION CARDIAC OUTPUT DETERMINATION & STATE CLASS
Date 6/29/84   Time 11: 5   Intervention No. 18
Patient:B   M   MIEMSS # :016527-01
Age: 24 Yrs   Sex:M   Admitted: 6/ 4/84
Attending Physician: RODRIGUEZ
Height 72.0 in   Weight 95.0 kg   BSA 2.17 m2
Pat Class A State Dist To R   4.8 Dispersive Vol 627. ml   PT. ADDRESSOGRAPH

STRESS RESPONSE   METABOLIC DECOMP.

VpO2 38.7   CI 5.62
Co-vo2 3.3   HR 120
                           MAP 68

A State: 4.1   RAP 23.0   B State: 4.7
D/A Ratio: 1.82   C/B Ratio: 1.48
CARDIOGENIC   RESP. DECONP.
                           VpH 7.33
EjT 0.30
                           VpCO2 37.7
Td 3.1   TM 4.7

D State: 7.5   C State: 6.9

Diagnosis _____	Inj. Site **Right Atrium**
	Art. Site **Radial Artery**
	fc **0.130** PB **756** Curve ____

Pre/Post Day 1	Ventilator:**Volume Cycle**
C.V. Drugs **Isuprel** 1.00 mcg/min	Mode: **CMV (vol. control)**
Dopamine 960.0 mcg/min	FIO2: 35.0 PEEP: 5 TEMP: 36.2
Dobutamine 1400.0 mcg/min	TV : 1330 Peak Press.: 60
Epinephrine 3.20 mcg/min	Rate: 12 Total Rate:
	pHa : 7.37 pHv : 7.33 Co-vo2: 3.3
	PaCO2: 32.8 PvCO2: 37.7 VO2 : 397
CO: 12.2 td : 3.1 BP :118/ 45 HR : 120	HaCO3: 18.4 HvCO3: 19.2 VO2/m2: 182
CI: 5.6 tm : 4.7 MAP: 68 TPR: 444	PaO2 :131.3 PvO2 : 38.7 AoD2 : 79
DV: 627. SV :101.8 RAP:23.0 VTI: -8.5	SaO2 : 95.8 SvO2 : 76.2 RI : 0.6
MV: 962. EjT:.30 PLP:15.0 EFx: 76	Hgb : 10.8 VA/QT: 0.6 QS/QT : 21
CW: 11.3 LW:134.0 NPA:26.0	Bs Ex:-10.2 VD/VT: 0.5

A

FIG. 15-52 (A) Physiologic consultation from 24-year-old multiple injury patient in A state hyperdynamic septic pattern with increased oxygen consumption ($\dot{V}O_2/m^2 = 182$ ml/min/m²). See text for details. Variables and circle diagram as in Fig. 15-2. (*Figure continues.*)

index had declined, so that oxygen consumption fell from a normal hypermetabolic level of 182 ml/min/min² to 126 ml/min/m². In association with this metabolic abnormality there was a marked further decrease in vascular tone, so that the TPR remained low in spite of the decrease in cardiac output and the ventilation/perfusion maldistribution characteristic of sepsis also increased. The $\dot{V}A/\dot{Q}T$ declined from 0.6 to 0.4 as the dead space to tidal volume ratio (VD/VT) increased from 0.5 to 0.6. The

transition from the A to B state is clearly demonstrated by the physiologic pattern shown in Figure 15-52B. Although the clinical condition remained much the same, it seemed clear that a further physiologic metabolic insufficiency had occurred. During this period repeated computed axial tomographic (CAT) scans demonstrated no evidence of intra-abdominal abscess or fluid collection and his pulmonary status also remained constant.

Since the only remaining area involved in

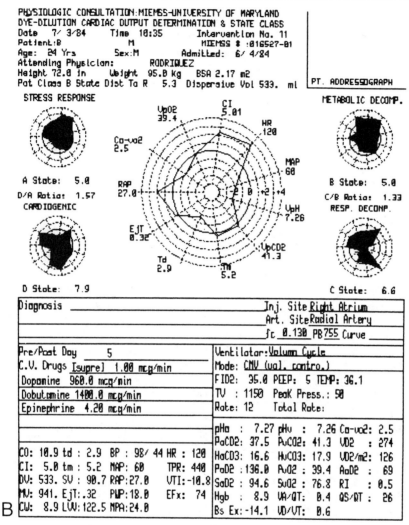

PHYSIOLOGIC CONSULTATION:MIEMSS-UNIVERSITY OF MARYLAND
DYE-DILUTION CARDIAC OUTPUT DETERMINATION & STATE CLASS
Date 7/ 3/84   Time 18:35   Intervention No. 11
Patient:B   M   MIEMSS # :016527-01
Age: 24 Yrs   Sex:M   Admitted: 6/ 4/84
Attending Physician: RODRIGUEZ
Height 72.0 in   Weight 95.0 kg   BSA 2.17 m2
Pat Class B State Dist To R 5.3 Dispersive Vol 533. ml

PT. ADDRESSOGRAPH

STRESS RESPONSE

METABOLIC DECOMP.

A State: 5.0
D/A Ratio: 1.57

CARDIOGENIC

B State: 5.0
C/B Ratio: 1.33

RESP. DECOMP.

D State: 7.9

C State: 6.6

Diagnosis _____	Inj. Site Right Atrium
	Art. Site Radial Artery
	ʃc 0.130 PB 755 Curve _____

Pre/Post Day 5	Ventilator: Volume Cycle
C.V. Drugs [supre] 1.00 mcg/min	Mode: CMV (vol. contro.)
Dopamine 960.0 mcg/min	FIO2: 35.0 PEEP: 5 TEMP: 36.1
Dobutamine 1400.0 mcg/min	TV : 1150 Peak Press.: 50
Epinephrine 4.20 mcg/min	Rate: 12 Total Rate:

	pHa : 7.27 pHv : 7.26 Ca-vo2: 2.5
	PaCO2: 37.5 PvCO2: 41.3 VO2 : 274
CO: 10.9 td : 2.9 BP : 98/ 44 HR : 120	HaCO3: 16.6 HvCO3: 17.9 VO2/m2: 126
CI: 5.0 tm : 5.2 MAP: 60 TPR: 440	PaO2 :136.0 PvO2 : 39.4 AaO2 : 69
DV: 533. SV : 90.7 RAP:27.0 VTI:-10.8	SaO2 : 94.6 SvO2 : 76.8 RI : 0.5
MV: 941. EjT:.32 PLP:18.0 EFx: 74	Hgb : 8.9 VA/QT: 0.4 QS/QT : 26
B CW: 8.9 LW:122.5 MPA:24.0	Bs Ex:-14.1 VD/VT: 0.6

FIG. 15-52 (B) *(Continued).* Patient transitions to B state septic metabolic insufficiency with hyperdynamic cardiovascular state and fall in oxygen consumption ($\dot{V}O_2/m^2$=126 ml/min/m²). See text for details. Legend as in Fig. 15-2. *(Figure continues.)*

the trauma was the right lower extremity, it was decided that this change in physiologic state represented a categoric imperative for re-exploration of the limb. Surgery showed that a major deep muscle group had progressed to necrosis and seemed to be the focus for the septic process. As a result, an above-knee guilotine amputation was carried out. In the study carried out the next day (Fig. 15-52C), it can be seen that the patient has returned to an adequate hyperdynamic A state, the arteriovenous

oxygen content difference has widened to 3.1 volume percent in spite of an increase in cardiac output to 12 L/min, and the oxygen consumption has risen from 126 ml/min/m² in the B state to 172 ml/min/m² in the A state. The pH has corrected itself and while the percent shunt remains the same there has been an increase in the $\dot{V}A/\dot{Q}T$ to 0.7 and a corresponding fall in the V_D/V_T to 0.5, indicating a more effective redistribution of pulmonary blood flow. While a significant base deficit remains

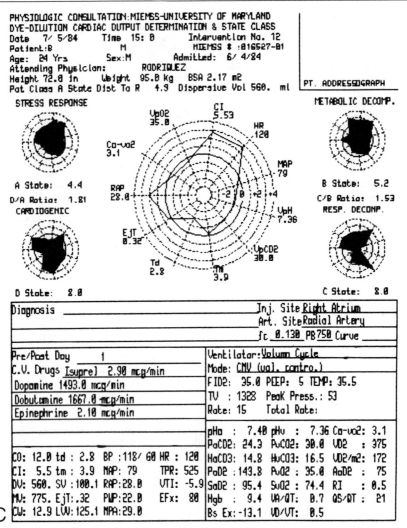

```
PHYSIOLOGIC CONSULTATION:MIEMSS-UNIVERSITY OF MARYLAND
DYE-DILUTION CARDIAC OUTPUT DETERMINATION & STATE CLASS
Date  7/ 5/84    Time  15: 0      Intervention No. 12
Patient:B              M              MIEMSS # :016527-01
Age: 24 Yrs        Sex:M            Admitted: 6/ 4/84
Attending Physician:        RODRIGUEZ
Height 72.0 in     Weight 95.0 kg    BSA 2.17 m2
Pat Class A State Dist To R   4.9 Dispersive Vol 560. ml    PT. ADDRESSOGRAPH
```

STRESS RESPONSE   METABOLIC DECOMP.

A State: 4.4
D/A Ratio: 1.81
CARDIOGENIC

B State: 5.2
C/B Ratio: 1.53
RESP. DECOMP.

D State: 8.0   C State: 8.0

Diagnosis	Inj. Site Right Atrium
	Art. Site Radial Artery
	fc 0.130 PB 750 Curve

Pre/Post Day 1	Ventilator: Volume Cycle
C.V. Drugs Isuprel 2.90 mcg/min	Mode: CMV (vol. contro.)
Dopamine 1493.0 mcg/min	FIO2: 35.0 PEEP: 5 TEMP: 35.5
Dobutamine 1667.0 mcg/min	TV : 1328 Peak Press.: 53
Epinephrine 2.10 mcg/min	Rate: 15 Total Rate:

	pHa : 7.40 pHv : 7.36 Ca-vo2: 3.1
	PaCO2: 24.3 PvCO2: 30.0 VO2 : 375
CO: 12.0 td : 2.8 BP :118/ 60 HR : 120	HaCO3: 14.8 HvCO3: 16.5 VO2/m2: 172
CI: 5.5 tm : 3.9 MAP: 79 TPR: 525	PaO2 :143.8 PvO2 : 35.0 AaO2 : 75
DV: 560. SV :100.1 RAP:28.0 VTI: -5.9	SaO2 : 95.4 SvO2 : 74.4 RI : 0.5
MV: 775. EjT:.32 PUP:22.0 EFx: 80	Hgb : 9.4 VA/QT: 0.7 QS/QT : 21
CW: 12.9 LW:125.1 MPA:29.0	Bs Ex:-13.1 VD/VT: 0.5

FIG. 15-52 (C) *(Continued).* Patient return to hyperdynamic metabolic A state with adequate oxygen consumption ($\dot{V}O_2/m^2$=172 ml/min/m²) following amputation of necrotic septic lower extremity. Legend as in Fig. 15-2.

(−13.1 mEq/L), the metabolic status appears more secure. It is important to emphasize, however, that throughout this entire process the patient required significant inotropic support with a variety of inotropic agents having both α- and β-adrenergic activity to control the septic myocardial contractile depression identified prior to this sequence of metabolic inadequacy. This sequence of physiologic studies shows that as septic processes manifested by severe metabolic insufficiency progress, a transition from the A to B state with progressive meta-

bolic acidosis is a physiologic clue to the underlying oxidative failure that can be reversed by drainage, or excision, of the septic focus.

Inotropic Support of Cardiovascular Function

The hyperdynamic cardiovascular response to sepsis is a fundamental aspect of the adaptation to sepsis. Clowes and his col-

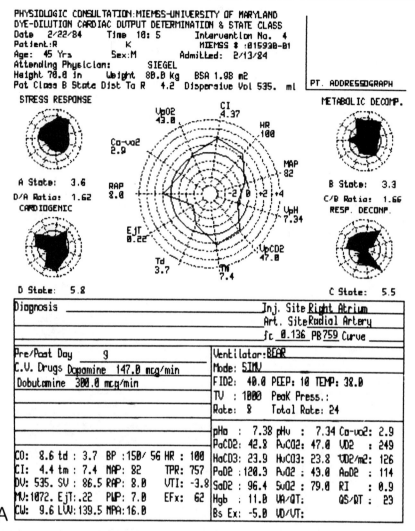

```
PHYSIOLOGIC CONSULTATION:MIEMSS-UNIVERSITY OF MARYLAND
DYE-DILUTION CARDIAC OUTPUT DETERMINATION & STATE CLASS
Date  2/22/84   Time  10: 5      Intervention No.   4
Patient:R          K             MIEMSS # :015938-01
Age:  45 Yrs      Sex:M          Admitted: 2/13/84
Attending Physician:      SIEGEL
Height 70.0 in    Weight  80.0 kg    BSA 1.98 m2
Pat Class B State Dist To R   4.2  Dispersive Vol 535. ml
```

PT. ADDRESSOGRAPH

STRESS RESPONSE

METABOLIC DECOMP.

CARDIOGENIC

RESP. DECOMP.

A State: 3.6   D/A Ratio: 1.62

B State: 3.3   C/B Ratio: 1.66

D State: 5.8

C State: 5.5

Diagnosis _____	Inj. Site Right Atrium
	Art. Site Radial Artery
	ʃc 0.136 PB 759 Curve ____

Pre/Post Day 9	Ventilator: BEAR
C.V. Drugs Dopamine 147.0 mcg/min	Mode: SIMV
Dobutamine 300.0 mcg/min	FID2: 40.0 PEEP: 10 TEMP: 38.0
	TV : 1000 Peak Press.:
	Rate: 8 Total Rate: 24
	pHa : 7.38 pHv : 7.34 Ca-vo2: 2.9
	PaCO2: 42.8 PvCO2: 47.0 VO2 : 249
	HaCO3: 23.9 HvCO3: 23.8 VO2/m2: 126
CO: 8.6 td : 3.7 BP :150/ 56 HR : 100	PaO2 :120.3 PvO2 : 43.0 AaO2 : 114
CI: 4.4 tm : 7.4 NAP: 82 TPR: 757	SaO2 : 96.4 SvO2 : 79.0 RI : 0.9
DV: 535. SV : 86.5 RAP: 8.0 VTI: -3.8	Hgb : 11.8 VA/QT: QS/QT: 29
MV:1072. EjT:.22 PLP: 7.0 EFx: 62	
CW: 9.6 LVW:139.5 NPA:16.0	Bs Ex: -5.0 VD/VT:

A

FIG. 15-53 (A) Physiologic consultation from 45-year-old male sustaining major hepatic trauma with development of the septic hepatic abscess. Development of hyperdynamic B state with evidence of reduced oxygen consumption ($\dot{V}O_2/m^2$=126 ml/min/m^2) and myocardial depression with fall in ejection fraction (EFx=62 percent). Legend as in Fig. 15-2. (*Figure continues.*)

leagues,[29] Siegel et al.,[125,129,130,133] and MacLean and his associates[86] have demonstrated that the hyperdynamic syndrome with increased cardiac output and oxygen consumption is necessary for a successful compensation for a prolonged or severe septic episode. As noted earlier, it is important to recognize that the incidence of clinical myocardial depression increases as the septic process continues, especially if evidence of metabolic insufficiency is present.[125,145,162] Although common, this myocardial depression may be hidden by the development of a high-output cardiac failure syndrome in response to the fall in peripheral resistance. However, if this is not recognized and treated, it is likely that the myocardial depression will deteriorate into an overt low-cardiac-output failure. Unless corrected, such low-flow acute myocardial decompensation is generally fatal, since it combines the oxidative

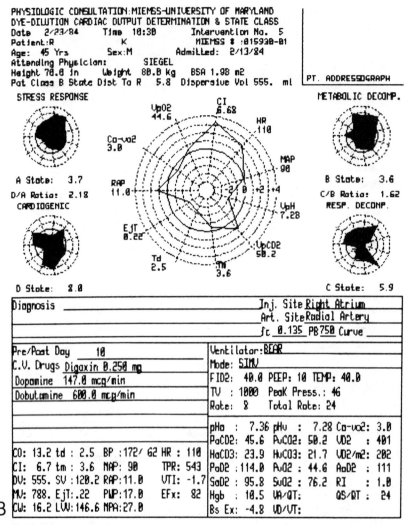

PHYSIOLOGIC CONSULTATION:MIEMSS-UNIVERSITY OF MARYLAND
DYE-DILUTION CARDIAC OUTPUT DETERMINATION & STATE CLASS
Date 2/23/84   Time 10:30   Intervention No. 5
Patient:R   K   MIEMSS # :015930-01
Age: 45 Yrs   Sex:M   Admitted: 2/13/84
Attending Physician: SIEGEL
Height 70.0 in   Weight 80.0 kg   BSA 1.98 m2
Pat Class B State Dist To R   5.8 Dispersive Vol 555. ml

PT. ADDRESSOGRAPH

STRESS RESPONSE

METABOLIC DECOMP.

VpO2 44.6
Co-vo2 3.0
CI 6.68
HR 110
MAP 90

A State: 3.7

B State: 3.6

D/A Ratio: 2.18
RAP 11.0

C/B Ratio: 1.62

CARDIOGENIC

RESP. DECOMP.

EjT 0.22
VpH 7.28
VpCO2 50.2
Td 2.5
TM 3.6

D State: 2.0

C State: 5.9

Diagnosis	Inj. Site Right Atrium
	Art. Site Radial Artery
	Jc 0.135 PB 750 Curve

Pre/Post Day 10	Ventilator:BEAR
C.V. Drugs Digoxin 0.250 mg	Mode: SIMV
Dopamine 147.0 mcg/min	FIO2: 40.0 PEEP: 10 TEMP: 40.0
Dobutamine 600.0 mcg/min	TV : 1000 Peak Press.: 46
	Rate: 8 Total Rate: 24

	pHa : 7.36 pHv : 7.28 Co-vo2: 3.0	
	PaCO2: 45.6 PvCO2: 50.2 VO2 : 401	
CO: 13.2 td : 2.5 BP :172/ 62 HR : 110	HaCO3: 23.9 HvCO3: 21.7 VO2/m2: 202	
CI: 6.7 tm : 3.6 MAP: 90 TPR: 543	PaO2 :114.0 PvO2 : 44.6 AoO2 : 111	
DV: 555. SV :120.2 RAP:11.0 VTI: -1.7	SaO2 : 95.8 SvO2 : 76.2 RI : 1.0	
MV: 788. EjT:.22 PLP:17.0 EFx: 82	Hgb : 10.5 VA/QT: QS/QT : 24	
CW: 16.2 LW:146.6 NPA:27.0	Bs Ex: -4.8 VD/VT:	

FIG. 15-53 (B) *(Continued)*. Response in hyperdynamic B state to increased inotropic support compensating for myocardial depression (EFx increased to 82 percent). Legend as in Fig. 15-2. *(Figure continues.)*

debt of ischemic hypoperfusion with that of the septic metabolic impairment of oxygen consumption.

The marked reduction in vascular tone produced by the by-products of septic metabolic failure may be a protective measure, since the reduction in vascular tone and the resultant reduced TPR that is a consequence of the B state pathologic vasodilatation reduces afterload. This in turn permits even a poor-quality myocardium to maintain a higher velocity of ejection and therefore to shift its ejection frac-

tion to a more favorable point on a depressed force–velocity curve. Nevertheless, such compensation is seldom sufficient if the Vmax is markedly decreased, the administration of synergistic nonvasoconstricting cardiac inotropic agents is essential if contractile dynamics and adequate peripheral perfusion are to be restored.

The interrelationship of the sequence of myocardial depression and its recovery by inotropic support with the metabolic failure of sepsis is demonstrated in Figure 15-53 for the pa-

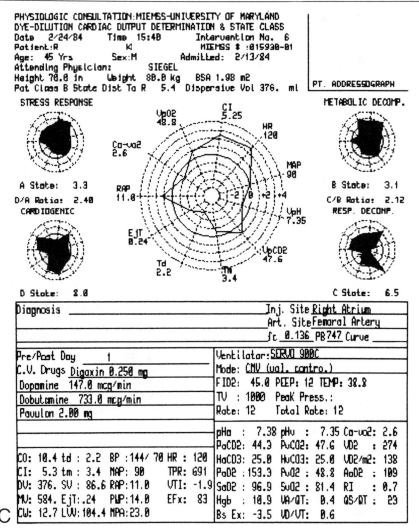

```
PHYSIOLOGIC CONSULTATION:MIEMSS-UNIVERSITY OF MARYLAND
DYE-DILUTION CARDIAC OUTPUT DETERMINATION & STATE CLASS
Date  2/24/84     Time 15:48      Intervention No.  6
Patient:R          K              MIEMSS # :015930-01
Age:  45 Yrs       Sex:M          Admitted: 2/13/84
Attending Physician:       SIEGEL
Height 70.0 in    Weight 80.0 kg  BSA 1.98 m2
Pat Class B State Dist To R  5.4  Dispersive Vol 376. ml
```

PT. ADDRESSOGRAPH

STRESS RESPONSE

METABOLIC DECOMP.

```
VpO2
48.8

CI
5.25

Co-vo2
2.6

HR
120

MAP
90
```

A State: 3.3

D/A Ratio: 2.40

CARDIOGENIC

RAP
11.0

B State: 3.1

C/B Ratio: 2.12

RESP. DECOMP.

```
VpH
7.35

EJT
0.24

VpCO2
47.6

Td
2.2

TM
3.4
```

D State: 8.0

C State: 6.5

Diagnosis	Inj. Site Right Atrium
	Art. Site Femoral Artery
	Jc 0.136 PB 747 Curve

Pre/Post Day 1	Ventilator: SERVO 900C
C.V. Drugs Digoxin 0.250 mg	Mode: CMV (vol. contro.)
Dopamine 147.0 mcg/min	FIO2: 45.0 PEEP: 12 TEMP: 38.8
Dobutamine 733.0 mcg/min	TV : 1000 Peak Press.:
Pavulon 2.00 mg	Rate: 12 Total Rate: 12

				pHa : 7.38	pHv : 7.35	Ca-vo2: 2.6
				PaCO2: 44.3	PvCO2: 47.6	VO2 : 274
				HaCO3: 25.0	HvCO3: 25.0	VO2/m2: 138
CO: 10.4	td : 2.2	BP :144/70	HR : 120	PaO2 :153.3	PvO2 : 48.8	AaDO2 : 109
CI: 5.3	tm : 3.4	MAP: 90	TPR: 691	SaO2 : 96.9	SvO2 : 81.4	RI : 0.7
DV: 376.	SV : 86.6	RAP:11.0	VTI: -1.9	Hgb : 10.9	VA/QT: 0.4	QS/QT : 23
MV: 584.	EjT:.24	PLP:14.0	EFx: 83			
CW: 12.7	LVW:104.4	MPA:23.0		Bs Ex: -3.5	VD/VT: 0.6	

FIG. 15-53 (C) *(Continued)*. Improvement in B state hyperdynamic response following incision and drainage of hepatic abscess on day prior to physiologic consultation. Legend as in Fig. 15-2. *(Figure continues.)*

tient shown in Figures 15-7 and 15-8. This 45-year-old man had sustained a major hepatic fracture following a fall from a ladder and underwent emergency surgery for a large stellate fracture of the right lobe of the liver. At operation, major hepatic bleeding was controlled by suture, with resectional debridement of the obviously devitalized liver at the time of primary surgery. Forty-eight hours following initial surgery the patient had a acute hemorrhage from a subsegmental arterial branch in the depths of the stellate fracture, which was controlled nonoperatively by angiographic embolization. Following this he became progressively septic and by the ninth postoperative day demonstrated the pattern shown in Figure 15-53A. As can be seen in this figure, which corresponds to INT 4 in Figure 15-8, the patient manifested a hyperdynamic cardiovascular state with a cardiac output of 8.6 L/min (CI, 4.37 L/min/m²). Oxygen consumption, however, was markedly reduced because of an inappropriately narrowed arteriovenous oxygen content difference (Ca-$\bar{v}O_2$, 2.9 volume percent) with a con-

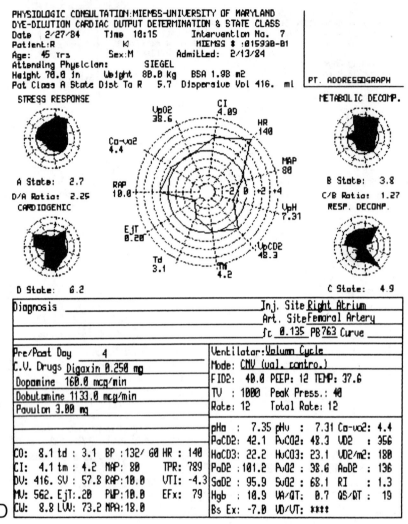

FIG. 15-53 (D) (*Continued*). Return to hyperdynamic compensated metabolic A state 4 days after drainage of hepatic abscess ($\dot{V}O_2/m^2$=180 ml/min/m²). Legend as in Fig. 15-2.

sequent reduction in oxygen consumption ($\dot{V}O_2/m^2$, 126 ml/min/m²) and a metabolic acidosis was present. There was also a reduction in vascular tone as evidenced by a fall in TPR disproportionate to the increase in cardiac output and a reduction in ejection fraction to 62 percent. Thus, the patient manifested a septic B state with septic high-output cardiac failure, in spite of inotropic support with dopamine (2µg/kg/min) and dobutamine (4 µg/kg/min).

To compensate for the metabolically induced myocardial depression, the level of inotropic support was increased by raising the dobutamine dosage to 8 µg/kg/min and the patient received digoxin 0.25 mg/day. As can be seen in Figure 15-53B, this therapy resulted in a substantial increase in cardiac output to 13.2 L (CI, 6.68 L/min/m²), which permitted an increase in oxygen consumption ($\dot{V}O_2/m^2$, 202 ml/min/m²). However, metabolic acidosis persisted and the patient continued to demonstrate features that placed him in the septic B state. Since his temperature continued to rise to 40°C, it was decided that surgical re-exploration was necessary to determine whether an abscess that could be satisfactorily drained was present. This surgical procedure was carried out immediately following the physiologic study shown in Figure 15-53B.

On the following day (postoperative day 1 after abscess drainage) the patient still manifested a B state (Fig. 15-53C). However, the studies suggested that compensation was being achieved. The cardiac output had decreased slightly to 10.4 L/min (CI, 5.25 L/min/m²) oxygen consumption had fallen to 138 ml/min, but there was now a reduction in the metabolic acidosis and the ejection fraction remained high (EFx, 83 percent).

Over the next 3 days, the pattern progressively improved and the various features of the septic process were noted to shift toward a more satisfactory compensation. The oxygen consumption remained high ($\dot{V}O_2$/m², 180 ml/min/m²) even though the cardiac output decreased to 8.1 L/min (CI = 4.09 L/min/m²). The temperature decreased to 37.6°C, the shunt was reduced from 24 percent prior to incision and drainage of the hepatic abscess to 19 percent afterward, and the $\dot{V}A/\dot{Q}T$ rose from 0.4 to 0.7, suggesting a better distribution of blood flow in the lung. Though the metabolic acidosis persisted, this cleared over the next few days. However, as is seen in Figure 15-53D, it was necessary to maintain the patient on high levels of inotropic support to assist cardiovascular compensation during this period.

The correlation of these events with improvement in the leucine/tyrosine (LT) clearance ratio is shown in Figure 15-54 in which the patient's time course after trauma is compared to the LT clearance ratio. As can be seen, because of the patient's precarious hemodynamic status during the first few days following his injury, he was maintained on only a low level of amino acid infusion. With the institution of standard TPN, the leucine/tyrosine ratio markedly increased as the patient manifested the B state metabolic failure culminating in the myocardial depression shown previously in Figure 15-53A. Surgical drainage of the hepatic abscess was followed shortly thereafter by improvement in the physiologic status with return to the A state as the leucine/tyrosine ratio fell. This demonstrated that the oxidative abnormalities and refractory myocardial depression

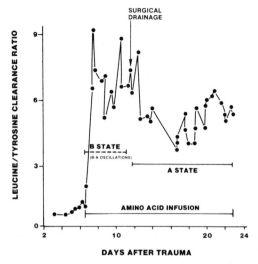

**KR.
159   SURVIVOR
HEPATIC LACERATION WITH DEVELOPMENT
OF HEPATIC ABSCESS**

FIG. 15-54 Time course of leucine/tyrosine clearance ratio in patient shown in Fig. 15-53 following evolution and drainage of hepatic abscess. Shown are the leucine/tyrosine clearance ratio during TPN (amino acid infusion) at time of B state metabolic decompensation showing response to surgical drainage with improvement in the hepatic decompensatory phase and return to septic A state. Leucine/tyrosine infusion ratio during TPN constant, although quantity of amino acid given per day varied by clinicians in order to help control patient's degree of hyperglycemia.

were paralleled by evidence of hepatic decompensation and that these physiologic abnormalities improved parallel with the improvement in hepatic function as MOFS cleared. This patient went on to have a complete resolution of his septic process and full recovery.

This case makes clear that even though an adequate cardiac output may be maintained as metabolic failure ensues, the cardiac force–velocity relationship and ejection fraction may be decreased. These must be carefully evaluated since failure to maintain an increased cardiac ejection fraction in hyperdynamic sepsis is an indication for the use of inotropic support. In those cases where a prolonged hyperdynamic state is anticipated due to the presence of major intra-abdominal sepsis, abscess formation, or another slowly resolving septic process, or in cases where pre-existing myocardial disease is present, acute digoxin therapy is also indicated. Since the failure to recognize that myocardial depression is occurring may have severe and fatal consequences, continuous inotropic support should be initiated in any severely hyperdynamic patient prior to the demonstration of acute failure in order to prevent sudden cardiovascular collapse and be continued as long as the pathophysiologic hyperdynamic state persists.[123,125-127,133]

The inotropic agents most commonly utilized are dopamine at a nonvasoconstricting dosage (2 to 5 μg/kg/min), dobutamine at a similar low-dose inotropic level (3 to 5 μg/kg/min), or low-dose isoproterenol (0.25 to 1.0 μg/min total dose). At the lower level, isoproterenol has virtually no chronotropic toxicity and appears to be most effective in increasing cardiac output. It is a good agent to use in conjunction with inotropic levels of dopamine and dobutamine. The use of two or three of these agents together in low dosages appears to be synergistic in maximizing cardiac inotropic activity without excessive chronotropic toxicity. In some patients we have utilized low-dose dopamine, dobutamine, and/or isoproterenol for more than 50 days with complete recovery and no evidence of residual myocardial damage.

With regard to the use of digoxin, it has been demonstrated that an inotropic effect occurs at approximately 75 percent of the normal digitalizing dose,[123] provided serum potassium levels are maintained at approximately 4.0 mEq/L. The use of digitalization in the absence of overt failure has also been demonstrated to be of value in the hyperdynamic septic patient since it provides an additional inotropic background drug without excessive chronotropic activity. It is especially valuable in the older patient who may have some degree of pre-existing intrinsic myocardial disease, since it prevents excessive cardiac dilatation that may place the heart in an unfavorable position with regard to its force–velocity relationship. By helping to maintain a low end-diastolic volume, it also tends to reduce the oxygen consumption of the myocardium in the hyperdynamic state.

In general it is not advisable to use vasoconstrictor agents, either dopamine at dosages greater than 8 to 10 μg/kg/min, or true vaso-

constrictor catecholamines, such as norepinephrine or methoxamine. There is virtually no indication for the use of norepinephrine in these patients, since the excessive vasoconstriction and reduction of flow to critical organs appears to magnify pathologically the pre-existing septic oxidative insufficiency. On rare occasions, when it is necessary to maintain a higher level of pressure then can be achieved with a combination of dopamine, dobutamine, and isoproterenol (for instance, where dialysis or hemofiltration must be maintained with a reasonable perfusion pressure) we have used low dosages of epinephrine (1 to 4 μg/min total dose), although this tends to increase further the hyperglycemia associated with the septic process. In any event, such agents should be used extremely sparingly during the period of frank hypotension and their use should be reduced or eliminated as soon as possible thereafter.

Afterload Reduction by Use of Vasodilator Agents

In patients with pre-existing disease, or where low-output myocardial failure is present as a complication of the septic process in the presence of intercurrent myocardial disease, an active vasodilator agent such as nitroglycerine paste, or, in severe cases, intravenous nitroglycerine or nitroprusside, may be of value. It has been demonstrated that the use of these agents can produce a marked improvement in both increasing flow and oxygen consumption in the low-output septic patient.[18] Vasodilatation will also permit the patient with overt myocardial failure to accept the volume loading necessary to produce compensation. This is demonstrated in Figure 15-55A.

This 72-year-old patient with severe intra-abdominal sepsis following a traumatic injury to the bowel, was demonstrated to be in a D cardiogenic decompensation state with a reduced ejection fraction (EFx, 62 percent) and a cardiac output of only 4.5 L/min/m² (CI, 2.4 ml/m²). Oxygen consumption ($\dot{V}O_2$/m²) was markedly reduced to 106 ml/min/m² and although the vascular tone index (VTI) was also

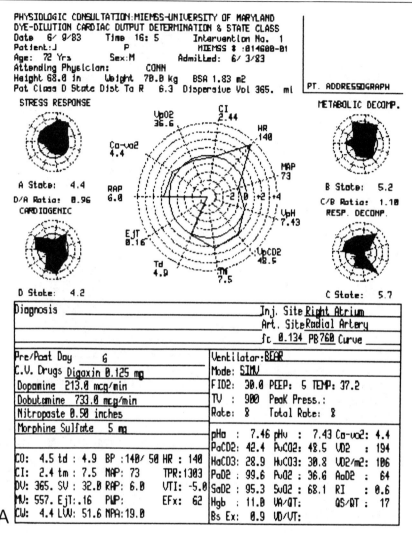

PHYSIOLOGIC CONSULTATION:MIEMSS-UNIVERSITY OF MARYLAND
DYE-DILUTION CARDIAC OUTPUT DETERMINATION & STATE CLASS
Date 6/ 9/83   Time 16: 5   Intervention No. 1
Patient:J   P   MIEMSS # :014600-01
Age: 72 Yrs   Sex:M   Admitted: 6/ 3/83
Attending Physician: CONN
Height 68.0 in   Weight 70.0 kg   BSA 1.83 m2
Pat Class D State Dist To R 6.3 Dispersive Vol 365. ml

PT. ADDRESSOGRAPH

STRESS RESPONSE

METABOLIC DECOMP.

VpO2 36.6
CI 2.44
HR 140
Co-vo2 4.4
MAP 73
A State: 4.4
RAP 6.0
B State: 5.2
D/A Ratio: 0.96
C/B Ratio: 1.18
CARDIOGENIC
VpH 7.43
RESP. DECOMP.
EJT 0.16
VpCO2 48.5
Td 4.9
TM 7.5
D State: 4.2
C State: 5.7

Diagnosis	Inj. Site Right Atrium
	Art. Site Radial Artery
	Jc 0.134 PB760 Curve

Pre/Post Day	6	Ventilator:BEAR
C.V. Drugs Digoxin 0.125 mg		Mode: SIMV
Dopamine 213.0 mcg/min		FIO2: 30.0 PEEP: 5 TEMP: 37.2
Dobutamine 733.0 mcg/min		TV : 900 Peak Press.:
Nitropaste 0.50 inches		Rate: 8 Total Rate: 8
Morphine Sulfate 5 mg		

pHa : 7.46 pHv : 7.43 Ca-vo2: 4.4
PaCO2: 42.4 PvCO2: 48.5 VO2 : 194
HaCO3: 28.9 HvCO3: 30.8 VO2/m2: 106
PaO2 : 99.6 PvO2 : 36.6 AaDO2 : 64
SaO2 : 95.3 SvO2 : 68.1 RI : 0.6
Hgb : 11.0 VA/QT: QS/QT: 17
Bs Ex: 0.9 VD/VT:

CO: 4.5 td : 4.9 BP :140/ 50 HR : 140
CI: 2.4 tm : 7.5 MAP: 73   TPR:1303
DV: 365. SV : 32.0 RAP: 6.0   VTI: -5.0
MV: 557. EjT:.16 PWP: EFx: 62
CW: 4.4 LW: 51.6 NPA:19.0

A

FIG. 15-55 (A) Combination of inotropic support of vasodilitation in hypodynamic septic patient with cardiac decompensation (D state). Hypodynamic cardiogenic D state sepsis (EFx=62 percent) with reduced oxygen consumption ($\dot{V}O_2/m^2$=106 ml/min/m²) due to atrial fibrillation. Physiologic consultation carried out immediately following initial dose of digoxin and application of ½ inch nitropaste and after start of combined inotropic support with dopamine and dobutamine. See text for details. Legend as in Fig. 15-2. (*Figure continues.*)

reduced, the TPR was still increased to a degree greater than could be compensated for by the patient's poor myocardial function. In addition, the patient demonstrated an atrial arrhythmia with a heart rate of 140. As a result the patient was digitalized and begun on inotropic support with dopamine 3 μg/kg/min and dobutamine 10 μg/kg/min. A small nitroglyce-

rine patch was placed on the interior chest wall (nitropaste, ½ inch).

Because of the arrhythmia as shown in Figure 15-55B, quinidine was begun and the dopamine was discontinued to enhance the relative vasodilatation, while the patient was maintained on dobutamine. On this therapy and chronic digitalization, the heart rate was re-

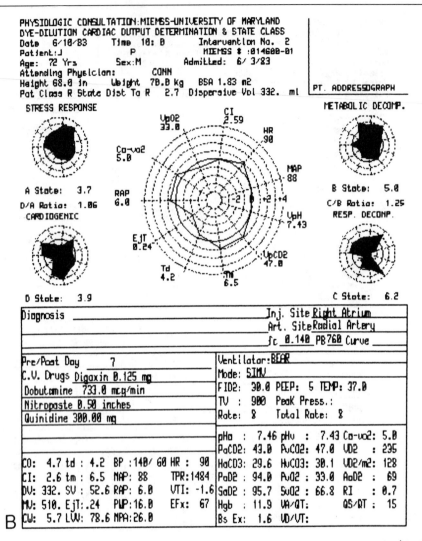

PHYSIOLOGIC CONSULTATION:MIEMSS-UNIVERSITY OF MARYLAND
DYE-DILUTION CARDIAC OUTPUT DETERMINATION & STATE CLASS
Date 6/10/83   Time 10: 0   Intervention No. 2
Patient:J   P   MIEMSS # :014600-01
Age: 72 Yrs   Sex:M   Admitted: 6/ 3/83
Attending Physician: CONN
Height 68.0 in   Weight 78.0 kg   BSA 1.83 m2
Pat Class R State Dist To R   2.7 Dispersive Vol 332. ml   PT. ADDRESSOGRAPH

STRESS RESPONSE   METABOLIC DECOMP.

VpO2 33.0   CI 2.59
                   HR 90
Co-vo2 5.0
                   MAP 88
A State: 3.7   RAP 6.0   B State: 5.0
D/A Ratio: 1.06   C/B Ratio: 1.25
CARDIOGENIC   RESP. DECOMP.
                   VpH 7.43
EJT 0.24
                   VpCO2 47.0
Td 4.2   TM 6.5
D State: 3.9   C State: 6.2

Diagnosis	Inj. Site Right Atrium
	Art. Site Radial Artery
	Jc 0.140 PB 760 Curve

Pre/Post Day 7	Ventilator:BEAR
C.V. Drugs Digoxin 0.125 mg	Mode: SIMV
Dobutamine 733.0 mcg/min	FIO2: 30.0 PEEP: 5 TEMP: 37.0
Nitropaste 0.50 inches	TV : 900 Peak Press.:
Quinidine 300.00 mg	Rate: 8 Total Rate: 8

pHa : 7.46 pHv : 7.43 Co-vo2: 5.0
PaCO2: 43.0 PvCO2: 47.0 VO2 : 235
HaCO3: 29.6 HvCO3: 30.1 VO2/m2: 128
PaO2 : 94.0 PvO2 : 33.0 AaDO2 : 69
SaO2 : 95.7 SvO2 : 66.8 RI   : 0.7
Hgb : 11.9 VA/QT: QS/QT : 15
Bs Ex: 1.6 VD/VT:

CO: 4.7 td : 4.2 BP :140/ 60 HR : 90
CI: 2.6 tm : 6.5 MAP: 88   TPR:1484
DV: 332. SV : 52.6 RAP: 6.0   VTI: -1.6
MV: 510. EjT:.24 PLP:16.0   EFx: 67
CW: 5.7 LW: 78.6 NPA:26.0

B

FIG. 15-55 (B) *(Continued)*. Slight improvement in cardiac output and oxygen consumption ($\dot{V}O_2/m^2$=128 ml/min/m²) following stabilization on maintenance digoxin and quinidine with control of atrial fibrillation. Legend as in Fig. 15-2. *(Figure continues.)*

duced to 90/min, cardiac output increased slightly to 4.7 L/min (CI, 2.6 L/min/m²). The ejection fraction (EFx) also increased slightly to 67 percent and oxygen consumption ($\dot{V}O_2/m^2$) rose to 128 ml/min/m².

Since this still represented an inadequate level of oxygen consumption, even when age-corrected (see Chapter 9), the nitropaste was increased to 1 inch and the dobutamine was maintained, although the dosage was reduced slightly to 7 µg/kg/min (Fig. 15-55C). There was a reduction in vascular tone shown by

the fact that the peripheral vascular resistance (TPR) fell from 1484 to 738 dyne·sec·cm⁻⁵, permitting the ejection fraction to rise to 72 percent. The patient was now able to accept an appropriate volume infusion preload, raising his pulmonary blood volume (DV) from an inadequate level of 181 ml/m² (DV, 332 ml) to 264 ml/m² (DV, 484 ml). This allowed the depressed myocardium to operate at a higher point on its ventricular volume curve (LVV) without an increase in afterload. Thus left ventricular volume increased from 78.6 to 120 ml

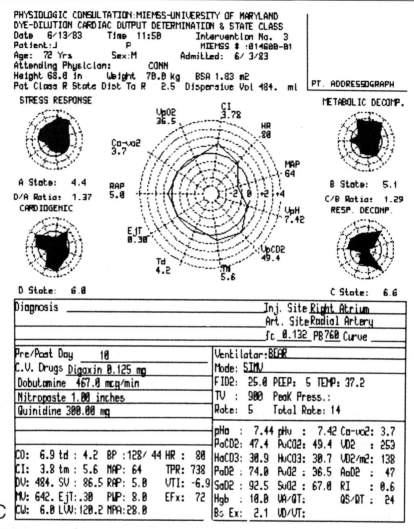

```
PHYSIOLOGIC CONSULTATION:MIEMSS-UNIVERSITY OF MARYLAND
DYE-DILUTION CARDIAC OUTPUT DETERMINATION & STATE CLASS
Date  6/13/83    Time 11:50       Intervention No.  3
Patient:J           P           MIEMSS # :014600-01
Age:  72 Yrs      Sex:M          Admitted:  6/ 3/83
Attending Physician:        CONN
Height 68.0 in    Weight  70.0 Kg   BSA 1.83 m2
Pat Class R State Dist To R  2.5  Dispersive Vol 484.  ml
```
PT. ADDRESSOGRAPH

STRESS RESPONSE

VpO2 36.5
Co-vo2 3.7

CI 3.78
HR 80
MAP 64
VpH 7.42
VpCO2 49.4

METABOLIC DECOMP.

A State: 4.4
D/A Ratio: 1.37
RAP 5.0

B State: 5.1
C/B Ratio: 1.29
RESP. DECOMP.

CARDIOGENIC

EJT 0.30
Td 4.2
TM 5.6

D State: 6.0

C State: 6.6

Diagnosis	Inj. Site Right Atrium
	Art. Site Radial Artery
	Jc 0.132 PB760 Curve

Pre/Post Day 10	Ventilator:BEAR	
C.V. Drugs Digoxin 0.125 mg	Mode: SIMV	
Dobutamine 467.0 mcg/min	FIO2: 25.0 PEEP: 5 TEMP: 37.2	
Nitropaste 1.00 inches	TV : 900 Peak Press.:	
Quinidine 300.00 mg	Rate: 5 Total Rate: 14	

pHa : 7.44	pHv : 7.42	Co-vo2: 3.7
PaCO2: 47.4	PvCO2: 49.4	VO2 : 253
CO: 6.9 td : 4.2 BP :128/ 44 HR : 80	HaCO3: 30.9	HvCO3: 30.7	VO2/m2: 138
CI: 3.8 tm : 5.6 MAP: 64 TPR: 738	PaO2: 74.0	PvO2: 36.5	AaD2 : 47
DV: 484. SV : 86.5 RAP: 5.0 VTI: -6.9	SaO2: 92.5	SvO2: 67.0	RI : 0.6
MV: 642. EjT:.30 PLP: 8.0 EFx: 72	Hgb : 10.0	VA/QT:	QS/QT : 24
CW: 6.0 LW:120.2 NPA:28.0	Bs Ex: 2.1	VD/VT:

C

FIG. 15-55 (C) *(Continued)*. Increase in vasodilitation, nitropaste increased to 1 inch with elimination of vasoconstrictor inotropic agents and use of dobutamine only to produce rise in cardiac index, EFx, and oxygen consumption ($\dot{V}O_2/m^2$=138 ml/min/m^2) to compensated physiologic response levels. Legend as in Fig. 15-2.

without substantial alteration in estimated myocardial oxygen consumption. As a result the cardiac output increased to 6.9 L/min (CI, 3.8 ml/m^2) and oxygen consumption ($\dot{V}O_2/m^2$) rose to an appropriate age-corrected figure of 138 ml/m^2.

These physiologically analyzed cases demonstrate the degree of subtlety with which this problem must be considered and how each aspect of the septic cardiovascular compensation (preload, afterload, and contractile state) must be addressed therapeutically in an at-

tempt to optimize flow to meet the estimated metabolic needs as reflected in oxygen consumption.

Support of Respiratory Complications

The septic process is frequently associated with the development of an acute respiratory insufficiency syndrome that has been designated septic ARDS (see Chapter 19). Under these circumstances the increased pulmonary blood flow produced by the peripheral hyperdynamic cardiovascular state is associated with evidence of an increase in pulmonary capillary permeability with resultant interstitial edema, alveolar collapse, and a gravitationally related maldistribution of ventilation relative to perfusion.[28,122,130] These two related phenomenon not only increase perfusion of the dependent low $\dot{V}A/\dot{Q}T$ segments of the lung with an increase in physiologic shunt and dead space, but also tend to alter the pulmonary compliance in a nonuniform fashion.

As shown in Chapter 19, the pressure–flow–volume relationships of the septic ARDS lung are pathophysiologically altered by a reduction in lung compliance so that the airway pressure rises rapidly after inspiration of very small increments in lung volume.[134] This tends to activate pulmonary distention reflexes and forces the spontaneously breathing patient with ARDS to take many small breaths that ventilate only relatively small volume of lung parenchyma. Since the functional residual capacity of the lung is reduced as the compliance falls while the anatomic dead space remains nearly normal, the dead space to tidal volume ratio rises as the patient manifests increasing hypoxemia of sepsis. The details of management of septic ARDS are discussed in Chapter 19. However, the relevant aspects for discussion here are that the therapeutic indications for intubation and ventilation with increased PEEP and mean airway pressures are present in any septic patient who manifests an increased pulmonary shunt ($\dot{Q}S/\dot{Q}T$), especially if there is evidence that impaired gas exchange (quantified by the Respiratory Index) is increased disproportionately to the increase in ($\dot{Q}S/\dot{Q}T$), as shown in Chapter 19. Failure to appreciate the meaning of this relationship [RI/($\dot{Q}S/\dot{Q}T$)] and its therapeutic implication will permit progressive alveolar collapse with alveolar flooding to occur without interference.

The development of alveolar exudates provides a medium in which bacterial growth can occur with destruction of alveoli. Thus the appropriate therapy to increase ventilation must be chosen with regard to enhancing the maintenance of an adequate functional residual capacity by expanding partially closed or incom-

pletely ventilated alveoli. This means that the characteristics of mechanical ventilation must be carefully matched to the patient's specific pattern of airway resistance and compliance and an appropriate level of positive end-expiratory pressure (PEEP) and an adequate level of mean airway pressure must be used to maintain open small airways in low-compliance alveoli. Alterations in the inspiratory/expiratory ratio can be used to improve the dynamic characteristics of ventilation. On occasion, the use of high frequency ventilation or simultaneous independent lung ventilation[134] is of value in selected patients where there is nonuniformity of the ARDS process with marked disparity between the two lungs (see Chapter 19). The choice and timing of the use of these advanced ventilatory modalities may be essential to permit adequate gas exchange to occur while one is attempting to resolve the cause of the septic process by surgery and antibiotic therapy.

Therapeutic Implications of Impaired Metabolic Control

The alterations in metabolic control that occur in the severely septic patient are enhanced by the marked protein proteolytic and catabolic processes activated to compensate for the septically altered pattern of skeletal muscle and liver fuel–energy utilization. In addition, the competitive requirements for an increased hepatic synthesis of critical acute host defense proteins and an increased fuel oxidation of some of the amino acids released by muscle proteolysis makes it mandatory that an adequate level of metabolic support be administered to the hyperdynamic septic patient, as soon as the diagnosis of sepsis is likely.

The goal of this nutritional support is to enable all of the critical organ functions to be carried out under circumstances of metabolic impairment. Fortunately, under most circumstances the myocardium appears to be able to metabolize a wide variety of metabolic fuels. Glucose, fatty acids, ketone bodies, and branched chain amino acids can be utilized by the myocardium, provided there is an adequate oxygen supply.[97] However, lipid and glucose sources appear to be favored. In addition the heart maintains a preferential ability to metabolize lactate over glucose as an oxidative source and does not appear to have the same glycolytic substrate limitations as skeletal muscle and liver under conditions of severe sepsis. The defects in pyruvate dehydrogenase activity demonstrated in these latter tissues have not been shown to occur in myocardium. In contrast to liver and skeletal muscle, PDH activity appears to be increased in the septic heart. Nevertheless the markedly increased work requirements as shown in Figure 15-3 demonstrate the need for a high level of energetic support that must be provided by exogenous nutritional sources if myocardial nutritional decompensation is to be avoided.

The nature of the preferred fuel for septic skeletal muscle is related to the degree of septic blockade of glucose oxidation and the resultant dependence of these tissues on the oxidation of nonglucose fuels. The reduction in glucose oxidation appears to be secondary to a postinsulin receptor blockade and may be at the level of PDH control.[151,153] Under these circumstances as glucose utilization is reduced in skeletal muscle, there appears to be a fall in respiratory quotient (RQ) that reflects the increased dependence of the septic patient on the utilization of lipid fuels.[95,143] This is a particularly prominent feature of the septic A state in which oxygen consumption has been demonstrated to be increased by increased lipid administration.[95] As shown earlier in this chapter, the increased oxygen consumption and energy generation produced by administration of a glucose-plus-lipid TPN, in contradistinction to the use of glucose fuel alone, indicates that the nutritional support for the patient with severe sepsis should include between 25 and 40 percent of the calories as lipid computed from the estimated metabolic rate (MR) derived from the deWeir equation[32] (MR = 3.9 [$\dot{V}O_2$] + 1.1 [$\dot{V}CO_2$]).

Another reason for the inclusion of lipids in the program of nutritional support is the recent evidence by Schlag and his co-workers[4] that dietary essential fatty acids may enhance the synthesis of pulmonary surfactant. This was of assistance in improving lung function after experimental multiple injury with shock.

Late in the septic process, when the metabolic insufficiency of the septic B state is accompanied by a fall in oxygen consumption, there is suggestive evidence that the oxidative metabolism of long chain fatty acids, as well as that of glucose, may be impaired even though lipogenesis with hypertriglyceridemia continues. Under these conditions, the septic patient appears to become increasingly dependent on the ketoacids of the branch chain amino acids for nutritional support. Evidence is increasing that the use of branched chain amino-acid-enriched solutions containing up to 50 percent of the total amino acids as BCAA may be better tolerated then a balanced amino acid TPN.[12,19] The development of the B state can be strongly suspected from the increased slope of the leucine to tyrosine clearance ratio when the patient is receiving at least 50 g/day of standard amino acid TPN mixture. While no studies have proven that the use of branched chain-enriched TPN mixtures in this type of patient improves outcome,[12,19] preliminary studies do suggest that BCAA ketoacids induce nitrogen sparing in starvation.[116] Branched chain-enriched mixtures given to septic patients may partially reverse the protein reprioritization that occurs with the development of the septic state, so that certain critical nutritional carrier proteins such as transferrin may not suffer the marked decrease seen in septic patients in whom conventional TPN support is used.[12,19]

Experimental studies showing that ketone synthesis is inhibited in severe sepsis, at the same time as the acetyl-CoA precursors are being increasingly diverted to triglyceride synthesis,[98,104,152] suggest that fuel sources that increase the effective delivery of ketone bodies may be of value in reducing septic proteolysis. At present, no study has been carried out in humans using infusion of ketone bodies as the main energy source. This is partly because of the need to infuse large amounts of sodium salt as the ketone anion and also because there is no clear experimental study to demonstrate that sufficient quantities of ketones can be given as TPN to suppress septic proteolysis. However, recent experimental studies[177] and some clinical work[114,115] have suggested a potential use for medium-chain triglycerides, which do not undergo lipogenesis and bypass the regulating enzyme system of carnitine acyl CoA transferase I (Fig. 15-44). These are directly converted to acetyl-CoA, can increase ketone body formation, and may potentially provide an alternative fuel source under septic conditions.[87,177] There is some controversy concerning the value of this fuel in terms of enhancing protein synthesis[141] and these experimental and preliminary observations in normal subjects must be tested in a prospective clinical sepsis study. Nevertheless, the interest in this area reflects the broadbased sense that an energetic substrate more easily utilizable by the peripheral tissues in the septic patient may be of value in reducing muscle proteolysis. The effectiveness of medium chain triglycerides in enhancing hepatic protein synthesis of critical host defense proteins must also be tested.

Other studies of the role of suppressing the stress-induced hormonal response as a means of modulating the septic metabolic process have been carried out. Wilmore and his colleagues[156] have demonstrated that certain aspects of the pattern of septic fuel utilization may be suppressed by the use of the glucagon- and insulin-inhibiting agent somatostatin with replacement of insulin. However, other studies[78] have shown that the septic picture is not mimicked by infusion of a pattern of hormones including epinephrine, glucagon, and corticosteroids, indicating that other factors that enhance proteolysis and stimulate protein synthesis may be necessary components of the septic host response. The mechanism of control of these factors, which may include interleukin I, or PIF, and their relationship to mediators of hepatic and skeletal muscle protein synthesis, have not been elucidated to a sufficient degree to allow us to advocate a specific therapeutic approach at the present time.

Many studies have indicated that both protein catabolism and protein synthesis are enhanced in sepsis. As a result there is some question as to whether the increased oxidative requirement for specific amino acids (specifically the branched chain amino acids) may interfere with the endogenous amino acid balance required for adequate protein synthesis, since this requires that all necessary amino acids be present at the replicating site at the same time. As a result, it is generally believed that it is critical to maintain increased nutritional

support with adequate levels of exogenously administered nonessential amino acids as well as essential amino acids to permit sufficient building blocks for protein synthesis to be available, while fuel utilization energetic needs are also supported by an adequate calorie input. Recently, these studies have focused on the role of nutritional support in enhancing specific host defense proteins, rather than in increasing total nitrogen balance, since the latter may continue to be negative while the critical host defense mechanisms that will ultimately determine survival appear to be enhanced by improved nutritional support.

While there appears to be a general agreement about the importance of nutritional support, the precise nature of the best fuel mixture to be used is still under considerable investigation. At present, the best evidence is that a balanced daily fuel mixture of 1400 to 1500 kcal/m² (28 to 30 kcal/kg) including a relatively low quantity of glucose with at least 30 to 40 percent of the calories as lipid and a complete amino acid profile are essential. We believe that under circumstances of progressive sepsis, especially in the presence of the physiologic B state, or when there is clinical evidence of MOFS with a hepatic component, the amino acid support may need to be tailored toward an increased quantity of branched chain amino acids. In general, parenteral nutritional support should be begun as soon as cardiovascular stability is achieved after major injury in all patients and unquestionably TPN should be begun at the earliest evidence of sepsis in any patient in whom full enteral support is not possible. (For a fuller treatment see Chapter 17.)

When enteral feeding is possible, recent studies suggest an advantage to feeding by gut, provided that diarrhea and aspiration can be prevented. This is based on the fact that the first passage of substrate from the gut is to the liver and duodenal and small bowel stimulation may also involve activation of normal pancreatic hormonal regulation. There is also suggestive evidence that the presence of intraluminal nutrients may also protect the integrity of the bowel mucosa. This has lead to the increased utilization of needle-catheter jejunostomy, or an endoscopically placed feeding catheter past the pylorus into the duodenum or upper jejunum. Some clinicians have advocated the use of an obstipating balloon to prevent regurgitation of the enteric mixture into the stomach and from there into the esophagus with aspiration, especially in the severely ill septic patient with gastric ileus.

Unfortunately there are still many circumstances in which effective bowel function cannot be maintained. In patients with severe intra-abdominal sepsis and septic MOFS with a hepatic component, there is some question as to whether enteric bacteria contribute to the MOFS through their enhanced growth in the bowel, with unrestricted passage into the portal blood under circumstances where bowel lymphoid and hepatic reticuloendothelial function may be impaired.[16] Under these circumstances parenteral nutrition may still remain a necessity and at least one prospective study

is in progress in which TPN is being combined with antibiotic gut sterilization to inhibit portal venous invasion by gut organisms.

Finally, during the transition from parenteral to enteral nutrition, diarrhea may be produced despite optimization of osmotic characteristics of the enteric fuel mixture. These circumstances make it critical that an adequate nutritional transition from TPN to full enteral feeding be effected. During this period the responsible physician or surgeon must demonstrate that the nutritional support being given enterically is in fact being absorbed. This transition may be prolonged and usually requires a period of combined enteric and parenteral nutrition to ensure that adequate caloric levels and amino acids are continued during the critical phase in recovery (see Chapter 17).

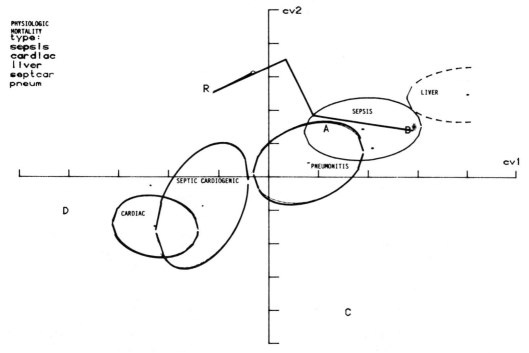

FIG. 15-56 Application of Bayesian statistical principles to development of a physiologic trajectory in which a patient's time course is evaluated with regard to its similarity to previously studied groups of patients who died in various clinical-physiologic conditions. Shown in this figure are the nonsurvivor elipses in a physiologic hyperspace developed by dimensional reduction from the original 11 physiologic variables shown in Fig. 15-2. Shown are the areas of nonseptic cardiac decompensation, septic cardiogenic decompensation, pneumonitis (ARDS), sepsis and liver decompensation with the time course of a 52-year-old cirrhotic patient who developed fatal sepsis following portacaval shunt. The patient had a hyperdynamic cardiovascular response, bilateral pneumonia and hepatic encephalopathy associated with clinical hepatic failure and the multiple organ failure syndrome (MOFS) and died in B state MOFS. (Siegel JH, Coleman B. Computers in care of the critically ill patient. Urol Clinics N Amer 13(1): 101, 1986. Reprinted with permission from WB Saunders Co., Philadelphia.)

New Techniques for Quantification of the Host Response to Therapy of Sepsis

Finally, it is important to emphasize that septic processes affect virtually every organ system, not only by direct invasion and activation of host-defense mechanisms that produce the septic syndrome, but also, and more importantly, by altering the cellular metabolic fuel control and interorgan fuel-energy transfers in a differential fashion as a function of the stage and severity of the disease process. This implies that the critical care specialist must be alert to subtle changes in each organ function as well as in the nature of the interactions between them at cardiovascular, respiratory, renal, hepatic, and immunologic levels. This re-

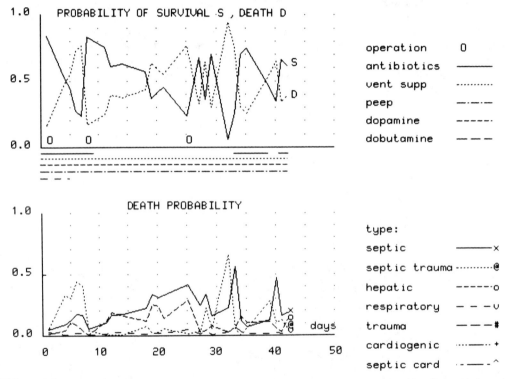

FIG. 15-57 Serial probabilities of survival and death during time course of a 26-year-old patient with hepatic trauma who developed a septic hepatic abscess requiring repeated surgical drainage (O) with changing probability of death (D) as survival (S) probability decreases with deteriorating clinical status and increases with responses to surgery and appropriate antibiotic therapy. Also shown are the individual probabilities that death could occur from each of the various clinical conditions investigated. Note that early in the time course the death probability from a septic trauma response is important. In the mid-course the death probability from a combination of hepatic failure and progressive sepsis are a relatively large proportion of the total death probability. However, late in the course as septic MOFS intervenes, the probability of hepatic decompensation falls, but that of septic death rises as the total probability of death increases. During the time course, repeated surgical drainage reduces the death probability from sepsis and increases the probability of survival. However by the 32nd postinjury day the overall death (D) probability rises due to an uncontrolled cholangitis due to enterococcus infection. At this time appropriate antibiotic therapy with gentamycin and ampicillin was begun with improvement in survival (S) probability and fall in septic death probability. Premature cessation of antibiotics (day 38) resulted in rise in septic death probability, but resumption of therapy (day 40) caused survival probability improvement with eventual patient recovery and discharge from the hospital.

quires careful and continued monitoring of the relevant physiologic and biochemical variables that reflect each organ's functional parameters during the evolution and recovery form a septic process. It also focuses on the need for techniques of multivariable data analysis to be used to quantify the relative interactions of these various systems as an index of severity. Recently, studies have been carried out by Tacchino et al.[146] on the use of a Bayesian statistical approach to enable pattern recognition of an individual patient's similarity to each of the various abnormal physiologic states that represent adaptive patterns most likely to be associated with recovery or death from the septic process. As is shown in Figure 15-56, at each study period a new septic patient's trajectory of movement through such a physiologic hyperspace can be compared in terms of his or her "distance" from regions of adaptive patterns characteristic of previously studied surviving or dying patients with various aspects of the septic or other organ failure processes. This has permitted the computation of a *posterior* probability of death based on the *likelihood ratio* of death to survival and an *a priori* probability of death that can be modified by evidence derived from the patient's immediately previous time course. This *posterior* probability of death can be used to delineate quantitatively an index of severity as a means of determining how well the patient is responding to a given therapeutic modality. In addition, because of the relationship of an individual patient's pattern of physiologic abnormalities to previously defined patterns seen in previously studied groups of patients with various forms of septic and nonseptic illness, it is also possible to gain some insight into the relative importance of one type of organ dysfunction over another in determining the overall probability of death and survival. The time course of a posttraumatic patient with hepatic injury and severe sepsis who evolved into a B state with a severe hepatic metabolic insufficiency is shown in Figure 15-57. This figure also demonstrates the response of the serial probabilities to surgical drainage and to the institution of specific antibiotic therapy. With appropriate therapy, there was a marked improvement in the probability of survival correctly predicting eventual complete recovery. These types of studies offer the possibility that the patient's response to a variety of therapeutic measures can be accurately quantified with a high degree of sensativity and specificity at the time that therapy is administered. In the near future this may provide an overall picture of the physiologic and metabolic response that can be used as a sophisticated guide to therapy.

REFERENCES

1. Altura M: Pharmacologic effects of alpha-methyldopa, alpha methyl-norepinephrine and octopamine on rat arteriolar, arterial and terminal vascular smooth muscle. Circ Res 36(Suppl): 233, 1975
2. Ashour B, Hansford RG: Effect of fatty acids and ketones on activity of pyruvate dehydrogenase in skeletal muscle mitochondria. Biochem J 214: 725, 1983
3. Babior BM, Kipnes RS, Curnutte JT: Biologic defense mechanisms. The production of superoxide—a potential bactericidal agent. J Clin Invest 52: 741, 1973
4. Bahrami S, Gasser H, Strohmaier W et al: Influence of parenteral nutrition on the composition of lung phospholipids and lung function on the traumatized rat. Proc. First Vienna Shock Forum p. 57, 1986
5. Baracos V, Rodemann HP, Dinarello CA, Goldberg AL: Stimulation of muscle protein degradation and prostaglandin E_2 release by leukocyte pyrogen (Interleukin-1). N Engl J Med 308: 553, 1983
6. Baue AE: Multiple, progressive, or sequential system failure. Arch Surg 110: 779, 1975
7. Beisel WR, Sobocinski PZ: Endogenous mediators of fever-elevated metabolic and hormonal responses. p. 39. In Lipton JM (ed): Fever. Raven Press, New York, 1980
8. Black PR, Brooks DC, Bessey PQ et al: Mechanism of insulin resistance following injury. Ann Surg 196: 420, 1982
9. Blackmore PF, Brumley FT, Marks JL, Exton JH: Studies on α-adrenergic activation of glucose output. J Biol Chem 253: 4851, 1978
10. Blair E, Cowley RA, Tait MK: Refractory shock in man: role of lactate and pyruvate metabolism and acid-base balance in prognosis. Ann Surg 31: 537, 1965

11. Border JR, Chenier R, McMenamy RH et al: Multiple systems organ failure: multiple systems organ failure: muscle fuel deficit with visceral protein malnutrition. Surg Clin North Am 56: 1147, 1976

12. Bower RH, Muggia-Sullam M, Vallgren S et al: Branched chain amino acid-enriched solutions in the septic patient. Ann Surg 203: 13, 1986

13. Brownsey RW, Edgell NJ, Hopkirk T, Denton RM: Studies on insulin stimulated phosphorylation of acetyl-CoA carboxylase, ATP citrate lyase and other proteins in rat epididymal adipose tissue. Biochem J 218: 733–743, 1984

14. Buse MG, Ried SS: Leucine: a possible regulator of protein turnover in muscle. J Clin Invest 56: 1250, 1975

15. Carpenter GA, Askanazi J, Elwyn DH: Effects of hypercaloric glucose infusion on lipid metabolism in injury and sepsis. J Trauma 19: 649, 1979

16. Carrico JC, Meakins JL, Marshall JC et al: Multiple-Organ-Failure-Syndrome. Arch Surg 121: 196, 1986

17. Cerra FB, Caprioli J, Siegel JH et al: Proline metabolism in sepsis, cirrhosis and general surgery. Ann Surg 190: 577, 1979

18. Cerra FB, Hassett J, Siegel JH: Vasodilator therapy in clinical sepsis with low output syndrome. J Surg Res 25: 180, 1978

19. Cerra FB, Mazuski JE, Chute E et al: Branched chain metabolic support. Ann Surg 199: 286, 1984

20. Cerra FB, Siegel JH, Border JR et al: The hepatic failure of sepsis: Cellular vs substrate. Surgery 86: 409, 1979

21. Cerra FB, Siegel JH, Coleman B et al: Septic autocannibalism. Ann Surg 192: 570, 1980

22. Chernow B, Roth BL: Pharmacologic manipulation of the peripheral vasculature in shock: clinical and experimental approaches. Circ Shock 18: 141, 1986

23. Cherrington AD, Assimacopoulos FD, Harper SC, Corbin JD, Park CR, Exton JH: Studies on the α-adrenergic activation of hepatic glucose output. J Biol Chem 251: 5209, 1976

24. Christou NV, Meakins JL, MacLean LD: The predictive role of delayed hypersensitivity in preoperative patients. Surg Gynecol Obstet 152: 297, 1981

25. Clowes GHA, George BG, Ryan NT: Induction of accelerated proteolysis and amino acid release from skeletal muscle by a potent non protein factor in the plasma of septic patients. p. 327. In McConn R (ed): Role of Chemical Mediators in the Pathophysiology of Acute Illness and Injury. Raven Press, New York, 1982

26. Clowes GHA, George BC, Villee CA, Saravis CA: Muscle proteolysis induced by a circulating peptide in patients with sepsis or trauma. N Engl J Med 308: 545, 1983

27. Clowes GHA, Hirsch E, George BC et al: Survival from sepsis: the significance of altered protein metabolism regulated by proteolysis inducing factor, the circulating cleavage product of Interleukin-I. Ann Surg 202: 446, 1985

28. Clowes GHA, Hirsch E, Williams L et al: Septic lung and shock lung in man. Ann Surg 181: 681, 1975

29. Clowes GHA, Vucinic M, Weidmer MG: Circulatory and metabolic alterations associated with survival or death in peritonitis. Ann Surg 163: 866, 1966

30. Clutter WE, Bier DF, Shah SD, Cryer PE: Epinephrine plasma metabolic rates and physiologic thresholds for metabolic and hemodynamic actions in man. J Clin Invest 66: 94, 1980

31. Davies CL, Newman RJ, Molyneaux SG, Grahme-Smith DG: The relationship between plasma catecholamines and severity of injury in man. J Trauma 24: 99, 1984

32. deWeir VJB: New methods for calculating metabolic rate with special reference to protein metabolism. J Physiol 109: 1, 1949

33. Deutschman C, Konstontinides FN, Tsai M et al: Metabolism on isolated viral sepsis: further support for an organism-independent response. Arch Surg (in press) 1986

34. Dinarello CA: Interleukin-1. Rev Infect Dis 6: 51, 1984

35. Evans OB, Stackpoole PW: Prolonged hypolactatemia and increased total pyruvate dehydrogenase activity by dichloroacetate. Biochem Pharmacol 31: 1295, 1982

36. Exton JH, Park CR: The role of cyclic AMP in control of liver metabolism. Adv Enzyme Reg 6: 391, 1968

37. Faist E, Baue AE, Dittmer H, Heberer G: Multiple organ failure in polytrauma patients. J Trauma 23: 775, 1983

38. Fantania HR, Law KS, Randle PJ: Activation of phosphorylated branched chain 2-oxoacid. FEBS Lett 147: 35, 1982

39. Fatania HR, Law KS, Randle PJ: Inactivation of purified ox kidney branched chain 2-oxoacid dehydrogenase complex by phosphorylation. FEBS Lett 132: 285, 1981

40. Fearon DT, Ruddy S, Schur PH et al: Activation of the properdin pathway of complement in patients with gram-negative bacteremia. N Engl J Med 292: 937, 1975

41. Felig P, Wahren J: Protein turnover and amino acid metabolism in regulation of gluconeogenesis. Fed Proc 33: 1092, 1974

42. Fischer JE, Horst WD, Kopin IJ: Beta hydroxyl-

ated sympathomimetic amines as false neuro-transmitters. Br J Pharmacol 24: 477, 1965

43. Flaim KE, Liao WS, Peavy DE et al: The role of amino acids in regulation of protein synthesis in perfused rat liver. J Biol Chem 257: 2939, 1982

44. Frayn KN, Little RA, Maycock PF, Stoner HB: The relationship of plasma catecholamines to acute metabolic and hormonal responses to injury in man. Circ Shock 16: 229, 1985

45. Freund HR, Ryan JA, Fischer JE: Amino acid derangements in patients with sepsis: treatment with branched-chain amino acid rich effusions. Ann Surg 188: 423, 1978

46. Friedman HP, Goldwyn RM, Siegel JH: The use and interpretation of multivariable methods in the classification stages of serious infectious disease processes in critically ill. p. 81. In Elashoff R (ed): Perspectives in Biometrics. Academic Press, New York, 1975

47. Fry DE, Garrison RN, Heitch RC et al: Determinants of death in patients with intra-abdominal abscess. Surg 89: 517, 1980

48. Fry DE, Pearlstein L, Fulton RL et al: Multiple organ failure: the role of uncontrolled infection. Arch Surg 115: 136, 1980

49. Fulks RM, Li JB, Goldberg AL: Effects of insulin, glucose and amino acids on protein turnover in rat diaphragm. J Biol Chem 250: 290, 1975

50. Fuller SJ, Randle PJ: Reversible phosphorylation of pyruvate dehydrogenase in rat skeletal muscle mitochondria. Biochem J 219: 635, 1984

51. Goodman MN, Ruderman NB, Aoki TT: Glucose and amino acid metabolism in perfused skeletal muscle: effect of dichloroacetate. Diabetes 27: 1065, 1978

52. Gorin AB, Weidner WJ, Demling RH: Non invasive measurement of pulmonary transvascular protein flux in sheep. J Appl Physiol 45: 225, 1978

53. Gregolin C, Ryder E, Lane MD: Liver acetyl CoA carboxylase I. isolation and catalytic properties. J Biol Chem 243: 4227, 1968

54. Guynn RW, Velosco P, Veech RL: The concentration of malonyl-coenzyme A and control of fatty acids synthesis in vivo. J Biol Chem 247: 4421, 1972

55. Hagg SA, Taylor SI, Ruderman NB: Glucose metabolism in perfused skeletal muscle. Biochem J 158: 203, 1976

56. Harlan JM, Harken LA: Hemostasis, thrombosis and thromboembolic disorders: the role of arachidonic acid metabolites in platelet vessel wall interactions. Med Clin North Am 65: 855, 1981

57. Haymond MW, Miles JM: Branched chain amino acids as a major source of alanine nitrogen in man. Diabetes 31: 86, 1982

58. Hechtman HB, Huval WV, Mathieson MA et al: Prostaglandin and thromboxane mediation of cardiopulmonary failure. Surg Clin North Am 63: 263, 1983

59. Holland R, Witters LA, Hardie DG: Glucagon inhibits fatty acid synthesis in isolated hepatocytes via phosphorylation of acetyl-CoA carboxylase by cAMP-dependent protein kinase. Eur J Biochem 140: 325, 1984

60. Holloway PAH, Alberti KGMM: Phentormin-induced lactic acidosis: prevention with dichloroacetate. Clin Sci Mol Med 50: 33, 1976

61. Ichihara K, Neely JR, Siehl DL, Morgan HE: Utilization of leucine by working rat heart. Am J Physiol (Endocrinol Metab 2) E: 430, 1980

62. Jefferson LS: Role of insulin in the regulation of protein synthesis. Diabetes 29: 487, 1980

63. Keller U, Chaisson JL, Liljenquist JE et al: The roles of insulin, glucagon, and free fatty acids in regulation of ketogenesis in dogs. Diabetes 26: 1040, 1977

64. Kelly NH, Burks H: Relative vasoconstrictor potencies of norepinephrine and octopamine. J Pharmacol Exp Ther 171: 413, 1974

65. Kerbey AL, Randle PJ: Pyruvate dehydrogenase kinase/activator in rat heart mitochondria. Biochem J 206: 103, 1982

66. Kerbey AL, Randle PJ, Cooper RH: Regulation of pyruvate dehydrogenase in rat heart. Biochem J 154: 327, 1976

67. Koj A: Acute phase reactants: their synthesis, turnover and biologic significance. p. 73. In Allison AC (ed): Structure and Function of Plasma Proteins. Plenum Press: New York, 1974

68. Krausz MM, Utsunomiya T, Feuerstein G et al: Prostacyclin reversal of lethal endotoxemia in dogs. J Clin Invest 67: 1118, 1981

69. Krebs HA, Lund P: Aspects of regulation of branched chain amino acids. Adv Enzyme Reg 15: 375, 1977

70. Krebs HA, Lund P, Stubbs M: Interrelations between gluconeogenesis and urea synthesis. p. 269. In Hanson RW, Mehlman MA (eds): Gluconeogenesis: Its Regulation in Mammalian Species. Wiley, New York, 1976

71. Lang CH, Bugby GJ, Spitzer JJ: Carbohydrate dynamics in hypermetabolic septic rat. Metabolism 33: 959, 1984

72. Lanser ME, Brown G, Mora R et al: Trauma serum suppresses superoxide production by normal neutrophils. Arch Surg 121: 157, 1986

73. Lanser ME, Mao P, Brown GE, Siegel JH: Serum mediated depression of neutrophil chemiluminescence following blunt trauma. Ann Surg 202: 111, 1985

74. Lanser ME, Saba TM, Scovill WA: Opsonic glycoprotein (plasma fibronectin) levels after burn injury. Ann Surg 192: 776, 1980

75. Lardy HA, Foster DO, Young JW et al: Hormonal control of enzymes participating in gluconeogenesis and lipogenesis. J Cell Comp Physiol 66: (Suppl 1) 39, 1965

76. Lau KS, Fatania HR, Randle PJ: Inactivation of rat liver and kidney branched chain 2-oxoacid dehydrogenase complex by adenosine triphosphate. FEBS Lett 126: 66, 1981

77. Lefer A: Eicosinoids as mediators of ischemia and shock. Fed Proc 44: 275, 1985

78. Liddell MJ, Daniel AM, MacLean LD et al: The role of stress hormones in the catabolic metabolism of shock. Surg Gynecol Obstet 149: 822, 1979

79. Linn TC, Pettit FH, Reed LJ: α-ketoacid dehydrogenase complexes and regulation of activity of pyruvate dehydrogenase complex from beef kidney mitochondria by phosphorylation and dephosphorylation. Proc Natl Acad Sci USA 62: 234, 1969

80. Livesey G, Lund P: Enzymatic determination of branched chain amino acids and 2-oxoacids in rat tissues. Biochem J 188: 705, 1980

81. Loda M, Clowes GHA, Dinarello CA et al: Induction of hepatic protein synthesis by a peptide in blood plasma of patients with sepsis and trauma. Surgery 96: 204, 1984

82. Long CL, Kinney JM, Geiger JW: Nonsuppressibility of gluconeogenesis by glucose in septic patients. Metabolism. 25: 193, 1976

83. Long CL, Spenser JL, Kinney JM: Carbohydrate metabolism in man: effect of elective operations and major injury. J Appl Physiol 31: 110, 1971

84. Marchuk JB, Finley RJ, Groves AC et al: Catabolic hormones and substrate patterns in septic patients. J Surg Res 23: 177, 1977

85. Marshall JC, Lee C, Meakins JL, Christou NV: In vivo hepatic and Kupffer cell-mediated modulation of the systemic immune response. Arch Surg (in press) 1986

86. MacLean LD, Mulligan WG, McLean APH, Duff JH: Patterns of septic shock in man. Ann Surg 166: 543, 1967

87. McGarry JD, Foster D: Regulation of hepatic fatty acid oxidation and ketone body production. Annu Rev Biochem 49: 395, 1980

88. McIrvine AJ, Mannick JA: Lymphocyte function in the critically ill surgical patient. Surg Clin North Am 63: 245, 1983

89. Mendes-Mourao J, McGiven JD, Chappell JB: The effects of L-leucine on synthesis of urea, glutamate and glutamine by isolated rat liver cells. Biochem J 146: 457, 1975

90. Miller G, Silverberg M, Kaplan AP: Autoactivatability of human Hageman factor (Factor XII). Biochem Biophys Res Commun 92: 803, 1980

91. Morgan HE, Chua B, Beinlich CJ: Regulation of protein degradation in heart. p. 87. In Wildenthal K (ed): Degradative Processes in Heart and Skeletal Muscle. Elsevier/North-Holland, 1980

92. Moss J, Lane MD: Acetyl-CoA carboxylase III. Further studies on relation of catalytic activity to polymeric state. J Biol Chem 247: 4944, 1972

93. Munster AM, Winchurch RA, Birmingham WJ et al: Longitudinal assay of lymphocyte responsiveness in patients with major burns. Ann Surg 192: 772, 1980

94. Nanni G, Pittiruti M, Giovannini I et al: Plasma carnitine levels and urinary carnitine excretion in sepsis. JPEN 9: 483, 1985

95. Nanni G, Siegel JH, Coleman B et al: Increased lipid fuel dependence in the critically-ill septic patient. J Trauma 24(1): 14, 1984

96. Neely AN, Cox JR, Fortney JA et al: Alterations of lysosomal size and density during rat liver perfusion. Suppression by insulin and amino acids. J Biol Chem 252: 6948, 1977

97. Neely JR, Denton RM, England PJ, Randle PJ: The effect of increased heart work on the tricarboxylate cycle and its interaction with glycolysis in the perfused heart. Biochem J 128: 147, 1972

98. Neufeld HA, Pace JG, White L: Effect of bacterial infections on ketone concentrations in rat liver and blood and on free fatty acid concentrations in rat blood. Metabolism 25: 837, 1976

99. Ninnemann JL, Stein MD: Bacterial endotoxin and the generation of suppressor T cells following thermal injury. J Trauma 21: 959, 1980

100. Ninnemann JL, Stockland AE: Participation of prostaglandin E in immunosuppression following thermal injury. J Trauma 24: 201, 1984

101. Numa S, Bortz WM, Lynen F: Regulation of fatty acid synthesis at acetyl-CoA carboxylase step. Adv Enzyme Reg 3: 407, 1965

102. Oliva PB: Lactic acidosis. Am J Med 48: 209, 1970

103. Oram JF, Bennetch SL, Neely JR: Regulation of fatty acid utilization in isolated perfused rat hearts. J Biol Chem 248: 5299, 1973

104. Pace JG: Fatty acid metabolism and ketogenesis during a streptococcus pneumonia injection in the rat. Dissertation; Graduate School of Arts and Sciences, George Washington University, 1980, p. 1

105. Pearl R, Clowes GHA, Hirsh EF et al: Prognosis and survival as determined by visceral amino acid clearance in severe trauma. J Trauma 25: 777, 1985

106. Peavy DE, Taylor JM, Jefferson LS: Correlation of albumin production rates and albumin in RNA in living normal and, diabetic and insulin-treated diabetic rats. Proc Natl Acad Sci USA 75: 5879, 1978

107. Pekala PH, Kawakami M, Angus CW et al: Selective inhibition of synthesis of enzymes for de novo fatty acid biosynthesis by an endotoxin-induced mediator from exudate cells. Proc Natl Acad Sci USA 80: 2743, 1983

108. Pittiruti M, Siegel, JH, Sganga G et al: Increased dependence on leucine in post traumatic sepsis: leucine/tyrosine clearance ratio as indicator of hepatic impairment in septic multiple organ failure syndrome. Surgery 98(3): 378, 1985

109. Pittiruti M, Siegel JH, Sganga G et al: Muscle catabolism, TPN and hepatic clearance of amino acids as determinant of urea production in sepsis. Arch Surg (submitted) 1986

110. Randle PJ, Fuller SJ, Kerbey AL et al: Molecular mechanisms regulating glucose oxidation in insulin deficient animals. p. 139. In Durmont JE, Nunet J (eds): Hormones and Cell Regulation INSERN European Symposium, 1984.

111. Randle PJ, Garland PB, Hales CN et al: Interactions of metabolism and the physiological role of insulin. Rec Prog Hormone Res 22: 1, 1966

112. Randle PJ, Sugden PH, Kerbey AL et al: Regulation of pyruvation oxidation and conservation of glucose. Biochem Soc Symp 43: 47, 1981

113. Robert JJ, Bier DM, Zhao XH et al: Glucose and insulin effects on de novo amino acid synthesis in young men studies with stable isotopes labelled alanine, glycine, leucine and lysine. Metabolism 31: 1210, 1982

114. Ruppin DC, Middleton WRJ: Clinical use of medium chain triglycerides. Drugs 20: 216, 1980

115. Sailer D, Muller M: Medium chain triglycerides in parental nutrition. JPEN 5: 115, 1981

116. Sapir DG, Walser M: Nitrogen sparing induced in starvation by infusion of branched-chain ketoacids. Meta Clin Exp 26: 302, 1977

117. Scholl RA, Lang CH, Bagby GJ: Hypertriglyceridemia and its relation to tissue lipoprotein lipase activity in endotoxemic, escherichia coli bacteremia and polymicrobial septic rats. J Surg Res 37: 394, 1984

118. Sganga G, Siegel JH, Brown G et al: Reprioritization of hepatic plasma protein release in trauma and sepsis. Arch Surg 120: 187, 1985

119. Shaw JHF, Klein FS, Wolfe RR: Assessment of alanine, urea and glucose interrelationships in normal subjects and in patients with sepsis with stable isotopes tracers. Surgery 97: 557, 1985

120. Shaw JHF, Wolfe RR: Energy and substrate kinetics and oxidation during ketone infusion in septic dogs. Circ Shock 14: 63, 1984

121. Sherwin RS: Effect of starvation on the turnover and metabolic response to leucine. J Clin Invest 1471, 1978

122. Sibbald WJ: Pulmonary capillary permeability in cell injury. In Cowley RA, Trump BF (eds): Shock, Anoxia and Ischemia, Pathophysiology, Prevention and Treatment. Williams & Wilkins, Baltimore, 1981

123. Siegel JH: Pattern and process in the evolution and recovery from shock. p. 381. In Siegel JH, Chodoff P (eds): The Aged and High Risk Surgical Patient: Medical, Surgical and Anesthetic Management. Grune & Stratton, New York, 1976

124. Siegel JH: Relations between circulatory and metabolic changes in sepsis. Annu Rev Med 32: 175, 1981

125. Siegel JH, Cerra FB, Coleman B et al: Physiological and metabolic correlations in human sepsis. Surgery 86: 163, 1979

126. Siegel JH, Cerra FB, Moody EA et al: The effect on survival of critically ill and injured patients of an ICU teaching service organized about a computer based physiologic CARE system. J Trauma 20: 558, 1980

127. Siegel JH, Cerra FB, Peters D et al: The physiologic recovery trajectory as the organizing principle for the quantification of horomonometabolic adaptation to surgical stress and severe sepsis. p. 177. In Schumer W, Spritzer JJ, Marshall BE (eds): Advances of Shock Research. Alan R Liss, New York, 1979

128. Siegel JH, Farrell EJ, Goldwyn RM, Friedman HR: The surgical implications of physiologic patterns in myocardial infarction shock. Surgery 72: 126, 1972

129. Siegel JH, Farrell EJ, Miller M et al: Cardiorespiratory interaction as determinant of survival and the need for respiratory support in human shock states. J Trauma 13: 602, 1973

130. Siegel JH, Giovannini I, Coleman B: Ventilation: perfusion maldistribution secondary to the hyperdynamic cardiovascular state as the major cause of increased pulmonary shunting in human sepsis. J Trauma 19: 432, 1979

131. Siegel JH, Giovannini I, Coleman B et al: Pathologic synergistic modulation of the cardiovascular, respiratory and metabolic response to injury by cirrhosis and/or sepsis: a manifestation of a common metabolic defect? Arch Surg 117: 225, 1982

132. Siegel JH, Goldwyn RM, Friedman HP: Pattern and process in evolution of in human septic shock. Surgery 70: 232, 1970

133. Siegel JH, Greenspan M, DelGuercio LRM: Abnormal vascular tone, defective oxygen transport and myocardial failure in human septic shock. Ann Surg 165: 504, 1967

134. Siegel JH, Stoklosa J, Borg U et al: Quantification of asymmetric lung pathophysiology as a guide to the use of simultaneous independent lung ventilation in post traumatic and septic ARDS. Ann Surg 202: 425, 1985

135. Solomkin JS, Bauman MP, Nelson RD et al: Neutrophil dysfunction during the course of intraabdominal infection. Ann Surg 194: 9, 1981

136. Solomkin JS, Jenkins MK, Nelson RD et al: Neutrophil dysfunction in sepsis. II. Evidence for the role of complement activation products in cellular deactivation. Surgery 90: 319, 1981

137. Solomkin JS, Simmons RL: Cellular and subcellular mediators of acute inflammation. Surg Clin North Am 63: 225, 1983

138. Stackpoole PW, Harman EM, Curry SH et al: Treatment of lactic acidosis and dichloroacetate. N Engl J Med 309: 390, 1983

139. Stackpoole PW, Moore GW, Kornhauser DM: Metabolic effects of dichloroacetate in patients with diabetes mellitus and hypolipoproteinemia. N Engl J Med 298: 526, 1978

140. Staub NC: State of the art review. Pathogenesis of pulmonary edema. Am Rev Respir Dis 109: 358, 1974

141. Stein TP, Presti ME, Leskin MJ et al: Comparison of glucose, LCT and LCT plus MCT as calorie sources for parentally nourished rats. Am J Physiol 246(Endocrinol. Metab 9): E277, 1984

142. Stephan RN, Kupper TS, Geha AS, Chaudry IH: Hemorrhage without tissue trauma produces immunosuppression and enhances susceptibility to sepsis. Arch Surg (in press) 1986

143. Stoner HB, Little RA, Frayn KN et al: The effect of sepsis on the oxidation of carbohydrate and fat. Br J Surg 70: 32, 1983

144. Sugden MC, Sharples SC, Randle PJ: Carcass glycogen as a potential source of glucose during short-term starvation. Biochem J 160: 817, 1976

145. Tacchino RM, Siegel JH, Emanuele T et al: Incidence and therapy of myocardial depression in critically ill post trauma patients. Circ Shock 18: 360, 1986 (abst)

146. Tacchino RM, Siegel JH, Goodarzi S, Giovannini I: Predicting death and illness severity in surgical and post traumatic ICU patients by Bayesian probability statistics: study and validation in 585 patients. J Trauma (submitted) 1986

147. Tranbaugh RF, Lewis FR, Christensen JM et al: Lung water changes after thermal injury. Ann Surg 192: 479, 1980

148. VandeWerve G, Proietto J, Jeanrenaud B: Control of glycogen phosphorylase interconversion by phorbolesters, diocylglycerol, Ca^{2+} and hormones in isolated rat hepatocytes. Biochem J 231: 511, 1985

149. Vary TC, Randle PJ: The effect of ischemia on the activity of pyruvate dehydrogenase complex in rat heart. J Mol Cell Cardiol 16: 723, 1984

150. Vary TC, Reibel DK, Neely JR: Control of energy metabolism of heart muscle. Annu Rev Physiol 43: 419, 1981

151. Vary TC, Siegel JH, Nakatani T et al: Regulation of glucose metabolism by altered pyruvate dehydrogenase activity in sepsis. JPEN 10, 1986

152. Vary TC, Siegel JH, Nakatani T et al: A biochemical basis for depressed ketogenesis in sepsis. J Trauma 26: 419, 1986

153. Vary TC, Siegel JH, Nakatani T et al: Effect of sepsis on activity of pyruvate dehydrogenase complex in skeletal muscle and liver. Am J Physiol 250 (Endocrin Metab 13), E634, 1986

154. Vary TC, Siegel JH, Tall BE, Morris JG: Altered glucose regulation in sepsis revealed by partial reversal of PDH inhibition by dichloroacetate. Circ Shock 18: 372, 1986 (abst)

155. Vito L, Dennis RC, Weisel RD et al: Sepsis presenting as acute respiratory insufficiency. Surg Gynecol Obstet 138: 896, 1974

156. Walters JM, Bessey PQ, Dinarello CA et al: Both inflammatory and endocrine mediators stimulate host responses to sepsis. Arch Surg 121: 179, 1986

157. Wannemacher RW, Klainer AS, Denterman RE et al: The significance and Mechanism of increased serum phenylalanine–tyrosine ratio during infection. Am J Clin Nutr 29: 997, 1976

158. Wannemacher RW, Pace JG, Beall FA et al: Role of the liver in regulation of ketone body production during sepsis. J Clin Invest 64: 1565, 1979

159. Wannemacher RW, Pekarek RS, Thompson WL et al: A protein from polymorphonuclear leukocytes (LEM) which affects the rate of hepatic amino acid transport and synthesis of acute-phase globulins. Endocrinology 96: 651, 1975

160. Webb DR, Rogers TJ, Nowowiejski I: Endogenous prostaglandin synthesis and the control of lymphocyte function. Ann NY Acad Sci 332: 262, 1979

161. Webb PJ, Westwick J, Scully MF et al: Do prostacyclin and thromboxane play a role in endotoxin shock. Br J Surg 68: 720, 1981

162. Weisel RD, Vito L, Dennis RC et al: Myocardial depression during sepsis. Am J Surg 133: 512, 1977

163. Whitehouse S, Cooper RH, Randle PJ: Mechanism of activation of pyruvate dehydrogenase by dichloroacetate and other halogenated carboxylic acids. Biochem J 141: 761, 1974

164. Wicks WD, Barnett CA, McKibbin JB: Interaction between hormones and cyclic AMP in regulating specific hepatic enzyme synthesis. Feb Proc 33: 1105, 1974

165. Wiles J, Cerra FB, Siegel JH et al: The systemic response: does the organism matter? J Crit Care Med 8: 55, 1980

166. Williamson DH: Regulation of ketone body me-

tabolism and effects of injury. Acta Chir Scand Suppl 507: 22, 1981

167. Williamson DH, Farrell R, Kerr A et al: Muscle-protein catabolism after injury in man as measured by urinary excretion of 3-methylhistidine. Clin Sci Mol Med 52: 527, 1977

168. Wilmore DW, Aulick, LH, Masin AP, Jr, Pruitt BA: Influence of burn wound on local and systemic response to injury. Ann Surg 186: 444, 1977

169. Wilmore DW, Goodwin CW, Aulick LH et al: Effect of injury and infection on visceral metabolism and circulation. Ann Surg 192: 491, 1980

170. Wilmore DW, Long JM, Mason AD et al: Catecholamines: mediators of the hypermetabolic response to thermal injury. Ann Surg 180: 653–669, 1974

171. Winn B, Harlan J, Nadir B et al: Thromboxane A$_2$ mediates lung vasoconstriction, but not permeability after endotoxin. J Clin Invest 12: 911, 1983

172. Witters LA, Kowaloff EM, Auruch J: Glucagon regulation of protein phosphorylation identification of acetyl-coenzyme A carboxylase as substrate. J Biol Chem 254: 245, 1979

173. Witters LA, Tipper JP, Bacon GW: Stimulation of site-specific phosphorylation of acetyl-coenzyme A carboxylase by insulin and epinephrine. J Biol Chem 258: 5643, 1983

174. Wolfe RR, Burke JF: Glucose and lactate metabolism in experimental septic shock. Am J Physiol 235: R219, 1978

175. Wolfe RR, Jahoor F, Peters E et al: Substrate cycling in severely burned patients. Circ Shock 18: 359, 1986 (abst)

176. Wolfe RR, O'Donnell TF, Stone MD et al: Investigation of factors determining the optimal glucose infusion rate of total parenteral nutrition. Metabolism 29: 892, 1980

177. Yamazaki K, Maiz A, Sobrado J et al: Hypocaloric lipid emulsion and amino acid metabolism in injured rats. JPEN 8(4): 361, 1984

16

Antibiotic Therapy in Critical Illness

Ellis S. Caplan

INTRODUCTION

Antibiotics constitute over one half of most major hospitals' pharmaceutical budgets and much of the use of these agents is in critically ill patients. The agents are used both prophylactically as well as therapeutically in a variety of patients and constitute a major expense during the patient's hospitalization. On the other hand, infection is a leading cause of complications in the critically ill surgical patient, especially patients in the intensive care unit. Infection is often the cause of mortality or severe morbidity. In recent years there has been a marked increase in the number of agents available, and each new agent has a small but definite advantage over prior agents. However, there is also some disadvantage to the new agents. All have certain things in common, particularly the increase in cost over prior antibiotics. In this chapter we will describe some of the principles of antibiotic use as they relate to critically ill postsurgical and posttrauma patients.

PROPHYLACTIC USE OF ANTIBIOTICS

The indications for prophylactic use of antibiotics have been expanded in recent years. However certain basic principles are important in understanding the use of prophylactic antibiotics. Prophylactic antibiotics, even when appropriate, are only one of many modalities that must be utilized to reach the expected goal of decreased infections. Prophylactic antibiotics are only used in situations where the risk of infection is substantial or, even though the risk is relatively small, the results of infection would be devastating. One problem is that the definition of substantial or devastating differs in different situations and even among physicians in the same situation. Prophylactic antibiotics have been shown to be most effective in preventing infection in situations where specific organisms cause the majority of the infections and a narrow-spectrum antibiotic is available given at an appropriate route, at an appropriate time, in an appropriate dose. The use of broad-spectrum antibiotics to cover all possible organisms has been shown to be ineffective and leads to increased adverse effects. Table 16-1 details the generally acceptable uses of prophylactic antibiotics and the antibiotic shown to be effective for this purpose.

Theoretically, wider-spectrum antibiotics should offer the same protection as those that are more organism-specific, but in practice their use may lead to increased adverse effects and superinfections. These wide-spectrum antibiotics should not be substituted where a narrower-spectrum antibiotic has been shown to be effective. There has always been great diffi-

culty in the design and execution of studies looking at the effectiveness of prophylactic antibiotics, as detailed in the review by Chodak and Plaut.[25] The authors criticize the design of the majority of studies that look at the use of antibiotics in the prophylactic setting. In addition, the reader is referred to a recent review of the use of prophylactic antibiotics.[56]

However, it is clear that to be effective the antibiotic must be present at the desired site at the time of bacterial invasion. Thus in the prophylactic setting, the antibiotic must be present at the time the surgery is undertaken. The pharmacokinetics of the antibiotics are very important since it has been found that many antibiotics given "on call" were not present when the surgical incision was made.[51,65,89] The recent introduction of antibiotics with prolonged half-lives may result in amelioration of many of these timing problems. In addition, the time necessary to continue antibiotics in the prophylactic situation has also been somewhat controversial. Clearly the most important

TABLE 16-1.   Indications for Prophylactic Antibiotics in Surgery: Organisms Involved and Antibiotics Used

Type of Surgery	Potential Infecting Organism	Antibiotic
Orthopedic		
Joint replacement	*Staphylococcus aureus*	1st-generation cephalosporin
	Staphylococcus epidermidis	β-lactamase-resistant penicillin
		Vancomycin
Open fracture	*Staphylococcus aureus*	1st generation cephalosporin
		β-lactamase resistant penicillin
		Vancomycin
Gynecologic		
Cesarean section	*E. coli*, anaerobes	Cephalosporin
Vaginal hysterectomy	*E. coli*, anaerobes	Cephalosporin
Abdominal hysterectomy	*E. coli*, anaerobes	Cephalosporin
Gastrointestinal		
Biliary	*E. coli, Enterococcus*	Cephalosporin in high-risk patients
Stomach–duodenum	Upper respiratory flora Occasional *S. aureus*	1st generation cephalosporins in high risk patients
Intestinal	*E. coli*, anaerobes including *B. fragilis, Enterococcus*	Oral neomycin plus erythromycin or cefoxitin or clindamycin and gentamicin
Thoracic		
Cardiac prosthesis	*Staphylococcus aureus*	1st generation cephalosporin
	Staphylococcus epidermidis	Penicillinase-resistant penicillin
		Vancomycin
Otolaryngologic		
Head and neck	*Staphylococcus aureus*	Cefazolin
	Upper respiratory anaerobe	Aqueous penicillin G
	Streptococcus	

dose is the first, so that the antibiotic will be present at the time of the possible bacterial invasion. Subsequent doses are far less important and in most studies where this has been looked at, one or a few doses have been as effective if not more effective than prolonged use of antibiotics.[56]

THERAPEUTIC USE OF ANTIBIOTICS

Assessment of the Patient

One can expect an adequate therapeutic response to appropriate antibiotics only when they are used to treat infections caused by susceptible organisms. The vast majority of therapeutic antibiotics are instituted because the patient is febrile. It must be remembered that there are many other reasons for fever in the postoperative and critically ill patient. While these are well known to most surgeons, it must be continually reemphasized that a thorough search for the source of the elevated temperature must be undertaken prior and subsequent to the institution of antibiotics and such factors as retained blood, obstruction of hollow viscus, pulmonary embolus, presence of necrotic tissue, and inflammation due to foreign objects must be ruled out. These may be associated with infection but all can cause fever by themselves. In addition, leukocytosis is a reflection of an inflammatory response and, as with fever, there are many other reasons for an inflammatory response besides infection, particularly in the stressed postsurgical patient. In addition to fever and leukocytosis there should be evidence of organ dysfunction, to point the physician to the site of infection. Thus, the patient with fever, leukocytosis, and pulmonary infiltrate who does not have any change in pulmonary functions is unlikely to have an active infection. Frequently, the hemodynamic effects of infection manifested by a hyperdynamic car-

diovascular state with increased cardiac output, reduced vascular resistance, and increased oxygen consumption can be identified very early as signs of sepsis with the use of hemodynamic monitoring. All of these clues must be taken into consideration when dealing with the possibilities of infection.

One must always attempt to define either the infecting organism or the site of infection before instituting antibiotics in the septic patient. The presence of an organism at a site is not sufficient evidence for infection, since these patients are frequently colonized with the endemic flora of the intensive care unit. This colonization may take place at any site in a patient, particularly those invaded with tubes, such as the trachea, urinary tract, sumps, drains, and intravenous (IV) sites. In our experience it is not at all uncommon that patients are put on an antibiotic simply because urinalysis showed greater than 100,000 gram-negative rods. This is not sufficient to make a diagnosis of a urinary tract infection. One must have the clinical symptoms of infection and an active urinary sediment to make this particular diagnosis. One must remember that antibiotics are used to treat infections and not to treat organisms identified by the laboratory.

Factors to Consider

In addition to the susceptibility of the infecting organism to the selected antibiotics, other factors must be taken into consideration to ensure a therapeutic response. The antibiotic selected must get into the appropriate tissue, thus the degree of binding, the route of administration, and the dose of the antibiotic all must be taken into account to ensure that adequate concentration of the active agent enters the desired tissue. In selecting the dose of the antibiotic, sufficient drug must be given to achieve a therapeutic concentration in the desired tissue. Half the dose of an antibiotic will not kill half the organisms. In addition, antibiotics must be given time to exert their antibacterial effect. Patients with pneumococcal pneumonia who are given penicillin will not defervesce for about 36 hours.[40] A patient who is on an appropriate antibiotic in a critical situation cannot really be expected to defervesce in any less time; expecting immediate responses usually entails daily changes of antibiotics, all to no avail.

The need for ancillary measures, particularly surgical drainage, cannot be overemphasized. Frequently an abscess must be drained, a line must be removed, a tube position changed, necrotic tissue removed, or some other manipulation is necessary in the vast majority of patients with nosocomial infections to attain the maximum therapeutic response.

The length of time for therapy of most infections has never been adequately studied. It is known that 10 days of penicillin is necessary to reduce significantly the chances of rheumatic fever in patients with group A β-hemolytic streptococci.[21] The length of treatment required for any other infection is extremely speculative. In general, with adequate antibiot-

ics and adequate ancillary measures in the appropriate host, the vast majority of infections should respond within 7 days. Most experienced infectious disease physicians would treat nosocomial pneumonia and intraabdominal abscesses for 14 days, or occasionally longer. However, it must be remembered that the possibility of superinfection and complications of the antibiotics and their administration, such as thrombophlebitis, increase substantially with increasing length of antibiotic use. If, after the appropriate length of time, an adequate response has not been obtained then all antibiotics should be discontinued, and reevaluation and reculturing undertaken. Almost without exception, attempts to add other antibiotics to increase the spectrum of effectiveness, without a careful investigation or some clear evidence that this change in therapy is necessary, are likely to fail. Table 16-2 lists the various antibiotics used in clinical practice

TABLE 16-2. Dosage of Antibiotics in Patients with Normal Renal Function and Life-Threatening Infection

Antibiotic	Initial Dose	Subsequent Dose and Interval
Penicillins		
Azlocillin	3–6 g	3–6 g q 4 hr
Carbenicillin	3–6 g	3–6 g q 4 hr
Mezlocillin	3–5 g	3–5 g q 4 hr
Nafcillin	1.5 g	1.5 g q 4 hr
Oxacillin	1.5 g	1.5 g q 4 hr
Penicillin	5 million units	3–5 million units q 4 hr
Piperacillin	3–5 g	3–5 g q 4 hr
Ticarcillin	3–6 g	3–6 g q 4 hr
Cephalosporins		
Cefamandole	2 g	2 g q 4 hr
Cefazolin	1 g	1 g q 8 hr
Cefoperazone	2 g	2 g q 8–12 hr
Cefotaxime	2 g	2 g q 4–6 hr
Cefoxitin	2 g	2 g q 4 hr
Ceftazidime	2 g	2 g q 8 hr
Cephalothin	2 g	2 g q 4 hr
Moxalactam	2 g	2 g q 8 hr
Aminoglycosides		
Amikacin	7.5 mg/kg	
Gentamicin	1.7–2 mg/kg	Adjust dose to obtain peak levels in therapeutic range
Netilmicin	2 mg/kg	
Tobramycin	1.7–2 mg/kg	
Others		
Amphotericin B	1 mg test dose	0.6 mg/kg per day
Clindamycin	600 mg	600 g q 6 hr
Metronidazole	500 mg	500 g q 6 hr
Trimethoprim–Sulfamethoxazole	5 mg/kg	15–20 mg/kg/day in 4 doses
Vancomycin	2 g	2 g q 6 hr

and the dosage used for patients with life-threatening infection and normal renal function.

over one-half of the cost of most hospital formularies; by using less expensive antibiotics, substantial savings in health care can be realized.

Cost

In this age of cost containment the expense of any medical manipulation must be taken into account. The cost of bringing a new compound to the market place has risen to astronomically high levels in recent years. As a result, the price of these new compounds reflects this. Table 16-3 shows a cost comparison of parenteral antibiotics that considers not only the cost of the compound but also the expense incurred for pharmaceutical mixing as well as the IV bag and tubing. One can see that the true cost of different antibiotics with the same or similar spectrum of activity varies a great deal and substantial savings can be achieved by selecting an equally effective, but less expensive, antibiotic. Currently antibiotic costs constitute

Use of Combination Antimicrobial Agents

In clinical practice, antimicrobial agents are frequently used in combination. Several reasons, at least theoretically, support the use of combination antibiotic therapy. One is to enhance the spectrum for a particular infection. This is frequently true for selecting combination antibiotics when an organism has not been identified, or if a gram-negative rod is identified and a mixed infection is suspected. Since no one currently available agent has a sufficiently broad spectrum to cover all of the wide variety of organisms that may be present in a given patient, the use of combination antibiotics may be necessary to cover gram-positive cocci, par-

TABLE 16-3. Antibiotic Costs

	Dosage for Seriously Ill Patients with Normal Renal Function	Cost to Hospital per Dose ($)	Cost per Day as Ordered $ (March 1985)[a]
Ampicillin	1.5 g q 4 hr	1.40/g	42.57
Penicillin	3 MU q 4 hr	0.48/million units	41.04
Amikacin	500 mg q 6 hr	17.04/500 mg	85.56
Gentamicin	80 mg q 6 hr	0.55/80 mg	19.60
Tobramycin	80 mg q 6 hr	4.88/80 mg	36.42
Clindamycin	600 mg q 6 hr	10.87/600 mg	60.88
Chloramphenicol	1 g q 6 hr	2.01/g	25.44
Cefoxitin	2 g q 4 hr	13.59/2-g vial	106.64
Metronidazole	500 mg q 6 hr	3.99/500 mg	31.96
Ticarcillin	3 g q 4 hr	7.23/3-g vial	68.78
Mezlocillin	3 g q 4 hr	11.04/4-g vial	76.70
Pipercillin	3 g q 4 hr	13.21/4-g vial	84.85
Cephalothin	2 g q 4 hr	4.47/2-g	53.33
Cefamandol	2 g q 4 hr	11.08/2-g vial	91.88
Cefazolin	2 g q 8 hr	3.15/g	32.30
Nafcillin	1.5 g q 4 hr	3.09/2 g	49.95
Vancomycin	500 mg q 6 hr	17.49/500-mg vial	87.36
Cefaperozone	2 g q 8 hr	19.00/2-g vial	70.40
Moxalactam	2 g q 8 hr	20.95/2-g vial	76.25
Cefotaxime	2 g q 4 hr	17.00/2-g vial	127.40
Trimethoprim–Sulfamethoxazole	1050 mg	3.65/80 mg	65.30

[a] Includes cost of preparation and IV administration for all doses (MIEMSS: University of Maryland Medical System).

ticularly *Staphylococcus* and/or *Enterococcus,* as well as gram-negative rods. Frequently a decision will have to be made as to whether the infection is more likely to be caused by a *Klebsiella* and/or *Pseudomonas* as the gram-negative component. These two-gram negative rods will usually require a different antibiotic in combination with an aminogycoside. For example, the aminopenicillins are much better for *Pseudomonas* infections than are most of the cephalosporins, which are usually better for *Klebsiella*. With the recent introduction of some of the newer antibiotics one can cover both *Klebsiella* and *Pseudomonas* infections with one antibioic. In addition, an infection may frequently include both aerobic and anaerobic organisms and in some circumstances this combination will require more than one agent.

The second common reason for using combination antibiotics is to achieve bactericidal synergy. This approach is probably most advantageous when used in the immunosuppressed host, particularly the granulocytopenic patient. However, there is no hard evidence to suggest that this is absolutely necessary. Many combinations of an aminoglycoside and a β-lactam antibiotic are synergistic for a wide variety of gram-negative rods including *Klebsiella, Enterobacter,* and *Pseudomonas* species. In this case, both agents to be used should have sufficient activity to be used as a single agent, but show in vitro evidence of more rapid killing of the organism when combined.[68] Whether this laboratory phenomenon has any relevance in the clinical situation has yet to be adequately proven.

In some instances in infections involving gram-positive organisms, particularly *Enterococcus,* only combination antibiotics will provide adequate killing. Thus, an *Enterococcus* that is resistant to penicillin and sensitive to aminoglycosides will be susceptible to synergistic killing when both penicillin and the aminoglycoside are used together. However, in general if the organism is resistant to the aminoglycosides then little or no synergy can be expected with the introduction of a β-lactam antibiotic.[67] This holds true both for *Enterococcus* and gram-negative rods.

Another reason for the use of combination antibiotics is to prevent emergence of resistant organisms. This perhaps is best known in the treatment of *Mycobacterium tuberculosis* infection, particularly those in abscess cavities where the concentration of the organism is known to be extremely large. Since there is a high likelihood that a single tuberculous bacillus may be resistant to one or more agents, a combination of drugs (e.g., isoniazid and rifampin) is necessary to be sure that a resistant population will not emerge during therapy. While this is probably an uncommon event with ordinary types of bacterial infections, it has been advocated by some authorities[83] as a reason to use combination agents.

Another reason for using combination antibiotics is that by giving more than one antimicrobial compound the pharmacokinetics of both compounds can be used to maximal advantage, particularly in patients in whom the pharmacokinetics may be somewhat different. For example, in young trauma patients who have rapid excretion of many compounds, the individual antibiotic's administration can be staggered to ensure a continuous therapeutic level in the blood or tissue.

When using combination antibiotics, keep in mind that certain combinations, that of a bactericidal antibiotic and a bacteristatic antibiotic may have an antagonistic effect. This problem is always discussed in patients with meningitis in whom the combination of chloramphenicol and ampicillin is frequently used. Although these drugs are antagonistic in the laboratory setting, true drug antagonisms have never been definitely shown to occur in the clinical situation. Table 16-4 lists various antibiotic combinations and shows what organisms can reasonably be expected to be "covered" by these combinations.

Laboratory Methods

The normal approach to antimicrobial therapy of human infections is based on the isolation and identification of the infecting organism and its in vitro susceptibility to antimicrobial agents. Since antimicrobial therapy is often initiated on an empiric basis in patients with serious infections, the results of cultures

TABLE 16-4. Combination Antibiotics and Organisms Covered

Antibiotics	Enterococcus	S. aureus Methicillin Sensitive/ Resistant	Enterobacteriaceae	Pseudomonas	B. fragilis	Other Anaerobes
Penicillin + aminoglycoside	Y	A/N	Y	Y	N	Y
1st generation cephalosporin + aminoglycoside	N	Y/N	Y	Y	N	Y
Cefoxitin + aminoglycoside	Y	A/N	Y	Y	Y	Y
Mezlocillin or pipercillin + aminoglycoside	Y	A/N	Y	Y	Y	Y
Ticarcillin + aminoglycoside	N	A/N	Y	Y	Y	Y
3rd generation cephalosporin + aminoglycoside	N	Y/N	Y	B	C	Y
Trimethoprim–sulfamethoxazole	N	A/A	Y	N	N	N

A, some activity but may not be adequate for serious infection.
B, moxalactam + cefaperazone–Ceftazidime has antipseudomonal activity.
C, moxalactam has adequate *B. fragilis* activity.
N, not adequate.
Y, yes.

and susceptibility tests permit more precise selection of agents and dosage after identification of the organism. A Gram's stain, however, is a quick, simple, and inexpensive test that can be done by any laboratory at any time and, if properly interpreted, can greatly enhance the physician's ability to select appropriate therapy. Table 16-5 outlines the method. The entire process can be done in less than 1 minute after the slide is dried. The specimen selected for Gram's stain should preferably be fresh and

TABLE 16-5. The Gram's Stain Procedure

1. Using a clean glass slide, smear a small amount of the specimen over the center portion of the slide.
2. Air dry.
3. Heat fix by quickly passing the slide through the flames of a bunsen burner.
4. Flood the slide with crystal violet stain and allow to stay on slide about 10 seconds. Specimen should be blue.
5. Wash with water.
6. Flood the slide with Gram's iodine solution and allow to remain on the slide for 10 seconds. Specimen should be black.
7. Wash with water.
8. Decolorize by flooding slide with decolorizing solution until the blue color stops coming off the slide. This should take only a few seconds. Do not try to get all the blue off the slide: this depends on the thickness of the specimen; if it is too thick you will not be able to get the blue off without overdecolorizing the rest of the slide.
9. Wash with water.
10. Flood the slide with the counterstain. The slide should now appear red.
11. Wash with water.
12. Air dry or dry using special drying papers.

uncontaminated with other tissue or fluids. A thin amount should be put on the slide and allowed to air dry. The slide should be stained as quickly as possible, and again allowed to dry, though it can now be patted dried with appropriate absorption paper. The slide should be examined first under lower power and then under high power in a search predominantly for polymorphonuclear cells. If the slide is properly stained they will appear pink, including their nuclei. If the nuclei are blue, there has been inadequate decolorization and subsequent interpretation may be erronous. Once identification of the proper cells is made, the physician can decide whether the specimen is adequate for subsequent interpretation. For example, if squamous epithelial cells are seen in the sputum specimen then one suspects that it is not sputum, but is contaminated with saliva.

The same is true for peritoneal fluid. Peritoneal macrophages and polymorphonuclear cells should be present to make an adequate determination. Once it is determined that adequate material is present, the physician looks for gram-negative organisms that stain red or pink. They frequently will blend into the background with serious fluids from the body, particularly peritoneal and pleural fluid in which the protein level is high. After a thorough search for gram-negative organisms is undertaken; gram-positive organisms, which stain a dark blue, should be sought. If one just looks for the gram-positive organisms, one frequently will miss the gram-negatives seen in the background. The structure of the organisms and their appearance on gram stain will frequently lead the astute physician to the proper identification of the organism and then subsequent selection of appropriate antibiotics. Table 16-6 is a guide for the most common organisms and their morphology as seen using Gram's stain. It cannot be emphasized sufficiently how important an adequate Gram's stain is in selecting initial and subsequent antibiotic therapy and in determining the site of an infection. In many situations the Gram's stain may give better information than subsequent cultures.

Once the specimen is sent to the laboratory, depending on the method used, various antibiotic susceptibility tests will be performed. These fall into two major groups; disc diffusion and tube dilution. The disc diffusion tests have been the standard for many years. However, with the advent of more automated equipment, microtiters are being used in increasing numbers of laboratories. The tube dilution test is the principal method to determine the minimum concentration of antimicrobial agent that inhibits the growth of an organism. The test is performed by serially diluting the antimicrobial agents in agar or broth and inoculating the mixture with a standardized suspension of the organism according to established procedures. The results are expressed as the minimum inhibitory concentration (MIC) in micrograms per milliliter. In general, the lower the MIC, the more susceptible the organism is to the antibiotic. The organism is considered to be susceptible when the MIC is one

half to one quarter the safely obtainable peak or mean blood level of the antimicrobial agent tested. The minimum bactericidal concentration (MBC) is the least amount of antimicrobial agents that kills 99.9 to 100 percent of a standard inoculation of the organisms. Among the few indications for performing MBC testing are infections at sites where host defenses may be impaired. Usually this occurs in endocarditis and osteomyelitis.

The disc diffusion test is still the more frequently used method for susceptibility testing. Its principle is that the diameter of a zone of inhibition about an antimicrobial impregnated paper disc relates approximately linearly to the log to the base 2 of the organism's MIC. Zone diameters of inhibition are intrepreted according to published criteria and the results are usually reported as susceptible, intermediate susceptible, or resistant to the appropriate antimicrobial agent. It must be remembered that both these tests are in vitro methods and do not take into account the white cell killing function of the patient, the diffusion of antibiotics into the appropriate site of infection, or the protein binding of the antibiotics in question. Generally, however, antibiotics determined to be susceptible by either of these sensitivity methods will usually cure the infections if other basic principles of treatment are adhered to.

Other laboratory methods available to the physician include the use of drug levels. Levels are usually obtained for drugs that have a very narrow toxic therapeutic ratio, particularly the aminoglycosides. Because of their wide use in clinical medicine and their rather narrow ther-

TABLE 16-6.   Appearance on Gram's Stain of Some of the More Common Organisms Causing Disease in the Critically Ill Surgical Patient

Organism	Appearance on Gram's Stain
Gram-positive	
Streptococci	Gram-positive cocci in chains, or single cocci
Staphylococci	Gram-positive cocci in clusters or single cocci
Clostridia	Gram-positive rods, fat with square ends, may stain, gram-variable
Listeria monocytogenes	Gram-positive rods thin, may appear as "chinese letters"
Gram-negative	
Neisseria sp.	Gram-negative cocci in pairs and singly
E. coli, Enterobacter spp.	Gram-negative rods cannot be distinguished among this group
Klebsiella spp., *Pseudomonas* spp.	
Serratia spp., *Citrobacter* spp.	
Proteus spp., *Salmonella* spp.	
H. Influenzae	Gram-negative organism in cocci; small cocobacillary rods; pleo-
Acinetobacter spp.	morphism is the rule

apeutic ratio, a number of tests have been devised to measure the levels of these drugs in the blood. One hopes to prevent use of too much, or too little, drug in the individual patient. While there are limits set on aminoglycosides usually a peak of somewhere between 6 μg/ml and 8 μg/ml and a trough of between 1 μg/ml and 2 μg/ml is usual for gentamicin and tobramycin. These are very broad limits. At this time, adequate data are not available to suggest that maintenance of aminoglycoside levels in these ranges will result in cure of the infection, or that this will prevent toxicity. In general, aminoglycoside levels should be used as a broad guide to therapy with these drugs, to be sure that, because of the various excretion rates in different patient populations, the patient is receiving what most would consider an adequate concentration. On the other hand it is equally important to be sure that adequate but not toxic drug levels are being maintained in the blood. While other drugs besides aminoglycosides can be measured, because of their high therapeutic ratio they frequently are not measured, and thus there is even less information available about the blood levels one would expect or should try to maintain with nonaminogycloside antibiotics. Table 16-7 shows the therapeutic levels for the most commonly measured antibiotics.

PRINCIPLES OF ANTIBIOTIC USE IN SPECIAL SITUATIONS

Burns

Infections have always been a serious problem in burn patients. Modern therapy has drastically reduced the incidence of infection in these patients from 80 percent in patients with greater than 40 percent body surface burns to less than 50 percent in patients with 65 percent body surface burns. However, if one excludes those due to smoke inhalation, 50 to

TABLE 16-7. Therapeutic Levels of Antibiotics in Blood for Serious Infections

Drug	Desired Peak Level (μg/ml)		Desired Trough Level (μg/ml)
Aminoglycoside			
Amikacin	20–25		8
Gentamicin	6	8	1.5
Tobramycin	6	8	1.5
Netilmicin	8	10	2
Vancomycin	20–30		10
Sulfamethoxazole	15		

75 percent of inhospital deaths in a burn unit are secondary to infection.[30] Previously, *Streptococcus* and *Staphylcoccus* were the predominant pathogens. Currently, gram-negative rods and fungi are responsible for the majority of infections in burn patients. Sixty percent of burn wounds are colonized by *Pseudomonas* by day 5 after surgery.[90] This organism is by far the major pathogen causing infection in today's burn units. Empiric treatment of burn patients should be avoided since fungi have emerged as superinfecting pathogens in many burn units where empiric therapy is frequently employed.[102] A quantitative biopsy has been useful in differentiating colonization and invasion of the burn wound. Greater than 10^5 organisms per gram of tissue is used as an indicator for tissue invasion. Repeat biopsy of the wound at 48-hour intervals allows constant monitoring of the patient so that therapy can be instituted prior to the onset of systemic sepsis. Prophylactic topical therapy has been useful in limiting bacterial proliferation at the burn site and compounds such as mafanide sodium, silver nitrate, and silver sulfadazine have been used frequently with good success. In addition to the burn wound, that other sites may be the cause of the systemic infection in these immunocompromised patients. Pneumonia and IV-line-associated phlebitis have been major problems in various units. Because burn patients characteristically have an increased volume of distribution, most antibiotics must be given in doses greater than one is accustomed to in order to obtain sufficient therapeutic levels in serum and the infected site. The aminoglycosides must be given at dosages of 100 mg 4 to 6 hr in patients with normal renal function to achieve therapeutic levels. Antibiotic moni-

toring is almost uniformly necessary in these patients to achieve these high levels and yet avoid toxic levels. Penicillins must also be given in larger than usual doses. Accordingly we would advocate the use of 40 g carbenicillin or ticarcillin and 30 g mezlocillin or piperacillin per day to achieve the needed therapeutic levels in young patients with normal renal function.

Trauma

Infection is the second leading cause of death in the multiply injured patient, only surpassed by severe head injury. The infections that occur in the trauma patient have been described.[19] Because of the vast amount of invasive procedures these patients undergo it is not surprising that 81 percent of all infections are related to the use of invasive equipment.[19] Because of the wide variety of infections that these patients are subject to, prophylactic antibiotics are not advisable and should only be used in specific situations that have been rather well defined: open fractures, penetrating abdominal wounds, and, possibly, through and through fractures of the oral cavity. The trauma

patient has an intensive inflammatory response secondary to the injury and care must be taken in differentiating fevers caused by this inflammatory response from those caused by infections. Since a large majority of these patients are relatively young and have large volume of distribution, antibiotics frequently have to be given in much higher than "normal" doses to achieve therapeutic levels. In addition, because these patients frequently have multiple injuries and multiple invasive lines it is not infrequent for successive and even simultaneous infections to be taking place at different sites. Thus, careful reappraisal of the infections, the organisms, and, of course, the patient must be undertaken in treating these patients. Table 16-8 shows the site of infection in a large number of trauma patients treated at the Maryland Institute for Emergency Medical Services Systems.

Postsplenectomy

The syndrome of overwhelming postsplenectomy sepsis was described by Schumacher and King in 1933 and recently this syndrome has been reported in adults.[11] While the inci-

TABLE 16-8. Percent of Infections (n = 1199), Bacteremic Infections (n = 529), and Mortalities (n = 137) Occurring by Site in 5,000 Patients at the Maryland Institute for Emergency Medical Services Systems, 1979–1983

Site	% Infections Occurring at Site	% Bacteremic Infections Occurring	% of Mortality from Infections Occurring at Site
Primary bacteremia	9	21	9
Vascular			
Arterial	2	5	0
Phlebitis	11	15	1
Sinusitis	7	0	0
Lower respiratory			
Pneumonia	16	19	33
Empyema	10	10	18
Urinary tract	16	3	0
Central nervous system	5	4	7
Intra-abdominal abscess	10	12	24
Surgical wound	9	6	1
Others	4	5	8
N	1199	529	137

dence of infection varies with the indications for the splenectomy it is clear that all patients with a splenectomy are at increased risk over the normal population.[74] The organisms involved are usually encapsulated organisms and rarely is this risk present while the patient is still in the hospital.[108] Much more commonly, infections occurring in the splenectomized patient who is still in the hospital are the nosocomial infections secondary to the intraveneous lines or the operation itself. Antibiotic therapy, therefore, is very different in the patient with postsplenectomy infection while still in the hospital from that in the patient who is under consideration or overwhelming postsplenectomy sepsis. In the latter, *Pneumococcus* is the offending organism in about half the cases with *Hemophilus influenzae*, *Neisseria meningitidis*, *Staphlococcus*, and *E. coli* causing the remainder of the infections. In the former the site of infection must be identified and antibiotics and surgical procedures that will address infection in these sites must be instituted. The syndrome of overwhelming postsplenectomy sepsis is distinct in its rapidity of onset and overwhelming nature of the infection as evidenced by the ability to see organisms on a Gram's stain of the buffy coat of peripheral blood. *Pneumococcus* is still a very common organism, causing infections in all types particularly of the lower respiratory tract, only infrequently will it cause an overwhelming infection in this type of patient.

Renal Failure

Most of the parenteral antibiotics used today to treat critically ill patients are dependent upon adequate renal function for their elimination. Thus, patients with impaired renal function may need substantial changes in an antibiotic dose depending upon the renal function and the particular antibiotic used. Table 16-9 outlines dose adjustments necessary for various degrees of renal failure for the more commonly used antibiotics.

TABLE 16-9.   Doses of Antibiotics in Various Degrees of Renal Impairment

Drug	Creatinine Clearance (ml/min)		
	≤ 50 > 25	≤ 25 > 10	≤ 10
Penicillin G	1.5 million units q 4 hr	800,000 units q 6 hr	500,000–800,000 units q 6–8 hr
Oxacillin	1.5 g q 4 hr	N/C	N/C
Nafcillin	1.5 g q 4 hr	N/C	N/C
Carbenicillin	2 g q 6 hr	2 g q 8 hr	2 g q 12–18 hr
Ticarcillin	2–5 g q 6 hr	2–5 g q 8 hr	2–5 g q 12 hr
Mezlocillin	3–5 g q 6 hr	3–5 g q 8 hr	3–5 g q 12 hr
Piperacillin	3–5 g q 6 hr	3–5 g q 8 hr	3–5 g q 12 hr
Gentamicin	Initial dose: 1.7 mg/kg, then adjust dose to maintain therapeutic level.		
Tobramycin	Initial dose: 1.7 mg/kg, then adjust dose to maintain therapeutic level.		
Amikacin	Initial dose: 7.5 mg/kg, then adjust dose to maintain therapeutic level.		
Metronidazole	500 mg q 6 hr	N/C	N/C
Chloramphenicol	1 g q 8 hr	N/C	N/C
Vancomycin	500 mg q 1–3 days	500 mg q 3–7 days	9–10 days
Trimethoprim– Sulfamethoxazole	2.5–5 mg/kg q 12 hr	q 18	Avoid
Cephalothin	1 g q 4 hr	1 g q 6–8 hr	1 g q 8–12 hr
Cefazolin	500 mg q 8 hr	1 g q 12 hr	1 g q 24 hr
Cefamandole	2 g q 8 hr	1 g q 8 hr	1 g q 12 hr
Cefoxitin	2 g q 12 hr	1 g q 12 hr	1 g q 24 hr
Cefuroxime	500 mg–1.5 mg q 8 hr	500 mg q 12 hr	500 mg q 24 hr
Moxalactam	1 g q 8 hr	1 g q 12 hr	1 g q 18 hr
Cefotaxime	2 g q 8 hr	2 g q 12 hr	2 g q 18 hr
Cefaperazone	1–2 g q 12 hr	N/C	N/C

N/C, no change.

Immunocompromised Host

While critically ill patients are frequently exposed to immunocompromising events the factor contributing most to infection is the absolute magnitude of the granulocyte count. It has been well shown that with granulocyte counts below a 1,000 cells/ml and even more particular below 500 cells/ml the risk of infection rises dramatically. Thus, patients who have white cell dysfunction or severe granulocytopenia either secondary to intensive chemotherapeutic agents, reactions to medications, or for whatever reason when the total granulocyte count is less than 500 cells/ml must be considered to be at a very high risk of bacterial infection. In studies on the infections that take place in these immunologically impaired patients, five organisms predominate: *Staphylococcus aureus, Pseudomonas aeruginosa, E. coli, Klebsiella pneumoniae,* and *Candida albicans.* The majority of infections in the granuloctyopenic patient take place in five sites[33]: the upper alimentary tract, mouth and lower esophagus; the lower alimentary tract, particularly perirectal lesions; the skin; lungs; and occasionally the urinary tract. Unfortunately, the granulocytopenic patient frequently does not show the typical inflammatory response. Infiltrates are frequently not present early with pneumonia, and purulence is not found at sites of infection.

In addition, because of the lack of granulocytes, the patient frequently will become bacteremic and the infection can become overwhelming in a very short period of time. It is for this reason that these patients are empirically started on broad-spectrum antibiotics that have been shown to be quite effective at both preventing complications and increasing survival.[38] Among the patients thought to have infection, 40 percent will turn out not to have an infection. Forty percent will have a probable or possible infection and 20 percent will be indeterminate.[99] Of the patients who subsequently turn out to have an infection, however, the organism usually becomes evident within the first 72 hours. Therefore while empiric broad-spectrum antibiotics are indicated to cover these organisms, if the site or the organism cannot be found within 4 to 5 days then

it is usually prudent to stop the antibiotics and reevaluate the patient. On the other hand, if the patient continues to do poorly one must suspect infection with organisms that are not covered with the empiric regimen, and frequently an antifungal agent such as amphotericin B will be added. The initial spectrum must include agents active against *Staphylococcus,* as well as gram-negative rods, and should be synergistic against these organisms. For this reason single agent therapy has not been successful in the treatment of these patients. Results of trials with some of the new compounds with exceedingly broad spectrums in treating infections in these patients are eagerly awaited. The combination chemotherapy regimens have been quite varied, but usually include a β-lactam broad-spectrum antibiotic to cover *Pseudomonas* and an aminoglycoside. Recently, combination β-lactam antibiotics have been used, however there is some speculation that increased resistance may become a problem with this regimen. The length of therapy in the granulocytopenic patient has not been determined. If the patient is doing well, generally 7 to 10 days seem to be adequate, however the biggest factor determining ultimate outcome is the return of the granulocyte level to greater than 500 cells/ml. If the patient remains profoundly granulocytopenic in spite of all efforts, the outcome is usually fatal. It must be emphasized that in these patients one cannot wait to determine the site nor the organism. Empiric therapy should be instituted at the first suspicion of infection, which is almost always marked by fever and/or by the patient's reporting that he or she does not feel well.

Gas-Forming Infections

While a variety of organisms are implicated in infections that produce gas, clearly the most feared are those due to clostridia. However while gas gangrene, anaerobic necrotizing cellulitis, synergistic necrotizing cellulitis, Meleny's gangrene, Fournier's gangrene, which are all synonyms for different types of infection, are handled with the same approach, on clinical inspection one can not distinguish the type of organisms involved. All require extensive surgical debridement and early biopsy and culture to make a definitive diagnosis. Clearly the history is helpful in identifying the probable organism, but frequently in these infections multiple organisms are isolated. After extensive and thorough surgical wound debridement, the institution of broad-spectrum antibiotics aimed at covering clostridia should be begun, if identified as large positive rods by Gram's stain. Other gram-positive anaerobic such as anaerobic streptococcus, gram-positive aerobes such as *Staphylococcus,* and the β-hemolytic *Streptococcus,* and a variety of gram-negative rods including *E. coli* and *Klebsiella* are also commonly present in these situations. In addition, *Enterococcus* is a frequently isolated organism although its exact role in these diseases is not clear. Broad-spectrum antibiotics consisting of penicillin, clindamycin, or metronidazole and an aminoglycoside, usually gentamicin, are instituted pending identification of the exact pathogens. This combination offers maximum coverage for clostridia (penicillin), *Enterococcus* (penicillin plus the aminoglycoside), gram-negative rods, (aminoglycosides), and anaerobes (clindamycin or metronidazole). We generally use high doses: 12 million units of penicillin per day to be given in equal doses every 4 hours, 600 mg clindamycin every 6 hours, or 500 metronidazole every 6 hours and adequate gentamicin to achieve a peak therapeutic level of at least 6 μg/ml. After surgical debridement the wounds are left open and followed very closely. Usually by 7 to 10 days the antibiotics can start to be tapered or discontinued completely. Of course once the appropriate organisms are identified, adjustment of the antibiotics is indicated. For clostridial infections, we would treat for at least 10 days. Contrary to popular opinion these patients do not have to be isolated. These organisms will not infect normal healthy wounds in other patients and other patients are at no greater risk than any other patient of acquiring organisms from a patient with a gas-forming infection. Clearly, adequate infection control procedures should be instituted when handling all wounds.

The role of hyperbaric oxygen remains controversial (see Chapter 37). Hyperbaric oxygen can halt toxin production of clostridial organisms and has been used in patients with gas gangrene infection.[53] Although many anecdotal reports attest to its efficacy, a well-controlled trial remains to be performed.

ANTIBIOTIC USE AT SPECIFIC SITES

Surgical Wound Infections

The incidence of surgical wound infections has been studied extensively by many authors.[2,24,53,79,112] It is clear that the major factor in determining the development of an infection at the surgical wound site is the type of surgical wound. The standard classification of surgical wounds defines four types according to their prospective risks of postoperative infections: clean, clean contaminated, contaminated, and dirty.[1] A clean wound is one made during elective surgery with primary closure and no drains used. There is no entry into a contaminated area, no break in sterile technique during the operation, and the wound is nontraumatic. The expected infection rate in such procedures is less than 5 percent and in one large study[29] it was 1.8 percent. In clean contaminated wounds, the alimentary or respiratory tract is entered without significant spillage or mechanical drainage. Appendectomy wounds and procedures involving entry into the vagina or the uninfected urinary or biliary tract are also classified as clean contaminated. These wounds have an expected postoperative wound infection rate of about 10 percent. Contaminated wounds include all fresh traumatic wounds, operations with a major break in sterile technique, gross spillage from the gastrointestinal tract, entry into an infected biliary or urinary tract, or incisions encountering acute nonpurulent inflammatory reaction. The anticipated infection rate here is approximately 20 percent. Finally, dirty wounds include traumatic wounds with retained devitalized tissue, fecal contamination, foreign body wounds requiring delayed treatment, and wounds from a dirty source such as those occurring from farm machinery contaminated by manure. This category also includes operations involving acute purulent material obtained during the operation, operation on perforated viscus, or a transection of clean tissue for surgical access to a collection of pus. In these wounds, organisms are already present and infection is ongoing; the postoperative wound infection rate is about 30 percent and higher in many studies. Thus, the type of wound is very important in determining the expected infection rate and because of this problem many studies looking at prophylactic antibiotics have been undertaken, especially in the wounds with higher infection rates.

When determining the choice of antibiotics for the patient who has a surgical wound infec-

tion it is imperative to be aware of which prophylactic antibiotics may have been used or whether there has been any previous antibiotic therapy, since it is less likely for the organisms causing the wound infection to be sensitive to any of the prior antibiotics. The predominant organism in the clean and clean contaminated wounds is almost always a *Staphylococcus* from the skin, whereas in the traumatic or operative wounds involving viscera it is frequently the organism encountered during the operative procedure. Thus, in biliary tract or enteric surgery one would worry more about gram-negative aerobic or anaerobic organisms, whereas in colorectal or vaginal surgery one has to worry about the anaerobic organisms of the vagina or large bowel (Table 16-10).

Many wound infections can be handled simply by local treatment of drainage and debridement. However if there are systemic signs

TABLE 16-10. Most Likely Organisms Causing Infections of Surgical Wounds at Specific Body Sites and Empiric Antibiotics Most Likely to be Effective

Site	Most Likely Organisms	Empiric Antibiotic Likely to be Effective
Face	*Staphylococcus aureus*	Nafcillin 1st generation cephalosporin
Oral cavity	Not *Bacteroides fragilis* Anaerobes	Penicillin Clindamycin
Paranasal sinuses, hospital-acquired	Variety of gram-negative rods Staphylococcus	Mezlocillin–aminoglycoside
Pleura	*Staphylococcus aureus* Gram-negative rods	Cephalosporin + Aminoglycoside
Abdominal Abscess	*E. coli;* anaerobes including *B. fragilis;* other negative rods; occasional *Staphylococcus aureus*	Clindamycin–aminoglycoside or Metronidazole–aminoglycoside
Biliary Tract	*E. coli* *Enterococcus* *Klebsiella*	Ampicillin + aminoglycoside
Colon	*B. fragilis* and other anaerobes; *E. coli*	Clindamycin–aminoglycoside Metronidazole–aminoglycoside
Urinary Tract	*E. coli,* other negative rods	Aminoglycoside or cephalosporin

Skin
  Nonburn
  Burn
	
	Staphylococcus aureus
	Staphylococcus aureus
	Streptococcus pyogenes
	Pseudomonas
		
		Nafcillin
		Nafcillin
		Mezlocillin–aminoglycoside

Decubitus ulcer	Anaerobes, *Staphylococcus*	Clindamycin Cefoxitin
Vagina	Gram-negative rods Anaerobes	Clindamycin–aminoglycoside

such as leukocytosis or fever, then frequently antibiotics will be necessary. Use of the Gram's stain to define the type of organisms present of the wound before culture and sensitivity analysis are available will greatly facilitate the selection of appropriate antibiotics. The color of pus is not due primarily to the organism, but to the number of white cells in the wound. With few exceptions, the organism cannot accurately be identified by the presence of creamy yellow, or green purulent material. A simple Gram's stain will identify whether antibiotic coverage should be aimed primarily at gram-positive organisms, gram-negative organisms, or both. Most systemic antibiotics will get into the wounds in sufficient concentrations to be therapeutic.

bic laboratories it may take several days to weeks to identify many of the organisms present in purulent material. For this reason, patients considered at risk, or those who develop a secondary infection, should be started on antibiotic combinations to cover both the aerobic and the anaerobic flora of the body. In infections that occur secondary to operative procedures, the prior use of prophylactic antibiotics must be taken into account when selecting the initial antimicrobial therapy. In general antibiotics should be chosen that will cover organisms that may be resistant to the previous antibiotics used, pending full identification and sensitivity. However the effectiveness of any antibiotic is secondary to the provisions of adequate surgical drainage and debridement of an infected wound or abscess.

Abdomen

With very few exceptions, all suspected infections of the abdomen should be treated as if a combination of anaerobic and aerobic organisms are involved. With the recent introduction of simplified anaerobic culturing methods, it has become quite apparent to most authors that the luxuriant anaerobic flora in the gastrointestinal tract frequently participate in a major way in most infections that occur in the abdomen.[47] Certainly, any infection that takes place following instrumentation or operation on a hollow viscus should be considered to contain anaerobes until proven otherwise. Since many hospitals have difficulty in fully identifying anaerobic organisms it has been suggested that all infections resulting from surgery or trauma to the gut or other intra-abdominal organs be treated as if anaerobes are involved, whether they are isolated or not.

In this type of infection the utility of the Gram's stain cannot be overemphasized. If a mixture of types of organisms is seen on Gram's stain, this is almost pathognomonic of an anaerobic infection, even though subsequent cultures do not confirm the presence of culturable anaerobes. It is suggested that one rely more on the Gram's stain of the material removed from the abdomen than on the subsequent culture results. Also, in the best anaero-

Sinusitis

Infections of the paranasal sinuses have been reported to cause a substantial number of postsurgical infections.[20] These usually occur during the second week of hospitalization in patients who have indwelling nasogastric or nasotracheal tubes in place. In addition, these patients are receiving heavy sedation for respiratory control or have some intracranial pathologic condition that decreases their mental status. It is thought that the patient's lack of mobility in conjunction with the intranasal tube interferes with the ventilation of their sinuses and leads to sinusitis. The presence of sinusitis is identified in a critically ill patient with a portable x-ray study of the paranasal sinuses looking for complete opacification or for an air-fluid level. On aspiration of the sinuses, the organisms involved are frequently the nosocomial flora of the intensive care unit and are not the normal colonizing organisms of the upper respiratory tract: *Pneumococcus* and *Hemophilus influenzae*. Therefore the treatment of this acute nosocomial sinusitis is with broad-spectrum antibiotics whose effectiveness includes the nosocomial organisms present. Because of the thick mucus-laden pus containing a large spectrum of organisms it is frequently necessary to drain the sinuses either by aspiration through the sinus wall via the nasal passage or by a modified Cauldwell-Luc procedure. In addition to the use of antibiotics, the removal of any nasal tube is indicated; it may be replaced through the oral cavity if still necessary. These patients usually respond fairly rapidly with a reduced temperature and white cell count. They should be continued on antibiotic therapy for approximately 10 days.

Lower Respiratory Infections

Lower respiratory tract infections have the highest mortality and morbidity of any infection that occurs in seriously ill postoperative patients.[109] A major reason for this lethality is that frequently these infections occur in patients with already compromised pulmonary function who are undergoing mechanical ventilation; contamination of the lower respiratory tract may lead to subsequent intrapulmonary infection. While a nosocomial pneumonia must be treated extremely vigorously, it is, unfortunately, also a difficult diagnosis to make. The postoperative critically ill patient frequently has a number of reasons besides pneumonia for the presence of pulmonary infiltrates, such as retained secretions, atelectasis, decreased pulmonary excursion, pulmonary embolus, and congestive heart failure, among others. Thus, all patients with fever and a pulmonary infiltrate may not have pneumonia and a vigorous work-up must be undertaken to decide which patients require antimicrobial therapy. The use of bronchoscopy and aggressive physical therapy is helpful in defining those patients who will require antibiotics.

Aggressive antibiotic therapy is indicated in patients in whom pulmonary x-ray findings do not improve after these forms of pulmonary therapy and who have a predominant organism on Gram's stain. Prior cultures may be helpful but cannot always be relied upon, since rapid colonization and infection with new pathogens can occur in these critically ill patients. Because of these facts, careful examination of the Gram's stain is mandatory before instituting antibiotic therapy. Although the Gram's stain

can be misinterpreted, it is still the best immediate guide to the type of therapy instituted, particularly in the patient who is not granulocytopenic. Specific antibiotic therapy for gram-positive nosocomial pneumonia is generally successful. Gram-negative infections, on the other hand, are extremely difficult to treat. In spite of high-dose combination antibiotics given early,[23] the mortality in these patients exceeds 50 percent. The mortality is even higher in those patients with subsequent bacteremia. Bacteremia is a frequent accompaniment of nosocomial pneumonia, particularly in the postsurgical and posttrauma patient. In granulocytopenic patients one has to consider opportunistic organisms such as fungi, yeast, protozoa, mycobacteria, and viruses. In these patients early use of open lung biopsy is frequently required to identify the infecting organism.

Primary Bacteremia

Primary bacteremia is defined as two positive blood cultures with the same organism, without a known sight of infection having that organism. This accounts for approximately 10 percent of the infections in the multiply traumatized patient. Because of this phenomenon and because intra-abdominal or reptroperitoneal abscess may first present as bacteremia it is extremely important to draw blood cultures whenever the critically ill patient is suspected of having an infectious process. While gram-positive bacteremia with no other source is frequently considered to be endocarditis, it is very difficult to prove in these patients. In our experience few of the posttrauma or postsurgical patients will have any clinical signs of endocarditis or any risk factors for this disease. However, if positive blood cultures are obtained it is prudent to treat these patients for 4 weeks with antibiotics considered bactericidal for the recovered organisms. Frequently it will be impossible to continue intravenous antibiotics for the full course because of limited venous access. Oral therapy can then be instituted; one should monitor the blood bactericidal levels to ensure that oral therapy is being absorbed and that adequate therapeutic levels are obtained in these patients.

For primary gram-negative bacteremia the correct length of treatment is unclear, since gram-negative organisms causing endocarditis are extremely uncommon. We would suggest that treatment consist of the intravenous use of a combination of antibiotics active against the organism for 2 weeks. The source of most of these infections is probably the intravenous lines, but this has not been shown to be true in all cases.

Fungal Infections

By far the most common fungal infection encountered in clinical practice is secondary to *Candida albicans*. It is generally believed that the presence of *Candida* in the blood (candidemia) may be a benign condition and that simply removing the lines and reculturing the patient until persistent negative cultures are seen may be all that is necessary. While this is a prevailing opinion, it is quite hard to document this and should not be assumed to be true. The only definitive signs of *Candida* infection are the presence of an endophthalmitis, which presents as white raised plaques in the retina or of skin lesions that, on biopsy, are shown to be *Candida*. However, it is quite unusual to find these early in the course of candidemia.

Patients with candidemia usually have been exposed to multiple antibiotics and frequently are in renal failure. So it is with some reluctance that the treating physician will put the patient on amphotericin B, because of its renal toxicity. However, in our experience the finding of candidemia is associated with active disease and it is our strong feeling that immediate therapy is warranted in the majority of patients while one awaits results of subsequent cultures, after having removed or changed all indwelling vascular access lines. It is not at all unusual for candida to take 5 to 7 days to grow out in blood cultures. As a result, frequently one finds that the patient is quite well

along into the disease before appropriate therapy is instituted. If antibiotics have been selected appropriately for specific situations, and not given for prolonged periods of time, the finding of *Candida* in the blood is unusual.[19] The dosing time of amphotericin is controversial. We would begin with a 1 mg test dose followed by 0.6 mg/kg and treat the patient for 14 to 21 days. Continued surveillance is required, looking for the onset of possible *Candida* endocarditis, which characteristically has large vegetations on the aortic valve and may be detected by echocardiography.[46,48] The presence of this disease frequently means that surgical intervention with replacement of the aortic valve is necessary, since antifungal therapy alone is often unsuccessful.

Vascular Lines

The incidence of vascular-line-related infections has been increasing in recent years, as more and more invasive lines have become commonly used in the hospital setting. While occasionally the problem is due to contamination of the infusing fluid, this is relatively rare. If an unusual organism appears in the blood of a patient, contamination of the intravenous fluid should be considered, as was demonstrated in a nationwide outbreak of contaminated albumin in which a *Pseudomonas cepacia* was identified.[104] However, the vast majority of infections are due to the intravenous device itself and more specifically to infection beginning at the insertion site.

There are two types of infections recognized. One is a suppurative phlebitis, almost always caused by *Staphylococcus aureus*. About half of the time, patients with this infection will be bacteremic. Careful examination of the insertion site will reveal purulent material that can be either aspirated from the vein or milked from the vein. These infections can frequently be treated with antibiotics alone, although in about 10 percent of the time removal of the infected vein will be required. However, in burn patients excision of the suppurating vein is mandatory since these patients must be considered as compromised hosts. Occasionally a perivascular abscess may be found around a stitch or even at the skin site itself. This often requires incision and drainage in addition to administration of appropriate antibiotics.

The second type of infection associated with venous catheterization is the nonsuppurative septic thrombophlebitis. This is usually heralded by the identification of a gram-negative rod, usually a *Klebsiella* species in the blood of a patient with no other obvious site of infection. Even after appropriate antibiotics are instituted, the patient may continue to be bacteremic when infected with these organisms. This then will strongly suggest the diagnosis of nonsuppurative septic thrombophlebitis and calls for removal of the infected venous segment. There is frequently only mild erythema and some induration of the infected site. No factors distinguish the involved vein from the others and frequently these patients have received numerous infusions through many different veins. Usually, however, the vein through which the infusion is currently running is affected. Therapy requires incision and removal of the infected venous segment, in addition to administration of antibiotics. These patients should then be treated for approximately 10 days after removal of the segment to ensure that no bacterial seeding has occurred. While originially described in burn patients, this condition has now been seen in many other settings in patients who have multiple intravenous fluids and multiple lines.

Urinary Tract

The urinary tract is characteristically the most common site for nosocomial infection in most populations studied. The vast majority of these infections occur in patients who have indwelling urinary catheters. The urethral catheter is by far the leading prediposing cause of urinary tract infections. However, the isolation of organisms from a catheterized specimen, particularly in a specimen obtained from an indwelling Foley catheter, is not sufficient to make a diagnosis of a urinary tract infection.

We would recommend that when an organism is isolated in large numbers a careful urinalysis be undertaken to look for inflammatory cells in the urinary sediment. This provides better evidence that a significant infection is taking place at this site, since it is not infrequent for a patient with an indwelling catheter to be colonized with organisms and not have an infection.

Almost all antibiotics given systemically will reach a sufficient achievable concentration in the urine to treat most of the infections that occur in the urinary tract. Even as a nosocomial infection, *E. coli* is the most common organism isolated from this site. However, the bacteria involved in a particular patient cannot be anticipated in patients with underlying urinary pathologic conditions who have been frequently exposed to multiple antibiotics. The infecting organism can be defined only by culturing the urine. The treatment of urinary tract infections in the patient who has other organ injuries or disease has not been well delineated. Clearly, short-course therapy is not indicated since the majority of these infections involve the upper urinary tract. The available methods for delineating upper and lower urinary tract infections are frequently not feasible and are generally not used in treating postsurgical patients. It is wise to assume that any infection of the urinary tract in the critically ill surgical patient will involve the upper tract. Systemic antibiotics are indicated when there are signs of the systemic stress response to infection. We recommend aggressive antibiotic treatment for 7 to 10 days with an agent demonstrated by culture to be specific for the infecting organisms; certainly if the indwelling Foley catheter can be removed, it should be. If the catheter must remain in place, the goals of therapy may have to be changed. In this situation, the therapeutic aim is to decrease the number of organisms rather than to maintain a sterile urinary tract; the latter is impossible for any length of time in patients with a chronic indwelling catheter. To chase the organisms by changing antibiotics soon becomes futile, since they change as rapidly as the antibiotics. Thus, in catheterized patients with bacteriuria, systemic signs of infection and an inflammatory sediment in the urine are required before they are treated for a urinary tract infection.

Central Nervous System

Central nervous system infection is a rare complication of critically ill surgical patients, with the notable exception of patients who have sustained head trauma or undergone neurosurgical procedures. The major risk factor for infection of patients with head injury is a defect in the dural membrane. Patients with closed head injury almost never develop subsequent CNS infections unless there is a break in the cribriform plate and dura with access to the subarachnoid space. The diagnosis of central nervous system infection may be very difficult to make in head trauma patients. Many of these patients have fever secondary to posttraumatic CNS inflammation and are already comatose or obtunded. As a result the major clinical sign that one would look for, namely deterioration of mental function, frequently cannot be evaluated.

Traditional diagnostic tests are not very helpful and it is frequently impossible, or at least extremely dangerous, to obtain cerebrospinal fluid in head-injured patients because of the possiblity of an increased cerebral pressure and the risk of subsequent brain herniation if the spinal fluid pressure is reduced. Thus the diagnosis of infection in these patients is difficult to make. In patients with localized findings, computer assisted tomography has proved invaluable in helping to make the diagnosis of brain abscess.

In addition to the difficulty of making a diagnosis in CNS infections, the organisms recovered are quite varied. *Staphylococcus aureus* is still the most common organism; however, many other gram-positive and gram-negative organisms have been found. Because of the wide variety of organisms that can occur, the use of antibiotics for prophylaxis after head injury with cerebrospinal fluid leak has been very controversial. At present, there are no adequate studies to support their use. The treatment of gram-negative CNS infections, when they do occur, is also hindered by the inability of many of the antibiotics with adequate gram-negative spectrum to enter the CSF and control the infection adequately.

The selection of antibiotics must be based on the knowledge of the nosocomial organisms present in a particular intensive care unit. In addition, antibiotics must be chosen that will enter the cerebrospinal fluid via the blood brain barrier in therapeutic levels. Until recently, this entailed the use of multiple antibiotics to cover most of the suspected organisms. The therapy of CNS septic processes has been substantially facilitated by the introduction of the third-generation cephalosporins (Table 16-11), which have a broad spectrum and a very low minimum inhibitory concentration (MIC) for many of the organisms responsible for CNS infections. However, there are still limitations to this type of therapeutic approach. Organisms such as *Acinetobacter* or *Pseudomonas,* as well as many of the gram-positive organisms, may frequently not be adequately coverd by the use of third-generation cephalosporins. In many of these cases, because of the increased cerebrospinal fluid pressure, adequate culture material cannot be obtained prior to the institution of therapy. If therapy was begun empirically, the patient must be very carefully watched for any sign of deteriorating mental function, at which point the choice of antibiotics must be altered empirically, or an attempt must be made to obtain cerebrospinal fluid by insertion of an intraventricular catheter or by asternal puncture if spinal tap is contraindicated. In particular, head-injured patients with cerebral contusion who develop signs of CNS infections should be repeatedly scanned by contrast-enhanced computed tomogaphy (CT) to search for evidence of an intracerebral abscess.

β-LACTAM ANTIBIOTICS

Mechanisms of Action

β-Lactam antibiotics are all cell-wall-active antibiotics. They interfere with the enzymes necessary to build peptidoglycan links within the bacterial cell wall. β-Lactam antibi-

TABLE 16-11. Useful Antibiotics in the Treatment of Central Nervous System Infections

Agent	Comments	Dosage
Chloramphenicol	Enters CSF well even in uninflamed meninges, good for *Streptococcus pneumonia, N. meningitidis, H. influenzae.* Has activity against many other gram-negative rods	1–2 g q 4–6 hr, initially, then 1 g q 6 hr
Penicillins	Enters CSF poorly except when inflamed. Drug of choice for *Pneumococcus, N. meningitidis*	20 million units per day given in divided doses, q 4 hr
Vancomycin	Fair penetration into CSF but adequate for treatment of *Staphylococcus* in penicillin-allergic patients or in methicillin-resistant *Staphylococcus*	500 mg q 6 hr
Aminoglycosides	Poor entrance into CNS: may be used in combination with other agents particularly bacteremic CNS infections. Questionable efficacy when given only intravenously	Gentamicin–tobramycin: 60–100 mg q 4–6 hr. Amikacin 500 mg q 6 hr
3rd generation cephalosporins	Enters fairly well, but adequate for treatment of sensitive organisms, particularly gram-negative rods. Data on *Pseudomonas* are sparse but ceftazidime appears best	Moxalactam: 2 g q 6 hr. Cefotaxime: 2 g q 4 hr

otics bind to bacterial cells through penicillin-binding proteins, which are enzymes active in the biosynthesis of the peptidoglycan component of the bacterial cell wall.[12]

Mechanisms of Bacterial Resistance

The major mechanism of bacterial resistance to penicillin is hydrolysis of the β-Lactam bond by β-lactamases with loss of antibiotic activity. This is plasmid-mediated in gram-positive bacteria where the enzymes are present in the surrounding media. Thus the enzymes can deactivate penicillin in the environment before they reach the cell surface. Gram-negative β-lactamases may be either chromosome- or plasmid-mediated. In gram-negative bacteria the β-lactamases are located in the periplasmic space, protecting the target area from the binding proteins. Another mechanism of resistance is failure of the antibiotics to bind to penicillin-binding proteins, which are critical to cell-wall division.[54]

Penicillin

PHARMACOLOGY

Penicillin V, ampicillin, cloxacillin, and dixcloxacillin, when taken orally, are absorbed sufficiently to achieve therapeutic levels in a variety of tissues. Other penicillins are inactivated by gastric acidity and cannot be relied on to achieve therapeutic levels when given orally. All penicillins given intravenously distribute quickly to achieve high therapeutic concentrations in a variety of tissues. Most penicillins are excreted rapidly, unchanged by glomerular filtration and tubular secretion, with a half-life of about 1 hour or less. Therefore, in order to maintain therapeutic levels frequent (i.e., every 4 hour) administration is necessary in patients with normal renal function. Nafcillin is a notable exception in that 80 percent is excreted by the liver and dose adjustment is not recommended in patients with impaired renal function. This also allows nafcillin to achieve very high levels in billiary secretions.

ADVERSE EFFECTS

All penicillins can cause immediate anaphylaxis, serum sickness, rash, Coombs'-positive hemolytic anemia, panctyopenia, and nephritis. While immediate anaphylaxis is the most serious of the adverse reactions with the penicillins, it occurs in less than 0.04 percent of all patients receiving these drugs. In extremely high doses penicillins are neurotoxins and can cause seizures. This usually occurs when patients with renal failure receive full therapeutic doses of penicillin without adjustment. Most penicillins are sodium salts and therefore can cause hypernatremia and secondary hypokalemia, if this is not taken into account in the appropriate patient.

SPECTRUM OF ACTIVITY

In the patient with no known allergy, penicillin is the drug of choice for all infections caused by susceptible organisms. Most streptococci are extremely sensitive to penicillin, *Streptococcus pneumoniae* and *Streptococcus pyogenes*. *Streptococcus pneumoniae* resistant to penicillin have been reported, but are very rare in the United States. Enterococci are resistant to penicillin and may be sensitive to ampicillin; however, for serious infections with *Enterococcus* a combination of penicillin and an aminoglycoside is required to kill this organism adequately.

Most anaerobes mentioned above whose normal habitat is the diaphragm are sensitive to penicillin. Most gram-positive rods, either aerobic or anaerobic, are sensitive to these drugs, if they are given in sufficient dosage after removal of necrotic tissue.

Nafcillin, oxacillin, methicillin, dicloxacillin, and cloxacillin are resistant to the β-lactamses produced by *Staphylococcus* and are therefore used to treat infections with staphylococci. Methicillin seems to cause the most interstitial nephritis,[4] oxacillin the most hepatitis,[33] and nafcillin the most granulocytopenia. All of these reactions are transient and reverse with cessation of therapy. Staphylococci resistant to all β-lactam antibiotics have been reported with increasing frequency.[84] The mechanism of resistance is not known and currently only vancomycin seems to be adequate treatment for infections with these organisms, which are classified as methicillin resistant.

The recommended dosages for penicillins are:

Penicillin G aqueous	up to 2 million units/ 24 hours given every 4 hours
Ampicillin	500 mg to 2 g every 4 hours IV or orally
Methicillin	1 to 2 g every 4 hours IV
Nafcillin	1 to 2 g every 4 hours IV
Oxacillin	1 to 2 g every 4 hours
Dicloxacillin	250 to 500 mg orally every 6 hours
Cloxacillin	250 to 500 mg orally every 6 hours

Extended Spectrum Antipseudomonas penicillins

Indanyl carbenicillin, ticarcillin, mezlocillin, piperacillin, and azlocillin all fit into this group. All compounds of these have excellent activity against most strains of *Pseudomonas aeruginosa* and, with the exception of indanyl carbenicillin, are all given as an intravenous preparation. However, indanyl carbenicillin does not achieve adequate therapeutic levels in the blood and therefore should only be used for urinary tract infections with susceptible organisms. The primary utility of these specialized penicillins is in serious infections in which *Pseudomonas* is the identified pathogen. These compounds should always be used in combination with an aminoglycoside, since emergence of resistance has been encountered frequently when they are used alone for serious infections caused by a pseudomonas. The adverse reactions are similar to other penicillins with the addition of bleeding that has been reported principally with carbenicillin, ticarcillin, and piperacillin, since these drugs in high concentrations bind to adenosine diphosphate in platelets, preventing normal aggregation.[16,43] This is primarily a problem of the high concentrations achieved, particularly when the drug is not decreased in patients with renal failure.

In addition, because carbenicillin and ticarcillin are disodium salts each gram contains 4.6 mEq sodium; when they are administered in high doses greater than 20 g/24 hours, secondary hypokalemia may occur. There is a nonreabsorbable anion load presented to the distal tubular, thus potentiating the hypokalemia of these compounds.[18] Mezlocillin and piperacillin have less of a sodium load and therefore cause less sodium and potassium problems. In addition, these two compounds have increased activity against many strains of *Pseudomonas, Klebsiella,* and *Enterococcus.* Thus, mezlocillin or piperacillin in combination with an aminoglycoside can be used in mixed infections when *Enterococcus* is the suspected pathogen. Azlocillin has less activity against other gram-negative rods than does carbenicillin, but has much more activity against pseudomonas than carbenicillin or ticarcillin.[37] All three drugs have adequate activity against anaerobes with the high doses given to treat serious infections.

The recommended dosages for these agents are:

Carbenicillin	40 g in 24 hours given every 4 hours
Ticarcillin	30 to 40 g in 24 hours given every 4 hours
Mezlocillin	18 to 30 g in 24 hours given every 4 hours
Piperacillin	18 to 30 g in 24 hours given every 4 hours
Azlocillin	18 to 30 g in 24 hours given every 4 hours

Cephalosporins

Cephalosporins are a large class of β-lactam antibiotics that have been used extensively in a variety of clinical situations. Currently, more than 17 preparations are available and it is estimated that there are at least as many to be released in the next several years. For convenience's sake the cephalosporins are currently divided into three generations. The first generation cephalosporins basically have a narrow gram-negative activity and are the most active against staphylococci. No cephalosporins have adequate activity against methicillin-resistant staphylococci. The second-generation cephalosporins basically have an extended spectrum over the first generation to include *Hemophilus,* and a better activity against *Klebsiella* and a few other gram-negative organisms. Cefoxitin has excellent anaerobic activity. The third-generation cephalosporins have an even more extended spectrum than the aforementioned drugs, including some activity against *Pseudomonas,* and have particularly good activity against most of the enterobacteria. Some of the compounds are active against anaerobic organisms.

MECHANISMS OF RESISTANCE

The most prominent mechanism of resistance may be the inability of the antibiotic to reach the site of the binding proteins.[93] The second mechanism is that alterations in binding proteins take place and thus the antibiotics cannot bind.[97,98] Another mechanism is the production of β-lactamases or cephalosporinases that can open the β-lactam ring and render the cephalosporin molecule inactive.[39]

PHARMACOLOGY

Since there are a large number of types of cephalosporins, each has slightly different pharmacologic properties. Most are absorbed by mouth and most of them are excreted renally. They can also be given intravenously for serious infections or in patients in whom oral intake is not permitted. The dose must be adjusted in patients with renal insufficiency. Cefaperazone is a notable exception in that its primary route of excretion is through the liver; therefore, dose adjustment is not necessary in patients with renal insufficiency.

ADVERSE REACTIONS

The major advantages of the cephalosporins are the remarkably small number of side effects attributed to them. Certainly, all allergic reactions may occur, but they are less than reported with penicillins, even in patients who have a penicillin allergy. However, in patients with severe immediate penicillin allergy these drugs should be avoided. In addition to a maculopapular rash, anaphylatic reactions have been reported but are quite rare. Other adverse reactions include hemolysis in patients given long-term cephalosporins,[94] thrombocytopenia, and defects in platelet aggregation.[49] Some cephalosporins, particularly cephalothin, have been shown to be synergistically nephrotoxic when combined with an aminoglycoside.[8,110] Cefamandole, cefaperazone, and moxalactam have been implicated as causes of prolongation of the prothrombin time and clinical bleeding.[3]

USES

Cephalosporins have been used in a variety of clinical situations. They are the most commonly used antibiotics for prophylaxis in many different surgical procedures, particularly the first-generation compounds for orthopedic and skin infections, and cefoxitin is widely used for prophylaxis before abdominal surgery, particularly for penetrating abdominal injuries.[82] Because of their relatively low toxicity and their broad spectrum they are frequently used to treat a variety of infections due to susceptible organisms in many different tissues. While the majority of the cephalosporin compounds do not enter the cerebrospinal fluid in sufficient concentrations to treat meninigitis, some of the newer compounds, particularly cefotaxime, moxalactam, and cefuroxime, are approved for use in patients with meninigitis due to susceptible organisms, particularly gram-negative rods. There are limited data on the penetration of cefozperazone into the cerebrospinal fluid; however, this compound does achieve extremely high levels in the bile of the unobstructed gallbladder. Most of the other cephalosporins also will achieve therapeutic levels in most other tissues.

Table 16-12 compares the features of the cephalosporins and their dosage.

AMINOGLYCOSIDES

Aminoglycosides were first used in the therapy of tuberculosis and have now become the standard by which other drugs are measured for treatment of serious gram-negative infections. Currently, the compounds available include streptomycin, gentamicin, tobramycin, amikacin, and netilmicin. All except streptomycin and kanamycin are frequently used to treat serious gram-negative infections.

Pharmacology

These compounds are not absorbed by the gastrointestinal tract and must be given parenterally to assure therapeutic levels in the blood and tissues in normal patients. They are excreted unchanged in the urine and may be found in the urine weeks after administration of the drug. They enter the cerebrospinal fluid and the aqueous humor of the eye poorly and adequate concentrations cannot be obtained in the obstucted biliary tract. Penetation of the bronchial epithelium and bronchial secretions is variable and some investigators find that therapeutic concentrations are difficult to achieve for infections of the lower respiratory tract.[64]

Mechanism of Action

The aminoglycosides are bactericidal antibiotics. They bind primarily to the 30S subunit and possibly to the 50S subunit of the bacterial ribosome,[9,10] leading to inhibition of protein synthesis and the subsequent death of the organism.

Mechanism of Resistance

Three mechanisms of resistance to aminoglycosides have been identified. The most common type is due to extranuclear plasmids that code for a variety of aminoglycoside-modifing enzymes. Of the available compounds, amikacin is the most resistant to inactivation by most of the enzymes produced by this mechanism.[100]

TABLE 16-12. Features of Cephalosporins and Recommended Dosage

Cephalosporin	Major Advantage	Disadvantage	Dosage
Cephalothin Cephradine Cephapirin	Most active agents against *Staphylococcus*	Limited gram-negative spectrum	0.5–2 g IV q 4–6 hr
Cefazolin	Prolonged half-life allowing q 8 hr dosing	Limited gram-negative spectrum	0.5–1 g q 8 hr
Cefamandole	Active against *H. influenzae*	Cost and limited gram-negative spectrum	0.5–2 g q 4–6 hr
Cefonicid	Prolonged half-life allowing once-daily dose	Limited gram-negative spectrum	0.5–2 g q 24 hr
Cefixime	Prolonged half-life allowing once daily dose	Limited gram-negative spectrum	0.5–2 g q 24 hr
Cefoxitin	Active against *B. fragilis* and other anaerobes	Most *Enterobacter* are resistant	1–2 g q 4–6 hr
Cefuroxime	Active against *H. influenzae* and enters CSF	Limited gram-negative spectrum	1.5 g q 6–8 hr
Moxalactam	Very active against *Enterobacteriaceae,* some *Pseudomonas* and anerobes; enters CSF well	Hypoprothrobinemia Increased bleeding time	500 mg–2 g q 1 6–8 hr
Cefotaxime	Very active against *Enterobacteriaceae;* enters CSF well	Limited *Pseudomonas* and anaerobic coverage	500 mg–2 g q 4–6 hr
Cefoperazone	Active against many pseudomonal organisms; Good activity against *Enterobacteriaceae*	Minimal anaerobic activity Hypoprothrombinemia Increased bleeding time Diarrhea	500 g–4 g q 6–12 hr
Ceftizoxime	Very active against *Enterobacteriaceae* Including *Acinetobacter*	Minimal activity against anaerobes and *Pseudomonas*	1–2 g q 8–12 hr
Ceftazidime	Very active against all gram-negative bacteria including *Acinetobacter* and *Pseudomonas*	New; experience limited: some emergence of resistance has been reported	0.5–3 g q 8–12 hr
Ceftriaxone	Prolonged half-life, very active against *Enterobacteriaceae*	New; experience limited: expensive; no *Pseudomonas* or anaerobic activity	1–2 g q 12–24 hr

Another mechanism of resistance is alteration in the cell membrane of the bacteria that then resists drug penetration into the bacterial cell.[32] Transport across the cell membrane is an aerobic process, thus anaerobic bacteria are resistant because they lack the oxygen-dependent active transport system. The third type of resistance is mutation in the ribosomes that cause alteration in the aminoglycoside-binding sites.[31]

Adverse Effects

The aminoglycosides are toxic compounds and can cause serious ototoxicity and nephrotoxicity as well as neuromuscular blockade. Severe, irreversible, and permanent ototoxicity can appear suddenly and without warning in patients taking these compounds.[5] This has most commonly been noted in patients on concurrent loop diuretics and may be related to high serum levels. Vestibular damage is perhaps more common with gentamicin and tobramycin and cochlear damage is more common with amikacin.[14,60,80] Netilmicin may have less ototoxicity, but experience with frequent use of this newest animoglycoside is still rather limited.[52]

In general, renal toxicity occurs late in the course of aminoglycoside therapy and is usually reversible and frequently mild. However in an individual patient it may be early and profound. The damage is primarily to the proximal tubule and a reliably clinically useful prediction of this damage has not been found. However most clinicians follow the creatinine clearance and plasma aminoglycoside levels to ensure that a therapeutic level is maintained and also to avoid levels considered toxic. In general, a plasma level peak of 6 to 10 μg/ml has been found acceptable, with greater toxicity noted at higher levels. A trough level of between 1 and 2 μg/ml is generally desired for both gentamicin and tobramycin. Plasma peak levels of 25 to 30 μg/ml and trough levels of less than 8 μg/ml have generally been used for amikacin.

Apnea due to neuromuscular blockade following peritoneal lavage with large doses of aminoglycosides, as well as following rapid intravenous injection, has been reported.[87] However, these are uncommon reactions and may be reversed with the use of anticholinergic drugs and calcium.[88]

many gram-negative bacilli are resistant to kanamycin and streptomycin, the clinical utility of this drug is limited. Gentamicin, tobramycin, amikacin, and netilmicin are the compounds used in the United States. Unfortunately, most gram-negative organisms resistant to gentamicin will generally be resistant to tobramycin as well, with the exception of some *Pseudomonas* strains.[15] Netilmicin has recently been introduced and though the experience is limited, its spectrum seems to be very similar to gentamicin and tobramycin. Most gram-negative organisms resistant to both gentamicin and tobramycin are generally still sensitive to amikacin and amikacin resistance, even when this agent has been the primary aminoglycoside used, is uncommon.[61] On the other hand, resistance to gentamicin and tobramycin has been a problem in some areas. Frequently, however, this resistance is limited to a particular intensive care unit in the hospital and when it occurs, it is usually in patients who have been in the unit for some time and who have been treated previously with other antibiotics including other aminoglycosides. Most staphylococci are sensitive to the aminoglycosides, particularly gentamicin, although methicillin-resistant staphylococci are frequently resistant to all aminoglycosides.

For gram-negative bacilli, enterococci and staphylococci, the combination of an aminoglycoside and a β-lactam antibiotic is frequently synergistic and leads to very rapid killing of the organisms.[66,78,96] For this reason the majority of aminoglycoside use is frequently in combination with another antibiotic.

Spectrum of Activity

The aminoglycosides have been the mainstay of treatment for serious gram-negative infections for over 20 years. Most aerobic gram-negative rods are quickly killed by these compounds. As mentioned previously, all anaerobic organisms are resistant to aminoglycosides and in fact aminoglycosides are frequently used to isolate anaerobic organisms in culture. The use of aminoglycosides alone is a known predisposing factor to subsequent infection with anaerobic organisms. Because

Aminoglycoside Levels and Dose

While the aminoglycosides have been studied more extensively than any other group of antibiotics, the optimal dosage and blood levels are still very controversial. When the antibiotics are used in severe infections, the pharmacokinetics vary a great deal. In young trauma patients who have been resuscitated with large amounts of intravenous fluids, the volume of distribution of these drugs is very large compared to that in the elderly patient who is admitted to the hospital with a chronic problem. Since the therapeutic to toxic ratio is very narrow, it is prudent to measure blood levels in most patients to confirm that therapeutic levels have been obtained and also to attempt to limit toxic accumulation of these drugs. There are several methods of measuring the levels and each has its advocates and detractors. The therapeutic level necessary and the timing in obtaining these levels is also very controversial. We try to obtain a peak level concentration 30 minutes after estimated full distribution of the drug. Others have advocated obtaining a level 1 hour after a 30-minute infusion. We have found that it is difficult to obtain levels reliably, unless the timing is very closely related to the infusion of the drug, thus we would obtain our trough level just prior to infusion and our peak level just following infusion. We try to achieve a peak level of 6 μg/ml for tobramycin and gentamicin and a trough level of less than 1.5 μg/ml. With amikacin we would use a peak of 25 μg/ml and a trough of less than 8 μg/ml. However, these levels are extremely difficult to achieve in relatively young patients with large volumes of distribution. Dosing nomograms have been devised and seem adequate for stable patients with normal renal function. However, in patients who are critically ill or septic and who have changing renal function we find that only by monitoring blood levels frequently can we have any idea as to whether therapeutic or toxic levels are being achieved.

CLINDAMYCIN

Clindamycin is a lincosamide related to lincomycin, but not to erythromcin. It can be given by all three routes, oral, IV, and intramuscular. It is well absorbed after oral administration and distributes to all tissues except the central nervous system.

Mechanism of Action

Clindamycin binds to 50S ribosomal binding sites and also binds to macrolids and chloramphenicol. This binding inhibits protein synthesis of the cell.

Mechanism of Resistance

In gram-negative organisms there is a failure of clindamycin to enter the cell. In gram-positive organisms that are resistant, there is a mutation in binding sites of the 50S ribosome.

Pharmocokinetics

Clindamycin is rapidly absorbed and has a half life of about 2.4 hours. It is metabolized by the liver to a number of metabolic compounds, some more active than the parent compound. Bioactive metabolites are found in both bile and urine as the drug is excreted. The dose needs to be reduced only in patients with severe concomitant renal and hepatic disease.[55]

Spectrum of Activity

Clindamycin is active against most gram-positive cocci including *Staphylococcus*, *Streptococcus viridans*, *Streptococcus pneumoniae*, and *Streptococcus pyogenes*. Enterococci are uniformly resistant.[77] All gram-negative aerobic bacilli are resistant. Clindamycin is active against over 95 percent of anaerobic organisms including *Bacteroides fragilis*.[105] While most clostridia are sensitive to clindamycin some including *Clostridia welchi* and others that can cause gas gangrene, and *Clostridia difficile*, are resistant.[7]

Adverse Reactions

The most frequent side effect of clindamycin is diarrhea, although in prospective studies the incident of diarrhea has been very variable.[107] Antibiotic-associated colitis originally thought to be due to clindamycin has now been reported with essentially all other antibiotics and appears to be due to toxin production from the overgrowth of *Clostridia difficile.*[6] Other side effects are quite uncommon, with a few patients having transient reversible increases in transaminase and other liver enzymes.[113]

Uses

Clindamycin is predominantly used because of its anaerobic spectrum. Because it does not have activity against aerobic gram-negative rods and because anaerobes are frequently involved in polymicrobial infections, it is usually used in association with another antibiotic, most commonly an aminoglycoside. Recent evidence suggests that it may be the drug of choice for lower respiratory anaerobic infections as well.[72] Because it is well absorbed orally, it may also be used as an alternative agent in penicillin-allergic patients with staphylococcal and streptococcal infections when an oral agent is needed and the organism has been shown to be sensitive to clindamycin.

Dose

The usual dose is 300 to 600 mg every 6 hours or 900 mg every 8 hours.

CHLORAMPHENICOL

Chloramphenicol, one of the first truly wide spectrum antibiotics, was introduced in 1949. Since then this antibiotic has enjoyed a wide popularity for the treatment of numerous infections. A rare but irreversible aplastic anemia has limited its use; as a result it is often an available choice for some life-threatening infections by organisms resistant to more commonly used agents.

Mechanism of Action

Chloramphenicol inhibits protein synthesis by binding to the 50S ribosomal subunit of the bacterial cell.

Mechanism of Resistance

Most resistance is due to R factor-mediated enzymatic acetylation that inactivates the compound. Another mechanism of resistance is by permeability block of the bacteria to entry of the cell. This is particularly common among *Pseudomonas* species.

Pharmacokinetics

Chloramphenicol is reliably absorbed even in severely ill patients and it has been used orally in critically ill patients. It is not absorbed as an intramuscular preparation, but can be given intravenously. It is metabolized by the liver by glucuronide conjugation and about 10 percent of biologically active compound is excreted in the urine.

Adverse Reactions

The major side effects of chloramphenicol are hematologic reactions. There are two major types. The first is reversible bone marrow depression due to the direct pharmacologic effect of the antibiotic on the inhibition of mitochondrial synthesis. This is dose-dependent and reversible with cessation of the drug. The second type is an "idiosyncratic" irreversible aplastic anemia unrelated to dose and is generally fatal. It can occur after either oral or parenteral administration. It is estimated to occur in approximately 1:25,000 to 40,000 patients who receive the drug.[111] Another toxic manifestation of chloramphenicol is the gray syndrome, seen only in neonates because of their incapacity to detoxify chloramphenicol. This results in abdominal distention, vomiting, circulatory collapse, cyanosis, and death.[17,28] Because of this syndrome chloramphenicol should be avoided in neonates and the dose reduced to 25 mg/kg; frequent monitoring of antibiotic levels is necessary. Optic neuritis is another complication described in patients receiving prolonged chloramphenicol.[35] This is usually reversible, but has resulted in blindness. Chloramphenicol can also result in the inhibition of hepatic metabolism of drugs, particularly sodium warfarin and phenytoin.[27] The dose of these drugs must be reduced during chloramphenicol therapy.

Uses

Chloramphenicol has been used in a variety of situations. Since it is active against all rickettsial organisms it is the therapy of choice in many of these diseases, particularly if tetracycline cannot be used. In addition, chloramphenicol along with penicillin is considered the treatment of choice for brain abscesses and chloramphenicol alone can be used in the severely penicillin-allergic patient with bacterial meningitis, particularly when caused by *Hemophilus, Pneumococcus,* and *Neisseria meningitidis.* It has also been used in meningitis caused by aerobic gram-negative rods, usually, however, in combination with other antibiotics. It is the drug of choice for *Salmonella* infections, particularly typhoid fever.[103] Since the drug is so well absorbed it can frequently be given orally even for serious infections, particularly in situations where intravenous therapy may not be feasible.

Dose

The usual dose is 500 mg to 2 g every 8 hours. The usual maintenance dose is 3 to 4 g per day. Careful monitoring of complete blood count is necessary.

METRONIDAZOLE

While metronidazole has been available for some time and has been used for parasitic infections, particularly trichomoniasis and giardiasis, only recently has it enjoyed increase use as an antianaerobic agent. It is used as an oral as well as a parenteral drug.

Mechanism of Action

Metronidazole enters the bacterial cells well and then undergoes reduction of the nitrogroup, leading to toxic compounds that bind to bacterial DNA and inhibit cell synthesis.

Pharmacokinetics

Therapeutic concentrations of metronidazole can be reached when it is administrered either by the parenteral or oral route. Metronidazole enters all tissues in concentrations similar to that obtained in the serum and therapeutic concentrations can easily be achieved. Eighty-five percent of metronidazole is metabolized by the liver and the remainder is excreted in the urine.[59,92] It is completely removed by dialysis.[42] In severe renal failure dose adjustments are not necessary; however, a reduction in dose is necessary in severe hepatic impairment.

Adverse Effects

Anorexia, nausea, vomiting, and a metallic taste occasionally occur during metronidazole therapy.[22] Convulsions, encephalopathy, and polyneuropathy have occurred and are usually reversible in patients receiving high-dose metronidazole therapy.[69] A disulfiram-like relation has been noted in some patients taking alcohol; patients should be warned about this possiblity.[71] Experimental studies in animals have suggested that metronidazole may be both carcinogenic and mutagenic, however, there are no data to show that this occurs in humans.[13,95] Since metronidazole enters the placenta it is probably prudent to avoid its use during early stages of pregnancy, if possible.

Spectrum of Activity

Almost all gram-negative anaerobic bacilli and anaerobic cocci are sensitive to metronidazole.[26,76,106] Most clostridia are also sensitive to this compound.[26,34] But anaerobic non-spore forming gram-positive bacilli such as *Propionobacterium* spp., eubacteria and *Bifiodobacterium* are relatively resistant.[26,36] While metronidazole has been shown to be active against some aerobic gram-negative rods under experimental conditions, under normal clinical circumstances these organisms are resistant. Metronidazole has been used to treat anaerobic infections. It is the only antibiotic that is consistently bactericidal against *Bacteroides fragilis.*[91] It can be used in combination with other antibiotics aimed at aerobic gram-negative rods to cover the mixture of organisms frequently present in anaerobic infections. Since it enters the central nervous sytem and brain well it is useful in the treatment of brain abscesses caused by susceptible organisms.[44,58] *Clostridia difficile* is almost uniformly sensitive to metronidazole, which can be used to treat antibiotic-associated colitis.

Dose

The usual dose of 500 mg to 1 g as a loading dose, followed by 500 mg every 6 hours in either intravenous or oral preparation. The dose should be reduced in patients with severe hepatic disease.

TRIMETHOPRIM–SULFAMETHOXAZOLE

Trimethoprim–sulfamethoxazole is a fixed combination of the diaminopyrimidine trimethoprim and the sulfonamide sulfamethoxazole in a five to one ratio; 80 mg trimethoprim to 400 mg sulfmethoxazole.

Mechanism of Action

Trimethoprim–sulfamethoxazole inhibits sequential steps in the synthesis of folic acid of bacterial cells. Since mammalian cells do not produce folic acid, the sulfamethoxazole-induced inhibition does not take place in humans. In addition, trimethoprim has an affinity for bacterial folate reductase that is at least 10,000 times greater than that of the human cells.[62]

Mechanism of Resistance

Resistance has been described due to plasmid-mediated mechanisms leading to production of enzymes that reduce the affinity for these drugs and to strains that do not utilize the tetrahydrofolic pathway.[86]

Pharmacokinetics

Trimethoprim–sulfamethoxazole is well absorbed from the upper gastrointestinal tract and both compounds can be therapeutic in essentially all tissues including CNS, prostate, and the aqueous humor of the eye. Fifty percent of trimethoprim and 30 percent of sulfamethoxazole is excreted in the urine unchanged. The remainder is metabolized. Excretion is by both glomerular filtration and tubular secretion. The dose must be decreased in patients with renal impairment. In severe renal disease with a serum creatinine clearance of less than 15 ml/min, the use of trimethoprim–sulfamethoxazole should be avoided unless drug levels can be carefully monitored. Dialysis removes both compounds.

Adverse Reactions

A variety of side effects have been attributed to this drug, although, considering the wide spread use of this combination agent, most are uncommon and usually mild. Mild nausea, vomiting, and diarrhea may occur. Allergic manifestations from rash and serum sickness to an exfoliated dermatitis and Stevens-Johnson syndrome may also occur uncommonly.[41] Hematologic effects such as leukopenia, aplasia, and thrombocytopenia have been associated with the sulfonamides.[41] Hepatic necrosis and cholectasis are uncommon reactions reported.[41] There is significant interaction between trimethoprim–sulfamethoxazole and warfarin hypoglycemic compounds and phenytoin, which may produce prolongation of prothrombin time.[50]

Spectrum of Activity

Trimethoprim–sulfamethoxazole was first introduced as an oral agent and has achieved considerable utility in the management of a variety of urinary infections. The broad spectrum of activity that includes most gram-positive organisms, as well as most gram-negative enterobacteriaceae, has lead to increased use in a variety of serious infections. Of the commonly acquired hospital organisms *Pseudomonas aeruginosa* is consistently resistant.[45] Most *Klebsiella, Enterobacter, Serratia,* even *Acinetobacter* may be found to be sensitive in particular hospital situations.[45] Of particular note is that many *Klebsiella, Enterobacter* and *Serratia* resistant to many other compounds are frequently sensitive to trimethoprim–sulfamethoxazole. In addition, staphylococci including methicillin-resistant staphylococci are frequently sensitive to this compound, although clinical evidence of its efficacy are not yet available. Opportunistic organisms including *Nocardia* and *Pneumocystis carinii* have been treated with this compound.[57,63,70,75]

Dose

In serious infections a dose of 10 to 20 μg trimethoprim per 24 hours is given in four divided doses. Considerably lower doses (in the range of 5 μg/kg per 24 hours) are used in less severe infections, particularly those of the urinary tract.

VANCOMYCIN

Vancomycin is a complex glycopolypeptide and is not related to any other antibiotic. It is not absorbed by the oral route and is quite painful when given by intramuscular IM injection, therefore, it is usually given by the intravenous route. It is eliminated by the kidneys and dose adjustment must be made in patients with renal failure. It is not removed by either hemo- or peritoneal dialysis and in anuric patients its half-life is 9 to 10 days making it an ideal drug for susceptible organisms in renal dialysis patients, since it can be given every 10 days.[73]

Mechanism of Action

Vancomycin inhibits production of cell wall polymers and can also cause alteration in protoplasts cytoplasmic membranes.[85]

Mechanism of Resistance

Resistance is rare, if it occurs, and its mechanism has not yet been defined.

Adverse Reactions

When first introduced, vancomycin was not as purified as the current preparation and many more side effects were attributed to this drug than seem to occur today. The most frequent side effects are fever, chills, phlebitis, rash, and even hypotension when the drug is injected too rapidly, therefore, slow 30 to 40 minute infusions should be employed to limit this pseudoanaphylactic-type reaction.[81] With prolonged high levels, ototoxicity is the most serious adverse reaction, but is infrequent if levels are maintained at a peak below 30 μg/ml. Tinnitus and high tone hearing loss may be a sign of impending deafness. Hearing loss unlike that secondary to the aminoglycosides is sometimes reversible with vancomycin.

Nephrotoxicity seems to be much less common than originally found but it may be potentiated by concomitant use of other nephrotoxic antibiotics, particularly the aminoglycosides.

Uses

Vancomycin is most commonly used for serious infections caused by all *Streptococcus* species including *Enterococcus* and all *Staphy-lococcus* strains including methicillin-resistant staphylococci. It is the drug of choice for these infections in the penicillin-allergic patient. While its penetration into the central nervous system is poor in the uninflamed meninges, it has been useful in the treatment of staphylococcal meningitis in penicillin-allergic patients. Because it is not appreciably absorbed from the gastrointestinal tract, oral vancomycin has been used to treat antibiotic-associated colitis secondary to *Clostridia difficile,* which is quite sensitive to this drug. Many other gram-positive organisms are sensitive to this unique compound and it should be considered when a gram-positive organism is identified as the cause of infection. All gram-negative organisms are resistant to vancomycin.

Dose

The usual dose in an adult with normal renal function is 2 g a day given in four divided doses. This must be reduced for patients with decreased renal function; one should try to maintain peak serum levels below 30 μg/ml.

TREATING THE UNKNOWN ORGANISM AT THE UNKNOWN SITE

While it is certainly desirable to identify either an organism or a site of infection prior to beginning antibiotic therapy frequently one is faced with the problem of the infected patient with no obvious source or organism. A careful history and physical examination must be performed looking for clues to the possible site or organism. However, there are usually four basic questions that one must ask to select the most appropriate antibiotic: Can we exclude gram-positive organisms? Can anaerobic organisms be excluded? Can *Pseudomonas* be excluded? Can multiply drug-resistant gram negative rods be excluded?

Can We Exclude Gram-Positive Organisms?

Clearly *Staphylococcus* and *Pneumococcus* are common organisms causing nosocomial infections in a variety of sites and it is often difficult to exclude these organisms as possible pathogens. If we cannot exclude gram-positive organisms, which is by far the most frequent case, then in selecting empiric antibiotic coverage we must also consider these organisms in the antibiotic selection. This will usually entail use of a β-lactam antibiotic, usually a cephalosporin or a semisynthetic antistaphylococcal penicillin such as nafcillin.

Can We Exclude Anaerobic Organisms?

This question is somewhat easier to answer than the first question. Factors suggesting that anaerobes may be involved in the infection include: (1) infections with foul-smelling discharge; (2) infections near mucous membranes; (3) infections occurring after or during aminoglycoside use; (4) presence of necrotic tissue; (5) presence of gas in tissues; and (6) presence of pleomorphic organisms on Gram's stain, especially both gram-negative and gram-positive organisms. The history will usually reveal violation of a mucous membrane or that the patient has been previously on other antibiotics, particularly aminoglycosides, which lead to an increased possibility of an anaerobic infection. If there is any possiblity that the abdomen is the site of infection, anaerobes should be considered and appropriate antibiotics selected that have activity against these organisms. However, if there has not been any violation of the mucous membranes anaerobes would be very unlikely as a cause of an acute infectious process, unless one is suspecting a hollow viscus injury, which can be usually ascertained through the history and physical examination.

Can We Exclude *Pseudomonas?*

Since this particular organism seems to be the most difficult organism to tailor antibiotics for, and most antibiotics, particularly the cephalosporins, have minimal activity against *Pseudomonas aeruginosa,* this becomes a very pertinent question in modern therapy. Usually *Pseudomonas* is an uncommon organism in community-acquired infections no matter what the source or even in infections early in the hospital stay. However burn patients, patients with chronic catheters, patients who have been on previous antibiotics, and patients who have been in the intensive care unit for at least a week have a high probability of having *Pseudomonas* involved in their potential infection and this organism should be considered in antibiotic selection. This would necessitate specific antibiotics aimed at this particulr organism, usually an aminoglycoside and an extended-spectrum penicillin.

Can Multiply Drug-Resistant Gram-Negative Rods be Excluded?

Usually previous cultures from the patient or other patients in the unit would lead one to suspect this possibility. Therefore it is important to know the ecology of the particular unit in which the patient is being cared for and whether resistant organisms are prevalent in the environment. If this is the case, specific antibiotics must be used, again based on previous experience in the particular unit. Usually amikacin is the aminoglycoside selected in this case since it has the least organisms resistant to it, and extended-spectrum penicillins or cephalosporins may be used. Other drugs that may be useful are trimethoprim–sulfamethoxazole, particularly for some resistant *Enterobacteriaceae.* For gram-positive organisms the most troublesome organism currently seems to be methicillin-resistant *Staphylococcus;* vancomycin is the only antibiotic consistently effective against this particular organism. Figure

16-1 shows a flow diagram for selecting antibiotics without a source or known organism.

Obviously other questions are asked by the physician about to embark on empiric therapy but because of the nature of the antibiotics available and their spectrum and the organisms one is most concerned about, these are the main questions that have to be answered to allow one to pick an appropriate empiric antibiotic regimen. Once the regimen is chosen, as the culture results become known and as diagnostic studies become available the antibiotics should be tailored to cover the most likely organism present at the suspected site or the organism identified by the particular cultures or Gram's stains obtained.

If one cannot rule out anaerobes as a possible cause of the infection, antibiotic combinations such as clindamycin and an aminoglycoside or cefoxitin and an aminoglycoside are usually chosen to cover gram-positive aerobic organisms, anaerobic organisms, and gram-negative organisms. If one believes that the source is in the abdomen, gram-positive aerobic organisms such as *Staphylococcus* and *Pneumococcus* would be very unlikely and metronidazole and an aminoglycoside would be equally efficacious. When one cannot exclude *Pseudomonas* or anaerobes, an extended spectrum penicillin such as mezlocillin and an aminoglycoside provide coverage for this particular organism, as well as anaerobes and other gram-negative rods. If we can exclude anaerobes but need to cover for *Pseudomonas,* the newer cephalosporins do have some activity against *Pseudomonas*, particularly drugs such as ceftazidime, and can be used in this situation. However drugs such as ticarcillin, mezlocillin, or piperacillin plus an aminoglycoside are probably the best combination of therapy available for *Pseudomonas* infections at most sites and should be used for identified *Pseudomonas* infections. If *Pseudomonas* can be excluded and anaerobes can be excluded, empiric therapy with a cephalosporin and an aminoglycoside or even a third-generation cephalosporin alone has been found to be very efficacious in treating these infections.[101]

Again, one must remember that the toxicity of aminoglycosides occurs after multiple doses over a prolonged period of time and it is extremely uncommon for the first 24 or 48 hours of an aminoglycoside to cause any substantial problems. Initial therapy with these drugs therefore has minimal toxicity and maximal spectrum for the patient. Once the organism is identified, the aminoglycoside can be discontinued if other drugs are shown to be effective. If, after an extensive work-up, the patient is put on empiric antibiotics and all the cultures remain negative after 5 days and there is no therapeutic response, antibiotics should be stopped and the patient reevaluated. On the other hand, if the patient clearly has a dramatic response even though the cultures have not become positive, antibiotics should be continued for a therapeutic course of 7 to 10 days. If after initial empiric therapy is instituted the patient continues downhill and after careful reevaluation no site nor organisms can be found, serious consideration must be given to the addition of broader-spectrum therapy to cover fungi and more fastidious organisms such as *Legionella* or *Mycobacterium,* depending upon the clinical situation. This is particularly true in the granulocytopenic patient. In these patients it is frequently difficult to delineate the source of the infection early enough because these patients do not have the classic signs of inflammation during severe infection. Usually when these signs are present the infection is out of control. Therefore, these patients are frequently given empiric antibiotics. If they do not respond promptly, therapy is expanded to include therapy aimed at fungi and other organisms such as mycobacteria, *Legionella, Pneumocystis,* and others, depending on the underlying disease.

TREATING THE KNOWN ORGANISM AND UNKNOWN SITE

A common finding in treating critically ill patients is that the laboratory will report a positive culture in the blood, such as gram-positive coccus, but the physician will not be able to delineate the particular site. Antibiotic therapy in these patients is usually quite simple anad

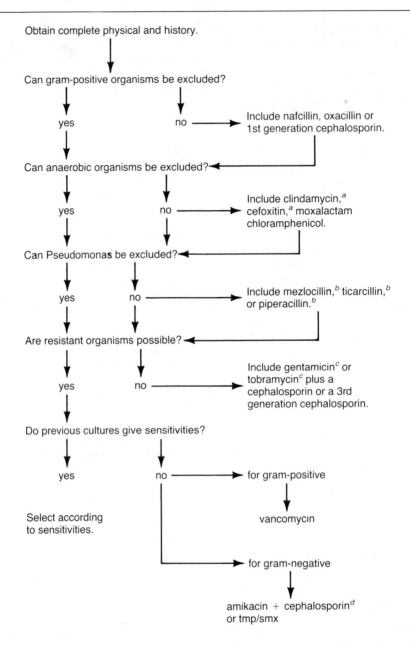

Obtain complete physical and history.

Can gram-positive organisms be excluded?

yes   no ──────► Include nafcillin, oxacillin or
                  1st generation cephalosporin.

Can anaerobic organisms be excluded?

yes   no ──────► Include clindamycin,[a]
                  cefoxitin,[a] moxalactam
                  chloramphenicol.

Can Pseudomonas be excluded?

yes   no ──────► Include mezlocillin,[b] ticarcillin,[b]
                  or piperacillin.[b]

Are resistant organisms possible?

yes   no ──────► Include gentamicin[c] or
                  tobramycin[c] plus a
                  cephalosporin or a 3rd
                  generation cephalosporin.

Do previous cultures give sensitivities?

yes   no ──────► for gram-positive
                         vancomycin
Select according
to sensitivities.
                  ──────► for gram-negative
                         amikacin + cephalosporin[d]
                         or tmp/smx

a, Select these if gram-positive cannot be excluded.
b, Drug has sufficient anaerobic activity to be used for anaerobes if they are still being considered in
   addition to *Pseudomonas*.
c, Select if *Pseudomonas* still in consideration.
d, Can omit if extended-spectrum penicillin included because of *Pseudomonas* consideration.

FIG. 16-1 Flow diagram for empiric antibiotic selection.

straightforward: if a gram-positive coccus is identified, treatment is begun for both *Staphylococcus* and *Streptococcus*. However, the real dilemma is the recent introduction of methicillin-resistant staphylococci as major pathogens. Prior to this organism becoming a notable pathogen, the use of a semisynthetic penicillin or a cephalosporin would cover gram-positive cocci in sufficient concentrations in all body sites. If, however, there are methicillin-resistant staphylococci in the community, empiric vancomycin therapy may be necessary until the sensitivity of the organism is known. Careful physical examination may reveal the site of infection. However, identification of the particular organism may help direct attention to the possible areas for the infection. Table 16-13 lists the most likely sites for some commonly encountered organisms in the intensive care unit. However, *Enterococcus* will not be adequately treated by the vancomycin therapy and will require penicillin, a substituted penicillin (mezlocillin), or cefoxitin and an aminoglycoside, if it is thought to be a serious pathogen.

If the laboratory reports a gram-negative rod from blood culture, it is important to determine if this organism is growing both in the aerobic and anaerobic bottles, or if it is growing in just the aerobic or the anaerobic bottle. Clearly, if it is growing in an anaerobic bottle alone, it is probably an anaerobic organism and one must institute antibiotics aimed particularly at anaerobic organisms. If, on the other hand, it is growing only in the aerobic bottle, or in both the aerobic and anaerobic bottles,

then, in all likelihood it is not an anaerobic organism and is probably aerobic. Antibiotics can be chosen that are used to treat aerobic gram-negative rods. *Pseudomonas* is a strict aerobic organism and will grow only in a properly inoculated aerobic bottle. Therefore, if the organism is growing in the aerobic and the anaerobic bottles and the jars have been inoculated properly, one can with some assuredness dismiss *Pseudomonas* as a possibility. Age of the patient, underlying renal disease, and length of stay in the intensive care unit all must be taken into consideration when selecting empiric therapy. In our unit, for example, organisms tht are gentamicin-resistant always occur after more than 2 weeks' stay in the intensive care unit. If an aminoglycoside is required to treat a patient during the first 2 weeks in the intensive care unit, gentamicin would be the most appropriate. However, since there is an increased chance of the organism being resistant to gentamicin if the patent has been in the unit for greater than 2 weeks, amikacin is the empiric aminoglycoside pending identification of the organism and its sensitivities. Once the organism is identified, antibiotics can be further tailored to provide the most inexpensive and most effective antibiotics for the individual patient.

TREATING THE KNOWN SITE AND UNKNOWN ORGANISM

In situations where the site of infection is identified because of the clinical characteristics, then the ecology of the particular infection as well as the anticipated organisms are relied upon in instituting antibiotic therapy. Table 16-14 reveals the most likely organisms at a particular site. In general, however this must be taken in the context of the type of unit under consideration, the type of patient, and the previous exposure to antibiotics of the particular patient. For example, a patient who develops a nosocomial pneumonia after being treated for a previous nosocomial infection may very

TABLE 16-13. Most Likely Sites to be Infected by Specific Organisms

Organism	Site
Staphylococcus aureus	Vascular lines
	Lungs
Staphylococcus epidermidis	Vascular lines
Escherichia coli	Urine
	Abdomen
Klebsiella	Vascular lines
	Lung
Enterobacter	Vascular lines
	Lungs
Serratia marcescens	Lungs
	Vascular lines
Pseudomonas aeruginosa	Lungs
	Urine
Anaerobes	Mucous membrane lesions

TABLE 16-14. Most Likely Organisms to Cause Infection According to Site

Site	Most Likely Organism
Primary bacteremia	*Staphylococcus aureus*
Vascular system	
Arterial	*Staphylococcus aureus*
Phlebitis	*Klebsiella*
Sinusitis	Various gram-negative rods
Lower respiratory system	
Pneumonia	*Staphylococcus aureus*
Empyema	*Pneumococcus, Klebsiella*
	Pseudomonas aeruginosa
Urinary tract	*E. coli*
Intra-abdominal infection	*E. coli,* anaerobes
Surgical wound	*Staphylococcus aureus*

well have an unusual organism and in this case the ecology is not helpful in delineating the organism that may be causing the infection.

REFERENCES

1. Ad Hoc Committee of the committee on Trauma, Division of Medical Sciences, National Academy of Sciences-National Research Council: Postoperative wound infections: the influence of ultraviolet irradiation of the operating room and various other factors. Ann Surg 160 (Suppl.) 1, 1964
2. Alexander JW: Nosocomial infections in current problems. Surgery 10: 1, 1973
3. Andrassy K, Koderisch J, Fritz S, Ritz E: New beta-lactam antibiotics and hemorrhagic diathesis: comparison of moxalactam and cefotaxime. Clin Ther 6 (1): 34, 1983
4. Appel GB, Neu HC: The nephrotoxicity of antimicrobial agents. N Eng J Med 296: 663, 1977
5. Appel GB, Neu HC: Gentamicin in 1978. Ann Intern Med 89: 528, 1978
6. Bartlett JG: Antibiotic-associated pseudomembranous colitis. Rev Infect Dis 1: 530, 1979
7. Bartlett JG, Chang TW, Gurwith M, et al: Antibiotic-associated pseudomembranous colitis due to toxic-producing clostridia. N Eng J Med 298: 531, 1978
8. Barza M: The nephrotoxicity of cephalosporins: an overview. J Infect Dis 137 (Supp): S60, 1978
9. Benewshe R, Davies J: Structure activity relationships among the aminoglycoside antibiotics: role of hydoxyl and amino groups. Antimicrob Agents Chemother 4: 402, 1973
10. Benveniste R, Davies J: Mechanisms of antibiotic resistance in bacteria. Annu Rev Biochem 42: 471, 1973
11. Bisno AL: Hyposplenism and overwhelming pneumococcal infection: a reappraisal. Am J Med Sci 262: 101, 1971
12. Blumberg PM, Strominger JL: Interaction of penicillin with the bacterial cell: penicillin binding proteins and penicillin sensitive enzymes. Bacteriol Rev 38: 291, 1974
13. Bost RG: Metronidazole: mammalian mutagenicity. p. 126. In Finegold SM (ed): Metronidazole. Proceedings of the International Metronidazole Conference. Excerpta Medica, Amsterdam, 1977
14. Boston Collaborative Drug Surveillance Program: Drug-induced deafness. A cooperative study. JAMA 224: 515, 1973
15. Brogden RN, Pender RM, Sawyer PR et al: Tobramycin: a review of antibacterial and pharmacokinetic properties and therapeutic use. Drugs 12: 166, 1976
16. Brown CH, III, Natelson EA, Bradshaw MW, et al: Study of the effects of ticarcillin on blood coagulation and platelet function. Antimicrob Agents Chemother 7: 652, 1975
17. Burns LE, Hodgman JE, Cass AB: Fatal circulatory collapse in premature infants receiving chloramphenical. N Eng J Med 261: 1318, 1959
18. Cabizuca SV, and Dresser KG: Carbenicillin associated hypokalemia. JAMA 236: 956, 1976
19. Caplan ES, Hoyt NJ: Infection surveillance and control in the severely traumatized patient. Am J Med 70: 638, 1981
20. Caplan ES, Hoyt NJ: Nosocomial sinusitis. JAMA 247: 639, 1982
21. Catanzaro FJ, Stetson CA, Morris AJ, et al: The role of the streptococcus in the pathogenesis of rheumatic fever. Am J Med 17: 749, 1954
22. Catteral RD: Fifteen years experience with metronidazole. p. 107. In Finegold SM (ed): Metronidazole: Proceedings of the International Metronidazole Conference. Excerpta Medica, Amsterdam, 1977
23. Centers for Disease Control: National Nosocomial Infections Study, Fourth Quarter 1973. April, 1974, p. 24
24. Centers for Disease Control, National Nosocomial Infection Study Report, 1977 (6 Month Summaries). November, 1979
25. Chodak GW, Plaut ME: Use of systemic antibiotics for prophylaxis in surgery. Arch Surg 112: 326, 1977
26. Chow AW, Bendnorz D, Guze LB: Susceptibility

of obligate anaerobes to metronidazole: an extended study of 1,054 clinical isolates. p. 286. In Finegold SM (ed): Metronidazole. Proceedings of the International Metronidazole Conference. Excerpta Medica, Amsterdam, 1977

27. Christensen LK, Stovsted L: Inhibition of drug metabolism by chloramphenicol. Lancet 2:1397, 1969

28. Craft AW, Brocklebank JT, Hey EN, et al: The "grey toddler": chloramphenicol toxicity. Arch Dis Child 49: 235, 1974

29. Cruse PJE, Foord R: A five-year prospective study of 23,649 surgical wounds. Arch Surg 107: 206, 1973

30. Curreri WP, Luterman A, Braun DW, Shires GT: Burn injury analysis of survival and hospitalization time for 937 patients. Ann Surg 192: 472, 1980

31. Davies J: Bacterial resistance to aminoglycoside antibiotics. J Infect Dis 124: S7, 1971

32. Davies J, Curvalin P: Mechanisms of resistance to aminoglycosides. Am J Med, 62: 868, 1977

33. Dismukes WD: Oaxacillin-induced hepatic dysfunction. JAMA 226: 861, 1973

34. Dornbusch K, Nord CE, Dahlback A: Antibiotic susceptibility of Clostridium species isolated from human infections. Scand J Infect Dis 7: 127, 1975

35. Editorial: Chloramphenicol blindness. Br Med J 1: 1511, 1965

36. Eykyn SJ, Philips L: Intravenous metronidazole in the treatment of anaerobic sepsis. p. 393. In Finegold SM (ed): Metronidazole. Proceedings of the International Metronidazole Conference. Excerpta Medica, Amsterdam, 1977

37. Eliopoulos GM, Moellering RC, Jr.: Azlocillin, mezlocillin, and piperacillin: new broad spectrum penicillins. Ann Intern Med 97: 755, 1982

38. EORTC, International Antimicrobial Therapy Project Group: Three antibiotic regimens in the treatment of infection in the febrile granulocytopenic patient with cancer. J Infect Dis 137: 14, 1978

39. Farrar WE, Jr., Kruse JM: Relationship between B-lactamase activity and resistance of Enterobacter to cephalothin. Infect Immun 2: 610, 1970

40. Fekety FR, Jr., McDaniel E: The fever index—an evaluation of the course of infectious diseases, with special reference to pneumococcal pneumonia. Yale J Biol Med 41: 282, 1968

41. Frisch JM: Clinical experience with adverse reactions to TMP/SMX. J Infect Dis 128: 607, 1973

42. Gabriel R, Page CM, Weller IVD, et al: The pharmacokinetics of metronidazole in patients with chronic renal failure. p. 105. In Phillips I, Collier J (eds): Metronidazole. Royal Society of Medicine, and Academic Press, London, 1979

43. Gentry LO, Jemsek JG, Natelson EA: Effects of sodium piperacillin on platelet function in normal volunteers. Antimicrob Agents Chemother 19: 532, 1981

44. George RH, Bint AJ: Treatment of a brain abscess due to Bacteroides fragilis with metronidazole. J Antimicrob Chemother 2: 101, 1976

45. Gleckman R, Alvarez S, Joubert DW: Drug therapy reviews: trimethoprim-sulfamethoxazole. Am J Hosp Pharm 36: 893, 1979

46. Gomes JAC, Calderon J, Lajam F, et al: Echocardiographic detection of fungal vegetations in Candida parapsiolosis endocarditis. Am J Med 61: 273, 1976

47. Gorbach SL: Treatment of intraabdominal sepsis. Management of anaerobic infections. Ann Intern Med 83: 377, 1975

48. Gottlieb S, Khuddus S, Balooki H, et al: Echocardiographic diagnosis of aortic valve vegetations in Candida endocarditis. Circulation 50: 296(A), 1974

49. Gralnick HR, McGinnis M, Halterman R: Thrombocytopenia with sodium cephalothin therapy. Ann Intern Med 77: 401, 1972

50. Griffin JP, D'Arcy PF: A Manual of Adverse Drug Interactions. John Wright and Sons, Bristol, 1975

51. Griffiths D, Simpson R, Shorey B, et al: Single-dose preoperative antibiotic prophylaxis in gastrointestinal surgery. Lancet 2: 325, 1976

52. Guay DRP: Netilmicin. Drug Intell Clin Pharm 17: 83, 1983

53. Hart GB, O'Reilly RR, Cave RH, Broussard ND: The treatment of clostridial myonecrosis with hyperbaric oxygen. J Trauma 14 (8): 712, 1974

54. Hartman B, Tomasz A: Altered penicillin-binding proteins in methicillin-resistant strains of staphylococcus aureus. Antimicrob Agents Chemother 19: 726, 1981

55. Hinthorn DR, Baker LH, Romig DA et al: Use of clindamycin in patients with liver disease. Antimicrob Agents Chemother 9: 498, 1976

56. Hirschmann JV, Inui TS: Antimicrobial prophylaxis: a critique of recent trials. Rev Infect Dis 2 (1): 1, 1980

57. Hughes WT, Feldman S Sanyal SK: Treatment of Pneumocystis carinii pneumonia with trimethoprim-sulfamethoxazole. Can Med Assoc J 112 (Suppl.): 47, 1975

58. Ingham HR, Selkon JB, Robxy CM: Bacteriological study of otogenic cerebral abscesses: chemotherapeutic role of metronidazole. Br Med J 2: 991, 1977

59. Ings RMJ, Law GL, Parnell EW: The metabolism of metronidazole. Biochem Pharmacol 15: 515, 1966

60. Jane AZ, Wright GE, Blair DC: Ototoxicity and

nephrotoxicity of amikacin. Am J Med 62: 911, 1977

61. Jauregul L, Cushing RD, Lerner AM: Gentamicin/amikacin resistant gram-negative bacilli at Detroit General Hospital, 1975–1976. Am J Med 62: 882, 1977

62. Kahn SB, Fein SA, Brodsky L: Effects of trimethoprim on folate metabolism in man. Clin Pharmacol Ther 9: 550, 1968

63. Katz P, Fauci AS: Nocardia asteroides sinusitis: presentation as a trimethoprim-sulfmethoxazole responsive fever of unknown origin. JAMA 238: 2397, 1977

64. Klastersky J, Cappel R, Noterman J et al: Endotracheal gentamicin for the prevention of bronchial infections in patients with tracheostomies. Int J Clin Pharmacol Biopharmacol 74: 279, 1973

65. Kluge RM, Calia FM, McLaughlin JS: Serum antibiotic concentrations pre and post-cardiopulmonary bypass. Antimicrob Agents Chemother 4: 270, 1973

66. Kluge RM, Standiford HC, Tatem B et al: Carbenicillin-gentamicin combination against Pseudomonas aeruginosa. Ann Intern Med 81: 584, 1974

67. Kluge RM, Standiford HC, Tatem B, et al: Comparative activity of tobramycin, amikacin, gentamicin alone and with carbenicillin against *Pseudomonas aeruginosa.* Antimicrob Agents Chemother 6: 422, 1974

68. Krogstad DJ, Moellering RC., Jr: Combinations of antimicrobial agents: Mechanisms of interaction against bacteria. In Lorian V (ed): Antibiotics in Laboratory Medicine. Williams & Wilkins, Baltimore, 1980

69. Kusumi RK, Plouffe JF, Wyatt RH, et al: Central nervous system toxicity associated with metronidazole therapy. Ann Intern Med 93: 59, 1980

70. Larter WE, John TJ, Sieber OF, et al: Trimethoprim-sulfamethoxazole treatment of Pneumocystis carinii pneumonitis. J Pediatr 92: 826, 1978

71. Lehman HE, Ban TA: Chemical reduction of compulsion to drink with metronidazole. New treatment modality in therapeutic program of alcoholic. Curr Ther Res 9: 419, 1967

72. Levinson ME, Mangura CT, Lorber B, et al: Clindamycin compared with penicillin for the treatment of anaerobic lung abscesses. Ann Intern Med 98 (4): 466, 1983

73. Lindholm DD, Murray JS: Persistence of vancomycin in the blood during renal failure and its treatment by hemodialysis. N Eng J Med 274: 1047, 1966

74. Lkhite VV: Immunological impairment and susceptiblity to infection after splenectomy. JAMA 236: 1376, 1976

75. Marcovitch H, Norman AP: Treatment of nocardiosis. Lancet 2: 362, 1970

76. Marrie TJ, Haldane EV, Swantee CA, et al: Susceptibility of anaerobic bacteria to nine antimicrobial agents and demonstration of decreased susceptibility of Clostridium perfringens to penicillin. Antimicrob Agents Chemother 19: 51, 1981

77. McGehee RF, Jr., Smith CB, Wilcox C, et al: Comparative studies of antibacterial activity in vitro and absorption and excretion lincomycin and clindamycin. Am J Med Sci 256: 279, 1968

78. Moellering RC, Jr., Wennersten C, Weinberg AN: Antibiotic synergism against enterococci. J Lab Clin Med 77: 821, 1971

79. Mulholland SG, Dieraufla J, Bruun JN, Blakemore WS: Analysis and significance of nosocomial infection rates. Ann Surg 188: 27, 1974

80. Neu HC, Bendush CL: Ototoxicity of tobramycin: a clinical overview. J Infect Dis (suppl) 1975

81. Newfield P, Roizen MF: Hazards of rapid administration of vancomycin. Ann Intern Med 91: 581, 1979

82. Nichols RL, Smith JW, Klein DB, et al: Risk of infection after penetrating abdominal trauma. N Engl J Med 311 (17): 1065, 1984

83. Parry MF, Neu HC: A comparative study of ticarcillin plus tobramycin versus carbenicillin plus gentamicin for the treatment of serious infections due to gram-negative bacilli. Am J Med 64: 961, 1978

84. Peacock JE, Jr., Moorman DR, Wenzel RP, Mandell GL: Methicillin-resistant Staphylococcus aureus: microbiologic characteristics, antimicrobial susceptibilities, and assessment of virulence of an epidemic strain. J Infect Dis 144 (6): 165, 1981

85. Perkins HR, Nieto M: the chemical basis for the action of the vancomycin group of antibiotics. Ann NY Acad Sci 235: 348, 1974

86. Pinney RJ, Smith T: Joint trimethoprim sulphamethoxazole resistance in bacteria infected with R factors. J Med Microbiol 6: 13, 1973

87. Pittinger CB, Eryasa Y, Adamson R et al: Antibiotic-induced paralysis. Anesth Analg. (Cleve) 49: 487, 1970.

88. Pittinger C, Adamson R: Antibiotic blockade of neuromuscular function. Annu Rev Pharmacol 12: 169, 1972

89. Polk H, Lopez-Mayor J: Post-operative wound infections: a prophylactic study of determinant factors and prevention. Surgery 66: 97, 1969

90. Pruitt BA, Jr: Infections of burns and other wounds caused by Pseudomonas aeruginosa. p. 55. In Sabath LD (ed): Pseudomonas Aeruginosa: The Organisms, Diseases It Causes and Their Treatment. Hans Huber, Berne, 1980

91. Ralph ED: The bactericidal activity of nitrofu-

rantoin and metronidazole against anaerobic bacteria. Antimicrob Agents Chemother 4: 177, 1978

92. Ralph ED, Clarke JT, Libke RD, et al: Pharmacokinetics of metronidazole as determined by bioassay. Antimicrob Agents Chemother 6: 691, 1974

93. Richmond MH, Sykes RB: The B-lactamases of gram-negative bacteria and their possible physiological role. Adv Microb Physiol 9: 31, 1973

94. Rubin KN, Burka ER et al: Cephalothin and Coombs'-positive hemolytic anemia. Ann Intern Med 86: 64, 1977

95. Salamanca-Gomez F, Castaneda G, Frafan J, et al: Chromosome studies of bone marrow cells from metronidazole-treated patients. Ann Genet 23: 63, 1980

96. Sande MA, Courtney K: Nafcillin-gentamicin synergism. J Lab Clin Med 88: 118, 1976

97. Sanders CC: Novel resistance selected by the new expanded spectrum cephalosporins: a concern. J Infect Dis 145: 585, 1983

98. Sanders CC, Sander WE, Jr.: Emergence of resistance during therapy with the newer B-lactam antibiotics: role of inducible B-lactamases and implications for the future. Rev Infect Dis 5: 639, 1983

99. Schimpff SC: Infections in patients with acute leukemia. p. 2263. In: Principles and Practice of Infectious Diseases. Wiley, New York, 1979

100. Shannon K, Phillips I: Mechanism of resistance to aminoglycosides in clinical isolates. Antimicrob Agents Chemother 9: 91, 1982

101. Smith CR, Ambinder R, Lipsky JJ, et al: Cefotaxime compared with nafcillin plus tobramycin for serious bacterial infections. Ann Intern Med 101: 469, 1984

102. Spebar M, Pruitt B: Candidiasis in the burned patient. J Trauma 21: 237, 1981

103. Standiford HC: Tetracyclines and chloramaphenicol. p. 273. In Mandell GL, Douglas RG, Bennett JE (eds): Principles and Practice of Infectious Diseases. Wiley, New York, 1979

104. Steere AC, Tenney JH, Mackel DC, et al: Pseudomonas species bacteremia caused by contaminated normal human serum albumin. J Infect Dis 135: 729, 1977

105. Sutter VL: In vitro susceptibility of anaerobes: comparison of clindamycin and other antimicrobial agents. J Infect Dis 135 (suppl): S7, 1977

106. Sutter VL, Finegold SM: In vitro studies with metronidazole against anaerobic bacteria. p. 279. In Finegold SM (ed): Metronidazole. Proceedings of the International Metronidazole Conference. Excerpta Medica, Amsterdam, 1977

107. Tedesco FJ, Barton RW, Alpers DH: Clindamycin-associated colitis. A prospective study. Ann Intern Med 81: 429, 1974

108. Torres J, Bisno AL: Hyposplenism and pneumococcemia: visualization of Diplococcus pneumoniae in the peripheral blood smear. Am J Med 55: 851, 855, 1973

109. Veazey J, Wenzel RP: Nosocomial Pneumonia. p. 2228. In Mandell GL, Douglas RG, Bennett JE (eds): Principles and Practice of Infectious Diseases. Wiley, New York, 1979

110. Wade JC, Petty BG, Conrad G, et al: Cephalothin plus an aminoglycoside is more nephrotoxic than methicillin plus an aminoglycoside. Lancet 604, 1978

111. Wallerstein RO, Condit PK, Kasper CK, et al: Statewide study of chloramphenicol therapy and fatal asplastic anemia. JAMA 208: 2045, 1969

112. Wenzel RP, Austrman CA, Hunting KJ: Hospital acquired infections. II. Infections rates by site, service and common procedures in the Univeristy Hospital. Am J Epidemiol 104: 645, 1976

113. Williams DN, Crossley K, Hoffman C, et al: Parenteral clindamycin phosphate: pharmacology with normal and abnormal liver function and effect on nasal staphylococci. Antimicrob Agents Chemother 7: 153, 1975

17

Nutritional Therapy in Trauma and Sepsis

Sheldon Randall
George L. Blackburn

Trauma is usually an affliction of previously healthy, free-living, and well-nourished members of society. Despite therapy directed at immediate resuscitation, emergency transport, and treatment of injury, a significant number of patients suffer a high morbidity and mortality.[98] This is a result of the close association between hypercatabolic states and starvation along with metabolic stress following injury. Since the discovery of increased losses of intracellular electrolytes from muscle, particularly potassium phosphates and sulfates, and increased excretion of urinary nitrogen following injury, considerable progress has been made in the nutritional management of the trauma victim.[10]

Many modalities of supportive care are required. While nutritional support is not usually part of initial care, it becomes one of the essential components for optimizing the long-term care of the trauma victim. Indeed, survival after the initial period of resuscitation and treatment is dependent on the understanding of the metabolic response to trauma.

The key role of nutritional support in trauma therapy is the prevention of sepsis. Sepsis ranks just after neurologic injury and acute exsanguination as a cause of injury-related morbidity and mortality. Trauma victims are susceptible to death from overwhelming systemic infection, culminating in multisystem failure. The metabolism accompanying sepsis differs significantly from uncomplicated traumatic catabolic states.

In sepsis there is an exaggerated stimulus to protein depletion and prolonged mobilization of amino acids. Depletion of body protein tissue, particularly after a loss of 100 to 150 g of nitrogen, is accompanied by deterioration of cellular structures, insufficient production of acute-phase reactant proteins, and impairment of the immune system, thus reducing the resistance to infection.[26]

The fundamental goals of nutritional support in trauma and sepsis are (1) early recognition, (2) understanding of the metabolic response, (3) control of the proteolytic stimulus, (4) replacement of essential macro- and micro-

543

nutrients, and (5) the key to prevention of infection and the rehabilitation of the injured state.

BIOCHEMICAL AND METABOLIC RESPONSE TO INJURY

The metabolic response to injury has been the subject of extensive research from studies of Cannon,[31] Cuthbertson and Tilstone[38] Moore,[78,79] and Kinney et al.[64] Normal body composition has the structural capacity for conversion to energy. Figure 17-1 depicts the body fuel stores available when energy needs cannot be met by diet, such as in trauma and sepsis.

Carbohydrate and glycogen are extremely limited and represent approximately 2,000 calories. Lean body mass (LBM) represents 75 percent of the total body weight; as such, LBM represents the protein-containing portion—the body weight without fat. Forty percent of LBM is composed of skeletal muscle, visceral organs, and the plasma proteins. These represent the actively metabolizing tissues referred to as body cell mass (BCM).

As seen, fat tissue is the largest fuel source containing in excess of 150,000 stored calories in most normal adults. Fat is the most abundant and efficient fuel in terms of energy available per gram of tissue.[15]

During the initial or acute phase of injury, significant changes take place in the hormonal milieu, resulting in a redistribution of the body structure for energy and metabolism. These changes in body composition secondary to trauma are characterized by a biphasic hormonal response, as illustrated in Figure 17-2.

The initial phase is characterized by local and systemic effects of the catabolic mobilizing hormones: catecholamines, growth hormone, glucagon, and glucocorticoids. These hormones released during the initial "ebb" phase of injury specifically antagonize the action of insulin. Insulin is the key anabolic hormone for skeletal

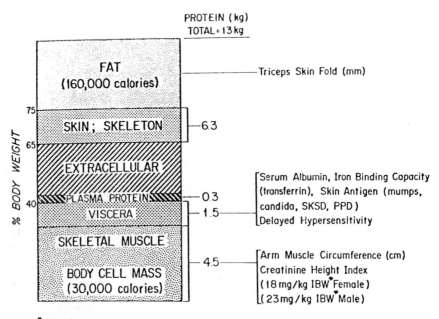

FIG. 17-1 Nutritional assessment for protein-calorie malnutrition based on the distribution of body tissue compartments. (Blackburn GL, Bistrian BR, Maini BS et al: Nutritional and metabolic assessment of the hospital patient. JPEN 1:11, 1977.)

NORMAL POST-OPERATIVE PATIENTS

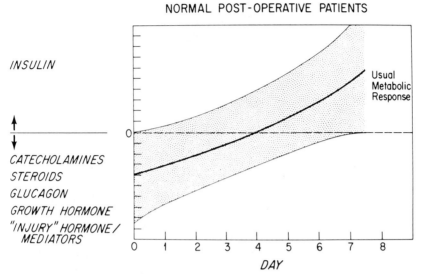

FIG. 17-2 Biphasic hormonal response to injury in the normal postoperative patient. The arrow refers to the net effect between the mobilizing hormones (e.g., catecholamines) and storage hormones (insulin), rather than absolute levels. This concept is related to the redistribution of body fat and muscle protein. The metabolic response to trauma includes an initial phase characterized by a predominant influence of mobilizing hormones. The adaptive phase that gradually follows is largely influenced by storage hormones. Homeostasis is preserved by this hormone–substrate interaction.

muscle and adipose tissue (Fig. 17-3). Glucocorticoids reduce the sensitivity of peripheral tissues to insulin, while the catecholamines inhibit the release of insulin from the peripheral tissues.[106]

The net effect is a loss of muscle tissue

- GLUCOSE UTILIZATION
- MUSCLE PROTEIN SYNTHESIS

(INCREASES)

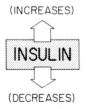

(DECREASES)

- PROTEOLYSIS
- GLUCONEOGENESIS
- LIPOLYSIS
- KETOGENESIS

FIG. 17-3 Physiologic effects of insulin.

(protein breakdown) and body fat in order to maintain adequate concentrations of amino acids for visceral protein synthesis and sufficient energy fuel substrates. In other words, the BCM apparently becomes sacrificed temporarily during the acute phase in order to maintain a relative abundance of circulating substrates, in order to meet working requirements at the cellular level. Of importance is the recognition that mobilization of body protein from skeletal muscle has purposes other than providing precursors for gluconeogenesis. Nutritional support must be designed for this purpose: to control the protein catabolic rate.

Protein kinetic studies have demonstrated many differences between elective surgery, trauma, and sepsis. Elective surgery is characterized by a period of decreased protein synthesis along with a mild degree of negative nitrogen balance (Fig. 17-4). Trauma is followed by an increase in protein synthesis and protein breakdown with a greater increase in the catabolic rate.

In sepsis, however, a much greater catabolic insult occurs. This leads to a marked increase in muscle breakdown and excessive ni-

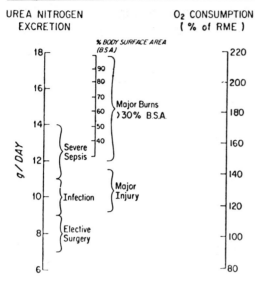

FIG. 17-4 Rates of hypermetabolism estimated from urinary urea nitrogen excretion.

trogen losses. The insulin resistance that develops in sepsis decreases glucose utilization. Plasma insulin levels remain sufficiently elevated and prevent lipolysis. A further energy deficit results, thereby limiting the availability of fuel sources. For substrate energy, the body must rely on a striking increase in muscle breakdown, gluconeogenesis, and amino acid oxidation.

Protein catabolic states in trauma and in sepsis are based on enhanced utilization of branched-chain amino acids (BCAA). This occurs secondary to the relative reduction in availability of the nonprotein fuels (fatty acids and glucose) as energy substrates for skeletal muscle. Glucose utilization is regulated by the pyruvate dehydrogenase enzyme complex. Its efficiency is reduced in trauma and sepsis. Fatty acids, the preferred fuel for skeletal muscle, are reduced by the hyperinsulinemia. Insulin fosters the re-esterification of free fatty acids within the adipocyte, thereby decreasing the net release and oxidation of free fatty acids. Carnitine acyl transferase activity is reduced in sepsis, and hepatic ketogenesis is impaired, contributing to an overall energy deficit in skeletal muscle. BCAAs regulate skeletal protein

dynamics in trauma and in sepsis. Increased oxidation of the essential BCAAs leucine, isoleucine, and valine reduces their availability and changes the kinetic pattern of skeletal protein from net anabolism to net catabolism. Administration of exogenous BCAAs is thus required to reduce the catabolism of skeletal protein while maintaining visceral protein synthesis (see Chapter 15).

The development of an effective nutritional plan at this time is limited to preservation of the patient's current nutritional status along with the appropriate cardiovascular support, fluid resuscitation, and surgery. The acute hypercatabolic phase of injury gives way to the so-called "adaptive" or "flow" phase. Effective nutritional support can occur during this adaptive phase, but the timing of the transition between phases is dependent on the severity of trauma, sepsis, and the associated nutritional depletion.

The adaptive phase is recognized by a reduction in both insulin and glucose concentrations. There is also a return to normal plasma concentrations of catecholamines and glucocorticoids. Body mechanisms now turn to different sources of energy.

NITROGEN METABOLISM

Nitrogen (gram proteins/6.25) necessary for tissue protein synthesis, erythropoiesis, wound healing, and cellular and humoral immune function is provided by this redistribution of muscle protein. This interrelationship entails catabolism of muscle protein along with the release of gluconeogenic precursors for utilization by the liver. The liver therefore meets the demands for visceral and secretory protein synthesis (Fig. 17-5). The efficiency of this mechanism is influenced by the extent of injury and the type of nutritional intake. It therefore becomes extremely important, when designing nutritional therapies, to keep these changes in

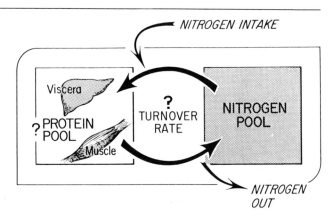

FIG. 17-5 The concept of nitrogen balance is illustrated. Nutritional support in the critically ill patient must provide a source of repletion of the visceral protein pool. A limitation exists because the turnover of the metabolic nitrogen pool and its various intracellular protein compartments differ.

mind so that the adaptation to the physiologic state of injury is enhanced.

OTHER ASPECTS OF INJURY METABOLISM

Shifts in body fluids and electrolyte compartments are an inevitable consequence of these physiologic hormonal and metabolic alterations. However, a decrease in the "functional" extracellular space produces a hypovolemic response, which entails conservation of water. This physiologic response is exaggerated by the activation of the renin–angiotensin system initiated by hypovolemia. Under the influence of aldosterone and glucocorticoids, retention of sodium and water occurs.[20]

Renal water retention, expressed as a negative free-water clearance, despite a decrease in plasma osmolarity, occurs secondary to the secretion of vasopressin, or antidiuretic hormone (ADH). Infused hypotonic solutions, particularly 5 percent dextrose in water or 0.45 percent saline solution, are major contributors to an inappropriate antidiuretic effect.

A considerable amount of fluid, rich in both colloid and crystalloid, is lost into the "third space," in the area traumatized and in other interstitial spaces. The fluid shift repre-sents a redistribution of the body's extracellular fluid (ECF) and therefore must be replaced appropriately.[21,97] Although one would expect glucocorticoids and aldosterone to increase renal excretion of potassium, the net effect during acute phase of injury (in the absence of excessive gastrointestinal losses) is that of maintaining normal serum potassium concentrations. Significant extrusion of intracellular potassium secondary to muscle injury, protein catabolism, blood transfusions, and absorption of blood from serous cavities is responsible for maintaining these levels. Once diuresis occurs (a sign of the adaptive phase of injury), renal potassium excretion increases and subsequent supplementation becomes necessary. The amount required can be quantitated by measuring 24-hour urinary potassium excretion.

Normal extracellular potassium and relative hyponatremia are present during the acute phase of injury. With added surgical intervention at this stage, an antagonistic affect of the high glucagon/insulin ratio teleologically counteracts this aldosterone mediated response.[28]

IMMUNOLOGIC RESPONSE

Severe immune depression after major trauma and sepsis has been recognized for many years; most recently, with the advent of newer immunologic techniques, the suppressive effect of trauma and sepsis on the immune system has been characterized as well.

Functional changes in the immune system have been observed in different aspects of host response, including neutrophil chemotaxis, intracellular killing, consumption of complement, cell-mediated immunity, and humoral immunity. Cell-mediated immunity is generally more suppressed than humoral immunity. The degree of suppression is dependent on the severity of injury and/or the degree of sepsis.[83,100] Recently, the use of monoclonal antibodies to identify T lymphocytes[94] demonstrated that immediately after a burn injury there is an inversion of the normal ratio between suppressor/cytotoxic (OKT8) and helper/inducer (OKT4) cells. In spite of all this, the total lymphocyte counts (OKT3) remain relatively unaltered.[3]

This reversal of the subsets of T lymphocytes was found to reach a peak at 5 to 7 days after injury and returned to normal levels within 10 days to 2 weeks.

Delayed reversal of the suppressor:helper ratio of T cells was also associated with episodes of systemic sepsis. Several studies on the effect of trauma on neutrophil function have been performed.[4,29,36] These studies showed the ability of neutrophils from patients with extensive trauma to kill ingested bacteria to be deficient. Defects in the chemotactic activity of polymorphonuclear leukocytes (PMNs) have been demonstrated after surgery,[35,71] and other investigators have failed to demonstrate defects in phagocytic and chemotaxic function of PMNs in surgical patients.[100] This may be partially explained by the severity of trauma.

The study of immunologic response to surgery is complicated, since it is modified by a variety of factors that include infection, malnutrition, disease associated with surgery, organ failure, age, and cancer. The most severe defect in phagocytic function of PMNs has been demonstrated to occur immediately before the onset of systemic sepsis[94] or in malnourished patients.[3,94] Defects may be found in the opsonic properties of serum after trauma and sepsis. This is usually associated with low levels of complement (CH_{50}), factor B, properdin,[2] and fibronectin.[25]

The presence of tissue damage in trauma activates the phagocytic mechanism. The activation of the immune system becomes triggered and must then be controlled or finely balanced in order to avoid immunologic problems. Excessive activation of the suppressor cells may lead to the development of opportunistic infections; conversely, excessive activation of helper/inducer subset may induce the development of autoimmune diseases. Although the mechanisms that cause this response are yet to be determined, it is known that the activation of these mechanisms serves to localize the lesion and clear from the bloodstream foreign bodies, such as bacteria or tissue debris. This leaves us to determine whether this overall response is pathologic or physiologic.

T-helper lymphocytes appear to congregate in the spleen, where important blood purification is accomplished and T-cell host-defense activity is initiated. The importance of the spleen to host defense against infection in recovery from surgery and trauma is compromised in previously splenectomized patients. Only when severe sepsis complicates surgical trauma do the physiologic and metabolic responses become pathologic. While in massive injury and/or systemic sepsis, a pathologic immune response may follow that will damage sensitive membranes of lung alveoli and tubules within the kidney, ultimately resulting in a multisystemic organ failure. This is not uncommon in today's intensive care (ICU) setting, thereby increasing the risk of morbidity and mortality.[96]

Most microorganisms are opsonized with complement (C3b, C5b) by either the alternative or classic pathway, if specific antibodies are present in the circulation. A defect in the complement system has been shown to be associated with an increased susceptibility to bacterial infection.[2]

Tissue debris, fibronectin degradation products, and some gram-positive organisms are opsonized by a nonspecific opsonic α_2-glycoprotein (fibronectin). Saba[3] describes that this opsonic glycoprotein facilitates the clearance of these substances both locally and from the bloodstream. The depletion of fibronectin has been associated with a reduction in reticuloendothelial activity and with multiple systemic organ failure.

Therapeutic repletion of fibronectin concentrations with cryoprecipitate in patients with sepsis and multiple organ failure have shown a significant reduction in pulmonary shunt and dead space after infusion of cryoprecipitate.[95]

Endogenous Mediators

Most of the immunologic events following the activation of leukocytes are in part mediated by lymphokinines. Lymphokinines are a family of soluble mediators that act on stimulated T lymphocytes. The lymphokinines were recently subdivided into two classes of similar or identical molecules: interleukin 1 (IL-1), also known as leukocyte endogenous mediator (LEM), and interleukin 2 (IL-2).[25] Interleukin 1 is a molecule that induces activation and proliferation of the helper-induced subset of lymphocytes. Interleukin 2, produced by activated helper lymphocytes, induces activation in and proliferation of cytotoxic suppressor subset lymphocytes.

LEM is a low-molecular-weight heat-labile protein released in response to phagocytosis by monocytic cells. Fever, secondary to bacterial infections or traumatic injuries, is associated with and probably mediated by LEM. Interleukin 1 activates B cells and T cells and induces the production of IL-2.

Current evidence from our laboratory suggests that many of the nonspecific metabolic sequelae associated with febrile states, such as increased skeletal protein catabolism, enhanced acute-phase protein synthesis, trace metal redistribution, and proliferation of certain leukocyte subpopulations, follow the administration of IL-1. Most recently, we have shown that the ability to induce an increase in whole-body amino acid flux, oxidation, and protein synthesis occurs after the administration of IL-1. We have also found that nutritional support in the critically ill can restore IL-1 production very rapidly in vitro, far earlier than other indices of nutritional repletion as cell-mediated immunity, serum albumin, and transferrin concentrations.[99]

NUTRITIONAL ASSESSMENT OF THE TRAUMATIZED PATIENT

In formulating the nutritional assessment of the traumatized patient it is important to address two fundamental issues: (1) the preexisting nutritional status of the individual, and (2) the degree of stress imposed by the disease process. Techniques such as anthropometry, biomechanical indices, immunologic testing, and the magnitude of the state of protein catabolism all offer insights and assist in identifying and categorizing patients with different degrees of malnutrition.[16,56] This relates to the risks of morbidity and mortality attending major stress such as trauma or sepsis in hospitalized patients. The variables mentioned above and others commonly used to address nutritional assessment, such as creatinine height index, serum albumin, serum transferrin, total lymphocyte count, and delayed hypersensitivity response to common intradermal skin antigen measurements, lose much of their value in the initial evaluation of the traumatized patient.[14,16,46,56]

Immediately after injury, there is a required fluid resuscitation for maintenance of cardiopulmonary stability. Thus, an increase rather than a decrease in weight follows the periods of resuscitation from injury, obviously related to fluid retention rather than to the accretion of lean body mass, thereby rendering the standard methods of nutritional assessment inaccurate.[46] Serum albumin, transferrin, and other secretory plasma proteins are dispersed by hemodilution after this resuscitation and by protein extravasation from the intravascular space into the interstitial space, the so-called buffer zone.[43] Serum protein values will be further lowered by any surgical intervention necessitated by the injury. The aforementioned fluid resuscitation is accompanied by a decline in albumin synthetic rate. This concomitant decline in serum albumin levels should not be viewed as a poor prognostic indicator, as it would be in other disease states.[1]

Measurement of presumed immune responsiveness as total lymphocyte count and of hypoanergy to skin-test antigens has been suggested as a guide to nutritional status. Trauma mediates an overall depression in neutrophil function as well in T-cell, B-cell, and macrophage competence. The underlying mechanism of these effects have yet to be clearly defined but may be attributed to a circulating immunosuppressive factor and an increased suppressor T-cell activity. Evidence now indicates that a rising total lymphocyte count correlates with an improved nutritional state.[72,73,80]

As the stress response is reduced, immune function testing will be improved and the shorter half-life visceral protein levels (i.e., transferrin, fibronectin, prealbumin, and retinol-binding protein) will usually increase within a 1- to 2-week period after injury. The initial depression in immune function and serum secretory protein levels truly denotes stress, while failure to return to normal reflects a continued catabolic state.

Skin testing should not be performed until 7 to 10 days after injury at which time it is important to begin serial skin testing every 10 to 14 days to assess immune status and response to nutritional support.[1,16] Multitest CMI, by Merieux Institute, Florida, is a more sensitive and specific index than the standard testing technique in measuring immunocompetence. The repletion of patients with protein calorie malnutrition does result in a return of delayed hypersensitivity,[67] while deficiencies of the micronutrients, including iron, zinc, folic acid, and vitamins A, C, B_6, and B_{12}, can lead to immunosuppression.[12] Thus, a rationale exists for the use of Multitest CMI serial skin testing for identifying the return of immunocompetence and the adequacy of continuing nutritional support.

The degree of metabolic stress produced by trauma is a crucial factor in the assignment of appropriate nutritional support. Resting energy expenditure in major injury is elevated 15 to 50 percent.[63] The hypermetabolism associated with injury is reflected in marked increases in energy expenditure. Unlike exercise, excitement, and feeding, which may result in only a transient increase in protein catabolism, the increase in energy expenditure after trauma is accomplished by sustained increased catabolism of not only fat and carbohydrate, but protein as well.[1,39,57]

An approximation of the energy needs for an injured patient may be obtained by multiplying the estimate calculated for the Harris-Benedict equation by a factor of 1.76.[93] The use of indirect calorimetry may also be used in intensive care settings, which accurately measures resting energy expenditure via expired carbon dioxide.

Protein catabolism is a hallmark of the metabolic response to trauma accounting for approximately 15 to 20 percent of the total energy expenditure after injury. Several methods have evolved to quantitate changes in protein metabolism.

Since the primary source of protein fuel for catabolism arises in skeletal muscle, the degree of breakdown of the skeletal muscle can be assessed by measurement of the excretion of 3-methylhistidine and 24-hour urine nitrogen collection.[109] It is important to recognize that 3-methylhistidine is an indicator of total rather than net breakdown of skeletal muscle protein, provided there is no recent intake of red meat.[1,23,37] The amino acid histidine may be posttranslationally modified to 3-methylhistidine in actin and myosin fibers. This methyl amino acid is not recycled, does not undergo further metabolism in the body, is quantitatively excreted in the urine, and has a low renal threshold. The 24-hour urine urea nitrogen excretion, the most easily accessible measurement, reflects the difference between whole-body protein synthesis and total-body protein catabolism (net protein degradation).[23,104]

The use of stable amino acid isotopes has become a major breakthrough reflecting the precursor pool for protein synthesis determination of whole-body protein turnover by the use of stable radioisotopes of individual amino acids represents an important technologic advancement for the study of protein kinetics. Its chief advantage is the more direct and more accurate measurement of protein synthesis and protein breakdown over short periods of time, as compared with nitrogen balance studies, which furnish only indirect information about the net effect of protein breakdown over long periods.[30,104]

The catabolic index formulated by Bistrian[13] is a practical approach to stratifying patients according to the degree of catabolic stress. It is useful in that it integrates the level of nitrogen intake and the degree of metabolic stress into a single number.

Catabolic index = urine urea nitrogen (g/day) − [½ dietary nitrogen (g/day + 3)] where a catabolic index of 0 represents no significant stress, 1–5 is mild stress, and 5 is moderate to severe stress. Protein turnover studies and catabolic indices have both been used successfully in predicting which patients would benefit from nutritional support that incorporates amino acid solutions enriched with BCAAs.

The adequacy of nutritional therapy in the traumatized patient remains complex. The development of sensitive prognostic indicators of wound healing and host-defense mechanisms is continually being investigated.

Despite the potential complexity arising in patient care, nutritional support can easily be reduced to an effective plan by considering the factors shown in Table 17-1.

NUTRITIONAL SUPPORT

The maintenance of cardiopulmonary stability and the restitution of acute external and third-space fluid losses preclude consideration of nutritional support for the first 24 to 48 hours after injury. Aggressive use of hemodynamic monitoring is essential in order to provide circulatory support.[1] The appropriate metabolic monitoring involves surveillance for starvation ketosis, which is associated with a lessening of stress-hormone signals and adaptation to caloric depreciation.

There is no evidence that 3 to 5 days of semistarvation in uncomplicated traumatic victims is detrimental to the previously well-nourished individual. In those patients who are malnourished before sustaining traumatic injury and in those whose clinical condition develops into a protracted "flow" phase in which the ongoing stress hormonal response results in a prolonged course of metabolic activity—aggressive nutritional supplementation is likely to be beneficial because these are the patients

TABLE 17-1. Nutrition Support for the Trauma Patient

I. Nutritional assessment
   a) Degree of depletion of body mass
   b) Visceral function
   c) Fat stores
II. Degree of hypercatabolism
   a) Disease categories and measured or estimated catabolic rates
   b) Inspection of the patient, presence of tachycardia
   c) Rate of weight loss and nitrogen excretion (urea nitrogen)
III. Gastrointestinal function
   a) History of dietary intake (adequate, insufficient, absent)
   b) High or low fistula output
   c) Use of a nasogastric, transpharyngeal, gastric, enteric, or transfistula feeding tube
IV. Appetite
   a) Solid or liquid food preference
   b) Taste preference (bland, fruits, sweet food groups)
V. Goal of nutritional support
   a) Fed
   b) Nonfed
   c) Combination
VI. Route of nutritional support
   a) Enteral
   b) Parenteral
   c) Combination
VII. Protein and calorie requirements
   a) Basal energy expenditure (BEE) according to Harris-Benedict standards
   b) Protein at 1:150 nitrogen/calorie ratio

(Blackburn GL, Bistrian BR: Nutritional care of injured and/or septic patient. Surg Clin North Am 56:1195, 1976. Reprinted with permission from WB Saunders Co., Philadelphia.)

in whom starvation ketosis does not develop in response to carbohydrate deprivation because of the ongoing muscle catabolism, hyperinsulinemia, high rates of gluconeogenesis, and suppression of free fatty acid release. Again, these patients require early aggressive nutritional support for maintenance of lean body mass and host-defense mechanisms while gaining time for recovery and to prevent systemic sepsis and eventual organ failure.[66,81]

In summary, to determine the optimal method of nutritional support to be used in an individual patient depends on the functional capability of the gastrointestinal (GI) tract, the degree of stress and hypermetabolism, the severity of preexisting malnutrition, and the relative risk of feeding complications.

ENTERAL FEEDING

A functional gastrointestinal (GI) tract should be used as the preferred route for nutritional support. The GI tract and liver occupy a regulatory role in body protein metabolism in addition to their involvement in more than one-half of the body's normal daily protein turnover.[60,89]

Absorbed nutrients pass into the portal vein and to the liver before entering the systemic circulation, permitting the initial hepatic processing of substrates to occur. Liver enzyme affinity constants are geared to portal vein concentrations whose tendency is to be higher than systemic levels. The regulatory role of the liver is clearly demonstrated by the marked alteration in amino acid profiles measured in the hepatic vein as compared to the portal vein.[44] Besides the physiologic considerations, enteral feeding has the advantages of greater safety and lesser expense in relationship to parenteral nutrition.[87,88]

Paralytic ileus often accompanies trauma and sepsis even if the peritoneal cavity has not been penetrated. If a laparotomy is conducted during the course of trauma management, the performance of a jejunostomy is easily accomplished.[34,40] Distal GI anastomoses are not a contraindication to early enteral nutrition and may in fact enhance anastomotic tensile strength and healing.[40] In traumatized patients who do not require abdominal surgical intervention, access to the GI tract may be required. A feeding tube with a guide wire can then be positioned under fluoroscopic control postpylorically. This procedure may be aided by the use of intravenously administered metachlopromide (Reglan) in 10-mg dosages. In patients in whom no gastric atony is present, the use of a nasogastric tube may be considered; however, stomach residuals should be checked every 4 hours and feedings withheld if the residuals exceed 100 ml. This minimizes the risk of tracheobronchial aspiration. The head of the bed should also remain elevated to at least 40 to 60 degrees.

A number of commercially prepared enteral feeding formulas are available. These formulas vary in composition. This is important in calculating the precise amount of protein, carbohydrate, and fat that is to be delivered. In some instances, an appropriate fuel mixture is not provided for the trauma patient. The use of specifically formulated modular feedings with appropriate additives to meet specific individual requirements is under investigation. Formulas with excessively high osmolarities should be avoided. This may be accomplished by the use of glucose polymers rather than monosaccharides. If fat digestion is impaired, medium-chain triglycerides may be substituted in place of long-chain triglycerides as the lipid source. Medium-chain triglycerides are not dependent on micella formation for transport and are rapidly transferred to the portal circulation, becoming metabolized immediately, unlike the long-chain triglycerides.[15,27,51,59]

The most common complication of enteral nutrition is profuse diarrhea. Because of this, it has become common practice to start a full-strength feeding formula at low rates (20 ml/hr) and to advance slowly over a 3- to 4-day period until the desired volume of delivery is attained. In cases of refractory diarrhea, stool specimens for the appropriate cultures (*C. dificili* and *C. + S.*) need to be obtained before treating the diarrhea aggressively (after negative culture reports). Several modalities have been instituted in controlling diarrhea. We prefer the use of Lomotil (5 to 10 ml) added directly to the enteral formula per each 250 ml and administered continuously as the best control. Most recently the bulk laxatives, Hydrocil Instant or Metamucil, have been found quite useful because the stool gels (water is absorbed) as it passes through the colon, facilitating care for sacral decubiti prevention. Feeding tubes must be cared for by a diligent nursing staff to prevent clogging of the tube.

PARENTERAL NUTRITION

Effective nutritional support with parenteral solutions requires an integrated team approach because of the increased risks afforded by limitations in fluid tolerance and by the metabolic changes associated with injury.

TABLE 17-2. **Glucose Oxidation During Total Parenteral Nutrition in Postoperative Patients**
(*N* = 5)[a]

Glucose Infusion Rate (mg/kg/min)	Glucose Oxidation Rate (mg/kg/min)	% of CO_2 from Glucose	RQ
4	1.87 ± 0.29	51.1 ± 5.0	0.94 ± 0.03
7	2.46 ± 0.09	54.6 ± 3.7	1.13 ± 0.16
9	3.16 ± 0.68	61.6 ± 13.5	1.12 ± 0.05

[a] To convert to mmol/kg/min divide mg/kg/min by 180.
(Wolfe RR, Allsop JR, Burke JF: Glucose metabolism in man: Responses to intravenous glucose infusion. Metabolism 28:210, 1979.)

Recent reports have substantiated the importance of an integrated team approach by pointing out several undesirable consequences of injudicious parenteral feedings in stressed patients. It has been well demonstrated that provision of hypertonic dextrose solutions far in excess of energy requirements results in respiratory quotients greater than one (Table 17-2). This results in increased carbon dioxide production, which is significant for patients requiring ventilatory support.[8,9]

During physiologic stress, glucose oxidation to carbon dioxide and water is not limited. Glucose infusions in excess of 4 mg/kg/min will not improve proportionately the oxidation of glucose but will result in increased glycogen synthesis and lipogenesis.[5,107] Fat synthesized from glucose in the liver is not adequately cleared. This is due to impairment of lipoprotein synthesis and is particularly true during infection and sepsis. This results in further lipid storage, hepatomegaly, and deranged morphology as well as secretory functions. The excessive lipogenesis, hepatic dysfunction, and carbon dioxide production are not desirable goals in the trauma and septic victim, leading to current concerns and controversies in overfeeding.

PROTEIN-SPARING THERAPY

Protein-sparing therapy provides 1.0 to 1.5 g protein per kilogram body weight intravenously without supplemental dextrose or fat (Fig. 17-6). This approach optimizes the meta-

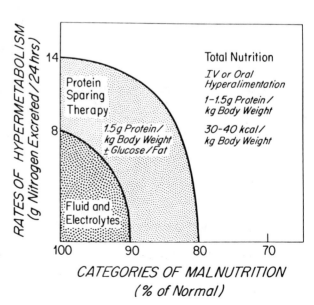

FIG. 17-6 In designing nutritional support therapy, the degree of stress and the extent of malnutrition must be known. The critically ill or septic patient with severe stress deserves full nutritional support providing adequate protein and calories. Patients with minimal short-term stress (5 to 7 days) who are immunocompetent will require only fluid and electrolyte replacement. Intermediate states will benefit from nutritional support by either protein or total parenteral nutrition therapy.

bolic response to injury and is useful in the moderately stressed reasonably well-nourished trauma victim who cannot be otherwise fed orally for 5 to 7 days.[18,19,60] The absence of glucose and the concomitant administration of hypocaloric amino acid lowers the blood glucose levels, relieving the hyperinsulinemia in trauma. This facilitates the mobilization of free fatty acids that can be used for energy production. Amino acids are conserved for the synthesis of proteins (acute-phase reactants) and other cells necessary for an appropriate response to injury. The clinical marker of effective protein-sparing therapy includes the development of ketonuria (this is best observed at frequent intervals) diuresis and a lowering of the respiratory quotient. Protein-sparing therapy has been shown to (1) improve protein synthesis, (2) minimize skeletal muscle catabolism, and (3) improve the metabolic response to postoperative infections.

Protein-sparing therapy becomes less beneficial in trauma victims presenting in severely stressed states. These individuals usually require fluid resuscitation and fail to develop ketonemia when administered protein-sparing therapy. The failure for ketonemia to develop within 48 hours implies ongoing hyperinsulinemia and persistent insulin resistance. It is therefore recommended that patients presenting with severe stress be treated with more aggressive measures.

PERIPHERAL INTRAVENOUS HYPERALIMENTATION

A mixed fuel system incorporating the use of fat emulsions to provide 30 to 60 percent of the total caloric input can be met through a peripheral vein for anabolic energy requirements and protein needs.[18,19] The proper use of peripheral veins is limited to solutions of less than 600 mmol and having potassium contents under 60 mEq/L. The commonly used solutions consist of 3.5 percent amino acids and 5 percent dextrose. Fat is infused via a Y connector directly into the peripheral hyperalimentation line, which also assists in decreasing the incidence of phlebitis because of its isotonicity. The intravenous fat emulsions are usually provided in 500-ml volumes (a 10 and 20 percent stock) and infused over a 10- to 12-hour period. Low-dose heparin, 1,000 units/L, and hydrocortisone, 5 to 10 mg/L, have been quite successful.

This type of delivery system is successful for patients receiving approximately 3 to 4 L/day, which will maintain their protein and energy requirements, but is contraindicated in patients with fluid restrictions, inadequate peripheral access, and type I or IV hyperlipidemia.[1]

CENTRAL INTRAVENOUS HYPERALIMENTATION

When the diagnosis of severe stress is present on initial assessment of the trauma victim, and use of the GI tract is not anticipated for at least 5 days, or if preexisting nutritional deficits are noted on a static nutritional assessment, central hyperalimentation will be required. This approach permits the infusion of hypertonic concentrations of protein, carbohydrates, and fat, in an effort to minimize skeletal muscle catabolism to maintain immunocompetence and, it is hoped, to prevent subsequent sepsis and multiple organ failure. This method of nutritional support provides an optimal fuel mixture of protein (1.5 g/kg/day), carbohydrate (3 to 5 mg/kg/min), and approximately 35 percent of the total caloric requirements as fat. The total caloric requirements should be measured by indirect calorimetry, which measures resting energy expenditure. In trauma the caloric requirements can be estimated at 35 to 40 kcal/kg/day, except in burns and head trauma. In these situations, it is best to maintain nitrogen balance instead of trying to replete caloric requirements with excessive administration of calories.

We recommend the use of the "3-in-1 admixture" method of infusion. This incorporates protein, carbohydrates, and fat into one admixture. This method is much more cost effective and lessens the number of line interruptions, thereby diminishing the septic complication rate of central line use. At our institution, the mortality associated with line sepsis is less than 1 percent.

This type of low-rate delivery of fat as a continuous 24-hour infusion, if no more than 100 g/day, has not been shown to be associated with the abnormal results in liver function tests, immune-deficiency states or worsening of stress-induced dyslipoprotenemias as reported with excessive administration of exogenous fat emulsions.

Because of concern about undesirable side effects of excessive dextrose administration in the critically ill, recent clinical trials have compared the use of a physical mixture of medium-chain and long-chain triglycerides (75/25 percent solution) with long-chain triglyceride (LCT) infusion alone. Safety and efficacy have clearly been established; the potential benefits of this physical mixture as a source of nonprotein calories include (1) faster rate of clearance and oxidation because carnitine is not required for medium-chain triglyceride (C8:10) as it is for LCT to enter into the mitochondria for β-oxidation (carnitine levels have been reported to be reduced in severe stress states), and (2) less impairment to the immune system, without flooding the reticuloendothelial system with lipid, facilitating clearance of bacteria by the liver and therefore avoiding sequestering in the lung tissue.

In addition, medications may be co-infused simultaneously (antibiotics) or may be directly incorporated in the 3-in-1 admixture (e.g., aminophylline, insulin steroids, cimetidine, albumin) without risk of incompatibility. We have shown that gastric pH levels are better maintained with a constant infusion of cimetidine (600 mg/24 hr). This method also permits continuous infusion of albumin, where the administration of 25 to 50 g albumin per day over a 4- to 5-day period results in a more sustained maintenance of albumin levels to the more desirable range of 2.0 to 2.4 g/day, which may benefit drug transport.

The metabolic response to injury increases the oxidation of BCAAs by the skeletal muscle, thereby lowering the serum levels of this amino acid. Evidence has convincingly documented the use of BCAA-enriched solutions for nutritional support in trauma patients by decreasing skeletal muscle breakdown, normalizing amino acid profiles, along with earlier improvement in nitrogen balance. Also, by incorporating these BCAAs, as compared with the standard essential and nonessential amino acids, there is a greater rate of protein synthesis and a greater preservation of hepatic nitrogen content. Investigations now include amino acid solutions with a greater concentration of BCAAs (Branchamine 45 percent, Travenol), formulated for the purpose of optimizing support of the metabolic response to injury.

Ideally, the use of a control catheter should be used exclusively for nutritional support. This ensures the constant and accurate infusion of the essential nutrients. With the present hemodynamic monitoring techniques (i.e., Swan-Ganz and multilumen catheters), access must be shared. Although a certain compromise is required, the meticulous management of the catheter is still mandatory in order to maintain the morbidity and mortality associated with line sepsis at a minimum.

MODIFICATION OF NUTRITIONAL SUPPORT SYSTEMS FOR SPECIFIC STATES OF ORGAN FAILURE

Nutritional management in trauma and sepsis may be complicated by coexisting organ dysfunction. Respiratory renal and liver failures are frequently associated with severe injuries, increasing the mortality of the trauma victim approximately two- to threefold. Each type of failure superimposes certain disturbances on the already altered metabolic profile of the trauma victim. Nutritional support must be modified appropriately to limit the biochemical alterations associated with organ failure while still providing an adequate supply of micro- and macronutrients to promote recovery.

carbohydrate calories lowers the production of carbon dioxide and the RQ, while maintaining oxygen consumption rates.

RESPIRATORY FAILURE

Acute respiratory insufficiency in the trauma victim frequently develops due to flail chest, pulmonary contusion, aspiration, resuscitation-induced pulmonary edema, fat embolism, or pneumonia.

Nutritional support has demonstrated substantial improvement in the ability to wean patients with acute respiratory failure (ARF) from mechanical ventilation.[11] Amino acid infusion produces an increase in both minute ventilation and oxygen consumption, thereby reversing the hypoxic and hypercapnic ventilatory responses in patients provided with hypocaloric dextrose infusion alone.[1,42,105] Particular care must be exercised to avoid overfeeding because extensive carbohydrate levels have been shown to precipitate or worsen the pulmonary mechanics. An understanding of the biomechanical rational for this is imperative. When the glucose administered equals the glucose oxidation rate, all the substrate then is used for the production of energy (Table 17-2). Thus, the complete catabolism of 1 mol glucose results in the production of 6 mol carbon dioxide for every 6 mol oxygen consumed, resulting in a respiratory quotient (RQ) of 1. If excess glucose (greater than 4 mg/kg/min) is given, it is then diverted to fatty acid synthesis, with 13.5 mol glucose, 3 mol of oxygen and input energy then producing 1 mol of fat and 26 mol carbon dioxide. This leads to an elevation of RQ to 8.7. The patient's adaptation to this increase in RQ and increased carbon dioxide is a hypercapnic ventilatory response that induces greater oxygen consumption ($\dot{V}O_2$), fatigue, and eventual respiratory failure. Phosphate balance must be carefully monitored and replaced along with the use of continuous intravenous aminophylline to assist with diaphragmatic muscle contractility.[84,85]

Provision of a mixed fuel system is safe and adequate. Substituting fat for some of the

RENAL FAILURE

Acute renal failure may develop in traumatized and septic patients primarily from direct parenchymal or renovascular trauma. ARF may also occur secondarily by hypovolemia or septic shock, myoglobinuria and by the use of nephrotoxic antibiotics. Oliguric renal failure, especially when combined with acute respiratory insufficiency severely limits the amount of fluid allotted to nutritional support, usually to a one liter infusion. Early frequent dialysis or hemo-ultrafiltration is deemed necessary because it not only reduces complications of uremia but also allows adequate nutritional support by controlling volume overload. The daily losses of 4 to 10 g amino acids with hemodialysis and 6 to 13 g protein with peritoneal dialysis further increases the already elevated protein requirements in these patients.[61,65]

Protein metabolism is profoundly altered by renal failure, resulting in an accumulation of the breakdown products of amino acid metabolism = urea, along with the inorganic ions (phosphate, sulfate, and potassium). Under these conditions, 1 to 1.5 g protein per kilogram per day should be provided as long as a serum urea nitrogen level under 100 is maintained. Nonoliguric acute tubular necrosis facilitates fluid management and has a lower mortality rate than that associated with oliguric renal failure.[7]

Clinical studies have been unable to demonstrate any difference in comparing both essential and nonessential amino acids.[17,47,53] An explanation for this is that the essential amino acids solutions, which provide approximately 20 g amino acids per day, have their metabolic benefits offset in stressed patients because of their inability to fulfill gluconeogenic and synthetic demands. Therefore, both essential and nonessential amino acids are required to prevent imbalance or deficits in nonessential amino acids. Different methods for administering nutritional support of traumatized and septic patients have been investigated, especially when the clinical situation is complicated by volume overload and/or a nonfunctioning gastrointestinal tract.

Hypertonic solutions of glucose may be infused via peritoneal dialysis for supplemental calories. The absorption of fat by the intraperitoneal route is, unfortunately, poor. Another modification is the infusion of hypertonic solutions of amino acids and glucose by the venous outflow tract in patients undergoing hemodialysis.[41,54]

Modification of amino acid formulas has been under clinical investigation in patients with renal failure. Valine levels have been found to be low in plasma specimens and in muscle biopsy samples. The administration of valine-enriched mixtures normalizes plasma tissue levels along with improvement in nitrogen balance. This raises the question of whether amino acids enriched with valine in excess of those quantities already used in BCAA solutions might prove beneficial; further investigation is warranted.[6]

The use of ketoacid analogues in patients with chronic renal failure has resulted in reduction of the urea pool while enhancing the supply of amino acids. Thus, protein requirements may be reduced, but further investigation is warranted for this possibility as well. Its usage seems quite beneficial in nontraumatized patients with acute renal failure by delaying their need for dialysis.

HEPATIC FAILURE

The close association of alcohol abuse with trauma has been highlighted by federal and state government legislation instituting strict penalties and jail sentences for drunken driving. Hepatic decompensation may be precipitated by direct injury itself, by sepsis, shock, hypotension, or anesthesia, or by preexisting liver dysfunction in the traumatized or septic patient.[45,86,101] The liver is an essential organ for the body's metabolic response to trauma. In the presence of hepatic dysfunction, gluconeogenesis, lipogenesis, ketone production, acute-phase protein synthetic rates, and removal of the normally occurring toxins are all potentially disturbed. Also affected is the regulatory role of the liver in the maintenance of micronutrient and amino acid concentrations. The most widely investigated complication of liver failure in trauma and sepsis has been hepatic encephalopathy.

The etiology of hepatic encephalopathy remains unanswered. One hypothesis concerns excess buildup of ammonia and related compounds, possibly through action as base products that form harmful chemical complexes within the brain.[103] Other investigations implicate an imbalance of amino acid profile as causing CNS depression. Clinical studies in cirrhotic patients have revealed elevation of the aromatic amino acids (phenylalanine, tyrosine, and tryptophan), while plasma concentrations of BCAAs are diminished.[49,82] Presumably, the damaged liver now is unable to catabolize the aromatic amino acids and, because of the inability of the damaged liver to remove excess insulin, BCAA uptake into muscle is activated. With the absence of BCAA and the increase in aromatic amino acid concentration, there is competition for the same transport mechanisms. This competition results in higher cerebral levels of tryptophan, phenylalanine, and tyrosine. Both the production of false neurotransmitters and the conversion of tryptophan to serotonin, a notable CNS depressant, may be responsible for hepatic encephalopathy.[48]

Several clinical investigations support this hypothesis by providing BCAA-enriched solutions. Improvement of hepatic encephalopathy is observed along with, enhancement of hepatic protein synthesis.[50,52] However, results of other studies have shown a normalization of amino acid profiles without demonstrating an improvement in encephalopathy with these modified formulas.[74] It remains to be resolved whether a subset of hepatic-induced encephalopathies in trauma and sepsis can be identified that may benefit from these BCAA-enriched formulas.

Commercially prepared enteral (Hepatic-Aid and Travasorb Hepatic) and parenteral (Hepatamine) mixtures are now available for use with an amino acid profile specifically tailored to hepatic insufficiency. Their use in trauma is problematic, however. Not only is their efficiency uncertain, but their depleted content of essential amino acids, phenylalanine and tryptophan, makes them unsuitable for support of adequate protein synthesis in the traumatized or septic patient. Cirrhotic livers are unable to convert (1) methionine to cysteine, and (2) phenylalanine to tyrosine, making these amino acids essential in this clinical setting.[92] Cysteine is the most insoluble amino acid, and adequate amounts can only be provided via the GI tract. Enterally administered casein hydrolysate has been shown to eliminate the problems of hypotyrosinemia and hypocysteinemia in cirrhosis.[70]

Even though altered lipid and carbohydrate metabolism exists in hepatic insufficiency, the provision of a mixed fuel system minimizes the dysfunction of the liver commonly associated with intravenous hyperalimentation.

Cyclic hyperalimentation involving the administration of hypertonic dextrose solution for only 14 to 18 hr/day promotes lipolysis. The elimination of glucose during the latter period decreases insulin secretion while promoting hepatic lipid and glycogen mobilization, thereby minimizing fatty infiltration of the liver.[69] Because of the increased energy demands that occur in severe trauma and sepsis, this approach is not recommended.

Parenteral administration of dextrose, 150 to 200 g, rarely causes any significant metabolic problems in this setting. Provision of 50 to 100 g fat, either continuously or intermittently, can be satisfactorily cleared by lipoprotein lipases and used by peripheral tissues in patients with hepatic insufficiency.[91]

complications and high mortality. Parenterally administered hyperalimentation is essential in supporting these patients through the acute phase.[22,55,58] Again, a mixed fuel may be administered. Enteral feeding is becoming increasingly used in pancreatic disease. Elemental diets distal to the ligament of Trietz either by fluoroscopically placed feeding tube or by a jejunostomy tube (Witzel or needle) have much the same effect on decreasing pancreatic secretions[61,102] as intravenous hyperalimentation and intestinal rest and can therefore be recommended.

CONCLUSION

Early provision of aggressive nutritional support is aimed at preventing the late mortality associated with trauma, sepsis, and multiple organ failure. Careful application of a specifically designed nutritional support regimen is geared to augment the metabolic response to injury, to provide substrates for acute-phase protein synthesis, to maximize immune function, and to potentiate wound healing, thereby improving survival. Although the techniques of nutritional support are individualized to meet fluid requirements and the metabolic rate of each patient, the benefits remain the same— to avoid the late and potentially lethal complications of sepsis and multiple organ failure.

PANCREATIC DISEASE

Pancreatic injury secondary to blunt or penetrating trauma has recognizably increased in the literature and is still fraught with serious

REFERENCES

1. Abbott WC, Echenique MM, Bistrian BR, et al: Nutritional care of the trauma patient. Surg Gynecol Obstet 157: 585, 1983
2. Alexander JW, McClellan MA, Ogle CK, et al: Consumptive opsoninopathy: possible pathogenesis in lethal and opportunistic infections. Ann Surg 184: 672, 1976

3. Alexander JW, Meakins JL: A physiological basis for the development of opportunistic infections in man. Ann Surg 176: 273, 1976

4. Alexander JW, Olge CK, Stennett JD, MacMilken BG: A sequential prospective analysis of immunologic abnormalities and infection following severe thermal injury. Ann Surg 182: 809, 1978

5. Allsop JA, Wolfe RR, Burke JF: Glucose kinetics and responsiveness to insulin in the rat injured by burn. Surg Gynecol Obstet 147: 565, 1978

6. Alvestrand A, Ahlberg M, Bergstrom J, et al: The effect of nutritional regimens on branched chain amino acid antagonism in uremia. p. 605. In Walser M, Williamson JR (eds): Metabolism and Clinical Implications of Branched Chain Amino and Keto Acids. Elsevier/North Holland, New York 1981

7. Anderson RJ: Nonoliguric acute renal failure. N Engl J Med 196: 1134, 1977

8. Askanazi J, Nordenstrom J, Rosenbaum SH, et al: Nutrition for the patient with respiratory failure: Glucose vs fat. Anesthesiology 54: 373, 1981

9. Askanazi J, Rosenbaum SH, Hyman AI, et al: Respiratory changes induced by the large glucose load of total parenteral nutrition. JAMA 243: 1980

10. Baker CC, Oppenheimer L, Stephens B, et al: Epidemiology of trauma deaths. Am J Surg 140: 144, 1980

11. Bassilii HR, Dietal M: Effect of nutritional support on weaning patients off of mechanical ventilators. JPEN 5: 161, 1981

12. Beisel WR, Edelman R, Nauso K, et al: Single nutrient effects on immunologic function. JAMA 245: 53–58, 1981

13. Bistrian BR: A simple technique to indicate the severity of stress. Surg Gynecol Obstet 148: 675, 1979

14. Bistrian BR: Assessment of protein energy malnutrition in surgical patients. p. 39. In Hill GL (ed): Nutrition and the Surgical Patient. Churchill Livingstone, Edinburgh, 1981

15. Blackburn GL, Bistrian BR: Nutritional care of injured and/or septic patient. Surg Clin North Am 56: 1195, 1976

16. Blackburn GL, Bistrian BR, Maini BS, et al: Nutritional and metabolic assessment of the hospitalized patient. JPEN 1: 11, 1977

17. Blackburn GL, Etter G, MacKenzie T: Criteria for choosing amino acid therapy in acute renal failure. Am J Clin Nutr 31: 1541, 1978

18. Blackburn GL, Flatt JP, Clowes GH, et al: Peripheral intravenous feeding with isotonic amino acids solutions. Am J Surg 125: 447, 1973

19. Blackburn GL, Flatt JP, Clowes GH, et al: Protein sparing therapy during periods of starvation with sepsis and trauma. Ann Surg 177: 588, 1973

20. Blackburn GL, Maini BS, Pierce Jr EC, et al: Nutrition in the critically ill patient. Anesthesiology 47: 181, 1977

21. Blackburn GL, Miller JDB, Bistrian BR, et al: Amino acids: Key nutrients in response to injury. In Richards J, Kinney J (eds) Nutritional Aspects of the Care of the Critically Ill. Churchill Livingstone, Edinburgh, 1977

22. Blackburn GL, Williams LF, Bistrian BR, et al: New approaches to the management of severe acute pancreatitis. Am J Surg 131: 114, 1976

23. Blimazes C, Kien CL, Rohrbaugh DK, et al: Quantitative contribution by skeletal muscle to elevated rates of whole body protein breakdown as measured by N-methyl histidine output. Metabolism 27: 671, 1978

24. Blumenkrantz MJ, Kopple JD, Moran JK, et al: Metabolic balance studies and dietary protein requirements in patients undergoing continuous ambulatory peritoneal dialysis. Kidney Int 21: 849, 1982

25. Blumenstock FA, Sabat M, Roccario E, et al: Opsonic fibronectin after trauma and particle injection determined by peritoneal macrophage monolayer assay. J Reticuloendothelial Soc 30: 61, 1981

26. Border JR, Chenia R, McMenamy RH, et al: Multiple systems organ failure: Muscle fuel deficit with protein malnutrition. Surg Clin North Am 56: 1147, 1976

27. Bothe A, Wade JE, Blackburn GL: Enteral nutrition: An overview. p. 76. In Hill GL (ed): Nutrition and the Surgical Patient. Churchill Livingstone, Edinburgh, 1981

28. Boulter PR, Spark RF, Acky RA: Effect of aldosterone blockade during fasting and refeeding. Am J Clin Nutr 26: 394, 1973

29. Bowers TK, O'Flaherty, Simmons RL, et al: Post surgical granulocyte dysfunction: Studies in healthy kidney donors. J Lab Clin Med 90: 720, 1977

30. Brikhan RH, Long CL, Fitkin D, et al: Effects of major skeletal trauma in whole body protein turnover in man measured by L-[1-14C]Leucine. Surgery 90: 294, 1980

31. Cannon WB: Bodily Changes in Pain, Hunger, Fear and Rage. Appleton, New York, 1929

32. Cerra FB, Mazuski JE, Chute E, et al: Branch chain metabolic support. Ann Surg 199: 286, 1984

33. Cerra FB, Upson D, Angelico R, et al: Branched chain support postoperative protein synthesis. Surgery 92: 192, 1982

34. Cobb ML, Cartmill AM, Gilsdorf RB: Early postoperative nutritional support using the serosal tunnel jejunostomy. JPEN 5: 397, 1981

35. Christou NV, Makin JL: Neutrophil adherence

and chemotaxis. Ann Surg 190: 557, 1979

36. Christov NV, Meakins JC: Neutrophil function in surgical patients. Two inhibitors of granulocyte chemotaxis associated with sepsis. J Surg Res 26: 355, 1979

37. Cuthbertson DP: The metabolic response to injury and its nutritional implications: Retrospect and prospect. JPEN 3: 108, 1979

38. Cuthbertson DP, Tilstone WJ: Metabolism suring the post injury period. Adv Clin Chem 12: 1, 1969

39. Danielson N, Arturson G, Wennberg L: Variations of metabolic rate in burned patients as a result of the injury and care. Burns 5: 169, 1978

40. Delany M, Carnevale N, Guavey JW, Moss CM: Postoperative nutritional support using needle catheter feeding jejunostomy. Ann Surg 186: 165, 1977

41. Desanto NG, Capodicasa G, Senatore T, et al: Glucose utilization from dialysate in patients on continuous ambulatory peritoneal dialysis. Int J Artif Organs 2: 119, 1979

42. Doekel RC, Zwillich CW, Scoggin CH: Clinical semistarvation; Depression of hypoxic ventilatory response. N Engl J Med 295: 358, 1976

43. Elwyn DH, Bryan-Brown CW, Shoemaker WC: Nutritional aspects of body water dislocation in postoperative and depleted patients. Ann Surg 182: 76, 1975

44. Elwyn DH, Parikh HC, Shoemaker WC: Amino acid movement between gut liver and periphery in unanaesthetized dogs. Am J Physiol 215: 1210, 1968

45. Evans C, Evams M, Pollock AV: The incidence and causes of postoperative jaundice, a prospective study. J Anesthesiol 46: 520, 1974

46. Faintuch J, Faintuch, JJ, Machado MCC, Raia AA: Anthropometric assessment of nutritional depletion after surgical injury. JPEN 3: 369, 1979

47. Feinstein EI, Blumenkrantz MJ, Mealy M, et al: Clinical and metabolic response to parenteral nutrition in acute renal failure. Medicine (Baltimore) 60: 124, 1981

48. Fischer JE, Baldessarini JR: False neurotransmitters and hepatic failure. Lancet 2: 75, 1971

49. Fischer JE, Funovics M, Aguire A, et al: The role of plasma amino acids in hepatic encephalopathy. Surgery 78: 276, 1975

50. Fischer JE, Rosen HM, Ebeid AM, et al: The effect of normalization of plasma amino acids on hepatic encephalopathy in man. Surgery 80: 77, 1976

51. Freeman JB, Egan MC, Willis BJ: The elemental diet. Surg Gyn Obstet 142: 925, 1976

52. Freund H, James JH, Fisher JE: Nitrogen sparing mechanisms of singly administered branch chain amino acids in the injured rat. Surgery 90: 237, 1981

53. Furst P, Anberg M, Bergstrom J: Principles of essential amino acid therapy in uremia. Am J Clin Nutr 21: 1744, 1978

54. Giordano C, Capodicasa G, Desanto NG: Artificial gut for total parenteral nutrition through the peritoneal cavity. Int J Artif Organs 3: 326, 1980

55. Goodgame JT, Fischer JE: Parenteral nutrition in the treatment of acute pancreatitis. Ann Surg 186: 651, 1977

56. Grant JP, Custer PB, Thurlow J: Current techniques of nutritional assessment. Surg Clin North Am 61: 434, 1981

57. Gump FE, Martin P, Kinney JM: Oxygen consumption and caloric expenditure in surgical patients. Surg Gyn Obstet 137: 499, 1973

58. Hamilton RF, Davis WC, Stephenson DV, McGee DF: Effects of parenteral hyperalimentation on upper gastrointestinal tract secretions. Arch Surg 102: 348, 1971

59. Heymsfeld SB, Betral RA, Ansley JD, et al. Enteral hyperalimentation; an alternative to central venous hyperalimentation. Ann Intern Med 90: 63, 1979

60. Hoover HC, Frant JP, Gorschboth C, et al: Nitrogen sparing intravenous fluids in postoperative patients. N Engl J Med 293: 172, 1975

61. Kamdar AV, Blumenkrantz MJ, Knutson DW, et al: Loss of serum protein during maintenance peritoneal dialysis. Kidney Inst 12: 483, 1973

62. Kelly GA, Nahrwold DL: Pancreatic secretion in response to an elemental diet and intravenous nutrition. Surg Gynecol Obstet 143: 87, 1976

63. Kinney JM: Energy expenditure and nutritional assessment. p. 21. In Levenson SM (ed): Nutritional Assessment: Present Status, Future Directions and Perspectives. Report of the Second Ross Conference on Medical Research. Ross Laboratories, Columbus Ohio, 1981

64. Kinney JM, Duke JH, Long C, et al: Carbohydrate and nitrogen metabolism after injury. J Clin Pathol 4: 65, 1970

65. Kopple JD, Swendseid ME, Shinberger JM, et al: The free and bound amino acids removed by hemodialysis. Trans Am Soc Artif Int Organs 19: 309, 1979

66. Kudsk KR, Ston JM, Sheldon GF: Nutrition in trauma and burns. Surg Clin North Am 61: 183, 1982

67. Law DK, Dudrick SJ, Abdou NI, et al: Immunocompetence of patients with protein calorie malnutrition. The effects of nutritional repletion. Ann Intern Med 79: 545, 1973

68. Lickley HLA, Tieck NS, Vranic M, Bury KD; Metabolic responses to enteral and parenteral nutrition. Am J Surg 135: 172, 1978

69. Maini BS, Blackburn GL, Bistrian BR, et al: Cyclic hyperalimentation, optimal technique for the preservation of visceral protein. J Surg Res 20: 515, 1976

70. McGhee A, Henderson JM, Millikan WJ Jr, et al: Comparison of the effects of hepatic-aid and a casein modular diet on encephalopathy, plasma amino acids and nitrogen balance in cirrhotic patients. Ann Surg 197: 42, 1983

71. McIrvine AJ, Mahony JB, Saporoschetz I, Mannick JA: Depressed immune response in burn patients. Ann Surg 196: 297, 1982

72. McIrvine AJ, Mannick JA: Lymphocyte function in the critically ill surgical patient. Surg Clin North Am 90: 245, 1983

73. Miller SE, Miller CL, Trunkey DD: The immune consequences if trauma. Surg Clin North Am 62: 167, 1982

74. Millikan WJ Jr, Henderson JM, Warren DW, et al: Total parenteral nutrition with F080ᴿ in cirrhotics with subclinical encephalopathy. Ann Surg 197: 295, 1983

75. Mitch WE: Amino acid analogues, metabolism and use in patients with chronic renal failure. p. 439. In Blackburn GL, Grant JP, Young VR (eds): Amino Acids, Metabolism and Medical Applications. John Wright, Boston, 1983

76. Moldawer LL, Echenique MM, Bistrian BR: The importance of study design to the demonstration of efficacy with branched chain amino acid enriched solutions. In Second Bermuda Symposium on Total Parenteral Nutrition. Plenum Press, New York, 1982

77. Moldawer LL, Sakamoto S, Blackburn GL, Bistrian BR: Alterations in protein kinetics produced by branched chain amino acid administration during infection and inflammation. p. 533. In Walser W, Williamson JR (eds): Metabolism and Clinical Implications of Branched Chain Amino and Ketoacids. Elsevier/North Holland, Amsterdam, 1981

78. Moore FD: Metabolic Care of the Surgical Patient. WB Saunders, Philadelphia, 1959

79. Moore FD, Brennan MG: Surgical injury: Body composition, protein metabolism, and neuroendocrinology. p. 169. In Ballinger WF (ed): Manual of Surgical Nutrition. American College of Surgeons–SB Saunders, Philadelphia, 1975

80. Mullin TJ, Kirpatrick JR: The effect of nutritional support on immune competence in patients suffering from trauma, sepsis or malignant disease. Surgery 90: 610, 1981

81. Mullen JL, Buzby GP, Matthews DC, et al: Reduction of operative morbidity and mortality by combined preoperative and postoperative nutritional support. Ann Surg 192: 604, 1980

82. Munro HN: Metabolic integration of organs in health and disease. JPEN 6: 271, 1982

83. Munster AM: Post-traumatic immunosuppression is due to activation of suppressor T-cells. Lancet 1: 1329, 1976

84. Murciano D, Aubier M, Lecolguic Y, Pariente R: Effects of theophylline on diaphragmatic strength and fatigue in patients with chronic obstructive pulmonary disease. N Engl J Med 311: 349, 1984

85. Newman JH, Neff TA, Ziporin P: Acute respiratory failure associated with hypophosphatemia. N Engl J Med 296: 1101, 1977

86. Norgenstern L. Postoperative jaundice; an approach to a diagnostic dilemma. Am J Surg 128: 255, 1974

87. Padberg FT, Ruggerrio J, Blackburn GL, Bistrian BR: Central venous catheterization for parenteral nutrition. Ann Surg 193: 264, 1981

88. Page CP, Carlton PK, Androssy RJ, et al: Safe, cost effective postoperative nutrition. Am J Surg 138: 940, 1979

89. Piccone VA, Leveen HH, Gloss P, et al: Prehepatic hyperalimentation. Surgery 87: 263, 1980

90. Ragins H, Levenson SM, Signer R, et al: Intrajejunal administration of an elemental diet at neutral pH avoids pancreatic stimulation. Am J Surg 126: 606, 1973

91. Rossmer S, Johansson C, Walldivs G, Aly A: Intralipid clearance and lipoprotein pattern in men with advanced alcoholic liver cirrhosis. Am J Clin Nutr 32: 2022, 1979

92. Rudman D, Kutner M, Ansley JD, et al: Hypertyrosinemia, hypocysteinemia and failure to retain nitrogen during total parenteral nutrition of cirrhotic patients. Gastroenterology 81: 1025, 1981

93. Rutten P, Blackburn GL, Flatt JP, et al: Determination of optimal hyperalimentation infusion rates. J Surg Res 18: 477, 1975

94. Schopfer K, Douglas SD: Neutrophil function in children with kwashiorkor. J Lab Clin Med 88: 450, 1976

95. Scovill WA, Annest ST, Saba TM, et al: Cardiovascular hemodynamic after opsonic alpha-2-surface binding glycoprotein therapy in injury patients. Surgery 86: 284, 1979

96. Sewitt S: Preview of the complications of burns, their origin and importance for illness and death. J Trauma 19: 358, 1979

97. Shizgal HM, Solomon S, Gutelius JR: Body water distribution after operation. Surg Gynecol Obstet 144: 35, 1977

98. Silverberg E: Cancer statistics. CA 29: 6, 1979

99. Blackburn GL, Sobrado J, Moldawer LL: Immunological abnormalities in the malnourished trauma patient. Infect Surg 9, 1983

100. VanDijk WC, Verbough HA, VanRijswijk REN, et al: Neutrophil function, serum opsonic activ-

ity and delayed hypersensitivity in surgical patients. Surgery 92: 21, 1982

101. VanThiel, DH, Lester R: Postoperative jaundice. Surg Clin North Am 55: 409, 1977

102. Voitk A, Brown RA, Echave U, et al: Use of an elemental diet in the treatment of complicated pancreatitis. Am J Surg 125: 223, 1973

103. Walser M: Urea cycle disorders and other hyperammonemic syndromes. p. 402. In Stanbury J, Wyngaorden JB, Frederickson DS, Goldstein JL, Brown MS (eds): The Metabolic Basis of Inherited Diseases. McGraw-Hill, New York, 1983

104. Wartlow JC, Jackson AA: Nutrition and protein turnover in man. Br Med Bull 37: 5, 1981

105. Weissman C, Askanazi J, Rosenbaum S, et al: Amino acids and respiration. Ann Intern Med 98: 41, 1983

106. Willmore DW, Long JA, Skreen R, et al: Catecholamines: Mediator of the hypermetabolic response following thermal injury. Ann Surg 180: 653, 1974

107. Wolfe RR, Allsop JR, Burke JF: Glucose metabolism in man: Responses to intravenous glucose infusion. Metabolism 28: 210, 1979

108. Wolfson M, Jones MR, Kopple JD: Amino acid losses during hemodialysis with infusion of amino acids and glucise. Kidney Int 21: 500, 1982

109. Young VR, Munro HN: N^t-methylhistidine (3-methylhistidine) and muscle protein turnover: An overview. Fed Proc 37: 2291, 1978

SECTION VI

THE ADULT RESPIRATORY DISTRESS SYNDROME

18

Humoral Mediators in Adult Respiratory Distress Syndrome

Herbert B. Hechtman
Shlomo Lelcuk
Frederick Alexander
David Shepro

INTRODUCTION

The principal function of the lungs is respiratory gas exchange, that is, the uptake of oxygen and excretion of carbon dioxide. Proper performance of this task requires that the entire cardiac output (CO) pass through the pulmonary vasculature and be distributed in a manner to match ventilation. Total blood flow must be sufficient to provide oxygen delivery to satisfy the body's metabolic requirements.

The lungs are richly endowed with smooth muscle surrounding the pulmonary vasculature and bronchi. This muscle is under neural control as well as under the control of circulating and locally produced humoral mediators. Variations in muscle tone induced by these mediators regulate perfusion and ventilation. These modifications in tone are frequent and have as their purpose the efficient uptake of oxygen and excretion of carbon dioxide.

It is the purpose of this chapter to review metabolic functions of circulating cells and the lungs themselves, which might give rise to vasoactive metabolites, directly or indirectly influencing the fine coordination of ventilation with perfusion. Second, since several of the vasoactive agents may be vasotoxic as well, the relationship of these metabolic events to the development of permeability or high protein pulmonary edema is discussed.

PLATELETS AND SEROTONIN RELEASE

Platelet activation can lead to release of the vasoactive amine serotonin, 5-hydroxytryptamine (5-HT). Experimentally, an intravenous infusion of 5-HT into a dog causes constriction of peripheral airways[23]. The resultant physiologic defect is a fall in lung compliance, that is, a rise in inspiratory pressure at fixed tidal volume. Surprisingly, there is little change in measured airways resistance, probably because of the peripheral nature of the airways constriction. This closure of bronchi leads to regions of the lungs that are poorly ventilated, accounting for the prominence of hypoxia. In addition, 5-HT causes pulmonary arteriolar constriction and pulmonary hypertension.

An intravascular clot in the form of a pulmonary embolism activates platelets[30]. The mechanism is via thrombin stimulation of platelet surface receptors. Platelets may then cause clot propagation. The entrapment and activation of platelets in the lungs following embolization set the stage for the release and local action of 5-HT. The salutary effects of heparin after embolization may in part be related to prevention of this platelet entrapment and 5-HT release.

Platelets need not aggregate or be entrapped in the lungs to undergo 5-HT release. After experimental pulmonary embolization, 5-HT levels in circulating platelets declined 36 percent[15]. Similar findings of activation of circulating platelets evidenced by 5-HT release have been noted after experimental acid aspiration[10] and experimental endotoxemia[14]. Our clinical experience substantiates these observations. Early in the course of acute respiratory failure (ARF) associated with a variety of illnesses, such as sepsis and aspiration, platelets are activated in the lungs and perhaps elsewhere to release 5HT. A variety of stresses that predispose to the development of ARF lead to platelet entrapment and 5-HT release. It is likely that this amine leads directly to smooth muscle constriction around the pulmonary vasculature and bronchi. Evidence to support this hypothesis is largely based on the use of antagonists to 5-HT. Currently, the most selective agent is ketanserin, a 5-HT receptor inhibitor that acts principally on S_2 sites located in blood vessels, bronchi, and platelets. The drug also exhibits moderate α-antagonism.

After pulmonary embolism, mechanical obstruction of the pulmonary vasculature occurs with resultant pulmonary hypertension. That the increase in pulmonary arterial pressure is due in part to a vasospastic component can be seen by the significant reduction in the mean pulmonary arterial pressure (MPAP) following ketanserin therapy as compared with untreated control animals (Fig. 18-1).

Embolization also leads to hypoxemia, an event not readily explained by simple obstruction of the pulmonary vasculature. Bronchoconstriction with diminished alveolar ventilation to perfused, nonembolized lung regions is the most logical explanation of the defect in oxygenation. The importance of 5-HT in experimental embolization is shown by the ability of ketanserin to reverse physiologic shunting completely (Fig. 18-2). Restoration of arterial oxygenation to baseline conditions by 5-HT inhibition emphasizes the fact that simple mechanical obstruction by the embolus is not responsible for the hypoxia.

OXYGENATION PRODUCTS OF ARACHIDONIC ACID

Phospholipase A_2

Platelet activation by pulmonary emboli or other intravascular clot leads not only to 5-HT release but to stimulation of the arachidonic acid cascade as well (Fig. 18-3). One of the major rate-limiting steps of this metabolic sequence is cleavage of arachidonic acid from its esterified form in the cell membrane by phospholipase A_2, a step requiring Ca^{++}. It has been postulated that the calcium-binding protein calmodulin exerts some regulatory control by stimulation of calcium transport.

A variety of drugs are inhibitory to phospholipase A_2, the most important of the enzymes that cleave the phospholipids. Such agents include bromophenacylbromide, mepacine, chlorpromazine, indomethacin, imipramine, and propanolol[3]. They act in a variety of ways: (1) directly on the enzyme; (2) by interfering with binding of the substrate; or (3) by interfering with Ca^{++} binding. Another class

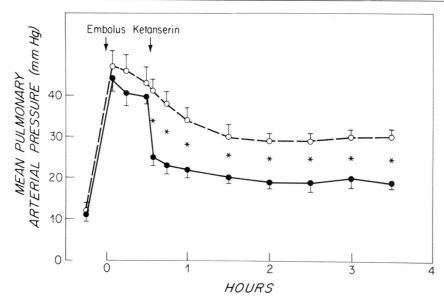

FIG. 18-1 Embolization leading to obstruction of the pulmonary vascular bed with pulmonary hypertension. The importance of 5-HT-induced vasospasm is illustrated by the reduction in mean pulmonary arterial pressure after infusion of the 5-HT receptor antagonist ketanserin. (○--○) control; (•—•) ketanserin; (⊥) SEM. (Huval WV, Lelcuk S, Allen PD et al: Determinants of cardiovascular stability during abdominal aortic aneurysmectomy. Ann Surg 199: 216, 1984.)

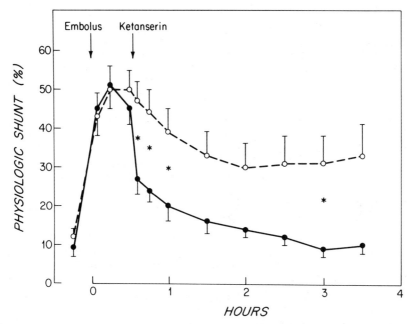

FIG. 18-2 Hypoxemia and increased physiologic shunt after embolization indirectly related to the clot. Platelet 5-HT-induced bronchospasm has been postulated to be of importance. The ability of ketanserin to reverse physiologic shunting is strong support for this thesis. (○--○) control; (•—•) ketanserin; (⊥) SEM. (Huval WV, Lelcuk S, Allen PD et al: Determinants of cardiovascular stability during abdominal aortic aneurysmectomy. Ann Surg 199: 216, 1984.)

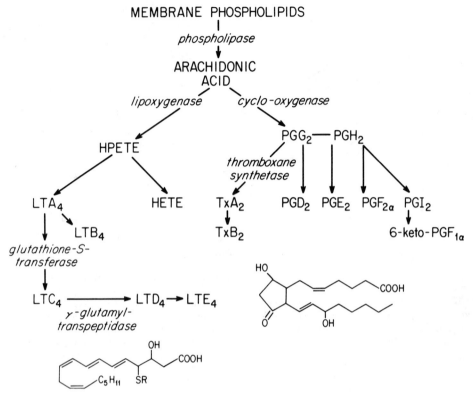

FIG. 18-3 Membrane-derived arachidonic acid processed to a variety of cyclo-oxygenase derivatives, such as thromboxane A_2 and PGI_2. The end product depends on cell type. Leukotrienes (LT) C, D, and E are the prominent spasminogens resulting from 5-lipoxygenase activity. HETE, hydroxyeicosatetraenoic acid; HPETE, hydroperoxyeicosatetraenoic acid. (Hechtman HB, Huval WB, Mathieson MA: Prostaglandin and thromboxane mediation of cardioplumonary failure. Surg Clin NA 63: 263, 1983. Reprinted with permission from WB Saunders Co., Philadelphia.)

of anti-inflammatory agents, the steroids, exert their effects by inducing synthesis of proteins that possess antiphospholipase properties.

Products of Cyclo-oxygenation

Two of the most potent agents that regulate platelet aggregation and thrombosis are thromboxane (Tx)A_2 and prostacyclin (PGI_2). These prostanoids are produced by the oxidation of arachidonic acid by cyclo-oxygenase to form endoperoxides, followed by the action of selective synthetases. In platelets, leukocytes, and the media and adventitia of blood vessels and lung fibroblasts, the endoperoxide

PGH_2 is converted by Tx synthetase to TxA_2. By contrast, endothelium possesses PGI_2 synthetase; PGI_2 is the product of the arachidonic acid cascade in these cells.

In normal settings, cyclo-oxygenase activity tends to be limited both by the availability of the arachidonic acid substrate in a nonesterified form and by the presence of a lipid peroxide activator[40]. Hydroperoxides such as 15-hydroperoxyeicosatetranoic acid (15-HPETE) or PGG_2 at low concentrations of less than 1 μmol/L are potent activators of arachidonic acid oxygenation. At concentrations greater than 1 μmol/L, they are effective inhibitors of prostacyclin synthetase while still stimulating cyclo-oxygenase. Thus, lipid hydroperoxides are necessary to activate cyclo-oxygenase to convert arachidonic acid to PGH_2. At low concentration, PGI_2 synthesis is not impeded, while at high hydroperoxide concentrations, PGH_2 is directed to TxA_2 synthesis. It is likely that the antioxidants and tissue peroxidases tend to keep the hydroperoxide concentration below micromolar levels, thereby determining the ratio of PGI_2/TxA_2 production. Increased levels of TxA_2 relative to PGI_2 will generally leads to a positive feedback because of enhanced platelet aggregation and migration of peroxide, producing leukocytes into the TxA_2-forming region. This cycle is hypothesized to underlie arteriosclerosis.

Lipoxygenation

Arachidonic acid may be metabolized by lipoxygenases to generate hydroperoxy derivatives. The lipoxygenases are a group of iron-containing dioxygenases that have achieved considerable attention during the last few years because of the ability of 5-lipoxygenase to lead to the formation of leukotrienes (LT), a family of biologically active substances. Initial steps of hydroperoxidation lead to the generation of a peroxy radical[33]. This is simlar to oxidizing intermediaries formed early in the cyclo-oxygenase reaction[2]. If uncontrolled, these highly reactive radicals may cause cell injury. The experimental use of antioxidants in the setting of leukocyte activation may result in cytoprotection not only because such treatment scavenges free radicals but possibly because these agents prevent formation of oxygenation products of arachidonic acid as well.

The first hydroperoxy product of lipoxygenase, HPETE, is rapidly reduced to HETE or converted to LTA_4 (Fig. 18-3). HETE is chemotactic. It also may help regulate cyclo-oxygenase and PGI_2 synthetase activities. Its physiologic role still remains to be defined. A product of major importance is LTB_4. This agent is equal to C5a and platelet activating factor in chemotactic ability and is more than 100 times as potent as HETE. It is a potent white blood cell (WBC), but not platelet, aggregator. Furthermore, LTB_4 activates WBCs to degranulate and to release lysosomal enzymes and oxygen-free radicals[25]. In parallel with its ability to stimulate accumulation of WBCs,

LTB_4 leads to increase in peripheral vascular permeability in a variety of experimental animals. When stimulated, polymorphonuclear leukocytes are themselves a rich source of LTB_4. More than 95 percent of WBC biologic activity after exposure to a calcium ionophore relates to LTB_4. Finally, LTB_4 contracts guinea pig lung parenchymal strips at doses as low as 10^{-12} M, an event attributable to the induction of TxA_2 synthesis.[25]

LTA_4 can be hydrolyzed enzymatically to produce LTB_4 or with glutathione transferase to form LTC_4. Furthermore, action of α-glutamyltransferase splits off an amino acid residue to form LTD_4. Loss of one more amino acid residue, cysteine, leads to LTE_4. These LT are formed by leukocytes as well as lung tissue. Indeed, the first demonstration of these substances was in 1938 when Feldberg and Kellaway[8] noted that lungs perfused with snake venom, rich in phospholipase A_2, led to the generation of slow-reacting substances now known as LT.

Leukotrienes display a marked action on smooth muscle, being thousands of times more active than histamine. The potency is in the order LTD_4, LTC_4, and LTE_4. The smooth muscle effect has been observed in a variety of bioassay preparations, including stomach, ileum, and bronchus. LTC_4 and LTD_4 have a selective action on the small airways of the lung and cause a reduction in compliance that is long lasting. The prolonged duration of the LT effects resembles that observed in asthma. LT activity is probably modulated by vasodilator prostaglandins, since indomethacin has been reported to potentiate the constrictive response to LTC_4 of bronchioles markedly[20].

Leukotrienes are at least 1,000 times as potent as histamine in causing plasma leakage after intradermal injection. Again, LTC_4 and LTD_4 are more potent than LTE_4. LTB_4 is less active in provoking permeability and does so at least in part because of its chemoattraction of leukocytes. Intravenous injection of LTC_4 results in a vasoconstrictive pulmonary response, but there is no evidence of increased permeability in the lungs. It is possible that the route of administration determines the biologic effect and that the pulmonary interstitial introduction or generation of LT may lead to increased permeability.

Prostacyclin

This potent vasodilator and antiaggregator is thought to function locally under physiologic conditions, since its concentration in plasma is below 2 pg/ml. The lowest concentration of PGI_2 that produces measurable effects on adenosine diphosphate (ADP)-induced platelet aggregation in vitro is 100 to 200 pg/ml. Vasodilation manifest by facial flush is seen at a PGI_2 level of about 200 pg/ml. At a concentration of 800 pg/ml, diastolic pressure is reduced by about 15 mmHg.

Prostacyclin production by endothelium can be stimulated by a variety of techniques, such as infusion of hypertonic dextrose, venous distention, or thrombin from an intravascular clot. An important physiologic regulatory mechanism is angiotensin stimulation. Platelets produce TxA_2 but also have the ability to control local PGI_2 synthesis via the secretion of platelet-derived growth factor, an event amplified by 5-HT[6]. It is possible that the circulating plasma agent that has been described as stimulating PGI_2 synthesis is also platelet-derived growth factor. The clinical importance of a circulating stimulus to PGI_2 synthesis becomes apparent during surgery. Within 10 to 30 minutes of surgical incision, a prominent rise in levels of 6-keto-$PGF_{1\alpha}$, the stable hydrolysis product of PGI_2, to levels above 400 pg/mg is noted and is associated with a modest but significant decrease in systemic blood pressure compared with aspirin-treated patients.[35] Transpulmonary assay of 6-keto-$PGF_{1\alpha}$ just after surgical incision shows that arterial values are higher than those in pulmonary arterial blood, indicating that the lungs are a principal source of this prostaglandin.[13]

On a theoretical basis, the antiaggregating properties of PGI_2 may serve as a useful therapeutic adjunct in settings in which platelet and/or leukocyte activation occurs. Unfortunately, no convincing patient studies exist to document a unique benefit of PGI_2 aside from vasodilation and afterload reduction in such conditions as angina, peripheral vascular disease, or thrombotic thrombocytopenic purpura. There is a diversity of opinion regarding the benefits of PGI_2 in the setting of cardiopulmonary bypass. Our own experience in a prospective study of 50 patients indicates that in doses of 25 ng/kg/min, which produces severe hypotension, there is a failure to maintain the platelet count or suppress TxA_2 synthesis. Indeed, in several canine models, PGI_2 appears to cause a paradoxical rise in Tx. This was seen during perfusion of an isolated lung lobe[19] and during experimental cardiopulmonary bypass surgery.[1] Furthermore, PGI_2 infusions after experimental acid aspiration were found to lead to a sustained rise in TxB_2 in contrast to a decrease in TxB_2 in untreated controls.[37] These increases in Tx levels are not innocuous and are associated with decreases in myocardial performance and increases in microvascular permeability.

In addition, to its antiaggregating and vasodilating abilities, PGI_2 possesses other properties that may be beneficial. After experimental pulmonary embolism in dogs, an infusion of PGI_2 led to a significant reduction in pulmonary hypertension, as well as to reversal of physiologic shunting. PGI_2 is not known to vasodilate the pulmonary vasculature selectively, although the effects of PGI_2 were much more prominent than those of PGE_1 or nitroprusside. The beneficial effect of PGI_2 was subsequently related to its ability to inhibit the transport of 5-HT across the endothelium and to stimulate platelet 5-HT uptake.[38] It is likely that this was the mechanism whereby PGI_2 reversed 5-HT-induced bronchoconstriction and physiologic shunting.

Another unique feature of PGI_2 is its ability to induce primary fibrinolytic activity, that is, to stimulate the release of plasminogen activator. In the presence of intravascular clot, PGI_2 leads to accelerated clot lysis. All these separate functions of PGI_2 act to enhance flow in the microvasculature. Finally, in other studies, PGI_2 has been shown to have various therapeutic advantages in animals given lethal endotoxin infusions.[17] Its mechanism of action in this setting is unknown.

Thromboxane

Platelet activation is probably one of the most common events leading to TxA_2 synthesis. Agents that activate platelets include thrombin, adenosine diphosphate, epinephrine, collagen fibrils exposed by endothelial cell damage, and foreign surfaces. These agents will trigger arachidonic acid mobilization in platelets with subsequent synthesis of TxA_2. Two other agents may be important, depending on the clinical setting: (1) platelet activating factor (PAF), which has a rich source in the alveolar macrophage, and (2) an intermediary LT, formed via the lipoxygenase pathway in many cells, including circulating leukocytes and lung mast cells.

PAF is itself a potent smooth muscle constrictor, an inducer of increased permeability, and a strong chemoattractant. PAF not only stimulates platelets but also serves as a potent activator of WBCs. Because alveolar macrophages are so prominent in the synthesis of PAF and are located in contact with the airways, it is possible that PAF has a local pulmonary homeostatic function. For example, in pathologic settings, such as acid aspiration, secretion of PAF may stimulate lung interstitial cells to form chemoattractants such as LTB_4. These agents may then act together with PAF to activate circulating platelets and WBCs. The net effect is the recruitment of an inflammatory reaction.

Leukotrienes can be potent constrictors of bronchial smooth muscle, but their mechanism of action varies according to the route of administration. When given intravenously to anesthetized guinea pigs, LTC_4 or LTC_4 causes bronchoconstriction that is slow in onset, long lasting, and inhibited by indomethacin.[24] However, aerosol administration of LT induces bronchoconstriction that is not reversed by indomethacin. In perfused guinea pig lungs, LTC_4, LTD_4, and LTE_4 cause release of TxA_2. The involvement of TxA_2 in LT-induced responses does not occur in human bronchial strips or in rabbit or human parenchyma. Species specificity appears to be a likely determinant of the LT effect in addition to the technique of LT application. The ultimate role of TxA_2 as an intermediary in determining both the vasospasticity and bronchospasticity of LT remains to be defined.

One of the most common clinical events, aside from intravascular thromboembolism, that stimulates Tx synthesis is ischemia. Abdominal aortic clamping during aneurysm surgery leads to pulmonary production of TxA_2. After 30 minutes, TxB_2 values have risen from 89 to 193 pg/ml.[13,35] Apparently, platelets are not activated by lower torso ischemia and do not increase their Tx synthesis. The mechanism whereby the lungs are stimulated by hypoxia to generate Tx is unknown.

Application of a tourniquet to the arm for 10 minutes produces a doubling of TxB_2 levels. Similarly, clamping the femoral artery during peripheral vascular surgery results in elevation in plasma Tx concentration. Ischemic tissues in these settings appear to be largely responsible for the Tx synthesis. The metabolic function of the lungs was not measured in these studies. Similarly, coronary sinus blood has been found to be rich in TxB_2 after pacing-induced anginal episodes in human subjects.

The local sources of Tx synthesis after ischemia may be the media and adventitia of blood vessels, as well as parenchymal cells.[26] If localized ischemia induces Tx synthesis, it might be anticipated that a generalized ischemic stress, such as that accompanying major hemorrhage, should do the same. However, after hemorrhagic hypotension in sheep to 50 mmHg for more than 1 hour, there was simply a doubling of plasma and lymph values of TxB_2. It appears that hypotension with severe flow restriction is only a modest stimulus. Complete flow restriction to an extremity for the same period of time resulted in a rise in plasma TxB_2 concentrations to 1,000 pg/ml.[19a]

Thrombin infusions were used experimentally in sheep to mimic intravascular clotting. Platelets and WBCs were thus activated, causing thrombocytopenia and leukopenia. After an intravenous infusion of thrombin in sheep, TxB_2 concentrations rose to 1,400 pg/ml.[31] Arterial Tx levels were higher than pulmonary arterial blood, indicating a pulmonary source. The fact that lymph TxB_2 levels did not rise strongly suggests that entrapped platelet and WBC microaggregates and not the pulmonary interstitium were responsible for TxB_2 synthesis. In association with the rise in TxB_2 levels, lymph flow and protein content rose, indicating enhanced permeability. Inhibition of Tx synthetase with dazoxiben prevented the rise in TxB_2 as well as the leukopenia and increased permeability, but not the thrombocytopenia. These data suggest a central permeability role for both Tx and WBCs.

A simple rise in Tx levels does not cause permeability; WBC involvement appears necessary. Thus, there is an absence of heightened permeability after experimentally induced pulmonary embolism, even though TxB_2 values rise from 100 to 500 pg/ml.[34] It appears that WBCs are not activated in this setting, since neither leukopenia nor lung entrapment occurs. This finding is in contrast to experimentally induced microembolism caused by small beads, which leads to pulmonary leukosequestration and edema.[9] The mechanism whereby differential activation of WBCs and platelets occurs is unknown. The involvement of Tx, particularly in WBC-mediated inflammatory events, appears likely.

The sequence and dependence of Tx synthesis and WBC-mediated edema remain unclear. Thus, minutes after experimental infusion of endotoxin, thrombocytopenia and leukopenia occur with pulmonary entrapment of platelet and WBC macroaggregates. At the same time, plasma levels of TxB_2 reach 750 pg/ml.[16] In this setting, Tx is responsible for pulmonary hypertension, which rapidly develops during the first several minutes after administration of endotoxin. Use of a selective Tx synthetase inhibitor prevents the rise in TxB_2 as well as the pulmonary hypertension. However, the development of protein-rich edema several hours after endotoxemia is not altered by inhibiting Tx synthesis. It is quite possible that in this setting WBCs have been activated by events that also led to Tx synthesis, such as the complement cascade. Therapy of experimentally induced endotoxemia with PGI_2 is effective, even though TxB_2 levels and the initial WBC entrapment in the lungs are scarcely altered. By contrast, aspirin reduces Tx values but does not reverse the lethal effects of endotoxin.[18]

Whether endotoxin leads to the initial platelet and WBC sequestration by means of complement activation with generation of the fragment C5a is debatable. Other methods of complement activation, such as the experimental infusion of zymosan-activated plasma, lead to selective activation and pulmonary entrapment of WBCs and not of platelets. In sheep, the infusion of zymosan-activated plasma results in a rise in TxB_2 and pulmonary hyperten-

sion as well as evidence of increased permeability of the lungs. Pretreatment with imidazole inhibits Tx synthesis and attenuates the pulmonary hypertension. Thus, the increased microvascular permeability, but not the WBC entrapment, is prevented.[28]

We interpret these observations as indicating that Tx synthesis and/or WBC entrapment are often, but not necessarily, related. Second, WBC entrapment appears to be a requisite for enhanced microvascular permeability, but another event must also occur to activate these cells to release permeability factors. It is likely that the many stimuli to arachidonic acid metabolism also stimulate mechanisms that influence WBC chemotaxins, intravascular aggregation, and activation. Synergism of TxA_2 with WBC events is likely but does not appear to be necessary for the expression of permeability.

LEUKOCYTES

WBCs are capable of generating three classes of agents that can injure the pulmonary microvasculature: (1) the oxygenation products of arachidonic acid, which have already been described; (2) neutral proteases, particularly elastolytic proteases, which have been shown to be particularly toxic; the elastases are normally held in check by naturally occurring protease inhibitors; and (3) oxygen free radicals, which are now appreciated to have a fundamental role in cellular injury.

Proteases are often considered important as direct or indirect mediators of acute lung damage. Thus, complement, especially C5a, is thought to act via neutrophil aggregation or by directly injuring the microvasculature.[7] The intermediary role of WBCs in C5a, endotoxin, acid aspiration, and other events that trigger ARF is probably of importance.[11] When activated, a variety of plasma factors may lead to permeability. Contact activation of Hageman factor (HF) yields a product (HFa) that converts prekallikrein to kallikrein, which in turn can activate WBCs[27] or lead to plasmin generation and release of a potential permeability factor, bradykinin, from high-molecular-weight kininogen. HFa itself will promote vascular permeability in quantities as low as 3 ng, which is 1/10,000th the amount of HF present in 1 ml plasma.[22]

Proteases can injure lung tissues by direct action on the vascular basement membranes, elastin, collagen, or structural elements of the pulmonary tissues. Elastase can cause permeability either directly or by activating components of the contact and/or complement systems. The importance of leukocyte elastase in ARF is now appreciated. For example, bronchoalveolar lavage fluid from patients with ARF usually contains elastase activity.[22] If the lavage fluid does not exhibit free enzyme, an inhibitor of elastase, either α_1-antiproteinase inhibitor or α_2-microglobulin, is demonstrable.

The extracellular space contains high concentrations of proteinase inhibitors that normally prevent tissue damage by released leukocyte proteinases. In order for proteolytic injury to be produced by elastase, either the quantity of proteinase present must exceed the proteinase-inhibitor capacity or effectiveness, or the inhibitors must be impaired. Evidence from several laboratories indicates that the elastase inhibitory capacity of α_1-proteinase inhibitor is lost when this inhibitor is exposed to oxidants such as those that might originate from WBCs.[21] This opinion is not shared by everyone.[4]

Activated neutrophils may not only release proteolytic activity but may generate oxygen metabolites, including superoxide (O_2^-) and H_2O_2 as well. The experimental infusion of cobra venom factor activates the complement system and neutrophils. These WBCs are then sequestered in the pulmonary capillary bed. Subsequent vascular injury may be prevented by infusing superoxide dismutase (SOD) and catalase, providing strong evidence that production of O_2^- and H_2O_2 is related to vascular injury.[32] SOD is the primary defense against O_2^- and very efficiently catalyzes the reaction

$$O_2^- + O_2^- + 2\,H^+ \rightarrow H_2O_2 + O_2$$

Some investigators postulate that damage by free radicals may relate not only to the generation of oxygen radicals but to inadequate levels of SOD as well. Other free radicals and their inhibitors also play a role. Thus, in the absence of catalase, H_2O_2 may be reduced to the hydroxyl radical (OH $\cdot$), a very reactive species that may be neutralized by antioxidants such as dimethylsulfoxide. Despite clear evidence that these free radicals may themselves be very toxic, it is still not certain whether treatment with antioxidants exerts salutary effects directly or indirectly by inhibiting formation of vasotoxic oxygenation products of arachidonic acid.

The lungs contain abundant numbers of mast cells. These cells are LT factories that may be triggered by events such as immunologic reactions and probably by alveolar macrophage-generated PAF as well. It is likely that the oxygenation products of arachidonic acid may themselves induce severe vasoconstriction and bronchoconstriction and increased microvascular permeability. In addition, the chemotactic abilities of LTB_4 and PAF will recruit circulating WBCs into the lungs. An inflammatory response follows that, if sufficiently intense, can obscure the initiating agent. This is probably the reason why the final pulmonary pathologic picture of patients with ARF is seldom diagnostically specific. It is likely that a number of events associated with ARF activate the arachidonic acid cascade in pulmonary parenchymal cells. Likely stimuli are acid aspiration, smoke inhalation, pulmonary contusion, bacterial or viral pneumonias, and fat microembolism.

The fact that the lungs contain the capillary bed draining systemic organs means that circulating agents and cells stimulated by systemic events will first contact the pulmonary vasculature. A vascular–humoral mechanism is proposed to explain the frequency of ARF in association with severe systemic disease. Thus, a transfusion reaction is likely to lead to the release of complement fragment C5a. This fragment can lead to intravascular aggregation of WBCs and their mechanical sieving by the lungs. In addition, C5a will activate WBCs so that toxic products may be released in the pulmonary microvasculature and cause increased vasomotor and bronchomotor tone, as well as protein-rich edema. Although complement is an attractive mechanism, its role is difficult to prove.[28] Thus, assays of circulating levels of C5a fail to predict the development of, or relate to, the severity of ARF. However, the thesis that an aggregator or activator of WBCs, released by one or more systemic organs, may trigger an intense and generalized inflammatory response in the lungs is attractive. Other initiating agents that might gain access to the vasculature include the arachidonic acid products TxA_2 and LT, as well as PAF. Such agents may mediate the ARF associated with systemic sepsis, bowel infarction, or pancreatitis.

ACID ASPIRATION

Major aspiration of gastric contents is lethal. The incidence of aspiration is probably high. However, most episodes are likely to involve small volumes of acid and to be subclinical. For example, despite intubation with a cuffed endotracheal tube, most patients have pharyngeal secretions appear in the tracheal aspirate.[5.]

Experimental acid aspiration has been a convenient preparation to study the evolution of ARF. Within 5 to 10 minutes after aspiration of 3 ml/kg 0.1 N HCl in dogs, platelets are entrapped in the lungs and are an important source of the elevated TxB_2 concentrations.[36] Lung parenchyma may also be an early source of this prostanoid. Pulmonary hypertension gradually develops. The slowly developed and prolonged increase in pulmonary pressure suggests that TxA_2, an agent with a 30-second half-life, is not the responsible mediator. Indeed, cyclo-oxygenase and Tx synthetase inhibitors do not alter the pulmonary hypertension.

Minutes after acid aspiration, severe thrombocytopenia develops in association with platelet aggregates observed in smears of peripheral blood (Fig. 18-4). Platelet aggrega-

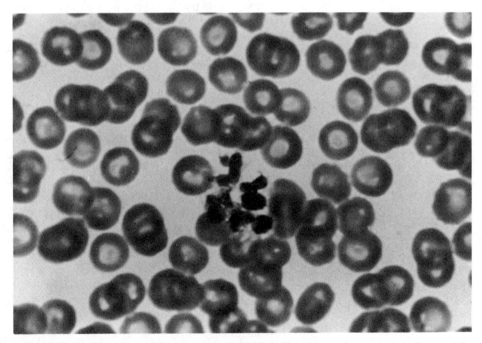

FIG. 18-4 Peripheral blood smear showing frequent platelet microaggregates, 5 minutes after experimental aspiration of one lung. Systemic response to localized injury is illustrated. Within 30 minutes, the aggregates are no longer noted, and the severe thrombocytopenia is slowly being reversed.

tion and entrapment are temporary and, within 30 to 60 minutes, the platelet count is restored almost to normal. These platelets show evidence of activation in that they have been stimulated to synthesize TxA_2. Furthermore, platelet 5-HT levels decrease from 2.09 to 0.82 $\mu g/10^9$ platelets, indicating release (unpublished data). Although the initial lung injury following aspiration may be primarily to bronchi, the early transpulmonary entrapment of platelets and later, after 1 to 2 hours of WBCs, indicates involvement of the capillary–alveolar regions. Furthermore, the pulmonary edema that develops in association with WBC entrapment is sensitive to variations in the perfusion pressure of the pulmonary vascular bed. Thus, either nitroprusside or the 5-HT receptor antagonist, ketanserin, will reduce the pulmonary perfusion pressure, an event that is directly related to the volume of edema fluid formed (Fig. 18-5). The fact that ketanserin reduces pulmonary hypertension so effectively while minimally lowering systemic pressure, in contrast to the effect of nitroprusside indicates that 5-HT is an important, if not principal, mediator of the increase in pulmonary arterial pressure.

The improvement in oxygenation with ketanserin is probably largely due to the reduction in the volume of pulmonary edema. It is also possible that ketanserin reverses 5-HT-induced bronchoconstriction, an event of great importance after embolization.[15] In the setting of aspiration, however, bronchospasm may be less significant. This would be more in accord with the observation that nitroprusside is also partially effective in reducing the physiologic shunt. Nitroprusside usually worsens oxygenation by abolishing the hypoxic pulmonary vasoconstrictor response. It appears that the ability of nitroprusside to reduce the volume of edema formation by lowering capillary hydrostatic pressure is of paramount importance.

Coincident with WBC entrapment in the lungs is their activation to produce TxA_2.[36] The formation of TxA_2 by WBCs and/or lung parenchyma appears to be an event closely related to WBC sequestration. Treatment of the experimental animals as late as 1 hour after aspiration with either the cyclo-oxygenase inhibitor, ibuprofen, or the Tx synthetase inhibitor ketoconazole, a 1-substituted imidazole derivative, prevents WBC entrapment and significantly reduces the volume of edema formation.[12,37]

The ability of ketoconazole to reduce edema may be related to several mechanisms. Neither pulmonary arterial nor pulmonary arterial wedge pressure changes, indicating that simple reductions of hydrostatic pressure are not operative. The pulmonary entrapment of WBCs containing damaging agents, however, appears to be dependent on Tx synthesis, since ketoconazole will prevent leukosequestration. TxA_2 may lead to the intravascular formation of microaggregates and to their mechanical sieving by the lungs. Although this can occur,

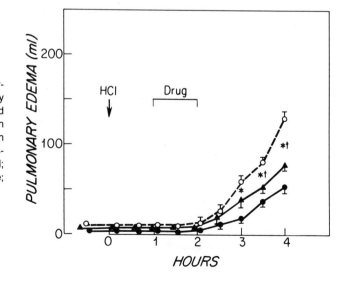

FIG. 18-5 Reduction of pulmonary hypertension after acid aspiration, directly related to decreased edema collected from the endotracheal tube. Ketanserin was more effective than nitroprusside in reducing mean pulmonary arterial pressure as well as edema. (○--○) control; (•—•) ketanserin; (▲—▲) nitroprusside; (⊥) SEM.

the failure to find WBC clumps by smear, and the apparent lack of relationship of the delayed WBC sequestration and early rise in TxB_2 levels, indicate that TxA_2-induced aggregation is apt to be of minor importance. On the other hand, TxA_2 may act directly or indirectly as a chemotactic agent(s).[29] Other chemotactic agents, such as PAF and LTB_4, may also be operative in acid aspiration. Both can be produced by lung parenchyma. PAF operates by a mechanism that cannot be inhibited by blocking cyclo-oxygenase. The potent chemoattractant LTB_4 owes some of its properties, such as contraction of guinea pig lung parenchyma, to TxA_2 synthesis.[25] LTB_4 will also stimulate cultured bovine endothelial cells to synthesize TxA_2. LT dependency on cyclo-oxygenase products may be species specific and related to the mode of introduction of the LT.

genase inhibitor ibuprofen or the Tx synthetase inhibitor imidazole. These data indicate the importance of Tx in LTB_4- or C5a-mediated chemotactic events. It is likely that the ability of ibuprofen or ketoconazole to prevent WBC entrapment in acid aspiration is based on a Tx mechanism such as LTB_4-induced endothelial synthesis of TxA_2.

Without WBC entrapment in the lungs, the formation of pulmonary edema is lessened, but not abolished, indicating that acid induces other injuries. These injuries might include direct microvascular damage via protein denaturation, as well as the production and release of vasotoxic agents from lung parenchyma itself.

CHEMOTAXIS

The topical application of the chemoattractants LTB_4 or C5a to abraded patches of skin in rabbits leads to accumulations of WBCs. Similar events occur after intradermal injection of the same chemoattractants. The accumulation of WBCs can be modified by pretreating the animal with either the cyclo-oxy-

PERMEABILITY

The LT are prominent in their ability to provoke permeability. Thus, treatment of the acid aspirated dog with the LTC_4, LTD_4, and LTE_4 receptor antagonist FPL 55712 reduced the volume of edema. This finding, taken with the above considerations, indicates that both LT and TxA_2 are involved in permeability edema after aspiration.

Edema fluid itself, taken from untreated control animals, leads to enhanced microvas-

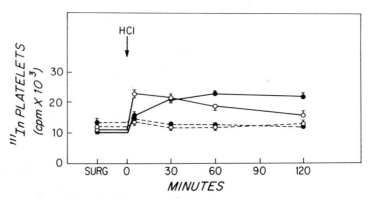

FIG. 18-6 After aspiration localized to one lung,[111] In platelets are observed to be entrapped in both lungs. (•) aspirated lung; (○) nonaspirated lung; (—) lower lobe; (--) upper lobe.

cular permeability when bioassayed on a hamster cheek pouch or in guinea pig skin. The end points of the bioassays are the extravasation of fluorescein-labeled dextran, 150,000 molecular weight, into the cheek pouch or of Evans blue dye into the injected skin regions. Permeability was noted even after the edema fluid specimens were held for 1 to 2 hours, a time when all TxA_2 should have hydrolyzed to the inactive species TxB_2. This observation was surprising and led to a series of in vitro studies using human polymorphonuclear leukocytes. Following activation with a Ca^{++} ionophore, these cells secreted permeability agents that could be separated from the intact cells by centrifugation. The supernatant retained its permeability activity after 1 hours at a time when neither TxA_2 nor free radicals could have been directly involved. Treatment of the bioassay animal with a Tx synthetase or Tx receptor inhibitor prevented permeability. We postulate that a relatively stable LT is liberated into the edema fluid after aspiration as well as into the stimulated WBC supernatant. The role played by the LT was thought to be as an intermediary. Supportive evidence for this thesis was the finding that when LTC_4 or D_4 was applied to the cheek pouch or injected into the skin, the edema that formed could be prevented by pretreatment with imidazole. Thus, it appears that in these settings of permeability, an LT could act as an intermediary and express its biologic activity via TxA_2. This is similar to the previous findings, in which LTB_4 required Tx synthesis in order for chemotaxis to be manifest.

The permeability mediated by LT and TxA_2 represents a reversible event. Following application of edema fluid or LTD_4 to the cheek pouch, permeability sites appeared in minutes and were in maximum numbers at 10 minutes. By 1 hour, there was no longer any evidence of increased permeability. The importance and frequency of such reversible microvascular effects in ARF are unknown. It is plausible to believe that they are early phenomena in the course of any inflammatory reaction.

Under certain circumstances, a local injury triggers a generalized response. For example, acid aspiration involving one lung will recruit a systemic inflammatory reaction. Indium-labeled platelets will be entrapped in both aspirated and nonaspirated lungs (Fig. 18-6). Microscopic evaluation shows WBC invasion bilaterally. Edema is present in the nonaspirated lung as well as in systemic organs. Despite large volumes of crystalloid infusions to maintain filling pressures of the heart, the hematocrit rises, indicating a generalized increase in microvascular permeability. Such large-scale activation of the inflammatory response is self-destructive, much as in autoimmune disease. The therapeutic modulation of such inflammatory events is the goal.

THERAPY OF ARF

Tracheal intubation, supplementary oxygen, and mechanical ventilatory support remain the undisputed key elements in respiratory management. These supportive techniques provide time to explore the nature of, and to treat the problem underlying, ARF. In most cases, the ultimate cause of ARF is sepsis, which is usually, but not necessarily, secondary to an extrathoracic focus of infection.[39]

Systemic blood pressure tends to be low, generally forcing the use of large fluid infusions, particularly if the CO is low as well. Lesser circuit pressures, both pulmonary arterial and pulmonary arterial wedge, are high in ARF. They may be raised even higher with fluid infusion, an event that magnifies fluid transudation across the damaged pulmonary microvasculature by increasing hydrostatic forces. Pharmacologic attempts to stabilize systemic pressure and flow using inotropes such as dopamine and dobutamine are frequently successful. However, the high pulmonary pressures are usually resistant to pharmacologic agents.

Cyclo-oxygenase derivatives, particularly TxA_2, appear to have a role in WBC-mediated permeability, as well as in cardiac function. In a variety of settings in which myocardial performance is impaired, such as after experimental acid aspiration or during abdominal aortic aneurysm surgery, inhibition of TxA_2 synthesis has salutary effects, manifest by an increase in cardiac output and reduction in fluid requirements. In theory, reduced fluid requirements lead to lower cardiac filling pressures and reduced pulmonary capillary pressures. The effect is to reduce edema formation. No reports have yet been published regarding the application of cyclo-oxygenase or Tx synthetase inhibitors in clinical ARF. One of the many difficulties in conducting such a study is the fact that no cyclo-oxygenase inhibitors are available for parenteral use.

Since platelets interact during the first 1 to 2 days with the lungs of patients suffering from ARF, 5-HT may have a significant role at this time. Indeed, not only do the transpulmonary platelet counts indicate lung entrapment, but circulating platelets have discharged 81 percent of their 5-HT. A 30-minute infusion of ketanserin improved oxygenation in patients suffering from early ARF (Fig. 18-7). Mean pulmonary arterial pressures fell an average of 3 mmHg at a time when there was no change in systemic arterial pressure. This significant, although very modest, reduction in pulmonary

pressure may have been one mechanism for decrease in the physiologic shunt by reducing lung edema. Alternatively, ketanserin may have reversed 5-HT-induced constriction of small bronchi, thereby improving alveolar ventilation.

These tentative pharmacologic approaches suggest new directions of investigation. The inflammatory reaction is central. Control of stimuli that aggregate and activate platelets and WBCs appears promising. An alternative approach is to modify the secretion and toxicity of the many vasoactive agents carried by these cells. This chapter has concentrated on the vasoactive oxygenation products of arachidonic acid and 5-HT, but serious consideration should also be directed toward oxygen free radicals and proteolytic enzymes.

REFERENCES

1. Aznavoorian S, Utsunomiya T, Krausz MM, et al: Prostacyclin inhibits 5-hydroxytryptamine release but stimulates thromboxane synthesis during cardiopulmonary bypass. Prostaglandins 25: 537, 1983
2. Bakhle YS: Synthesis and catabolism of cyclo-oxygenase products. Br Med Bull 39: 214, 1983
3. Blackwell GJ, Flower RJ: Inhibition of phospholipase. Br Med Bull 39: 260, 1983
4. Campbell EJ, Senior RM, McDonald JA, Cox DL: Proteolysis by neutrophils: Relative importance of cell substrate contact and oxidative inactivation of proteinase inhibitors in-vitro. J Clin Invest 70: 845, 1982
5. Cameron JL, Reynolds J, Zuidema GD: Aspiration in patients with tracheostomies. Surg Gynecol Obstet 136: 68, 1973
6. Coughlin SR, Moskowitz MA, Antoniades HN, Levine L: Serotonin receptor-mediated stimulation of bovine smooth muscle cell prostacyclin synthesis and its modulation by platelet-derived growth factor. Proc Natl Acad Sci USA 78: 7134, 1981
7. Craddock PR, Fehr J, Brigham KL, et al: Complement and leukocyte mediated pulmonary dysfunction in hemodialysis. N Engl J Med 296: 769, 1977
8. Feldberg W, Kellaway CH: Liberation of hista-

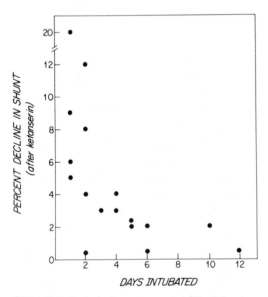

FIG. 18-7 Early in the course of ARF, defined as the first 1 to 2 days of intubation and mechanical ventilatory support, infusion of the 5-HT receptor antagonist, ketanserin, significantly reduces physiologic shunting. (Huval WV, Lelcuk S, Shepro D, Hechtman HB: Role of Serotonin in patients with respiratory failure. Ann Surg 200: 166, 1984.)

mine and formation of lysolecithin-like substances by cobra venom. J Physiol (Lond) 94: 187, 1938

9. Flick MR, Perel A, Staub NC: Leukocytes are required for increased lung microvascular permeability after microembolism in sheep. Circ Res 48: 344, 1981

10. Hechtman HB, Huval WV, Lelcuk S, et al: Platelet serotonin mediates respiratory failure after aspiration. Ninth Annual International Congress for Thrombosis and Haemostasis, Proceedings Stockholm, Sweden July 1983. Thromb Haemost

10a. Hechtman HB, Huval WV, Mathieson MA: Prostaglandin and thromboxane mediation of cardiopulmonary failure. Surg Clin NA 63: 263, 1983

11. Heflin AC, Brigham KL: Prevention by granulocyte depletion prevents of increased lung vascular permeability after endotoxemia in sheep. Clin Res 27: 399A, 1979

12. Huval WV, Dunham BM, Lelcuk S, et al: Thromboxane mediation of cardiovascular dysfunction following aspiration. Surgery 94: 259, 1983

13. Huval WV, Lelcuk S, Allen PD, et al: Determinants of cardiovascular stability during abdominal arotic aneurysmectomy. Ann Surg 199: 216, 1984

14. Huval WV, Lelcuk S, Hechtman HB, Demling RH: Serotonin content of lung lymph and plasma and endotoxemia in sheep. Fed Proc 42: 490, 1983

15. Huval WV, Mathieson MM, Stemp LI, et al: Therapeutic benefits of 5-hydroxytryptamine inhibition following pulmonary embolism. Ann Surg 197: 220, 1983

16. Krausz MM, Utsunomiya T, Dunham B, et al: Thromboxane response to prostacyclin and aspirin treatment in lethal endotoxemia. Fed Proc 40: 619, 1981

17. Krausz MM, Utsunomiya T, Feuerstein G, et al: Prostacyclin (PGI$_2$) reversal of lethal endotoxemia in dogs. J Clin Invest 67: 1118, 1981

18. Krausz MM, Utsunamiya T, Feuerstein G, et al: Prostacyclin reversal of lethal endotoxemia in dogs. J Clin Invest 67: 1118, 1981

19. Krausz MM, Utsunomiya T, Levine L, et al: Adverse effects of prostacyclin used to perfuse isolated lung lobe. Am J Physiol 242: H745, 1982

19a. Lelcuk S, Alexander F, Valeri CR et al: Chromboxane A$_2$ Moderates permeability after limb ischemia. Ann Surg 200: 642, 1985

20. Leitch AG, Corey EJ, Austen KF, Drazen JM: Indomethacin potentiates the pulmonary response to aerosol leukotriene C$_4$ in the guinea pig. Am Rev Respir Dis 128: 639, 1983

21. Matheson NR, Wong PS, Schuylen M, Travis J: Interaction of human α_1-proteinase inhibitor with neutrophil myeloperoxidase. Biochemistry 20: 331, 1981

22. McGuire WW, Spragg RG, Cohen AB, Cochrane CG: Studies in the pathogenesis of the adult respiratory distress syndrome. J Clin Invest 69: 543, 1982

23. Nadel JA, Colebatch HJH, Olsen CR: Location and mechanism of airway constriction after barium sulfate microembolism. J Appl Physiol 19: 387, 1964

24. Piper PJ: Pharmacology of leukotrienes. Br Med Bull 39: 255, 1983

25. Piper PJ, Samhoun MN: Stimulation of arachidonic acid metabolism and generation of thromboxane A$_2$ by leukotriene B$_4$, C$_4$ and D$_4$ in guinea pig lung in-vitro. Br J Pharmacol 77: 267, 1982

26. Serneri GGN, Abbate R, Gensini GP, et al: TxA$_2$ production by human arteries and veins. Prostaglandins 25: 753, 1983

27. Shapiro M, Despland E, Scott CF, et al: Purified human plasma kallikrein aggregates human blood neutrophils. J Clin Invest 69: 1199, 1982

28. Solomkin JS, Cotta L, Hurst JM, Joffe SN: Does complement activation in acute pancreatitis result in respiratory failure? Surg Forum 34: 17, 1983

29. Spagnuolo PJ, Ellner JJ, Hassid A, Dunn MJ: Thromboxane A$_2$ mediates augmented polymorphonuclear leukocyte adhesiveness. J Clin Invest 66: 406, 1980

30. Stein M, Hirose T, Yasutake T, Khan MA: The effects of platelet amines on airway function. In Bouhuys A (ed): Airway Dynamics. Charles C Thomas, Springfield, Illinois 1970

31. Tahamant MV, Malik AB: Granulocytes mediate the increase in pulmonary vascular permeability after thrombin embolism. J Appl Physiol 54: 1489, 1983

32. Till GO, Johnson KJ, Kunbel R, Ward PA: Intravascular activation of complement and acute lung injury: Dependency on neutrophils and toxic oxygen metabolites. J Clin Invest 69: 1126, 1982

33. Taylor GW, Morris HR: Lipoxygenase pathways. Br Med Bull 39: 219, 1983

34. Utsunomiya T, Krausz MM, Dunham B, et al: Circulating negative inotropic agents following pulmonary embolism. Surgery 91: 402, 1982

35. Utsunomiya T, Krausz MM, Dunham B, et al: Maintenance of cardiodynamics with aspirin during abdominal aortic aneurysmectomy. Ann Surg 194: 602, 1981

36. Utsunomiya T, Krausz MM, Dunham B, et al: Modification of the inflammatory response aspiration with ibuprofen. Am J Physiol 243: H903, 1982

37. Utsunomiya T, Krausz MM, Shepro D, Hechtman HB: Treatment of aspiration pneumonia with ibuprofen and prostacyclin (PGI$_2$). Surgery 90: 170, 1981

38. Utsunomiya T, Krausz MM, Shepro D, et al:

Treatment of pulmonary embolism with prostacyclin. Surgery 88: 25, 1980

39. Vito L, Dennis R, Weisel RD, Hechtman HB: Sepsis presenting as acute respiratory insufficiency. Surg Gynecol Obstet 138: 896, 1974

40. Warso MA, Lands WEM: Lipid peroxidation in relation to prostacyclin and thromboxane physiology and pathophysiology. Br Med Bull 39: 277, 1983

19

Cardiorespiratory Management of the Adult Respiratory Distress Syndrome

John H. Siegel
Joan C. Stoklosa
Ulf Borg

INCIDENCE AND OUTCOMES

The adult respiratory distress syndrome (ARDS) is a perplexing and serious complication of traumatic injury, aspiration, inflammation, sepsis, and a variety of other predisposing factors.[5,16,19,25,36,37,63,122,131,154,202,213] It has been characterized as a form of noncardiac pulmonary edema with increased permeability characteristics occurring primarily in the lung and has been noted to have a rapid and progressive course frequently associated with a fatal outcome.[5,16,25,37,63,66,89] In a recent study of 993 patients at risk for the development of ARDS, Fowler and his colleagues[63] found an overall incidence of 6.8 percent, ranging from 1.7 percent following cardiopulmonary bypass to 35.6 percent in patients having pulmonary aspiration. In addition, they noted that both the incidence and the resultant mortality rose as the number of risk factors to which a patient was exposed increased. In their study, patients who

developed ARDS had a mortality rate that ranged from 44 percent when the predisposing factor was hypertransfusion (with 10 or more units of whole blood or packed cells) to 94 percent following documented pulmonary aspiration, for a mean mortality rate from all causes after the onset of the syndrome of 64.8 percent. The time from the occurrence of the predisposing event to the need for endotracheal intubation for respiratory failure ranged from 1 hour to more than 300 hours, with approximately 90 percent of the patients being intubated within 72 hours of the predisposing insult and two-thirds of the patients requiring intubation within 24 hours after onset of the syndrome. Respiratory insufficiency appeared to be the major cause of death in 75 percent of the fatal cases and was usually related to a combination of hypoxemia and nosocomial pneumonia. The median survival time for patients who died with the ARDS syndrome was 13.3 days after the onset of ARDS. Their study also noted that increased age and pre-existent sepsis were statistically significant factors predisposing to mortality.

Other studies of this syndrome have shown that the initiating mechanism can be related to either major thoracic or nonthoracic trauma, burns, hemorrhagic shock with volume replacement, severe systemic sepsis, usually with abscess formation, and certain non-specific inflammatory diseases, such as acute pancreatitis, or transplantation rejection crisis.[1,19,36,63,89,131,149] It has been noted that the severity, lethality, and duration of the pulmonary syndrome are greater in sepsis than after major traumatic or hemorrhagic shock and that a prior episode of massive hemorrhage or trauma may predispose to subsequent ARDS when sepsis supervenes after injury.[5,16,37,46,130,202]

Clinical Diagnosis

In order to diagnose ARDS, certain criteria need to be met. As indicated earlier, the clinical problem occurs after a variety of catastrophic events that can be either pulmonary or nonpulmonary, but acute respiratory insufficiency arising from decompensated chronic pulmonary disease and left heart failure with hydrostatic pulmonary edema are generally excluded from this diagnosis. The degree of respiratory distress is usually judged clinically, but in the spontaneously breathing patient who develops ARDS there is usually a tachypnea with a rate greater than 20 and labored breathing, as evidenced by the use of the accessory muscles of respiration. In quantitative terms, Peters and Hiberman showed that spontaneously breathing surgical patients with early respiratory insufficiency had increased inspiratory work (> 0.08 kg/L/min) and that mechanical ventilatory support was always indicated when the level of inspiratory work rose to greater than 0.18 kg/L/min.[143,144] Initially the chest radiograph may be normal, but later there is radiographic evidence of diffuse pulmonary infiltrates. When first seen, these generally have an interstitial character, but as the syndrome develops an alveolar pattern appears. Pathophysiologically, ARDS is characterized by

interstitial lung edema with decreased lung compliance and increased bronchiolar air flow resistance. Alveolar and small airway closure produces decreased functional residual capacity (FRC) and persistent hypoxemia.[25,27,42,46,73,80,149,177] The usual physiologic criteria for diagnosis include an arterial oxygen tension (PaO$_2$) of less than 50 mmHg on an inspired oxygen concentration (FiO$_2$) greater than 0.6, and a total respiratory compliance of less than 0.05 L/cm H$_2$O (50 ml/cm H$_2$O), but which is generally less than 0.03 L/cm H$_2$O. More sophisticated studies show an increased physiologic shunt fraction ($\dot{Q}S/\dot{Q}T$) and there is frequently increased physiologic dead space (VD/VT).[41,43,44,80,130,148,166-168] It is postulated that in ARDS increased alveolar capillary permeability leads to increased interstitial fluid, which is usually accompanied by microatelectasis and alveolar edema and these factors account for the observed decrease in FRC.[8,19,25,26,28,73,113,183,184]

Pathologic Anatomy

Pathologic examination of the lungs of ARDS victims reveals that this syndrome is due to more than just permeability pulmonary edema. In addition to the pulmonary edema the lungs are noted to be stiff and, on gross pathologic examination, are heavy, airless, sink in water, and the cut surfaces have the appearance of liver (Fig. 19-1). Microscopic examination[8,36,131] shows congestive atelectasis, which presents as airless collapsed alveoli with debris. Hyaline membranes, which are organized proteinaceous material with abundant fibrinogen and fibrin, are usually formed within 24 to 48 hours. Early collagenation of the lung occurs, usually beginning at 72 to 96 hours and extensive fibrosis in association with alveolar cell necrosis and white cell infiltration is characteristic in progressive ARDS[8,36,214] (Fig. 19-2). Lamy et al.[109] correlated the pathologic picture found on lung biopsy or postmortem examination with the physiologic abnormalities and defined three types of patients. In his group I, the patients had the most severe hypoxemia with a minimal response to positive end-expi-

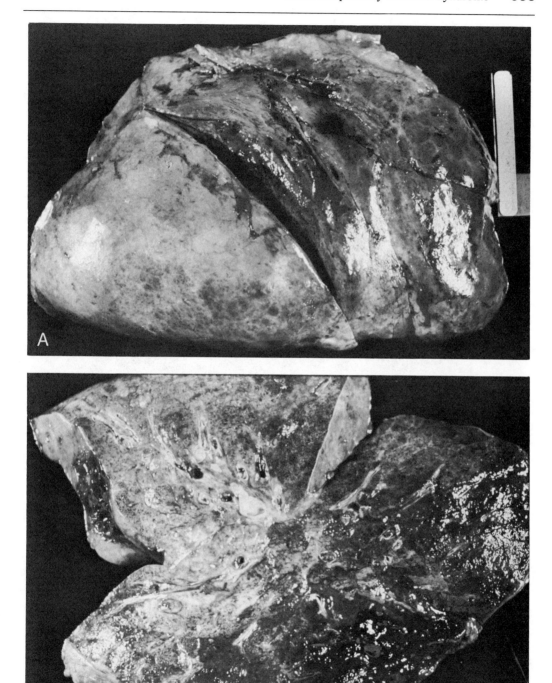

FIG. 19-1 (A) Lateral view of ARDS lung at postmortem. **(B)** Hilar view of ARDS lung with cut surface demonstrating hepatization of the pulmonary parenchyma.

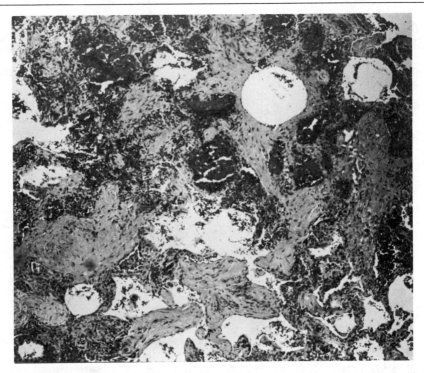

FIG. 19-2 Microscopic section of the ARDS lung. Notice hyalinization and fibrosis of alveoli with round cell infiltration and some hemorrhage. The few remaining alveoli are distended.

ratory pressure (PEEP) and a fixed shunt fraction with all concentrations of inspired oxygen. These patients showed edema, exudation, and massive intra-alveolar hemorrhage which included areas of consolidation as judged by autopsy or open lung biopsy.

Group II patients had less hypoxemia and a moderate arterial blood gas improvement with PEEP, but this improvement was achieved slowly, over 30 minutes to several hours. These patients had extensive fibrosis. Group III patients had the least amount of hypoxemia, a rapid and marked improvement with PEEP, and a good increase in arterial oxygen tension as FiO_2 was increased. Lung specimens from this group showed edema and exudation with hemorrhage, but these abnormalities were not as severe as in the first group described. This third group also had less fibrosis. There were 2 survivors out of 11 patients in group I, 3 of 13 in group II, and 10 of 21 in group III. These data suggested that early fibrosis can resolve during

the healing phase, if sufficient respiratory exchange can be maintained to permit recovery to occur.

PATHOPHYSIOLOGIC MECHANISMS

Humoral Mediators Initiating ARDS

The fundamental initiating mechanisms of this syndrome have been much debated. The studies of Blaisdell[19] and Lindquist et al.[116] contended that the common initiating event in shock or, after endotoxin release into the circulation,[47,61,186] was a formation of platelet microaggregation in the pulmonary capillary bed, which produced early microvascular obstruction and was associated with a release of vasoactive substances.[46-48,60,76,132,185] A thorough discussion of the humoral mediators of the adult respiratory distress syndrome is presented in Chapter 18. This excellent review demonstrates the complexity of the process, but suggests that many of the initiating factors lead to release of vasoactive products such as serotonin,[38,78,79,91,185,186] which causes smooth muscle constriction around the pulmonary vasculature and bronchi. In addition, these same initiating factors appear to cause stimulation of the arachidonic acid–lipoperoxidase cascade,[77,147,203] which stimulates cyclo-oxygenase activity and the production of endoperoxide PGH_2, which is converted[90] to thromboxane A_2. These factors initiate pulmonary vasoconstriction[211] and platelet aggregation and thrombosis,[61,77-79,175] as well as initiating leukocyte migration and adhesiveness[175,179] and complement-mediated aspects of the injurious inflammatory response.[194]

Additional important factors appear to be the generation of leukotrienes,[147] which cause white cell activation with degranulation and release of superoxides and lysosomal enzymes.[62,175,194] These latter factors, rather than[211] thromboxane A_2, alter the ultrastructure of the alveolar capillary membrane with resulting increased permeability.[28,46-48,62,77,79,132] Also, leukotrienes have been demonstrated to have vasoconstrictor actions on smooth muscle,[50] which may be related to the decrease in lung compliance and the increased small airway resistance that occur as early features of this disease.[39,177,183] Other factors discussed in greater detail in Chapters 3 and 18 are related to the liberation of proteases that may lead to alterations in permeability and to the activation of Hageman factor, which converts prekallikrein to kallikrein with the eventual formation of bradykinin, which has major vascular permeability-altering effects.[19] The proteases released may in themselves act to damage the vascular basement membranes, as well as elastin, collagen, and other structural elements of the pulmonary tissues. Finally, the activation

of neutrophils through this inflammatory process has been demonstrated to generate superoxides that have a major capability for producing vascular injury.[62,178,194] The relative importance of each of these factors is not clearly delineated nor is it definitively known whether a different sequence, or relative importance of one set of factors over another, is characteristic of the ARDS syndrome developing in trauma as opposed to that occurring in sepsis, after massive transfusion, or following pulmonary aspiration.

Role of Capillary Permeability Changes and Altered Transcapillary Fluid Flux in Early ARDS

Nevertheless, the alteration in capillary permeability produced by these mediators has been unequivocally demonstrated as a major initiating event in the development of this syndrome.[25-28,47,48,62,74,95,183,184] An increase in the rate of pulmonary capillary protein leak occurring prior to the fall in arterial oxygen tension (PaO_2) has been shown by Sugerman and his colleagues to occur after experimental ARDS initiated by oleic acid[189,190] and also following the experimental ARDS produced by hydrochloric acid aspiration.[29] These findings and others[25-28,48,79,183,184] related to the development of vascular permeability changes in patients and animals with the ARDS syndrome have provided a basis for understanding the evolution of the physiologic abnormalities in the development of this syndrome. Considerable evidence has been marshalled by Levine et al.[112] by Staub,[183,184] and by Brigham[25] to support the fundamental validity of using the Starling equation[182] for the transcapillary movement of fluid as a means of explaining and understanding the interactions of these various humoral mediators in initiating and enhancing the pathologic process producing ARDS.

While this physiologic relationship was originally developed by Starling[182] in 1896 as a result of experiments in normal skeletal muscle on the direction of transfer of extracellular fluid between plasma in the capillary bed and fluid in the interstitial space, more contemporary studies have demonstrated that this hypothesis also applies to the movement of intravascular and extravascular water in the lung.[112,119] Furthermore, the classic experiments of Landis[110] and Landis and Papenheimer,[111] which confirmed and quantified Starling's theory, also demonstrated that the permeability or filtration of the capillary bed could be altered by anoxia. Current work has shown that many other noxious stimuli such as bacteremia, endotoxin, or heroin administration, platelet aggregation, and the action of various vasoactive polypeptides, kinins, and prostaglandins may also change capillary permeability characteristics.[46,47,79,182,183]

Briefly stated, the Starling hypothesis indicates that the flow of fluid ($\dot{Q}_f$) from the alveolar capillary to the pulmonary interstitium is a function of the filtration coefficient of the capillary membranes (K_f) times the intramicrovascular (P_{IV}) to the extramicrovascular (P_{EV}) pressure gradient minus the reflection coefficient (σ), expressing the relative permeability of the membrane to solute as opposed to water, times the intramicrovascular (Π_{IV}) to extramicrovascular (Π_{EV}) osmotic pressure gradient.

$$\dot{Q}_f = K_f (P_{IV} - P_{EV}) - \sigma(\Pi_{IV} - \Pi_{EV}) \qquad (1)$$

At any given pulmonary capillary membrane permeability (K_f), the values for the intramicrovascular to extramicrovascular pres-

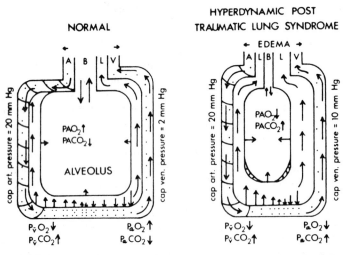

LYMPH FLOW = Permeability · (Hydrostatic Press. Grad.) − (Osmotic Press. Grad.)

$$\dot{Q}_f = K_f \quad (P_{IV} - P_{EV}) \quad - \sigma(\Pi_{IV} - \Pi_{EV})$$

Cap. Permeability	Increased
Cap. Hydrostatic Pressure	Increased
Colloid Oncotic Pressure	Reduced
Pulmonary Lymph Flow	Increased
Alveolar Surface Tension	Increased
Lung Compliance	Reduced
Airway Resistance	Increased
Alveolar Volume	Reduced
A-$_a$DO$_2$ Gradient	Increased
Cap. A-V Pressure Gradient	Reduced
Functional Residual Capacity	Reduced
%Shunt (Venoarterial Admixture)	Increased

FIG. 19-3 Effect of alterations in Starling's law of capillary action on transcapillary fluid loss, pulmonary gas exchange, compliance, resistance, and pulmonary shunting. Hyperdynamic posttraumatic lung syndrome produces interstitial edema with distention of lymphatics and venules and narrowing of respiratory bronchioles producing partial obstruction of alveoli. (Siegel JH, Farrell EJ: The management of the acute respiratory distress syndrome in the aged or high risk surgical patient. p. 457. In Siegel JH, Chodoff P (eds): The Aged and High Risk Surgical Patient. Grune and Stratton, New York, 1976, by permission.)

sure gradient $(P_{IV} - P_{EV})$ and the corresponding osmotic pressure gradients $(\Pi_{IV} - \Pi_{EV})$ change continuously along the length of the alveolar capillary surface from the inflow to the outflow end (Fig. 19-3). At each point along the capillary, this is altered as a function of the relative difference between the pulmonary arterial and left atrial pressures, as well as the extravascular tissue pressures, and the net flow of osmotically active solutes and intravascular protein molecules (primarily albumin) across the alveolar capillary. From this equation one can see how alterations in each of the factors, or a combination of any, can enhance the flow of capillary fluid into the pulmonary alveolar interstitial space at the arterial side and can also retard the flow of pulmonary interstitial fluid back from the interstitium into the venous side of the pulmonary capillary bed. If this balance is altered from normal so as to exceed the capacity of the pulmonary lymphatics to drain the interstitial space, pulmonary interstitial fluid accumulation occurs.

Role of Increased Colloid Movement in the Evolution of ARDS

Understanding the importance of the transcapillary pressure gradient is not difficult. However, the importance of the net transcapillary flow of large protein molecules that exert the intravascular oncotic pressure needs further explanation to clarify the pathologic implications of colloid deficits and increased protein flow into the pulmonary interstitial space in the genesis of this syndrome. The net flow of plasma proteins across the alveolar capillary membrane is a separate but related factor governing the rate of fluid transport from alveolar capillary to pulmonary interstitial space. This colloid flow $(\dot{Q}_p)$ a function of the permeability of the capillary membrane to the protein molecule in question (ω), times the transcapillary osmotic pressure gradient $(\Pi_{IV} - \Pi_{EV})$, plus 1 minus the reflection coefficient (σ) times the membrane concentration of the same protein (C_p), times the net transvascular flow of fluid $(\dot{Q}_f)$.

$$\dot{Q}_p = \omega(\Pi_{IV} - \Pi_{EV}) + [(1 - \sigma)C_p]\dot{Q}_f \qquad (2)$$

As a result of these fundamental relationships, when an increase in pulmonary alveolar capillary permeability occurs, there is an increased net flow of both crystalloid-containing plasma fluid and protein molecules (mostly albumin, but also fibrinogen and other acute phase plasma proteins, as well as kinins, circulating proteases, interleukins and other molecules) into the pulmonary interstitial space and eventually into the alveoli. This increased flow of these specific acute phase proteins, inflammatory reactants, and albumin may account for the hyaline deposits, cellular necrosis, accelerated fibrosis, and collagen deposition seen on microscopic pathologic examination of lung tissues from ARDS patients (Fig. 19-2).

The absolute rate of the interstitial fluid flux and its direction are functions of the pulmonary intravascular hydrostatic pressure, which determines the value for P_{IV} in Equation 1. Pulmonary intramicrovascular hydrostatic pressure is increased by a rising pulmonary venous pressure (PVP), due to cardiac failure or to a cardiac hyperdynamic state with high left atrial pressures (both of which increase cardiac intraventricular volume to a higher point on the left ventricular end-diastolic pressure–volume relationship). Therefore at any given level of capillary blood flow, the net transfer of both fluid and plasma proteins from capillary lumen to pulmonary interstitial space will increase at a *normal* alveolar capillary permeability.[75] This fluid transfer into the interstitium will be markedly enhanced if capillary permeability is *increased*. Such changes in pulmonary capillary permeability have been described as occurring with shock,[19,25,26,74,113] sepsis,[28,36,37] and after the administration of certain toxic drugs, such as heroin[95] or alloxan.[183]

In a similar fashion, reduction in the oncotic colloid concentration of the plasma, either by nutritional dysfunction (cirrhotic liver disease, malnutrition, cancer), or by the acute iatrogenic replacement with non-colloid-containing fluids of intravascular losses due to inflammatory loss of intravascular colloid with a low oncotic plasma refill (pancreatitis, burn, peritonitis), or any combination of these events, will reduce the intravascular colloid oncotic pressure. This will reduce the effectiveness of the intravascular osmotic pressure (Π_{IV}) in modifying the intravascular–extravascular pressure gradient ($P_{IV} - P_{EV}$) and in determining the level and direction of fluid flow ($\dot{Q}_f$) from the pulmonary capillary to the interstitial space (Equation 1). The increased movement of albumin and water into the lung interstitum has been demonstrated clinically by the radioalbumin studies of Sugerman and his group[189,190] as well as by the direct measurement of lung water by Chinard,[34] Lewis,[113] Gump,[73,74] and others.[26,27,45,183,184] These data are consistent with the Starling hypothesis of capillary transfer (Equation 1), as is the relationship between a reduced serum oncotic pressure and the development of pulmonary edema at low intravascular hydrostotic pressures, which has been noted experimentally by Guyton and Lindsey.[75]

Relation of Fluid Flux and Gas Exchange Abnormalities

Recent studies have shown that the correlation of a decreased alveolar–arterial oxygen gradient is primarily with the vascular permeability surface area alterations rather than with the lung water changes.[26] This is probably due to the fact that it takes only an extremely small change in the rate of fluid transfer to alter oxygen diffusion gradients and to produce the compliance and resistance changes secondary to alveolar–capillary interstitial and peribronchial edema.[177,184] However, the sensitivity of the lung water method is low enough that very substantial changes in extravascular fluid must be produced before this can be detected by the double-indicator technique.[26,27] Consequently, as shown by Brigham and his colleagues,[27] Dauber and Weil,[45] and by Sugerman et al.[189,190] techniques that can measure this pulmonary capillary fluid flux are far more sensitive to early ARDS changes than those that measure static extravascular lung water.[34,74,113] Thus fluid flux and labeled protein loss into the lung parenchyma are more highly correlated to alterations in the alveolar–arterial oxygen gradient (A–aDO_2) than are increases in lung water.[26,189,190]

Role of Pulmonary Lymphatic Clearance

A number of pathophysiologic and ultramicroscopic studies have demonstrated the permeability changes in the alveolar capillary membrane and suggested that this alteration is the initial and key pathophysiologic lesion in ARDS.[8,112,183,205] However, it is clear from the Starling equation and from a variety of experimental studies that the reduction in the colloid oncotic pressure of the plasma caused by dilutional hypoalbuminemia with crystalloid fluid replacement,[1,74,75,158] or diminution of the capillary arteriovenous differential pressure gradient because of myocardial depression or failure,[27,85,96,166,168] will exaggerate the effects of any pulmonary capillary permeability alteration. These factors will reduce the rate of tissue fluid return to the venous side of the capillary bed and thus will place a greater demand on the clearance capacity of the pulmonary lymphatics.

In the lung, the special nature of the air-filled alveolus that supports the capillary bed and its ventilation-related function of gas exchange, requiring expansion for exchange of this gas-filled structure, present special pathophysiologic problems related to the ability of the lung lymphatics to handle the increased flow of fluid into the pulmonary interstitial space (Fig. 19-3). Although pulmonary lymph flow through the thoracic duct increases markedly,[48,183,184] as the alveolar capillary permeability changes there is accumulation (and perhaps relative stasis) of fluid in the alveolar capillary interstitial space. This tends to reduce alveolar compliance in that the pressure needed to distend the alveolus becomes greater for a given volume of gas, much as filling a balloon under water takes more distending pressure than filling it at atmospheric pressure. In addition, as demonstrated by Staub,[184] the interstitial edema tends to extend to the peribronchial area and since these narrow-lumen air-filled structures are the only compressible structures in the area relative to the fluid-filled pulmonary arterioles, venules, and lymphatics, the bronchioles tend to be reduced in size, thus increasing the resistance to airflow (Fig. 19-3). Late in the process when interstitial edema is marked, Staub[184] has shown that there appears to be a breakthrough at the junction between the respiratory bronchiole and the alveolus, so that alveolar flooding occurs with the appearance of pulmonary edema. This not only interferes with gas exchange but also results in alveolar instability due to increased surface forces.

Pulmonary Surfactant Alterations and Their Significance

With pulmonary venous stasis and reduction in capillary exchange, there is suggestive evidence that the nutrition of the surfactant secreting alveolar type II lining cells is impaired. The net result is cellular injury with a loss of the ability to produce surfactant.[8,145,146,205] Once surfactant is damaged or inactivated there is a loss of alveolar stability, which has been speculated to result in hydrostatic tissue forces that increase capillary transmural pressure and thereby encourage more edema formation.[145,146] It also appears likely that these surfactant abnormalities contribute to lung stiffness, since the interfascial tensions of wet and folded alveolar surfaces require high inflation pressures (increased opening pressures) to recruit these alveolar units.

Evolution of Microatelectasis and Pathologic Anatomic Shunting

The absence of this important surface-tension-lowering phospholipid makes alveolar distention more dependent on the sum of the intra-alveolar gas partial pressures, especially when, as noted earlier, there may be some degree of narrowing of the respiratory bronchioles because of peribronchial edema with resultant increased airway resistance to gas flow. When the patient breathes atmospheric air ($FiO_2 = 0.21$), the sum of the partial pressures of mixed venous oxygen ($P\bar{v}O_2$) and carbon dioxide ($P\bar{v}CO_2$) are low. The partially occluded alveolus equilibrates to a greater degree than normal with the mixed venous gas partial pressures and thus *the partial pressure of nitrogen (N_2) becomes of key importance as an alveolar scaffolding to hold open alveoli that have a reduced compliance and impaired gas exchange with the atmosphere.* Because of the reduction in gas exchange, converting some areas of the lung to physiologic shunts, such patients generally have a fall in arterial oxygen tension to clinically unsafe levels. As a result, the FiO_2 is therapeutically increased and the partial pressure of the inert structural gas (N_2) is reduced, further reducing alveolar volume. Under these conditions in ARDS where surfactant production is impaired, the surface tension factors collapsing the alveolus become greater than the intra-alveolar gas distending pressure and microatelectasis and true pulmonary venoarterial shunting will occur.

In this regard, it is important to emphasize that there is a shunt both in *space* and in *time*. The former of course is a function of the completely atelectatic or destroyed alveoli. The latter occurs when the sum of the collapsing forces is such that alveolar expansion occurs later than normal in the respiratory cycle, when a greater pressure–volume ratio is achieved. This means that in each ventilatory cycle the cardiac output perfuses a nonventilating alveolus for a longer than normal period of time, even at the same alveolar minute ventilation, because the time course and the pattern of ventilation have been altered unfavorably in the direction of a reduced inspiratory/expiratory (I/E) ratio in time.

Role of Ventilation/Perfusion Abnormalities in the Generation of Physiologic Shunting

Finally, it is important to emphasize that the relative perfusion ($\dot{Q}$) and ventilation ($\dot{V}A$) of individual alveoli are not uniform in different regions of the lung. A large number of physiologic studies in normal erect men have shown that perfusion per unit lung volume is increased in the dependent alveoli at the base of the lung and reduced in the apex alveoli, which are superior to the effective level of perfusion pressures[4,13,57,58,96,209,210] (Fig. 19-4). The total volume of ventilation per unit lung volume in the erect position is also greater in the basal lung segments[4,13,57,58,125,208] (Fig. 19-5). However, the relative ventilation to perfusion ratio of alveoli at the apex is greater than at the base. This can be seen by computing the gradient estimate value of the normalized $\dot{V}A/\dot{Q}$ in Figures 19-4 and 19-5. The $\dot{V}A/\dot{Q}$ estimate ranges from 1.7 at the apex to 0.56 at the base. A less steep relation is present in the aged patient[96] than in the young.[4,13,126,208] As these data show, under normal circumstances there is a wide range of ventilation/perfusion ratios ($\dot{V}A/\dot{Q}$),

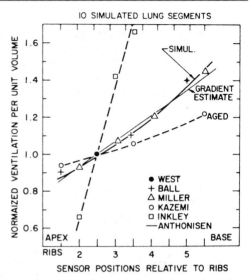

FIG. 19-5 Normalized ventilation per unit lung volume in normal erect men. Comparison of data from six authors together with gradient estimate of difference from apex to base along 10 simulated lung segments data. (Farrell EJ, Siegel JH: Investigation of Cardiorespiratory abnormalities through computer simulation. Computer Biomed Res 5: 161, 1973.)

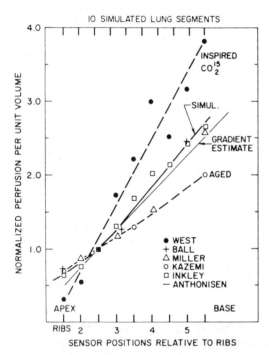

FIG. 19-4 Demonstration of normalized perfusion per unit lung volume in normal erect men. Comparison of data from six investigators together with gradient of estimate from apex to base derived from these data along 10 simulated lung segments. (Farrell EJ, Siegel JH: Investigation of cardiorespiratory abnormalities through computer simulation. Computer Biomed Res 5: 161, 1973.)

but in ARDS an increase in the number of lung units with very low ventilation/perfusion ratios (0.02 to 0.1) was suggested by the work of Markello et al.,[118] who showed a significant alveolar–arterial difference in nitrogen. In progressive late-stage ARDS this disparity may become greater, with larger numbers of alveoli with low $\dot{V}A/\dot{Q}$ occurring and being responsible for the increase in physiologic shunting ($\dot{Q}S/\dot{Q}T$). This is supported by the work performed by Lamy et al.,[109] who showed that in patients with ARDS whose lung biopsies showed predominant fibrosis, changing the concentration of inspired oxygen (FIO_2) led to an increase in PaO_2. This increase would not occur if the hypoxemia was caused by right-to-left shunting alone, as is seen in ARDS patients whose biopsy showed predominant alveolar edema, where there was a fixed PaO_2 with changing FIO_2.

The role of low $\dot{V}A/\dot{Q}$ areas of lung as a cause of the increased $\dot{Q}S/\dot{Q}T$ seen in ARDS have been contested by Dantzker,[41-43] whose studies using the multiple inert gas method have been interpreted as showing that blood flow in ARDS is distributed mainly to two types of lung units: those normally ventilated and those unventilated. Since the spectrum of changes in ARDS is very wide, ranging from early interstitial edema through alveolar flooding to late fibrosis with diminished alveolar dynamics, it is likely that the relative degree of importance of low $\dot{V}A/\dot{Q}$ lung regions to that of areas of fixed shunt (where only right-to-left perfusion occurs) varies as a function of the disease state and the nature of the ventilatory support used. However, regardless of the stage of the disease, when an ARDS patient lies supine, the relative volume of ventilation allocated to the more dependent lung is reduced compared to that in the erect position, thus further compounding the effects of any ventilation/perfusion mismatching or nonuniform fixed shunt mechanisms.

FACTORS INFLUENCING THE DISTRIBUTION OF PULMONARY BLOOD FLOW

Blood flow to the normal lung is modified by a number of factors. As noted by Minor and Gonzales,[127] Permutt et al.,[140,141] Riley and his colleagues,[153] and Bannister and Torrance,[14] the distribution of flow through the lung can be considered as being modified by a series of Starling resistances. At any right heart output, inflow to a given lung segment is mainly determined by the relative pulmonary vascular resistance of that segment, compared to its intra-alveolar pressure.[14,24,140] Structural changes in the configuration of lung arterioles with inflation also appear to play a role, which may become increased in importance when alveolar collapse and hypoxemia occur.[88,193] Also, direct pulmonary arteriolar vasoconstriction may occur with hypoxemia,[59] acute burns,[48] or septic bacteremia or endotoxemia.[33,47,61,162,212] Pulmonary outflow however, is largely a function of the level of pulmonary venous pressure, which is in turn dependent on the left atrial pressure (LAP) and the left ventricular end-diastolic (LVED) pressure/volume relations, which are in turn functions of the total cardiac output, as determined by venous return (preload), peripheral vascular resistance (afterload), and myocardial contractility[24,69,85,93,96,103,166,181,209,210] (see Chap. 9).

However, plumonary segmental blood inflow depends on the relative net pulmonary artery pressure exerted at the level of the superior and dependent lung segments compared to the input resistance effects.[209,210] In the more superior lung segments, the effective pressure in the pulmonary arteries and veins is less than that in the more dependent lung. In what has been called zone I of the lung, the intra-alveolar pressure in the superior portion of the lung is greater than the effective pulmonary artery pressure during a significant portion of the respiratory cycle, especially in patients with decreased compliance in the dependent lung segments and those on higher levels of positive end-expiratory pressure (PEEP).[9–12,81,150] Under these circumstances these alveoli are ventilated, but not perfused and therefore are essentially converted to physiologic dead space and thus increase the dead space to tidal volume ratio (V_D/V_T).

In the intermediate portion of the lung there is a region (zone II) where the pressure in the pulmonary artery (PAP) is greater than the intra-alveolar pressure, but alveolar pressure is in turn greater than the PVP and LAP. In this region, the mean capillary flow is determined by the intra-alveolar pressure, which exerts a Starling resistance effect against the alveolar capillary bed. Under normal airway pressures, this region of lung has the most favorable relationships between alveolar ventilation ($\dot{V}A$) and pulmonary blood flow ($\dot{Q}$). In each alveolus in zone II, the absolute magnitude of the blood flow is proportional to its specific pressure gradient between the pulmonary arterial pressure and the intra-alveolar pressure. The ARDS patient is usually treated with high PEEP and mean airway pressures. As a result in many alveoli the intra-alveolar pressure may be much higher than PVP and LAP in this region of the lung. If these pressures are transmitted to the alveolus, the Starling resistance effect reduces the percent of the total pulmonary blood flow perfusing zone II compared to that occurring through regions of partially occluded, or collapsed, alveoli where the alveolar pressure is less than the PVP (zone III). In zone II also, the alveolar capillaries although open, will be somewhat compressed because of the higher alveolar pressure in relation to the PVP. This tends to increase the surface to volume ratio of the capillary and produces a greater potential exchange surface per unit flow. However, because of the sudden pressure drop of the capillary blood leaving the alveolus to the pressure level of PVP, there is an acceleration of the blood (Bernoulli effect) which is proportional to the difference between the alveolar pressure and the PVP. Therefore the lower the LAP and consequently the PVP relative to the alveolar pressure,[140,209,210] the greater will be the velocity of blood flowing through this alveolar capillary bed region. Since velocity rises inversely as the square of the vessel radius decreases,

in some hyperdynamic patients with extremely high pulmonary blood flows the velocity of blood flow caused by the alveolar-pulmonary venous "Water-fall" effect may exceed the alveolar–capillary transfer rate of oxygen, especially in alveoli somewhat reduced in volume or with diminished gas washout. This will result in pulmonary venous desaturation and thus contribute in some degree to the magnitude of the physiologic shunt.

However, the major area of physiologic shunting is in the more dependent lung (zone III) where PAP, PVP, and LAP all exceed alveolar pressure and there is distention of the alveolar capillaries. The mean flow in this case is totally dependent on the pressure gradient between PAP and PVP–LAP. This region has the highest mean flow, and will receive the greatest fraction of the distribution of the total pulmonary blood flow. Unfortunately, since the PVP–LAP exceeds alveolar pressure, alveolar volume is reduced and in some instances alveoli collapse, forming a fixed right-to-left shunt.

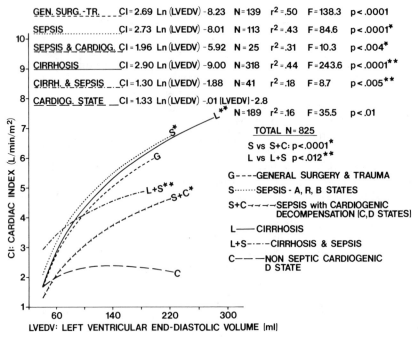

FIG. 19-6 Ventricular function mean slopes labeled by clinical condition and various states of critical illness. N, number of studies. (Siegel JH, Giovaninni I, Coleman B et al: Pathologic synergy modulation of the cardiovascular, respiratory and metabolic response to injury by cirrhosis and/or sepsis: a manifestation of a common metabolic defect? Arch Surg 117: 225, 1982. Copyright 1982 American Medical Association.)

Thus the net $\dot{V}A$ in this area will be less than the net $\dot{Q}$. Consequently, functioning alveoli in this region will have a low $\dot{V}A/\dot{Q}$ ratio, which forms the main contribution to the physiologic shunt.[209,210]

Influence of the Hyperdynamic Cardiovascular State on the Development of Gas Exchange Abnormalities

All of these effects that contribute to the development of $\dot{V}A/\dot{Q}$ distribution abnormalities and the resultant increase in venoarterial shunt ($\dot{Q}S/\dot{Q}T$) are exaggerated by the hyperdynamic states that occur after injury, following acute nonseptic inflammation such as pan-creatitis, and are present in hyperdynamic liver disease, or severe sepsis.[163-168] In these conditions there is a reduced vascular tone and a lowered outflow resistance to cardiac ejection (afterload). These prominent features of all hyperdynamic states are particularly pronounced in sepsis and hyperdynamic liver disease, which have the highest cardiac outputs.[166,167] Combined with the sympathetically mediated increase in myocardial contractility,[165-168] the reduced afterload allows a shift to the left in the cardiac ventricular function relationship (Chap. 9), with a rise in cardiac index (CI) at the same time as there is a reduction in LVEDV (Fig. 19-6), LAP, and PVP. These outflow factors, which in themselves cause a redistribution of pulmonary blood flow, are exaggerated by the increased venous return that contributes to the increased cardiac output. This in turn increases the mean pulmonary artery pressure and thus the PAP–LAP gradient. The net result (Fig. 19-7) is an increase in the

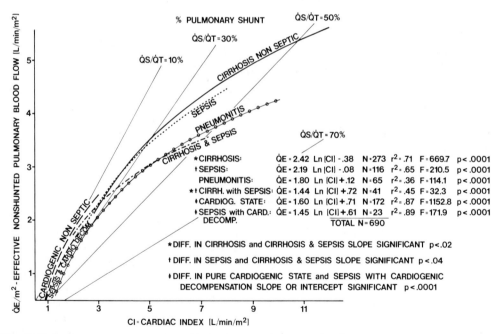

FIG. 19-7 Effect of cardiac index (CI) and percent pulmonary shunt ($\dot{Q}S/\dot{Q}T$) on effective, nonshunted pulmonary blood flow ($\dot{Q}E/m^2$). Lines represent mean slope and intercept data for patients with various clinical conditions. Note that in patients with cirrhosis or sepsis, and especially in those with cirrhosis and sepsis, or those with pneumonitis, increased flow (CI) is necessary to maintain effective pulmonary blood flow because of high $\dot{Q}S/\dot{Q}T$. N = number of studies. (Siegel JH, Giovaninni I, Coleman B et al: Pathologic synergy modulation of the cardiovascular, respiratory and metabolic response to injury by cirrhosis and/or sepsis: a manifestation of a common metabolic defect? Arch Surg 117: 225, 1982. Copyright 1982 American Medical Association.)

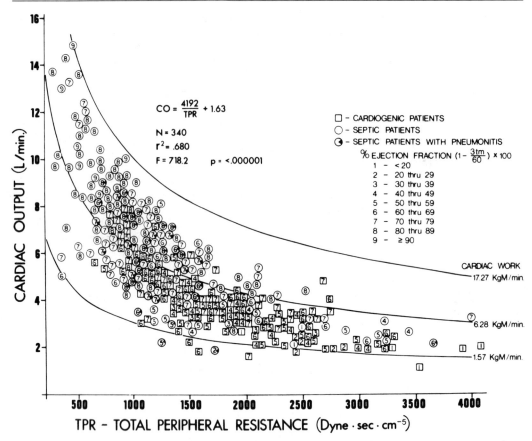

$$CO = \frac{4192}{TPR} + 1.63$$

N = 340

r^2 = .680

F = 718.2   p = <.000001

□ – CARDIOGENIC PATIENTS
◯ – SEPTIC PATIENTS
◑ – SEPTIC PATIENTS WITH PNEUMONITIS

% EJECTION FRACTION $(1 - \frac{3tm}{60}) \times 100$

1 – < 20
2 – 20 thru 29
3 – 30 thru 39
4 – 40 thru 49
5 – 50 thru 59
6 – 60 thru 69
7 – 70 thru 79
8 – 80 thru 89
9 – ≥ 90

CARDIAC WORK
17.27 KgM/min.

6.28 KgM/min.

1.57 KgM/min.

FIG. 19-8 Relationship of cardiac output and total peripheral resistance in 340 studies. Individual points labeled by percent cardiac ejection fraction. Lines of constant cardiac work are shown. (Siegel JH, Giovaninni I, Coleman B: Ventilation: perfusion maldistribution secondary to the hyperdynamic cardiovascular state as the major cause of increased pulmonary shunting in human sepsis. J Trauma 19: 432, 1979; © 1979 The Williams & Wilkins Co., Baltimore.)

percent pulmonary shunt, so that a higher cardiac index is necessary to achieve any given level of effective pulmonary blood flow ($\dot{Q}_E$). This effect becomes more prominent when cirrhosis and sepsis occur together, producing a further synergistic reduction in vascular tone, or when pneumonitis with alveolar infiltration adds a pathologic right-to-left shunt to the physiologic shunt.

As a further explanation of the relationship between cardiovascular function and shunt, Figure 19-8 shows the relation between cardiac output, peripheral resistance, and cardiac ejection fraction (EFx) in patients with septic and nonseptic pathologic conditions. It

is clear from this study that the septic patients (circles) and many of the hyperdynamic nonseptic patients (squares) studied following injury or acute inflammation have increased cardiac outputs and reduced total peripheral resistance. *These patients also have the highest cardiac ejection fractions.* As a result the left ventricular end-diastolic volume tends to be reduced relative to the increase in flow as the ventricular function (VF) relationship is shifted to the left.

The effect of this VF shift on the pulmonary shunt is shown in Figure 19-9. It demonstrates, in patients with hyperdynamic sepsis in whom pneumonitis was not present, that those pa-

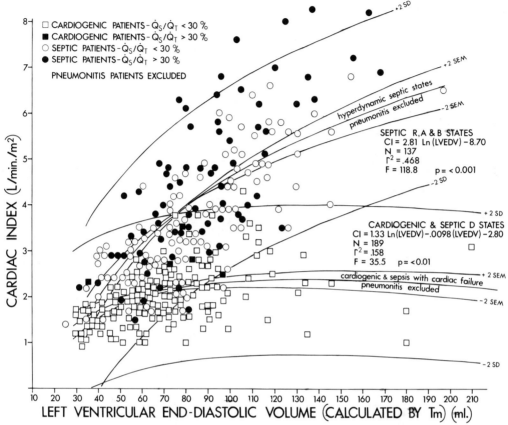

FIG. 19-9 Relation between cardiac index and left ventricular end-diastolic volume (LVEDV) for septic and cardiogenic patients. The regression mean and confidence limits for septic R-, A-, and B-state patients show them to be on a different range of Starling relationships than the regression and confidence lines for cardiogenic and septic D state patients. The regression slopes of these two groups are significantly different (F ratio 191.3, P < 0.0001). Hyperdynamic septic patients with large CI/LVEDV tend to have $\dot{Q}S/\dot{Q}T > 30$ percent. (Siegel JH, Giovaninni I, Coleman B: Ventilation: perfusion maldistribution secondary to the hyperdynamic cardiovascular state as the major cause of increased pulmonary shunting in human sepsis. J Trauma 19: 432, 1979; © 1979 The Williams & Wilkins Co., Baltimore.)

tients with the most left-shifted curves (where the increase in cardiac index was great compared to the relative rise in left ventricular end-diastolic volume) not only had the highest flows but also tended to have the highest percent shunt. In these patients left ventricular end-diastolic volume was normal or low, so that the LAP and PVP would be expected to be reduced and pulmonary blood flow redistributed. This supports the contention that a major early component of the blood gas abnormalities seen with the initiation of the acute

ARDS physiopathology may be related to functional alterations in ventilation/perfusion distribution before the development of observable intrinsic lung pathology.[58,163-165]

This observation has been made by Clowes and his colleagues[36] as well as by Siegel et al.,[166] who found that with the development of the hyperdynamic state of sepsis the earliest manifestations of ARDS (arterial hypoxemia accompanied by increased venoarterial shunting) were usually associated with normal chest x ray findings. Only later in the

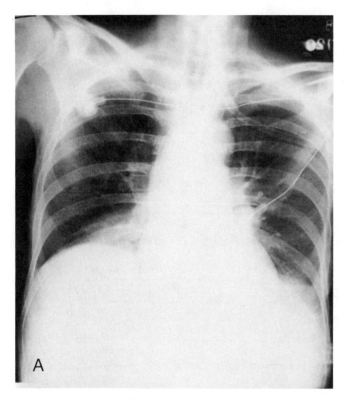

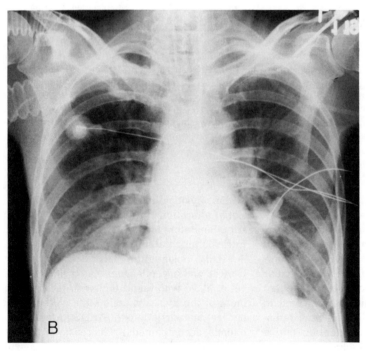

FIG. 19-10 **(A)** Chest radiograph during initial hyperdynamic respiratory distress syndrome (10:00 A.M. postop day 5). FiO_2, 0.40; in vivo PaO_2, 56 mmHg; $PaCO_2$, 33 mmHg pH, 7.53; $\dot{Q}S/\dot{Q}T$, 33 percent. **(B)** Chest radiograph following inotropic resuscitation from patient shown in (A) (postop day 6) MA-1 respirator. FiO_2 , 0.60 with 3 cmH_2O PEEP; in vivo PaO_2, 163 mmHg; $PaCO_2$, 37 mmHg; pH, 7.56; $\dot{Q}S/\dot{Q}T$, 15 percent. (Siegel JH, Giovaninni I, Coleman B: Ventilation: perfusion maldistribution secondary to the hyperdynamic cardiovascular state as the major cause of increased pulmonary shunting in human sepsis. J Trauma 19: 432, 1979; © 1979 The Williams & Wilkins Co., Baltimore.)

TABLE 19-1. Development of Postseptic ARDS

	Day and Time	
	Postoperative Day 5, 10:00 A.M.	Postoperative Day 6, 13:31 P.M.
Chest x-ray	Clear (see Fig. 19-10A)	Early ARDS [see Fig. 19-10(B)]
Physiologic state	A	B
Cardiac index (L/min/m²)	6.37	5.05
Ejection fraction (%)	83	80
FIO_2	0.40	0.60
PEEP (cmH$_2$O)	0	3
PaO$_2$ (mmHg)	56	163
P$\bar{v}$O$_2$ (mmHg)	38	43
PaCO$_2$ (mmHg)	33	37
apH	7.53	7.56
A − aDO$_2$	191	220
RI	3.4	1.4
$\dot{Q}$S/$\dot{Q}$T (%)	33	15
RI/($\dot{Q}$S /$\dot{Q}$T)	0.10	0.09

development of the ARDS syndrome did the characteristic radiologic features appear. This is shown in Figure 19-10 and Table 19-1.

This patient was a young woman who developed acute hyperdynamic ARDS secondary to severe sepsis on her fifth postoperative day following drainage of an infected pancreatic pseudocyst. At the time that the hyperdynamic state occurred with a CI of 6.37 L/min/m² and an EFx of 83 percent. Abnormal blood gases also developed in which a reduced PaO$_2$ of 56 mmHg (FIO$_2$ of 0.40) was associated with an increased A–aDO$_2$ gradient of 191 mmHg, an elevated respiratory index (3.4), and an increased shunt (33 percent). Not until twenty-four hours later on ventilatory support (Fig. 19-10B), when the blood gases had actually improved to a PaO$_2$ of 163 mmHg with a reduction in the respiratory index to 1.4 and the percent shunt to 15 percent, did the characteristic radiographic picture of ARDS appear, reflecting the altered permeability phase of the disease. This radiologic evidence of ARDS occurred despite the fact that the patient was now on volume-controlled ventilation with a PEEP of 3 cm H$_2$O. It is also worth noting that during the initial period (Fig. 19-10A) when the patient was breathing spontaneously, the arterial hypoxemia stimulated a tachypnea with a reduction in PaCO$_2$ to 33 mmHg and a rise in arterial pH to 7.53.

Cardiopulmonary Flow Dynamics and Mean Ventilation Perfusion Ratio ($\dot{V}$A/$\dot{Q}$T), VD/VT, and $\dot{Q}$S/$\dot{Q}$T Alterations

These observations further support the concept[166] that not only is a major cause of arterial hypoxemia in the early stage of hyperdynamic nonseptic and septic respiratory insufficiency due to ventilation/perfusion maldistribution, but also that this may be secondary to the development of the hyperdynamic cardiovascular state related to the reduction in vascular tone. The fall in peripheral resistance, by reducing afterload, allows a more complete left ventricular ejection to lower left ventricular end-diastolic volume and pressure, as well as LAP and PVP. This reduction in PVP shifts a higher percentage of the now increased cardiac output (pulmonary blood flow) to the more dependent portion of the lung, thus reducing the ventilation/perfusion ratio. This is demonstrated in Figure 19-11, which shows the overall $\dot{V}$A/$\dot{Q}$T ratio as a function of the cardiac index in a group of patients on controlled ventilation. The septic (circles) and nonseptic (squares) patient points are labeled by the percent ejection fraction (EFx). As can be seen by this study, those septic patients with

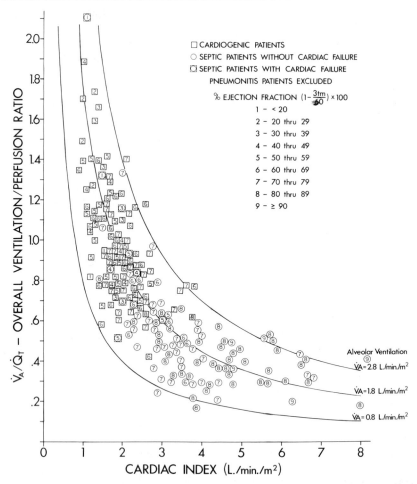

FIG. 19-11 Relation of the V̇A/Q̇T to cardiac index. Points labeled by percent ejection fraction. Lines of constant alveolar ventilation are shown. Note that the septic patients have lower V̇A/Q̇T, higher CIs, and larger ejection fractions than cardiogenic patients. (Siegel JH, Giovaninni I, Coleman B: Ventilation: perfusion maldistribution secondary to the hyperdynamic cardiovascular state as the major cause of increased pulmonary shunting in human sepsis. J Trauma 19: 432, 1979; © 1979 The Williams & Wilkins Co., Baltimore.)

the highest cardiac indices and the greatest cardiac ejection fractions are also those with the lowest V̇A/Q̇T. These patients also turn out to be patients in the septic B state (Chap. 15) of hyperdynamic metabolic insufficiency in whom the vascular resistance per unit flow (vascular tone), and therefore the afterload, are most reduced, thus allowing for a disproportionately high cardiac ejection fraction (Fig. 19-8).

This pattern is in marked contradistinction to that seen in normal exercise, in which an increase in cardiac ejection fraction is associated with a rise in V̇A/Q̇T. However in normal exercise in conditioned athletes, the increased flow is largely produced by an increase in cardiac stroke volume, rather than by an increase in heart rate, since vagal tone is heightened.[54] Consequently, in normal exercise, the LVEDV tends to rise with an increase in LAP and PVP, with a more uniform distribution of blood flow through the lung. Such an increase in V̇A/Q̇T occurs in cardiogenic patients (Fig. 19-11), but in this pathologic situation the rise in

LAP is due to left ventricular failure with a rise in the left ventricular end-diastolic volume and pressure.[54,166]

That this reduction in $\dot{V}A/\dot{Q}T$ in hyperdynamic septic and cirrhotic patients is a major cause of their increased venoarterial admixture ($\dot{Q}S/\dot{Q}T$) is shown in Figure 19-12, where the septic and nonseptic hyperdynamic patients, without pneumonitis, who had the highest percent shunt are also seen to have the lowest $\dot{V}A/\dot{Q}T$ ratios. (When pneumonitis occurs with alveolar consolidation then additional pathologic anatomic shunting is present for a given $\dot{V}A/\dot{Q}T$.) All of these relationships are highly significant and have been confirmed in a large number of patient studies.[163-167]

As also shown in Figure 19-12, studies by Siegel and colleagues[166,167] have revealed that

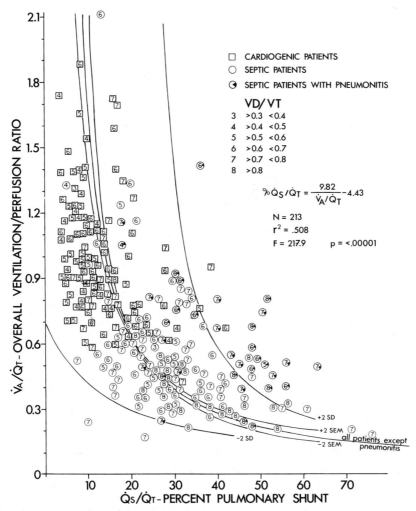

FIG. 19-12 Relation of $\dot{V}A/\dot{Q}T$ to $\dot{Q}S/\dot{Q}T$ with points labeled by VD/VT level. Note that septic patients *without* pneumonitis tend to have a lower $\dot{V}A/\dot{Q}T$ and higher VD/VT for a given level of $\dot{Q}S/\dot{Q}T$, and that the highest $\dot{Q}S/\dot{Q}T$ and lowest $\dot{V}A/\dot{Q}T$ occur in septic patients. However, septic patients *with* pneumonitis have a higher shunt for a given $\dot{V}A/\dot{Q}T$, and fall outside of the 95 percent confidence limits of the regression for nonpneumonitis patients, indicating the additive effect of the pathologic anatomic shunt produced by alveolar infiltration, exudates, and necrosis superimposed on the physiologic shunt produced by increased perfusion of dependent low $\dot{V}A/\dot{Q}$ lung segments. (Siegel JH, Giovaninni I, Coleman B: Ventilation: perfusion maldistribution secondary to the hyperdynamic cardiovascular state as the major cause of increased pulmonary shunting in human sepsis. J Trauma 19: 432, 1979; © 1979 The Williams & Wilkins Co., Baltimore.)

the fall in of $\dot{V}A/\dot{Q}T$ in hyperdynamic septic ARDS, which is directly related to a rise in cardiac ejection fraction, is also associated with an increase in respiratory dead space (VD/VT). These data further suggest that in sepsis and other abnormal hyperdynamic states, the pathophysiologic hyperdynamic increase in cardiac output is increasing perfusion to a smaller region of dependent low $\dot{V}A/\dot{Q}$ lung with increased physiologic shunting while at the same time reducing perfusion to the supe-

rior high $\dot{V}A/\dot{Q}$ lung segments, thus converting them to dead space. In contrast with cardiac failure[96,157] or volume loading,[103] the LAP rises and perfusion is shifted upwards to superior, better-ventilated lung with a higher $\dot{V}A/\dot{Q}$, generally decreasing shunt and VD/VT unless pulmonary edema with alveolar flooding occurs.

This is shown in Figure 19-13, which proposes a model of the cardiovascular determinants of pulmonary $\dot{V}A/\dot{Q}T$, $\dot{Q}S/\dot{Q}T$ and VD/VT in hyperdynamic sepsis (A and B states)

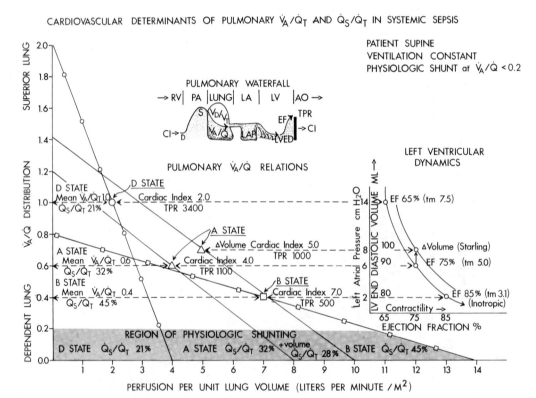

FIG. 19-13 Cardiovascular determinants of pulmonary $\dot{V}A/\dot{Q}$ distribution and $\dot{Q}S/\dot{Q}T$ in septic ARDS. This diagram shows the hypothetical relationship of the $\dot{V}A/\dot{Q}$ relationship, $\dot{V}A/\dot{Q}T$, and $\dot{Q}S/\dot{Q}T$ as functions of left ventricular dynamics and the pulmonary "waterfall." Examples are shown of selected relationships for hyperdynamic A- and B-state septic patients and for cardiogenic D-state septics. Note the relationship of the mean $\dot{V}A/\dot{Q}T$ point to the LVEDV and ejection fraction in the left ventricular dynamic relationship diagram. Values below 0.2 in $\dot{V}A/\dot{Q}$ are assumed to represent the main region of physiologic shunting. The effect of increasing LVEDV with volume in an A-state hyperdynamic patient is contrasted with the pathologic effect of increasing the ejection fraction because of reduced afterload in the B-state septic patient. (Siegel JH, Giovaninni I, Coleman B: Ventilation: perfusion maldistribution secondary to the hyperdynamic cardiovascular state as the major cause of increased pulmonary shunting in human sepsis. J Trauma 19: 432, 1979; © 1979 The Williams & Wilkins Co., Baltimore.)

compared to that which occurs with cardiogenic decompensation (D state). The hypothesis for the control and interaction of these physiologic functions in the development of the hypoxemia and ARDS syndrome of hyperdynamic sepsis and other hyperdynamic states is that the Starling ventricular function relationship of the heart and its inotropic control mechanisms set the slope of the $\dot{V}A/\dot{Q}$ distribution function. In this way cardiac function sets the mean $\dot{V}A/\dot{Q}T$ point, by establishing the specific cardiac index to left ventricular end-diastolic volume (LVEDV) relation at any given moment. The LVEDV sets the LVED pressure, the mean LAP, and the mean pulmonary venous pressure (PVP) by virtue of the left ventricular length/tension relationship (Chap. 9). Thus, the magnitude of the ratio of pulmonary inflow (cardiac index) to the LVEDV is the primary determinant of the pulmonary artery pressure (PAP) to LVEDP gradient. The LVEDV is in turn determined by the inotropic contractile mechanisms and afterload factors produced by the alterations in vascular tone, which are reflected in the ejection fraction (EFx). Thus from a given baseline LVEDV an EFx increase reduces LVEDV, raises cardiac index, and thus increases total pulmonary flow ($\dot{Q}T$). The pulmonary dispersive blood volume (DV/m^2) and its mean distribution of transit times (t_d) are functions of the inflow cardiac output and its gravitational distribution and the outflow pressure "waterfall" effect (PAP–PVP–LAP–LVEDP). Thus these hemodynamic factors set the level of effective $\dot{V}A/\dot{Q}$ distribution for a given ventilation ($\dot{V}E$) and thereby influence the inverse physiologic component of VD/VT (VA/VT).

Total shunt ($\dot{Q}S/\dot{Q}T$), however, is largely determined by two factors, the fixed anatomic and pathologic anatomic shunt, representing collapsed, consolidated, or absent alveoli, and the physiologic shunt, representing flow through the alveoli of very low $\dot{V}A/\dot{Q}$. The basic lung pattern and distribution of alveolar capillary and pulmonary interstitial and alveolar changes are set by the initiating factors in the ARDS process and by the degree of secondary bronchopneumonic invasion. However, at any given stage in the ARDS process, the number of alveoli with low $\dot{V}A/\dot{Q}$ ratios in the physiologic shunt range is determined by the inflow rate to outflow pressure control of $\dot{V}A/\dot{Q}$ distribution at a given minute ventilation ($\dot{V}E$). Once a particular $\dot{V}A/\dot{Q}$ distribution and thus a mean $\dot{V}A/\dot{Q}T$ and VD/VT are established, the absolute level of flow (cardiac output) will set the magnitude of flow through the physiologic and fixed pathologic right-to-left shunts as a volumetric distribution function. This is seen in Figure 19-7, which demonstrates that in septic and cirrhotic hyperdynamic patients *without pneumonitis* a progressive increase in cardiac output produces an increase in the percent shunt ($\dot{Q}S/\dot{Q}T$). Septic patients *with pneumonitis*, where alveolar infiltration produces a fixed shunt component, and patients with the pathologic synergistic vascular tone abnormalities produced by a combination of sepsis and cirrhosis are shifted to a greater $\dot{Q}S/\dot{Q}T$ to flow relationship by their intrinsic disease processes, but have a similar increase in the percent shunt as cardiac output is increased.

ASSESSMENT OF THE ADEQUACY OF GAS EXCHANGE

The adequacy of ventilation is assessed by analysis of arterial blood for oxygen tension (PaO_2), carbon dioxide tension ($PaCO_2$), and pH. The alveolar CO_2 tension ($PACO_2$) is directly related to carbon dioxide production ($\dot{V}CO_2$) and inversely related to alveolar ventilation ($\dot{V}A$). For practical purposes $PaCO_2$ can be substituted for $PACO_2$ and thus:

$$PaCO_2 = \frac{\dot{V}CO_2 \times K}{\dot{V}A}$$

(K is a constant converting L to mmHg = 0.863)

It is apparent that $PaCO_2$ can increase if alveolar ventilation decreases or if CO_2 production increases.

Alveolar ventilation can be decreased as a result of a decrease in total ventilation ($\dot{V}E$) or as a result of a ventilation/perfusion mismatching resulting in an increased dead space (VD)

$$\dot{V}A = \dot{V}E - \dot{V}D$$

The volume of dead space can be measured by collecting mixed expired gas over a period of time and measuring minute ventilation ($\dot{V}E$) and the carbon dioxide tension of this mixed expired gas ($P\bar{E}CO_2$) as well as the $PaCO_2$:

$$\dot{V}D = \frac{PaCO_2 - P\bar{E}CO_2}{PaCO_2} \times \dot{V}E$$

This value represents the physiologic dead space, which includes the alveolar as well as the anatomic dead space volume. The VD/VT ratio, which represents the fraction of ventilation that is dead space ventilation, can be obtained by obtaining a mixed expired gas sample as well as arterial blood sample and measuring the PCO_2 of both.

$$VD/VT = \frac{PaCO_2 - P\bar{E}CO_2}{PaCO_2}$$

A normal VD/VT ratio is 0.20 to 0.40.

Carbon dioxide production ($\dot{V}CO_2$) can be calculated from the formula:

$$\dot{V}CO_2 = \dot{V}E \times F\bar{E}CO_2$$

or

$$\dot{V}CO_2 = \dot{V}E \times \frac{P\bar{E}CO_2}{(PB-47)}$$

where $F\bar{E}CO_2$ is fractional concentration of mixed expired carbon dioxide and PB is barometric pressure.

The end-tidal carbon dioxide tension ($PETCO_2$) is an approximation of the alveolar ($PACO_2$) and, in turn, of the arterial $PaCO_2$. It can be monitored using infrared sensors or a mass spectrometer. In normal individuals the $PETCO_2$ (or $PACO_2$) is only 1 to 4 mmHg below the $PaCO_2$. However, when the distribution of ventilation becomes more uneven, as in obstructive lung disease, pulmonary emboli, or ARDS, where significant venoarterial shunting occurs, the gradient widens. We have seen differences of up to 20 mmHg in some patients with ARDS. If one correlates the $PETCO_2$ ($PACO_2$) with a simultaneously drawn arterial blood sample it can be of value in alerting one to changes in the patient's status since in an intubated patient the $PETCO_2$ ($PACO_2$) can be monitored continuously and noninvasively, in contrast to the $PaCO_2$ which is only monitored

sporadically by blood gases, or by an indwelling arterial sensor. The CO_2 content can be calculated.[98]

Skin sensors are now available that allow for the measurement of transcutaneous carbon dioxide tension ($PTCCO_2$) and transcutaneous oxygen tension ($PTCO_2$). The $PTCCO_2$ gives a value slightly higher than $PaCO_2$ due to venous or tissue CO_2 concentrations. It is also useful as a trend monitor and is especially valuable when one is making changes in ventilator settings in normodynamic or hyperdynamic posttrauma patients breathing increased levels of FIO_2 (> 0.28), since in these cases there is a close relationship between $PaCO_2$ and $PTCCO_2$ when one is using heated sensors[187]:

$$PaCO_2 = 0.81 \, (PTCCO_2) + 8.2$$
$$N = 79, \; r^2 = 0.652, \; F_{2.76} = 143, \; P < 0.0001$$

In general the $PTCCO_2$ is less sensitive to changes in hemodynamic states of the patient than is the transcutaneous oxygen tension ($PTCO_2$), but this relationship is also useful[187]:

$$PaO_2 = 1.22 \, (PTCO_2) + 21.8$$
$$N = 79, \; r^2 = 0.804, \; F_{2.76} = 294, \; P < 0.0001$$

The arterial oxygen tension (PaO_2) is dependent upon the FIO_2, the alveolar ventilation, ventilation/perfusion inequality, the degree of shunting, and diffusion limitations for oxygen in the interstitial fluid separating the alveolus from the alveolar capillaries. However, abnormalities in diffusion are likely to be only a very minor component of the causes of hypoxemia in ARDS patients.

Alveolar hypoventilation as a cause for hypoxemia can be ascertained by calculating the alveolar-arterial oxygen tension gradient $P(A-a)DO_2$ ultizing the alveolar gas equation to calculate PAO_2 and the measured PaO_2

$$PAO_2 = FIO_2(PB - PH_2O)$$
$$- \frac{PACO_2}{R} + FIO_2 \times PACO_2 \frac{(1 - R)}{R}$$

where PB is barometric pressure, PH_2O is water vapor pressure (47 mmHg at 37°C), FIO_2 is fractional concentration of inspired oxygen, R is respiratory quotient (assumed to be 0.8), and $PACO_2$ is alveolar carbon dioxide (assumed to equal $PaCO_2$). For simplicity's sake, the last term [$FIO_2 \times PACO_2 (1 - R)/R$] is usually ignored and a value of 0.8 is used for R, thus $PAO_2 = FIO_2(PB-47) - PACO_2/0.8$ and

$$P(A - a)DO_2 = PAO_2 - PaO_2$$

The normal gradient is 5 to 10 mmHg and may be as high as 20 mmHG in the aged individual.[124] If hypoxemia is present and the $P(A - a)DO_2$ is normal, then alveolar hypoventilation with its resultant increase in $PACO_2$ and $PaCO_2$ is the cause since all other causes of hypoxemia result in a widened $P(A - a)DO_2$.

The respiratory index, which is the alveolar arterial O_2 gradient divided by the PaO_2:

$$RI = \frac{[(PB - PH_2O) FIO_2 - PaCO_2] - PaO_2}{PaO_2}$$

$$= P(A - a)DO_2/PaO_2$$

helps to normalize for the effect of increasing FIO_2 in critically ill patients.[159,165] As will be shown later, this index is a useful method of quantifying the severity of abnormalities in oxygen exchange that has been used to assess overall respiratory oxygen exchange in trauma,[71] sepsis or hepatic failure syndromes,[159] in pneumonitis,[83,159] and cardiogenic decompensation.[159,165] When evaluated as a function of the simultaneously obtained total shunt (QS/QT), it can provide diagnostic information concerning the type of clinical process producing the oxygen exchange limitations and the importance of raising cardiac output to a level greater than that needed to support VO_2 as a mechanism to increase the level of mixed venous O_2 (PvO_2) as a therapeutic modality that permits an increase in PaO_2 at any[159] given FIO_2.

The total cardiac output (QT) is made up of two major components: QC, which is the portion of the blood flow that exchanges perfectly with alveolar air, and QS, the shunt component, or that portion of blood flow that does not exchange at all with alveolar air:

$$QT = QC + QS$$

Shunting of blood can occur as a result of a large-vessel or intracardiac anatomic shunt where a portion of the cardiac output is returned to the left ventricle without entering the pulmonary capillary vasculature, a capillary shunt where blood enters a pulmonary capillary adjacent to an unventilated alveolus and returns to the left ventricle without under-

going gas exchange, or to a physiologic shunt where VA/Q inequality (perfusion [Q] in excess of ventilation [V] as a result of either a poorly ventilated alveolus or an excessive rate of blood flow) causes blood leaving the alveolar–capillary unit to have a lower oxygen content than blood leaving a normal unit. The total shunt (QS) is made up of the anatomic, capillary, and physiologic shunt components. The sum of the anatomic and capillary components is the "true" or "absolute" shunt and usually does not respond to manipulations of inspired oxygen concentration (FIO_2). The physiologic shunt component, which is secondary to VA/Q inequality, is responsive to changes in FIO_2 and often small changes in FIO_2 result in large changes in blood oxygen content.

The PaO_2 and $P(A-a)DO_2$ are abnormal in ARDS patients. However, they are relatively insensitive indicators of the degree of abnormality in gas exchange since they are altered not only by the level of overall ventilation[18] but also by such nonpulmonary causes as changes in cardiac output,[51,57,67,85,159] reductions in hemoglobin concentration,[57,164] shifts in the oxygen dissociation curve,[56,97,121,126] and changes in oxygen consumption[40] that can affect the mixed venous oxygen content (CvO_2). This can be seen by examining the Fick equation, which relates oxygen consumption (VO_2), cardiac output (QT), arterial O_2 content (CaO_2) and mixed venous O_2 content (CvO_2).

$$VO_2 = QT(CaO_2 - CvO_2)$$

$$CvO_2 = CaO_2 - \frac{VO_2}{QT}$$

Changes in CaO_2 may be due to changes in PaO_2, percent O_2 saturation (SaO_2), or hemoglobin concentration (Hb).

$$CaO_2 = Hb \times 1.39 \times \frac{SaO_2}{100} + 0.0031 \, PaO_2$$

therefore

CvO_2

$$= \left[Hb \times 1.39 \times \frac{SaO_2}{100} + 0.0031 \, PaO_2 \right] - \frac{VO_2}{QT}$$

Under normal circumstances any perturbations causing a decrease in CvO_2 will be accompanied by compensatory changes in cardiac output or minute ventilation. In the critically ill individual, however, these compensatory mechanisms may not be fully operative and a decrease in $C\bar{v}O_2$ will lead to a decrease in PaO_2 and widened $P(A-a)DO_2$. Changes in inspired O_2 may also lead to changes in PaO_2 and $P(A-a)DO_2$ that are unrelated to changes in lung function. Patients with a fixed shunt will have an increasing $P(A-a)DO_2$ as FIO_2 is increased toward 1.0. Patients with $\dot{V}A/\dot{Q}$ inequality have a curvilinear change with $P(A-a)DO_2$ first increasing and then decreasing as FIO_2 is increased. Therefore, in order to follow changes in lung function both PaO_2 and $P(A-a)DO_2$ must always be measured at the same FIO_2, or a normalizing function such as the respiratory index (RI) must be used to compare O_2 exchange from one time to the next.

Quantification of gas exchange efficiency can be accomplished by the assessment of total shunt ($\dot{Q}S/\dot{Q}T$). The admixture of mixed venous blood from the shunt compartment with the fully saturated pulmonary capillary blood is assumed to lower the PaO_2. A simple mixing equation is used to quantify the percent of blood flow being shunted and thus not undergoing gas exchange.

$$\dot{Q}T(CaO_2) = \dot{Q}S(C\bar{v}O_2) + (\dot{Q}T - \dot{Q}S)(CiO_2)$$

This equation states that the total amount of oxygen in the arterial blood that is a function of both total cardiac output and arterial oxygen content is the sum of the oxygen in the shunt component and the oxygen from the matched alveolar–capillary compartment. CiO_2 is the content of oxygen at full saturation in the end-capillary blood of the alveolar compartment. The arterial and mixed venous bloods are sampled directly and their pH, PCO_2, PO_2, Hb, and SO_2 are analyzed and oxygen contents are calculated, utilizing the formula:

$$CaO_2 = Hb \times 1.39 \times \frac{SaO_2}{100} + 0.0031\, PaO_2$$

$$C\bar{v}O_2 = Hb \times 1.39 \times \frac{S\bar{v}O_2}{100} + 0.0031\, P\bar{v}O_2$$

The oxygen content of the alveolar-capillary compartment must be calculated using the alveolar air equation to determine the correct alveolar PO_2 (PAO_2). When high FIO_2 mixtures are breathed, resulting in an alveolar $PAO_2 \geqslant$ 150 mmHg, one can assume that blood leaving this alveolar capillary unit is essentially completely saturated and CiO_2 can be calculated as:

$$CiO_2 = [Hb \times 1.39] + 0.0031\, PaO_2$$

At levels below a PaO_2 of 150 mmHg the true saturation must be calculated using a mathematical algorithm.[56,97] Shunt flow as a percentage of the total cardiac output is calculated as:

$$\dot{Q}S/\dot{Q}T = \frac{CiO_2 - CaO_2}{CiO_2 - C\bar{v}O_2}$$

Factors other than true right-to-left shunt influence the calculated value of shunt when room air is being breathed. These include $\dot{V}A/\dot{Q}$ inequality, diffusion, and the nonpulmonary factors that influence mixed venous oxygen content. As FIO_2 is increased, the contribution of these other factors diminishes, but the rate at which their influence is diminished is variable and depends upon the underlying pathophysiology. At an FIO_2 of 1.0 (100 percent) breathed for a sufficient time to wash out nitrogen, the calculation will reflect the level of the true shunt.[18] Therefore, if factors other than true right-to-left shunt alone contribute to hypoxemia there will be a linear fall in the calculated total shunt ($\dot{Q}S/\dot{Q}T$). In patients in whom true right-to-left shunt is the mechanism for the observed hypoxemia, the measured $\dot{Q}S/\dot{Q}T$ will be constant at any FIO_2, unless the actual shunt has changed. Some studies have shown that shunt does indeed increase when FIO_2 is increased and this phenomenon has been attributed to the reversal of compensatory hypoxic pulmonary vasoconstriction in areas with extremely low $\dot{V}A/\dot{Q}$ ratios and reabsorption microatelectasis as a result of denitrogenation of these lung units.[49,161] Dantzker[42,43] claims that this effect may only be theoretical, especially in patients with ARDS, where his anatomic and physiologic data suggest that lung units are either well-ventilated with normal or high $\dot{V}A/\dot{Q}$ ratios or totally collapsed. He believes that if there are areas with low $\dot{V}A/\dot{Q}$ ratios their contribution is small and they are only intermittently ventilated at peak inspiration. However, other studies suggest that a bimodal distribution of $\dot{V}A/\dot{Q}$ exists in ARDS with some very low $\dot{V}A/\dot{Q}$ regions that may be collapsed if high FIO_2 levels are used.[118] In practice most workers, including the authors, have utilized shunt calculations based on the patient receiving an $FIO_2 > 0.40$ (> 40 percent), which should yield a PAO_2 in excess of 240 mmHg to avoid potential problems with a FIO_2 of 1.0.

When interpreting shunt one must be aware that the level of the intrapulmonary shunt can be affected by the level of the cardiac output and that an increase or decrease can cause similar changes in $\dot{Q}S/\dot{Q}T$.[44,166,167,174] The mechanism for this dependence (Fig. 19-11) may be related to the relative increase in perfusion of more dependent low $\dot{V}A/\dot{Q}$ lung segments so that physiologic shunt rises (Fig. 19-12) as flow increases.[166] This phenomenon and its physiologic effects are discussed later. However, regardless of mechanism, as a result of this dependence one must always interpret changes in the level of the shunt in conjunction with concomitant changes in cardiac output.[44,167,174]

Reformatting the shunt equation (adding and subtracting CaO_2 to the denominator of the content equation) brings out the important role cardiac output plays in altering the result of shunted cardiac output and arterial hypoxemia. One can demonstrate this effect on this new form of the classic shunt equation mathematically by increasing or decreasing $C\bar{v}O_2$, which widens or narrows the arteriovenous oxygen content difference consistent with a change in cardiac output at a constant body oxygen consumption.

$$\frac{\dot{Q}S}{\dot{Q}T} = \frac{CiO_2 - CaO_2}{[CaO_2 - C\bar{v}O_2] + [CiO_2 - CaO_2]}$$

Gas Exchange/Shunt Relations

Since the peripheral vascular tone alterations that influence the cardiac ejection fraction by reducing afterload are the earliest and most prominent feature of the physiologic response to stress and the subsequent development of a septic process,[165-168] it seems clear why vascular tone reduction produces early physiologic changes in gas exchange. Even though the alterations in permeability produced by sepsis and other causes of the humoral ARDS response are undoubtedly occurring at the same time, when measured with sensitive functional indicators such as the γ-scintigraphic technique developed by Sugerman et al.[189,190] the permeability changes produced by these factors appear to have a longer time constant than the hemodynamically induced $\dot{V}A/\dot{Q}$ changes before their direct effects on gas exchange become clinically manifest. Nevertheless, it is clear that the interaction of hyperperfusion and altered permeability will synergistically potentiate the process of interstitial fluid accumulation and accelerate the time course over which the microscopic picture of interstitial edema, leukocyte septal invasion, and intravascular congestion (stage I of Clowes) progresses to that of diffuse alveolar collapse, hyaline deposition, alveolar cell necrosis, and interstitial fibrosis (stage II of Clowes).[37] This explains the observations of Hechtman[80] that there was a lack of correlation between shunt and either lung water or pulmonary compliance in the early phases of the ARDS process, and those of Demling[46-49] that increased alveolar capillary fluid flow in the absence of thromboxane-A_2-mediated injury did not increase lung water or lower PaO_2. However, as the process of pulmonary perfusion maldistribution continues in the presence of altered capillary permeability (K_f), the increased tissue pressure in the dependent lung segments (caused by an increase in $\dot{Q}_f$ relative to the increase in lymph flow) will result in a reduction of alveolar size and the $\dot{V}A$ and FRC will fall producing the relationship between FRC and shunt noted by Powers[130,149] and Hechtman.[80]

When complete alveolar collapse, infiltration, or consolidation occurs, the functional $\dot{V}A/\dot{Q}$ disparities are converted to a pathologic anatomic shunt, which is added to the remaining $\dot{Q}S/\dot{Q}T$ physiologic shunt. This is seen in hyperdynamic patients with late ARDS and those with sepsis and pneumonitis, who have a greater increase in the percent of pulmonary shunt for a given level of $\dot{V}A/\dot{Q}T$ then do septic patients *without* pneumonitis (Fig. 19-12).

When the relationship between the percent shunt ($\dot{Q}S/\dot{Q}T$), which calculates the total percentage of cardiac output passing through the lung without being effectively oxygenated, and the respiratory index (RI), which represents the relationship of the gas exchange factors (the alveolar-arterial oxygen gradient to PaO_2 ratio) is examined systematically, it also can be seen that the septic pneumonitis patients have a higher $A\text{-}aDO_2/PaO_2$ (respiratory index) for a given shunt than do septic patients without pneumonitis. There are thus different slopes in the various pathophysiologic clinical conditions. This is shown in Figure 19-14, which demonstrates that there are significant differences in the relationship between the RI and $\dot{Q}S/\dot{Q}T$ as a function of different disease states. In hyperdynamic sepsis and cirrhotic liver disease without a pneumonitis component, there is a relatively small increase in RI for a large increase in percent shunt, reflecting the primary $\dot{V}A/\dot{Q}T$ maldistribution and resultant physiologic shunting that is the underlying cause of this abnormality. In contrast, in septic pneumonitis and/or late ARDS, there is a relatively large RI increase for an increase in shunt percentage, reflecting the direct impairment of gas exchange due to alveolar exudates and interstitial edema, infiltration, and fibrosis characteristic of this disease (Fig. 19-2). In contrast

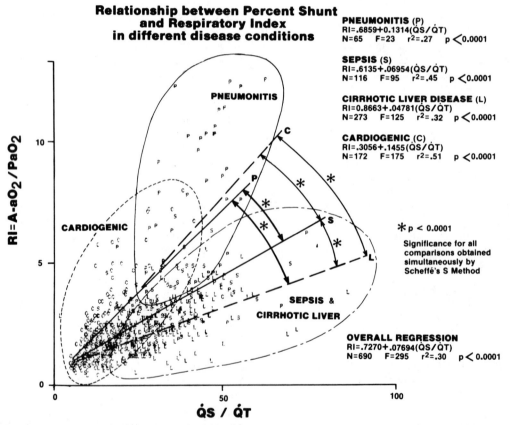

FIG. 19-14 Relationship between percent shunt and respiratory index in different disease conditions. Note that the increase in respiratory index (RI) per unit $\dot{Q}S/\dot{Q}T$ is greater in patients *with* pneumonitis ARDS than in those with hyperdynamic sepsis or cirrhotic liver disease *without* pneumonitis. Cardiogenic patients have a similar slope because of the more uniform ventilation perfusion relationship with alveolar flooding due to pulmonary edema, but do not maintain the high levels of $\dot{Q}S/\dot{Q}T$ seen in septic patients with ARDS and pneumonitis. (Sganga A, Siegel JH, Coleman B et al: The physiologic meaning of the respiratory index in various types of critical illness. Circ Shock 17: 179, 1985.)

to low V̇A/Q̇T states such as sepsis and cirrhosis, in patients with cardiogenic pulmonary edema the relationship between RI and Q̇S/Q̇T is also steep, although the flow range is more limited. In cardiogenic conditions the relatively high RI per unit shunt is secondary to the fact that although there is a more uniform distribution of ventilation and perfusion in this disease condition,[96,157,166] the high venous pressure also promotes pulmonary edema and alveolar flooding with direct impairment of alveolar gas exchange.

The evolution of the ARDS process from a stage where ventilation/perfusion disparities

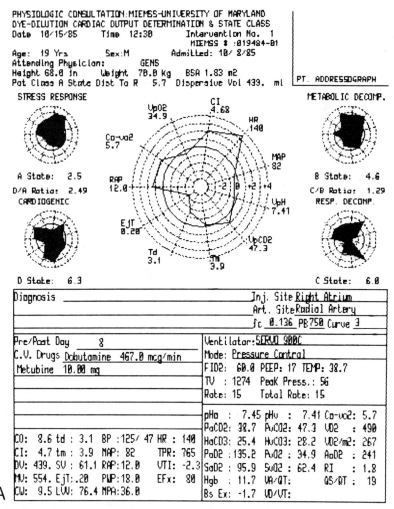

FIG. 19-15 (A) Pattern of physiologic accommodation in a 19-year-old patient with posttraumatic and septic ARDS. DV, pulmonary dispersive blood volume; MV, mixing volume; CW, cardiac work; BP, blood pressure, systolic and diastolic; MAP, mean arterial pressure; RAP, right atrial pressure; PWP, pulmonary wedge pressure; MPA, mean pulmonary artery pressure; HR, heart rate; TPR, total peripheral resistance; VTI, vascular tone index; pHa, arterial pH; aHCO₃, arterial bicarbonate; SaO₂, arterial oxygen saturation; Hgb, hemoglobin concentration; BsEx, base excess; PHv̄, venous pH; Pv̄CO₂, venous CO₂; Pv̄O₂, venous O₂; Sv̄O₂, mixed venous saturation; V̇O₂, oxygen consumption; V̇O₂/m², oxygen consumption per meter square. Note hyperdynamic state and low RI to Q̇S/Q̇T ratio early in development of ARDS. See text for other abbreviations. (*Figure continues.*)

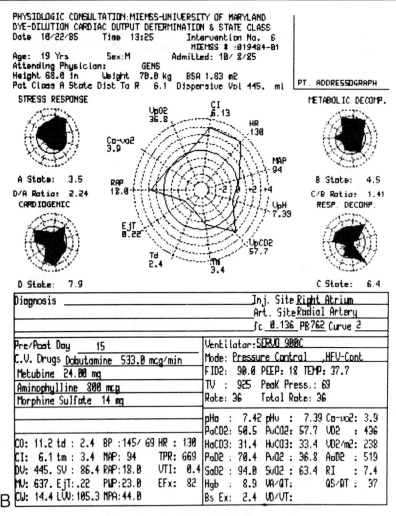

FIG. 19-15 *(Continued)* **(B)** Continued development of ARDS syndrome in patient shown in (A) 7 days later. Hyperdynamic state is increased and the RI to $\dot{Q}S/\dot{Q}T$ ratio has increased disproportionately to the increase in cardiac output. Abbreviations as in (A). *(Figure continues.)*

and fixed shunt caused by collapsed alveoli, magnified by the hyperdynamic cardiovascular response, are the major cause of the total shunt (identified by a low RI to $\dot{Q}S/\dot{Q}T$ ratio), to that where more uniformly distributed alveolar gas exchange limitations (caused by alveolar flooding or necrosis) produce a high RI to $\dot{Q}S/\dot{Q}T$ ratio, as well as CO_2 retention, is shown in Figure 19-15. This figure also shows the endogenous physiologic response to this degree of gas exchange limitation in ARDS, namely, that of a heightened hyperdynamic response.

This may be seen as an attempt to increase perfusion of the few remaining alveolar exchange surfaces, as well as a mechanism to sustain a high enough $P\bar{v}O_2$ to allow a favorable position on the hemoglobin dissociation curve so that a near-normal arterial saturation can be maintained.

This patient was a 19-year-old man who suffered a fractured femur, a closed head injury with hemiparesis, and bilateral pulmonary contusion in a motor vehicle accident. Severe ARDS developed complicated by a gram-nega-

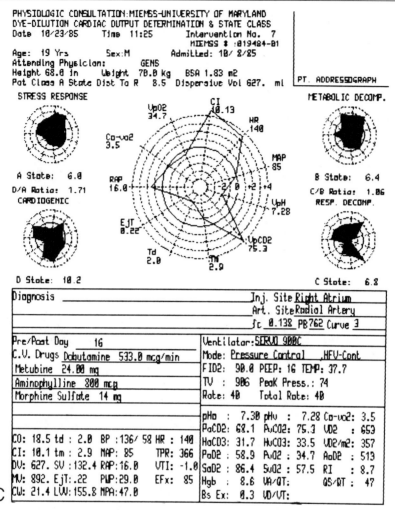

PHYSIOLOGIC CONSULTATION:MIEMSS-UNIVERSITY OF MARYLAND
DYE-DILUTION CARDIAC OUTPUT DETERMINATION & STATE CLASS
Date 10/23/85   Time 11:25   Intervention No. 7
                                  MIEMSS # :019484-01
Age: 19 Yrs   Sex:M   Admitted: 10/ 8/85
Attending Physician: GENS
Height 68.0 in   Weight 78.0 kg   BSA 1.83 m2
Pat Class A State Dist To R   8.5 Dispersive Vol 627. ml   PT. ADDRESSOGRAPH

STRESS RESPONSE   METABOLIC DECOMP.

VpO2 34.7   CI 10.13
                   HR 140
Co-vo2 3.5
                              MAP 85
A State: 6.0   RAP 16.0   B State: 6.4
D/A Ratio: 1.71   C/B Ratio: 1.86
CARDIOGENIC   VpH 7.28   RESP. DECOMP.

EjT 0.22
Td 2.0   TM 2.9   VpCO2 75.3

D State: 10.2   C State: 6.8

Diagnosis	Inj. Site Right Atrium
	Art. Site Radial Artery
	Jc 0.138 PB 762 Curve 3

Pre/Post Day 16	Ventilator: SERVO 900C
C.V. Drugs Dobutamine 533.0 mcg/min	Mode: Pressure Control ,HFV-Cont
Metubine 24.00 mg	FID2: 90.0 PEEP: 16 TEMP: 37.7
Aminophylline 800 mcg	TV : 906 Peak Press.: 74
Morphine Sulfate 14 mg	Rate: 40 Total Rate: 40

		pHa : 7.30 pHv : 7.28 Co-vo2: 3.5
		PaCO2: 68.1 PvCO2: 75.3 VO2 : 659
CO: 18.5 td : 2.0 BP :136/ 58 HR : 140		HaCO3: 31.7 HvCO3: 33.5 VO2/m2: 357
CI: 10.1 tm : 2.9 MAP: 85 TPR: 366		PaO2: 58.9 PvO2: 34.7 AoDO2 : 513
DV: 627. SV :132.4 RAP:16.0 VTI: -1.0		SaO2 : 86.4 SvO2 : 57.5 RI : 8.7
MV: 892. EjT:.22 PWP:29.0 EFx: 85		Hgb : 8.6 VA/QT: QS/QT : 47
CW: 21.4 LW:155.8 MPA:47.0		Bs Ex: 0.3 VD/VT:

FIG. 19-15 *(Continued)* **(C)** Continued progression of the ARDS syndrome 8 days after the physiologic pattern shown in (B). Progressive increase in cardiac output and cardiac index with increased RI to $\dot{Q}S/\dot{Q}T$ ratio demonstrating progression of disease. Now also there is a respiratory acidosis superimposed on the hyperdynamic state with rise in $PaCO_2$ and fall in pH. Note also that in spite of the increased respiratory insufficiency the progressive hyperdynamic state has produced an increased $P\bar{v}O_2$ between 36.8 and 34.7 mmHg, thus permitting a higher PaO_2 and arterial saturation to be maintained in spite of the increasing shunt and respiratory exchange failure. Abbreviations as in (A).

tive pneumonia. As the course of the patient's ARDS evolved from the stage I response seen in Figure 19-15A, where a normal hyperdynamic cardiac index response (CI = 4.7 L/min/m²) with a high EFx of 80 percent was associated with RI of 1.8 at a $\dot{Q}S/\dot{Q}T$ of 19 percent to the stage II response (Fig. 19-15B,C) due to progressive pneumonitis infiltrating the

ARDS lung, the cardiac index progressively rose from 6.1 L/min/m² to 10.1 L/min/m². The gas exchange limitations are seen in the increase in RI to 7.4 (Fig. 19-15B) and then to 8.7 (Fig. 19-15C) as the $\dot{Q}S/\dot{Q}T$ rose to 37 and 47 percent respectively. Although the PaO_2 fell to 58.9 mmHg on 0.90 FIO_2 (90 percent) and the $PaCO_2$ rose to 68.1 mmHg (despite the use of continuous high-frequency ventilation to re-duce the effective respiratory dead space by lowering the $PECO_2$ levels). As a result of the cardiac compensation to the ARDS produced gas exchange limitations, oxygen delivery was increased more than needed to meet the sepsis imposed body oxygen consumption needs, as shown by the rising $\dot{V}O_2$ (see Chap. 9). Thus the rise in cardiac output from 8.6 L/min (Fig. 19-15A) to 18.5 L/min (Fig. 19-15C), by increas-ing oxygen delivery from 2.6 to 2.9 times the required oxygen consumption, maintained $P\bar{v}O_2$ fairly constant between 34 and 37 mmHg. While aggressive tailoring of the nature and mode of ventilatory support was able to main-tain this patient for 40 days after his accident and initiation of posttraumatic and septic

ARDS, he eventually died due to the exten-sive pulmonary alveolar necrosis and intersti-tial fibrotic process characteristic of stage II ARDS.[36,37,109]

CARDIOVASCULAR THERAPEUTIC MEASURES

This relationship between increasing car-diac output and rising $P\bar{v}O_2$ (Fig. 19-16) also explains why adjusting the cardiovascular fac-

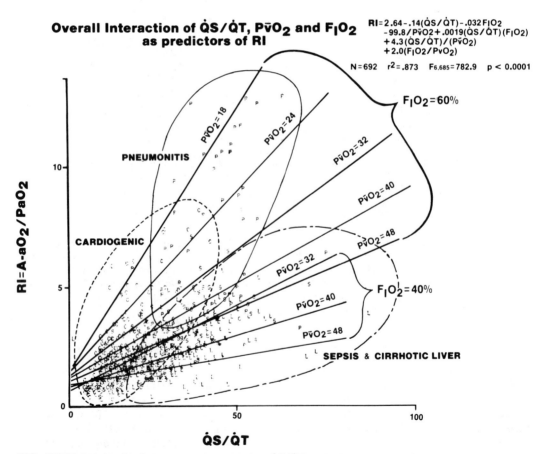

FIG. 19-16 Relationship between respiratory index, $\dot{Q}S/\dot{Q}T$ and mixed venous PO_2 ($P\bar{v}O_2$) in permitting a lower FIO_2 to be administered for any given level of respiratory insufficiency in various disease states.

tor becomes an important therapeutic maneuver for use in compensation for severe ARDS. This figure shows the same regions of the RI to $\dot{Q}S/\dot{Q}T$ relationship as shown in Figure 19-14, but also plots lines of constant pulmonary artery oxygen tension ($P\bar{v}O_2$). It demonstrates that for any given $\dot{Q}S/\dot{Q}T$ it is possible to increase the effective mixed venous gas delivery to exchanging alveoli and thereby to reduce the RI, by raising the $P\bar{v}O_2$. As noted above, this can be done by increasing the cardiac output to a higher level than required by the body's oxygen consumption needs (see Chap. 9). The physiologic mechanism is shown in Figure 19-17, where a computer simulation example has been constructed, assuming a constant $\dot{V}O_2$ of 300 ml/min at a constant shunt ($\dot{Q}S/\dot{Q}T = 30$ percent). By increasing the cardiac output (CO) from 5 L/min to 10 L/min at a given F_IO_2, systemic oxygen delivery increases at any given level of arterial hemoglobin saturation. Consequently, the mixed venous saturation also rises, if $\dot{V}O_2$ is constant. Because of the shape of the oxyhemoglobin dissociation curve, the $P\bar{v}O_2$ is increased as the arterial venous oxygen content gradient ($Ca-\bar{v}O_2$) difference narrows and the PaO_2 increases to a greater extent than the $P\bar{v}O_2$ as the arterial saturation rises to the flat portion of the curve.[108,121,126] Thus increasing CO helps to compensate for any given shunt. More important, since for any F_IO_2 in-

creasing $P\bar{v}O_2$ raises PaO_2 at a given $\dot{Q}S/\dot{Q}T$ level, increasing cardiac output becomes an important therapeutic maneuver to allow the critical care physician or surgeon to *lower* the F_IO_2 (Fig. 19-16). This reduces the potential for microatelectasis in partially obstructed alveoli[41,161,164] and also diminishes the chance of direct oxygen toxicity to the cells of the alveolar–capillary bed.[8,101,133]

As one assists the patient with ARDS to compensate for the underlying respiratory dysfunction by increasing cardiac index, it also is possible to capitalize on the relationship between the cardiac function and pulmonary perfusion to obtain a more uniform ventilation/perfusion ratio, provided the proper balance between infusion preload and cardiac inotropic stimulation is achieved.[103,166] This is shown in Figure 19-18, which demonstrates the effect of manipulating cardiac index by either the Frank-Starling mechanism of raising left ventricular end-diastolic volume, or the inotropic mechanism of increasing cardiac ejection fraction by the use of a cardiac inotropic agent that increases myocardial contractility. This figure shows that patients (numbers 1 and 2) who had an increase in cardiac index by virtue of use of the inotropic mechanism without volume loading (solid line) also showed an increase in percent shunt as the left ventricular end-diastolic volume decreased. In these same

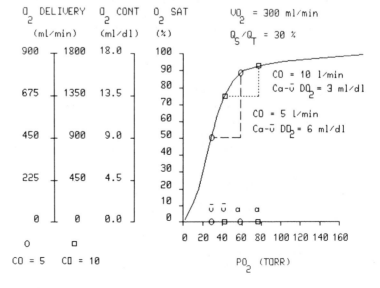

FIG. 19-17 The role of the oxygen hemoglobin disassociation curve in mediating the effect of an increased oxygen delivery on the level of arterial PO_2 and arterial oxygen content.

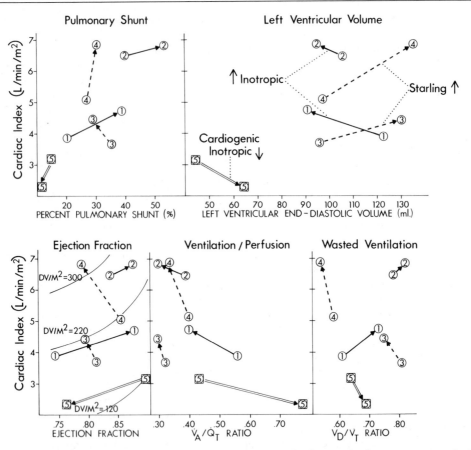

FIG. 19-18 Differential effect of increasing cardiac output by the Starling mechanism versus a pure inotropic increase in flow on percent shunt (QS/QT) left ventricular end-diastolic volume (LVEDV), cardiac ejection fraction (EFx), ventilation perfusion ratio (VA/QT), and VD/VT ratio. Note that pure inotropic increases (which do not raise end-diastolic volume) result in an increase in percent shunt, a reduction (or no change) in the pulmonary blood volume, and a reduction in VA/QT with an increase in VD/VT, demonstrating in ARDS the increased disparity in VA/Q relationships under these conditions.

cases, it can also be seen that the decrease in end-diastolic volume as associated with an increase in EFx, which facilitates an increase in flow without substantial increase in total pulmonary blood volume (DV/m²). At the same time, the area of lung converted to dead space, reflected by the VD/VT ratio, also increased. Although the ventilation/perfusion ratio increased as well, this increase in VA/QT was much smaller than that caused by a comparable increase in cardiac output due to volume infusion (patients number 3 and 4), which raised the ventricular end-diastolic volume under the Frank-Starling mechanism (dashed

line). In this case, the rise in flow (cardiac index) was associated with either a negligible increase, or an actual decrease, in percent shunt as the left ventricular end-diastolic volume rose. Under the Starling mechanism using volume infusion, the ejection fraction fell slightly and as a result the pulmonary blood volume (DV/m²) increased, reflecting a more uniform distribution of blood flow in the lung. This was associated with a significant rise in the ventilation/perfusion ratio as the flow increased. In contrast to the inotropic increase in flow, with volume infusion the VD/VT was decreased. A negative inotropic effect as with cardiogenic failure (patient number 5) acts like the flip side of the Starling mechanism with a fall in $\dot{Q}S/\dot{Q}T$, and a rise in $\dot{V}A/\dot{Q}T$ as LVEDV and pulmonary blood volume increase.

The therapeutic manipulation of all of these factors (ventilation/perfusion distribution and the level of $P\bar{v}O_2$ presented to the alveolar capillary exchange surface) in achieving respiratory compensation after severe injury is shown in Figure 19-19. These physiologic patterns were obtained from the study of a 27-year-old man who had sustained a major fracture of the right lobe of the liver associated

with multiple rib fractures after being crushed under a heavy piece of construction equipment. He underwent a major surgical procedure for hepatic debridement and control of hemorrhage with multiple transfusions before, during and after surgery. Figure 19-19A demonstrates his physiologic pattern immediately after surgery (Day 1 postoperatively). Postoperatively he had edematous swelling in the remaining injured liver producing a functional inferior vena caval obstruction with partial obstruction of venous return from the lower half of the body. To assist in maintaining venous return,

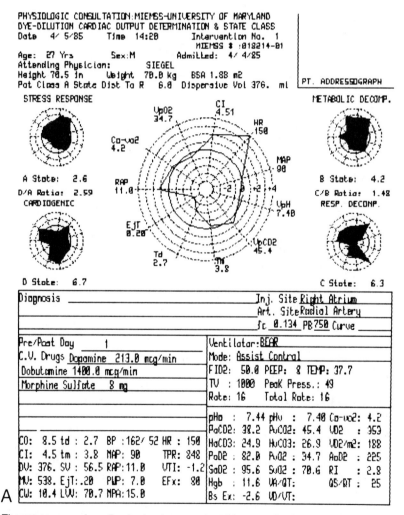

FIG. 19-19 The proper use of cardiac inotropic support and increased pulmonary blood volume by infusion in maintaining a high level of oxygen delivery and permitting improved PaO_2 as a result of the rise in $P\bar{v}O_2$ **(A)** Inotropic support alone. Abbreviations as in Figure 19-15(A). (*Figure continues.*)

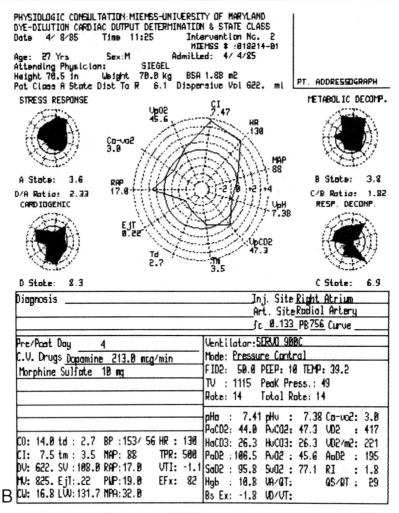

PHYSIOLOGIC CONSULTATION:MIEMSS-UNIVERSITY OF MARYLAND
DYE-DILUTION CARDIAC OUTPUT DETERMINATION & STATE CLASS
Date 4/ 8/85   Time 11:25   Intervention No. 2
                                     MIEMSS # :018214-01
Age: 27 Yrs   Sex:M   Admitted: 4/ 4/85
Attending Physician: SIEGEL
Height 70.5 in   Weight 70.0 kg   BSA 1.88 m2
Pot Class A State Dist To R   6.1 Dispersive Vol 622. ml

PT. ADDRESSOGRAPH

STRESS RESPONSE

A State: 3.6
D/A Ratio: 2.33
CARDIOGENIC

D State: 8.3

METABOLIC DECOMP.

B State: 3.8
C/B Ratio: 1.82
RESP. DECOMP.

C State: 6.9

Diagnosis	Inj. Site Right Atrium
	Art. Site Radial Artery
	fc 0.133 PB 756 Curve

Pre/Post Day	4	Ventilator:SERVO 900C
C.V. Drugs Dopamine 213.0 mcg/min	Mode: Pressure Control
Morphine Sulfate 10 mg	FIO2: 50.0 PEEP: 10 TEMP: 39.2
	TV : 1115 Peak Press.: 49
	Rate: 14 Total Rate: 14

		pHa : 7.41 pHv : 7.38 Co-vo2: 3.0	
		PaCO2: 44.0 PvCO2: 47.3 VO2 : 417	
CO: 14.0 td : 2.7 BP :153/ 56 HR : 130		HaCO3: 26.3 HvCO3: 26.3 VO2/m2: 221	
CI: 7.5 tm : 3.5 MAP: 88 TPR: 500		PaO2 :106.5 PvO2 : 45.6 AoO2 : 195	
DV: 622. SV :108.0 RAP:17.0 VTI: -1.1		SaO2 : 95.8 SvO2 : 77.1 RI : 1.8	
MV: 825. EjT:.22 PLP:19.0 EFx: 82		Hgb : 10.8 VA/QT: QS/QT : 29	
CW: 16.8 LW:131.7 NPA:32.0		Bs Ex: -1.8 VD/VT:	

B

FIG. 19-19 *(Continued)* **(B)** Combination of inotropic support and volume infusion. Abbreviations as in Figure 19-15(A).

an inotropic support program was utilized which increased cardiac output while lowering right atrial pressure to 3 cm H_2O above PEEP. On this program he had a normal stress A state cardiovascular response (see Chap. 9) with an increase in cardiac index to 4.5 L/min/m² (cardiac output 8.5 L/min) on inotropic support (dopamine 3 μg/kg/min and dobutamine 20 μg/kg/min). There was a resulting increase in cardiac ejection fraction (EFx = 80 percent) but because of the marked tachycardia his left ventricular volume was relatively low (LVV = 70.7 ml). The posttraumatic ARDS pulmonary flow disparity resulted in a PaO_2 of only 82 mmHg

on an FIO_2 of 0.5 (50 percent) with a respiratory index of 2.8 at a total shunt ($\dot{Q}S/\dot{Q}T$) of 25 percent. These values suggest that a flow distribution disparity, rather than alveolar flooding, was the cause for the shunt.

To assist in respiratory compensation while still providing cardiac inotropic support to allow for the needed increase in cardiac output, the pulmonary reservoir blood volume (DV/m²) was increased by transfusion from the normal level of 200 ml/m² (DV = 376 ml) to an increased level of 330 ml/m² (DV = 622 ml) and dobutamine was withdrawn, leaving the patient on dopamine (3μg/kg/min) alone. The resulting volume plus inotropic-agent-supported stress response increase in cardiac index to 7.5 L/min/m² (cardiac output = 14.0 L/min) increased the P$\bar{v}O_2$ from 34.7 mmHg to 45.6 mmHg by increasing body flow in excess of body oxygen consumption needs as the LVV rose to 131.7 ml, inducing a better pulmonary perfusion distribution. The $\dot{V}O_2$/m² rose from 188 ml/min to 221 ml/min as Ca-$\bar{v}O_2$ narrowed and minute ventilation remained essentially unchanged (16 L/min to 15.6 L/min), as did the FIO₂ of 0.5 (50 percent). However, the PaO₂ increased from 82 to 106 torr and the RI decreased to 1.8, even though $\dot{Q}S/\dot{Q}T$ rose slightly to 29 percent.

These responses in individual patients tend to confirm the basic hypothesis that at any given ARDS stage the distribution of blood flow in the lung and the relative ventilation/perfusion mismatch is largely controlled by the relationship between total pulmonary flow and cardiac ejection fraction. This is due to the left ventricular end-diastolic volume and pressure relationship, which sets the perfusion of the lung relative to the three zones of hemodynamic and alveolar pressure relationships.[209,210] Within the limitations imposed by these relationships, at any FIO₂ the PaO₂ can be raised by cardiovascular support measures that will increase P$\bar{v}O_2$ by raising cardiac output higher than required by body oxygen consumption needs. In addition experimental studies suggest that β-inotropic support may directly attenuate lung edema and improve pulmonary function.[128,129]

PHARMACOLOGIC THERAPY DIRECTED AT MODIFYING ALVEOLAR CAPILLARY PERMEABILITY

While there have been a number of reports of improvement in experimental ARDS syndromes by the pretreatment with prostaglandin,[2,17,79,105,200] serotonin,[48,78,79,92] and thromboxane or superoxide-inhibiting agents,[33,48,79,104,152,178,198] other important research efforts demonstrate that these agents produce no significant alteration in the pulmonary permeability and albumin leak induced by either oleic acid or acid infusion ARDS syndromes.[29] The pharmacotherapy of the humoral response awaits both experimental verification of its efficacy as well as controlled clinical trials such as are now being carried out with prostacycline PGI₂.

The role of steroids in this syndrome is even more confusing.[134,162,180] Ashbaugh and his colleagues[6] have reported methylprednisolone amelioration of late ARDS patients with refractory clinical courses who had idiopathic pulmonary fibrosis on lung biopsy. However, a recent study by Weigelt et al.[206] in a randomized double-blind study of 81 patients at risk demonstrated an increased incidence of ARDS (64 percent) in the methylprednisolone-treated group, compared to only 33 percent in the placebo group. More importantly septic complications occurred in 77 percent of the steroid group and only 43 percent in the controls. At present there is *no* statistically significant, clinically validated indication for steroids in either the prophylaxis for or the treatment of patients with ARDS.

Consequently, the major therapy for this difficult disease process remains the proper utilization of ventilatory support with the adjunct of therapeutic modalities directed toward maintaining a high cardiac output, to compensate for the increased shunt seen in these conditions. This is demonstrated in Figure 19-7, which shows that in sepsis and hyperdynamic liver disease and especially when these are complicated by pneumonitis, as opposed to nonseptic syndromes, the maintenance of an effective ventilation requires a progressive increase in cardiac output due to the increase in shunt occurring as the hyperdynamic state occurs, such that a larger increase in flow is necessary to allow effective ventilatory exchange to occur. The pattern of cardiovascular and respiratory parameters that characterizes each of these clinical conditions is shown in Figure 19-20, as standard deviations from a control group of nonstressed general surgical patients.

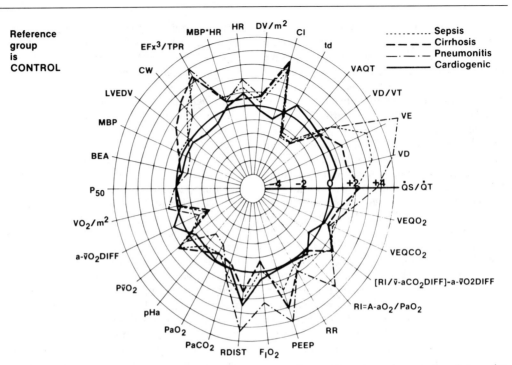

FIG. 19-20 Cardiorespiratory patterns in different disease conditions; TD, pulmonary mean transit time; V̇E, minute ventilation; V̇D, minute dead space ventilation; VEQ O_2, ventilatory equivalent for oxygen; VEQ CO_2, ventilatory equivalent for CO_2; RI/v̄-a CO_2 Diff (a-v̄O_2 Diff), relation between oxygen extraction and CO_2 production; RR, respiratory rate; R distance, relative degree of patient pattern disparity between that of normal control; PHa, arterial pH; Pv̄O_2, mixed venous O_2; AvO_2 Diff, arterial venous oxygen content difference; V̇O_2/m^2, oxygen consumption per square meter; p50, p50 of oxygen hemoglobin dissociation curve; BEA, arterial base excess; MBP, mean blood pressure; CW, cardiac work; EFx³/TPR, relationship of ejection fraction to resistance as an index of combined effect of reduction in vascular tone and increased contractility on cardiac ejection; MBP × Heart Rate, indication of oxygen consumption; HR, heart rate; DV/m^2, pulmonary dispersive blood volume. (See text for other abbreviations.) All values are normalized to the mean and standard deviation of a control group of preoperative unstressed general surgical patients (R state). Note the increase in ventilatory response of patients with cirrhosis or sepsis ARDS modified by pneumonitis, compared to those with cardiogenic insufficiency. Major features in the ARDS response are increase in ventilation with a proportionate increase in dead space secondary to an increase in physiologic shunt. The ventilatory equivalents of oxygen and CO_2 rise, as does the respiratory index. As therapeutic response varies, the patients have increased PEEP and are generally administered a higher FiO_2 in attempt to compensate for the respiratory insufficiency. The influence of the hyperdynamic state is shown by the increased EFx³/TPR and cardiac work relationships, as CI is also increased with a shorter more restricted pulmonary mean transit time and a reduction in V̇A/Q̇T. (Sganga A, Siegel JH, Coleman B et al: The physiologic meaning of the respiratory index in various types of critical illness. Circ Shock 17: 179, 1985.)

AIM OF RESPIRATORY THERAPY

The earliest mechanical feature noted in the development of the posttraumatic or postseptic ARDS syndrome appears to be an increase in the pressure required to dis- tend the lung (reduction in pulmonary compliance), which takes the form of an increase in the critical opening pressure when the abnormal lung segments are expanded. This can be seen by examining the dynamics of ventilation.[20,23,120,135,144,149,169,170] These abnormalities reflect the development of localized areas of interstitial perialveolar and peribronchial edema.[8,37] As ARDS develops, it is characterized by a decrease in the alveolar volume as manifested by a decrease in the functional residual capacity (FRC) of the lung. The alveolar volume measured by the FRC is dependent upon transpulmonary pressure and compliance. They also can be reduced by destruction or necrosis of alveoli. Transpulmonary pressure is the distending pressure across the lung and equals the difference between alveolar pressure and intrapleural pressure. The compliance is a measure of the elastic forces acting on the lung. At a given compliance, in order to increase lung volume either the pleural pressure must be decreased or the alveolar pressure increased. To increase the volume of the FRC one must increase the distending pressure at end-expiration, by maintaining PEEP. Understanding the mechanical and gas exchange abnormalities is the key to administering the proper mode and degree of ventilatory support. To achieve this end, precise quantification of lung function must be done for each patient as the extent of ARDS pathophysiology changes during the course of the disease. This quantitative analysis should also extend to the

evaluation of each substantial change in ventilatory therapy to determine the patient's response in terms of its effects on lung mechanics, cardiac output, and gas exchange. The aim of respiratory therapy in ARDS is to maintain the exchange of oxygen and carbon dioxide by opening and stabilizing closed lung units without compromising cardiac function and circulation. In achieving this goal, the ventilation must be tailored to the underlying abnormalities in lung physiology.

QUANTIFICATION OF RESPIRATORY MECHANICS

Bone[20] described a method of generating pressure/volume (P-V) curves by plotting volume against peak pressure and plateau pressure to obtain both a dynamic characteristics curve and a static compliance curve. Automated systems are now available that can gen-

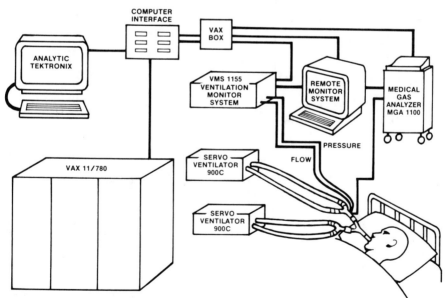

FIG. 19-21 Computer-based respiratory monitoring and evaluation system, set for use with two Servo ventilators for simultaneous independent lung ventilation. Under normal circumstances, only a single ventilator is used.

erate P-V curves from each breath. We have developed a computer-based analytic system (Fig. 19-21) that allows us to evaluate respiratory pressures (P), flows (F), and volumes (V) in intubated and ventilated patients[169,170] as a means of quantifying respiratory mechanics and adjusting the characteristics of ventilatory support therapy (Fig. 19-22).

Analysis of P-F-V curves can be used to define the area of best ventilation by determining the tidal volume and PEEP level that result in the maximum compliance value. To determine this maximum compliance value, a compliance curve is generated by varying the delivered tidal volume at a set PEEP level and measuring the actual tidal volume delivered (Insp. vol.), the plateau pressure, and the PEEP (Fig. 19-23). The PEEP level is then varied in

3-cmH$_2$O increments above and below the initial set support level and the compliance curve again measured as shown in Figure 19-23.

The Pmax, or peak pressure required to deliver a given tidal volume, is dependent upon the resistive forces and the elastic properties of the respiratory system. Figure 19-24A shows the dynamic characteristics of two mechanical breaths, one generated as a result of a fixed inspiratory flow rate mode of ventilation (volume control) and the other as a result of a decelerating rate of inspiratory flow (pressure control). Both (Fig. 19-24B) are superimposed on the total static compliance curve generated as described by Figure 19-23. Figure 19-24B also shows the dynamic compliance characteristics produced by the elastic resistance factors of the total respiratory system (lung and chest

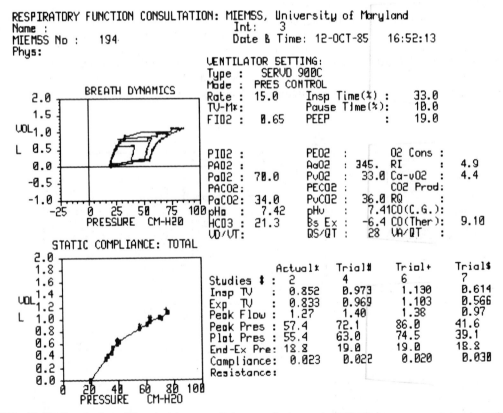

FIG. 19-22 Standard graphic output from respiratory monitoring system showing pressure–volume dynamics of four breaths of varying tidal volumes, static compliance curve, and blood gas data. Actual ventilator setting data (*) can be compared with trial settings at different volumes (#, +, $), with regard to breath dynamics and where they fall on the static compliance curve. Blood gas data is from actual setting.

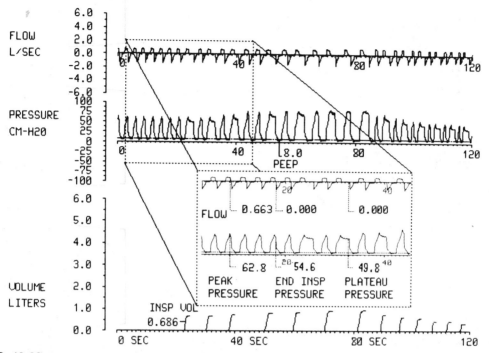

FIG. 19-23 Primary respiratory flow and pressure data showing method used to determine total static compliance curve. Volume is obtained from integration of area under the inspiratory and/or expiratory flow curve. When using the Servo ventilator 900C in volume control mode and a constant minute volume, varying the respiratory rate produces a series of breaths at different tidal volumes. An inspiratory pause hold is used to obtain the plateau pressure.

wall) compared to that of the frictional or non-elastic resistance factors of the lung alone.

Determination of Dynamic Compliance Characteristics

The plateau pressure, or pressure at zero flow, is dependent upon the elastic force. The peak pressure-plateau pressure difference (Fig. 19-23) relates to the resistive component (Fig. 19-24B). In patients without obstructive airway disease maintained at optimal flow rates this difference is usually less than 10 cmH$_2$O. A difference greater than 10 cmH$_2$O indicates an increase in airway resistance, whether due to a small-bore endotracheal tube, increased secretions, or clotted blood in the tube or airway, or bronchospasm. *When flow rates are exces-*

sive, there also will be a large gradient between peak and plateau pressure. By altering the characteristics of ventilatory flow (Fig. 19-24A), by changing from a steady-state high inspiratory flow (volume-controlled ventilation) to a decelerating inspiratory flow (pressure-controlled ventilation), it is possible to change the dynamic characteristics of the breath so as to reduce the peak–plateau pressure gradient and obtain a larger ventilatory volume delivery for a given peak pressure response.

Compliance is a measure of the elasticity of the lung and is usually obtained by determining the slope of the pressure/volume curve, or the change in volume per unit change in pressure (Fig. 19-25A). The compliance of the normal human lung is about 0.2 L/cmH$_2$O (200 ml/cmH$_2$O). To measure lung compliance one needs a measure of both the intrapleural pressure and the intra-alveolar pressure. In humans it is difficult to measure the intrapleural pres-

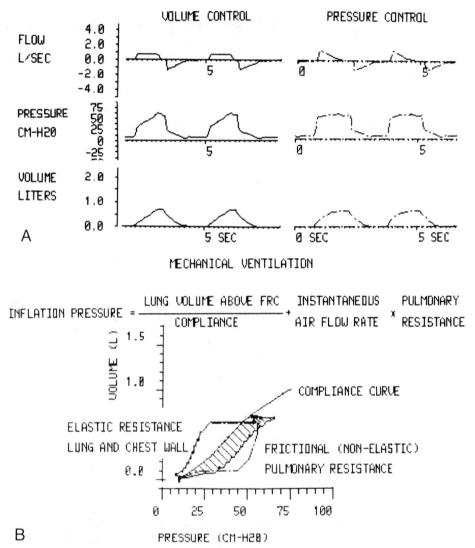

FIG. 19-24 **(A)** Flow, pressure, and volume data from two different modes of ventilation: volume control (-) where inspiratory flow is constant (square wave) and pressure control (---), where the inspiratory flow is initially high and then decreases as the pressure limit is reached (decelerating). **(B)** Dynamic pressure–volume curves for two different modes of ventilation, volume control (-) and pressure control (---), superimposed on the total static compliance curve, illustrating the factors that determine the inflation pressure required to deliver the mechanical breath. The area to the left of the compliance curve represents the pressure required to overcome the elastic resistance of the lung and chest wall. The area to the right of the compliance curve represents the pressure required to overcome the frictional (airway) resistance. The hatched area shows that as volume increases the pressure component required to overcome the frictional resistance is equal throughout the inspiratory cycle when the constant flow pattern is utilized. In contrast, when a decelerating flow pattern is used, the pressure component required to overcome the frictional resistance is initially high and then decreases as the flow rate decreases.

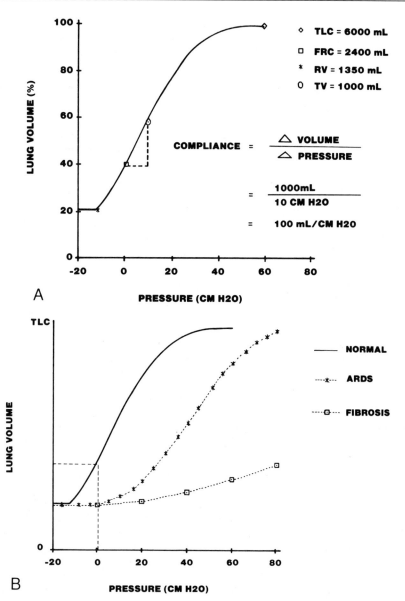

FIG. 19-25 (A) Measurement of compliance. (See text for explanation of abbreviations.) (B) Static compliance curve: Lung and chest wall. Change in compliance curve with progression of ARDS from early interstitial edema phase to late fibrosis stage of the disease.

sure, and the esophageal pressure is usually substituted. The esophageal pressure, while not equal to pressure in the intrapleural space, does reflect the changes in pressure, except in supine subjects where the weight of the me-diastinal structures interferes with the accuracy of measurement.

To obtain an assessment of the lung compliance of patients with ARDS it has now become standard to measure total static respiratory compliance (CST), which is the sum of the lung compliance (CL) and the compliance of the thoracic cage (CT). Under equilibrium conditions at FRC the chest wall is pulled inward while the lung is pulled outward, these two forces balancing each other. The normal total CST is approximately 0.1 L/cmH$_2$O (100 ml/cmH$_2$O) and ranges from 0.040 to 0.140 L/cmH$_2$O. It is affected by age, body size, and the total lung capacity.

$$\frac{1}{CST} = \frac{1}{CL} + \frac{1}{CT}$$

Where
$$CT = \frac{V_T}{\Delta Paw}$$

$$CL = \frac{V_T}{\Delta PL} = \frac{V_T}{\Delta Paw - \Delta PpL}$$

$$CT = \frac{V_T}{\Delta PpL}$$

where Paw is airway pressure; Ppl is pleural pressure; and V$_T$ is tidal volume.

Total static respiratory compliance (CST) can be decreased as a result of a decrease in the compliance of the lung, of the thorax, or because of a decrease in both.

As is also evident from Figure 19-25A, the compliance range during normal breathing is a function of where on the total lung pressure/volume curve the tidal volume excursion occurs. It is obvious that as the FRC point is raised from residual volume (RV) to total lung capacity (TLC) the slope of the pressure/volume relationship varies. Even in a normal lung and chest wall system as the FRC level is increased above the normal tidal volume range toward the TLC, the compliance decreases. In ARDS and especially in the late fibrosis phase of ARDS (Fig. 19-25B) the pressure/volume curve of compliance relations is shifted to the right compared to the normal curve.

The change in transpulmonary pressure (Paw minus Ppl) that produces a given tidal volume is similar whether it is generated by spontaneous breathing or mechanical breathing. The total CST can be measured in patients with ARDS, who are intubated and are on a ventilator, by measuring the tidal volume and the distending pressure required to deliver this volume. The distending pressure is determined by measuring the airway pressure at the points of zero airflow on both inspiration and expiration (the plateau pressure minus the end-expiratory pressure).

$$CST = \frac{Tidal\ volume}{Plateau\ pressure - PEEP}$$

An example of how this can be done in ARDS is shown in Figure 19-23. The sedated or paralyzed patient was placed on a mechanical ventilator with a set tidal volume of 0.800 L, a PEEP of 8.0 cmH$_2$O with an inspiratory hold, or pause, of 10 percent and a rate of 20/min. During the period of inspiratory pause the ventilator does not deliver any volume, as demonstrated by the zero airflow (Fig. 19-23) and there is an equalization of pressure between the alveoli and the point of measurement of the intra-airway pressure at the proximal end of the endotracheal tube. This is the *plateau pressure* and can be read from the manometer on the ventilator. Exhalation then occurs and the pressure at which expiratory airflow becomes zero is the *end-expiratory pressure,* in this case the set PEEP level of 8.0 cmH$_2$O. The actual inspired *tidal volume* of 0.686 L is less than the set exhaled tidal volume of 0.800 L, since a certain amount is always "lost" in the compressible volume of the ventilator system. This "lost" volume is dependent upon the type of ventilator tubing used, the presence of heated humidifiers and the level to which they are filled, and the *peak pressure* required to deliver the set tidal volume. A rough approximation of this "lost" volume can be obtained by multiplying the peak pressure times a correction factor, usually 3.0 ml/cmH$_2$O, as shown in Table 19-2. The computer-based system described above measures the actual inspired tidal volume (V$_T$) at the endotracheal tube rather than at the expiratory valve of the mechanical ventilator.

What is also apparent is that as peak pressure increases the magnitude of the "Lost" volume increases, thus further reducing the V$_T$ actually delivered to the patient. If one fails to measure the actual V$_T$ the derived compliance value will be higher than the true level.

Using an end-inspiratory pause to hold the inspiratory volume until equilibration with the lung elastic factors can occur may result in

TABLE 19-2. Comparison between Set Tidal Volume and Actual Volume Delivered

Exhaled (Set Tidal Volume)	Peak Pressure	"Lost"	Volume Delivered (Inspired Tidal Volume: V_T)
800	20	60	740
800	40	120	680
800	60	180	620
800	80	240	560
800	100	300	500

some of this "lost" volume being delivered to the patient, thus increasing the actual inspired tidal volume. The pressure measured at the point of zero airflow at the end of inspiration may not accurately reflect the "true" alveolar equilibrium pressure, and thus compliance, if there are different time constants for alveolar expansion in the lung as are seen in patients with airway disease. In this situation, flow may still be occurring within the lung when it has ceased at the proximal airway, causing a continuing redistribution of volume from lung units with normal time constants to lung units with prolonged time constants located behind partially obstructed airways. These lung units may continue to fill when the rest of the lung has begun to empty, the so-called "pendeluft" effect. As the rate of ventilation is increased, the portion of the tidal volume that goes to these partially obstructed regions becomes less and less. As a consequence, the lung appears to become less compliant since a smaller portion of the lung is participating in the tidal volume changes. By increasing the inspiratory pause time, one can see a continuing fall in plateau pressure until a true plateau pressure is reached. This may take up to 2 to 4 seconds to equilibrate in some individuals. This effect is demonstrated in Figure 19-23 where the end-inspiratory pressure is 54.6 cmH₂O measured at the end-inspiratory pause pressure point where air flow rate is 0.000 L/sec, and the calculated dynamic compliance is 0.013 L/cmH₂O. If the inspiratory hold time is extended by forestalling the onset of expiration (flow remains 0.000 L/sec), the pressure equilibrates to the actual plateau or alveolar pressure of 49.8 cmH₂O and the true static compliance is 0.014 L/cmH₂O. However, it must be remembered that a continuing fall in the plateau pressure can also be caused by air leaks in the system,

whether they be at the site of the cuff of the endotracheal tube or because of the presence of a bronchopleural fistula. In this case there will be a marked discrepancy between the measured inspiratory and expiratory tidal volumes.

Determination of Total Static Compliance Relationships

It is possible to generate a total static compliance curve by varying the tidal volume and measuring the plateau pressure at each new tidal volume level. This is demonstrated in Figures 19-23 and 19-24A,B, which show the data from a 30-year-old man admitted following a motor vehicle accident. The patient sustained a ruptured thoracic aorta, fractured left fibula, fractured right ulna, and right retroperitoneal hematoma. He developed posttraumatic ARDS complicated by *Pseudomonas* and *Streptococcus* D septicemia. The patient was ventilated using a Servo Ventilator 900 C. The tidal volume was varied from 0.3 L to 1.2 L, by maintaining the inspired minute volume constant and adjusting the respiratory rate. The tidal volume was not increased beyond 1.2 L because at this level the patient's compliance decreased below (0.014 L/cmH₂O) and the peak plateau pressures markedly increased (> 80 cmH₂O) at the higher tidal volumes. The measured tidal volume and its associated plateau pressure were automatically plotted on a volume–pressure diagram by our computer system to produce the total static compliance curve shown in Figure 19-24B. Analyzing this curve shows that the compliance initially increased from a value of 0.012 L/cmH₂O at an actual delivered tidal volume (VT) of 0.229 L, to 0.014 L/cmH$_2$O at a VT of 0.686 L and then decreased to < 0.012 L/cmH$_2$O at VT above 0.985 L. Since any attempt to increase his actual delivered tidal volume above 0.700 L resulted in excessively high airway pressures, this patient was ventilated by increasing the respiratory rate from 12/min to 20/min and reducing the set tidal volume to 0.8 L (producing an actual delivered volume of 0.686 L).

The conventional method of calculating total static compliance using the mechanically set PEEP as reflecting the end-expiratory pressure may also be in error. Jonson and his co-workers[94] as well as Pepe and Marini[139] showed that a positive alveolar pressure can be present throughout the breathing cycle when the patient is being mechanically ventilated, even though PEEP is *not* being applied. Pepe and Marini[139] demonstrated the presence of what they termed "auto-PEEP" by occluding the airway at end-expiration and delaying the onset of the next breath (Fig. 19-26). Rossi et al.[155] showed the effect of what they termed "intrinsic positive end-expiratory pressure" or "PEEP$_i$," on the measurement of the static compliance of the total respiratory system (CST). They studied 14 mechanically ventilated patients with acute respiratory failure. Measurement of air flow, airway pressure, and volume changes were made. The pressure at end-expiration "auto PEEP" was determined using the occlusion method of Pepe and Marini.[139] The CST was determined using the conventional method (using the mechanically set PEEP), by using the "auto-PEEP" determined by occluding

the expiratory port at end-expiration, and by determining PEEP from the flow and pressure tracings (using the airway pressure at which inspiratory airflow begins).

Figure 19-26 demonstrates this effect in a patient who was being ventilated at a rate of 18/min using an I/E ratio of 1:1 and a PEEP of 13.6 cmH$_2$O. Note that at the end of the period set for exhalation the pressure was 13.6 cmH$_2$O, which was equivalent to the PEEP set on the ventilator, and expiratory flow was not complete as shown by the expiratory flow rate of −0.222 L/sec. (Since a bidirectional flow sensor is being used, inspiratory airflow is shown as positive and expiratory airflow as negative). The fourth breath shows the effect of occluding the expiratory port at the end of the expiratory period. Airflow is now essentially zero (−0.009 L/sec) and the airway pressure is 15.6 cmH$_2$O and represents the *actual* PEEP. Also shown is the pressure at which inspiratory airflow begins: 16 cmH$_2$O. The difference between the set PEEP of 13.6 cmH$_2$O and the pressure at the onset of inspiratory airflow represents the pressure the ventilator must generate to overcome the elastic recoil pressure producing expiratory airflow during passive exhalation. If expiration is not complete when the ventilator cycles to inspiration, then the pressure required for delivery of the volume is equal to the plateau pressure minus the pressure at the point at which inspiratory airflow actually begins and *not* the difference between the plateau pressure minus the mechanically set PEEP level.

Rossi et al.[155] found that 10 of the 14 pa-

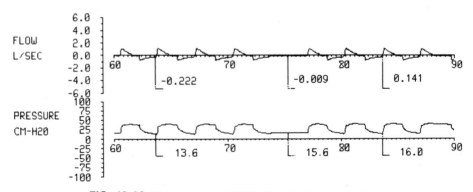

FIG. 19-26 Measurement of PEEP. (See text for explanation.)

tients studied were still exhaling at the point at which the ventilator started to increase airway pressure and that up to 7.5 cmH₂O of positive pressure above the set PEEP level had to be applied before inspiratory airflow began. In their series, using the set PEEP to calculate total static compliance led to an *underestimation* in calculated compliance of up to 48 percent. Eight of their patients had chronic obstructive pulmonary disease (COPD), but two patients (one with pneumonia and the other a patient with ARDS following barbiturate overdose and aspiration, without evidence of COPD) also showed a higher intrinsic PEEP than the mechanically set PEEP. The level of PEEP was also found to vary with change in time for expiration.

When using the airway occlusion method to determine PEEP, care must be taken to see that occlusion of the expiratory port occurs *precisely* at end-expiration. Some ventilators, such as the Servo Ventilator 900C, which was used in Figure 19-23, have the capability to occlude the expiratory port automatically at end-expiration and thus provide a true static measurement of intrinsic PEEP.

When obtaining a measurement of total static compliance (CST), the patient must be fully relaxed or paralyzed and in synchrony with the ventilator. Any respiratory efforts made at the time of measurement, whether inspiratory or expiratory, will change the compliance of the thoracic cage and thus affect the measurement of total compliance. Another factor that must be considered is the lung volume at which the compliance is measured (Fig. 19-25A). As shown in this figure, when the FRC alone or FRC plus the tidal volume approaches the level of total lung capacity, the compliance begins to decrease.

The compliance measured when a tidal volume of 1000 ml is delivered to an 80-kg, 72-inch, 20-year-old man with a TLC of 6.0 L will be much larger than the compliance measured when this same tidal volume is delivered to a 20-year-old, 50-kg, 60-inch woman who has a TLC of 3.0 L. If total lung volume is decreased from 6 to 3 L in our 20-year-old man, for example as a result of pneumonectomy, the total compliance measured utilizing the same delivered tidal volume (1,000 ml) will decrease to approximately one-half of the prepneumonectomy value (Fig. 19-27). This does not mean that the subject has developed a true decrease in lung compliance, but only that the entire 1,000 ml volume is being delivered to one lung where previously it was divided between two. Lung compliances are additive. If one were to measure a total compliance of 0.100 L/cmH₂O (100 ml/cmH₂O) for both lungs and then selectively intubate each lung and measure the compliance of the right and left lungs separately

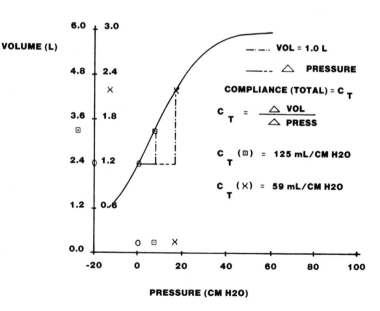

FIG. 19-27 Static total compliance at different lung volumes. Effect of delivering the same volume (1.0 L) to two subjects who have a normal static total compliance (CT) but with differing total lung capacities of 3.0 L (□) and 6.0 L (x).

one would find that the compliance of the right lung was approximately one-half of the total. Because of this effect of lung volume on compliance one must take into account the patient's size when selecting the tidal volume to be used.

Pleural Pathology as a Factor in Decreasing Respiratory Compliance

Extrapulmonary factors may also be important in reducing static lung compliance and in altering the dynamic breath characteristics to produce an increased pressure/volume relationship. This is demonstrated in Figure 19-28, taken from an 18-year-old woman who had been admitted 2 months earlier after a severe motor vehicle accident with bilateral chest contusion associated with multiple injuries including pelvic and left femoral fractures, splenic laceration with hemoperitoneum and shock,

and a mild closed head injury. After stabilization and surgery she developed severe ARDS complicated by *Staphylococcus* and *Enterococcus* pneumonia with recurrent pneumothoraces and right-sided pneumatoceles, which altered the pressure/volume characteristics of the lungs. This can be seen both in the prethoracotomy breath dynamics of 12/12/84, which show an elevated plateau pressure at a low tidal volume, and in the right shifted total static compliance curve.

Because of the pleural pathologic condition and recurrent pneumothoraces on the right, a decortication with closure of the bronchial segment leaking into the pneumatocele was carried out immediately after the study discussed above. The post-thoracotomy study after release of multiple visceral to parietal pleural adhesions and removal of a chronically atelectatic right lateral segment of the middle lobe showed an improved compliance relations. These show an increase in tidal volume from 0.554 to 0.650 L, with essentially no change in plateau pressure (34.8 to 36.9 cmH₂O). The

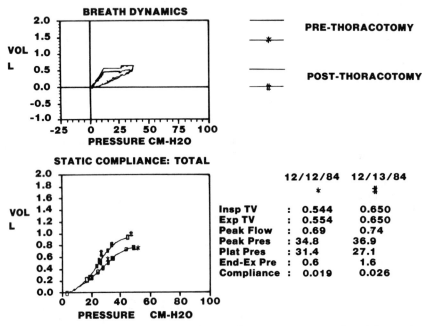

FIG. 19-28 Pressure–volume loops and total static compliance curves pre- and post thoracotomy at Pt# 301.

total compliance has improved from 0.019 to 0.026 L/cmH$_2$O and the static total compliance curve has shifted to the left with a higher tidal volume possible for any given plateau pressure developed. Subsequent to this decortication, the patient recovered and was discharged with nearly normal lung function and blood gas values. Quantification of shift in static compliance in the presence of persistent recurrent pneumothoraces and pneumatoceles helped to assess the severity of the pleural process and enabled a rational decision for operative decortication to be made.

APPLICATION OF PHYSIOLOGIC PRINCIPLES IN VENTILATORY MANAGEMENT

Influence of Altering Lung Dependency

The interrelationship between the nonuniform alterations in capillary permeability and the maldistribution of the pulmonary blood flow in the hyperdynamic state produces some of the unique features of ARDS. This important feature of ARDS is often concealed by the apparent uniformity of the radiographic findings. In many cases, the interstitial and alveolar infiltrates appear to be fairly uniformly distributed throughout the upper and lower lung fields on posteroanterior or anteroposterior film (Fig. 19-29A). However, on computed tomographic (CT) scan (Fig. 19-29B) or at autopsy, it can be clearly seen that the most involved segments of the lung are in the dependent portions, which in the case of the severely ill supine patient are the *posterior* aspects of both upper and lower lobes. Since the PA film does not distinguish the anterior from posterior lung segments but rather projects them, one on the other, what is really a gravitationally influenced process appears to a large extent to be pathologic change uniformly distributed

throughout the lung fields. The implication of this observation is that no segment of the lung should be allowed to be dependent for any great length of time, and that frequent change in position represents an important modality of therapy. The influence of changing position on improving blood gases by altering the relative $\dot{V}A/\dot{Q}$ distribution is shown in Figure 19-30 and Table 19-3, which show data from a patient who sustained a closed head injury and bilateral pulmonary contusion as a result of a motor vehicle accident. He developed pneumonia and ARDS and his chest radiographs revealed greater involvement of his left lung than right lung. The use of the noninvasive transcutaneous monitor allowed identification of a significant deterioration in the patient's respiratory status with the change in position from sitting 60° to left side down and with suctioning. Note the improvement when the patient was placed in the right lateral position (right side down). The transcutaneous data generally correlated with the measured arterial carbon dioxide and oxygen tensions (Table 19-3), if adjusted by regression coefficients shown earlier.

This case also makes the point that the transcutaneous monitor is useful as a trend monitor and is especially valuable when one is making changes in ventilator settings in normodynamic or hyperdynamic posttrauma patients. Since the maldistribution of ventilation/perfusion accentuates this process, early intubation and ventilation with a maintenance of increased PEEP as recommended by Ashbaugh[7] and others[150,160,196] has been advocated as a mechanism of combatting this ventilation/perfusion maldistribution, especially when combined with attempts to maintain the erect chest position for as much of the day as possible.

Role of Positive End-Expiratory Pressure

The clinical use of PEEP was first described in 1938 by Barach et al.[15] in the treatment of pulmonary edema secondary to congestive heart failure. Its use in ARDS as a means of supporting oxygenation was first re-

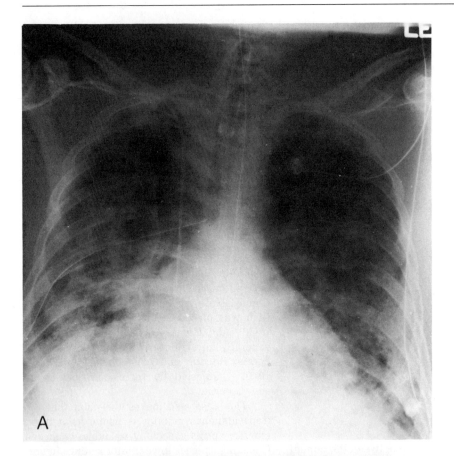

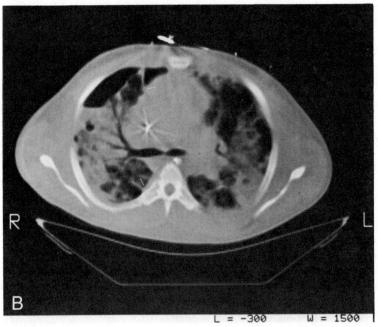

FIG. 19-29 (A) Antero-posterior chest radiograph of patient with severe ARDS. (B) The same patient's CT scan.

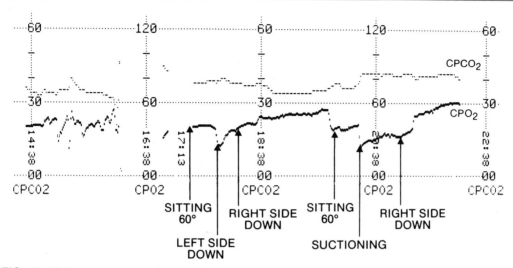

FIG. 19-30 Transcutaneous oxygen (CPO₂) and carbon dioxide (CPCO₂) partial pressure data for patient EP:194, showing effect of changes in position and of suctioning. (See Table 19-3 for concomitant arterial blood gas data of 10/12. For regressions relating transcutaneous to blood gas tensions, see p. 602.)

ported by Ashbaugh and colleagues[7] in 1969. Since that time PEEP has become the primary therapeutic maneuver for improving oxygenation in patients with ARDS. However, it should be emphasized that the recent studies of Pepé and his colleagues[138] demonstrate that *the early application of PEEP does not influence the incidence of ARDS,* even though there was improvement in the PaO_2/FiO_2 ratio during PEEP in patients who developed ARDS. This is as would be expected, since the time course of the initiating humoral response would not be expected to be influenced by a strictly mechanical therapy, which though not useful in preventing ARDS alterations may help to compensate for the altered permeability and venti-

lation/perfusion ratio induced by this disease process.

Ideal gas exchange occurs when there is an even match of ventilation and perfusion in all lung units. Ventilation in excess of perfusion leads to an increase in wasted ventilation, as manifested by an increase in the V_D/V_T ratio, an increase in the arterial-end-tidal carbon dioxide gradient, and, in patients who are on controlled ventilation, a decrease in alveolar ventilation with a subsequent increase in the arterial $PaCO_2$. Perfusion in excess of ventilation results in a decrease in PaO_2 because of a rise in venoarterial admixture in low $\dot{V}A/\dot{Q}$ alveoli, or due to an increase in flow through fixed right-to-left shunts.

TABLE 19-3. Gas Exchange Values

E.P:194 Date	10/12				10/13		
Time	1745	1900	2110	2220	0315	0445	1030
FiO₂	.65						
PEEP (cmH₂O)	20						
Position	SIT60	RT LAT	SIT 60	RT LAT	RT LAT	SIT 60	RT LAT
PaCO₂(mmHg)	34	29	41	37	35	32	32
PaO₂(mmHg)	70	85	63	84	119	73	122
RI	5.0	4.0	5.5	4.0	2.5	4.8	2.5
QS/QT (%)	29			24			
CO (L/min)	9.1			7.4			

The postulated mechanisms for the improvement in oxygenation by PEEP as manifested by an increase in PaO_2 include holding open respiratory bronchioles with the prevention of alveolar collapse. In addition, direct measurement[150,196] has demonstrated that PEEP leads to an increase in FRC, which will be discussed later as the most important effect. However, compliance may be either increased or decreased by PEEP and ventilation/perfusion relationships in the lung and PaO_2 and $PaCO_2$ can be improved, unchanged, or can deteriorate when PEEP is used. Positive end-expiratory pressure can have varying effects on the volume of dead space. There can be a decrease in dead space if the application of PEEP leads to a more even distribution of a constant tidal volume, as a result of a re-expansion of previously collapsed alveoli. Dead space can increase if the size of conducting airways is increased, normal alveoli are overexpanded, or if there is a reduction in the amount of perfusion to normal alveoli due to increased intra-alveolar pressure that exceeds that in the alveolar capillary bed. In unilateral lung disease generally applied PEEP can cause a redistribution of perfusion from the normal lung to the diseased lung, leading to an increase in the amount of venous admixture or shunt.[9,10,80] This occurs when the application of PEEP leads to an overexpansion of alveoli in the normal lung and an increase in pulmonary capillary vascular resistance compared to that in the abnormal lung. These differences may account for the sometimes divergent results obtained when using compliance and oxygen delivery to determine optimal or "best" PEEP level.

At normal atmospheric pressures (zero PEEP), the vascular resistance of the collapsed lung is greater than that of the expanded lung. Permutt et al.[141] and Howell et al.[88] showed that further expansion of the lung, after initial increase in vascular volume, with inflation is characterized by an increase in the volume of the larger vessels and a decrease in the volume of the smaller vessels and capillaries. It has been proposed that the smaller interalveolar arterioles in the lung may respond like the airways, in that radial tension on them produced by expanding lung structures causes them to enlarge and thus resistance to blood flow decreases. However, when the lung is overdistended, the transmitted intra-alveolar pressure on the capillary bed tends to counteract the pressure–volume increase on the larger vessels. Finally, as the lung is further stretched, as it approaches total lung capacity, the resistance to flow in both large and small vessels increases.

One might postulate that as long as areas of collapsed lung are being reinflated by PEEP, pulmonary vascular resistance will fall and compliance will increase. However, to maintain venous return, venous pressure also must increase. Reflex mechanisms induced by raising the intrathoracic pressure cause peripheral venoconstriction, which under normal circumstances will compensate for modest decreases in venous return.[84] As long as lung compliance increases as PEEP increases, the circulation can cope with the PEEP effect. However, when the PEEP (or mean airway pressure) exceeds the level needed to overcome the compliance effects, this excess pressure will be transmitted transpleurally and will raise intrapleural pressure from its normal negative values closer to the level of the extrathoracic venous pressure. This will reduce the caval to atrial pressure gradients and impede venous return to the heart. Thus there will be a diminished right heart filling and a reduced cardiac preload with a consequent fall in cardiac output. This mechanism can be of major significance in the posttrauma patient where residual systemic hypovolemia may be masked by arterial vasoconstriction with maintenance of blood pressure (see Chap. 9).

While the most common cause for a reduced cardiac output occurring with the application of PEEP is reduced right heart venous return, another cause is ventricular dysfunction. This is assumed to occur when significant reduction in cardiac output persists despite reasonable intravascular volume augmentation. Part of this dysfunction has been ascribed to a change in left ventricular compliance due to a leftward intraventricular septal deviation caused by increased right ventricular pressure, as the right heart dilates to increase developed tension because of pulmonary arteriolar vasoconstriction (see Chap. 9). Acute pulmonary arterial hypertension may occur immediately after traumatic injury, or with the initiation of a septic insult with bacteremia or endotoxin release into the pulmonary circulation.[33,36,46,48,61,76,90] However, direct humoral or septic depression of myocardial contractility may also be a factor.[163,168] Unfortunately these two mechanisms may occur together in the posttrauma patient who develops ARDS.

As discussed earlier, the ARDS process is associated with an increase in lung water, presumably due to interstitial edema. However, the immediate improvement in arterial oxygenation and lung compliance after PEEP therapy is not secondary to a decrease in lung water. The overwhelming balance of evidence suggests that PEEP results in either no change in extravascular lung water or a significant increase due to an alteration in the transcapillary to interstitial pressure gradient as collapsed alveoli are expanded.[25,138,177,190] In the presence of atelectasis it is necessary to achieve a critical opening pressure to re-expand collapsed alveoli.

While the predictable effects of PEEP in opposing small airway closure are conflicting,[7,9,10,150,160,177] the best documented and most important effect of PEEP on the lung is to increase the functional residual capacity (FRC).

This is accomplished by an increase in both alveolar size and alveolar recruitment, the latter occurring when ARDS-induced alveolar atelectatic pathology is present.[138,150,156,160,172,177] Figure 19-31 illustrates the effect of increasing the PEEP at end-expiration from 0.5 to 25.3 cmH_2O. Displayed are the inspiratory and expiratory flows, airway pressure, and, from integration of the flow, the inspiratory and expiratory volumes. The pressure level was increased on the third breath. Note that while inspired volume remained constant for the subsequent breaths, its expiratory volume was less than inspired until the seventh breath when the inspired and expired volume again became equal. This difference in volume amounted to 0.817 L and *is equivalent to the increase in the FRC level.*

However, an increase in the FRC level by the use of PEEP does not necessarily indicate recruitment of collapsed alveoli; it may represent overdistention of relatively normal lung. Figure 19-32 shows the total static compliance curve obtained at the zero PEEP level. This curve was obtained by varying the inspired volume delivered by the ventilator from 0.3 to 1.9 L and using an inspiratory pause hold to

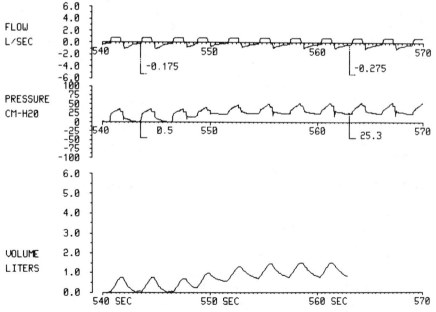

FIG. 19-31 Effect of increasing positive end-expiratory pressure (PEEP) from 0.5 cmH_2O to 25.3 cmH_2O on level of functional residual capacity (FRC).

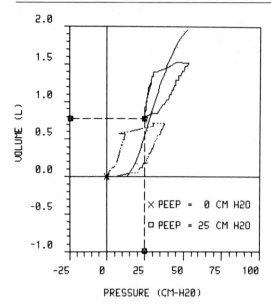

PRESSURE (CM-H2O)

FIG. 19-32 Total static compliance curve obtained by increasing inspired volume from zero to 2.0 L at a PEEP of 0 cmH₂O. Superimposed are two breaths, one starting at a PEEP level of 0 cmH₂O (x) and the other at a PEEP level of 25 cmH₂O (□).

obtain the plateau pressure. Superimposed on this curve are a pre-PEEP breath at 0.5 cmH₂O (zero) PEEP and the seventh breath at 25 cmH₂O PEEP from the previous figure. The change in the end-expiratory pressure and volume level is readily apparent.

Note that on the breath originating at *zero* PEEP there is essentially no volume change until a pressure of 6 cmH₂O is reached and that the compliance curve is flat until a pressure of 12 cmH₂O is achieved. At zero PEEP the total respiratory static compliance was 0.026 L/cmH₂O while at a PEEP level of 25 cmH₂O the total respiratory static compliance (CST) was 0.032 L/cmH₂O. In actuality the highest CST (0.040 L/cmH₂O) occurred at a PEEP of 12 cmH₂O, which was the point at which there was a change in the slope of the static compliance curve from that obtained at zero to just under 12 cmH₂O PEEP.

Suter et al.[191,192] showed that when the FRC decreased the most initially, patients required the highest levels of PEEP to maximize gas exchange. It appears to be necessary to overdistend those alveoli operating on a favorable portion of their pressure/volume curve to

recruit fluid-filled or atelectatic areas. Below a certain critical volume, alveoli tend to collapse and expand only at a much higher pressure than that originally needed to maintain expansion, because for any level of airway pressure the volume of each alveolus and of the lung as a unit is determined by the *distending pressure multiplied by the compliance.* As a result, the markedly compliant alveoli have more volume. A sudden lapse in PEEP can immediately and substantially decrease PaO₂ as FRC decreases. *Because the time necessary for FRC to respond to a PEEP increase correlates highly with total compliance, subjects with the least compliant lungs are least able to tolerate a sudden loss of PEEP,* which frequently occurs when patients with severe ARDS are suctioned for aspiration of tracheal secretions or bag breathed during transport to radiologic facilities or to the operating room, or for respiratory toilet maneuvers. This is shown in Figure 19-33, which demonstrates that the loss of PEEP in the patient with severe ARDS even for a brief period of time during airway toilet results in the collapse of alveoli with a reduction in small airway compliances. This is only revealed after determining the static compliance curve (CST) at the higher lung volumes, since the large airway and relatively normal alveoli fill identically at lower tidal volumes. The implications of this observation are that PEEP should be maintained as continuously as possible and bag breathing as is commonly done during suctioning should be done with a continuous positive airway pressure (CPAP) valve or by minimal interruption of the mechanical ventilator system with PEEP adjustment.

Determination of the "Best" PEEP

The generation of a family of compliance curves at varying PEEP levels can aid in determining the "best" or "optimal" PEEP level to be used when ventilating patients with ARDS. This level can be considered to be the PEEP value that results in a balance between the pressure needed to prevent airway and alveo-

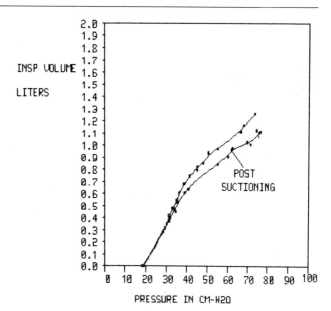

INSP VOLUME

LITERS

FIG. 19-33 Total static compliance curves from pt EP:194 showing the effect of suctioning the airway for removal of secretions and the subsequent decrease in FRC due to the loss of PEEP.

PRESSURE IN CM-H2O

lar collapse and promote alveolar recruitment and that which causes overexpansion of the more compliant areas in the lung. Such overdistention can result in hemodynamic compromise and worsening of $\dot{V}A/\dot{Q}$ relationships due to the transmission of high airway pressures to the alveolar capillary vasculature, which acts as a Starling resistance to blood flow with diversion of blood flow away from the well-ventilated areas.

Suter et al.[191,192] showed that systemic oxygen transport (arterial oxygen content times cardiac output) was maximal when total static compliance was highest. To determine the maximal compliance value, the PEEP level is varied by 3-cmH2O increments, maintained at the new level for 15 to 30 minutes, and then data for a new P-V curve are generated as shown in Figure 19-23. Three representative P-V curves taken from evaluation of an ARDS patient in whom the PEEP level was varied from zero to 23 cmH2O are shown in Figure 19-34. The curves shown were obtained at PEEP values of 0, 12, and 23 cmH2O.

Inspection of the curve at a PEEP level of zero shows that the pressure must rise to 6 cmH2O before there is any increase in volume and there is an inflection point or area where there is a change in slope after which the P-V curve becomes essentially linear. The pres-

ence of an inflection point was first demonstrated by Cook et al.[39] in dogs with pulmonary edema and Slutsky et al.[173] showed this same phenomenon in oleic-acid-induced pulmonary edema. Matanis and his colleagues[120] correlated the patterns seen on sequential P-V curves measured at zero PEEP with the stage of ARDS and the pattern of the chest radiograph. They demonstrated the presence of an inflection at low pulmonary volumes when alveolar opacities were seen on the chest x-ray study. No specific pressure of inflection was identified, but there was a zone where the slope increased abruptly. This is demonstrated in Figure 19-34, where the point of inflection occurs at about a pressure of 12 cmH2O and above 17 cmH2O the P-V curve becomes grossly linear.

Glaister et al.[68] explained the inflection in the inflation curve, which they demonstrated in excised lungs, as being the result of the reopening of lung units that had closed during the period of deflation. If this is the explanation for this inflection point, *the level of PEEP should be set above this pressure level to prevent distal airway collapse at the end of expiration.*

The P-V curves obtained when PEEP was increased to 12 cmH2O and then 23 cmH2O show an immediate increase in volume. Figure 19-32 is a plot of the dynamic inspiratory and

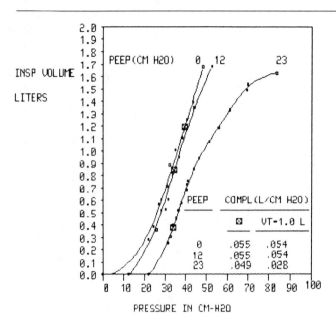

FIG. 19-34 Total static compliance curves obtained during determination of "best" or optimal PEEP level. Shown are curves obtained at 0, 12, and 23 cmH₂O. The point at which the lung volume is the same is indicated by the marker (⊠) on each of the compliance curves.

expiratory P-V loops obtained at PEEP levels of 0 and 25 cmH₂O superimposed on the total static compliance curve. This figure also demonstrates a lack of volume change until a pressure of 6 cmH₂O is reached. This is in contrast to the P-V loop obtained at 25 cmH₂O, where there is a small but immediate change in volume as the inspiratory pressure is increased.

When comparing the P-V curves in Figure 19-34, it can be seen that the curve obtained at zero PEEP was essentially linear above an inspired volume of 0.3 L, while at a PEEP of 12 cmH₂O it was linear up to a volume of 1.4 L and at a PEEP of 23 cmH₂O the linear portion extended only to an inspired volume of 0.8 L. It should be recalled that when the end-expiratory pressure level is increased there is an associated increase in the volume of the FRC. When the PEEP level was increased from zero to 12 cmH₂O, the FRC increased by 0.38 L and at a PEEP level of 23 cmH₂O by an additional 0.82 L above the FRC volume at zero PEEP.

A frequent concern is overdistention of lung units as PEEP and thus FRC is increased. With the institution of PEEP there is a movement of the end-expiratory point from the lower flatter portion of the P-V curve to the steeper portion (Fig. 19-32). As the FRC level approaches the total lung capacity (TLC), ventilation now occurs on the upper flatter portion

of the curve (Fig. 19-25A). If the compliance, which is a measurement of the slope of the P-V curve at a given point, is increasing or remains the same it is assumed that overdistention is not occurring. This movement up the P-V curve is further demonstrated in Figure 19-34, where *equivalent lung volumes* are indicated by the square markers placed at an inspired volume of 1.2 L on the zero PEEP curve, 0.85 L on the curve at a PEEP level of 12 cmH₂O, and at 0.38 L on the curve at 23 cmH₂O. The slopes of the P-V curves at these points, as represented by the compliance values, are 0.055, 0.055, and 0.049 L/cmH₂O, respectively. However, if one were to use an *equivalent inspired tidal volume* (VT) of 1.0 L to ventilate the patient at each of these PEEP levels (Fig. 19-34), one would see that at the PEEP levels of 0 and 12 cmH₂O ventilation is still occurring on the linear portion of the curve and the compliance is essentially unchanged: 0.054 L/cmH₂O. In contrast, at a PEEP level of 23 cmH₂O, the end-inspiratory point has moved from the steep portion toward the flatter upper portion of the P-V curve and the compliance has fallen to 0.028 L/cmH₂O, indicating that some alveoli have reached their distensible limits.

As a final caution, determination of "best PEEP" from the static compliance curve and

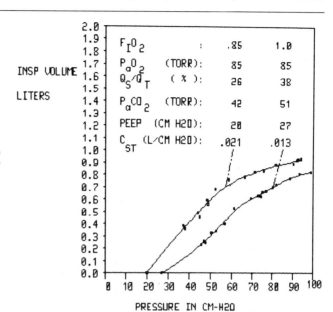

FIG. 19-35 Total static compliance curves from pt MM:193 obtained at PEEP levels of 20 cmH₂O and 27 cmH₂O.

the parameters of respiratory gas exchange clearly demonstrates that *more PEEP is not necessarily better* and super PEEP levels, by markedly increasing FRC, frequently force the already poorly compliant ARDS lung to operate at an even less favorable point on the lung pressure/volume curve. This is seen in the patient whose static compliance and blood gas data are shown in Figure 19-35. This patient sustained severe posttraumatic ARDS following a motor vehicle accident. Because of difficulties in maintaining her PaO_2 she was placed on an FIO_2 of 1.0 (100 percent) and, as is the usual tendency in the absence of quantification of the response to PEEP, the PEEP level was progressively increased to 27 cmH₂O in response to the increased shunt (38 percent), high $PaCO_2$ levels (51 mmHg), and respiratory acidosis (pH 7.29). Examination of the static compliance curve done at this point showed that it was shifted far to the right and at the tidal volume chosen (0.668 L) had a CST of 0.013 L/cmH₂O.

By utilizing the best PEEP technique it became evident that reducing PEEP to 20 cmH₂O enabled a marked shift to the left in the CST curve to a more favorable compliance (CST = 0.021 L/cmH₂O) at the same operational tidal volume (0.669 L) and permitted the maintenance of PaO_2 (85 mmHg) at a lower FIO_2 (0.85), a reduction in $\dot{Q}S/\dot{Q}T$ to 26 percent, and a reduction of $PaCO_2$ to 42 mmHg with an increase in pH to 7.39. This demonstrated that the higher PEEP level in this patient was acting to divert flow from exchanging alveoli to nonexchanging or low $\dot{V}A/\dot{Q}$ alveoli so that respiratory dead space, with increased $PaCO_2$, rose as $\dot{Q}S/\dot{Q}T$ increased. This example demonstrates how tailoring the PEEP characteristics of ventilatory support to match the static compliance curves of the ARDS lung can improve respiratory gas exchange.

Continuous Positive Airway Pressure in the Spontaneously Breathing Patient

Continuous positive airway pressure (CPAP) is a means of maintaining a PEEP in the spontaneously breathing patient. It was developed by Gregory and co-workers[72] for the treatment of infants with the idiopathic respiratory distress syndrome and has become an accepted method of treatment in adults who develop ARDS. It is delivered utilizing a breathing circuit with a threshold resistor or underwater seal on the expiratory limb to maintain the selected PEEP and a source of gas to provide inspiratory flow when airway pressure falls below the PEEP level on the inspiratory limb.

The use of PEEP in the spontaneously breathing patient significantly increases the work of breathing since the patient must generate a greater negative pressure to initiate inspiration. The use of a CPAP system should require less work since a positive inspiratory pressure is maintained utilizing a source of continuous gas flow. However, work may still be greater than that without the use of PEEP unless there is a significant improvement in compliance as a result of the use of PEEP.

The cardiopulmonary effects of PEEP and CPAP in the spontaneously breathing patient were assessed by Sturgeon and associates.[188] They found no differences in expiratory transpulmonary pressures but an increase in inspiratory effort with PEEP. There was a decrease in effective cardiac filling pressures without a change in stroke volume with CPAP while with PEEP effective cardiac filling pressures were not modified but stroke volume was increased.

MECHANICAL VENTILATION

The use of position and PEEP can help improve gas exchange abnormalities that are largely related to alteration in the static compliance relations of the respiratory system. However compliance abnormalities reflected in the dynamic characteristics of ventilation can be compensated by a proper choice of the type and mode of mechanical tidal ventilation above the optimal PEEP level. When the mouth pressure is raised during inspiration it is opposed by the two forms of resistance (Fig. 19-24B), the elastic resistance of lungs and chest wall and the frictional nonelastic pulmonary resistance (airway resistance + pulmonary tissue resistance)

Inflation pressure = pressure required to overcome elastic resistance + pressure required to overcome pulmonary resistance

$$\text{Pressure required to overcome elastic resistance} = \frac{\text{lung volume above FRC}}{\text{compliance}}$$

Pressure required to overcome the pulmonary resistance

$$= \text{pulmonary resistance} \times \text{instantaneous air flow rate}$$

$$\text{Inflation Pressure} = \left(\frac{\text{lung volume above FRC}}{\text{compliance}}\right) + \left(\begin{matrix}\text{instantaneous} \\ \text{air flow rate}\end{matrix} \times \begin{matrix}\text{pulmonary} \\ \text{resistance}\end{matrix}\right)$$

When the lung volume is equal to FRC (at start of inspiration) the first term on the right is equal to zero and the inflation pressure is acting solely against the pulmonary resistance to airflow. When gas flow ceases (at end of inspiration) the second term is zero and the inflation pressure is acting solely against elastic recoil.

During inspiration the component opposed by elastic forces (which equals alveolar pressure) increases in proportion to the lung volume, while the component opposed by air flow resistance is proportional to the instantaneous air flow rate (which equals the slope of the plot of the lung volume against time).

With a square pressure wave, flow is maximal at first and then declines exponentially: the component of the inflation pressure opposed by airway resistance is maximal at first and also declines exponentially (Fig. 19-24A). Since the successful ventilation of the trauma patient with ARDS must accommodate to a number of pathophysiologic mechanisms ranging from decreased compliance and reduced FRC (due to alveolar collapse) to major bronchopleural or parenchymal air leaks, the types of ventilator function must be fully understood and their characteristics matched to the patient.[100]

Types of Ventilators

There are three basic types of ventilators:

Time cycled: inspiration terminated after a preset time

Volume cycled: inspiration terminated after delivery of a preset volume

Pressure cycled: inspiration terminated after a preset pressure is attained at the mouth or elsewhere in the apparatus

More than one method of cycling can be included in one apparatus.

Characteristics of Operation

TIME-CYCLED VENTILATION

In time-cycled ventilators a pressure generator will deliver a smaller volume in the face of an increased resistance. A true flow generator will deliver almost the correct volume, provided the raised mouth pressure does not exceed the setting of the safety volume.

If compliance is diminished the flow generator should again deliver the correct tidal volume while the pressure generator would deliver a reduced tidal volume in proportion to the reduction in compliance.

VOLUME-CYCLED VENTILATION

A flow generator should deliver the correct tidal volume in the normal time. The minute volume should therefore be independent of moderate changes in compliance and resistance.

PRESSURE-CYCLED VENTILATION

Only flow generators can be pressure-cycled and a constant-pressure generator must be cycled by either time or volume.

Cycling by pressure has the disadvantage that if the resistance increases or the compliance decreases, the mouth pressure will reach the set or critical level at a smaller tidal volume than with normal respiratory function.

In an effort to determine optimal ventilator settings for critically ill or injured patients with ARDS, airway pressures should be routinely measured as well as the flow rates and volumes delivered. From the data obtained one can as- sess the effect of manipulations of these pressures and flows on lung mechanics (as reflected in changes in compliance and/or, airway resistance) cardiac output, and gas exchange (as demonstrated by blood gas analysis) (Fig. 19-22).

PATIENT-ASSISTED VENTILATION

The usual practice when choosing the appropriate ventilator setting at which to begin therapy is to use a tidal volume of 12 to 15 ml/kg and a rate sufficient to maintain $PaCO_2$ between 36 and 44 mmHg. If the *control* mode of ventilation is utilized, this rate is usually between 10 and 16/min and all ventilation is provided by the ventilator. In the control mode the patient is unable to initiate a breath and, unless paralyzed or anesthetized, will "fight" the ventilator if the settings are inadequate to provide for optimal gas exchange (Fig. 19-36).

In the *assist-control* mode the patient initiates the machine breath by generating pressure that is negative in relation to the baseline or end-expiratory pressure and thus controls the rate and minute volume delivered. In this mode of ventilation the tidal volume remains constant and if the patient's ventilatory rate falls below a set level, the ventilator will automatically deliver the number of breaths set as the "back-up" rate.

Two modes of ventilation that can be used not only for control mode but also for spontaneous breathing are *intermittent mandatory ventilation* (IMV) and *synchronized intermittent mandatory ventilation* (SIMV). For the IMV mode a control mode ventilator with attached circuitry that allows the patient to breathe spontaneously gas of the same temperature, humidity, and FIO_2 as provided by the ventilator is used. At preset intervals a volume-controlled breath is delivered by the ventilator. To ensure unimpeded spontaneous ventilation, a continuous gas flow with a flow rate at least four times the patient's minute ventilation must be provided and care must also be taken that the circuitry does not cause any increase in resistance to breathing.

The SIMV mode (Fig. 19-37) utilizes a ventilator in the assist/control mode with circuitry that also allows the patient to breathe sponta-

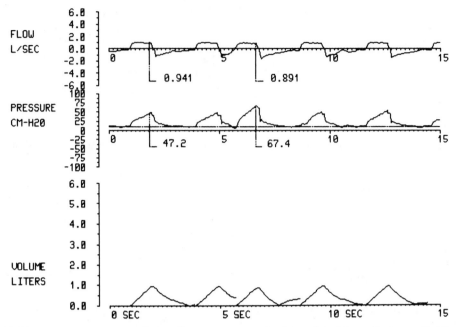

FIG. 19-36 Volume-controlled ventilation: flow, pressure, and volume data. The patient was "fighting" the ventilator and inspiration began before expiration was completed as shown by the second and third breaths. The pressure required to deliver a volume of 0.96 L was 47.2 cmH$_2$O. As indicated by the failure of the volume tracing to return to 0 on the second breath, expiration was not completed and the pressure required to deliver the set tidal volume increased to 67.4 cmH$_2$O since this volume was being stacked upon part of the previously delivered breath. Note that for the third breath not only was the total inspired volume expired but an additional volume, representing the volume left in the lung from the previous breath, was expired.

neously. Unlike the IMV mode, however, the ventilator breath is initiated by the patient's inspiratory effort. As in the assist/control mode, if the patient does not initiate the breath the ventilator will automatically deliver it. A demand flow system for the spontaneous breath is used in SIMV since a continuous-flow system does not allow for generation of the subbaseline pressure necessary for this means of synchronizing volume delivery by the ventilator to the patient's inspiratory effort.

The SIMV mode was developed due to concerns that using the IMV mode would result in "stacking" of a ventilator breath on top of a machine-initiated breath, with production of excessively high airway pressures and their subsequent effect on cardiorespiratory function. In actuality "stacking" does not have any significant effect on function and there is no demonstrable physiologic advantage of SIMV over IMV. One practical advantage, however,

is that one can more easily monitor the minute ventilation of the patient as well as his or her spontaneous tidal volume using the SIMV mode.

When rates of greater than 8/min are used in the IMV or SIMV mode, the ventilator is essentially providing controlled ventilatory support. At rates below this the patient is providing a significant portion of his or her ventilatory requirement.

There is much controversy concerning the reputed advantages of the IMV or SIMV mode of mechanical ventilation over the controlled or assist-controlled mode of ventilation. Weisman et al.[207] discuss the "putative" advantages and disadvantages of intermittent mandatory ventilation and readers may wish to consult this article to come to their own conclusions regarding the value of these techniques on ARDS patient management. Assist-control modalities are of value in weaning the patient

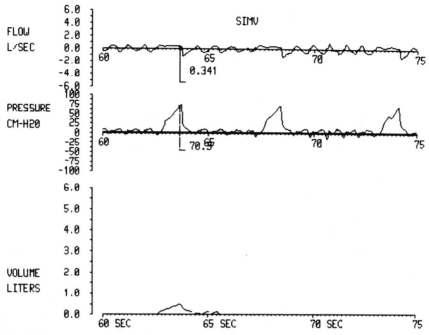

FIG. 19-37 SIMV mode of ventilation: flow, pressure, and volume data. The patient was being mechanically ventilated at a rate of 12 and tidal volume of 0.6 L. Breaths 4, 9, 15 are the ventilator breaths and it required a peak pressure of 70.5 cmH₂O to deliver a volume of 0.48 L. The spontaneous breaths had a volume of 0.1 L. The total rate was 60/min.

from ventilatory support, especially if the patient has been on some form of controlled ventilation for a prolonged period and may have wasting of the accessory muscles of respiration so that he or she tires easily after a brief period of spontaneous breathing. However, as discussed later, gradually decreasing levels of pressure support have also been used to wean this type of patient from ventilator dependence and may be a more reliable method with less chance of allowing muscle weakness respiratory failure due to hypoventilation, with CO_2 retention and respiratory acidosis.

VOLUME-CONTROLLED VENTILATION

In this mode of ventilation (Fig. 19-38), a set volume is delivered to the patient. The volume to be delivered is determined by selecting the rate, and tidal volume, or the rate and minute ventilation. The pressure required to deliver each tidal volume is dependent upon the patient's compliance and resistance. A pressure limit is set on the ventilator to guard against excessively high airway pressures. If this pressure limit is exceeded the volume actually delivered will be less than the set tidal volume. As noted earlier, the volume delivered to the patient is also dependent upon the amount of gas compressed within the ventilator itself and its tubing and humidification system.

Volume controlled ventilators are either time-cycled or volume-cycled. Time-cycled ventilators terminate inspiratory gas flow at a predetermined time, thus allowing for adjustments of inspiratory/expiratory time (I/E) ratios. Volume-cycled ventilators stop gas flow when a predetermined volume (as signaled by a measuring device such as a flow sensor, potentiometer, or bellows) has been delivered. The I/E ratio is dependent upon the inspiratory flow rate. Some ventilators have the ability to set a period of inflation-hold at the end of the inspiratory period; this phase is usually considered a part of inspiration. Inflation-hold is used to improve gas distribution when lung areas have

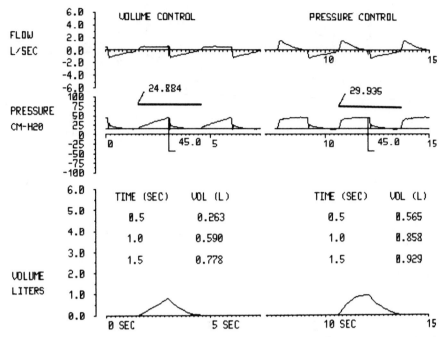

FIG. 19-38 Volume control and pressure control. Ventilation comparison: Flow, pressure, and volume data. See text for explanation.

differing time constants. Varying inspiratory flow patterns are also available on many ventilators now used in critical care. Flow can be either constant or nonconstant (i.e., sine wave, accelerating, or decelerating). These different patterns of flow are especially useful in ventilating patients who have markedly dissimilar time constants in different lung areas because of the asymmetrical distribution of their disease process.

PRESSURE CONTROLLED VENTILATION

In this mode (Fig. 19-38) gas is delivered at a constant pressure and for a set period of time. The flow rate is a decelerating pattern, that is, flow is initially high and decreases throughout the inspiratory cycle. The volume delivered is determined by the set inspiratory pressure, the rate, and the time for inspiration.

In the pressure-controlled mode, the volume delivered will vary dependent upon the patient's compliance and airway resistance and close monitoring of the actual volume delivered is essential. Any increase in airway resistance caused by bronchospasm, or a decreased lumen of the endotracheal tube due to secretions, will result in a decrease in the tidal volume actually delivered since these will result in a decrease in the flow rate delivered by the ventilator.

Gas flow rate = pressure gradient

$$\times \left(\frac{\text{II (radius of tube)}^4}{8 \times \text{length of tube} \times \text{gas viscosity}} \right)$$

Gas flow rate is proportional to the fourth power of the radius. Therefore, with a constant pressure gradient, halving the tube radius or diameter results in a 16-fold decrease in flow. If the time for inspiration is constant there will be a concomitant decrease in the volume delivered. If the inspiratory pressure level is constant and there is an increase in the elastance of the lung (leading to an increase in the recoil pressure and a subsequent decrease in compliance), there will be a decrease in the pressure gradient. This will result in a decrease in the gas flow rate and a resultant decrease in the volume delivered, since under conditions of laminar flow the pressure gradient is directly proportional to gas flow rate.

$$\frac{\text{Pressure gradient}}{\text{Flow rate}} = \text{Resistance}$$

$$\text{Resistance} = \frac{8 \times \text{length of tube} \times \text{gas viscosity}}{\Pi \, (\text{radius of tube})^4}$$

Resistance is constant only during laminar flow.

Under conditions of turbulent flow

1. The pressure gradient required to produce a given flow rate is proportional to the square of the gas flow rate.
2. Since resistance is defined as pressure gradient divided by flow rate, "resistance" is not constant but rises in proportion to the flow rate.

When flow is both laminar and turbulent

$$\text{Pressure gradient} = K_1 \, (\text{flow}) + K_2 \, (\text{flow})^2$$
$$\qquad\qquad\quad (\text{laminar}) \quad\ (\text{turbulent})$$

where K_1 contains all the constant factors of the Hager-Poiseuille equation for laminar flow (gas viscosity, tube radius, etc.) and K_2 contains all the constant factors in the equation for turbulent flow (gas density, tube radius, etc.).

Figure 19-38 shows the actual pressure and flow data utilizing two different modes of ventilation, volume control (VC) and pressure control (PC), from a patient who sustained a closed head injury (CHI), brain contusion, hemopneumothorax, right lung contusion, myocardial contusion, left diaphragmatic rupture, gastric contusion, and a hepatic contusion as a result of a motor vehicle accident. While on *volume control* (VC) ventilation utilizing a PEEP of 12 cmH$_2$O and an FiO$_2$ of 1.0, his blood gas measurements showed a PaO$_2$ of 53 mmHg, PaCO$_2$ of 39 mmHg, and pH of 7.38. At this point, without changing the FiO$_2$ it was decided to place the patient on *pressure control* (PC) ventilation utilizing the same peak inspiratory pressure (45 cmH$_2$O) as that used while on volume control. His blood gases at this time showed a PaO$_2$

of 60 mmHg, P$\bar{\text{v}}$O$_2$ of 24 mmHg, PaCO$_2$ of 26 mmHg, and pH of 7.52. The cardiac output was 4.04 L/min and the mean airway pressure was increased from 24.9 to 29.9 cmH$_2$O. The PEEP level was then increased to 14 cmH$_2$O and the inspiratory peak pressure level was decreased to less than 45 cmH$_2$O, resulting in a decrease in mean airway pressure. Blood gas measurements on an FiO$_2$ of 0.85 showed a PaO$_2$ of 125, P$\bar{\text{v}}$O$_2$ of 33, and the cardiac output rose to 6.24 L/min. The patient was being hyperventilated because of his closed head injury with increased intracranial pressure and his PaCO$_2$ was kept between 25 and 30 mmHg. The total compliance at this time was 0.034 L/cmH$_2$O.

The pressure, flow, and volume data shown in Figure 19-38 also demonstrate the important differences in the two modes of ventilation, VC and PC. In the critical care setting it is conventional practice to utilize volume-controlled ventilation. We have found, however, that in selected cases the use of time-cycled, pressure-controlled ventilation is more effective in ventilating patients with ARDS. When contrasting these two modes of therapy by looking at the pressure and flow wave forms generated by these two modes, the difference between them is readily apparent. Ventilator rate, PEEP, and I/E ratio were held constant. In PC the inspiratory flow rate is initially high and then decreases, a decelerating pattern. A constant flow was used in the VC mode as shown by the square wave pattern of the flow data. During the PC mode the inspiratory pressure control limit was set to the same peak pressure level (45.0 cmH$_2$O), which resulted from setting the tidal volume to 1.0 L while on the VC mode. The VC ventilation had resulted in a delivered tidal volume of only 0.778 L. The mean airway pressure in the VC mode was 24.9 cmH$_2$O, but in the PC mode it *increased* to 29.9 cmH$_2$O.

The increased mean airway pressure with PC produced an increase in the actual amount and a more favorable time pattern of volume delivery than with the VC mode. For the same peak airway pressures, 19 percent more volume was delivered using the PC mode (0.929 L). In addition, with PC a greater amount of the total tidal volume was delivered at each time interval: 0.565 L versus 0.263 L (61 percent versus 34 percent) at 0.5 sec; 0.858 L versus 0.590 L

(92 percent versus 70 percent) at 1.0 sec; and 0.929 L versus 0.778 L at 1.5 sec.

The increase in mean airway pressure (Pam) with PC is significant and in hypovolemic conditions can adversely affect cardiac output and thus oxygen delivery, as well as result in an increased risk for barotrauma, and these must be monitored when it is used. When the peak inspiratory pressure (PIP) is decreased so as to decrease the tidal volume delivered and thus increase the $PaCO_2$, the Pam also decreases. In ARDS patients, we have consistently found that utilizing the pressure control mode, with its decelerating flow pattern, results in a higher tidal volume at any given peak inspiratory pressure when compared to the VC mode constant flow pattern. Part of this effect may be due to a reduction in airway resistance, since that component of resistance due to turbulence is not constant, but rises in proportion to the flow rate. In the decelerating flow pattern, the flow rate is initially high but decreases throughout inspiration. There is therefore a reduction in the pressure gradient required to deliver a given volume of gas. A recent study by Al-Saady and Bennett[3] comparing these two inspiratory wave-forms, at constant tidal volume, I/E ratio, and rate, found that PC had statistically significant reductions in peak airway pressure, total respiratory resistance, work of inspiration, ratio of dead space to tidal volume, and alveolar–arterial gradient for oxygen. There also was a significant increase in total static and dynamic compliances and PaO_2 with no significant changes in cardiac output or other hemodynamic measurements.

Using the PC mode with its decelerating flow pattern, earlier delivery of the greatest percentage of the tidal volume, as well as higher initial airway pressure has resulted in improved gas exchange in our patients with ARDS when compared to volume-controlled ventilation with a constant inspiratory flow rate. This is in agreement with the studies of Al-Saady and Bennett.[3] The mechanism for this improvement probably lies in the availability of a longer time period for gas redistribution to occur from areas with shorter time constants to those with longer time constants, the so called pendeluft effect, as well as the higher Pam achieved.

Importance of Mean Airway Pressure

The mean airway pressure (Pam) is a reflection of all pressures transmitted to the airways. Factors that affect the Pam include peak inspiratory pressure (PIP), PEEP, inspiratory time including inflation hold or end-inspiratory pause (EIP), rate of ventilation, and the pressure wave-form created by the ventilator. Recent studies[23,35,64,142] have shown that improvement in oxygenation is directly correlated with changes in mean airway pressure irrespective of how the increase in Pam was achieved, whether by increasing PEEP, changing the inspiratory pressure wave-form, increasing inspiratory time by decreasing inspiratory flow rate, or using an inflation hold.

Creating PEEP is conventionally used to improve oxygenation in patients with ARDS. However, increasing the level of PEEP will also result in an increase in the mean airway pressure. In neonates with severe lung disease including hyaline membrane disease or aspiration of meconium or blood, Boros[23] showed that when FIO_2, tidal volume, respiratory rate, and PEEP remained constant, increasing the inspiratory/expiratory (I/E) ratio to increase Pam resulted in improved oxygenation. This could be achieved by either decreasing inspiratory flow rate thus producing a triangular pressure pattern as seen with constant flow, volume-controlled ventilation, or by adding an end-inspiratory pause (EIP) resulting in an inspiratory plateau or square pressure wave. When looking at the same I/E ratio (1:1) using these two different pressure patterns while maintaining PEEP constant, there was a significantly greater PaO_2/FIO_2 value using the squared pressure wave-form than the triangular wave-form. However, if the PEEP level was increased when using the triangular pressure wave-form, to the same level of Pam as resulted from the use of the squared pressure wave-form, there was no significant difference in the mean PaO_2/FIO_2 value using these two different pressure patterns. Gallagher and Banner,[64] in a study in patients with acute respiratory failure requiring PEEP greater than 15 cmH_2O, showed that decreasing PEEP level by 40 percent and peak inflation pressure by 33 percent, but increasing inspiratory time from 1 second to 4 seconds *to maintain the same Pam* as in the baseline study had no effect on oxygenation or cardiac output.

In achieving the desired level of mean airway pressure, it is better to utilize the effect of increasing the I/E ratio than to increase Pam by raising PEEP, providing the critical opening pressure level (Pflex) has been reached. This was shown by Pesenti et al.[142] who studied the effects of both PEEP and Pam on gas exchange in lambs subjected to lung lavage to induce severe respiratory insufficiency. The animals were mechanically ventilated at constant tidal volume, respiratory rate, and FIO_2. The Pflex, the point at which there is a major change in the inflation limb of the respiratory system's pressure-volume curve (Fig. 19-34), was obtained by manually plotting the airway pressures resulting from the step-by-step inflation of the lungs using 50-ml increments of air. The PEEP level was selected as −5, +5, and +10 cmH2O relative to Pflex for each lamb and the Pam was set by varying the I/E ratio. In each animal, the effects of the three PEEP levels were studied at two Pam levels differing by 5 cmH2O. When the PEEP level was greater than Pflex, both PaO_2 and $\dot{Q}S/\dot{Q}T$ were significantly better then the control level (PEEP: 5 cmH2O below Pflex). However, there was no significant improvement in oxygenation when the PEEP was raised further above Pflex. Increasing the Pam significantly improved PaO_2 and $\dot{Q}S/\dot{Q}T$ regardless of the PEEP level. For all PEEP increases, $PaCO_2$ increased. In contrast, increasing Pam caused a decrease in $PaCO_2$ at any given level of PEEP.

However, as noted in the case study presented earlier, changes in cardiac output must be considered when using increases in mean airway pressure to improve oxygenation, since the increase in Pam may also reduce cardiac output, thus producing an undesirable decrease in peripheral oxygen delivery. Presenti's studies[142] showed that cardiac output was not significantly affected by changes in PEEP but was significantly reduced by the Pam increase. PEEP increased central venous pressure (CVP) especially at the higher Pam but there was no significant change in either mean pulmonary

pressure (PAP) or mean systemic artery pressure. However, there was a significant negative interaction for PAP; increasing PEEP above Pflex decreased PAP at low Pam while it had an opposite effect at higher Pam.

High-Frequency Ventilation

Since the introduction of high-frequency ventilation (HFV) two types of systems have been used clinically, high-frequency positive pressure ventilation (HFPPV)[171,172] and high-frequency jet ventilation (HFJV).[102] The rationale for HFV is that by delivering a small tidal volume (smaller than physiological dead space) with a high rate, the peak airway pressure and sometimes the mean airway pressure may be lowered, thereby lowering the risk for barotrauma and cardiocirculatory embarrassment. Both experimental[22,87,197] and clinical[30,204] studies have not shown firm evidence to support this supposition. However, it has been shown that both HFPPV[204] and HFJV[30] are as efficient as the conventional modes of ventilation and in some cases (major bronchopleural fistula) HFV may be the only method that can achieve an adequate minute ventilation.[32,211] Other clinical areas of use include bronchoscopy, laryngoscopy, special cases of thoracic and upper abdominal surgery, and neurosurgery,[21,52,117,176,201] since in the latter case it does not increase intracranial pressure.[195]

A new method of HFV was introduced[53] in 1983, in which a combination of conventional ventilation and HFV was used, this was called combined high-frequency ventilation (CHFV). The theory of this method is to enhance gas mixing in the conducting airways[55] with the aid of high-frequency pulses and thereby increase the efficiency of the conventional breaths. We have modified this approach by developing a flexible purpose, multicomponent high-frequency system by which the HFV pulses can be superimposed during any part of the ventilatory cycle (Fig. 19-39). By superimposing on the expiratory phase with a low frequency (1 to 4 Hz) (Fig. 19-40), an improved washout of carbon dioxide in the conducting

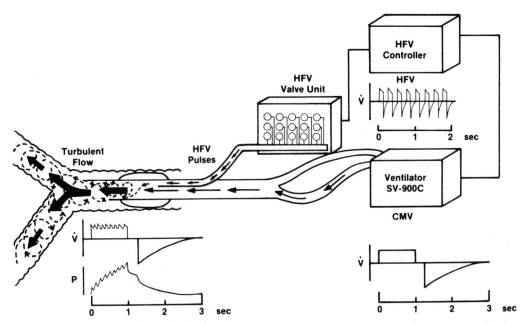

FIG. 19-39 Schematic layout for the combined high-frequency ventilation system. The HFV-controller is electronically connected to the SV 900C. The SV 900C generates trigger pulses regulating the start and stop of the superimposed high-frequency pulses. The high-frequency volume is delivered by the value unit consisting of a number of precalibrated valves. The flow patterns for the SV 900C and the HFV controller, as well as the combined flow pattern, are illustrated in the figure.

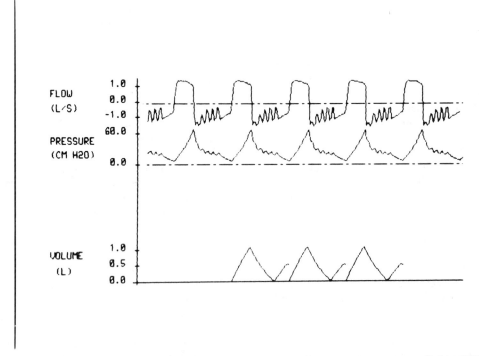

FIG. 19-40 Example of flow and pressure waveforms during combined high frequency ventilation (CHFV). High-frequency pulses are superimposed during expiration. The volume integration curve shows a second upswing representing the volume delivered by the high-frequency pulses.

airways may be achieved. This is shown in Table 19-4 from a patient with severe stage ARDS in whom marked CO_2 retention with rising $PaCO_2$ and respiratory acidosis occurred. The CHFV with the HFV component given in expiration (Fig. 19-40) reduced $PaCO_2$ and increased pH while also increasing PaO_2. This effect on $PaCO_2$ was most likely due to increased washout of the dead space. Mean airway pressure was increased from 26.9 on VC to 30.1 cmH_2O on CHFV without increase in PEEP or peak airway pressure. This resulted in an increase in PaO_2 from 66 to 96 mmHg and a reduction in $\dot{Q}S/\dot{Q}T$ from 39 to 27 percent without lowering cardiac output. The higher mean airway pressure can be assumed to have resulted in recruitment of perfused but underventilated areas of the lung, thus leading to an improvement in oxygenation. The fall in $PaCO_2$ may be due to improved washout of and a reduction in, end-tidal CO_2 ($PETCO_2$) so that near-atmospheric gas concentrations were effectively brought to the respiratory bronchioles leading to the alveoli.

However, one must be careful when using rates higher than 1 to 4 Hz during the expiratory phase, since in some patients this may create an unwanted PEEP effect and retention of carbon dioxide. In patients with a markedly re-

duced compliance due to ARDS and an increased demand for minute ventilation, due to hypermetabolic increases in $\dot{V}CO_2$,[99] superimposition of the HFV pulses during both inspiration and expiration may prove to be the only way to achieve adequate minute volumes without increasing the peak airway pressure. In these patients, oxygenation may sometimes be improved by superimposing the HFV pulses on the inspiratory phase with rates ranging from 10 to 20 Hz (Fig. 19-39). This improvement is probably due to the enhanced convection of oxygen-enriched gas into the conducting airways achieved by the HFV pulses.

The results of CHFV therapy given over a limited period of the ventilatory cycle in 27 patients with severe ARDS who had reached the limits of conventional mechanical ventilation (CMV) are shown in Table 19-5 over an average of 96 hours after initiation of CHFV. The tendency for mean airway pressure (Pam) to decrease during CHFV was most likely due to the prevention of high spikes in peak pressure, since there was no reduction in PEEP. By 96 hours, PaO_2 had increased significantly ($P < 0.05$) although in some individual patients major improvements in PaO_2 could be effected earlier. The RI fell but was not significant due to the wide standard deviation over all patients. However, compared to the control period of CMV support, the percent shunt ($\dot{Q}S/\dot{Q}T$) was significantly reduced ($P < 0.05$) at 24, 72, and 96 hours after initiation of CHFV.

While the results of CHFV are encouraging, based on our recent experience the most promising way to use CHFV seems to be by superimposing HFV pulses continuously during the entire respiratory cycle (CHFVC) at a single frequency (10 to 20 Hz) as is demonstrated in Figure 19-41. The patient shown was a 22-year-old woman admitted with a gunshot wound to her left chest. She developed septic ARDS which resulted in decreasing compliance and rising airway pressures. An impairment in arterial oxygenation and carbon dioxide retention were also noted. It was thus decided to try CHFVC in an early stage of ARDS to improve oxygenation without increasing the airway pressures. At this time she was on a PEEP level of 8 cmH_2O and an improvement in arterial oxygenation might have been achieved by increasing the PEEP. However, it was feared that

TABLE 19-4. Comparison of Gas Exchange and Respiratory Mechanics Parameters with Change from Volume Control (VC) to Combined High-Frequency Ventilation, in Expiration (CHFV—EXP)

Mode	VC	CHFV-EXP
Rate (br/min)	22	22
FiO_2	0.70	0.70
PEEP (cmH_2O)	10	10
VTI-CMV (L)	1.130	1.296
VTI-HFV (L)		.435
VTE (L)	1.166	1.731
PK Press (cmH_2O)	70.2	69.8
MN Press (cmH_2O)	26.9	30.1
Compliance (L/cmH_2O)	0.023	0.026
pHa	7.28	7.35
$PaCO_2$ (mmHg)	54	42
PaO_2 (mmHg)	66	96
RI	5.4	3.5
$\dot{Q}S/\dot{Q}T$ (%)	39	27
CO (L/min)	12.2	13.8

TABLE 19-5. Mean Values for 27 ARDS Patients on CHFV

	CMV	Hour 3	Hour 24	Hour 48	Hour 72	Hour 96
Paw	53.9	57.1	48.0	60.6	55.2	54.7
Pam̄	20.5	18.6	17.6[a]	17.2	18.7	14.8[a]
PEEP	14.1	15.4	13.7	17.6	14.0	17.0
PaCO₂	46	43	37	44	41	49
VTI	756	644	437	420	553	504
HFV[c]		347(35%)	351(55%)	473(53%)	411(43%)	380(43%)
VTE	724	991[b]	788	893[a]	964[a]	884[a]
FiO₂	0.71	0.69	0.71	0.64	0.68	0.66
PaO₂	77	79	81	86	78	93[a]
RI	5.6	5.5	4.9	4.2	4.7	3.6
Q̇S/Q̇T	34	33	29[a]	28[a]	34	26[a]

CMV, conventional Mechanical Ventilation; hour 3, 3 hours of HFV; Hour 24, 24 hours of HFV; Hour 48, 48 hours of HFV; Hour 72, 72 hours of HFV; Hour 96, 96 hours of HFV. Index, $(PAO_2 - PaO_2)/PaO_2$, Q̇S/Q̇T = Intrapulmonary Shunt (%).

[a] $P < 0.05$.

[b] $P < 0.001$.

[c] Includes patients with air leaks due to bronchopleural fistulae; HFV component averaged 392 ml (44 percent of VTE).

Superscripts *a* and *b* show significance of value at that hour compared to CMV.

this would result in an airleak through the lung penetration tract of the gunshot wound. Therefore, CHFVC was commenced and HFV pulses were superimposed throughout the entire respiratory cycle initially with a frequency of 18 Hz, which was later decreased to 10 Hz. As illustrated, the arterial oxygenation (PaO₂) increased (Fig. 19-42) as the intrapulmonary shunt (Q̇S/Q̇T) decreased (Fig. 19-43). On this mode of ventilation, her pulmonary status improved. After 25 days CHFVC was discontinued and the patient was managed on pressure-supported ventilation alone while being weaned from the mechanical ventilator. During the entire CHFVC period no pneumothorax occurred. This patient demonstrates the potential of CHFVC as an alternative to conventional ventilation in patients with ARDS related to

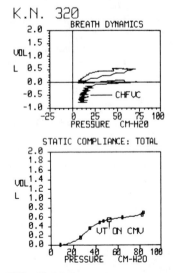

K.N. 320	CMV	CHFVC			
		1	10	25	Days
VTcmv	0.526	0.142	0.261	0.338	L
VThfv		0.765	0.561	0.632	L
FIO2	.60	.50	.55	.35	
pHa	7.35	7.35	7.44	7.42	
PaCO2	48	47	38	39	TORR
PaO2	87	122	215	175	TORR
PvO2	44	40	48	42	TORR
RI	3.3	1.5	.7	.2	
CO	8.2	8.4	8.2	8.1	L/MIN
Qs/Qt	31	21	23	14	%
PCWP	20	19	18	19	TORR
COMPL	.013	.013	.013	.016	L/CM H2O

FIG. 19-41 Breath dynamics, total static compliance, ventilation volumes, and circulatory and gas exchange parameters for a patient (K.N.:320 ventilated with CMV and CHFC.)

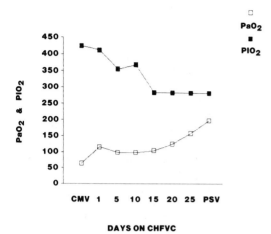

FIG. 19-42 Time course of PIO_2 and PaO_2 in patient with severe ARDS and high peak airway pressures maintained on CHFVC. (Also see Figure 19-41.)

trauma and/or sepsis, especially where there is a potential or actual air leak. Unfortunately no controlled experimental or clinical studies have been performed using CHFVC ventilation, although a few cases reported in the literature indicate the possible beneficial use of CHFV.[17] However, some form of combined high-frequency ventilation seems to be promising for the ventilatory management of patients with traumatic and/or septic ARDS.

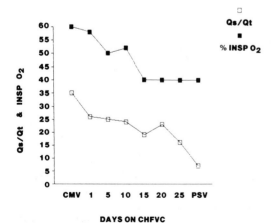

FIG. 19-43 Time course of percent inspired O_2 and percent shunt ($\dot{Q}S/\dot{Q}T$) during CHFVC in patient shown in Figure 19-42.

Simultaneous Independent Lung Ventilation

Respiratory failure in patients with asymmetrical lung disease is not well treated by conventional methods of ventilatory support, which apply their volume and pressure characteristics indiscriminately to all lung regions. This has led to a resumption of interest in techniques of independent lung ventilation.[11,31,65,151,169]

Recent studies of patients with acute unilaterally asymmetrical lung disease have suggested the use of independent lung ventilation employing a greater level of PEEP in the diseased lung to overcome the reduced compliance and effect better ventilation of partially collapsed alveoli.[11,31,65,151,169] Experimental studies[136] have suggested that pulmonary contusion that reduces ventilation and pulmonary compliance also increases the percent shunt ($\dot{Q}S/\dot{Q}T$) in the injured lung, but that the resulting increased hypoxic vasoconstriction diverts blood flow to the uninjured side, thus minimizing the effects of the injury. However, the application of PEEP, which appears to be effective in opening small airways and alveoli, may also alter the balance of perfusion by shifting blood flow back to the low $\dot{V}A/\dot{Q}$ and shunt areas. This occurs as a function of its relative effectiveness in opening closed alveoli and because of its effect in reducing perfusion to more compliant alveoli by transmitting the PEEP pressure to the normal alveolar capillaries, thus acting as a Starling resistance at the capillary level.[70,150,210] West[209] and Hedenstierna[81] have shown that the normal dependent lung has the greatest degree of perfusion. However with generalized PEEP the relative perfusion of the dependent lung increased. In the clinical setting both trauma and sepsis appear to induce a hyperdynamic cardiovascular state in which perfusion to dependent (zone III) lung regions is increased.[159,166] As a consequence, there is a total flow increase relative to the available ventilation to the contused or dependent edematous ARDS lung that tends to increase the magnitude of the $\dot{Q}S/\dot{Q}T$ as a function of the increase in cardiac index.[166]

There is a therapeutic paradox imposed by this pathophysiologic problem: controlled volume ventilation with generalized PEEP may increase flow through low-$\dot{V}A/\dot{Q}$, low-compliance lung while reducing that through high-compliance, high-$\dot{V}A/\dot{Q}$ lung. This occurs even though the PEEP effect assists in opening underventilated alveoli by raising mean airway pressures above the now increased critical opening pressures in the injured lung. This pathophysiologic sequence has suggested that a technique of independent ventilation in the normal compared to the injured lung may be beneficial.[12] The SILV technique has been applied with some success to unilateral lung contusion,[65,169] lobar pneumonia,[151] and refractory unilateral atelectasis.[156,169] More recently, it has been suggested that even acute asymmetrical bilateral lung pathology may be treated by independent lung ventilation in the lateral position,[9,10,12,169] thus artificially creating a situation of one lung with increased perfusion (the dependent lung) and the other lung (nondependent) with increased ventilation. Then by using selective PEEP and pressure- or volume-controlled ventilation it may be possible to shift perfusion upwards to the hyperventilated nondependent lung while simultaneously increasing ventilation to the hy-

perperfused dependent lung thereby effecting a more even $\dot{V}A/\dot{Q}$ matching.[9,10,12]

The difficulties in achieving an optimal ventilatory solution to this set of clinical problems have been in three areas. The first has been the need for an easily insertable double-lumen bronchial catheter for separation of the two lungs. The second is the development of a suitable dual-ventilator system with sufficient flexibility to accommodate all of the variations in PEEP, volume, flow, I/E ratio, and modalities of pressure- and volume-controlled support required to meet all possible clinical situations. The third need has been for a simple clinically applicable bedside technique of ventilatory assessment whereby the magnitude of the asymmetrical pathologic lung condition can be rapidly assessed, criteria for the initiation of SILV established, and management of this therapy effected.

In unilateral ARDS or atelectatic lung disease there is a mismatch of ventilation to perfusion between the two lungs. Compared to normal (Fig. 19-44), hypoxic vasoconstriction in the atelectatic portion of the diseased lung has a tendency to shift perfusion to the more normally ventilated lung (Fig. 19-45). However, in

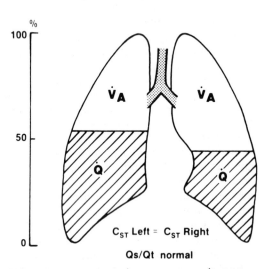

FIG. 19-44 Ventilation ($\dot{V}A$) to perfusion ($\dot{Q}$) distribution in normal lungs in supine position during spontaneous breathing. Total static compliance (CST) is approximately equal in each lung and intrapulmonary shunt ($\dot{Q}S/\dot{Q}T$) is normal.

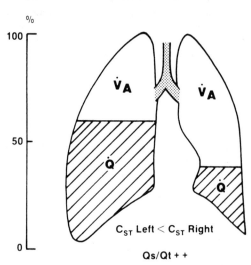

FIG. 19-45 Unilateral ARDS at 0 PEEP resulting in a shift in blood flow from the involved (left) to the uninvolved (right) lung. Hypoxic vasoconstriction accounts for this shift, which is a protective measure trying to keep the $\dot{V}A/\dot{Q}$ relation normal. $\dot{Q}S/\dot{Q}T$ is slightly elevated. Tidal volume is distributed freely. The patient is nonseptic with atelectasis.

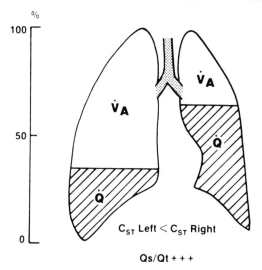

come this vasoconstrictive response so that increased perfusion of dependent lung segments with low ventilation/perfusion ratios occurs with a resulting large percentage of pulmonary venoarterial admixture[166] (Fig. 19-46).

The therapeutic doctrine in these instances has been to use controlled inspiratory volumes at increased PEEP[7,106] to overcome the pathologically increased small airway resistance (SAR) and reduced alveolar compliance that together alter the time constant for expansion of the diseased lung.[137] While this technique has generally been effective in bilaterally equal lung disease, applied generally in asymmetrical or unilateral lung pathologic conditions (Fig. 19-47), it may produce a compounding of the ventilation/perfusion ($\dot{V}A/\dot{Q}$) mismatch.[11,31,65,114,136,151] This occurs because of the differing time constants for expansion in normal compared to diseased lung which cause the gas volumes and pressures not to be uniformly distributed between the two lungs.[169] The result of this maldistribution of tidal volume is to overdistend the more compliant lower SAR lung, with transmission of the high PEEP and mean airway pressures to the distended normal alveolar capillary beds. This increases effective capillary resistance and diverts a share of the normal lung's perfusion to the

FIG. 19-46 In unilateral ARDS at 0 PEEP with superimposed inflammatory process and/or sepsis, the hypoxic vasoconstriction is abolished. This gives a maldistribution of perfusion to the involved lung thereby increasing the $\dot{Q}S/\dot{Q}T$. Tidal volume is distributed freely. The patient has septic ARDS on left.

areas of lung with inflammatory pneumonitis[115] or with posttraumatic or postseptic ARDS, local vasodilation and the hyperdynamic systemic cardiovascular response tend to over-

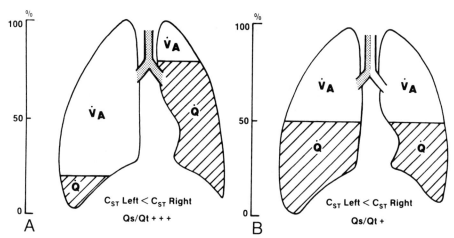

FIG. 19-47 Unilateral ARDS supine position. **(A)** When general PEEP is applied to increase FRC above closing volume in the involved lung, a further compounding of the $\dot{V}A/\dot{Q}T$ matching is seen. This is due to the overexpansion of the uninvolved lung. General PEEP > 10 cmH$_2$O. Tidal volume is distributed freely. **(B)** By instituting SILV with differential PEEP, with independent lung ventilation, the $\dot{V}A/\dot{Q}$ relation may be normalized. Higher PEEP is used in the involved (left) lung compared to the uninvolved (right) lung.

pathologic alveolar capillary beds, which have a low $\dot{V}A/\dot{Q}$ ratio. As a consequence, the parameters of gas exchange that reflect pulmonary venoarterial admixture (alveolar-arterial O_2 gradient, respiratory index, and percent shunt) may be worsened and arterial oxygen tension (PaO_2) falls at any inspired oxygen concentration (FIO_2).

This problem is also seen in bilateral ARDS when there is a marked disparity in disease severity between lung segments. Consequently the $\dot{V}A/\dot{Q}$ mismatch is distributed nonuniformly within both lungs due to regional differences in compliance and resistance. Under these circumstances the application of PEEP to prevent small airway closure and alveolar collapse also unintentionally may result in a greater $\dot{V}A/\dot{Q}$ mismatch, for the same reasons as are noted to occur in unilateral asymmetrical lung disease.[11,65]

In acute unilateral asymmetrical lung disease, it has been proposed that the technique of SILV could be used to match better the ventilatory volume to the perfusion of each lung.[31,151,169] This technique is designed to result in a better gas exchange by tailoring the ventilatory pressures and time patterns of the volume delivery to each lung so as to alter perfusion to obtain better $\dot{V}A/\dot{Q}$ distribution and

interfere less with cardiac filling and cardiac output levels[9,150] (Fig. 19-47).

The SILV technique has also been advocated for nonuniform bilateral ARDS. It has been suggested that the asymmetrical aspects of the pathophysiologic ARDS phenomena may be better isolated by placing the patient in the lateral position.[10] In this circumstance, gravity will redistribute most of the perfusion to the dependent lung regardless of whether the patient is spontaneously breathing or mechanically ventilated on zero PEEP (Fig. 19-48). This change in posture leads to a change in the functional residual capacity (FRC) level for each lung. In the dependent lung there will be a reduction in FRC, due to airway closure, in comparison to FRC in the nondependent lung. When mechanical ventilation is used there will be an increase in ventilation to the nondependent lung at the expense of the dependent lung, thus creating a situation more like that of unilateral asymmetrical lung disease. This is exaggerated when general PEEP is applied with overdistention of the nondependent lung (Fig. 19-49). Under favorable conditions such patients also can be more effectively treated by SILV which balances the $\dot{V}A/\dot{Q}$ for each lung (nondependent versus dependent) by enabling one to raise PEEP and ventilatory volume in

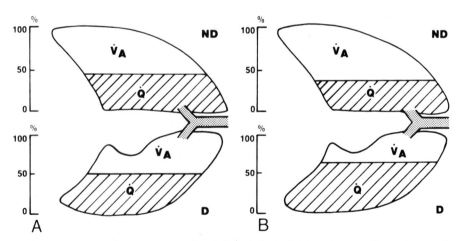

FIG. 19-48 **(A)** Ventilation ($\dot{V}A$) to perfusion ($\dot{Q}$) relationship in the left lateral posture in spontaneous breathing. Perfusion is slightly greater in the dependent lung due to gravity. **(B)** Bilateral ARDS. During mechanical ventilation in left lateral position at 0 PEEP the distribution of perfusion will increase to the dependent lung. Ventilation is distributed to the nondependent lung due to the decrease in compliance in the dependent lung. This creates a simulated unilateral pathologic lung condition with increased $\dot{Q}S/\dot{Q}T$.

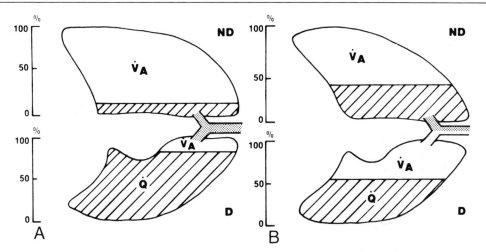

FIG. 19-49 Bilateral ARDS. Lateral position. **(A)** When applying general PEEP in the lateral position the perfusion will be forced, almost completely, to the dependent lung while ventilation will be distributed to the nondependent lung. This will compound the $\dot{V}A/\dot{Q}$ mismatch with markedly increased $\dot{Q}S/\dot{Q}T$. Tidal volume is freely distributed. **(B)** Independent lung ventilation. By using SILV in the lateral position with differential PEEP the perfusion may be forced back into the nondependent lung, thereby normalizing the $\dot{V}A/\dot{Q}$ matching. Higher PEEP is used in the dependent lung.

the dependent lung, forcing more perfusion to the nondependent better ventilated lung (Fig. 19-49).

Decisions for Using SILV

While clinical use of SILV techniques has become possible due to the commercial development of an easily placed double-lumen endobronchial tube that can atraumatically isolate the right and left lungs,[86,169] no clear and easily applied guidelines have been established for initiating and quantifying the need for SILV. Different approaches to diagnosis have been suggested, including the use of radioisotopic[12] or inert gas[81] studies of $\dot{V}A/\dot{Q}$ distribution, or the evaluation of lung capillary perfusion using radiopaque contrast injected through a pulmonary artery catheter.[31] Unfortunately, while valuable, these methods are cumbersome, expensive, and often require the transport of a critically ill patient from an intensive care unit to a radiologic facility. Also, they cannot be repeated frequently to permit fine tuning of ventilatory control on an hour-by-hour basis.

To address this problem, the computer-based pulmonary evaluation technique[169,170] described earlier has been applied. The computer is linked to the use of a Servo Ventilator 900 C for quantifying the mechanical properties of each lung, so as to assess the static and dynamic compliance changes by the delineation of flow, pressure, and volume relationships (Fig. 19-21). These measurements can be easily repeated without interrupting ventilatory support, as frequently as desired, to ensure that ventilator adjustment produces the best possible gas exchange. This technique provides a set of quantitative criteria for determining when SILV should be instituted and for assessing the optimal ventilatory techniques which should be applied to each lung.

Figure 19-50 shows the graphic output of the analytic system in a patient with nonuniform unilateral ARDS. The dynamic data from single breaths taken at the actual and trial ventilator settings, the entire static total compliance curve obtained by spline fit of the individual volume and pressure data points, and the blood gases, pH, cardiac output (CO), and computed variables (RI = alveolar-arterial O_2 difference/PaO_2, percent shunt = $\dot{Q}S/\dot{Q}T$, etc.) at the actual ventilator setting are also shown.

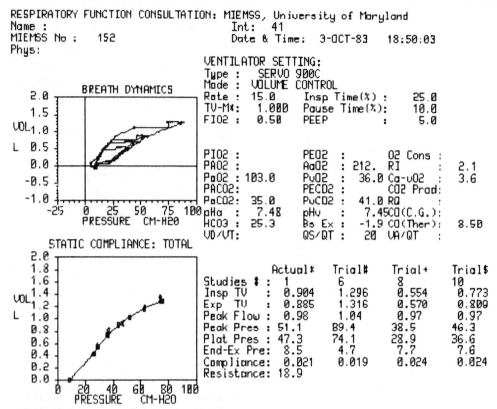

```
RESPIRATORY FUNCTION CONSULTATION: MIEMSS, University of Maryland
Name :                              Int:   41
MIEMSS No :    152                  Date & Time:  3-OCT-83    18:50:03
Phys:
                          VENTILATOR SETTING:
                          Type :    SERVO 900C
         BREATH DYNAMICS  Mode :    VOLUME CONTROL
   2.0                    Rate :   15.0    Insp Time(%) :    25.0
   1.5                    TV-M% :   1.000  Pause Time(%):    10.0
VOL 1.0                   FIO2 :    0.50   PEEP        :      5.0
 L 0.5
   0.0                    PIO2 :           PEO2 :          O2 Cons :
  -0.5                    PAO2 :           AaO2 : 212.   RI      :   2.1
                          PaO2 : 103.0     PvO2 :  36.0  Ca-vO2  :   3.6
  -1.0                    PACO2:           PECO2:         CO2 Prod:
      -25  0   25  50  75 100 PaCO2: 35.0   PvCO2 : 41.0 RO      :
         PRESSURE  CM-H2O pHa  :   7.48     pHv  :   7.45 CO(C.G.):
                          HCO3 :  25.3      Bs Ex :  -1.9 CO(Ther):   8.50
     STATIC COMPLIANCE: TOTAL  VD/VT:       QS/QT :   20  VA/QT   :
   2.0
   1.8                             Actual*  Trial#  Trial+  Trial$
   1.6                    Studies # :   1      6       8      10
VOL 1.4                   Insp TV   : 0.904  1.296   0.554   0.773
    1.2                   Exp  TV   : 0.885  1.316   0.570   0.809
 L 1.0                    Peak Flow : 0.98   1.04    0.97    0.97
   0.8                    Peak Pres : 51.1   89.4    38.5    46.3
   0.6                    Plat Pres : 47.3   74.1    28.9    36.6
   0.4                    End-Ex Pre:  8.5    4.7     7.7     7.6
   0.2                    Compliance: 0.021  0.019   0.024   0.024
   0.0                    Resistance: 18.9
      0   20  40  60  80 100
         PRESSURE   CM-H2O
```

FIG. 19-50 Graphic output of the analytic system in a patient with nonuniform unilateral ARDS (MC:152). Shown are the ventilator settings, the actual inspired (Insp TV) and expired (Exp TV) tidal volume, peak pressure (Peak Pres), plateau pressure (Plat Pres), end-expiratory pressure (End-Ex Pre), compliance and resistance values for the set breath delivered by the ventilator (actual x), as well as the arterial and mixed venous (v) pH and blood gases ($PaCO_2$, $P\bar{v}CO_2$, PaO_2, $P\bar{v}O_2$), the percent shunt ($\dot{Q}S/\dot{Q}T$), respiratory index (RI), arterial-venous oxygen content difference (Ca-$\bar{v}O_2$), and cardiac output (CO) whether measured using the dye-dilution (CO[CG]) or thermal dilution (CO[Ther]) method. Also shown is the total static compliance curve and three trial breaths plotted with the actual set breath as pressure–volume loops to show the breath dynamics as well as where these individual breaths fall on the static compliance curve.

This standard plot allows for the integration of all data and also allows the physician to see the point on the static total compliance curve at which the present ventilatory support setting is maintained (actual setting versus trial settings) so as to optimize ventilation for the particular lung mechanics demonstrated by the patient. Analysis of the static pressure–volume curve shown (Fig. 19-51) shows the typical multicomponent static compliance, reflecting nonuniformity of the ARDS process. When this pattern is associated with a radiographic picture of unilateral ARDS or atelectatic lung disease following chest contusion, extrathoracic trauma, aspiration, or sepsis, the SILV technique should be considered.

OPTIMIZATION OF PEEP AS A TEST FOR INITIATING SILV

Before SILV is carried out, the optimization of generalized PEEP, as described previously, should be re-evaluated to ensure that the apparent multicomponent nature of the static compliance curve, and the blood gas abnormal-

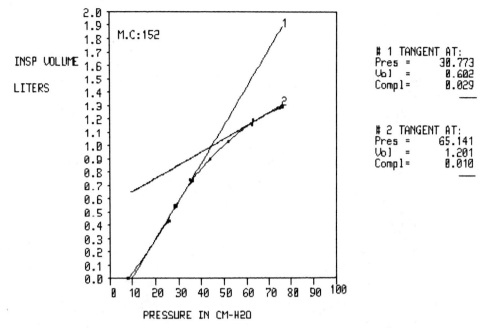

FIG. 19-51 Total static compliance curve in a patient with nonuniform unilateral ARDS (MC:152) with tangents drawn at inspired volumes of 0.6 L and 1.2 L showing a typical multicomponent static compliance curve that reflects nonuniformity of the disease process.

ities, are not the result of insufficient or excess PEEP that is positioning the patient at an unfavorable pressure–volume point between FRC and TLC on the static compliance curve.

THERAPEUTIC SYSTEM FOR SILV

The system to carry out SILV is shown in Figure 19-52. In this therapeutic system two advanced Servo ventilators are synchronized to start of inspiration. Each complete system is connected to one lumen of a dual-lumen Broncho-cath (National Catheter Corp., Argyle, N.Y.) catheter. *Regardless of the side of greatest pathologic change, the long arm of a left angled Broncho-cath is placed in the left mainstem bronchus to avoid obstruction to the right upper lobe segmental bronchus.* The proximal balloon occludes the trachea, providing a closed system, and when the distal balloon is inflated the right and left lungs can be independently ventilated by the two Servo ventilators using different tidal volumes, PEEPs, I/E ratios, pause times, and, in some instances, totally different ventilatory modes (i.e., volume-con-

trolled in one lung and pressure-controlled in the other). To start the SILV process, initially the total tidal volume is divided in half, the pressures monitored, and a compliance curve created for each lung. Then adjustment to an appropriate pressure–volume point for each lung is carried out. The value of this approach is seen in Figure 19-53, in which the different static total compliance curves of the right and left lungs mandate two different volume optimization points at different PEEPs.

In using this technique, the cardiac output (CO) should be measured by thermodilution or cardiogreen dye dilution at frequent intervals and after all major ventilatory changes (Fig. 19-50). Arterial and mixed venous oxygen saturations and the blood partial pressures of respiratory gases (PO_2, PCO_2) and pH should also be measured at the same time and the oxygen content difference ($Ca\text{-}\bar{v}O_2$), percent pulmonary venoarterial admixture ($\dot{Q}S/\dot{Q}T$), and the respiratory index (alveolar-arterial O_2 gradient/PaO_2 ratio) computed to permit accurate quantification of physiologic changes in response to SILV therapy.[18,165]

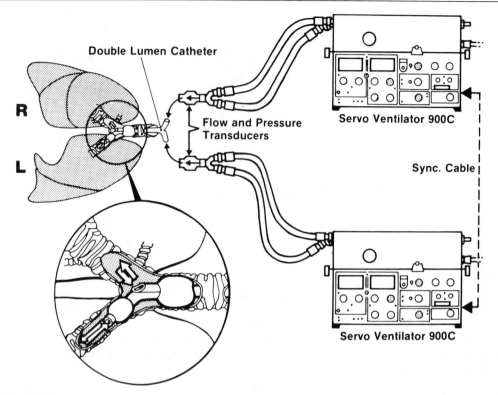

FIG. 19-52 Therapeutic system for simultaneous independent lung ventilation (SILV). (Siegel JH, Stoklosa J, Borg U et al: Quantification of asymmetric lung pathophysiology as a guide to the use of simultaneous independent lung ventilation in posttraumatic and septic ARDS. Ann Surg 202: 425, 1985.)

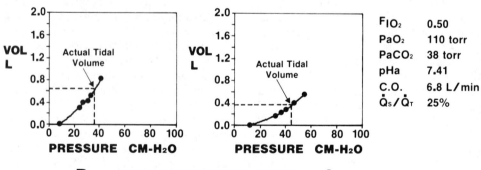

FIG. 19-53 Total static compliance curves for right (R) and left (L) lungs showing optimization points at different tidal volumes and PEEP levels. (Siegel JH, Stoklosa J, Borg U et al: Quantification of asymmetric lung pathophysiology as a guide to the use of simultaneous independent lung ventilation in posttraumatic and septic ARDS. Ann Surg 202: 425, 1985.)

Role of SILV in Asymmetrical Pathologic Lung Conditions

In addition to providing a physiologically directed therapy aimed at the reduction of posttraumatic ventilation–perfusion abnormality, the use of SILV in selected instances can reverse persistent atelectatic changes associated with ARDS even late in the clinical course, provided irreversible fibrotic or necrotic changes

have not occurred. This result occurred in the patient in Figure 19-50, in whom a persistent ARDS pattern was seen despite the continuous use of PEEP and high tidal volumes with conventional ventilation. Attempts to re-expand the left lung while on conventional ventilation resulted in marked increases in airway pressure to the right lung as well, resulting in overdistention barotrauma (Fig. 19-54B). There was also a diversion in blood flow from the relatively compliant area, which produced an in-

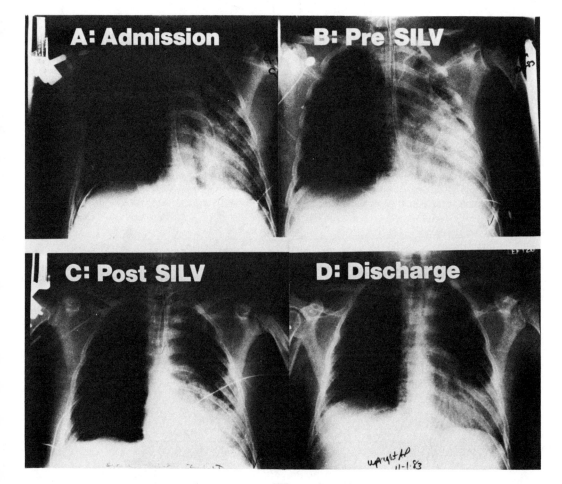

FIG. 19-54 Radiologic examination of posttraumatic unilateral atelectasis (patient MC:152). **(A)** 9–14–83: Admission, postresuscitation, postinjury to left lung. **(B)** 10–3–83: Persistent atelectatic ARDS with hyperexpansion of right lung on conventional ventilation, immediately prior to SILV. **(C)** 10–5–83: Improvement in aeration of left lung on SILV. **(D)** 11–1–83: Sustained resolution of ARDS, immediately before patient's discharge from hospital. (Siegel JH, Stoklosa J, Borg U et al: Quantification of asymmetric lung pathophysiology as a guide to the use of simultaneous independent lung ventilation in posttraumatic and septic ARDS. Ann Surg 202: 425, 1985.)

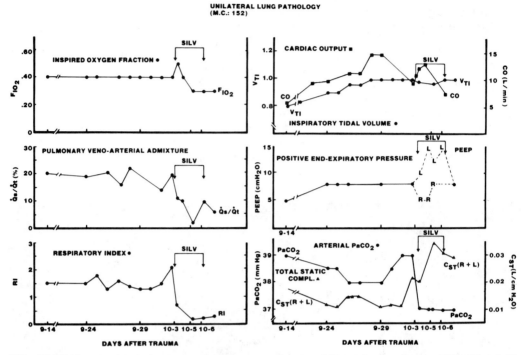

FIG. 19-55 The physiological aspects of time course of patient MC:152 in response to SILV. (Siegel JH, Stoklosa J, Borg U et al: Quantification of asymmetric lung pathophysiology as a guide to the use of simultaneous independent lung ventilation in posttraumatic and septic ARDS. Ann Surg 202: 425, 1985.)

crease in shunt fraction (Table 19-6, Fig. 19-55). With the initiation of SILV (Table 19-6, Fig. 19-55) there was improvement as the shunt fraction fell from 20 to 10 percent and the RI from 2.1 to 0.3.

A comparison of the static compliance relations for the total lung and the individual right and left lung compliances are shown for the period corresponding to the start of SILV (Fig. 19-56A) on 10/3/83 and the period at the

end of SILV (Fig. 19-56B) on 10/6/83. The quantitative gas exchange and compliance data are presented in Table 19-6. The initial study before SILV (10/3/83) demonstrated marked difference in the mechanical properties of the right and left lung. The chest radiograph (Fig. 19-54B) at this time showed a marked dissimilarity in aeration between the lungs. This correlated with the total compliance curve for both lungs obtained immediately before initiation

TABLE 19-6. Response to SILV Therapy

	Start ⟶	SILV		⟶ End
	10/3/83	10/4/83	10/5/83	10/6/83
FiO₂	0.50[a]	0.34	0.34	0.30
PaO₂ (mmHg)	103[a]	135	175	122
QS/QT (%)	20[a]	13	5	10
RI	2.1[a]	0.2	0.1	0.3
CST (Rt) (L/cmH₂O)	0.020	0.020	0.018	0.020
CST (Lt) (L/cmH₂O)	0.005	0.013	0.011	0.012

[a] Gas values immediately prior to SILV therapy.

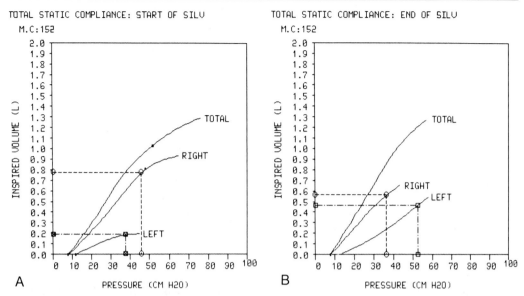

FIG. 19-56 (A) Comparison of static compliance relations in right and left lungs of patient MC:152 immediately upon institution of SILV. Also shown is the total static compliance curve for both lungs immediately before SILV. **(B)** Comparison of static compliance relations in the right and left lungs of patient MC:152 immediately before termination of SILV. Also shown is the total static compliance curve of both lungs after termination of SILV. (Siegel JH, Stoklosa J, Borg U et al: Quantification of asymmetric lung pathophysiology as a guide to the use of simultaneous independent lung ventilation in posttraumatic and septic ARDS. Ann Surg 202: 425, 1985.)

of SILV, which had two distinct slopes (Fig. 19-51) with tangents equivalent to compliances of 0.029 at a VT of 0.6 L and 0.010 L/cmH₂O at a VT of 1.2 L, indicating unilateral or asymmetrical pathologic lung condition. Initially the compliance of the left lung was 0.005 L/cmH₂O and only a VT of 0.2 L could be delivered to this lung (Fig. 19-56A). Attempts to increase this volume led to marked increases in airway pressure with minimal improvement in amount of volume actually delivered as evidenced by the plateau in the compliance curve for this lung. A VT of 0.8 ml delivered to the right lung was required to maintain gas exchange. This resulted in hyperinflation even though low PEEP was applied. The left lung was reexpanded by using a PEEP level of 12 cmH₂O and gradually increasing the tidal volume delivered. It was thus possible to reduce the VT to the right lung and thereby lower the distending pressures in this lung to more reasonable levels (Fig. 19-56B). The compliance in the left lung improved from 0.005 to 0.012 L/cmH₂O and there was marked improvement in the chest

radiograph (Fig. 19-54C). The improvement was sustained and the atelectasis continued to resolve upon discontinuation of SILV (Figs. 19-54D, 19-55).

Therapy of Bilateral Asymmetrical ARDS

The use of SILV along with lateral positioning is shown for a patient with diffuse bilateral posttraumatic and septic ARDS with an associated bronchial air leak decompressed by a chest tube on the left side (Table 19-7). Initially the patient was placed on SILV and was kept in the supine position; this led to deterioration of the patient's pulmonary status, even though many adjustments were made over a 12-hour period (18:35 P.M. to 7:00 A.M. studies) to optimize ventilation settings. It was decided to place the patient in the left lateral position at 9:00 A.M., with results as shown in the 10:45

TABLE 19-7. Response to SILV Therapy

	Supine	SILV Supine (18:35 P.M.)		SILV Supine (7:00 A.M.)		SILV Lt Lateral (10:45 A.M.)	
FiO$_2$	1.0	1.0		1.0		1.0	
PaO$_2$ (mmHg)	66	70		43		88	
RI	9.1	8.4		14.8		5.9	
Q̇S/Q̇T (%)				63		36	
Lung	Both	R	L	R	L	R	L
Mode	PC	PC	PC	PC	PC	PC	VC
PEEP (cmH$_2$O)	12	6	14	10	10	13	12
Mean press (cmH$_2$O)	24	17	24			28	33
VtI (L)	0.795	0.490	0.412			0.588	0.563
VtE (L)	0.663	0.456	0.305			0.557	0.502
Compliance (L/cmH$_2$O)	0.026	0.023	0.014			0.015	0.016

R, right; L, left; PC, pressure control; VC, volume control.

study in Table 19-7. Both lungs were ventilated with *pressure-controlled* ventilation in the supine position. However, when the patient was placed in the left lateral position the dependent lung was ventilated with *volume-controlled* ventilation to ensure a constant volume with a higher mean pressure in the dependent lung. This change in position with pressure adjustment to favor increased perfusion of the superior lung resulted in an apparent improvement in V̇A/Q̇ distribution. The change in PaO$_2$ with positioning was from 43 to 88 mmHg on FiO$_2$ 1.0. Over the next 24 hours, there was a further increase in PaO$_2$ to 129 mmHg on FiO$_2$ 0.80. The shunt decreased from 63 to 36 percent initially with further improvement to 27 percent and the RI fell from 14.8 to 5.9 and then to 3.1 during the following 24 hours.

It is important to emphasize that in complex respiratory management problems various combinations of techniques often must be used to obtain the optimal results for any given clinical situation. This situation is demonstrated by this case at the point where sufficient improvement had occurred after ventilation in the lateral position to allow us to place the patient back in the supine position. As shown earlier (Fig. 19-38), using pressure-controlled ventilation results in a more rapid lung volume expansion at a declining flow pattern. This type of expansion will frequently bring the lung parenchyma in apposition to the chest wall earlier in inspiration, tending to reduce parenchyma-

tous lung air leaks. Consequently, because of the persistent air leak the left lung was again placed on pressure-controlled ventilation. This led to a more uniform pressure profile as volume expansion occurred compared to the previous volume-controlled ventilatory mode. This also stopped the air leak. The three-dimensional pressure–flow–volume curves shown in Figure 19-57 demonstrate the differences between pressure and volume control in the left lung in the supine position (the right lung was maintained on pressure control throughout). By applying a pressure sufficient to overcome the critical airway opening pressure during the early phase of inspiration, a more even volume distribution and more complete expansion of the lung was achieved during pressure-controlled ventilation, which resulted in better control of the air leak. This can be seen in Figure 19-57, where the gap in the pressure–volume plane, representing the nonexpired volume (air leak), is reduced.

In eight patients 20 hours of SILV produced a significant ($P < 0.05$) increase in the net tidal volume that could be delivered to the two lungs if the separate tidal volumes were combined compared to what could be delivered by conventional therapy to the two lungs considered as a unit (Fig. 19-58). This occurred while maintaining lower plateau and peak pressures in the less damaged lung and generally produced a higher combined total (right plus left) compliance. The PaCO$_2$ was essentially unchanged

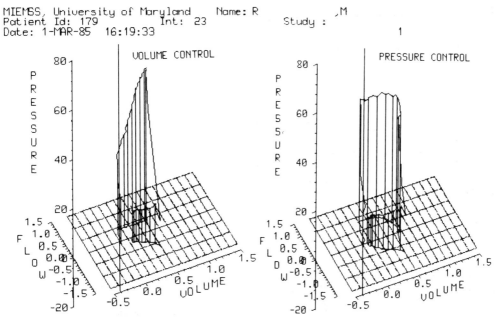

FIG. 19-57 Comparison of dynamic pressure–flow–volume relations of the left lung in patient MR:179 while on SILV. Graph shows a reduction in air leak from 164 to 69 ml in response to the change from volume control to pressure control ventilation to the left lung while in the supine position. The right lung was being ventilated using the pressure control mode. (Siegel JH, Stoklosa J, Borg U et al: Quantification of asymmetric lung pathophysiology as a guide to the use of simultaneous independent lung ventilation in posttraumatic and septic ARDS. Ann Surg 202: 425, 1985.)

while the respiratory index (and shunt) tended to fall and the PaO_2 to rise at any FiO_2.

The use and limitations of this technique are still being explored in the severely impaired ARDS patient with nonuniform disease. However, a number of recent studies[11,169] suggest that sufficient progress has now been achieved in the SILV technique to make it a clinically relevant method for early, safe, and effective therapy in selected patients with either unilateral or bilateral asymmetrical ARDS.

Quantitative Basis for Therapeutic Decision-making in Severe Complicated Posttraumatic ARDS

Perhaps the most difficult aspect of the therapy of the patient with severe posttraumatic ARDS is the proper choice of the optimal modes of ventilatory therapy either interactively or on a sequential basis as the ARDS process improves or worsens. The key to this type of decision-making is a quantification of the patient's lung mechanics and gas exchange characteristics at each phase of the process and an understanding of how each mode of ventilatory therapy is likely to affect the basic pathophysiology. Then, after choosing the modality of ventilatory support and the exact characteristics of ventilation, repeat quantification on a serial basis must be carried out to ensure that the practical implications of the theoretically chosen ventilatory support program are beneficial. Finally, since the condition of the patient with severe posttraumatic and/or septic ARDS is likely to change rapidly, this assessment and readjustment process must be repeated frequently to ensure continued optimization of ventilatory support.

An example of this interactive process is the case of a 17-year-old boy who was in a head-on motor vehicle collision on 6/6/85. He

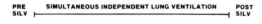

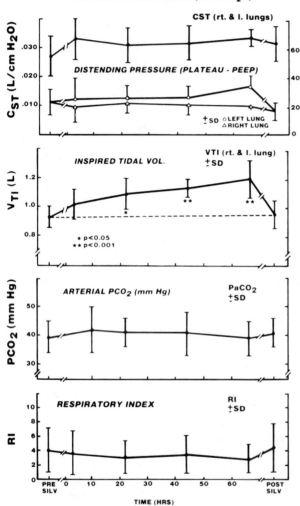

FIG. 19-58 A summary of the physiologic effects of SILV in eight patients. There is a significant increase in total inspired tidal volume (right and left lung) with no increase in distending pressure (P_{DIST}). Also shown are a trend for improvement in combined (right and left) compliance and respiratory index, suggesting improvement in ventilation perfusion distribution. (Siegel JH, Stoklosa J, Borg U et al: Quantification of asymmetric lung pathophysiology as a guide to the use of simultaneous independent lung ventilation in posttraumatic and septic ARDS. Ann Surg 202: 425, 1985.)

sustained severe chest contusion with a left pneumothorax and pneumomediastinum for which left chest tubes were placed, and also had a probable cardiac contusion. In addition there were major maxillofacial fractures and pulmonary aspiration. A closed head injury with basilar skull fracture and coma occurred, as did splenic rupture requiring emergency splenectomy. A fracture of the left femur was treated by internal fixation following the sple-

nectomy. The facial fractures were also stabilized. Following surgery and while the patient was in the critical care unit, the pneumomediastinum developed into a tension pneumopericardium and an emergency pericardial window was performed producing a gush of air. This was drained with a pericardial tube. Over the next 3 postoperative days the patient developed worsened ARDS. Higher airway pressures were required for ventilation and there was progressive subcutaneous emphysema as a result of the bronchial air leak into the mediastinum. Because of these circumstances, quantified by the static total compliance curve of 6/10/85 (Fig. 19-59A), combined high-frequency ventilation (CHFV) in both inspiration and expiration was begun on 6/10/85 and maintained until 6/17/85. On this therapy (Table 19-8), it was possible to increase the tidal volume from 0.870 L to between 1.2 and 1.3 L, with a reduced peak and mean airway pressure while maintaining a $PaCO_2$ below 35 mmHg, as required by the hypocapnia therapy for his severe closed head injury. On this therapy the PaO_2 was maintained as FiO_2 was reduced and the RI fell from 3.6 at the

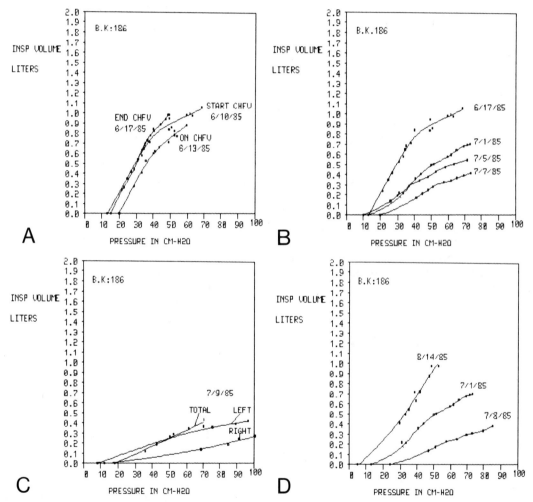

FIG. 19-59 Total static compliance curves in a patient (BK:186) with severe complicated ARDS treated with combined high frequency ventilation (CHFV), simultaneous independent lung ventilation (SILV), and a combination of SILV with CHFV to one lung. **(A)** 6/10/85–6/17/85: Initial use of CHFV. **(B)** 6/17/85–7/7/85: Progression of ARDS. CHFV was reinstituted on 7/3/85. On 7/7/85, clinical evidence showed that the right lung was more involved than the left. **(C)** 7/9/85: SILV begun. Shown are the compliance curves for both lungs and for the right and left lungs, which were being ventilated at different PEEP levels. **(D)** 7/1/85–8/14/85: Return of total static compliance curve toward normal. Patient was maintained on SILV with CHFV to the left lung between 7/10/85 and 7/27/85. See Table 19-8.

TABLE 19-8. Response to CHFV Therapy

	ON CHFV									
					X	□				
Date	6/10	6/10	6/11	6/13	6/14	6/14	6/14	6/16	6/17	6/17
FiO₂	0.60	0.60	0.60	0.50	0.80	0.60	0.50	0.40	0.40	0.40
PEEP (cmH₂O)	13	7	19	20	20	20	20	10	16	10
pHa	7.42	7.40	7.41	7.44	7.31	7.43	7.42	7.38	7.37	7.36
PaCO₂ (mmHg)	25	33	32	32	42	33	34	29	35	38
PaO₂ (mmHg)	100	69	94	113	81	112	106	88	88	91
PvO₂ (mmHg)	32	32	32	32	34	33			40	
RI	2.3	3.6	2.6	1.5	4.4	2.0	1.5	1.6	1.5	1.4
QS/QT (%)	21	25	20	18	32	24			25	
Compliance (L/cmH₂O)	0.032	0.029	0.028	0.028	0.028	0.026	0.031	0.028	0.036	0.030
Pk Press (cmH₂O)	46	50	47	51	49	55	49	50	43	45

X Pneumothorax.
□ Postchest tube insertion.

beginning of CHFV to 1.5 at the termination of CHFV on 6/17/85.

Unfortunately as a complication of the initial aspiration at the time of injury and the severe posttraumatic ARDS, a secondary septic process evolved with the patient spiking temperatures to 104° F and white counts as high as 23,000/mm³. This septic process was treated with antibiotics but responded poorly and the patient developed a septic hyperdynamic state with cardiac outputs ranging from 8.0 to 10.0 L/min and the Q̇S/Q̇T rose as high as 43 percent with an increased RI, as FiO₂ was increased from 0.55 to 0.90 (Table 19-9).

These findings are characteristic of an infiltrative septic process in the lung. During this period (Fig. 19-59B) from 6/17/85 to 7/7/85 the static total compliance shifted markedly down and to the right. The peak and mean airway pressures rose as the compliance fell (Table 19-9) and it was necessary to reinstitute CHFV during inspiration and expiration to permit an adequate total tidal volume (> 0.8 L) without excessively raising airway pressures further. During this period the HFV tidal volume component was always larger than the CMV tidal volume. Nevertheless, despite the marked hyperdynamic septic ARDS deterioration, an ade-

TABLE 19-9. Response to CHFV and SILV Therapy

	CHFV									SILV	
	7/1	7/2	7/3		7/4	7/5	7/7	7/8		7/9	
Mode	PC	PC	PC	PC	PC	PC	PC	PC	PC	VC-R	VC-L
Rate (Br/min)	26	26	28	26	26	26	38	36	36	36	
FiO₂	0.55	0.50	0.70	0.65	0.55	0.65	0.80	0.90	0.90	0.80	
PEEP (cmH₂O)	13	10	5	8	8	10	20	24	18	12	8
VtI-CMV (L)	0.677	0.556	0.630	0.379	0.350	0.385	0.296	0.243	0.347	0.233	0.365
VtI-HFV (L)				0.502	0.472	0.459	0.515	0.482	0.378		
VtE (L)	0.681	0.554	0.595	0.831	0.822	0.844	0.811	0.725	0.725	0.193	0.343
Pk Press (cmH₂O)	81.0	73.2	68.9	56.8	63.4	67.2	79.2	80.4	71.5	86.8	77.9
Mn Press (cmH₂O)	30.0	31.5	29.8	26.5	28.5	30.3	33.4	32.6	25.1	40.5	30.0
Compliance (L/cmH₂O)	0.012	0.011	0.010	0.012	0.011	0.009	0.008	0.007	0.008	0.003	0.005
pHa	7.37	7.25	7.39	7.38	7.44	7.41	7.38	7.38	7.38	7.29	
PaCO₂ (mmHg)	39	48	41	40	38	41	53	51	47	63	
PaO₂ (mmHg)	150	105	116	106	94	103	77	80	117	166	
RI	1.4	1.9	2.9	2.8	2.5	2.9	5.3	5.9	3.7	1.7	
QS/QT (%)	23	22		31	28	33	31	36	43	34	
CO (L/Min)	8.5	8.6	8.0	10.5	8.5	9.1	8.7	7.4	10.0	11.5	

↑ Start CHFV-Cont   ↑ Stop CHFV   ↑ Start SILV

quate gas exchange was maintained as evidenced by an acceptable PaO₂ and PaCO₂ with a normal pH.

By 7/9/85 this process had progressively deteriorated (Fig. 19-59C) and there was now clinical evidence that the right lung was more involved than the left (Fig. 19-60). The need for an increased FiO₂ and difficulties in maintaining an acceptable PaCO₂ and pH (Table 19-9) led to the decision to initiate SILV using volume-controlled ventilation in each lung. To enhance CO₂ exchange, CHFV was added to the better (left) lung (Table 19-10) on 7/10/85. The need for this CHFV-L component was demonstrated by a brief cessation of CHFV to the left lung on 7/12/85, when PaCO₂ rose to 100 mmHg and PaO₂ fell to 65 mmHg. Reinstitution of CHFV-L returned arterial gases to acceptable values and enabled a slow reduction in

FiO₂ to 45 percent by 7/29/85 when SILV and CHFV-L were discontinued.

Over the next 15 days lung compliance (Fig. 19-59D) and gas exchange gradually improved (Table 19-10). The Q̇S/Q̇T fell to 26 percent as RI declined to 0.9, which suggested that the major component of the shunt was due to the high cardiac output (15.4 L/min) associated with the hyperdynamic state. The return of the static total compliance curve toward more normal relations allowed ventilation at lower peak and mean pressures. Also, as FiO₂ was reduced to 0.40 there was good maintenance of PaO₂ at 112 mmHg and PaCO₂ at 42 mmHg with a pH of 7.43 on SIMV plus pressure support. However, even though the PEEP was now reduced to 5 cmH₂O, the flattened shape of the compliance curve of 8/14/85 compared to that of 6/10/85 suggests that a considerable fibrosis

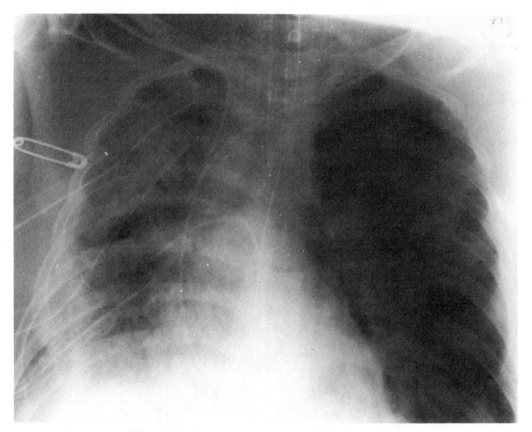

FIG. 19-60 Chest radiograph of patient BK:186 on 7/7/85.

TABLE 19-10. Response to SILV Plus CHFV to Left Lung (CHFV-L)

Date	7/10		7/12 (SILV)			7/16		7/23		7/29	8/14
Mode	VC-R	CHFV-L	VC	VC-R	CHFV-L	VC-R	CHFV-L	VC-R	CHFV-L	VC	SIMV + PS
Rate (br/min)	40			26			26		26	20	18
FiO_2	0.70		0.65		0.60		0.50		0.50	0.45	0.40
PEEP (cmH_2O)	23	21	8	8	12	14	19	12	20	18	5
VtI-CMV (L)	0.213	0.237		0.246	0.250	0.264	0.247	0.260	0.259	0.676	0.726
VtI-HFV (L)		0.245			0.871		0.692		0.641		
VtE (L)	0.214	0.482		0.213	1.121	0.207	0.939	0.179	0.900	0.719	0.715
Pk Press (cmH_2O)	79.9	119.2		84.8	99.9	78.1	97.1	75.0	79.9	80.0	51.1
Mn Press (cmH_2O)	34.3	32.6		21.8	24.0	17.8	25.6	21.0	21.2	26.7	19.3
Compliance (L/cmH_2O)	0.004	0.006				0.004	0.008	0.004	0.010	0.014	0.020
pHa	7.34		7.15		7.40		7.40		7.36	7.40	7.43
$PaCO_2$ (mmHg)	52		100		47		47		49	52	42
PaO_2 (mmHg)	98		65		82		101		119	130	112
RI	3.1		4.2		3.2		2.0		1.4	0.8	0.9
QS/QT (%)	38				31		35		28		26
CO (L/min)	12.4				11.6		11.5		13.1		15.4
	Start CHFV-E,L	Off CHFV		Start CHFV-Cont,L					7/27 Off SILV/CHFV		

component had developed as the late result of the ARDS process, even though bronchiolar–alveolar patency and gas exchange parameters had improved.

The use of prolonged SILV therapy is not without the risk of complications. Late in this patient's course, as he was recovering from his other injuries, it was noted that his chest expansion appeared asymmetrical. Tomography of the left mainstem bronchus (Fig. 19-61) and bronchoscopy demonstrated a localized stricture due to granulation tissue, undoubtedly a consequence of long intubation of the left mainstem bronchus and the high cuff pressures used for left lung ventilation. This required repeated bronchial dilatation with good results and a normal blood gas reading was obtained and

maintained by the time the patient was discharged on 12/12/85.

The sequence of static compliance and gas exchange relations under the different ARDS disease stages and ventilatory support programs shown by the cases demonstrated in this chapter makes two points. The first is that quantification of lung compliance and gas exchange abnormalities permits rational decisions to be made regarding application of the various modes of ventilatory support. It also allows the tailoring of each mode to suit the nature of the respiratory insufficiency pattern. The second point is that ARDS is frequently a time-limited process, if sepsis can be controlled. Recovery from ARDS is possible if ventilatory support can be maintained at a level

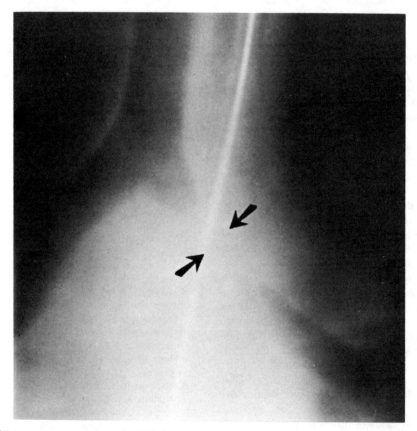

FIG. 19-61 Tomogram of patient BK:186 demonstrating localized stricture of the left mainstem bronchus (arrows).

sufficient to permit adequate gas exchange to occur during the healing process, so that the patient does not suffer irreversible hypoxemic injury.[107,109,214] These two factors provide justification for the use of sophisticated measurement techniques to quantify lung function and for the aggressive use of ventilatory support measures to match the abnormalities revealed by this analysis.

Indeed our most recent clinical experience supports this conclusion.[66] From June, 1984, to July, 1985, the MIEMSS Clinical Center admitted 2,104 patients of whom 1,768 had acute traumatic injuries. Of these trauma victims with a distribution of injuries and ISS scores similar to that shown in Chapter 1, 337 patients (19 percent) were considered to be at serious risk for ARDS by virtue of requiring more than 36 hours of ventilatory support, having abnormal chest radiographic findings, and at least one of the following abnormal physiologic measures: PEEP > 10 cmH$_2$O, FiO$_2$ > 0.5, PaO$_2$/FiO$_2$ < 300, or $\dot{Q}S/\dot{Q}T$ > 15 percent. Within the at-risk group there were 115 trauma patients (34 percent) who had at least one set of observations in which all four of the above criteria were met and who were thought to have had clinical ARDS. This group (6.5 percent of all trauma admissions) represents a similar incidence of ARDS to that reported by Fowler[63] in his studies. However, the overall mortality from all causes for the MIEMSS posttraumatic ARDS patients, treated by the methods outlined in this chapter, was only 39.1 percent compared to the mean mortality rate of 64.8 percent for ARDS reported by Fowler,[63] or to similarly high death rates noted by others.[6,7,16,89,162,206] These data are not offered as any sort of statistical comparison, since the groups may not be comparable for a variety of reasons, but they do point out that aggressive physiologic management of patients with severe posttraumatic and septic ARDS can produce good results in terms of patient outcomes. This is especially important since alternative measures of gas exchange support by partial extracorporal mechanical circulation (ECMO) have not proven effacious in adults with ARDS,[213] although they have been shown to be of great value in infant respiratory distress due to hyaline membrane disease, or meconium aspiration. Perhaps the future will hold a completely satisfactory technique for adult ECMO, but at present well-planned, carefully monitored, and physiologically adjusted ventilatory support remains the best method of treating this difficult disease process.

REFERENCES

1. Abrams JS, Deane RS, Davis JH: Adverse effects of salt and water retention on pulmonary function in patients with multiple trauma. J Trauma 13: 788, 1973
2. Adams T, Traber DL: The effects of a prostaglandin synthesis inhibitor, ibuprofen, on the cardiopulmonary response to endotoxin in sheep. Circ Shock 9: 481, 1982
3. Al-Saady N, Bennett ED: Decelerating inspiratory flow waveform improves lung mechanics and gas exchange in patients on intermittent positive-pressure ventilation. Intensive Care Med 11: 68, 1985
4. Anderson FL, Jubiz W, Tsagaris J, Kiuda H: Endotoxin induced prostaglandin E and F release in dogs. Am J Physiol 228(2): 410, 1979
5. Anthonisen NR, Milic-Emili J: Distribution of pulmonary perfusion in erect man. J Appl Physiol 21: 760, 1966
6. Ashbaugh DG, Bigelow DB, Petty TL, Levine BE: Acute respiratory distress in adults. Lancet 2: 319, 1967
7. Ashbaugh DG, Petty TL, Bigelow DB, Harris TM: Continuous positive pressure breathing (CPPB) in adult respiratory distress syndrome. J Thorac Cardiovasc Surg 57: 31, 1969
8. Bachofen M, Weibel ER: Structural alterations of lung parenchyma in the adult respiratory distress syndrome. Clin Chest Med 3: 35, 1982
9. Baehrendtz S: Differential ventilation and selective positive end-expiratory pressure. Opusc J Med Suppl 61, 1983
10. Baehrendtz S, Bindslev L, Hedenstierna G, Santesson J: Selective PEEP in acute bilateral lung disease: effect on patients in the lateral posture. Acta Anaesth Scand 27: 311, 1983
11. Baehrendtz S, Hedenstierna G: Differential ventilation and selective positive end-expiratory pressure: effects on patients with acute bilateral lung disease. Anesthesiology 61: 511, 1984
12. Baehrendtz S, Santesson J, Bindslev L et al: Differential ventilation in acute bilateral lung dis-

ease: influence on gas exchange and central hemodynamics. Acta Anaesth Scand 27: 270, 1983

13. Ball WC, Stewart PB, Newsham LGS et al: Regional pulmonary function studied with Xenon. J Clin Invest 41: 519, 1962

14. Banister J, Torrance RW: The effects of tracheal pressure upon flow:pressure relations in the vascular bed of isolated lungs. Q J Exp Physiol 45: 352, 1960

15. Barach AL, Marin J, Eckman M: Positive pressure respiration and its application to the treatment of acute pulmonary edema. Arch Intern Med 12: 754, 1938

16. Bauman WR, Jung RC, Koss M et al: Incidence and mortality of adult respiratory distress syndrome: a prospective analysis from a large metropolitan hospital. Crit Care Med 14: 1, 1986

17. Begley CJ, Ogletree ML, Meyrick BO: Modification of pulmonary responses to endotoxemia in awake sheep by steroidal and nonsteroidal antiinflammatory agents. Am Rev Respir Dis 130: 1140, 1984

18. Berggren SM: The oxygen deficit of arterial blood caused by nonventilating parts of the lung. Acta Physiol Scand Suppl II, 1942

19. Blaisdell FW: Pathophysiology of the respiratory distress syndrome. Arch Surg 108: 44, 1974

20. Bone RC: Diagnosis of causes for acute respiratory distress by pressure-volume curves. Chest 70: 740, 1976

21. Borg U, Eriksson I, Sjostrand U: High frequency positive pressure ventilation (HFPPV): a review based upon its use during bronchoscopy and for laryngoscopy and microlaryngeal surgery under general anesthesia. Anesth Analg 59: 594, 1980

22. Borg U, Eriksson I, Sjostrand U, Wattwil M: Experimental studies of continuous positive pressure ventilation and high frequency positive pressure ventilation. Resuscitation 9: 1, 1981

23. Boros SJ: Variations in inspiratory:expiratory ratio and airway pressure wave form during mechanical ventilation: the significance of mean airway pressure. J Pediatr 94: 114, 1979

24. Borst HG, McGregor M, Whittenberger JL: Influence of pulmonary arterial and left atrial pressures on pulmonary vascular resistance. Circ Res 4: 393, 1956

25. Brigham KL: Mechanisms of lung injury. Clin Chest Med 3: 9, 1982

26. Brigham KL, Kariman K, Harris TR et al: Correlation of oxygenation with vascular permeability-surface area but not with lung water in humans with acute respiratory failure and pulmonary edema. J Clin Invest 72: 339, 1983

27. Brigham KL, Snell J, Marshall S et al: Indicator dilution lung water and vascular permeability in humans: effects of pulmonary vascular pressure. Circ Res 44: 523, 1979

28. Brigham KL, Woolverton WC, Staub NC: Increased pulmonary vascular permeability after pseudomonas aeruginosa bacteremia in unanesthetized sheep. Fed Proc 32: 440, 1973

29. Buchman SR, Sugerman HJ, Tatum JL et al: Failure of methylprednisolone, ibuprofen, or prostacyclin to reduce HCL-induced pulmonary albumin leak in dogs. Surgery 96: 163, 1984

30. Carlon GC, Groeger JS: High frequency jet ventilation compared to volume-cycled ventilation: a prospective randomized evaluation. In Scheck PAE, Sjostrand UH, Smith RB (eds): Perspectives in High Frequency Ventilation. Martinus Nijhoff, The Hague, 1983

31. Carlon GC, Kahn R, Howland WS et al: Acute life-threatening ventilation-perfusion inequality: an indication for independent lung ventilation. Crit Care Med 6: 380, 1978

32. Carlon GC, Ray C, Jr., Klain M, McCormack PM: High frequency positive-pressure ventilation in management of a patient with bronchopleural fistula. Anesthesiology 52: 160, 1980

33. Casey L, Fletcher JR, Zmudka MI, Ramwell PW: Prevention of endotoxin-induced pulmonary hypertension in primates by the use of a selective thromboxane synthetase inhibitor, IKY 1581. J Pharmacol Exp Ther 222: 441, 1982

34. Chinard F, Enns T, Nolan M: Pulmonary extravascular water volumes from transit time and slope data. J Appl Physiol 17: 179, 1962

35. Ciszek TA, Modanlou HD, Owings D, Nelson P: Mean airway pressure-significance during mechanical ventilation in neonates. J Pediatr 99: 121, 1981

36. Clowes GHA, Jr., Hirsch E, Williams L et al: Septic lung and shock lung in man. Ann Surg 181: 681, 1975

37. Clowes GHA, Jr., Zuschneid W, Dragacevic S et al: The nonspecific pulmonary inflammatory reactions leading to respiratory failure after shock, gangrene and sepsis. J Trauma 8: 899, 1968

38. Comroe JH, Van Longer B, Strand RC et al: Reflex and direct cardiopulmonary effects of 5-OH tryptamine (serotonin). Am J Physiol 173: 379, 1953

39. Cook CP, Mead J, Schreiner GL et al: Pulmonary mechanics during induced pulmonary edema in anesthetized dogs. J Appl Physiol 14: 177, 1959

40. Danek SJ, Lynch JP, Weg JS, Dantzker DR: The dependence of oxygen uptake on oxygen delivery in the adult respiratory distress syndrome. Am Rev Respir Dis 122: 387, 1980

41. Dantzker DR: Gas exchange in the adult respira-

tory distress syndrome. Clin Chest Med 3: 57, 1982

42. Dantzker DR: Mechanisms of hypoxemia and hypercapnia. In Bone RC (ed): Critical Care: A Comprehensive Approach. American College of Chest Physicians, Park Ridge, Ill, 1984

43. Dantzker DR, Brook CJ, Dehart P et al: Ventilation-perfusion distributions in the adult respiratory distress syndrome. Am Rev Respir Dis 120: 1039, 1979

44. Dantzker DR, Lynch JP, Weg JG: Depression of cardiac output is a mechanism of shunt reduction in the therapy of acute respiratory failure. Chest 77: 636, 1980

45. Dauber IM, Weil JV: Noninvasive radioisotopic assessment of pulmonary vascular protein leak. Clin Chest Med 6: 427, 1985

46. Demling RH: The pathogenesis of respiratory failure after trauma and sepsis. Surg Clin North Am 60: 1373, 1981

47. Demling RH, Smith M, Gunther R et al: Pulmonary injury and prostaglandin production during endotoxemia in conscious sheep. Am J Physiol H348-H353, 1981

48. Demling RH, Worg C, Jim LS et al: Early lung dysfunction after major burns: role of edema and vasoactive mediators. J Trauma 25: 959, 1985

49. Douglas ME, Downs JB, Dannemiller FJ et al: Change in pulmonary venous admixture with varying inspired oxygen. Anesth Analg 55: 688, 1976

50. Drazen JM, Austen KF, Lewis RA et al: Comparative airway and vascular activities of leukotrienes C-1 and D in-vivo and in-vitro. Proc Natl Acad Sci 77: 4354, 1980

51. Edelman NH, Gorfinkel HJ, Lluch S et al: Experimental cardiogenic shock: pulmonary performance after acute myocardial infarction. Am J Physiol 219: 1723, 1970

52. El-Baz N, El-Ganzouri A, Gottschalk W, Jensik R: One-lung high frequency pressure ventilation for sleeve pneumonectomy: an alternative technique. Anesth Analg 60: 683, 1981

53. El-Baz N, El-Ganzouri A, Invahovich A: Combined high frequency ventilation for treatment of severe respiratory failure. In Scheck PAE, Sjostrand UH, Smith RB (eds): Perspectives in High Frequency Ventilation. Martinus Nijhoff, The Hague, 1983

54. Epstein SE, Beiser GD, Stampfer M et al: Characterization of the circulatory response to maximal upright exercise in normal subjects and in patients with heart disease. Circulation 25: 1049, 1967

55. Eriksson I: The role of conducting airways in gas exchange during high frequency ventila-

tion—a clinical and theoretical analysis. Anesth Analg 61: 483, 1982

56. Farrell EJ, Eberhart R, Siegel JH: Accuracy of O_2 and CO_2 blood content computations based on a computer model. IBM, Thomas J. Watson Research Center RC4449, 1973

57. Farrell EJ, Siegel JH: Investigation of cardiorespiratory abnormalities through computer simulation. Computers Biomed Res 5: 161, 1973

58. Farrell EJ, Siegel JH: Cardiorespiratory simulation for the evaluation of recovery following coronary artery bypass surgery. Computers Biol Med 11(3): 105, 1981

59. Ferrer MI, Enson Y, Harvey RM: The hydrogen ion and pulmonary vasomotricity. Am Heart J 78: 692, 1969

60. Feuerstein N, Ramwell PW: In vivo and in vitro effects of endotoxin on prostaglandin release from rat lung. Br J Pharmacol 73: 511, 1981

61. Fletcher JR, Ramwell PW, Harris RH: Thomboxane, prostacyclin and hemodynamic events in primate endotoxin shock. Adv Shock Res 5: 143, 1981

62. Flick MR, Perel A, Staub NC: Leukocytes are required for increased lung microvascular permeability after microembolization in sheep. Circ Res 48: 344, 1981

63. Fowler AA, Hamman RF, Good JT et al: Adult respiratory distress syndrome: risk with common predispositions. Ann Intern Med 98: 593, 1983

64. Gallagher TJ, Banner MJ: Mean airway pressure as a determinant of oxygenation. Crit Care Med 8: 244, 1980

65. Geiger K: Differential lung ventilation. Int Anesthesiol Clin 21: 83, 1983

66. Gens D, Siegel JH: Incidence predisposing factors and prognosis of ARDS after major trauma. J Trauma, September, 1986 (abst.)

67. Gerst PH, Rottenborg C, Holaday DA: The effects of hemorrhage on the pulmonary circulation and respiratory gas exchange. J Clin Invest 38: 524, 1958

68. Glaister DH, Schroter RC, Sudlow MF, Milic-Emili J: Transpulmonary pressure gradient and ventilation in excised lungs. Respir Physiol 17: 365, 1973

69. Glauser FL, Dingledein G, Rhodes R et al: Minimal increases in pulmonary wedge pressure associated with improved PaO_2 in dogs. Respiration 32: 415, 1975

70. Glazier JB, Hughes JMB, Maloney JE, and West JB: Measurement of capillary dimensions and blood volume in rapidly frozen lungs. J Appl Physiol 26: 65, 1969

71. Goldfarb MA, Ciurej TF, McAslan TC et al:

Tracking respiratory therapy in the trauma patient. Am J Surg 129: 255, 1978

72. Gregory GA, Kitterman JA, Phibbs RH et al: Treatment of the idiopathic respiratory distress syndrome with continuous positive airway pressure. N Engl J Med 284: 1333, 1971

73. Gump FE, Mashima Y, Ferenczy A, Kinney JM: Pre- and post mortem studies of lung fluids and electrolytes. J Trauma 11: 474, 1971

74. Gump FE, Mashima Y, Jorgensen S: Simultaneous use of three indicators to evaluate pulmonary capillary damage in man. Surgery 70: 262, 1971

75. Guyton AC, Lindsey AW: Effect of elevated left atrial pressure and decreased plasma protein concentration on the development of pulmonary edema. Circ Res 7: 649, 1959

76. Hales CA, Sonne L, Peterson M et al: Role of thromboxane and prostacyclin in pulmonary vasomotor changes after endotoxin in dogs. J Clin Invest 68: 497, 1981

77. Harlan JM, Harken LA: Hemostasis, thrombosis and thromboembolic disorders: the role of arachidonic acid metabolites and metabolites in platelet-vessel wall interactions. Med Clin North Am 65: 855, 1981

78. Hechtman HB, Huval WV, Lelcuk S et al: Platelet serotonin mediates respiratory failure after aspiration. IXth Annual International Congress for Thrombosis and Haemostasis. Stockholm, Sweden July 1983. Thromb Haemost p. 67

79. Hechtman HB, Valeri CR, Shepro D: Role of humoral mediators in adult respiratory distress syndrome. Chest 86: 623, 1984

80. Hechtman HB, Weisel RD, Vito L et al: The independence of pulmonary shunting and pulmonary edema. Surgery 74: 300, 1973

81. Hedenstierna G, White FC, Mazzone R, Wagner PD: Redistribution of pulmonary blood flow in the dog with PEEP ventilation. J Appl Physiol 46: 278, 1979

82. Hedley-Whyte J, Pontoppidan H, Jocelin Morris M: The response of patients with respiratory failure and cardiopulmonary disease to different levels of constant volume ventilation. J Clin Invest 45: 1543, 1966

83. Hegi T, Hiatt IM: Respiratory index: a simple evaluation of severity of idiopathic respiratory distress syndrome. Crit Care Med 7: 500, 1979

84. Helmholz HF, Jr.: Editorial: Static total compliance and "best PEEP." Respir Care 26: 637, 1981

85. Higgs BE: Factors influencing pulmonary gas exchange during the acute stages of myocardial infarction. Clin Sci 35: 115, 1968

86. Hillman KM, Barber JD: Asynchronous independent lung ventilation (AILV). Crit Care Med 8: 390, 1980

87. Hoff BH, Robotham JL, Smith RB, Cherry D, Bunegin L: Effects of high frequency ventilation (300–2400/min) on cardiovascular function and gas exchange in dogs. Anesth Analg 60: 256, 1981

88. Howell JBL, Permutt S, Proctor DE, Riley RL: Effect of inflation of the lung on different parts of the pulmonary vascular bed. J Appl Physiol 16: 71, 1961

89. Hudson LD: Courses of the adult respiratory distress syndrome—clinical recognition. Clin Chest Med 3: 195, 1982

90. Huttenmeier PC, Watkins W, Peterson MB, Zapol WM: Acute pulmonary hypertension and lung thromboxane release after endotoxin infusion in normal and leukopenic sheep. Circ Res 50(5): 688, 1982

91. Huval WV, Lelcuk S, Hechtman HB, Demling RH: Serotonin content of lung lymph and plasma and endotoxemia in sheep. Fed Proc 42: 490, 1983

92. Huval WV, Mathieson MM, Stemp LI et al: Therapeutic benefits of 5-hydroxytrptamine inhibition following pulmonary embolism. Ann Surg 197: 220, 1983

93. Iliff LD, Greene RE, Hughes JMB: Effects of interstitial edema on distribution of ventilation and perfusion in isolated lung. J Appl Physiol 33: 462, 1972

94. Jonson B, Nordstrom L, Olsson SG, Akerback D: Monitoring of ventilation and lung mechanics during automatic ventilation. A new device. Bull Eur Physiopathol Respir 11: 729, 1975

95. Katz S, Aberman A, Frand V, Stern I: Heroin pulmonary edema: evidence for increased pulmonary capillary permeability. Am Rev Respir Dis 106: 472, 1972

96. Kazemi H, Parsons EF, Valenca LM et al: Distribution of pulmonary blood flow after myocardial ischemia and infarction. Circulation 41: 1025, 1970

97. Kelman GR: Digital computer subroutine for conversion of oxygen tension into saturation. J Appl Physiol 21: 1375, 1966

98. Kelman GR: Digital computer procedure for the conversion of PCO_2 into blood CO_2 content. Respir Physiol 3: 111, 1967

99. Kinney JM, Askanazi J, Gump FE et al: Use of the ventilatory equivalent to separate hypermetabolism from increased dead space ventilation in the injured or septic patient. J Trauma 20: 111, 1980

100. Kirby RR, Smith RA, Desautels DA (eds): Mechanical Ventilation. Churchill Livingstone, New York, 1985

101. Kistler GS, Caldwell PRB, Weibel ER: Development of fine structural damage to alveolar and

capillary lining cells in oxygen poisoned rat lungs. J Cell Biol 32: 605, 1967

102. Klain M, Smith RB: High frequency percutaneous transtracheal jet ventilation. Crit Care Med 5: 280, 1977

103. Krausz MM, Perel A, Eimerl D et al: Cardiopulmonary effects of volume loading in patients in septic shock. Ann Surg 185: 429, 1977

104. Krausz MM, Utsunomiya T, Dunham B et al: Inhibition of permeability edema with imidazole. Surgery 92: 299, 1982

105. Krausz MM, Utsunomiya T, Feuerstein G et al: Prostacyclin (PGI$_2$) reversal of lethal endotoxemia in dogs. J Clin Invest 67: 1118, 1981

106. Kumar A, Falke KJ, Geffin B et al: Continuous positive pressure ventilation in acute respiratory failure. N Engl J Med 24: 1430, 1970

107. Lakshminarayan S, Stanford RE, Petty TL: Prognosis after recovery from adult respiratory distress syndrome. Am Rev Respir Dis 113: 7, 1976

108. Lambertsen CJ, Bance PI, Drabkin DL et al: Relationship of oxygen tension to hemoglobin oxygen saturation in the arterial blood of normal man. J Appl Physiol 4: 873, 1952

109. Lamy M, Fallat RJ, Koeniger E et al: Pathologic features and mechanisms of hypoxemia in adult respiratory distress syndrome. Am Rev Respir Dis 114: 267, 1976

110. Landis EM: The effect of the lack of oxygen on the permeability of the capillary wall to fluid and to the plasma proteins. Am J Physiol 83: 528, 1928

111. Landis EM, Pappenheimer JR: Exchange of substances through the capillary walls. p. 961. In Hamilton WF (ed): Handbook of Physiology (Section 2) Circulation, vol. 2. American Physiological Society, Washington, D.C., 1963

112. Levine OR, Mellins RB, Senior RM, Fishman AP: The application of Starling's law of capillary exchange to the lungs. J Clin Invest 46: 934, 1967

113. Lewis FR, Elings VB, Sturm JA: Bedside measurement of lung water. J Surg Res 27: 250, 1979

114. Light RB, Mink SN, Wood LDH: The effect of unilateral PEEP on gas exchange and pulmonary perfusion in canine lobor pneumonia. Anesthesiology 55: 251, 1981

115. Light RB, Mink SN, Wood LDH: Pathophysiology of gas exchange and pulmonary perfusion in pneumococcal lobar pneumonia in dogs. J Appl Physiol 50: 524, 1981

116. Lindquist O, Rammer L, Saldeen T: Pulmonary insufficiency, microembolism and fibrinolysis inhibition in post traumatic autopsy material. Acta Chir Scand 138: 545, 1972

117. Malina JR, Nordstrom SG, Sjostrand UH, Wattwil LM: Clinical evaluation of high frequency positive pressure ventilation (HFPPV) in patients scheduled for open chest surgery. Anesth Analg 60: 324, 1981

118. Markello P, Winter P, Olszowka A: Assessment of ventilation–perfusion inequalities by arterial-venous nitrogen differences in intensive care patients. Anesthesiology 37: 4, 1972

119. Mason GR, Effros RM, Uszler JM, Mena I: Small solute clearance from the lungs of patients with cardiogenic and non cardiogenic pulmonary edema. Chest 88: 327, 1985

120. Matamis D, Lemaire F, Harf A et all: Total respiratory pressure–volume curves in the adult respiratory distress syndrome. Chest 86: 58, 1984

121. McConn R, DelGuercio LRM: Respiratory function of the blood in the acutely ill patient and the effect of steroids. Ann Surg 174: 436, 1971

122. McGuire WW, Spragg RG, Cohen AB, Cochrane CG: Studies in the pathogenesis of the adult respiratory distress syndrome. J Clin Invest 69: 543, 1982

123. McNeill RS, Rankin J, Forster RE: The diffusing capacity of the pulmonary membrane and the pulmonary capillary blood volumes in cardiopulmonary disease. Clin Sci 17: 465, 1958

124. Mellemgard K: Alveolar-arterial oxygen differences: size and components in normal man. Acta Physiol Scand 67: 10, 1966

125. Milic-Emili J, Henderson JAM, Dolovich MB et al: Regional distribution of inspired gas in the lung. J Appl Physiol 21: 749, 1966

126. Miller LD, Oski FA, Diaco JF, Sugerman HJ: The affinity of hemoglobin for oxygen: its control and in vivo significance. Surgery 68: 187, 1970

127. Miner ME, Gonzales MC: Variations in pulmonary gas exchange due to changes in pulmonary artery pressure and flow. J Surg Res 18: 431, 1975

128. Mizus I, Summer W, Farrukh I et al: Isoproterenol or aminophylline attenuate pulmonary edema after acid lung injury. Am Rev Respir Dis 131: 256, 1985

129. Molloy DW, Lee KY, Jones D et al: Effects of noradrenaline and isoproterenol on acute cardiopulmonary function in a canine model of acute pulmonary hypertension. Chest 88: 432, 1985

130. Monaco V, Burdge R, Newell J et al: Pulmonary venous admixture in injured patients. J Trauma 12: 15, 1972

131. Moore FD, Lyons JH, Pierce EC et al: Post-Traumatic Pulmonary Insufficiency. WB Saunders, Philadelphia, 1969

132. Nachman RL, Webster B, Feries B: Characterization of human platelet vascular permeability-enhancing activity. J Clin Invest 51: 549, 1972

133. Nash G, Blennerhassett JB, Pontoppidan H: Pulmonary lesions associated with oxygen therapy

and artificial ventilation. N Engl J Med 276: 368, 1967

134. Nicholson DP: Glucocorticoids in the treatment of shock and the adult respiratory distress syndrome. Clin Chest Med 3:121, 1982

135. Nunn JF: Applied Respiratory Physiology. Butterworths, London, 1977

136. Oppenheimer L, Craven KD, Forkert L, Woods LDH: Pathophysiology of pulmonary contusion in dogs. J Appl Physiol 47: 718, 1979

137. Otis AB, McKerrow CB, Bartlett RA et al: Mechanical factors in distribution of pulmonary ventilation. J Appl Physiol 8: 427, 1956

138. Pepe PE, Hudson LD, Carrico CJ: Early application of positive end-expiratory pressure in patients at risk for the adult respiratory distress syndrome. N Engl J Med 311: 281, 1984

139. Pepe PE, Marini JJ: Occult positive end-expiratory pressure in mechanically ventilated patients with airflow obstruction: the auto-PEEP effect. Am Rev Respir Dis 126: 166, 1982

140. Permutt S, Bromberger-Barnes B, Bane HN: Alveolar pressure, pulmonary venous pressure and the vascular waterfall. Med Thorac 19: 239, 1961

141. Permutt S, Howell JBL, Proctor DE, Riley RL: Effect of lung inflation on static pressure volume characteristics of pulmonary vessels. J Appl Physiol 16: 64, 1961

142. Pesenti A, Marcolin R, Prato P et al: Mean airway pressure vs. positive end-expiratory pressure during mechanical ventilation. Crit Care Med 13: 34, 1985

143. Peters RM, Hilberman M: Respiratory insufficiency: diagnosis and control of therapy. Surgery 70: 280, 1971

144. Peters RM, Hilberman M, Hogan JS et al: Objective indications for respirator therapy in post-trauma and postoperative patients. Am J Surg 124: 262, 1972

145. Petty TL, Reiss OK, Paul GW et al: Characteristics of pulmonary surfactant in adult respiratory distress syndrome associated with trauma and shock. Am Rev Respir Dis 115: 531, 1977

146. Petty TL, Silvers GW, Paul GW, Stanford RE: Abnormalities in lung elastic properties and surfactant function in adult respiratory distress syndrome. Chest 75: 571, 1979

147. Piper PJ, Samhoun MN: Stimulation of arachidonic acid metabolism and generation of thromboxane A_2 by leukotriene B_4, C_4 and D_4 in guinea pig lung in-vitro. Br J Pharmacol 77: 267, 1982

148. Pontoppidan H, Hedley-Whyte J, Bendixen HH, Laver MD: Ventilation and oxygen requirements during prolonged artificial ventilation in patients with respiratory failure. N Engl J Med 273: 401, 1965

149. Powers SR, Burdge R, Leather R, Monaco V: Studies of pulmonary insufficiency in nonthoracic trauma. J Trauma 12: 1, 1972

150. Powers SR, Mannal R, Neclerio M et al: Physiologic consequences of positive end-expiratory pressure (PEEP) ventilation. Ann Surg 178: 265, 1973

151. Powner DJ, Eross B, Grenvik A: Differential lung ventilation with PEEP in the treatment of unilateral pneumonia. Crit Care Med 5: 170, 1977

152. Reines HD, Halushka PV, Olanoff LS, Hunt PS: Dazoxiben in human sepsis and adult respiratory distress syndrome. Clin Pharm Ther 37(4): 391, 1985

153. Riley RL, Permutt S, Said S et al: Effect of posture on pulmonary dead space in man. J Appl Physiol 14: 339, 1959

154. Rinaldo JE, Rogers RM: Adult-respiratory distress syndrome: Changing concepts of lung injury and repair. N Engl J Med 306: 300, 1982

155. Rossi A, Gottfried SB, Zocchi L: Measurements of static compliance of the total respiratory system in patients with acute respiratory failure during mechanical ventilation. The effect of intrinsic positive end-expiratory pressure. Am Rev Respir Dis 131: 672, 1985

156. Sachdeva SP: Treatment of post-operative pulmonary atelectases by active inflation of the atelectatic lobe(s) through an endobronchial tube. Acta Anaesth Scand 19: 65, 1974

157. Saunders KB: Physiological dead space in left ventricular failure. Clin Sci 31: 145, 1966

158. Schloerb PR, Hunt PT, Plummer JA, Cage GK: Pulmonary edema after replacement of blood loss by electrolyte solutions. Surg Gynecol Obstet 135: 893, 1972

159. Sganga G, Siegel JH, Coleman B et al: The physiologic meaning of the respiratory index in various types of critical illness. Circ Shock 17: 179, 1985

160. Shapiro BA, Cane RD, Harrison RA: Positive end-expiratory pressure therapy in adults with special reference to acute lung injury: a review of the literature and suggested clinical correlations. Crit Care Med 12: 127, 1984

161. Shapiro BA, Cane RD, Harrison RA, Steiner MC: Changes in intrapulmonary shunting with administration of 100 percent oxygen. Chest 77: 138, 1980

162. Sibbald WJ, Driedger AA, Finley RJ et al: High-dose corticosteroids in the treatment of pulmonary microvascular injury. Ann NY Acad Sci 384: 496, 1982

163. Siegel JH, Cerra FB, Coleman B et al: Physiologic

and metabolic correlations in human sepsis. Surgery 86: 163, 1979

164. Siegel JH, Farrell EJ: The management of the acute respiratory distress syndrome in the aged or high risk surgical patient. p. 457. In Siegel JH, Chodoff P (eds): The Aged and High Risk Surgical Patient. Grune & Stratton, New York, 1976

165. Siegel JH, Farrell EJ, Miller M et al: Cardiorespiratory interactions as determinants of survival and the need for respiratory support in human shock states. J Trauma 13: 602, 1973

166. Siegel JH, Giovannini I, Coleman B: Ventilation: perfusion maldistribution secondary to the hyperdynamic cardiovascular state as the major cause of increased pulmonary shunting in human sepsis. J Trauma 19: 432, 1979

167. Siegel JH, Giovannini I, Coleman B et al: Pathologic synergy modulation of the cardiovascular, respiratory and metabolic response to injury by cirrhosis and/or sepsis: a manifestation of a common metabolic defect? Arch Surg 117: 225, 1982

168. Siegel JH, Greenspan M, DelGuercio LRM: Abnormal vascular tone, defective oxygen transport and myocardial failure in human septic shock. Ann Surg 165: 504, 1967

169. Siegel JH, Stoklosa J, Borg U et al: Quantification of asymmetric lung pathophysiology as a guide to the use of simultaneous independent lung ventilation in post traumatic and septic ARDS. Ann Surg 202: 425, 1985

170. Siegel JH, Stoklosa J, Geisler FH et al: Computer-based evaluation of cardiopulmonary function for the optimization of ventilatory therapy in the adult respiratory distress syndrome. Int J Clin Monitor Comput 1: 107, 1984

171. Sjostrand U: Review of the physiological rationale for and development of high frequency positive pressure ventilation—HFPPV. Acta Anaesth. Scand (Suppl) 64: 7, 1977

172. Sjostrand U: Pneumatic systems facilitating treatment of respiratory insufficiency with alternative use of IPPV/PEEP, HFPPV/PEEP, and CPPB or CPAP. Acta Anaesth Scand (Suppl) 64: 123, 1977

173. Slutsky AS, Scharf SM, Brown R, Ingram RH: The effect of oleic acid-induced pulmonary edema on pulmonary and chest wall mechanics in dogs. Am Rev Respir Dis 121: 91, 1980

174. Smith G, Cheney FV, Jr., Winter PM: The effect of change in cardiac output on intrapulmonary shunting. Br J Anaesthesiol 46: 337, 1974

175. Smith M, Gunther R, Gee M, Demling R: Leukocytes, platelets and thromboxane A_2 in endotoxin induced lung injury. Surgery 99(1): 102, 1981

176. Smith RB, Lindholm CE, Klain M: Jet ventilation for fiberoptic bronchoscopy under general anesthesia. Acta Anaesth. Scand 20: 111, 1976

177. Snapper JR: Lung mechanics in pulmonary edema. Clin Chest Med 6: 393, 1985

178. Snapper JR, Hutchison AA, Ogletree ML et al: Effects of cyclooxygenase inhibitors on the alterations in lung mechanics caused by endotoxemia in unanesthesized sheep. J Clin Invest 72: 63, 1983

179. Spagnuolo PJ, Ellner JJ, Hassid A, Dunn MJ: Thromboxane A_2 mediates augmented polymorphonuclear leukocyte adhesiveness. J Clin Invest 66: 406, 1980

180. Stanley TH, Lunn JK, Wen-Shin L et al: Effects of left atrial pressure on pulmonary shunt and the dead space/tidal volume ratio. Anesthesiology 49: 128, 1978

181. Starling EH: On the absorption of fluids from the connective spaces. J Physiol (Lond) 19: 312, 1896

182. Staub N: Pulmonary edema. Physiol Rev 54: 678, 1974

183. Staub NC: State of the art review. Pathogenesis of pulmonary edema. Am Rev Respir Dis 109: 358, 1974

184. Staub NC, Nagano H, Pearce ML: Pulmonary edema in dogs, especially the sequence of fluid accumulation in the lungs. J Appl Physiol 22: 227, 1967

185. Stein M, Hirose T, Yasutake T, Khan MA: The effects of platelet amines on airway function. p. 283. In Bouhuys A (ed): Airway Dynamics; Physiology and Pharmacology. Charles C Thomas, Springfield, 1970

186. Stein M, Thomas DP: Role of platelets in the acute pulmonary response to endotoxin. J Appl Physiol 23: 47, 1967

187. Stokes C, Blevins S, Stoklosa JC et al: Prediction of arterial blood gas by transcutaneous O_2 and CO_2 in critically ill hyperdynamic trauma patients. Abstract submitted to the Society of Critical Care Medicine 1986

188. Sturgeon CL, Jr., Douglas ME, Downs JB et al: PEEP and CPAP: cardiopulmonary effects during spontaneous ventilation. Anesth Analg 56: 633, 1977

189. Sugerman HJ, Strash AM, Hirsch JI et al: Sensitivity of scintigraphy for detection of pulmonary capillary albumin leak in canine oleic acid ARDS. J Trauma 21: 520, 1981

190. Sugerman HJ, Strash AM, Hirsch JI et al: Scintigraphy and radiography in oleic acid pulmonary microvascular injury: effects of positive end-expiratory pressure (PEEP). J Trauma 22: 179, 1982

191. Suter PM, Fairley B, Isenberg MD: Optimum end-expiratory airway pressure in patients with

acute pulmonary failure. N Engl J Med 292: 284, 1975

192. Suter PM, Fairley HB, Isenberg MD: Effect of tidal volume and positive end-expiratory pressure on compliance during mechanical ventilation. Chest 73: 158, 1978

193. Thomas LJ, Jr., Roos A, Griffo ZJ: Relation between alveolar surface tension and pulmonary vascular resistance. J Appl Physiol 16: 457, 1961

194. Till GO, Johnson KJ, Kunbel R, Ward PA: Intravascular activation of complement and acute lung injury: dependency on neutrophils and toxic oxygen metabolites. J Clin Invest 69: 1126, 1982

195. Todd M, Toutant S, Shapiro H: The effect of high frequency positive pressure ventilation on intracranial pressure and brain movement in cats. Anesthesiology 54: 496, 1981

196. Tyler DC: Positive end-expiratory pressure: a review. Crit Care Med 11: 300, 1983

197. Tyson GS, McIntyre RW, Maier GW et al: The mechanical effects of high frequency ventilation on cardiac function in intact dogs. Crit Care Med 10: 212, 1982

198. Utsunomiya T, Krausz MM, Dunham B et al: Modification of the inflammatory response to aspiration with ibuprofen. Am J Physiol 243: H903, 1982

199. Utsunomiya T, Krausz MM, Shepro D, Hechtman HB: Treatment of aspiration pneumonia with ibuprofen and prostacyclin (PGI$_2$). Surgery 90: 170, 1981

200. Utsunomiya T, Krausz MM, Shepro D et al: Treatment of pulmonary embolism with prostacyclin. Surgery 88: 25, 1980

201. Versrchelen L, Rolly G, Kluyskens P, Vermeersch H: Anésthesie generale pour laryngoscopie et/ou bronchoscopie chez l' énfant. Anesth Analg Reanim 38: 463, 1981

202. Vito L, Dennis R, Weisel RD, Hechtman HB: Sepsis presenting as acute respiratory insufficiency. Surg Gynecol Obstet 138: 896, 1974

203. Warso MA, Lands WEM: Lipid peroxidation in relation to prostacyclin and thromboxane physiology and pathophysiology. Br Med Bulle 39: 219, 1983

204. Wattwil LM, Sjostrand UH, Borg UR: Comparative studies of IPPV and HFPPV with PEEP in critical care patients—a clinical evaluation. Crit Care Med 11: 30, 1983

205. Weibel ER: Lung cell biology. In Fishman AP, Fisher AB (eds): Handbook of Physiology: Respiration, vol. 4. American Physiological Society, Washington, 1984

206. Weisman IM, Rinaldo JE, Rogers RM, Sanders MH: Intermittent mandatory ventilation. Am Rev Respir Dis 127: 641, 1983

207. West JB: Regional differences in gas exchange in the lung of erect man. J Appl Physiol 17: 893, 1962

208. West JB, Dollery CT: Distribution of blood flow and the pressure-flow relations of the whole lung. J Appl Physiol 20: 175, 1965

209. West JB, Dollery CT, Matmark A: Distribution of blood flow in isolated lung: relation to vascular and alveolar pressures. J Appl Physiol 19: 713, 1964

210. Wilson EA, Hoff BH, Sjostrand UH et al: Conventional and high frequency ventilation in dogs with bronchopleural fistula. Crit Care Med 10: 232, 1982

211. Winn B, Harlan J, Nadir B et al: Thromboxane A$_2$ mediates lung vasoconstriction but not permeability after endotoxin. J Clin Invest 22: 911, 1983

212. Wynne JW: Aspiration pneumonitis. Clin Chest Med 3: 25, 1982

213. Zapol WM: Extracorporeal membrane oxygenation in severe acute respiratory failure. JAMA 242: 2193, 1979

214. Zapol WM, Trelstad RL, Coffey JW et al: Pulmonary fibrosis in severe acute respiratory failure. Am Rev Respir Dis 119: 547, 1979

SECTION VII

METABOLIC PROBLEMS

20

Acute Hypothermia, Local Cold Injury, and Acute Hyperthermia

Robert A. Margulies
Donald C. Arthur
Michael D. Burton

HYPOTHERMIA

Incidence

The application of cold to produce local analgesia and to reduce fever has been known since the dawn of history, and probably antedates the keeping of records. Though disorders of increased body temperature are more common, clinical disorders due to cold have always been present, and there has been confusion and disagreement as to appropriate therapies for these disorders.

Perhaps the most widely cited mass casualty associated with cold injuries is the destruction of the Grand Army of Napoleon in the retreat from Moscow in 1812. It has been stated that the history of scientific observation of cold injuries began then, with Baron Larrey and his observation of gangrene of frozen tis-

sues exposed to the heat of a fire. Warfare has always provided us with a plethora of hypothermic injuries; the tragedies of Washington's army at Valley Forge, the winter incidents of World War I in Europe, sailors and aviators exposed to cold water in World War II, and the heroism and heartache of U.S. Marines walking out of Chosin Reservoir in Korea. But combat is not the only source of hypothermic injury today. We are reminded of homeless people in our cities during the winter, the stories of campers and climbers in the mountains at almost any time of year, the presumed 20 percent or greater incidence of hypothermia in scuba diving fatalities,[31] and the incidence of hypothermia in the very young and the aged as energy conservation becomes an increasing focus of attention.[40]

An increased incidence of hypothermia is noted in older persons, but older age does not seem to be a determinant of survival in hypothermic victims. The Centers for Disease Control (CDC) reported in 1979 that 711 deaths

677

were attributed to cold in the United States,[34] though this is probably an underestimate. Persons aged 65 to 74 years accounted for 18 percent of these deaths, though they represented only 7 percent of the total U.S. population. The 75 years and older group accounted for 28 percent, though representing 4 percent of the population. There is further evidence that the elderly are now suffering a higher death rate due to hypothermia than in the recent past, and this trend is projected to continued. Individuals with an impaired perception of cold, decreased mobility, and/or inadequate nutrition, clothing, and heating systems represent a subgroup of the population including the poor, the elderly, and drug and/or alcohol abusers. Such individuals may develop chronic hypothermia from exposure to temperatures below 16° C over a prolonged period of time. This may occur indoors.[34]

Data published in *Morbidity Mortality Weekly Report* provide a different perspective.[33] Over a 9-year period, exposure-related hypothermia deaths (ERHD) per 100,000 person years were 1.91 for black males, 1.01 for white males, 0.17 for black females, and 0.12 for white females. In contradiction to the broader United States based study noted above, the highest age-specific death rate in this study was in the 50 to 54-year-old group: 3.0 deaths per 100,000 person years. These ERHD occurred in all months from October through April; 72 percent, however, occurred in December and January. Of those victims for whom the data were available, one third were undernourished, being described as less than the fifth percentile of weight for height. Of those in whom blood/alcohol levels were measured, 48 percent had levels greater than 0.15 g/dl, a level considered high enough to impair central thermoregulatory capacity. An additional 21 percent had lower levels of ethanol. A real danger is that intoxicated subjects may be taken to general hospitals or detoxification centers where their hypothermia may not be recognized. Thirty-seven percent were found either completely or partially undressed, and no victim was noted to have a hat. This phenomenon, paradoxical undressing,[29,53] has been previously described and has been noted in climbers, campers, and hunters. It is predicated on the hypothesis that as core temperature falls, there is a loss of vas-

cular control and vasoconstriction ceases. The resulting vasodilation is perceived as extraordinary warmth and the victim disrobes in an attempt to compensate.

Research in hypothermia has waxed and waned since the end of the 19th century and in the 1940s there were unsuccessful attempts to utilize the modality in the treatment of carcinoma and psychiatric disorders. In the 1950s, hypothermia again enjoyed a resurgence of interest as an adjunct in the surgical correction of intracardiac disease, but extracorporeal circulation proved to be a more technically and physiologically advantageous modality, except in the very small child. Further modifications were developed and, at present, hypothermia is used surgically in pediatric cardiac surgery, with metabolic inhibitors in adults, and for the preservation of organs for transplantation. Human research is fraught with difficulty, and is frequently terminated in the range of core temperatures of 35°C, before significant physiologic and pathophysiologic findings are demonstrable. Animal research in this arena, as in so many others, is of questionable value due to the significant differences in anatomy and physiology in all models. Nevertheless, much is known and should be used in the preparation of protocols for the treatment of victims of cold injury.

Pathophysiology

TEMPERATURE REGULATION

The body temperature of normal, healthy individuals remains nearly constant with a diurnal variation[8] of approximately 0.5 to 0.75°C. This results from the balance between metabolism that results in heat production and heat loss to the environment. Approximately 25 percent of the energy stored in food is used directly by the body, the remaining 75 percent results in heat production.[8] The determinant of the amount of heat produced is the metabolic rate. The basal metabolic rate (BMR) is the lowest normal metabolic rate of a given individual, and is specific for each person. It can be changed, however, by a number of factors.

The first variable is age. The BMR is highest in the young and decreases with age, but is relatively constant between the ages of about 18 and 50. The most dramatic effect on metabolic rate is that of exercise. Sustained exercise can increase the metabolic rate by perhaps five times.[21] Short bursts of maximum muscle activity will liberate as much as 10 times the usual amount of heat.[4,8,21] Shivering, which is a maximum muscle activity, will rapidly deplete available energy stores, and if this were the only heat-producing mechanism between normal thermal balance and hypothermia, exhaustion would rapidly occur and uncompensated heat loss would ensue.

Fortunately, the human organism has other methods of increasing heat production. Among these are hormonal effects. It is important to note that while the response to exercise is immediate, there is a lag between the stimulus and the secretion of a metabolically active hormone, and a further lag between the secretion and the eventual effect of that hormone on metabolic rate. Thyroid hormone is the most active metabolic hormone in the body; maximum stimulation of the thyroid can result in an increase in metabolic rate by up to five times the basal rate.[27,42,44,51] In contrast, loss of thyroid hormone effects would result in a decrease in the basal rate by only about 50 percent. Exposure to the cold can stimulate the sympathetic nervous system,[4,42] and this causes the release of other metabolically active hormones such as epinephrine, norepinephrine, and growth hormone. These can collectively double the basal metabolic rate.[4,21] This is small compared to the effect of thyroid hormone, but the effect on vasoconstriction by the sympathetic hormones is also of great importance.

MECHANISMS OF HEAT LOSS

It is usually noted that heat loss occurs by the mechanisms of radiation, conduction, convection, and evaporation; and by combinations thereof. The usual definitions of these all apply; however, it is helpful to understand the significance of combined effects in people. Thus, the conductive loss of body heat to the layer of air surrounding the body is very important, but it is made more important when that layer of air is moved away, a new layer of air replaces it, and the new cold layer must also be warmed. This is conduction/convection and we refer to this phenomenon as the wind chill.[9] For protection, it is just as important to provide a mechanism to prevent the convection as to provide an insulating layer.

Evaporation is a mechanism we readily appreciate in heat but which we tend to appreciate less well with regard to cold. Evaporation continues to occur and insensible loss of moisture and the associated cooling that occurs with this loss of moisture continues in the cold. In addition, the loss of moisture, and heat, associated with the humidification of inspired gases, such as in respiration, is very important. An individual exposed to a cold environment, even if properly dressed, loses a significant amount of moisture in normal respiration; this may result in the loss of a large amount of heat over a long enough period of time.[16]

Regulation of body temperature is controlled centrally in the preoptic anterior hypothalamus (POAH). This thermostat and its setting mediates the responses of the organism to the environment.[18] The balance of heat production/conservation versus heat loss involves vasoconstriction and is mediated primarily by hormonal effects, by shivering, which is mediated centrally, and by local spinal cord reflexes, which are involved in the abolition of sweating and piloerection. Most clinicians would agree that a measurement of rectal or other core temperature of approximately 35°C is consistent with hypothermia, and a temperature of 32°C is consistent with severe hypothermia. When core temperature decreases occur, the POAH thermostat is reset so that as the body generates more heat to return core temperature to normal, there is an overshoot and an increase in body core temperature beyond the basal norm.[21] In this way the body ensures adequate heat production and distribution.

CHANGES IN CLINICAL STATUS

Oxygen consumption decreases with decreasing core temperature. If 37°C is considered unity, then consumption at 28° is about 0.5 and at 22° is about 0.25 the usual rate.[6] With decreasing oxygen consumption, produc-

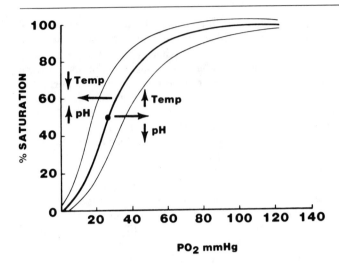

FIG. 20-1 Effects of temperature and pH on the oxyhemoglobin curve. (Redrawn from McConn R: The oxyhemoglobin dissociation curve in acute disease. Surg Clin North Am 55:627, 1975.)

tion of acid metabolites increases. Decreasing temperature also shifts the oxygen hemoglobin dissociation curve to the left, thus decreasing oxygen release to the tissues. A decreasing pH tends to shift the curve back to the right and compensation tends to occur.[32] (Fig. 20-1). In the central nervous system, decrements in arithmetic, logic, and recall functions are noted as core temperature begins to decrease and may be documented[5,25,38,49,50] before the temperature decreases to 35°C. Manual dexterity also begins to decrease and confusion and memory losses are found when the temperature is in the region of 32.5°C. Cold narcosis[38] is found beginning at approximately 29.5°C. Analgesia is noted at 32.5°C, and when the core temperature reaches 26.5°C obtundation and frank coma are usual.[38] Cerebral blood flow decreases with decreasing temperature,[43] but this change tends to be matched by decreasing metabolic requirements in the cold to 20°C. At this temperature, the brain receives a lower percentage of the cardiac output due to loss of vascular resistance.[55] Autopsy reports have indicated that clots are found in cortical regions and these may be associated with sludging due to dehydration as well as the vasospastic effects of calcium release, which is a general stress response.[54] Peripheral nerve conduction velocities decrease slowly, dropping to about half of normal at 24°C, then more rapidly to about 25 percent of normal at 21°C and may be essentially absent by 20°C.[2,12,38]

If the victim is suddenly exposed to cold water, there may be a marked and uncontrollable hyperventilation[20,30,44] to greater than 90 L/min. Abrupt exposure to dry cold leads to a lesser, but still notable, hyperventilation. In persistent exposure, decreasing carbon dioxide production secondary to decreased metabolism occurs with decreasing core temperature. Coupled with increased elimination of carbon dioxide due to hyperventilation, a decreasing respiratory drive yields a decreased respiratory frequency.[13,20,44] This contributes to a potentially profound metabolic acidosis as decreased oxygen is available for delivery,[52] and must be considered in therapy.

CIRCULATORY CHANGES

Circulatory parameters also change. Pulse rate drops with decreasing temperature and is approximately 50 percent of normal at 28°C. As the pulse rate drops, blood pressure may not be obtainable by palpation and auscultation; however, intra-arterial monitoring reveals pressures consistent with pulse rate.[47] Stroke volume remains constant[8,44] while cardiac output decreases; relative systole increases and coronary flow tends to decrease concomitantly. The arteriovenous (A-V) oxygen difference remains essentially constant at all levels of hypothermia, with oxygen utilization apparently matching oxygen delivery in the cardiac system. There is little evidence of progressive or permanent damage even during long periods of hypothermia to approximately 33°C; but anatomic evidence of damage becomes apparent after 6 hours at 25°C or lower.[6] Electrically, all intervals tend to prolong, consistent with the rate,[7] and both (A-V) dissociation and ventricular fibrillation become significant[35] at 28°C. There are differences of opinion as to the underlying mechanism of hypothermic ventricular fibrillation. There is a decreased incidence of ventricular fibrillation in children, and this is thought to be associated with the relative size of the myocardium. Small animals are refractory to ventricular fibrillation in hypothermia. This experiment, in conjunction with experiments showing that sections of hypothermic fibrillating heart would regain organized contractility, provide support for the explanation and observation in children.[6]

EFFECT ON OTHER ORGANS

Ileus occurs at approximately 35°C and decreasing blood flow, through the stomach in particular, occurs with decreasing temperature, leading to stasis and clotting. Necrosis and ulceration then occur.[2,3,12,38] Ileus and decreasing blood flow result in hypoxia and activation of proteolytic enzymes in the pancreas.[38] This is the usual explanation for the pancreatitis referred to in the literature on hypothermia, but which we have not often seen. Insulin production is probably decreased,[1] but the levels of blood glucose in hypothermic patients vary, with early hyperglycemia being the usual finding.[15] Prolonged or chronic hypothermia generally presents with hypoglycemia.[16] Hepatocytes are relatively resistant to the effects of hypothermia but glycogen depletion occurs within the first 2 hours of decreasing core temperature.[51] Other functional decrements in the liver also occur[23] and there is a significant decrease in the metabolism of drugs, further strengthening arguments against early pharmacologic intervention.

The kidneys are relatively resistant to the effects of cold; this may explain why the kidneys were the first organs to be successfully transplanted using hypothermic preservation. As in the heart and brain, there is an increase in vascular resistance with decreasing core temperature. Despite decreasing blood flow and decreasing oxygen utilization, the kidneys retain about 50 percent of their functional capacity at 28°C, about one sixth at 22°C, and some function[45] to as low as 10°C. The enzyme systems of ATPase, succinic dehydrogenase, and cytochrome oxidase initially retain much of their functional capability but as enzymatic function decreases, there is a loss of active resorption and, therefore, sodium is wasted. Potassium, which is normally actively excreted, then begins to accumulate.[26,36] There is marked variability, but hyponatremic hyperkalemia is the more common finding. Again, aggressive early correction is to be avoided and it is expected that frequent evaluation will demonstrate a trend to correction with increasing core temperature. Either cold or immersion can produce a significant diuresis and the combined effects of hypothermic immersion produce an initial massive diuresis.[8,26]

The most important responses in the endocrine system are those of the adrenal and thyroid which, as noted above, result in increasing production of epinephrine, norepinephrine, cortisol, and thyroxine with initially decreasing core temperature. These adaptive responses are also degraded with progressive hypothermia. The human organism, being homeothermic, tends to try to restore its internal milieu. However, the organism begins to become poikilothermic at 33°C and this is complete[24] at about 30°C. Therefore, the individual whose core temperature drops below 33°C may not have the ability to restore homoeostasis and therefore cannot survive in the absence of intervention.

As shown in Table 20-1, certain temperatures are key and provide points upon which we can pivot an understanding of therapy. Thus, at 35°C mental function is deteriorating and fine coordination is lost. Ileus and damage to the gastric mucosa, as well as the potential for pancreatitis, begin here. At 31°C shivering stops and at 30°C the J wave appears. At 28°C there is a 50 percent utilization rate of oxygen. Cardiac function decrements lead to a pulse rate of 50 percent of normal, which may not be palpable; and there is a marked increase in electrical sensitivity with susceptibility to ventricular fibrillation. Renal blood flow is down to 50 percent, with a glomerular filtration rate of approximately one third baseline. At

TABLE 20-1. Significant Temperatures and Events

Approximate Temperature		Event
°C	°F	
37.6	99.6	Normal rectal temperature
37.0	98.6	Normal oral temperature
36	96.8	Metabolic rate begins to increase
35	95.0	Moderate hypothermia Shivering maximal Mental functions (logic and discrimination) decreasing Fine coordination lost Ileus, gastric mucosal damage Pancreatitis
33	91.4	Severe hypothermia Poikilothermia begins
32.5	90.5	Wake from hypothermic coma
31	87.7	Shivering stops
30	86.0	J wave appears Poikilothermia complete Surgical anesthesia Cortical electrical activity decreases
28	82.4	75% aortic blood pressure 50% pulse rate 50% utilization of O_2 50% renal blood flow 33% glomerular filtrate rate Susceptibility to ventricular fibrillation
27	80.6	Deep tendon reflexes return
26	78.8	Hypothermic coma ensues Deep tendon reflexes lost
25	77.0	J wave (if not in ventricular fibrillation) frequent
22	71.6	Maximum risk of ventricular fibrillation
20	68	Asystole Peripheral nerve conduction ceases Flat EEG

26°C, coma ensues and reflexes are lost. The risk of ventricular fibrillation is maximal at 22°C. Below 20°C peripheral nerve conduction effectively ceases, the electroencephalogram (EEG) is flat, and asystole supervenes. In therapy, deep tendon reflexes return at 27°C and patients who have been in hypothermic coma tend to reawaken at 32.5°C.

Clinical Presentation

The clinical presentation of the hypothermic patient varies, of course, depending upon the temperature at which the patient pres-

ents, and may be complicated by underlying diseases. The hypothermic patient may be otherwise normal, but exposed to the cold, or an individual with underlying diseases who has been exposed to the cold, or one in whom disease process produces hypothermia.[6] Examples of each of these are presented in Table 20-2.

If one were able to observe an individual slowly becoming hypothermic, one would see an individual who begins to make mistakes. With decreasing core temperature and decreasing logic capacity, patients lose the ability to extract themselves from an environment that may cause further disease or injury. As cooling continues, the individual loses muscular strength and begins to shiver, thereby losing coordination. As shivering increases in intensity, the individual becomes unable to do anything else. During this time, respiration has increased, leading to loss of carbon dioxide, but with decreasing core temperature the decreasing utilization of oxygen leads to a high PO_2 level. Cold produces significant changes in arterial blood gas measurements; measurements must therefore be temperature-corrected.[30] A diagnostic problem that continues to occur with distressing frequency is the lack of adequate temperature measuring capability in many emergency departments. All too frequently, one hears of a patient whose core temperature was 94°F (34.4°C) but who just did not seem to respond. In reality, the thermometer did not respond. Low-reading thermometers are essential, not only in northern climates where people tend to think of hypothermia in the wintertime, but also anywhere that exposure to water temperatures below 33.3°C (92°F) or air temperatures below 10°C (50°F) is possible. A water temperature of 33.3°C (92°F) represents the point at which the body can maintain homeostasis. Below that water

TABLE 20-2. Categories of hypothermic patients

Status	Example
Healthy, exposed	Campers, divers, stranded motorists, accident victims
Diseased, exposed	Patients with diabetes mellitus, hypothyroidism, Addison's disease, or heavy alcohol ingestion
Hypothermia secondary to	Fulminant sepsis, trauma, cerebrovascular accident

temperature the body loses heat faster than it can generate it, and progressive hypothermia will ensue.[48] Certainly, the colder the water, the faster the hypothermia will occur. A long enough exposure to almost any available water temperature can produce hypothermia. This is consistent with the fact that most recreational cases of hypothermia occur when the temperature is not extremely low. When either the water or the air is very cold, people tend to reduce their exposure or protect themselves appropriately. It is when people do not expect to become hypothermic that they do not protect themselves. Certainly, persons who are chilled in relatively warm water, or who feel chilled when the air temperature is 40°F should either increase their insulation or decrease their exposure. But if this is not possible, or if someone is inadvertently exposed to very cold temperatures, we must prepare to treat them.

Treatment

Several excellent reviews[16,22,29] discuss prehospital care and specialized techniques for use in the prehospital setting. The reader is referred to them for specifics.

REWARMING

The sine qua non of therapy is rewarming. Those who are only moderately chilled (whose core temperatures are in the range of 35°C, perhaps down to 33°C) can be treated most often with little difficulty. Certainly if the temperature is up to 35°C, and if the patient is awake, passive rewarming is acceptable. Increasing insulation and providing adequate fluids and food will allow individuals to rewarm themselves. They may be rewarmed actively but there is little justification to expose these patients to anything more rigorous than warm water immersion or showers, hot packs at key points, or ingestion of heated food and fluids. Oral fluids should be started in very small quantities, and only if bowel sounds are present. Food is presented only after fluids are well tolerated and the core temperature is above 35°C. Generally, the individual whose core temperature is below 33°C requires active re-

warming. As noted, once poikilothermia begins, patients may have lost the capability to rewarm themselves and require assistance.

External rewarming may act to decrease the rate of core rewarming by eliminating shivering, thereby decreasing internal heat production.[11] Acute peripheral vasodilation, an effect of external warming, causes a relative hypovolemia and can result in complications. In addition, external rewarming is also associated with an afterdrop, the continuation of a decrease in core temperature even though rewarming is occurring. Afterdrop has frequently been attributed to the presentation of a bolus of cold, acidotic blood to the core, as a result of vasodilation in the periphery. An elegant study[19] has convincingly demonstrated that afterdrop is also a conductive phenomenon and has to do with more than boluses of cold blood. Nonetheless, afterdrop does occur, and must be watched for. In combination with acidotic peripheral blood, this can produce increased myocardial irritability, particularly if one is compelled to use external rewarming in a patient with a body temperature in the range of 28°C or lower.

If immersion rewarming is used, as in a Hubbard tank, patients in the usual head-up position will require specific support, which is less desirable from a hemodynamic point of view. In anticipation of the possible need to preform cardiopulmonary resuscitation (CPR), the patient cannot be left afloat. The patient must be placed on a litter locked in place and a backboard must be inserted.

COMATOSE PATIENTS

The patient who presents awake is of less concern and can most likely be handled in the emergency department and transferred to a regular ward. The patient who is not awake is of much greater concern. Though the patient is cold, and hypothermia is suspected, fundamentals in the care of the comatose patient must be followed. While the arterial blood gases (ABGs) are evaluated, an indwelling thermister is placed either 5 to 10 cm into the rectum, or 25 to 30 cm into the esophagus if the patient is intubated. As is done for other emergency and intensive care patients, a flow-sheet should be immediately established. If the airway is patent and respirations are present, they should be counted for at least a full minute since they may be irregular. If a palpable pulse is not readily apparent, a cannula should be placed in a radial artery, a specimen for blood gases obtained, and a pressure transducer connected. The results of the ABG measurement must be corrected for the patient's temperature (Table 20-3).

If the patient's core temperature is low, but a pulse and respirations are present, decisions as to diagnosis and therapy can then be made. If the temperature is low (below 33°C) and the patient is not awake, intubation, if not already done, should be performed by the nasotracheal technique; take care to avoid movement of the head and neck. A manually triggered volume respirator may then be used as needed. All clothing should be removed with as little manipulation of the patient as possible, and cardiac monitoring leads should be placed. In the absence of known specific injuries, and while active core rewarming techniques are used, the following should be done. With the airway secured, a nasogastric tube is passed since ileus due to hypothermia and/or occult disease may be present. Both peripheral and central venous lines should be started if the temperature is below 28°C. The central venous line may be converted to a Swan-Ganz catheter when the temperature rises above 28°C. Initial fluids should be only D5W and should be passed through a blood warmer and infused at a temperature of 40°C. Lactated Ringer's solution, which we so frequently use for resuscitation, should be avoided due to the hypothermic liver's inability to metabolize lactate. A Foley catheter is used both to decompress the bladder and to assist in monitoring fluid requirements. Venous blood is drawn and baseline values are obtained for levels of glucose, electrolytes, blood urea nitrogen (BUN), creatinine, calcium, creatine phosphokinase (CPK), isoenzymes, and a clotting profile. This last should include measurement of prothrombin time (PT), partial thromboplastin time (PTT), fibrinogen, and fibrin degradation product levels, and the platelet count should be part of a complete blood count. A cervical spine series, a chest radiograph, and a flat plate radiograph of the abdomen should be obtained.

TABLE 20-3. Corrections in Arterial Blood Gas Values Required at Decreasing Temperatures

Temperature		Correction		
(°F)	(°C)	$PaCO_2$	PaO_2	pH
108	42.2	1.25	1.35	−0.08
106	41.1	1.19	1.26	−0.06
104	40.0	1.14	1.19	−0.04
102	38.9	1.08	1.11	−0.03
98.6	37.0	1.00	1.00	0
95	35.0	0.92	0.89	+0.03
90	32.2	0.82	0.76	+0.07
88	31.1	0.78	0.72	+0.09
86	30.0	0.74	0.67	+0.10
84	28.9	0.71	0.63	+0.12
82	27.8	0.68	0.59	+0.14
80	26.7	0.64	0.56	+0.15
78	25.6	0.61	0.52	+0.17
76	24.4	0.59	0.49	+0.18
74	23.3	0.56	0.46	+0.20
72	22.2	0.53	0.43	+0.22

pH decreases 0.008 units/°F fall in temperature
PaO_2 increases 3.3%/°F fall in temperature
$PaCO_2$ decreases 2.4%/°F fall in temperature
(Wears R C: Blood gases in hypothermia. JACEP 8(1):247, 1979.)

While this diagnostic work is in progress, respirations, blood pressure, and the cardiac electrical activity must be carefully observed. If ventricular fibrillation is noted, even below 28°C, a single attempt at electrical defibrillation using 2 Wsec/kg is attempted. If this fails, further efforts are deferred until the temperature rises[9,46] above 28°C. In the presence of either asystole or ventricular fibrillation unresponsive to an initial electrical attempt, CPR is performed at approximately one half the usual rate below 28°C. The rate may be increased as 28°C is approached and at that point pharmacologic and electrical version is appropriate. Bretylium tosylate has been shown to be useful in dog studies and has been credited with a successful chemical defibrillation in human hypothermia.[17]

The use of heated intravenous fluids, as noted above, is termed *active internal rewarming*. The capability should then exist to proceed to core rewarming. While active core rewarming is being performed by whatever technique(s) available, arterial and venous blood gas samples should be obtained with every 2 to 3° rise in temperature. Again, ABGs must be corrected for temperature, and the temptation to correct electrolytes should be resisted until the trend associated with rewarming is evident. Volume replacement is based on the central venous pressure, and the pulmonary wedge pressure if a Swan-Ganz catheter is placed, and must be followed closely. Many patients respond to rewarming with marked vasodilation and relative hypovolemia.

AIRWAY WARMING

Obviously, core rewarming techniques are highly desirable and several measures should be available almost immediately. The first is the inhalation of warmed, humidified oxygen. This technique takes advantage of the large ventilatory circulatory interface, and is relatively simple. Any respirator system available with the capacity to have a controllable warmer placed in the line may be used. Of extreme importance is frequent, careful monitoring of the temperature of the inspired gas. The patient whose level of consciousness is depressed is effectively anesthetized, and the risk of heat injury to the airway must be considered. The temperature of the inspired gas should be in the range of 43.5 to 44°C. It is important to ensure that the inspired gas is fully saturated with water vapor, since this water vapor conducts most of the heat to the patient, and its condensation in the lung actually delivers the heat. Clinical experience also indicates that this condensation is valuable in maintaining, and in fact increasing, ciliary activity and pulmonary hygiene without evidence of causing pulmonary edema. The respiratory rate should be controlled to result in a PCO_2 in the expired air of approximately 40 mmHg until arterial blood gas values are returned. If necessary, carbon dioxide may be bled into the inspiratory loop as is necessary to maintain arterial PCO_2 levels in the range of 40 mmHg, while oxygenation is maintained as high as is possible.

Though this technique, and all other core rewarming techniques, may decrease shivering thermogenesis, this should not be considered to be all bad, since shivering, while generating large quantities of heat, also consumes large quantities of energy. With the patient under control, it is better to provide that heat exogenously.

GASTROINTESTINAL WARMING

Another technique that requires little technologic sophistication is irrigation of the gastrointestinal tract with warmed fluids. With a nasogastric tube in place, warm fluids may be instilled and then evacuated. A second tube may be passed and continuous irrigation performed. Concurrently, or instead, rectal fluids may be infused. In either case, a balanced salt solution without lactate should be used. The fluid temperature should be maintained in the range of less than 41°C. A minor complication of either of these techniques is that the temperature readings from the colorectal thermister will be invalid. Frequent monitoring of electrolyte status is essential, though there should be little risk of major shifts in either direction if balanced salt solutions are used.

Gastric or rectal and colonic balloons may be used instead of free fluids. The disadvantage is that the surface for heat exchange is markedly reduced, though the constituents of the fluids are inconsequential since there is no contact and exchange. Rupture of one of these balloons could be dangerous. In general, the use of gastric and/or colonic balloons adds nothing to the effectiveness of resuscitation.

Peritoneal lavage should be available in most institutions. Again, the large surface areas of the peritoneum and the bowel provide an advantage in terms of thermal exchange. The same considerations noted above apply to the temperature and constituents of the exchanged fluid. The frequency of exchange can be determined simply by the temperature of the fluid within the peritoneal space. Though the rate of cooling can be calculated, it is easiest simply to pass a thermister through the cannula and to exchange the fluid when the temperature is halfway between the temperature of the fluid infused and the temperature of the body at the starting point.

EXTRACORPOREAL WARMING

Hemodialysis and/or other forms of extracorporeal circulatory assistance are usually not necessary for rewarming. However, for the patient who has no mechanical cardiac activity, extracorporeal circulation provides an excellent method of warming, oxygenating, detoxifying (if necessary), and circulating that blood.

Extracorporeal circulating devices are most often primed with sterile dextrose in water with electrolytes added as necessary. This priming agent causes hemodilution, which may improve perfusion by reducing sluding, particularly in the hypothermic patient. The patient who presents with a decreased red cell mass, whether chronically or as a result of acute trauma, may require additional blood to maintain oxygen-carrying capacity. Each unit of blood, straight from the storage refrigerator at 4°C, requires 14.5 kilocalories and 3L oxygen to have its temperature raised to 37°C. Blood to be transfused should be warmed prior to or during infusion. Since red cells hemolyse in the range of 44 to 45°C, it is best to keep the water in the heat exchanger no warmer than 42°C. A large area for heat exchange is desirable so that rapid flow is possible.[10] A decision tree for resuscitation from hypothermia is shown in Figure 20-2.

Diathermy has been recommended as a method of rewarming but until better evidence of success is presented, the risk of providing point heat in areas that may have altered circulation constitutes too grave a danger. Microwave heating is in the research stage, but there are no clinical data upon which to base a recommendation. The danger is the same as for diathermy.

CIRCULATORY COMPLICATIONS

With rewarming and resuscitation in progress, other problems and complications should be sought. Arterial blood gas measurements should be performed frequently and the temperature-corrected information used to guide additional therapy. Though acidosis may be present, vigorous correction is contraindicated. The standard correction of half the calculated base deficit combined with the utilization of oxygen is the method of choice. If the hypothermic patient is not in ventricular fibrillation, other dysrhythmias may be noted. Bradydysrhythms are most often a direct response to the hypothermia, and the rate will tend to increase with rewarming. As noted above, drugs are contraindicated and the rhythm will be refractory to atropine. Intracardial pacing is contraindicated, because of both refractoriness and the potential to initiate ventricular fibrillation. Atrial tachycardias will usually have a slow ventricular response and pharmacotherapy with digitalis is unnecessary and inappropriate. Atrial fibrillation is throught to be due to acute atrial distention and to be more common in acute than in chronic hypothermia.[16]

Circulation may be hindered by sludging and rheologic changes. Low molecular weight dextran may be useful in enhancing flow characteristics.[9,37] Maintenance of blood pressure and perfusion as rewarming proceeds should preclude renal failure. Prophylactic diuretics are not indicated. Dopamine has been shown to be helpful in maintaining blood pressure and renal perfusion in hypothermic patients.[41]

During rewarming, blood glucose levels should fall as cellular metabolism increases. Persistent hyperglycemia should be considered as due to diabetes mellitus or pancreatitis. As the temperature rises, insulin and potassium should be infused cautiously to help in restoring intracellular energy substrates. Amylase levels should be obtained repeatedly. Hypoglycemia, if present, should be corrected, but cerebral function will not improve until the temperature rises.

Any tissue damage, including that of generalized or local thermal injury, may precipitate disseminated intravascular coagulation (DIC). This acquired disorder, in which the rate of depletion of hemostatic substances exceeds the ability of the body to restore them, can result in severe hemorrhage. The target protein is fibrinogen, which is attacked by both thrombin and plasmin. Thrombin also aggregates platelets, removing them from circulation. Plasmin fibrinolysis yields fibrinogen and fibrin degradation products that have anticoagulant properties.[39] Platelet and fibrinogen levels are decreased, fibrin degradation products are elevated, and PT and PTT levels are usually elevated, though the latter may be normal. Heparin, 400 to 600 IU/kg/day by intravenous drip or divided into 4-hourly doses may lead to replenishment of the hemostatic substances by

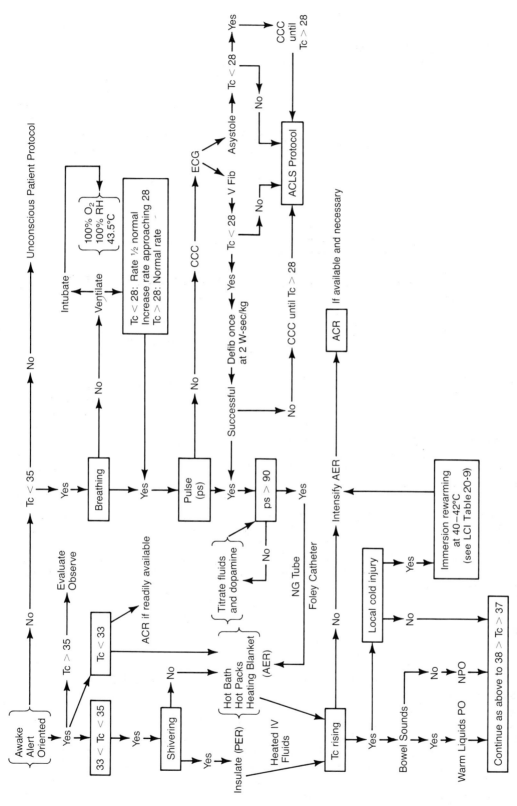

FIG. 20-2 Decision trees for resuscitation from hypothermia. Tc, core temperature (°C); PER, passive external rewarming; AER, active external rewarming; CCC, closed chest compression; ACR, active core warming; ps, systolic blood pressure.

TABLE 20-4. Complications of Hypothermia

Cardiac dysrhythmia
Disseminated intravascular coagulation
Stress ulcers
Pneumonia
Other infections
Renal failure
Hepatic failure
Pancreatitis
Diabetes-like syndrome
Hypoglycemia

inhibition of coagulation. Fresh frozen plasma, though frequently used, is considered by several authorities to be inadequate, and it is thought that concentrated fibrinogen, 3 to 6 g, is necessary for replacement. Unfortunately, this carries a high risk of transmitting hepatitis. Intensive treatment of the causative process is both mandatory and the best therapy.[14]

STEROIDS AND THYROID HORMONE

Though steroids have been recommended as treatment for practically every disease, there is no good documentation of a reason, other than the presence of hypoadrenalism, for its administration in hypothermia. Intracranial pressure, which is of immediate concern, was monitored in one case and remained normal during an entire resuscitation from severe hypothermia without the use of steroids.[28] Similarly, unless hypothyroidism is known to exist, or there is an inadequate response to rewarming, thyroid hormones should be withheld.

STRESS ULCERATION

During the recovery period, stress ulceration may occur. Though there are not yet controlled studies of prophylaxis, cimetidine, 300 mg q.i.d. orally or parenterally, or ranitidine should be considered. Histamine receptor blockers have been shown to be capable of producing a reversible psychosis-like syndrome. If this occurs, a mucosal coating agent (sucralfate, 1 g orally q.i.d.) should be substituted. If a nasogastric tube is in place, the tab-

lets of all the above agents may be crushed and administered in a water slurry. It is reported that pneumonia occurs frequently in patients recovering from hypothermia, and prophylactic antibiotics have been recommended.[28] In this, as in most other cases, we believe that antibiotics should be withheld until a causative organism can be documented. The complications resulting from hypothermia are listed in Table 20-4.

LOCAL COLD INJURY

Introduction

While hypothermia is a generalized cooling of the body, other local processes may result in injuries including chilblains, frostnip, trenchfoot (and immersion foot), and frostbite. It is important to note that an individual may suffer hypothermia with or without suffering specific local cold injury or vice versa. However, it is highly unlikely that an individual will suffer significant local cold injury without concomitant hypothermia. This has obvious therapeutic implications: all victims of local injury must be treated as if they were hypothermic until proven to be normothermic, or rewarmed. The local cold injuries can be further classified into those that are freezing and nonfreezing. Examples of the latter are trenchfoot (and immersion foot) and chilblain.

Chilblain

Chilblain seems to be restricted to individuals predisposed by excessively high vascular tone in peripheral extremities. In them, the normal physiologic response of vasoconstriction on exposure to cold is modified by a delay in release of vasoconstriction of some small vessels after the normal vasodilation of rewarming occurs. The phenomenon manifests as edema in the papillary dermis and there may be a mild vasculitis of the dermal vessels. Clinically, the injury most often occurs on the dorsal surfaces of the hands and feet and is most frequently reported in young women.[93] It frequently presents as patchy, pruritic, and edematous regions that are usually hyperemic and feel as if they are burning. Those who are susceptible frequently note that the phenomenon occurs in cold, damp climates and may recur perennially with the beginning of cold weather, resolving with the end of the wintry season.[78] Raynaud's disease, collagen diseases, and macroglobulinemias are among the disease processes associated with, and that may increase the risk of, chilblain.[67,93]

Trenchfoot

Trenchfoot and immersion foot are essentially the same disease, but are described differently depending on the environment in which they occur. Trenchfoot, which is thought of in a military setting,[93] is due to wet socks and shoes or boots worn in a temperature range[65,66] of just above freezing to approximately 10°C. Constriction from tight socks and/or boots and immobility and dependency exacerbate the problem.[66,67,74] Alcoholics, drug abusers, and individuals who may for other reasons be exposed to a similar set of circumstances will suffer the same effects. Immersion foot is usually considered the maritime equivalent of trenchfoot and has most often been described in survivors of wartime shipwrecks. It is caused by prolonged immersion of the extremities in chilly water. Much of the world's oceans in which commerce and troop movements occur have a water temperature in the range described as chilly: below 15.5°C. In addition to the immersion, significant factors are dependency and relative immobility due to the crowding of lifeboats and liferafts. In both situations, the disease begins with vasoconstriction, which proceeds to vasospasm and relative ischemia. If this persists for more than 8 hours, the prolonged hypoxemia and tissue hypoxia

result in vascular damage and edema. Sensations of numbness and heaviness are almost universally described. In trenchfoot, walking is painful, due to stiffness of the feet and ankles, and may become impossible because one falls as a result of the loss of proprioception. During both trenchfoot and immersion foot, persistence of the inciting conditions and the presence of minor skin injuries may result in severe cellulitis, which may affect the deeper tissues.

In the worst of situations, not only in wartime, but also in the case of a lost hunter or camper, or a driver stranded in a winter storm, the process can result in a wet gangrene.[70] When the patient is removed from the precipitating environment, and after rewarming, there is a hyperemic phase in which the skin becomes red and warm, with formation of bullae and vesicles, and ecchymosis that frequently delineates the areas subject to the greatest pressure. Areas that do not become hyperemic, but which remain pale and/or cyanotic, will tend to form dry gangrene. The hyperemic phase usually lasts 4 to 6 days but may persist for as long as 2 weeks. This period may be extremely painful, with sensations described as lightning or shooting pains, though they may begin as a continuous ache that worsens. Due to the neural damage that occurred in the anoxic phase, and depending upon the extent of that damage, muscle atrophy, usually of the intrinsic muscles of the feet, may occur.

If gangrene has occurred, it is usually superficial and affects only the skin. When the gangrenous skin sloughs, granulation tissue is usually exposed and then new skin forms. As sensation is recovered in the healing phase, hyperesthesia may be so severe that stockings and shoes are intolerable, and even contact with bed covers is unacceptable. Blanket cradles are mandatory. In recovery, depigmentation of the skin is not uncommon, and hypersensitivity to the cold and associated pain on weight bearing may persist almost indefinitely.

The most important points in treatment are careful air drying of the extremities, avoidance of further skin trauma, bed rest, early antibiotic treatment of infections with necessary debridement, and avoidance of amputation until adequate demarcation has occurred.[86] Cool air has been used to treat pain in the hyperemic phase,

TABLE 20-5. Treatment of Trenchfoot/Immersion Foot

Litter: patient to bed rest
Air dry the extremity
No friction
Systemic analgesia
Tetanus toxoid
Blanket cradle
Broad spectrum antibiotics if infection occurs
Debridement
Avoid amputation until demarcation occurs
Injection sympathectomy

but systemic analgesia is frequently necessary. With appropriate long-term physical therapy, muscular anatomy and function usually recover. Persistent cold sensitivity and hyperhidrosis may require sympathectomy.[59,95] Injection techniques may be used to confirm efficacy before surgical ganglionectomy is performed (Table 20-5).

Frostnip

Frostnip precedes frostbite; the affected areas do not actually become frozen. Frostnip most often occurs on the cheeks, the tip of the nose, and the ears, and progresses from a hyperemic, state to one of pallor and numbness. If these areas are rewarmed early in the latter state, actual freezing of tissue does not occur. There are then no sequelae. In delineating freezing injuries, it must be kept clear that the temperature of the tissue, not the ambient temperature, is the determining factor. If any portion of the body is allowed to cool to the point at which tissue freezing occurs, true frostbite has occurred.

Frostbite

Frostbitten tissues are pale, cold, and firm to palpation. They are frequently described as waxy white and woody feeling. Color changes are less obvious in patients with darker skin. Frostbite is the end result of several differ-

ent mechanism (Fig. 20-3). Vasoconstriction and changes in rheology yield intravascular stasis and sludging of the formed elements.[97] Cellular necrosis may then occur as a result of prolonged stagnant hypoxia. Ice crystal formation occurs in the chilled intravascular and interstitial extracellular spaces. Hypertonicity resulting from the sequestration of extracellular water draws out intracellular water, resulting in intracellular dehydration and hyperosmolarity.[69] Both of these processes are potentially reversible: the former, if flow can be restored before cellular anoxic death supervenes; the latter, if thawing and rehydration occur before anoxic death, or before about one third of the intracellular water is extracted, at which point cell death results from enzymatic disruption and failure of metabolic processes.[64]

Intracellular freezing with disruption of cellular membranes and spillage of lysozymes irreversibly results in necrosis. This will most likely occur when tissue freezing is very rapid,[78] such as during unprotected exposure to effective temperatures of −30°C or below. These temperatures are not uncommon in many parts of the United States, particularly at higher altitudes. Factors that affect the effective temperature to which the skin is exposed include the velocity of the wind, whether the exposed part is wet or dry, and contact with excellent heat conductors, such as metals. The wind chill index[8] (Table 20-6) is used to demonstrate the increased cooling power of any temperature with increases in wind velocity.

Water conducts heat about 25 times faster than dry air.[57,94] Anyone participating in cold weather activities should be aware that wet clothing can produce critical conditions in minutes. Contact of bare skin with metal can result in "sticking" and, depending on the temperature of the metal, an almost instantaneous injury. Minus 15°C is the point at which immediate injury occurs almost invariably.[57] Another significant danger is a group of petroleum products (gasoline, kerosene, and related substances) that do not freeze at 0°C as water does. These materials remain liquid at almost any ambient temperature humans can tolerate, and they achieve that ambient temperature. Pouring such cooled (below −15°C) petroleum products on exposed skin will result in instant frostbite.[57] Most people are not aware that get-

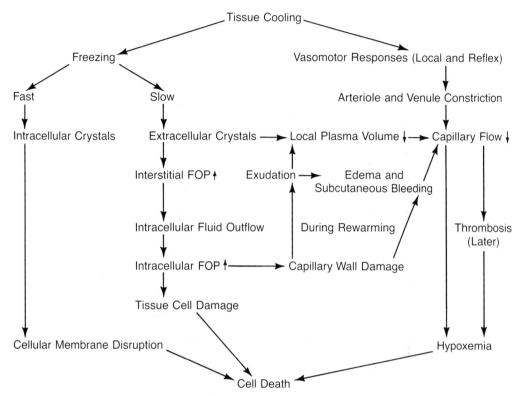

FIG. 20-3 Pathogenesis of frostbite. FOP, fluid osmotic pressure. (Modified from Goldman RF: Cold injuries. Presented at the Walter Reed Army Institute of Research August, 1982.)

ting gloves or trousers wet from such liquids can result in the same injury.

Demographic and Environmental Factors

Selected military campaigns—Napoleon's retreat from Moscow, the European winter campaigns of World War I and World War II, and the march from the Chosin Reservoir in Korea—are repeatedly used in the study of frostbite. Other physiologic and operational studies[61,79,83] have clarified demographic and environmental factors associated with frostbite, and demonstrated that cold weather exercises can take place without environmental casualties.[75,76] Other studies demonstrate that cold injuries in civilians are frequently associated with trauma, unexpected immersion or isolation, fatigue, ethanol, psychiatric disease, or extremes of age.[72,81,96] Healthy adults, properly attired to maintain an appropriate microclimate, do not suffer cold injury simply upon exposure.[65,68,91]

Two specific demographic points require explanation: the relationships between cold injuries in particular and racial and geographic background. Data from World War II and Korea indicated that U.S. troops from areas of the country with warmer winters, and black troops, had higher instances of cold injury.[58,90] There are interrelationships between these factors, but blacks had higher rates of injury than whites from similar climatic regions. Urban development (city versus rural area) was not taken into consideration in these studies. The racial variable is relatively straightforward. Though there are large individual differences, blacks as a population tend to have a less well directed cold-induced vasodilation (CIVD) response than whites, who suffer in comparison

TABLE 20-6. Cooling Power of Wind on Exposed Flesh Expressed as an Equivalent Temperature (Under Calm Conditions)

Estimated Wind Speed (in mph)	Actual Thermometer Reading (°F)											
	50	40	30	20	10	0	−10	−20	−30	−40	−50	−60
	EQUIVALENT TEMPERATURE (°F)											
Calm	50	40	30	20	10	0	−10	−20	−30	−40	−50	−60
5	48	37	27	16	6	−5	−15	−26	−36	−47	−57	−68
10	40	28	16	4	−9	−24	−33	−46	−58	−70	−83	−95
15	36	22	9	−5	−18	−32	−45	−58	−72	−85	−99	−112
20	32	18	4	−10	−25	−39	−53	−67	−82	−96	−110	−124
25	30	16	0	−15	−29	−44	−59	−74	−88	−104	−118	−133
30	28	13	−2	−18	−33	−48	−63	−79	−94	−109	−125	−140
35	27	11	−4	−21	−35	−51	−67	−82	−98	−113	−129	−145
40	26	10	−6	−21	−37	−53	−69	−85	−100	−116	−132	−148

(wind speeds greater than 40 mph have little additional effect).

LITTLE DANGER (for properly clothed person) Maximum danger of false sense of security.

INCREASING DANGER Danger from freezing of exposed flesh.

GREAT DANGER

Trenchfoot and immersion foot may occur at any point on this chart

(T B MED 81/NAUMED P-5052–29/AFP 161–11 USGPO 1970)

to native Alaskans (Eskimos). Thus, when an extremity is exposed to cold, CIVD will take longer in blacks; they will experience a lower skin temperature before CIVD occurs, and will have a smaller temperature rise during CIVD. Findings in whites are intermediate between those of blacks and Alaskan natives.[87] Blacks are therefore more liable to cold injury.

Geographically, the answer is less clearly defined. In the past, when there was less population shifting, persons from areas where winter temperatures do not fall below − 6°C had a higher risk of cold injury. This was most likely due to a lack of knowledge and experience in the cold, since acclimatization, while seeming to occur, takes about 6 weeks of exposure to appropriate conditions,[62] and is rapidly lost. There seem to be less clearly geographically defined subgroups today.

Most importantly, military experience has shown that, despite individuals' demographic predisposition, with proper training, clothing, and equipment, they can conduct extensive exercises with little, if any, cold injury.

Extent of Injury

The extent of tissue damage is related to the tissue temperature and the length of exposure, but tissue temperatures are not available in natural experiments. Reviews of the Korean war experience[58] revealed that, of frostbite injuries, 90 percent resulted from exposure to conditions of less than −7°C and for greater than 7 hours. In another clinical review, all patients exposed to less than −7°C for longer than 1 hour suffered tissue loss.[63] Wind velocity and moisture were not specifically correlated in these studies. Another study[72] indicated that all patients who had been exposed to temperatures of less than −1.7°C for longer than 1 hour, and were either wet or in contact with metal, had some tissue destruction. Clearly, the conductivity of water or metal enhanced the ability of the relatively benign temperature to extract heat more quickly than the affected region could be warmed.

Treatment

Though it is well documented that the extent of injury is directly related to the duration of freezing, and that the underlying muscle and osseous tissues are injured with prolongation of exposure, it is mandatory that attempts at rewarming not occur until definitive therapy can be provided. The military experiences noted above, and more recent Alaskan civilian experience,[80] confirm that when survival is in question, it is better to continue to walk on a frozen lower extremity than to attempt to thaw such an injury in the field. Because of the vascular instability and tissue damage, it is almost certain that re-exposure to the inciting conditions will result in a refreezing and more destructive situation. Slow, uncontrolled thawing may also result in high metabolic requirements at the surface, before the capacity of the underlying circulation to meet those requirements is restored.

In transporting a patient with frostbite, extreme care should be taken to avoid mechanical injury and, in light of the above, rewarming of a frozen extremity during transport is contraindicated.

REWARMING

Despite the above caveat, in most cases that occur in cities, slow rewarming of the affected part begins during transport of the patient to the treating facility. Whether or not slow rewarming has begun, upon arrival the treatment of choice is immersion of the affected part in water between 38 and 42°C; the optimum[80] is 40 to 42°C. The temperature of the water should be continuously monitored, additional warm water added to maintain the desired temperature range, and a whirlpool bath or other gentle agitator used to reduce local temperature differences. Extreme care must be taken to avoid allowing the water temperature to rise above 44°C, since the affected parts have no ability to circulate heat away and therefore are very easily burned.[60] Thawing continues until capillary circulation is documented in the nailbeds. As rewarming and reperfusion occur, the patient may experience pain that is quite severe. The patient should be forewarned of this and systemic analgesia should be provided.

Frostbite, once simply described as "frozen," is now modified by being classified into first through fourth degrees, much like burns. Though it frequently requires time for the final determination of extent to be made, and for some purposes a simpler classification will suffice, meticulous documentation of extent of injury is required for correlation with epidemiologic, pathophysiologic, and therapeutic information, to increase our knowledge.

DEGREES OF FROSTBITE

First degree frostbite progresses during rewarming through pallor, cyanosis, and then hyperemia. Edema forms, which tends to resolve in approximately a week. Though bullae do not form, desquamation may occur. Frostbitten extremities tend to develop recurrent cyanosis if left in a dependent position. In some cases, hyperhidrosis, pain, and/or paresthesias may develop. The duration of these signs and symptoms is unpredictable. Even if they resolve, reexposure to cold may cause recurrence. Though only skin loss is the rule in these cases, treatment consists of bed rest and avoiding dependency of the affected part.

In second degree frostbite, after the skin progresses through hyperemia and edema, bullae tend to appear, particularly on the dorsal aspects of affected digits. These bullae are nonhemorrhagic and, if not manipulated or debrided, tend to resorb and form an eschar. This eschar usually separates in about 3 weeks, revealing thin, pink skin. Permanent tissue loss does not occur, though sequelae such as in first degree frostbite are more common. Treatment is essentially the same as for first degree, though bullae that open spontaneously should be debrided. Antibiotic prophylaxis is considered inappropriate.

Third degree injuries are marked by the absence of bullae formation distally, while more proximal parts progress through the same stages as first and second degree burns. Proximal bullae may contain hemorrhagic as well as serous fluid. Lack of response in distal tissues is borne out by persistent coldness, cyanosis and hypesthesia. All of the sequelae to second degree injuries may occur in third degree injuries and in addition, there may be scarring of the skin and radiographic evidence of bone damage, particularly near painful joints.

Fourth degree injuries are defined as full thickness: the entire part is frozen and does not rewarm. There is a lack of bulla formation, with persistence of the cold, wooden (or waxy) feel. The skin may mottle but may also remain cyanotic, rapidly (in 2 or 3 days) mummifying. Surgery should be rigorously avoided until demarcation occurs, even though this may require as long as 3 months. If, on the other hand, the dry gangrene becomes a wet gangrene with ascending cellulitis, lymphangitis, and perhaps edema formation, or if systemic toxicity occurs, aggressive antibiotic therapy and possibly early amputation will be necessary to save the remainder of the limb and perhaps the patient's life.

PROGNOSIS

Though the final classification of the injury is made retrospectively, prognostic indicators in the first 24 to 48 hours allow one to predict accurately superficial (Table 20-7) versus deep (Table 20-8) injury.

SPECIFIC THERAPY

Regardless of the extent of injury, a portion of the therapy of frostbite after thawing is completed is relatively straightforward and standard. The parts are dried carefully and without rubbing, and should be elevated if possible,

TABLE 20-7. Indicators of Superficial Injury

Large bullae, filled with a clear fluid
Return of warmth (normal temperature)
Return of sensation
Pink or erythematous
Blanching on pressure
Rapid capillary refill after blanching

(Based on data in Fourt and Hollies.[68])

TABLE 20-8. Indicators of Tissue Loss

A hard consistency
No bullae or edema
Hemorrhagic bullae
Cold
Insensitive
White or cyanotic
No blanching
Superimposed trauma
Systemic signs of tissue necrosis
History of freeze, thaw, refreeze
History of contact with water or ice, subfreezing metal
  or petroleum products

(Based on data in Fourt and Hollies.[68])

without undue pressure. Creams, oils, and ointments should be avoided, except as noted below. Bullae should not be ruptured but, if broken, should be debrided. Cotton pledgets, foam plugs, or gauze fluffs are used to separate the digits initially, and after each debridement. Blanket cradles are necessary to prevent contact with covers. As in burns, open, sterile therapy in a comfortably warm (23 to 25°C) room is best. If the treating physician is not certain that the patient has received tetanus immunization within the past 2 years, tetanus toxoid should be administered. 0.5 ml IM. Prophylactic antibiotics are, in this as in most other cases, inappropriate. As therapy progresses, and open wounds are epithelialized, sterility may be relaxed to cleanliness.

The patient is treated at bed rest, and active physiotherapy is begun as soon as possible. For about the first 2 weeks, depending on the extent of injury, 20 to 25 minute whirlpool sessions are used for debridement. The water temperature[63] should be approximately 37°C, and the surgical scrub of choice is added to the water. Escharotomy is performed if encirclement occurs, and over joints in all cases, to enhance physical therapy. The patient should be encouraged to move the digits actively and frequently. Smoking is traditionally prohibited due to the well-known vasoconstrictive effects of nicotine. There has been question about whether the potential adrenergic surge associated with the stress of withdrawal from smoking could be physiologically more harmful for the patient. There is no evidence that this occurs.

Skin grafting to cover large areas of slough in third degree injuries should be considered.

The use of human skin versus artificial coverings will depend upon the practice and expertise of the surgeon and the availability of suitable material. Amputation should be avoided as long as possible to allow for extension of viability unless limb- or life-threatening infection supervenes.

RESTORING CIRCULATION

There is now little question in the mind of any practitioner that restoration of circulation, and protection—even enhancement—of that circulation is the sine qua non of tissue salvage. Radioisotopic and thermographic studies have shown that loss of perfusion occurs as a result of early thrombosis due to intravascular cellular aggregation, and later may be caused by inflammatory responses secondary to tissue injury and direct vascular injury. Much of this vascular damage occurs within minutes, and may be complete within several hours.[63,73,82] Experimental work in rabbits, in which adequate heparinization was performed early and maintained, indicated that tissue survival was enhanced.[56] Most clinical studies are from the Korean war era, when heparinization usually occurred late and was ineffective, but some reduction in tissue loss was reported[63] if heparinization was performed within 36 hours. Considering the difficulties in maintaining adequate anticoagulation in a patient who has cold injuries and may have other serious injuries as well, heparinization per se may be inadvisable. Low molecular weight dextrans have been considered in the same category as heparinization; there are only experimental, but no clinically documentable, benefits.[63,82,84] This may also be true because therapy is started after the critical first hour. Since there are fewer contraindications to the use of low molecular weight dextrans than to heparin and oral anticoagulants, early use of these agents and continuation for the first 5 days may be of benefit. Controlled studies of their value are indicated. Vasodilators such as nicotinic acid have been experimentally verified to be effective, but their clinical efficacy is unclear,[60] perhaps due to the resulting hypotension.[63]

Sympathectomy has been shown experimentally and clinically to be effective in the reduction of swelling and pain. There is evidence that the earlier the procedure is performed, the greater the benefit.[60,89] The discussion of surgical versus medical sympathectomy continues. As noted in the section on nonfreezing cold injuries, chemical sympathectomy is advisable prior to surgical ganglionectomy. One usually thinks of direct injection of either the stellate ganglion or the lumbar sympathetic plexus when one hears "sympathectomy." Certainly, the stellate ganglion is readily accessible and repeated direct injections are a suitable technique. The approach to the lumbar sympathetics is more painful for the patients and we recommend the consideration of an indwelling epidural catheter to avoid the need for such repeated injections. Use of intra-arterial reserpine[85] is a well known and tested technique, and intra-arterial tolazine[92] is also being used. Guanethidine, which is not available in a parenteral form in the United States, is used by Bier technique in Europe.[71] Though there is disagreement as to whether sympathectomy, despite the above benefits, results in tissue salvage,[80] it is hard to conceive of any situation in which improved circulation would be detrimental. We recommend early chemical sympathectomy in these cases. As in nonfreezing cold injury, sympathectomy may also be effective in the later treatment of hyperesthesias and causalgia.[89,92]

The effects of thromboxane and other breakdown products of arachidonic acid in the progression of dermal ischemia have been a subject of extensive discussion. Aspirin and indomethacin have been repeatedly shown to reduce the generation of prostaglandins. Aloe vera and other substances such as dipyridamole have been shown to block the generation of thromboxane.[77] Aloe vera was also found to have bacteriocidal effects against many organisms frequently cultured from hospitalized burn and frostbite patients. The authors of these studies express strong support for the early and extensive use of aloe, and claim uniform success in the treatment of frostbite patients.[77] This particular area of controversy may fall into the same category as that of sympathectomy, above. It is hard to argue in the face of experimental evidence that would tend

TABLE 20-9.   Initial Treatment of Frostbite

Litter patient if lower extremity is affected
Immersion of affected part at 40°–42°C
Maintain water temperature
Intravenous access
Low molecular weight dextran
IV analgesia
Tetanus toxoid
Protect bullae (debride if ruptured)
Injection sympathectomy
Oral acetylsalicylic acid
Topical Aloe vera

to support the enhancement of circulation (Table 20-9).

PSYCHOLOGICAL ASPECTS

In these patients, much as in those suffering from burns, a great deal of attention must be paid to their psychological status as well as physiologic status. There are many similarities between the burned and the frostbitten patient, not the least of which is the prolonged hospitalization required by those with second degree or more extensive injury. Perhaps the frostbite patient has an even greater problem because the extent of injury cannot be determined for a much longer period of time. It is essential that the patient, significant others, and the responsible physician recognize and accept this uncertainty. In the acute case, the physician must work rapidly yet avoid precipitous actions. The most serious, and not infrequent, case is the patient who presents in hypothermia and with evidence of frostbite. The complexity of this combined injury is analgous to the multiple trauma patient, for whom many things must be done simultaneously. There is no conflict in the initial treatment: salvage of life takes precedence over salvage of limbs, but the ability to save both exists. Preplanning is essential. Resuscitation must not be interfered with, but that does not preclude rapid rewarming, as above, if staffing is adequate and only the hands or feet are frostbitten. More extensive frostbite may tend to compromise resuscitation and the associated painful decisions must be made on an individual basis.

ACUTE HYPERTHERMIA

Introduction

The body's failure to balance heat loss with production and gain is responsible for the continuum of medical conditions described as heat edema, fatigue, cramps, syncope, exhaustion, and stroke.[111] Variations in age, pre-existing medical conditions, and presenting history make the rapid diagnosis of heat stroke potentially difficult for the emergency room practitioner. The wide range of environmental conditions that contribute to heat injury further obscures an easy diagnosis.[105] Heat stroke can occur in individuals who were healthy just a few hours prior to presentation, but who have overstressed their cardiovascular system in an environment that does not allow adequate body cooling. This can be seen in high school football players, military recruits,[111,130] and in well-trained marathon runners.[132,140] If environmental parameters are excessive, heat stroke can occur in the absence of exercise, as when infants or young children are left in automobiles that are closed and parked in the sun.[122,137]

Even when the environment would not be considered extreme, the extremes of age, alcoholism, diabetes, obesity, cardiovascular disease, prior heat stroke, and pre-existing medical problems that preclude adequate fluid intake and cooling have been shown to be factors increasing risk.[99,103,120,121,126] Phenothiazine tranquilizers and anticholinergic drugs are mong numerous other medications that can precipitate or aggravate heat illness.[117,126,130]

Normal Physiology

As the body's core temperature increases, the hypothalamus normally regulates the Benzinger reflex (increased sweating and dilation of peripheral cutaneous vessels) in an effort to dissipate heat.[98,111] Tachycardia and increased cardiac output enhance the transfer of core heat to the skin surface, where heat is dissipated by conduction, radiation, and convection, and accelerated by heat loss due to sweat evaporation.[123] In exercise, an increased proportion of cardiac output is shunted to skeletal muscles and peripheral vasculature, normally compensated for by splanchic vasoconstriction to prevent hypotension.[123] Fluid loss from sweating, which may exceed 1.5 L/hr in unclimatized individuals and up to 2.5 L/hr in acclimatized individuals,[123] helps in removing up to 900 kcal/hr of heat.[105] Sweat also accounts for varying amounts of electrolyte loss. For example, potassium loss varies from 5 mEq/L of sweat in the unacclimatized, decreasing to 2 mEq/L in the well-acclimatized athlete.

Pathophysiology

The body's ability to dissipate heat while maintaining vital tissue perfusion can be overridden, allowing injury to occur. Skin diseases, use of anticholinergic drugs, or occlusive clothing impair heat loss by the evaporation of sweat. Environmental conditions of high temperature and humidity may add to the body's heat burden. This is exacerbated in an individual who exercises and produces heat that the body's ability to maintain homeostasis cannot compensate for. Injury begins to occur at this point.

The mechanisms required for heat injury to occur are postulated to be combinations of organ failure of the sweat glands and altered set-point of the POAH, or other dysfunction of the hypothalmus.[98,106,123] The damage to organ systems is by protein denaturization due to the excessive heat and by hypoxia due to hypoperfusion.[102,123] Essentially every organ in the body is affected.

Definition

Several clinical conditions are described, brought about by the effects of excessive heat and the body's attempt to cope with that stress.

In heat cramps, the patient complains of pain in the abdomen and legs, with some degree of fatigue. The rectal temperature is usually less than 37.5°C, blood pressure and pulse are usually normal, and the ability to continue sweating remains. The cramping of voluntary muscles is most likely due to an acute loss of sodium in sweat, with adequate oral water replacement in the absence of salt.[123] This cramping may also be compounded by hyperventilation and subsequent respiratory alkalosis.[123] Correction of the hyponatremia usually promptly relieves the cramping.[104,123]

As heat stress progresses, heat exhaustion may occur. This may be a result of a fairly short duration of strenuous activity in a hot environment or several days of lesser insult.[104] Rectal temperatures of 38 to 40°C are recorded. Blood pressure is normal to low, with tachycardia. The patient's skin is warm, moist and pale. Symptoms of fatigue, possible cramps, dizziness, headache, nausea, vomiting, and diarrhea may occur.[104,123] This condition is differentiated from heat stroke by lesser severity of symptoms and retention of mental function without loss of consciousness or seizure activity. Some degree of temperature regulation remains. Two basic forms of heat exhaustion are described, due primarily either to water depletion or to salt depletion.[98,104] Primary water depletion exhaustion generally occurs with exercise in a hostile environment without replacement of the water lost from sweat. Salt depletion is perhaps a progression of the circumstances in heat cramps, where salt losses are replaced by adequate volumes of water without salts. The patient with this condition usually does not experience intense thirst.[123]

As the body's capacity to function under increasing heat stress diminishes, heat stroke ensues and has been divided into two major types, classic and exertional. Classic heat stroke is more commonly seen in infants, the medically compromised, and elderly patients. This form may develop over several days in which severe dehydration may exist. The hallmark is a triad of central nervous system dysfunction, rectal temperature in excess of 40.5°C, and anhidrosis.[98,104,123] Exertional heat stroke commonly occurs due to intense exercise in an uncompromising environment. It can develop within a few hours and hence dehydration is usually not profound. The triad for diagnosis remains the same except that 50 percent or more of patients with exertional heat stroke will be sweating profusely.[98,104]

Central nervous system symptoms in heat stroke include confusion, coma, stupor, combativeness, and seizures.[104,123] Rectal temperatures are 40.5°C or higher and may still be rising during transport to or after arrival at the emergency room. Sweating may be profuse or absent. High output cardiac failure generally is present, with a blood pressure that can be normal, but is usually low. However, hypodynamic responses are seen with low cardiac output and increased central venous pressure (CVP) values.[98,131] A tachycardia of 150 to 180 beats/min is not uncommon.[98,104]

Complications

Heat stroke represents a conclusion to many different sets of circumstances in medical conditions. Hence the medical complications of heat stroke are as variable as the type of presentation encountered.

Hypotension is common and is usually the result of dilated peripheral vasculature in the face of high cardiac output. Hypovolemia also secondary to dehydration is commonly profound and usually normalizes once the temperature is corrected.[110] Dehydration is more pronounced in the classic form, but even here, rarely are more than 1.5 L replacement fluid required within the first 2 hours of treatment, at which time laboratory values should be available to aid in determining therapy.[104,108]

Electrolyte abnormalities are extremely variable. Certain "hyper- and hypoelectrolyte" values are widely reported.[98] Most commonly, sodium and chloride values are elevated, while potassium levels may be low, normal, or elevated.[98,106,110,111,127,131] Hypokalemia is more commonly associated with classic heat stroke.[98] Potassium deficiency may have a role in the pathogenesis of exertional heat stroke,[123] as well as rhabdomyolysis. Total body potassium loss occurs in exercising, unacclimated volunteers exposed to high humidity and temperature rather than in those exercising in cool climates. Net body potassium losses are reported to be from 41 to 79 mEq/day from individuals in hotter environments.[123] Hypokalemia is not, however, a universal finding in heat stroke. Levels of BUN, creatinine, and serum osmolalities are usually elevated.[110] Mild hypoglycemia is occasionally found,[110] yet hyperglycemia is not uncommon, since diabetics seem to have an increased incidence of heat-related injury.[136]

Hypocalcemia is seen in exertional heat stroke due to metabolic acidosis with skeletal muscle injury.[97,123] Unless tetany occurs, correction of altered calcium values should be avoided.[98] Hypophosphatemia is not infrequent, and is partially attributed to respiratory alkalosis and increased cellular uptake.[136]

A metabolic acidosis secondary to increased lactic acid is common; acute hypoxemia, shock, increased metabolic demand, hypocapnia, and impaired hepatic function are thought to be responsible.[136] Respiratory alkalosis occurs with hyperventilation and is seen in heat exhaustion to a greater degree than in heat stroke.[98,136]

Levels of serum glutamic oxaloacetic transaminase (SGOT), serum glutamic pyruvic transaminase (SGPT), lactic dehydrogenase (LDH), and CPK are almost always elevated.[97,110,126] The skeletal muscle fraction of CPK is commonly reported.[110] The levels of these enzymes peak about 48 hours after insult and if not elevated, a diagnosis of heat stroke perhaps should not be made.[111] Some authors have used SGOT levels of greater than 1,000 units as an indicator of poor prognosis.[98]

Renal complications are common and due to several mechanisms. Prolonged tissue hypoxia, hypoperfusion, tubular occlusion by myoglobin, actual cellular damage by the increased temperature, and hyperuricemia result in acute renal failure in 10 to 30 percent of patients.[98,111,123,130] Hemodialysis should be instituted if oliguric renal failure occurs.[98] Urine output, specific gravity, osmolality, and levels of urea nitrogen and sodium should be monitored to allow one to anticipate and attempt to prevent acute tubular necrosis.[98]

Hepatic damage is probably a complication of hypoxemia, hemolysis, DIC, and high temperature.[119] Jaundice can occur and is typically seen in the more severe cases.[98,107] He-

patic dysfunction prolongs prothrombin time and decreases fibrinogen levels.[107,111] Coagulation changes seen in severe heat stroke are complex and resemble frank DIC.[100] In fatal cases, hemorrhagic conditions are present and are probably the result of hepatic failure as well as DIC.[133] The diagnosis of DIC may not be easily differentiated from the coagulation abnormalities found in acute liver failure. However, once the presence of DIC is established, as seen in cases of severe heat stroke, heparin should be administered.[100]

Central nervous system dysfunction is a primary criterion for diagnosis of heat stroke. On admission, marked euphoria, combativeness, disorientation, or coma may be present. Tonic–clonic seizures, fecal incontinence, and vomiting are not uncommon.[98,108] Coma especially for more than 10 hours, is associated with a poor prognosis.[113] Autopsy typically reveals cerebral edema, petechial hemorrhages, degeneration of Purkinje cells, and patchy congestion.[98,100,108,123]

Skeletal muscle damage due to the elevated temperature is always present to varying degrees and is demonstrated by elevated CPK levels. As severity increases, rhabdomyolysis, which contributes to tubular necrosis, is observed.[110,130] Plasma exchange with dialysis has been used to treat extensive rhabdomyolysis in an effort to prevent and treat ensuing renal failure.[124]

Myocardial damage is not common. Elevations in CPK levels do not reflect myocardial fraction elevations. However, many transient electrocardiogram recordings of nonspecific ST segment changes, prolonged Q-T intervals, and other conduction abnormalities are reported.[110]

Treatment

Treatment of heat-related illness must begin as soon as the diagnosis is suspected. At the site of injury, occlusive clothing should be removed. The patient's skin should be wetted with iced water, or wet sheets or towels and a fan, if available, should be used to increase convection.[128] Transportation to a definitive treatment center should be accomplished as soon as possible. The more severe the degree of heat injury, the more aggressive the medical treatment and support is required. The rapid assessment of vital signs, specifically including core temperature, is mandatory. Oral temperature readings are of no value.[141] A rectal temperature probe is required to monitor temperature and cooling continuously regardless of the cooling technique employed. If uncomplicated heat cramps are diagnosed, oral electrolyte solutions, rest, and stretching or massage of the cramping muscles may be all that is required. Lowering of the patient's temperature is not needed since the body is still capable of heat regulation. This condition usually occurs at rectal temperatures less than 38°C. Cramps can, however, be a component of more severe heat illness.

As the degree of heat stress increases and core temperatures are found to be in the range of 39 to 42°C, normal hypothalamic regulation is failing and assistance in cooling is needed. Two major treatment goals must be met: rapid cooling of the patient, which is the single most important action; and supportive care as indicated by close monitoring.

The techniques for lowering the body temperature for heat exhaustion and heat stroke are perhaps the single most disputed topic in heat related illness. Two major methods are currently advocated; variations of total or partial body immersion in ice water, and a warm water mist combined with a rapid exchange of air across the patient. Both techniques require prior preparation in the hospital emergency room. Both procedures produce a wet environment and cannot be immediately used unless the necessary tubs, baths, or hammocks are immediately available, and personnel are trained to operate electrical monitoring and support devices in the presence of water.

Advocates of ice water immersion remove occlusive clothing from the patient, who is then lowered into an ice bath, with the head and airway supported. This can range from a Hubbard tank to a bathtub, or even a rapidly inflatable child's pool filled with ice and water. Vigorous massaging of the patient's extremities is performed by staff in an effort to prevent peripheral vasoconstriction and enhance the transfer of heat from the core to the skin surface. Constant monitoring of vital signs is performed. Perhaps the single best argument for the ice tub technique for body cooling is that it appears to work. It is commonly employed with good success at some military training centers,[108,110,130] where medical personnel encounter heat stroke with a fair degree of regularity. The type of patient usually seen in this setting is frequently a young, healthy adult who was briefly undergoing stressful exercise in a high-temperature, high-humidity environment. This is a significant contrast to an elderly, hypertensive, diabetic who has been without air conditioning for 4 days in August.

Recent studies[139,141] on techniques for cooling patients with elevated temperatures convincingly propose the use of evaporation of finely atomized warm water sprayed over an unclothed patient. Water temperatures of 15°C[139] to 21°C[141] with an airflow rate of 0.5 meters per second have been shown to provide a more rapid cooling process than other tested techniques. Wyndham et al.[141] report that cooling patients at 21°C dry-bulb temperature and a wind velocity of 100 feet/min is more effective than ice water immersion techniques. The evaporative cooling with warm mist sprays does not produce the discomfort experienced while in ice water. The procedure also avoids both peripheral vasoconstriction, which decreases heat transfer from the core to the skin surface, and intense shivering, which increases metabolic heat production.

The advantages of evaporative cooling over ice water immersions are supported by numerous authors.[112,115,120,125,141] These are, however, disputed by those favoring ice water submersion procedures.[108,113,138] Whichever technique is employed, cooling should be stopped at a core temperature of approximately 38.8°C (102°F) to prevent rebound hypothermia.[108] Additional treatment for heat stroke is primarily supportive and requires careful monitoring of the patient's condition.

Hypoxemia and pulmonary shunting are not characteristic of heat stroke; however, oxygen supplementation is frequently overlooked and may be lifesaving, especially for a patient with a poorly perfused myocardium or hypoxic central nervous system.[115,119,128] Intravenous fluids should be initiated; however, dehydration, hypovolemia, and electrolyte abnormalities are not usually severe[108] and are frequently corrected when the temperature and the peripheral circulation return to normal levels.[110] The choice of solutions does not seem to be critical. Ringer's lactate or saline with glucose is frequently used.[108] Intravenous Valium may be necessary to control seizure activity.

Intravenous mannitol has been recommended to prevent cerebral edema, promote renal blood flow,[108] and reduce myoglobin accumulation in renal tubules.[116] However, renal perfusion is probably not increased by the use of osmotic diuretics in dehydration, and its actions could aggravate those complications of hypovolemia and electrolyte imbalances.[114,129] The evidence for cerebral edema is from autopsy results[133] and is not clinically pronounced. Certainly, if a diuretic is used, an indwelling bladder catheter should be placed and meticulous intake and output monitoring is essential. Dantrolene sodium, 4 mg/per kg IV has been used to treat heat stroke,[127] although it is recommended more for use in the treatment of malignant hyperthermia (See Chapter 27). Dantrolene may help reduce muscle injury[116]; however, it is not commonly used by the majority of authors.

Chlorpromazine or phenothiazine[108,128] is occasionally given to prevent the shivering that counteracts cooling efforts. Evaporative cooling procedures will minimize the incidence of shivering; other investigators find that chlorpromazine is unnecessary and may complicate hypotension.[110]

The use of peripheral vasoconstrictors to treat hypotension should be avoided, since hypotension usually indicates a need for fluids, and vasoconstrictors reduce heat exchange at the skin surface.

Laboratory studies of importance for prognosis and monitoring treatment complications should routinely include a complete blood count, measurement of platelets, PT, PTT, electrolytes, calcium, BUN, glucose, SGPT, CPK, LDH and serum LDH, serum osmolality and ABGs.[104] The choice of intravenous solution and rate of infusion should be adjusted in accordance with laboratory results after cooling is accomplished. Again, it is very important to note that cooling to near normal core temperatures often corrects abnormalities seen at elevated temperatures. Large volumes of fluids should not be administered prior to cooling unless needed for the treatment of trauma. As the temperature stabilizes at 39°C or lower, the patient can be transported to the intensive care unit for monitoring of possible complica-

TABLE 20-10. Diagnosis and Treatment of Heat Cramps, Heat Exhaustion, and Heat Stroke

	Heat Cramps	Heat Exhaustion	Heat Stroke
Symptoms	Skeletal muscle cramping	Possible cramping	Increased severity of symptoms found in heat exhaustion, especially those of CNS dysfunction
	Hyperventilation	Hyperventilation	
		Dizziness, nausea, fatigue, syncope	
Findings	Rectal temperature less than 37°C	Rectal temperature 38–40°C.	Rectal temperature greater than 40.5°C.
	Skin: moist, pale	Skin: warm, moist, pale	Skin: hot, may or not be sweating
	Blood pressure normal	Blood pressure low to normal	Blood pressure low
		Pulse: tachycardia	Pulse: tachycardia (150–180)
		Mental function intact	CNS dysfunction: confusion, coma, seizures
Treatment	Correct hyponatremia orally	Rapid cooling	Rapid cooling
	Massage affected muscles	Rest	After temperature control, adjust therapy based on obtained
		Hydration; if mild, oral electrolytes; if severe, IV solutions	laboratory values. Apply routine ICU monitoring of renal function, electrolytes, CNS status, cardiac monitoring

tions, including DIC, renal, hepatic, and central nervous system dysfunction.

A summary of the diagnostic criteria for distinguishing between heat cramps, heat exhaustion, and heat stroke, and guides for treatment of these conditions, are presented in Table 20-10.

Prognosis

Mortality rates from 10 to 80 percent are reported for heat stroke.[101,108,109] Fatal outcomes[134] are associated with coma lasting more than 10 hours and nearly all fatalities are complicated by DIC.[100] Reports indicate that SGOT levels greater than 1,000 U/ml are associated with high mortality rates.[118] Complete recovery without permanent disability has been reported in 1 case,[135] from a rectal temperature of 46.5°C (115°F). Rapid diagnosis and rapid lowering of temperature are the mainstays of a favorable prognosis.

REFERENCES

Hypothermia

1. Baum D, Dillard DH, Porte D: Inhibition of insulin release in infants undergoing deep hypothermic cardiovascular surgery. N Engl J Med 279: 1309, 1968
2. Beattie D: Physiologic changes in rats exposed to cold/restraint/stress. Life Sci 23: 2307, 1978
3. Beckman EL, Reeves E: Physiological implications as to survival during immersion in water at 75°F. Aerosp Med 37: 1136, 1966
4. Benet M, Hensel H, Lieberman H: The central control of shivering and nonshivering thermogenesis in the rat. J Physiol 283: 569, 1978
5. Biersner RJ: Motor and cognitive effects of cold water immersion under hyperbaric conditions. Hum Factors 18: 299, 1976
6. Brantigan CO, Paton BC: Clinical hypothermia, accidental hypothermia, and frostbite. In Byrne JJ (ed): Goldsmith Principles of Surgery. Harper and Row, Philadelphia, 1983
7. Brennan D, Ross BK, and Brumleve SJ: Electrocardiographic responses of ice diving scuba divers. Proc North Dakota Acad Sci 29(1): 3, 1975
8. Brobeck JR (ed): Best and Taylor's Physiologic Basis of Medical Practice. Williams and Wilkins, Baltimore, 1979
9. Cold injury: TB MED 81/NAVMED P-5052–29/AFP 161–11. Departments of the Army, the Navy, and the Air Force. USGPO, Washington, D.C. 1976-241-379-3005B, 1976
10. Collins JA: Blood transfusions and disorders of surgical bleeding. In Sabiston DC (ed): Davis-Christopher Textbook of Surgery. WB Saunders, Philadelphia, 1981
11. Collis ML, Steinman AM, Chaney RD: Accidental hypothermia, an experimental study of practical rewarming methods. Aviation Space Environ Med 48: 625, 1977
12. Coniam SW: Accidental hypothermia. Anesthesiology 34(3): 250, 1979
13. Cooper KD: Respiratory and thermal responses to cold water immersion. In: Proceedings of the Cold Water Symposium, Toronto, May 8, 1976. Royal Life Saving Society, Canada, Toronto, 1976
14. Corn M: Bleeding disorders. In Schwartz GR, Safar P, Stone JH, et al (eds): Principles and Practice of Emergency Medicine. WB Saunders, Philadelphia, 1978
15. Curry DL, Curry KP: Hypothermia and insulin secretion. Endocrinology 87: 750, 1970
16. Danzl DF: Accidental hypothermia. Rosen P (ed): Emergency Medicine, Concepts and Clinical Practice. CV Mosby, St. Louis, 1983
17. Danzl DF, Sowers MG, Vicario SJ: Chemical ventricular defibrillation in severe hypothermia. Ann Emerg Med Dec 1982
18. Gale CC: Neuroendocrine aspects of thermoregulation. Ann Rev Physiol 35: 391, 1973
19. Golden F, Hervey GR: The "after-drop" and death after rescue from immersion in cold water. In Adams JM (ed): Hypothermia ashore and afloat. Aberdeen University Press, Aberdeen, 1981
20. Goode RC: Acute responses in cold water. In: Proceedings of the Cold Water Symposium, Toronto, May 8 1976. Royal Life Saving Society, Canada, Toronto, 1976
21. Guyton AC: Textbook of Medical Physiology. WB Saunders, Philadelphia, 1978
22. Harnett RM, O'Brien EM, Sias FR, Pruitt JR: An experimental comparison of methods for rewarming from deep hypothermia in the field.

1980 International Hypothermia Conference and Workshop, University of Rhode Island, January, 1980

23. Henneman DH, Bunker JP, Brewster WR: Immediate metabolic response to hypothermia in man. J Appl Physiol 12: 164, 1958

24. Hervey GR: Physiological changes encountered in hypothermia. Proc R Soc Med 66: 1053, 1973

25. Hoar PF, Raymond LW, Langworthy HC, et al: Physiological responses in men working in 25.5°C. water breathing air or helium tri-mix. J Appl Physiol 40: 605, 1976

26. Kanter GS: Hypothermic hemoconcentration. Am J Physiol 214(4): 856, 1968

27. LeBlanc J, Physiological changes in prolonged cold stress, In: Proceedings of the Cold Water Symposium, Toronto, May 8 1976. Royal Life Saving Society, Canada, Toronto, 1976

28. MacLean D, Emslie-Smith D: Accidental Hypothermia. JB Lippincott, Philadelphia, 1977

29. MacInnes H: International Mountain Rescue Handbook. Charles Scribner's Sons, New York, 1972

30. Martin S, Diewold RJ, Cooper KE: The effect of clothing on the initial ventilatory response during cold water immersion. Can J Physiol Pharmacol 56(5): 886, 1978

31. McAniff J: The incidence of hypothermia in scuba diving fatalities. International Hypothermia Conference and Workshop, University of Rhode Island, June, 1980

32. McConn R: The oxyhemoglobin dissociation curve in acute disease. Surg Clin North Am 55: 627, 1975

33. Morbidity Mortality Weekly Report 31: 50, 669, 1982

34. Morbidity Mortality Weekly Report 32: 3, 46, 1983

35. Mouritzen CV, Andersen MN: Myocardial temperature gradients and ventricular fibrillation during hypothermia. J Thorac Cardiovasc Surg 49(6): 937, 1965

36. Moyer JH, Morris GC, DeBakey ME: Hypothermia: effect on renal hemodynamics and on excretion of water and electrolytes in dog and man. Ann Surg 145(1): 26, 1957

37. Mundth ED, Long DM, Brown RB: Treatment of experimental frostbite with low molecular weight dextran. J Trauma 4: 246, 1964

38. Naizi SA, Lewis FJ: Profound hypothermia in man. Ann Surg 147(2): 246, 1958

39. Nossel HL: Disorders of blood coagulation factors. In Isselbacker KJ, Adams RD, Braunwald E, et al (eds): Harrison's Principles of Internal Medicine. McGraw-Hill, New York, 1980

40. Rango NA: Action needed to prevent deaths from hypothermia in the elderly. JAMA 243: 407, 1980

41. Reheja R, Purick V, Schaeffer RC: Shock due to profound hypothermia and alcohol ingestion. Crit Care Med 9: 644, 1981

42. Reuler JB, Hypothermia: pathophysiology, clinical settings and management. Ann Intern Med 89(4): 519, 1978

43. Rosomoff HL: The effects of hypothermia on the physiology of the nervous system. Surgery 40: 328, 1956

44. Russell CJ, McNeill A, Evonuk E: Some cardiorespiratory and metabolic responses of scuba divers to increased pressure and cold. Aerospace Med 43: 998–1001, 1972

45. Sell KW, Small A, Benjamin JL: Renal function in the hypothermic perfused state. Transplant Proc 4: 617, 1974

46. Stine RJ: Accidental hypothermia. J Am Coll Emerg Phys 6(9): 413, 1977

47. Swan H: Clinical hypothermia: a lady with a past and some promise for the future. Surgery 73: 736, 1973

48. Trostle HS, Dully FE, Millington RA (eds): U. S. Naval Flight Surgeons Manual. USGPO, Washington, D.C., 1978

49. Vaughan WS, Jr.: Diver temperature and performance changes during long-duration cold water exposure. Undersea Biomed Res 2: 75, 1975

50. Vaughan WS, Jr.: Distraction effect of cold water on performance of higher-order tasks. Undersea Biomed Res 4: 103, 1977

51. Wang LCH, Rie P: Changes in plasma glucose, free fatty acids, corticosterones and thyroxine in HE-O₂ induced hypothermia. J Appl Physiol 42: 694, 1977

52. Wears RL: Blood gases in hypothermia. J Am Coll Emerg Phys 8(6): 247, 1979

53. Wedin B, Vanggaard L, Hirvonen J: Paradoxical undressing in fatal hypothermia. J Forensic Sci 24: 543, 1979

54. White BC, Weyerstein JG, Winegar CD: Brain ischemic anoxia. JAMA 251: 1586, 1984

55. Zarins CK, Skinner DB: Circulation and profound hypothermia. J Surg Res 14: 97, 1973

Local Cold Injury

56. Abramowicz M (ed): Treatment of frostbite. Med Lett 22: 112, 1980

57. Bangs CC, Burt CP, Fowler JC, et al (eds): Staying Alive in the Arctic. American Petroleum Inst, Washington, D.C., 1976

58. Blair JR: Follow-up study of cold injury cases from the Korean War. In Ferrer MI (ed): Cold Injury. Josiah Macy Jr. Foundation, New York, 1956

59. Blair JR, Schatski R, Orr KD: Sequelae to cold injury in one hundred patients. JAMA 163: 1203, 1957

60. Brantigan CO, Paton BC: Clinical hypothermia, accidental hypothermia, and frostbite. In Byrne JJ (ed): Goldsmith: Principles of Surgery. Harper and Row, Philadelphia, 1983

61. Campbell MR: Proceedings, Frostbite Symposium, Arctic Aeromedical Research Laboratory. Fort Wainwright, Alaska, February, 1964

62. Cavenaugh AJM: Cold acclimatization of the fingers. J Appl Physiol 19: 158, 1964

63. Cold Injury. T.B. Med. 81, NAVMED T5052–29, AFT 161–11. Departments of the Army, the Navy and the Air Force. Washington, D.C., USGPO, 1976

64. Dinep M: Cold injury: a review of current theories and their application of treatment. Conn Med 39: 8, 1975

65. Edholm OD, Bacharach AL (eds): The Physiology of Human Survival. Academic Press, New York, 1965

66. Emergency War Surgery. NATO Handbook, First United States Revision. USGPO, Washington, D.C., 1975

67. Fishlowitz MR: Environmental factors in cold injury. U.S. Army Medical Field Service School, Fort Sam Houston, Texas, 1973

68. Fourt L, Hollies NRS: Clothing Comfort and Function. Marcel Dekker, New York, 1970

69. Hanson HE, Goldman RF: Cold injury in man: a review of its etiology and discussion of its prediction. Milit Med. 134: 1307, 1969

70. Herman G: The problem of frostbite in civilian medical practice. Surg Clin North Am 43: 519, 1963

71. Kaplan R, Thomas P, Tipper H, Strauch BL: Treatment of frostbite with guanethidine. Lancet.² : 940, 1981

72. Knize DM, Weatherley White RCA, Paton BC, Owens JC: Prognostic factors in the management of frostbite. J Trauma 9: 749, 1969

73. Lang K, Boyd LJ: The functional pathology of experimental frostbite and prevention of subsequent gangrene. Surg Gynecol Obstet 80: 346, 1945

74. Marcus P: Trenchfoot caused by the cold. Br Med J 622, 1979

75. Margulies RA: Anorak Express 80: A USMC Exercise in Norway in Winter, Unpublished Notes, 1980

76. McCarrol JB, Denniston JC, Pierce DR, Farese LJ: Behavioral Evaluation of a Winter Warfare Training Exercise, Report T/78. U.S. Army Institute of Environmental Medicine, Natick, Massachusetts, 1977

77. McCauley RL, Hing DN, Robson MC, Heggers JP: Frostbite injuries: a rational approach based on the pathophysiology. J Trauma 23: 143, 1983

78. Merryman HT: Mechanics of freezing in living cells and tissue. Science 124: 515, 1956

79. Miller D, Bjornson DR: An investigation of cold injured soldiers in Alaska. Milit Med 127: 247, 1962

80. Mills WJ: Frostbite and hypothermia—current concepts. Alaska Med 15: 26, 1973

81. Mills WJ: Out in the cold. Emerg Med 8: 134, 1976

82. Mundth EE, Long DM, and Brown RB: Treatment of experimental frostbite with low molecular weight dextran. J Trauma 4: 246, 1964

83. Orr KD, Fainer DC: Cold injuries in Korea during the winter of 1950–51. Medicine 31: 77, 1952

84. Penn I, Schwartz SI: Evaluation of low molecular weight dextran in the treatment of frostbite. J Trauma 4: 784, 1964

85. Porter JM, Wesche DH, Rosch J, Baur GM: Intra-arterial blockade in the treatment of clinical frostbite. Am J Surg 132: 625, 1976

86. Steenburg RW: Cold Injury. In Ballinger WF, Rutherford RB, Zuidema GD (eds): The Management of Trauma. WB Saunders, Philadelphia 1968

87. Rennie DW, Adams T: Comparative thermoregulatory response of negroes and white persons to acute cold stress. J Appl Physiol 11: 201, 1957

88. Robson MC, Heggers JP, Hagstrom WJ: Myth, magic, witchcraft or fact? Aloe vera revisited. JBCR 3: 157, 1982

89. Schumacker HB, Kilman JW: Sympathectomy in the treatment of frostbite. Arch Surg 89: 575, 1964

90. Schuman G: Epidemiology of Frostbite, Korea, 1951–52. In Orr KD (ed): Report #113. Army Medical Research Lab., Fort Knox, 1953

91. Siple P: Clothing and climate. In Newburgh RW (ed): Physiology of Heat Regulation and the Sciences of Clothing. LH Hafner, New York, 1968

92. Snider RL, Porter JM: Treatment of experimental frostbite with intra-arterial sympathetic blocking drugs. Surgery 77: 557, 1975

93. Tring FC: Chilblains. Nursing Times 73: 1753, 1977

94. Trostle HS, Dully FE, Millington RA (eds): U.S. Naval Flight Surgeon's Manual. USGPO, Washington, D.C., 1978

95. Ungley CC, Channell GD, Richards RL: The immersion foot syndrome. Br J Surg 33: 17, 1946

96. Washburn B: Frostbite: what it is—how to pre-

vent it—emergency treatment. N Engl J Med 266: 974, 1962

97. Weatherly-White RCA, Sjostrom B, Paton BC: Experimental studies in cold injury: II. The pathogenesis of frostbite. J Surg Res, 4: 17, 1964

Acute Hyperthermia

98. Anderson RJ, Reed G, Knochel J: Heat Stroke. Year Book, Chicago, 1983

99. Bark NM: Heat stroke in psychiatric patients; two cases and a review. J Clin Psychiatry 43: 9, 1982

100. Beard ME, Hickton CM: Haemostasis in heat stroke. Br J Haematol 52: 269–274, 1982

101. Beller GA, Boyd AE: Heat stroke: a report of 13 consecutive cases without mortality despite severe hyperpyrexia and neurological dysfunction. Milit Med 140: 464–467, 1975

102. Benzinger TH: On physical heat regulation and the sense of temperature in man. Proc Natl Acad Sci USA 46: 645, 1959

103. Caldroney RD: Risk factors in heat stroke. JAMA 249: 193–194, 1983

104. Callahan ML: Emergency management of heat illness. Emergency Physician Series, Abbott Laboratories 1979

105. Canadian Association of Sports Sciences: Position paper on protection from exertional heat injuries. Can J Appl Sport Sci June 99–100, 1981

106. Carlson RW, Besso J, Carpio et al: Hyperoncotic state and hypovolemia associated with heat injury. Crit Care Med 9: 807–809, 1983

107. Chobanian SJ: Jaundice occurring after resolution of heat stroke. Ann Emerg Med 12: 2, 1983

108. Clowes GH, Jr., O'Donnell TF: Current concepts—heat stroke. N Engl J Med 291: 564–567, 1974

109. Cole D: Heat stroke during training with nuclear, biological and chemical protective clothing: case report. Milit Med 148: 624–625, 1983

110. Costrini AM, Pitt HA, Gustafson AB, Uddin DE: Cardiovascular and metabolic manifestations of heat stroke and severe heat exhaustion. Am J Med 66: 296–302, 1979

111. Ellis FP: Heat illness. Trans R Soc Trop Med Hyg 70: 402–425, 1976

112. Exertional heat injury. Med Lett 23: 63–64, 1981

113. Goldfrank L, Osborn H, Webman RS: Heat stroke. Physician Assist Health Pract July 43–56, 1982

114. Goodman LS, Gilman AG (eds): Osmotic diuretics. p. 819. In: The Pharmacological Basis of Therapeutics, 5th ed. MacMillan, New York, 1975

115. Hoagland RJ, Bishop PH: A physiological treatment of heat stroke. Am J Med Sci 241: 415–422, 1961

116. Jardon OM: Physiological stress, heat stroke, malignant hyperthermia—a perspective. Milit Med Vol 147: 8014, 1982

117. Johnson LW: Preventing heat stroke. Am Fam Physician 26: 137–139, 1982

118. Kew MC, Bershas I, Sefteh H: The diagnostic and prognostic significance of the serum enzyme changes in heat stroke. Trans R Soc Trop Med Hyg 65: 325, 1971

119. Kew MC, Minick OT, Bahu RM et al: Structured changes in the liver in heat stroke. Am J Pathol 90: 609–614, 1978

120. Khogali M, Weiner JS: Heat stroke: report on 18 cases. Lancet 2: 276–278, 1980

121. Kilbourne EM, Choi K, Jones TS, Thacker SB: Risk factors in heat stroke. JAMA 247: pp 3332–3336, 1982

122. King K, Negus K, Vance JC: Heat stress in motor vehicles: a problem in infancy. Pediatrics 68: 579–582, 1981

123. Knochel JP: Environmental heat illness. Arch Intern Med 133: 841–864, 1974

124. Kuroda M, Katsuki K, Uehara H et al: Successful treatment of fulminating complication associated with extensive rhabdomyolysis by plasma exchange. Artif Organs 5: 372–378, 1981

125. Lackin JT: Treatment of heat related illness. JAMA 245: 570–571, 1981

126. Lee DKH: Epidemic heat effects. JAMA 247: 3354–3355, 1982

127. Lydinett JS, Hill GE: Treatment of heat stroke with dantrolene. JAMA 246: 41–42, 1981

128. Management of Heat Stroke (Editorial): Lancet 2: 910–911, 1982

129. Mannitol, Merck Sharpe Dohme: package insert.

130. O'Donnell TF: Acute heat stroke; epidemiologic, biochemical, renal and coagulation studies. JAMA 234: 824–828, 1975

131. O'Donnell TF, Jr.: The hemodynamic metabolic alterations associated with acute heat stress injury in marathon runners. Ann NY Acad Sci 301: 262–269, 1977

132. Rose RC, Hughes RD, Yarbrough DR, Dewees SP: Heat injuries among recreational runners. South Med J 73: 1038–1040, 1980

133. Rubel LR: Case for diagnosis. Milit Med 148: 756–757, 1983

134. Shibolet S, Lancaster M, Danon Y: Heat stroke: a review. Aviation Space Med 47: 200–301, 1976

135. Slovis CM, Anderson GF, Casolano A: Survival in a heat stroke victim with a core temperature

in excess of 46.5°C. Ann Emerg Med 11: 269–271, 1982

136. Sprung CL, Portocarrero CJ, Fernaine AV, Weinberg PF: The metabolic and respiratory alterations of heat stroke. Arch Intern Med 140: 665–669, 1980

137. Surpure JS: Heat-related illness and the automobile. Ann Emerg Med 11: 61–63, 1982

138. Treatment of Heat Stroke. Med Lett 23: 76–77, 1981

139. Weiner JS, Khogali M: A physiological body cooling unit for treating heat stroke. Lancet 507–509, 1980

140. Whitworth JAG, Wolfman MJ: Fatal heat stroke in a long distance runner. Br Med J 287: 948, 1983

141. Wyndham CH, Strydon NB, Cooke HM et al: Methods of cooling subjects with hyperpyrexia. J Appl Physiol 14: 771–776, 1959

21

Fluid and Electrolyte Management In Critical Illness

Frank E. Gump

INTRODUCTION

Management of fluid and electrolyte problems in the critically ill patient constitutes one of the most important areas in intensive care medicine. Venipuncture provides access to the body fluids for both diagnosis and treatment and makes it possible for the physician to influence body composition in a very direct way. Disorders of fluid and electrolyte balance are manifested by functional abnormalities in multiple organ systems and treatment is designed to correct these defects. A thorough appreciation of the effects of injury on the metabolism of water, sodium, and the other electrolytes will prevent or minimize many of the fluid disorders seen in the intensive care unit.

The body fluid compartments and the principles governing normal fluid exchange will be discussed first. This leads to a discussion of the concept of balance, which is of great value in critically ill patients both in terms of water

and specific ions. Finally, fluid and electrolyte abnormalities will be considered in terms of volume, tonicity, and composition.

FLUID COMPARTMENTS AND TONICITY

A major portion of body weight is water. A knowledge of the various subdivisions of total body water is essential for both understanding and managing complex fluid and electrolyte problems. Unfortunately direct measurement of these fluid compartments is not possible in a clinical setting, with the possible exception of measurements of plasma volume. However, normal values have been reported by a number of investigators and the three major compartments that constitute total body water are shown in Figure 21-1. Although the concentration of ions in solution is readily determined with a flame photometer, it is important to remember that the volumes of the various fluid compartments are of even greater importance.[2] While total body water may not be the most important compartment for the clinician, it is worth examining in some detail because some degree of quantitation is available.

Total Body Water and its Subdivisions

Isotope dilution techniques (usually with tritiated water) have been used to measure total body water (TBW) in a variety of normal and pathologic states. The actual quantity varies among individuals depending upon their age, sex, and lean body mass, but in the average healthy male 60 percent of total body weight is water. Since fat is essentially water-free, the greater the body fat content, the lower the percentage of water. As lean body mass decreases for whatever reason and there is a relative increase in body fat, the contribution of water to total weight will decrease. While

these factors make it difficult to arrive at an absolute value for TBW from body weight measurements, the clinician can take advantage of the relationship between TBW and body weight to quantitate changes in TBW based on careful daily weights.

The subdivisions of body water are reasonably constant in health, in which the following values are representative. Intracellular fluid represents 40 percent of body weight and extracellular fluid (ECF) represents approximately 20 percent. The extracellular portion is subdivided into plasma volumes (about 5 percent of body weight) and interstitial fluid.[8] Blood volume can be measured, and when red cell volume and plasma volume are determined separately blood volume values are quite accurate. Even when blood volume is approximated from measured plasma volume and the hematocrit, reasonable accuracy can be achieved. While these measurements were widely used at one time, it became apparent that in critical illness the intravascular space could contract or expand. Under such circumstances a given value, even if in the normal range, might not reflect an important disparity between the measured volume and the vascular space that has to be filled. Hemodynamic measurements have been far more effective than static measurements in assessing patients' circulatory

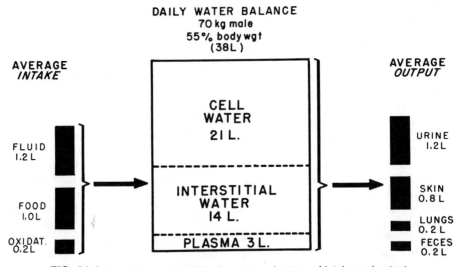

FIG. 21-1 Subdivisions of total body water and routes of intake and output.

status. However, the volume of total body water remains important in fluid and electrolyte management.

Each fluid compartment has its own unique composition. The major components of the ECF compartment are sodium and chloride with small amounts of potassium, magnesium, calcium, phosphate, bicarbonate, protein, and organic acids. The greater protein concentration of plasma constitutes its only difference with interstitial fluid. On the other hand, sodium is largely excluded from intracellular water by processes that require energy.[1] The importance of sodium relates to its control of the distribution of water throughout the body. The number of molecules of sodium per unit of water determines the osmolality of the ECF. If sodium is lost, water is excreted in an effort to maintain normal osmolality. If sodium is retained, water must also be retained in order to dilute it into the physiological range. While there are about 4000 mEq sodium in the body, this is misleading since much of this is in bone. Fluid and electrolyte dynamics revolve around the exchangeable sodium, which totals about 2800 mEq or 40 mEq/kg body weight. Control of this critical ion is primarily vested in the kidney since it regulates excretion. Fixed losses take place via the skin and the gastrointestinal (GI) tract but they are small under ordinary circumstances. However, one should remember the high sodium concentration of biliary, pancreatic, and small intestinal secretions if such losses are high and require replacement.

chloride dissociates into 1 equivalent of sodium ion and one of chloride so 1 molecular weight of sodium chloride produces 2 mOsm. On the other hand, glucose and urea remain in solution as such (they do not dissociate) and therefore provide only 1 mOsm. Proteins may have molecular weights in the thousands, with thousands of milligrams required to make 1 mOsm protein.

The cell wall is a semipermeable membrane since it is completely permeable to other substances. The limited passage of plasma proteins is responsible for the effective osmotic pressure, usually referred to as colloid osmotic pressure. Water can pass freely through all cell membranes and therefore movement of water will equalize the osmotic pressure inside and outside the cell. If osmotic pressure is altered in the extracellular fluid, it will result in a redistribution of water between the cellular and extracellular compartments. These shifts of body water result from changes in composition rather than volume so that intracellular water is far less affected by increases or decreases in extracellular fluid volume than in osmotic pressure.[12]

NORMAL EXCHANGE OF FLUID AND ELECTROLYTES

Permeability and Tonicity

If two solutions containing solutes at different concentrations are separated by a membrane that allows water to move freely from one solution to the other but does not permit the movement of solute across the membrane, water will move until the osmolality on the two sides is identical. Solutions have the same osmolality when the number of particles in solution per unit volume is the same. The unit 1 milliosmole (mOsm) is defined as the number of milligrams of a substance equal to its molecular weight dissolved in 1L of water. Sodium

Water Balance

Water balance is not a commonly employed term in clinical medicine but the concepts involved are widely applied. Body weight has become a critically important measurement in the intensive care unit because acute changes reflect increases or decreases in total body water. While the absolute value, 35 to 45 L in a 70 kg adult, is of little value because of the wide normal range, changes in total body water have clear clinical import. Water balance provides a means of quantitating these changes. Furthermore, when accurate weights are not available water balance measurements provide the only means of obtaining this information.

Serial measurements of water balance, or body weight, are important to the clinician because they provide information about the volume of fluid in which the body's electrolytes are dissolved. Such information is often critical in the diagnosis and management of complex electrolyte disorders.[6] Water balance requires the measurement of intake and output of water. Output consists of urine, stool water, and drainages that have to be measured as well as evaporative losses. Intake usually consists of IV fluids. Water balance measurements have received limited clinical application because of difficulties in measuring the water content of solid food, stool, and most important of all, evaporative water losses. Certain of these problems do not exist in the critically ill patient because there is no food intake and GI function is frequently absent. On the other hand, the presence of fever creates uncertainty about the estimate of evaporative losses. However, measurements have been carried out that make it possible to use realistic estimates.[6]

While 1,000 ml per 24 hours is generally accepted as the normal evaporative loss via skin and airway in an afebrile ambulatory patient, the figure is lower in patients restricted to bed. A value of 600 to 750 ml would be more accurate and while airway humidification might be expected to lower this further, it is not a major factor since two-thirds to three-quarters of the water loss is via the skin rather than the airway.[9] Febrile patients obviously have increased losses but measurements have been carried out at different temperatures.[6] Evaporative losses are not as dramatic as had been expected. In an air-conditioned environment, losses are still less than 2L/day in the usual febrile patient.[6] Major burns are the only important exception on a surgical service and the unique problems posed by such patients have been documented repeatedly.

The most serious limitation associated with measurements of water balance or body weight changes relates to sequestration of fluid in areas of injury or inflammation. These losses can be extensive and will contribute to weight gain or a positive water balance. Unfortunately, they cannot be measured and the physi-

cian's approximation based on the clinical situation is required.

Since sequestration is often a factor some estimate of *functional* volume becomes important. Plasma volume is the only clinically available volume measurement but it has been of limited value. Clinical evaluation of the patient is essential and certain signs point to the existence of abnormalities in body fluid volume. The cardiovascular system is the most sensitive indicator and a central venous pressure below 3 cmH_2O, tachycardia, and even orthostatic hypotension all indicate a volume deficit. Excess volume is the more common problem following resuscitation; increased venous pressure, increased cardiac output, a gallop or an increased pulmonary second sound, pulmonary congestion, or sometimes even edema are well-recognized signs of volume overload.[10]

The central nervous system may provide information in some patients. Apathy, decreased deep tendon reflexes, obtundation, or coma provide evidence of fluid deficit but isotonic excesses have little effect on central nervous system function. While tissue signs have long been used to assess the state of hydration they are slow to develop and require marked deviations from normal to become manifest.

Sodium and Potassium Concentration

Sodium is the major osmotically active substance in extracellular fluid and the basic sodium values in a 70 kg man are listed in Table 21-1. Osmolality can be measured directly but few clinicians are comfortable with either the results or the interpretation. Serum sodium level represents a reliable guide, provided that glucose or urea levels are not markedly elevated. Hyponatremia is common in critically ill patients and a variety of causes may be involved. Generally speaking, hyponatremia reflects loss of sodium or accumulation of water or a combination of the two. Dilutional hyponatremia will occur after any major injury or operation and is self-correcting when the diuresis of recovery takes place. While antidiuretic hor-

TABLE 21-1. Average Sodium Values for a 70 kg Man

Body composition	
Total body sodium	4,000 mEq
Exchangeable sodium	2,800 mEq or 40 mEq/kg
	250 mEq or 3.5 mEq/kg
Intracellular	1,600 mEq or 23 mEq/kg
Extracellular	
Balance	
Intake	100 mEq/day (or 6 g NaCl)
Output	80 mEq/day urine
	10 mEq/day stool
	10 mEq/day evaporation
Concentration	
Plasma	138–142 mEq/L
Cell	8 mEq/L
CSF	130 mEq/L

mone is undoubtedly involved in this response, inappropriate secretion has not been considered to be a major factor in surgical patients.

Internal shifts of ions also play a role in hyponatremia. The mechanisms designed to limit sodium penetration or accumulation in cells require energy and can easily be disturbed. The movement of sodium into cells will lower ECF sodium concentration.[13]

Infusion therapy is also a factor and the confidence that physicians have in the ability of the kidney to correct improper fluid replacement, while justified in the uncomplicated surgical patient, is misplaced in the critically ill. Most IV solutions are hypotonic in terms of salt content, especially in the case of dextrose and water. The dilutional effects of aminoacids, mannitol, salt-free albumin, and intravenous fat must also be considered. Such concerns are of great importance in critically ill or septic patients because large volumes of fluid are needed to support the circulation and additional (usually hypotonic) fluid is administered with medications and for nutritional support.

Potassium has many contrasts to sodium. The most important one is the difference is our ability to quantitate its concentration. We sample extracellular fluid for both sodium and potassium determinations. However, sodium is primarily an extracellular ion and measurements are reliable. Since potassium is intracellular, our sample is not a good reflection of true potassium concentration. This is shown in Table 21-2 which points out that of the ap-

proximately 4000 mEq potassium, only 60 mEq are in the extracellular fluid. This means that serum potassium values are meaningful only at the extremes of the concentration range. In other words, levels below 3 mEq/L or above 6 mEq/L provide a clear message. However, values between those figures, whether above or below normal, cannot be interpreted without careful study of the clinical situation. While the extracellular portion of total body potassium is small, it is important in neuromuscular and cardiac function. Symptoms may range from mild muscular weakness and paresthesias to flaccid paralysis. However, such problems are rare unless serum levels fall below 3 mEq/L. The cardiovascular effects of potassium are of special importance. Hypotension, bradycardia, and arrhythmias may result from low potassium levels and the diagnosis is usually made by the characteristic electrocardiographic (ECG) findings. T waves will be flat or inverted with depressed S-T segments and usually there will be prominent U waves. The ECG changes are especially important because they will often antedate low serum potassium values. Patients receiving digitalis are at special risk because low levels of potassium will accentuate or bring on digitalis toxicity.

Hyperkalemia is far less common and almost always indicates some degree of renal failure. The major concern, as with hypokalemia, is with cardiac function and similar findings of hypotension and bradycardia may be seen. Arrhythmias, especially ventricular fibrillation, are more common with high potassium levels and cardiac arrest may take place. Once

TABLE 21-2. Average Potassium Values for a 70 kg Man

Body composition	
Total body potassium	3,800 mEq
Exchangeable potassium	3,300 mEq or 46 mEq/kg
	3,240 mEq or 45 mEq/kg
Intracellular	60 mEq or 1 mEq/kg
Extracellular	
Balance	
Intake	80 mEq/day
Output	70 mEq/day urine
	10 mEq/day stool
Concentration	
Plasma	3.6–5.0 mEq/L
Cell	140 mEq/L
CSF	3 mEq/L

again, the ECG will herald these problems and the characteristic manifestations include peaked T waves, depressed S-T segments, prolonged P-R intervals, diminished P waves, and widened QRS complexes.

Potassium levels are affected not only by exogenous potassium but also by release of this ion from cells as the result of direct or catabolic injury. Acidosis has the same effect in that potassium competes with hydrogen ion in the exchange with sodium that takes place in the renal tubule.[7] Accelerated loss of cellular potassium results in movement of hydrogen ion into the cell. This also plays a role in metabolic alkalosis, which cannot be treated without potassium replacement.

FLUID AND ELECTROLYTE ABNORMALITIES

A rational approach to the management of fluid and electrolyte abnormalities requires that they be subdivided into manageable components. Despite their complexity, all derangements have three components: volume, concentration, and composition. As a rule two or even three patterns coexist in the same patient but management is clarified when they are considered individually. The order in which the three patterns are listed here reflects priorities as they exist in the body. The body will always defend volume over concentration or composition and the clinician must keep these priorities in mind when correcting complex derangements. Volume abnormalities are at the top of the list and will be considered first.

Abnormalities of Volume

Our ability to replace volume losses rapidly has had the desired effect in that volume deficits are now unusual in the critically ill patient. That ability has also made volume over-load the most common clinical disorder in the postoperative or postinjury patient. Management of such patients in the intensive care unit (ICU) requires that the clinician review the intake and output records associated with resuscitation and surgery. These figures should be checked against the weight change that has taken place since most patients (or their families) can give a preoperative or preinjury weight that can be contrasted with the weight recorded in the ICU, which will inevitably be greater. In other words, there has been an increase in total body water and some effort to quantitate this change is needed.

When we studied a consecutive series of patients presenting to our emergency room in shock, resuscitation according to standard guidelines resulted in a positive water balance in all patients. However, the positive balance[5] varied from 2.8 to 9.0 L. Diuresis is expected but is not inevitable and failure to excrete these large fluid loads constitutes an important threat to the critically ill patient. The hope that excess salt water will be excreted by the kidneys automatically is not realistic. The change in tonicity of extracellular fluid space allows the kidney to retain or excrete water and electrolytes as needed.

As a rule, resuscitation is characterized by an isotonic expansion of the extracellular fluid compartment because of the nature of the fluids employed. Such solutions do not affect the osmolality of the extracellular space, so no net shifts between compartments take place. Even more important, the usual laboratory measurements cannot detect or quantitate the excess. Serum electrolyte concentrations will be normal in isotonic expansion and there are no clinical tests to measure compartment volumes. Plasma volume measurement is certainly possible but normal values recorded for healthy volunteers are meaningless in a critically ill patient. Since body weights and water balance measurements represent the only approach, attention to these admittedly troublesome parameters is essential.

It is important to recognize that resuscitation is not the only problem. Volume abnormalities can be made worse during the patient's stay because the hormonal environment of the critically ill patient promotes water retention. A further and often insidious gain in weight is possible especially once the circulation is thought to be stabilized and attention is directed to other areas. Long-term mechanical ventilation may also contribute to water retention by stimulating volume receptors in the right atrium.[15]

While precise resuscitation can minimize a positive water balance, it will not abolish the problem of the fluid-overloaded patient. Fluid restriction can often be more severe than generally appreciated because of the excess water present, but in most patients oliguria will soon limit this approach. As a rule diuretics will be needed; furosemide and ethacrynic acid inhibit tubular reabsorption of sodium and are sufficiently potent that a diuresis can be stimulated even in the presence of renal hypoperfusion. Since body weight and water balance measurements do not distinguish between extracellular fluid that is sequestered as opposed to circulating, care must be taken to avoid using diuretics when the oliguria is due to unrecognized hypovolemia. A single intravenous dose of 50 to 100 mg represents an adequate amount of either agent. While dosages have been increased to far higher levels in oliguric patients this is not necessary when dealing with volume overload in patients who continue to have functioning kidneys. The goal is to achieve weight loss greater than the 200 to 400 g of tissue lost due to catabolism.

Albumin has been employed in an effort to mobilize excess fluid as a first step in renal excretion.[11] Unfortunately, the impaired capillary function characteristic of the sickest patients have limited the usefulness of this technique. Since albumin infusions often increase fluid intake, the balance that they create may be positive rather than negative and such efforts are becoming less commonplace.

Volume deficits require only brief mention because they are usually recognized and effec-

TABLE 21-3. Volume of Gastrointestinal Secretions (ml/day)

Gastric	2,500
Small intestine	3,000
Saliva	1,500
Pancreatic	700
Bile	500
Total	8,200

TABLE 21-4. Composition of Gastrointestinal Secretion (mEq/L)

	Na	K	Cl
Gastric	60–80	8–10	80–100
Small intestine	100–110	4–6	80–120
Saliva	10–12	20–28	10–12
Pancreatic	135–145	4–6	60–80
Bile	140–150	4–6	80–110

tively treated. Intestinal suction or fistulas may be responsible; Tables 21-3 and 21-4 provide information regarding losses and therefore the kind of replacement that might be required. The varying electrolyte content of the individual secretions should be noted since losses of potassium, hydrogen, and chloride are of special importance in acid–base balance.

Abnormalities of Concentration

SODIUM

Hyponatremia is the most common electrolyte abnormality seen on a surgical service. While hyponatremia may result in clinical signs, such signs have received little attention since the advent of the flame photometer which provides rapid and accurate information regarding the sodium ion concentration. Even though abnormalities of volume are more critical to body function than concentration, the ease of measuring sodium as opposed to the patient's volume status has given undue emphasis to this parameter.

The frequency with which hyponatremia is encountered should not be allowed to obscure the fact that it usually represents an error in management. While adrenal insufficiency or inappropriate secretion of antidiuretic hormone will result in hyponatremia, these are not usually responsible for the low serum sodium values seen in surgical patients. Rather, the problem relates to the loss of isotonic fluids and their replacement with dextrose and water or electrolyte solutions that are hypotonic. While proper management of IV fluid replacement will minimize hyponatremia, the critically ill patient does have certain problems that tend to drive down serum sodium levels. Free water is introduced into the ECF by oxidation of endogenous tissues (water of oxidation) and while this is only 200 to 250 ml a day in a normal state it is far greater in a catabolic patient. More than 1L of salt-free water may be produced from the oxidation of 1 kg fat, while 750 ml cellular water may be mobilized following the oxidation of 1 kg lean body mass. Hydrated protein contains between 73 and 82 percent water. In a severely catabolic patient, 750 g tissue may be catabolized daily and thereby produce approximately 500 ml free water.[10]

Another factor that contributes to hyponatremia was pointed out by Edelman and his co-workers.[3] Body potassium is an important and predictable determinant of daily changes in serum sodium concentration. Edelman expressed the relationship between sodium, potassium, and body water in the following way:

$$\text{Serum Na}^+ = K \times \frac{\text{total Na}^+ \text{ and total K}^+}{\text{total body water}}$$

This equation explains the tendency of critically ill patients to develop hyponatremia in the face of sodium retention. Hyponatremia is usually not due to a decreased quantity of sodium but the result of increases in total body water as well as potassium losses. The latter is hard to quantitate but is inevitable in depleted, septic, or badly injured patients. At times only vigorous potassium replacement will correct a persistent hyponatremic state.

The danger that hyponatremia poses is not so much in the ECF but in the intracellular compartment. Since the body will not allow osmotic gradients across the various compartments, water has to move into cells to preserve this equilibrium. This results in swelling of the cells and functional consequences in the bowel wall (ileus), the lung (decreased compliance), and, most importantly, the brain because it is enclosed in a confined space.

Water intoxication requires special consideration even though it is simply an extreme form of hyponatremia. It may occur when isotonic fluid losses are replaced by electrolyte-free solutions such as 5 percent dextrose and water. Actually physicians are well aware of this danger and this is no longer the usual mechanism. Rather, free water is introduced in other ways such as patients who drink liquids in large amounts or receive numerous tap water enemas. A sudden drop of the serum sodium concentration to below 120 mEq/L will produce symptoms, even though much lower levels have been recorded in patients whose hyponatremia took place over days or weeks. Correction can be gradual with isotonic solutions but if the patient exhibits confusion, muscle twitching seizures, or other CNS symptoms, more rapid correction with hypertonic saline is required. Although one can estimate the sodium deficit by multiplying the patient's estimated total body water by the difference between the observed and normal serum sodium concentration, it is not necessary to give this amount all at once. Half the deficit should be provided and given rapidly until the symptoms subside. At that point replacement should be with isotonic saline while one monitors the serum sodium concentration.

Hypernatremia is rare in critically ill patients and is inevitably iatrogenic. The one exception would be a major burn, where evaporative water loss will result in severe hypernatremia unless corrective measures are taken. More common causes relate to overly zealous salt replacement or poorly monitored nutritional support. It is worth remembering that hyperosmolar coma, which aroused great concern in the early days of total parenteral nutrition (TPN), was first described in a patient receiving tube feedings.[16] The hyperglycemia is dramatic but these patients are also hypernatremic. This is the more serious problem because insulin administration will control the elevated blood sugar level. The only way to deal with the hypernatremia is to administer free water (dextrose and water despite the high blood sugar) but it is important to realize that an expansion of extracellular fluid will follow.

POTASSIUM

Potassium has an intracellular concentration about 30 times greater than its plasma level. Maintenance of this differential requires metabolic energy-consuming activity by the cell membrane. For that reason injury, sepsis, and other factors that affect energy metabolism frequently result in the loss of cellular potassium. When this loss takes place, sodium will move into the cell to preserve osmotic equilibrium. There is little relationship between the concentration of potassium in the cell and in the plasma, making it difficult to diagnose potassium deficits. This means that the clinician must evaluate the patient to document either a low intake or increased losses of potassium. Outside the hospital setting, low intake may be associated with poor nutrition or alcoholism. When patients are hospitalized the problem may be aggravated by use of potassium-free intravenous solutions. Increased losses are often related to the GI tract whether vomiting, tube suction, or diarrhea. Bile has a potassium level, and this may at times be an overlooked route of loss. Pancreatic fistulas are sufficiently dramatic that these losses are usually recognized.

The kidneys may be an equally important route of loss. This is often the result of overenthusiastic use of diuretics but may also reflect steroid administration or a form of renal failure.

At times low serum potassium levels will be recorded without actual loss of potassium from the body. Alkalosis will result in a shift of additional potassium into the cells and a similar situation will arise when glucose-based TPN is administered.

The major clinical problem in this area relates to the difficulty in diagnosing a potassium deficiency. The surgeon must be alert to the factors in the patient's history or management that have been mentioned above. At times it is necessary to follow ECG changes or monitor urinary losses in addition to the serum concentration. The greatest danger of a low potassium state is its effect on the heart, with bradycardia and hypotension. The ECG changes are extremely important since they are thought to reflect intracellular rather than plasma levels. Muscle weakness is also characteristic and this includes both skeletal and smooth muscle. Some instances of persistent paralytic ileus will not resolve until potassium repletion has been accomplished.

Hyperkalemia is not complicated by the need to differentiate between plasma and total body levels because total body potassium cannot be increased if renal function is adequate. Obviously impaired renal function is the major cause of hyperkalemia and once again the heart is of major concern. Treatment should focus on the underlying cause but temporary measures are often employed if serum levels are dangerously high. Dextrose and insulin have been used to transport potassium into the cells as a temporary expedient until renal function improves or dialysis can be instituted. If acidosis is present, correction of this abnormality will result in a prompt drop in serum potassium levels. The close relationship between potassium and acid–base balance will be further discussed in the next section.

Acid–Base Abnormalities

The diagnosis of acid–base abnormalities has been greatly simplified by the availability of blood gas electrodes and a variety of systems have been introduced to aid in analysis of the underlying abnormality. This is especially important in the critically ill patient because the classic clinical syndromes are modified by special techniques used in treating organ failure.

It is worth looking at the concepts and terms currently in use in order to understand the laboratory data routinely provided to clinicians. Contemporary acid–base theory defines an acid as a substance that can denote a hydrogen ion; *pH* represents the concentration of free hydrogen ions in solution. The actual pH value is inversely proportional to the concentration of hydrogen ions in solution. The addition of strong acid to water will obviously lower the pH, but the presence of buffers will modify this effect.

In vivo, the pH values are held in the normal range primarily by maintaining plasma concentration of two substances: HCO_3 at 24 mmol/L and CO_2 near 1.2 mmol/L. This represents a 20:1 ratio of HCO_3 to CO_2 and while this buffer pair is but one of many in the plasma it has special physiologic importance because the body is able to control the concentrations of these substances independently. Pulmonary control of PCO_2 and the renal excretion of bicarbonate allow adjustment of both numerator and denominator; survival is dependent on these control mechanisms except over very short time periods when other buffers may play a role. Probably the most important role played by the other buffers consists of protection against sudden respiratory failure, which would cause an abrupt rise in pH. These buffers buy time since renal compensation requires many hours to be effective.

Analysis of any acid–base problem requires a detailed knowledge of the clinical situation but specific management depends on examination of the blood. The clinician wants to know three things about the patient: the pH of the blood, the role of the lung, and some quantitative estimate of the amount of nonvolatile (sometimes called fixed) acid or base present. Electrodes measure pH directly, making it possible to diagnose acidosis or alkalosis and, most importantly, to quantitate the severity of the abnormality. Electrodes designed to measure PCO_2 provide information on the role that the lung is playing in the disturbance. However, there is no way in which the nonrespiratory constituents in any abnormality of acid base composition can be measured in the direct way that can be applied to pH and PCO_2. Because the $HCO_3 : CO_2$ buffer pair exercises such a dominant role in acid–base homeostasis the plasma bicarbonate concentration is a useful index of the extent of accumulation of excess nonvolatile acid or base, but it does not constitute a quantitative measure.

For that reason much work has been expended in an effort to combine with the evaluations of arterial pH and PCO_2 an accurate estimate of the nonrespiratory component.[4] One of the first systems was derived by Van Slyke and called the CO_2 combining power. More recent variables based on CO_2 titration of whole blood have included the buffer base of Singer and Hastings, the standard bicarbonate of Jorgensen and Astrup, and the base excess of Astrup and Siggaard-Andersen. All of these derived measurements share a common objective, which is to compensate for errors that arise when one attempts to evaluate the accumulation of nonvolatile acid or base in the whole body from a blood sample that reflects only the vascular compartment.

Base excess is the derived variable that has been in use for the past few years. It represents the amount of acid or base needed to bring the HCO_3 of the blood sample to 25 mmol/L. The titration is carried out at a PCO_2 of 40 mmHg, the normal value, and since it is expressed in terms of mEq/L of blood it is theoretically possible to estimate how much mineral acid or alkali has to be given to achieve a neutral pH. In practice, this makes little sense because carbon dioxide titration of blood in vitro is not equivalent to the situation in the body, where multiple extravascular compartments contribute to buffering capacity. Therefore measurements of base excess or deficit should be regarded as an index rather than a measure of nonvolatile acid or base. No effortless rules can be applied; rather, the information made available by comprehensive acid–base analysis of blood must be applied in accordance with the patient's clinical problems.

Acidosis is the most alarming problem facing the critically ill patient because of its effects on the cardiovascular system. Decreased myocardial contractibility results in a decreased cardiac output. When this is coupled with decreased vasomotor responsiveness, severe hypotension will result. The most common cause of acidosis is poor tissue perfusion with accumulation of lactic acid but pulmonary insufficiency (carbon dioxide retention) is also a common problem. Less devastating causes include diabetic acidosis, loss of alkali from the gastrointestinal tract, and impaired renal function.

Respiratory acidosis in the postoperative period is readily correctable provided the clinician is aware of the problem. Unlike patients with carbon dioxide retention due to chronic pulmonary disease, postoperative patients require only improved alveolar ventilation. The solution may be as simple as an adjustment in pain medication or it may require intensive pulmonary therapy. Mechanical ventilation remains the last resort.

A variety of metabolic disorders result in acidosis. The kidneys normally regulate acid–base balance by resorption of bicarbonate and excretion of inorganic acids such as phosphate and sulfate. Abnormalities of renal function may prevent these adjustments and accumulation of acids may take place. Body buffers are able to limit acutal pH changes but if there is a rapid rise in potassium or total body water, these factors will pose an immediate threat to the patient.

When acidosis is due to poor perfusion,

resuscitation and restoration of the circulation is uniformly effective. Diabetic acidosis can also be corrected but the clinician should be aware that injury and the changes in intermediary metabolism brought about by severe catabolism will greatly complicate diabetic management.

Alkalosis may be less common but is certainly more difficult to correct than acidosis. A major factor is the overadministration of sodium-containing solutions in the initial management of the patient. This would include both sodium bicarbonate and sodium lactate. Transfused blood may also result in alkalosis, even though the pH of blood is low, by conversion of citrate to bicarbonate. Renal correction should correct such problems, but the required renal sodium excretion will not take place if there is impaired renal function.

Loss of acid from the stomach may result in alkalosis and the associated potassium depletion creates a special problem. Renal correction suffers since normally dependent sodium retention and increased renal potassium excretion override the ability of the kidneys to excrete bicarbonate and retain hydrogen ions to restore acid–base equilibrium. As losses of gastric secretions continue, the kidneys attempt to maintain intravascular volume and osmolality by retaining sodium. This results in increased potassium excretion in the urine and the urine is often acidic despite the patient's alkalotic state. The condition has been referred to as paradoxic aciduria and further aggravates the alkalotic state.[14]

The treatment of metabolic alkalosis is frustrating and the best advice would be to focus on preventing it. Once the condition is established, everyone is aware that vigorous potassium replacement is essential. The need for volume replacement must be stressed and it is important to avoid the common error of using lactated Ringer's solution. Instead, sodium chloride is needed and once vascular volume has been restored, tubular reabsorption of sodium will decrease making it possible for the kidneys to excrete excess bicarbonate. It is also necessary to specify the nature of the potassium supplementation. Potassium chloride should be used since potassium citrate or lactate will result in increased bicarbonate. Potassium replacement must be substantial and

may require ECG monitoring. It is often necessary to give 200 to 300 mEq potassium chloride in a 24 hour period in patients with refractory metabolic alkalosis.

Loss of alkali can take place from the kidney as well as the GI tract. This is common in critically ill patients because of the widespread use of diuretics. Adequate potassium replacement is also of value in this situation. The use of dilute hydrochloric acid to combat alkalosis directly has become less common over the years. This reflects not only the unavailability of commercial preparations suitable for IV use but also, and more importantly, a better understanding of the mechanisms underlying refractory alkalosis. This has made it possible to treat the underlying disturbance rather than simply the pH abnormality.

Acid–base problems have traditionally been considered in terms of metabolic, respiratory, and mixed disturbances as well as a variety of compensated or partially compensated states. While these classifications are still of value it is probably more useful to focus on specific abnormalities that can be identified and treated using modern systems of blood analysis and clinical evaluation of the patient. It is important to avoid excessive reliance on laboratory values; careful and repeated examination of the patient is essential. Furthermore, biologic systems react primarily to rate of change rather than absolute concentrations so abnormalities can be treated at a rate similar to their rate of development. Such clinical considerations must be taken into account in caring for the critically ill patient.

REFERENCES

1. Earley LE, Daugharty TM: Sodium metabolism. N Engl J Med 281: 72, 1969
2. Edelman IS, Liebman J: Anatomy of water and electrolytes. Am J Med 27: 256, 1959
3. Edelman IS, Liebman J, O'Meara MP, Birkenfeld LW: Interrelations between serum sodium concentration, serum osmolality and total exchange-

able sodium, total exchangeable potassium and total body water. J Clin Invest 37: 1236, 1958

4. Gump FE: Acid–base disturbances. In Berk JL (ed): Handbook of Critical Care. Little Brown, Boston, 1982

5. Gump FE, Kinney JM, Iles M, Long CL: Duration and significance of large fluid loads administered for circulatory support. J Trauma 10: 431, 1970

6. Gump FE, Kinney JM, Long CL, Gelber R: Measurement of water balance—a guide to surgical care. Surgery 64: 154, 1968

7. Hills AG: Acid–base Balance. Williams and Wilkins, Baltimore, 1973

8. Kleeman CR, Fichman MP: The clinical physiology of water metabolism. N Engl J Med 277: 1300, 1967

9. Kuno Y: Human Perspiration. Charles C Thomas, Springfield, Ill., 1956

10. Miller TA, Duke JH: Fluid and electrolyte management. In Dudrick SJ (ed): Manual of Preoperative and Postoperative Care. WB Saunders, Philadelphia, 1983

11. Poole GU, Meredith JW, Pennell T, et al: Comparison of colloids and crystalloids in resuscitation from hemorrhagic shock. Surg Gynecol Obstet 154: 577, 1982

12. Schrier RW, Leaf A: Effects of hormones on water sodium chloride and potassium metabolism. In Williams RH (ed): Textbook of Endocrinology, ed 6. WB Saunders, Philadelphia, 1981

13. Shires GT, Canizaro PD: Fluids, electrolyte and nutritional management of the surgical patient. In Schwartz SI (ed): Principles of Surgery, ed 3. McGraw-Hill, New York, 1979

14. Skillman JJ: Disturbances of body fluids, ions and acid–base balance. In Skillman JJ (ed): Intensive Care. Little Brown, Boston, 1975

15. Sladen A, Laver MB, Pontoppidan H: Pulmonary complications and water retention in prolonged mechanical ventilation. N Engl J Med 279: 448, 1968

16. Wilson WS, Meinert JK: Extracellular hyperosmolarity secondary to high protein nasogastric tube feeding. Ann Intern Med 47: 585, 1957

22

Management of Acute Renal Failure After Trauma

William M. Stahl

INTRODUCTION

Acute renal failure can be defined as a rapid decrease in previously adequate renal function, to levels that do not maintain stable or normal body chemistry. The onset of acute renal failure in critically ill patients is an indicator of a worsening of the state of illness and an indicator of a diminished chance of survival. With improved physiologic support of the injured patient or with the patient undergoing a major operation, pure hemorrhagic shock is rarely a cause of acute renal failure. Most patients now seen with acute renal failure have a combination of severe tissue injury and sepsis. The prognosis in such patients is necessarily guarded because of their underlying illness and because of the added metabolic insult of renal failure itself. Survival in such patients has not improved significantly over the past 20 years, despite advances in general supportive care, especially in the quality of dialysis

and nutritional support. This lack of improvement can be ascribed to the more critical state of illness in patients who now develop renal failure after tissue injury.[116]

INCIDENCE

The rate of occurrence of acute renal failure in critically ill surgical patients is related to several factors: diagnosis, age, severity and duration of hypotension and shock, type of operative procedure, amount of tissue injury, and the presence or absence of sepsis. In one study, acute renal failure occurred in 20 percent of 475 admissions to a general intensive care unit. These patients came from a total of 57,000 admissions to a general hospital.[129] A study of

719

the incidence of acute renal failure in the general population revealed an annual rate of 4.8 to 5.7:100,000 population, with a male/female preponderance[36] of 1.6. Renal failure occurring in young healthy individuals subjected to major trauma due to war injuries has been reported in 1:600 such patients.[127] Risk factors clearly include advanced age; presence of systolic hypotension; specific diagnostic categories including aortic surgery, cardiovascular surgery, burns, and biliary disease with jaundice; the presence of sepsis, predominantly abdominal and pulmonary; and the administration of nephrotoxic drugs, including antibiotics and contrast agents.

PATHOPHYSIOLOGY

It is obvious that acute renal failure results from injury to renal cells. The precise nature of this injury is gradually being clarified. Knowledge of the cellular damage is far from complete, however, and puzzling questions remain. Some of these relate to the fact that some patients develop renal failure without an equal degree of failure of other vital organs, whereas in other patients simultaneous failure of multiple organs seems to occur, or other organs fail initially followed by renal failure. It is generally believed that a similar cellular insult occurs in all tissues of the critically ill patient. The functional results, however, appear different in different settings.

In general, the injury to renal cells can be described as ischemic and toxic. This results from reduced blood flow and oxygen delivery, coupled with exposure to toxic material administered to the patient or manufactured by damaged local cells or other organ systems.

Ischemic Injury

Renal ischemia is produced when blood flow to the kidney decreases due to a severe fall in perfusion pressure, or from intense vaso-constriction. Such vasoconstriction is usually part of a general increase in total peripheral resistance as a response to a decrease in cardiac output. Alterations in systemic and intrarenal blood flow distribution occur in states of hepatic failure and sepsis diverting flow from the renal cortex. Direct interruption of renal arterial flow with suprarenal aortic or renal artery clamping, and removal of the kidney during renal transplantation produce total ischemia.

The cellular response to acute ischemia has been studied extensively. Oxygen deprivation appears to affect predominantly structures in the renal cortex, including glomerular capillary cells and the pars recta of the proximal renal tubule. Various segments of the nephron may be injured more easily than others but clearly an interruption of one vital portion of the nephron unit may cause failure of the entire nephron. Renal cell energetics seem to be affected more rapidly than those in cells of other organs, such as liver or heart, and renal tissue adenosine triphosphate (ATP) levels fall to 22 percent of normal within 2 minutes of renal artery interruption.[58,60,121] After 15 minutes ATP levels decrease further to 13 percent of control and lactate levels rise to 11 times normal.

The cell damage that results depends on the duration of the ischemic insult. Ischemia of 25 minutes or less at normothermia results in mild injury that is reversible.[121] Forty to 60 minutes of ischemia produces more severe damage with some recovery occurring over a period of 2 to 3 weeks. Forty minutes of ischemia in experimental animals caused loss of vascular control and the production of focal segmental necrosis in muscle cells and tubular endothelium.[86] Sixty minutes of ischemia in the rabbit kidney has been shown to decrease fluid transport in the proximal convoluted tubule to approximately 20 percent of normal and to produce back leakage in the medullary tubules.[55]

Cellular injury may continue to occur after restoration of systemic pressure and flow. Renal blood flow does not return to normal following resumption of circulation after a period of ischemia (the so-called "no reflow" phenomenon). Animal studies show that after an ischemic insult renal blood flow remains reduced by as much as 50 percent for many hours.[7] This interference with the resumption of normal renal blood flow distribution potentiates ischemic injury with further damage to glomerular cells and tubular epithelium.[12] Micropuncture studies have shown that a vascular abnormality persists even after restoration of normal blood pressure and flow in the intact animal and that this is due to increase in afferent arteriolar resistance.[33]

The cause of this lingering vasoconstriction has not been clearly proved. The most likely explanation is that an increase in proximal tubular sodium and chloride content occurs due to failure of function of tubular cells, and this increase stimulates vasoconstriction of the afferent arteriole via feedback through the juxtaglomerular apparatus.[132,134] This vasocontriction, plus damage to glomerular cells causing loss of surface area for filtration,[12] results in a profound fall in glomerular filtration rate which is perpetuated even after blood flow is restored (Fig. 22-1).

Tubular obstruction by hyaline, granular, and pigmented casts is found in animal models of acute renal failure due to ischemia. Such obstruction of the tubular lumen also contributes to the lack of excretion of filtrate in the ischemically damaged kidney.[28,43] Biopsies of human patients during acute renal failure have shown similar changes with collapsed glomeruli, alteration in tubular cells with necrosis and loss of the brush border, and tubular casts.[61] Ultrastructural studies of tubular cells show a profound decrease in luminal surface area due to loss of the brush border and other alterations of the cell surface that could lead to a decrease in sodium chloride filtration.

Other factors also potentiate ischemic injury in the kidney as in other organs. Failure of prostacyclin synthesis by glomerular endothelial cells has been suggested.[32,125] Intracellular increase in calcium concentration has also been postulated as a potentiating mechanism for cell injury both in systemic cells and in renal cells. Intracellular calcium has been shown to increase by 50 percent after 1 hour of renal ischemia.[120]

In summary, it appears that renal ischemic produced by vasoconstriction, hypotension, or arterial interruption causes a progressive lesion in glomerular and tubular cells that worsens with time. After resumption of blood flow, a varying degree of circulatory insufficiency persists. Cellular injury may continue depending on local factors related to cell integrity and

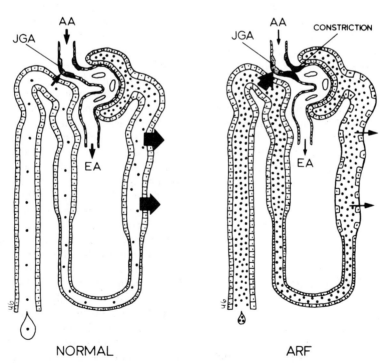

NORMAL   ARF

FIG. 22-1 Tubuloglomerular feedback. Failure of proximal absorption due to tubular cell injury produces feedback afferent arteriolar constriction.

on tubuloglomerular feedback phenomena potentiating the abnormal blood flow state.

Toxic Injury

The effect of toxic substances on renal cells has been studied in a variety of classic models, most of which are not directly applicable to the critically ill patient. Specific toxins such as aminoglycocides and contrast agents appear to affect renal blood flow and tubular function in a manner somewhat similar to ischemic injury. Renal failure in the critically ill patient usually occurs following the onset of sepsis and this lesion has not been well clarified in terms of renal cell functional integrity. All body cells suffer a metabolic insult in the presence of sepsis, manifested by impairment of function, cell swelling, and shift to anaerobic metabolism with production of lactic acidosis. Progressive renal damage occurs with oliguria in the presence of normal or even supranormal renal blood flow.

A fall in the cellular levels of ATP occurs rather rapidly after the administration of a variety of nephrotoxic substances,[119] but decrease in ATP levels alone may not cause renal failure without direct membrane injury. The persistance and aggravation of cell injury in toxic renal damage is thought to be due to a tubuloglomerular feedback mechanism similar to that in renal ischemic damage, with failure of flow to cortical glomeruli.[59,99] Similarly, interference with postaglandin synthesis may also contribute to lingering vasoconstriction and/or alteration in intrarenal blood flow distribution in septic states.

DIAGNOSIS

Attention is usually directed to the possibility of renal failure when urine output falls below normal levels, approximately 0.5 ml/kg/ hr, or when serum creatinine levels increase above the normal range. Primary attention should be directed toward the general state of the patient, especially to evaluate potential causes of prerenal failure. Thus, evidence of adequate cardiac output and circulating fluid volume must be obtained by the usual physical examination and monitoring methods. In addition, careful exclusion of causes of postrenal failure due to urinary tract obstruction must be carried out. Most renal failure occurring in hospitalized patients is due to intrinsic renal disease of the toxic/anoxic variety.[29]

Initial examination in a patient who is suspected of having acute toxic/anoxic renal failure should be directed toward examination of the urine. The urinary sediments in most patients with acute renal failure of this type are highly characteristic,[73] and usually contain numbers of tubular epithelial cells with cellular and granular pigmented casts. Pre- and postrenal acute renal failure states usually do not show significant changes in the urinary sediment.

Examination of the urine content of solute and of free water and the concentration of creatinine and urea is also very valuable. In the case of prerenal acute renal failure, the oliguric patient will excrete a concentrated urine. The ratio of urine to plasma concentration of solute will be high, thus the urine to plasma ratio of osmolality will be greater than 1.1, the urine to plasma ratio of urea will be greater than 10, and the urine to plasma ratio of creatinine will be greater than 2.5. If these ratios fall below these levels in the oliguric patient, renal damage is usually present. Renal sodium excretion is also a useful measurement, since the prerenal azotemic patient will be maximally conserving sodium, and the urinary sodium will usually be below 20 mEq/L. However, the damaged nephron will leak an increased amount of sodium into the urine thus raising the urine sodium concentration above 20 mEq/L.

The renal failure index[54] is an expression that combines these two tests, the urinary sodium content and the urine to plasma creatinine ratio, by dividing the urinary sodium concentration by the urine to plasma creatinine ratio. This index is approximately 1 in normal individuals. Use of the renal failure index can usually differentiate prerenal oliguric patients from those with acute renal failure.[39] Patients with acute renal failure have a renal failure index greater than 1. In the difficult case where there is a question between a prerenal oliguric patient normally conserving sodium and water, and a patient with acute renal failure, a careful test of volume expansion and/or increase in cardiac index by cardiotropic drugs can be tried while one monitors cardiac preload and function.

METABOLIC EFFECTS

When patients with tissue injury or sepsis develop acute renal failure, it is difficult to determine precisely which metabolic alterations are due to the underlying disease and which are due to the onset of renal failure. Metabolic alterations in chronic renal failure in humans have been studied extensively over the past 15 years. It is thought that these alterations reflect adaptation to a chronic state and that the studies of chronic renal failure cannot be transposed directly to the acute renal failure patient. Other information has come from experimental acute uremia produced in animal models, but there may be certain species differences. Thus, although it seems quite clear that the acute onset of the uremic state in a patient who already has serious disease produces additional metabolic defects, the precise nature of these defects is still not completely understood.

Certain abnormalities are clearly related to the inability to excrete water and solute and the direct results of build up of these substances in the plasma (Table 22-1). In the predialysis period the signs of uremia included overhydration and hyperkalemia as obvious results of the inability to excrete water and potassium. Such occurrence should now be controlled or reversed by adequate dialysis. Metabolic acidosis was frequently a serious problem in the predialysis period, due in part to the inability to excrete fixed acids, and in part to a more basic metabolic disturbance.

Other cellular malfunctions leading to malnutrition, gastrointestinal hemorrhage, and susceptibility to invasive infection clearly represent complicated responses to alterations in the internal milieu, the result of "uremic toxins."

The most consistent cellular abnormality detected is failure of active membrane sodium pumping, a function that utilizes ATP and requires sodium/potassium ATPase. Several studies have shown diminution in membrane transport with fall in sodium/potassium ATPase in uremic patients.[20,31] Decrease in activity of the membrane transport system decreases transmembrane potential,[2] with resulting alterations in intracellular/extracellular transport of ions and water.[136] With active sodium transport impeded, intracellular water, sodium, and chloride will increase, and potassium will leak from the cell. The few studies that have been done on intracellular composition and transmembrane potential indicate that the decrease in membrane potential is clearly related to the degree of uremia. Cotton and co-workers[31] reported that the potential difference remained normal until the creatinine clearance rate fell below 6.3 ml/min. Below that level, it was demonstrated that intracellu-

TABLE 22-1. Abnormalities Produced by Filtration Failure and Tissue Catabolism with Production of Fixed Acids

Abnormality	Effect
Metabolic acidosis	Intracellular acidosis Cerebral dysfunction Nausea, vomiting
Retention of nitrogen compounds and toxins	Decreased membrane transport Decreased cell energetics Insulin resistance
Overhydration	Hypotonicity Hyponatremia Cardiac overload Tissue edema
Hyperkalemia	Membrane instability Cardiac arrhythmias
Hypophosphatemia Hypocalcemia	Decreased cell energetics
Insulin resistance Glucose intolerance	Interference with substrate utilization

All abnormalities are improved by nutritional support and adequate dialytic therapy.

lar water and sodium content increased and potassium content decreased. Dialysis improved these abnormalities and returned the potential difference to normal. Bergstrom et al.[16] studied 15 patients with acute renal failure and found that 50 percent showed such abnormalities, with elevated levels of intracellular water and sodium. The rest showed normal levels of intracellular electrolytes. Studies[130] of experimental animals rendered acutely uremic indicate that intracellular electrolyte and water patterns remain normal over the first 24 hours. It would thus appear that cellular membrane transport mechanisms may be maintained for some time following the onset of acute renal failure, and are related to the level of renal function and the amount of abnormal substances accumulating in the blood.

The relationship of transmembrane potential alterations, clinical symptoms, and the production and excretion of uremic toxins was studied by Cotton et al.[31] These authors demonstrated that patients showed gastrointestinal symptoms of nausea, vomiting, and anorexia at the same point at which membrane potential alterations occurred: at a creatinine clearance rate below 6 to 7 ml/min. Reduction of dietary protein intake from 1.0 to 0.5 g/kg/day and the administration of essential amino acid mixtures improved both the symptoms and the muscle membrane potential defect in five of these six patients. These authors concluded that a dialyzable toxin that interfered with cellular ion transport seemed the most likely cause. They believed that this toxin derived from dietary protein and that increased endogenous protein catabolism occurring in the hypermetabolic state would clearly have a similar effect.

An abnormality in cellular function occurring relatively early in uremia is failure of cell reproduction. It has been shown[81] that cell division in the jejunal mucosa is decreased in the experimental animal when plasma urea concentrations reach 100 mg/dl. Similar alterations have been shown in red blood cells,[25] fibroblasts,[80] and esophageal epithelial cells.[79] Cell division and growth are clearly vital to maintenance of gastrointestinal mucosal integrity and to the satisfactory healing of wounds.[92] These alterations in cell function are reversed by adequate dialysis.

The level of resting energy expenditure in patients with acute renal failure has been extremely difficult to determine because most patients are acutely ill and the energy expenditure is more related to the underlying illness than to the acute renal failure. Bluemle et al.[24] studied eight patients in acute renal failure after gynecologic procedures and determined the daily caloric expenditure to be 2,405 calories. Studies by Feinstein et al.[42] also indicate that acute renal failure patients are hypercatabolic and require more than normal protein and calorie support. The energy requirements measured in their study averaged 50 kcal/kg/day. While this is approximately 50 percent greater than the requirement of unstressed persons, it is in the range of the hypercatabolic response to trauma and sepsis in patients who do not have renal failure. Thus, it is not clear whether acute renal failure in patients who are under stress adds significantly to the energy requirement.[126]

In general, it is thought that energy expenditure can be calculated for patients in acute renal failure using formulas similar to those for stressed patients without renal failure. The usual formula used estimates the energy requirement in calories per day as the basic metabolic requirement, multiplied by 1.25, multiplied by a stress factor, which for the severely injured or septic patient is equal to 1.3 to 1.55. Thus, a 70 kg individual with a basic metabolic requirement of 1694 calories, in acute renal failure with multiple trauma or severe infection, would utilize approximately 3176 calories, while an 80 kg individual with a basic metabolic requirement of 1872 calories would utilize approximately 3510 calories.[126]

Measurements of the "stress hormones", glucagon, catecholamines, and cortisol have shown that serum levels of these hormones increase markedly in patients with acute renal failure.[21,38,47] A recent study in human volunteers subjected to an infusion of levels of these hormones characteristic of the stress state showed that the experimental subjects developed hypermetabolism, negative nitrogen balance, and insulin resistance.[19] Increase in circulating levels of these hormones is undoubtedly due to several factors. First, many of these hormones are degraded as well as excreted by the kidney and decrease in metabolic clearance rates occurs in renal failure.[37] Also, clearance by tissue uptake appears to be impaired.[100] To complicate the picture there are questions regarding the value of the assay of circulating hormones in acute renal failure patients since heterogeneity of the molecules has been found, and the bioactivity of some of these substances is not known.[70]

Metabolic acidosis often occurs rapidly in patients with acute renal failure due to the hypercatabolic state. The increased metabolism of substrate releases more fixed acid, including sulfate, phosphate, and other organic anions. Failure of renal excretion of these fixed acids produces metabolic acidosis. Multiple adverse affects can occur from acidosis alone, including symptoms of nausea, vomiting, and cerebral dysfunction. The potentially harmful effects of severe acidosis include insulin resistance with interference in carbohydrate utilization, and a decrease in intracellular enzyme activity, especially phosphofructokinase with reduction in glycolysis.[102]

One of the major alterations in general body metabolism in acutely uremic patients appears to be a defect in carbohydrate metabolism with the development of insulin resistance. Studies by Kokot and Kuska[69] have shown that patients with acute renal failure are unable to metabolize glucose normally. In response to a glucose infusion, insulin levels were excessive and plasma disappearance was prolonged. This study suggested that insulin resistance in the tissues was the cause of the abnormality. Mondon and co-workers found a decrease in the insulin-enhanced uptake of glucose by muscle mass in the acutely uremic rat.[89] The role of hepatic gluconeogenesis in the uremic subject has not been clarified. Studies by Riegel and Stepinski and co-workers indicate that hepatocytes from acutely uremic rats show lower glucose production using pyruvate as a substrate, but unchanged glucose production from dyhydroacetone or serine.[104,105] The exact role of glucagon in altering hepatic gluconeogenesis has not been clarified.[90]

Water and mineral balance in acute renal failure patients is altered with the production of hyponatremia and hyperkalemia. Some of this alteration occurs[24] due to the hypercatabolic state of these patients, with release of endogenous tissue water in amounts up to 400 ml/day. Failure of the sodium pump, with intra-cellular sodium movement and leak of potassium, may occur. Also, release of large amounts of potassium results from the endogenous metabolism of protein. Acidosis itself can increase the leak of potassium into the extracellular fluid. The administration of hypertonic solutions with increase in extracellular tonicity induces water to flow from the cell into the extracellular fluid, bringing with it a certain amount of potassium due to solvent drag.[84] Hyperkalemia itself can stimulate release of catecholamines[64] and insulin.[106]

Disorders of calcium and phosphorus metabolism occur rapidly in the patient with acute renal failure. Hyperphosphatemia occurs for two major reasons; first, excretion of phosphorus in the urine is inadequate, and second, leak of phosphates from the intracellular locations occurs with cell injury, the rapidity and magnitude of the leak depending upon the degree of cell destruction. Patients with massive muscle damage such as that which occurs with crush injury or rhabdomyolysis[76] can show elevation of the serum phosphorous concentration to as high as 21 ml/dl. In the absence of major muscle destruction, hyperphosphatemia usually does not exceed 8 mg/dl. Elevations of phosphorus above this level in a patient without obvious tissue destruction may indicate undetected necrotic tissue masses.

Hypocalcemia occurs rapidly in these patients. In 10 patients studied by Massry et al., hypocalcemia, hyperphosphatemia, hypermagnesemia, and elevated levels of parathyroid hormone occurred in the oliguric phase.[85] In these patients, the fall in calcium occurred within the first 2 days. These authors found that the level of calcium bore little relationship to the phosphorus levels but was inversely proportional to the levels of parathyroid hormone. Also, there were no direct parallels with changes in magnesium. Protein binding of calcium did not change and therefore the level of ionized calcium was low. Other authors have more closely related the fall in serum calcium to the rise in serum phosphate,[62] and it would appear that the increase in parathyroid secretion is secondary to this hypocalcemia.[68]

Animal studies have shown that during the first few days of renal failure calcium is deposited in the tissues, including brain and muscle.[8,87] Calcium administered to animals in the acute uremic state deposited nine times as rapidly as normal in injured skeletal muscle.[87] This deposition of calcium in the muscle is dependent on parathyroid hormone.[124] Intracellular calcium levels rise under these conditions.[51] It has been demonstrated that increase in the concentration of calcium within cells may aggravate and potentiate cellular injury.[40] It would seem extremely important, therefore, not to administer extra calcium to patients in acute renal failure unless symptoms occur related to the level of hypocalcemia. Fortunately, this rarely occurs. In addition, the monitoring of the need for dialysis by measuring levels of serum phosphate would appear wise, since correction of the hyperphosphatemia can be achieved by this means and calcium abnormalities can be ameliorated.

Disturbances of other endocrine glands in the acute renal failure patient have not been well documented, although there is a large literature on patients in chronic compensated renal failure. Possible abnormalities may occur due to alteration of cellular response to specific hormones, to secretion of abnormal hormones, to overproduction of hormones in response to the alterations of uremia, and to diminished metabolism or excretion due to failure of renal cell function. Human growth hormone responses to insulin injection were found to be abnormal in patients with acute renal failure,[69] their response being three times greater than normal. Plasma renin activity and aldosterone levels are significantly elevated above the normal value in the renal failure patient. Elevation of parathyroid hormone levels and elevation of glucagon have been previously mentioned. In addition, levels of 1, 25-dihydroxy vitamin D3 are below normal and apparently aggravate the prevailing hypocalcemia.[76]

The search for the precise toxic substance(s) that produce these abnormalities in clinical uremia has continued for the past 50 years. Many substances originally suspected as the toxic elements have now been clearly shown not to be the cause of this syndrome. These include ammonia, creatinine, guanidine, indican, phenols, and urea. Uremic symptoms do not correlate with levels of blood urea nitrogen (BUN), phenol, guanidine, or creatinine except in a general way.[94] Attempts to isolate toxic substances from dialysis fluid continue

to suggest phenolic derivatives, aliphatic and aromatic amines, and guanidines as suspicious substances.[103] Red blood cell abnormalities appear to be caused by abnormally elevated levels of creatine, guanidinobutyric acid, and guanidinopropionic acid.[63] These compounds are capable of interfering with glucose 6-phosphate dehydrogenase, and thus interfering with the hexose monophosphate shunt.[18]

Even with intensive study the problem of identifying the precise uremic toxin resolves itself into a combined multifactorial one. As stated by Balestri and co-workers in 1970, "uremia is a syndrome resulting from the combined toxic affect of many (probably all) the metabolites retained because of renal failure. Each of them is likely to cause only a group (more or less important) of symptoms which, altogether result in the clinical syndrome of uremia."[11]

As previously reported, the mortality of acute renal failure occurring in the posttrauma or septic patient remains in the 40 to 50 percent range in spite of modern treatment techniques. This undoubtedly reflects the severity of the underlying illness. It also points up the extreme importance of preventing renal failure whenever possible. Since the injury to the kidney results from an anoxic and toxic insult, the prevention or reversal of anoxic and low flow states is critical to survival of the kidney and preservation of adequate function. Homer Smith showed in 1939 that renal blood flow responds with great sensitivity to circulating endogenous catecholamine, exogenous catecholamine, and decrease in cardiac index.[113] In these studies he demonstrated that hypovolemia with normotensive hypoperfusion resulted in a reduction in renal blood flow of over 50 percent (due to compensatory vasoconstriction), while mean arterial pressure remained in the normal range. This points up the absolute necessity of adequate monitoring of the traumatized or septic patient, using indices of perfusion rather than blood pressure levels. These studies also showed the effect of pyrogen on renal hemodynamics and renal tubular fluid flow.[113]

Lessons to be learned from these studies, and from others confirming them in subsequent years, are as follows. First, the trauma victim must be aggressively resuscitated with appropriate fluids to an adequate perfusion state.

This means monitoring indices of adequate cardiac index to ensure the completeness of resuscitation, rather than using blood pressure as an index. Arterial pressure may reach normal levels while a deficit in blood volume exists and cardiac index remains abnormally low. Invasive monitoring may be needed to measure cardiac preload, venous oxygen content, and cardiac output. Urine output is of value when time permits. Second, the condition of patients undergoing elective surgical procedures must be optimized prior to the traumatic insult of the operation. This includes adequate sedation to prevent fright and endogenous catecholamine release; adequate hydration to bring the patient to the operating room with an appropriate cardiac index, good renal blood flow, and a high tubular fluid flow; physiologic anesthesia; a minimally traumatic operative procedure; and adequate fluid replacement for blood loss and loss of extracellular fluid into the environment or third space. Monitoring of urine output throughout the procedure and adjustment of fluid therapy is vital. Third, the damaging effects of continuing sepsis have been demonstrated many times over. Aggressive therapy of the septic process by surgical drainage and appropriate antibiotic administration is vital. Until the septic process is controlled, renal cells will continue to suffer injury from toxins released from the infected area.

TREATMENT

Diuretics

Uncertainty still exists concerning potentially beneficial effects of diuretics in patients at risk for acute renal failure. Theoretically, diuretic agents could prevent or ameliorate renal tubular cell injury in a variety of ways. Both mannitol and loop diuretics are vasodilators under some conditions.[22,23] Furosemide has been shown to inhibit tubuloglomerular

feedback and possibly thus break the vasoconstrictor cycle.[133] Increase in tubular fluid flow may prevent tubular obstruction and thus maintain filtration and urine flow. Dilution of toxic molecules in the tubular fluid may ameliorate direct damage to the brush border of tubular cells. Osmotic swelling of tubular cell may be reduced by the action of an extracellular solute such as mannitol (Table 22-2).

A variety of animal studies have shown that diuretics protect the kidney when exposed to ischemic or toxic insult. Selkurt, in 1945, first showed that infusion of mannitol before total occlusion of the renal artery in dogs prevented anuria.[109] Most laboratory series since that time have shown protection by pretreatment with mannitol.[56,135] Recent studies have suggested that mannitol provides slightly more protection than furosemide.[56,135]

Diuretic therapy has been suggested for patients in three different situations: first, prophylactically to prevent acute renal failure in high risk situations; second, in incipient renal failure to test for the responsiveness of the kidney, or to perhaps ameliorate the renal cell damage; and third, to influence the course of established renal failure (Table 22-3).

Reported series utilizing mannitol and the loop diuretics, furosemide, or ethacrynic acid in high risk situations, such as open heart surgery, aortic surgery, and major trauma, have generally been uncontrolled and not prospective. It is thus extremely difficult to evaluate whether any improvement in renal function, or reduction in incidence of acute renal failure, is in fact due to the diuretic therapy or due to improved fluid management in general. Although the protective effects of diuretic agents remain essentially unproven, many surgeons use prophylactic infusions during open heart surgery or aortic surgery. The use of prophylac-

TABLE 22-2. Action of Diuretics in Acute Renal Failure

Diuretic	Effect
Mannitol	Must be filtered. Osmotic effects reduce tubular water resorption
Loop diuretics (ethacrynic acid, furosemide)	Need not be filtered. Act on tubular cells reducing sodium and water resorption

TABLE 22-3. **Effectiveness of Diuretics in Acute Renal Failure (ARF)**

Diuretic	Effect
Prophylactic	Not proved in patients with surgical or other trauma or hemorrhagic shock Valuable in: Patients with jaundice Contrast media Hemoglobinemia Nephrotoxic drugs (Amphotericin, Cisplatinum) ? Hyperuricemia
Amelioration of ARF (early therapy)	Lower mortality if diuresis occurs (? patient selection by drug, or real benefit)
Therapy of established ARF	Production of diuresis may decrease need for dialysis. No improvement in survival

tic diuresis in patients who are in mild renal failure or whose renal reserve is limited is generally accepted.[114]

The use of diuretic therapy to diagnose and/or reverse early acute renal failure has many adherents. Most investigators agree that diuretic therapy early in the course of clinical oliguric renal failure reverses the oliguria in about two thirds of the patients.[13,66,110,117] The change from oliguric to nonoliguric renal failure is also thought to indicate an improved prognosis and a lesser renal injury.[9,34,65] The use of diuretic agents seems to lessen the incidence of posttransplant oliguria.[3,78] However, as discussed by Levinsky et al., it is very difficult to tell whether the diuretic agents improved the state of the kidney or whether the patients who responded had a lesser degree of injury.[74]

Diuretic agents have also been tried in the treatment of established acute renal failure. At times, large doses of loop diuretics, such as 2,000 mg furosemide daily, have been used. Most studies have shown that diuresis may in fact be produced and that the need for dialysis may be slightly reduced, but that mortality remains unchanged. Levinsky, in summarizing 19 such studies, indicated that "the evidence against a beneficial effect of diuretics on patient survival is impressive."[74] This is similar to our opinion, and in our patients massive doses of diuretics following the diagnosis of acute renal failure are no longer employed. The spontaneous occurrence of nonoliguric renal failure as opposed to oliguric renal failure, however, does imply an improved prognosis.[5,88]

Once the diagnosis of renal failure has been made and a trial of diuretic therapy fails to produce urine flow, the treatment plan must include all measures required to continue maximal therapy for the underlying disease state, plus specific measures directed to provide support of the hypercatabolic patient, and to institute aggressive and adequate dialytic therapy.

Nutritional

Nutritional support of the stressed patient with acute renal failure follows the basic principles of surgical nutrition. The special problem is in providing adequate calories and nitrogen in a restricted volume of water to avoid fluid overload and hyponatremia. Protein must be administered to maintain neutral nitrogen balance. Additional protein may be needed because of losses due to dialysis. Sodium intake should balance sodium output unless water and sodium abnormalities exist in the patient. Potassium, calcium, magnesium, and phosphate levels must be monitored and adequate amounts administered to maintain normal serum concentrations. The need for caution in administering large amounts of calcium has already been mentioned. Insulin may be needed to control hyperglycemia.

The route of administration of nutritional support depends upon the condition of the patient and the ability of the gastrointestinal tract to function. If the patient can eat, oral feeding is the preferable route. If the patient cannot eat and the gastrointestinal tract is functional, nasogastric tube, gastrostomy, or jejunostomy feeding may be utilized. If gastrointestinal absorption is inadequate, intravenous nutrition must be instituted.[126]

Wesson et al. classified patients with acute renal failure into three groups depending on clinical characteristics: mild catabolism was found in acute renal failure due to drug toxicity, blood transfusion, and nontraumatic or septic events; moderate catabolism was found in patients following elective surgery with or without infection; and severe catabolism occurred in patients with renal failure associated with severe injury, burns, and sepsis. Patients in the mild category usually showed excess nitrogen loss of approximately 2 g/day, required at least 100 g carbohydrates, and very often could be managed conservatively without dialysis or prolonged nutritional support. The moderate group was seen to produce excess nitrogen, at a rate of 3 to 10 g/day. Nutritional support was usually required for these patients. Carbohydrates were needed for 60 to 70 percent of the total requirement and essential amino acids were required. In the severe group requirements often exceeded 3,000 calories per day and carbohydrate intake was needed for up to 60 to 100 percent of the energy requirement. Insulin was occasionally needed for control of hyperglycemia. Essential amino acids, 10 to 20 g/day, were required and dialysis was routinely needed on a frequent basis.

Guidelines for dietary therapy in acute renal failure indicate that all intake should be administered with a high percentage of glucose calories utilizing many satisfactory sources of carbohydrates. Protein should average 40 g/day. In patients who are markedly catabolic, protein intake must reach 1 to 1.5 g/kg/day. Supplementary vitamins should be administered. Gastrointestinal tube feedings can utilize a variety of prepared diets that include essential amino acids and glucose, to which electrolytes, minerals, and vitamins can be added. Fat emulsion or medium chain triglycerides can also be added. Some patients in renal failure cannot tolerate feedings into the stomach because of problems of gastric emptying but can tolerate feedings directly into the upper jejunum through a tube passed beyond the pylorus or through a jejunostomy. The sickest patients require intravenous nutritional support. Because of fluid limitations, concentrated solutions of up to 50 to 70 percent dextrose and 8.5 percent amino acid solution are frequently required. Intravenous fat emulsion can supply more calories per volume and may be needed on a frequent basis, especially in patients who become hyperglycemic due to insulin resistance. Several recent publications have indicated various treatment regimens for maintaining the nutritional integrity of the acute renal failure patient.[1,10,17,41,46,72,98]

Dialysis

It is widely accepted at present that dialytic therapy should be instituted and maintained at a level to prevent the occurrence of clinical uremia.[53,107] With rare exceptions, this means hemodialysis. The value of early and aggressive dialytic therapy in survival from acute renal failure has been debated since the 1960 publications of Teshan[118] and Scribner[108] urged aggressive dialysis. In subsequent years, clinical series have suggested benefits from dialysis designed to maintain relatively normal conditions as compared to dialysis to correct severe uremia. Kleinknecht reported a series of 500 patients, comparing a group of 279 patients treated prior to July 1968 and dialyzed only when urea levels reached 350 mg/dl, to a group of 221 patients treated after July 1968 and dialyzed to maintain the BUN below 200 mg/dl. This series, although sequential in nature, revealed a reduction in mortality in the surgical patients from 54 percent in the early group to 38 percent in the later group. The improvement was due to a decrease in the incidence of septicemia and gastrointestinal bleeding.[67]

Fisher and colleagues[44] similarly showed a decrease in mortality from 77 to 51 percent when dialysis was used to maintain the BUN below 150 mg/dl rather than 200 mg/dl. Parsons and co-workers reported similar results.[97] In the only prospective randomized study of posttrauma patients with renal failure, Conger was able to show a significant difference between the group aggressively dialyzed to maintain the BUN below 70 ml/dl and the serum creatinine below 5 mg/dl, as opposed to the "routine" group in which dialysis was instituted when the BUN reached 150 mg/dl or the creatinine reached 10 mg/dl. The mortality in the aggressively dialyzed group was 37 percent, and was 80 percent in the "routine" group.[30]

The difference in mortality in these two groups was primarily due to reduction in the incidence of septicemia and hemorrhage in the aggressively dialyzed group. In 1981, Rainford reported improved survival (71 percent), combining daily hemodialysis and total parenteral nutrition in 85 patients whose predialysis BUN level was maintained below 200 mg/dl. A previously treated group of 246 patients, also treated with daily dialysis and TPN whose predialysis BUN was above 200 mg/dl, showed a 58 percent survival rate. In Rainford's first group of 221 patients treated with interval dialysis and no nutritional support, only 42 percent survived. Again, it is difficult to describe the improvement to more aggressive dialysis since other factors of improvement may very well have been operating.[101]

Indications for dialysis therefore certainly should include the prevention of uremic signs and symptoms. Most authorities agree that dialysis should be instituted at BUN levels[53,107] of 80 to 100 mg/dl and creatinine levels of 8 to 11 mg/dl. The value of very aggressive dialysis with reduction of creatinine levels to 4 to 5 mg/dl as suggested by Congers remains to be proved. This author believes that this should be the goal.

Hyperkalemia remains an absolute indication for aggressive therapy. As mentioned, dialysis should be instituted before hyperkalemia occurs. However, in certain states of extreme catabolism or widespread muscle damage due to crush injury or ischemia, potassium may be liberated from injured cells into the plasma at a very rapid rate. Nondialytic means of reducing the serum potassium, such as the administration of hypertonic glucose and insulin intravenously, should be carried out immediately if potassium rises above 6 mEq/L or at lower levels if ECG changes occur. Cation exchange resins may be used to slow the rise in potassium while dialysis is being made available. Peritoneal dialysis can be used if hemodialysis is not immediately available. However, re-

moval of potassium by peritoneal dialysis rarely exceeds 12 mEq/hr and cation exchange[27] resin enemas may remove up to 30 mEq/hr. If extreme muscle injury is present and the potassium levels are rising rapidly, urgent hemodialysis is required.

Fluid overload is another frequent indication for hemodialysis, in which cases ultrafiltration of excess water should also be used. This may prove extremely valuable in the edematous septic patient. Hemodialysis by diffusion may be performed coincidently with ultrafiltration, or they may be used sequentially with good effect in some patients. The sequential use of ultrafiltration seems to produce less rapid metabolic and fluid volume disturbances and allows removal of up to 1 L/hr of excess fluid.[105] Continuous slow ultrafiltration using a small unit activated by the patient's arterial blood pressure has been used successfully to remove large quantities of fluid slowly over many hours.[96] Access to the vascular system in acutely ill patients can usually be achieved by the use of single needle catheterization in a major vein. This technique, however, may not always provide for adequate dialysis of at least 250 ml/min. Recirculation may be a problem. Double needle access may be required in hypercatabolic patients. In patients with established renal failure, the creation of an arteriovenous shunt may be necessary.

Peritoneal dialysis is an attractive possibility, since technically it is much simpler and can be instituted without the need to set up complicated equipment. In general, peritoneal dialysis is about 20 percent as effective as hemodialysis, and it will not provide a sufficiently high clearance rate to maintain acceptable biochemical levels in the hypercatabolic patient. It can be used for short periods while arrangements for hemodialysis are being made.

Drug Administration

Pharmacokinetics describe the relationship between the dose of a drug given and the blood level achieved. *Pharmacodynamics* describes the response of the organism to a given drug concentration in the plasma. Both of these functions are altered in the acute renal failure patient. Since intestinal absorption may be diminished, the effect of orally administered drugs cannot be predicted with certainty. In most surgical cases, due to the basic underlying illness, gastrointestinal alimentation is not available and the intravenous route must be used for drug administration. This removes the problems of impaired absorption and gives direct access to maintenance of a serum level using adjustments in dosage.

The bioavailability of a drug depends on the metabolism or alteration of the drug as it circulates through various organs, especially the liver. Some drugs are inactivated rapidly with up to 50 to 80 percent of the administered dose being altered by a single pass through the liver.[4] In uremia, bioavailability may be increased, because of a decrease in hepatic function and reduction of the first pass inactivation percentage.

The distribution of a drug in the body is determined by such factors as protein binding and lipid solubility. Alterations of these factors also occur in the acute renal failure patient, changing the distribution patterns of certain drugs. The accumulation of acid metabolites may decrease protein binding of acidic drugs due to competitive displacement. Also, changes in drug-binding sites on albumin may alter its affinity for certain drug molecules. Even the net effect of decreased albumin binding is not clear. On one hand, the increased amount of free drug should enhance the pharmacologic action. But, conversely, increased amounts of free drug may lead to greater and more rapid clearance from the body through residual renal function and/or dialysis. Reduction in the rates of drug metabolism in the kidney can clearly be related to renal cell disfunction. The activity of liver enzymes may also be reduced, interfering with drug metabolism in the liver as well.[6,52,75]

A major alteration in pharmacokinetics in acute renal failure is impaired elimination of drugs by the kidney. In general, renal excretion of drugs follows first-order kinetics and the amount of drug eliminated per unit of time is proportional to the level in the plasma. As the rate of excretion declines, the half-life of the drug within the plasma increases. This in turn produces an increasing level of drug in the serum if the usual administration schedules are followed, and may produce toxic overdose. Drugs that are excreted unchanged in their active form most clearly demonstrate this phenomenon. These include aminoglycoside antibiotics, digoxin, penicillins, tetracyclines, methotrexate, and ethambutol.[4]

Other drugs undergo transformation, with the production of drug metabolites that may in turn have bioactivity. These drug metabolites can also accumulate when excretory rates fall. Other untoward effects secondary to drug administration may occur in the patient with renal failure. Some patients become sensitive to central nervous system depressants and seem to have an increased response to normal dosages. This may be due to diminished protein binding of hypnotic drugs but also may be due to uremic alteration of the blood–brain barrier.

Alteration of serum electrolytes can occur due to the inadvertent administration of large amounts of cation when antacids or antibiotics are given. The amount of magnesium, sodium, and potassium that can be administered by this route is significant, and overdose with cation is a distinct risk.

To complicate further the problem of drug administration in the renal failure patient, dialysis removes many drugs along with other ions, and may thus rapidly change serum levels (Table 22-4). Commonly used drugs that are rapidly cleared by hemodialysis include aminoglycosides, cephalosporins, penicillins, and sulfonamides as well as procainamide and cimetidine. Digoxin and propranolol, on the other

TABLE 22-4. Clearance of Commonly Used Drugs by Dialysis

High Clearance	Low Clearance
Aminoglycosides	Cloxacillin
Penicillin G	Dicloxacillin
Carbenicillin	Cefazoline
Ticarcillin	Cefamandole
Amoxicillin	Vancomycin
Cephalothin	Clindamycin
Cephaloridine	Erythromycin
Cephaloxin	Digoxin
Water-soluble vitamins	Propranolol
Lithium	Lidocaine
Procainamide	Quinidine
	Phenytoin
	Insulin

hand, are changed very little by dialysis,[45,77] except for slight prolongation of the maximum period of action. Dialysis has little effect on insulin levels.[93] Although clearance rates are lower with peritoneal dialysis, drugs removed by hemodialysis are also removed by peritoneal dialysis, but at a slower rate.[50]

It is clear that proper administration of needed drugs to achieve appropriate therapeutic levels is a complex process in the patient with diminished renal function. In patients with acute renal failure secondary to trauma and sepsis, drug administration may be one of the most vital therapeutic requirements. Reference to publications containing detailed information on each drug should be made, and frequent blood levels obtained, in order to treat such patients optimally.[14,15,26,57,128]

New Approaches

In recent years drugs have been sought that might ameliorate the cellular injury produced by the ischemic and toxic insult to the kidney. Dopamine has been used to decrease renal vascular resistance and increase renal blood flow.[82,83] Clinically, the use of dopamine in incipient renal failure enjoys popularity. The precise effect on outcome is unknown. Other vasoactive agents investigated in animal models include isoproterenol, bradykinin, and various prostaglandins. A recent study of vasodilator drugs in the dog model indicated, however, that systemic effects predominated over renovascular effects, and the net result of administration of such drugs was usually a decrease in renal blood flow.[91] Human studies utilizing renal vasodilators after the onset of acute renal failure have shown an increase in renal blood flow, but no clinical improvement.[35,71,122,137]

Substances that are theoretically able to support cell energetics have also been studied experimentally. Administration of adenine nucleotide–$MgCl_2$ has been tried in an attempt to minimize cell injury and enhance cell survival. The administration of ATP-$MgCl_2$ improves results in animal models even when given after the renal insult.[111] This is true in a variety of experimental models of both ischemic and toxic renal injury.[48,112] The exact mode of action of ATP-$MgCl_2$ is not well understood. It is generally believed that ATP cannot pass cell membranes and thus it is not clear whether this substance enters the cell or interacts with the membrane. Alternatively, this substance may diminish adenine catabolism and thus reduce adenosine production, with reduction in the vasoconstriction that adenosine can produce.[95] Clinical studies have not been done with this substance. Nucleotides and magnesium chloride pose certain problems due to their vasoactivity.

Recognition of the damaging effects of increased intracellular calcium has led to studies on the use of calcium blocking agents, especially verapamil, on the damaged kidney. Experimental studies of the effect of verapamil in pre- and posttreatment of the ischemic injury model suggest that amelioration of the renal insult may be achieved by this method.[49,123] This may be due to prevention of mitochondrial injury.[131] Pharmacologic protection of some type appears to be the best hope for improved results in the future.

REFERENCES

1. Abel RM, Beck CH Jr., Abbott WM et al: Improved survival from acute renal failure after treatment with intravenous essential L-amino acids and glucose. N Engl J Med 288: 695, 1973
2. Akaike N: Operation of an electrogenic sodium pump in mammalian red muscle fibre. Life Sci 14: 141, 1974
3. Anderson CF, O'Kane HO, Shorter RG et al: Use of diuretic agents during oliguria after renal transplantation. Surgery 67: 249, 1970
4. Anderson RJ: Drug prescribing for patients in renal failure. Hosp Pract 145, 1983
5. Anderson RJ, Linas, SL, Berns, AS et al: Nonoliguric acute renal failure. N Engl J Med 269: 1134, 1977
6. Anderson RJ, Schrier RW (eds): Clinical Use of Drugs in Patients with Kidney and Liver Disease. WB Saunders, Philadelphia, 1981
7. Arendshorst WJ, Finn WF, Gottschalk CW:

Pathogenesis of acute renal failure following renal ischemia in the rat. Circ Res 37: 558, 1975

8. Arieff AI, Massry SG: Calcium metabolism of brain in acute renal failure. J Clin Invest 53: 387, 1974

9. Baek SM, Brown RS, Shoemaker WC: Early prediction of acute renal failure and recovery: II. Renal function response to furosemide. Ann Surg 178: 605, 1973

10. Baek SM, Makaboli GG, Bryan-Brown CW et al: The influence of parenteral nutrition on the course of acute renal failure. Surg Gynecol Obstet 141: 405, 1975

11. Balestri PL, Biagini M, Rindi P, Giovannetti S: Uremic toxins. Arch Intern Med 126: 843, 1970

12. Barnes JL, Osgood RW, Reineck HJ, Stein JH: Glomerular alterations in an ischemic model of acute renal failure. Lab Invest 45: 378, 1981

13. Barry KG, Malloy JP: Oliguric renal failure: evaluation and therapy by the intravenous infusion of mannitol. JAMA 179: 510, 1962

14. Bennett WM: Altering drug dosage in patients with diseases of the kidney and liver. p. 16. In Anderson RJ, Schreier RW (eds): Clinical Use of Drugs in Patients with Kidney and Liver Disease. WB Saunders, Philadelphia, 1981

15. Bennett WM, Muther RS, Parker RA et al: Drug therapy in renal failure: dosing guidelines for adults. Ann Intern Med 93: 62, 1980

16. Bergstrom J, Bittar EE: The basis of uremic toxicity. p. 495. In Bittar EE, Bittar N (eds): The Biological Basis of Medicine. New York, Academic Press, 1969

17. Bergstrom J, Furst P, Ahlberg M et al: Nutrition in renal failure. In Richards JR, Kinney JM (eds): Nutritional Aspects of Care in the Critically Ill. Churchill Livingstone, New York, 1977

18. Berlyne GM, Shaw AB, Nilwarangkur S: Low protein diet in renal failure. Nephron 2: 129, 1965

19. Bessy PQ, Watters JM, Aoki TT, Wilmore DW: Combined hormonal infusion simulates the matabolic response to injury. Am Surg Assoc 4/25/84, Toronto, Canada

20. Bilbrey GL, Carter NW, White MG et al: Potassium deficiency in chronic renal failure. Kidney Int 4: 423, 1973

21. Bilbrey GL, Faloona GA, White MG, Knochel JP: Hyperglucagonemia of renal failure. J Clin Invest 53: 841, 1974

22. Birtch AG, Zakheim RM, Jones LJ, Barger AC: Redistribution of renal blood flow produced by furosemide and ethacrynic acid. Circ Res 21: 869, 1967

23. Blantz RC: Effect of mannitol on glomerular ultrafiltration in the hydropenic rat. J Clin Invest 54: 1135, 1974

24. Bluemle LW Jr., Potter HP, Elkinton JR: Changes in body composition in acute renal failure. J Clin Invest 35: 1094, 1951

25. Bozzini CE, Devoto FCH, Tomio JM: Decreased responsiveness of hemopoietic tissue to erythropoietin in acutely uremic rats. J Lab Clin Med 68: 411, 1966

26. Brater DC: Handbook of Drug Use in Patients with Renal Disease. Improved Therapeutics, Dallas, 1983

27. Brown ST, Ahearn DJ, Nolph KD: Potassium removal with peritoneal dialysis. Kidney Int 4: 67, 1973

28. Brun C, Munck O: Lesions of the kidney in acute renal failure following shock. Lancet 1: 603, 1957

29. Bushinsky DA, Wish JB, Hou SH et al: Hospital acquired renal insufficiency. Proc Am Soc Nephrol 12: 105A, 1979

30. Conger JD: A controlled evaluation of prophylactic dialysis in post-traumatic acute renal failure. J Trauma 15: 1056, 1975

31. Cotton JR, Woodard T, Carter NW, Nnochel JP: Resting skeletal muscle membrane potential as an index of uremia toxicity. J Clin Invest 63: 501, 1979

32. Dach JL, Kurtzman NA: A scanning electron microscope study of the glycerol model of acute renal failure. Lab Invest 34: 409, 1976

33. Daugharty TM, Brenner BM: Reversible hemodynamic defect in glomeruler filtration rate after ischemic injury. Am J Physiol 228: 1436, 1975

34. Dayton DA, Anderson CR, Tucker RM: Use of diuretics in acute oliguria. The American Society of Nephrology, 1969, Washington, D.C.

35. Dollery CT, Goldberg LI, Pentecost BL: Effects of intrarenal infusions of bradykinin and acetylcholine on renal blood flow in man. Clin Sci 29: 433, 1965

36. Eliahou HE, Modan B, Leslau V et al: Acute renal failure in the community: an epidemiological study. In Friedman EA, Eliahou HE (eds): Proceedings, Acute Renal Failure Conference. Department of Health, Education and Welfare, Publication No. (NIH) 74–608, May 1973

37. Emmanouel DS, Lindheimer MD, Katz AI: Endocrine abnormalities in chronic renal failure: pathogenetic principles and clinical implications. Semin Nephrol 1: 151, 1981

38. Englert E Jr., Brown H, Willardson DG et al: Metabolism of free and conjugated 17-hydroxycorticosteroids in subjects with uremia. J Clin Endocrinol Metab 18: 36, 1958

39. Espinel CH, Gregory AW: Differential diagnosis of acute renal failure. Clin Nephrol 13: 73, 1980

40. Farber JL: The role of calcium in cell death. Life Sci 29: 1289, 1981

41. Feinstein EI, Blumenkrantz MJ, Healy M et al: Clinical and metabolic responses to parenteral

nutrition in acute renal failure. Medicine 6: 124, 1981

42. Feinstein EI, Blumenkrantz MJ, Healy M et al: Clinical and metabolic responses to parenteral nutrition in acute renal failure. Medicine 60: 124, 1981

43. Finckh ES, Jeremy D, Whyte HM: Structural renal damage and its relation to clinical features in acute oliguric renal failure. QJ Med (New Series) 31: 429, 1962

44. Fischer RP, Griffen WO, Reiser M, Clark DS: Early dialysis in the treatment of acute renal failure. Surg Gynecol Obstet 123: 1019, 1966

45. Funkelstein FO, Goffinat JA, Hendler ED, Lindenbaum J: Pharmacokinetics of digoxin and digitoxin in patients undergoing hemodialysis. Am J Med 58: 525, 1975

46. Freund H, Harmian S, Fischer JE: Comparative studies of parenteral nutrition in renal failure using essential and nonessential amino acid containing solutions. Surg Gynecol Obstet 151: 652, 1980

47. Giordano C, Bloom J, Merrill JP: Effect of urea on physiologic systems. I. Studies on monamine oxidase activity. J Lab Clin Med 259: 396, 1962

48. Glazier WB, Siegel NJ, Chaudry IH et al: Enhanced recovery from severe ischemic renal injury with adenosine triphosphate-magnesium chloride: administration after the insult. Surg Forum 29: 82, 1978

49. Goldfarb D, Iaina A, Serban I et al: Beneficial effect of verapamil in ischemic acute renal failure in the rat. Proc Soc Exp Biol Med 172: 389, 1983

50. Golper TA: Drugs and peritoneal dialysis. Dialysis Transplant. 8: 41, 1979

51. Guisado R, Arieff AI, Massry S: Muscle water and electrolytes in uremia and the effects of hemodialysis. J Lab Clin Med 89: 322, 1977

52. Gulyassy PF, Depner TA: Abnormal drug binding in uremia. Dialysis Transplant, 8: 19, 1979

53. Hakim RM, Lazarus JM: Hemodialysis in acute renal failure. In Brenner BM, Lazarus JM (eds): Acute Renal Failure. WB Saunders, Philadelphia, 1983

54. Handa SP, Morrins PAF: Diagnostic indices in acute renal failure. Can Med Assoc J 96: 78, 1967

55. Hanley MJ: Study of isolated nephron segments in a rabbit model of ischemic acute renal failure. Am J Physiol 239-F17, 1980

56. Hanley MJ, Davidson K: Prior mannitol and furosemide infusion in a model of ischemic acute renal failure. Am J Physiol 241, F556, 1981

57. Heel RC, Avery GS: Guide to drug dosage in renal failure. p. 1290. In Avery GS, Graeme S (eds): Drug Treatment—Principles and Practice of Clinical Pharmacology and Therapeutics. ADIS Press, Australia, 1980

58. Hems DA, Bronsnan JT: Effects of ischaemia on content of metabolities in rat liver and kidney in vivo. Biochem J 120: 105, 1970

59. Hollenberg NK, Adams DF, Oken DE et al: Acute renal failure due to nephrotoxins: renal hemodynamic and angiographic studies in man. N Engl J Med. 282: 1329, 1970

60. Jennings RB, Reiner KA: Lethal myocardial ischemic injury. Am J Pathol 102: 241, 1981

61. Jones DB: Ultrastructure of human acute renal failure. Lab Invest 46: 254, 1982

62. Kaplan MA, Canterbury JM, Gavellas G et al: Interrelationships between phosphorus, calcium, parathyroid hormone, and renal phosphate excretion in response to an oral phosphorus load in normal and uremic dogs. Kidney Int 14: 207, 1978

63. Kestenbaum RS, Giat Y, Berlyne GM: The toxicity of guanidino compounds in the red blood cell in uremia and the effects of hemodialysis. Nephron 31: 20–23, 1982

64. Kirpekar SM, Wakade AR: Release of noradrenaline from the cat spleen by potassium. J Physiol 194: 595, 1968

65. Kjellstrand CM: Ethacrynic acid in acute renal failure. The American Society of Nephrology 31, 1968

66. Kjellstrand CM: Ethacrynic acid in acute tubular necrosis. Nephron 9: 337, 1972

67. Kleinknecht D, Jungers P, Chanard J et al: Uremic and nonuremic complications in acute renal failure: evaluation of early and frequent dialysis on prognosis. Kidney Int 1: 190, 1972

68. Koffler A, Friedler RM, Massry SG: Acute renal failure due to nontraumatic rhabdomyolysis. Ann Intern Med 85: 23, 1976

69. Kokot F, Kuska J: The endocrine system in patients with acute renal insufficiency. Kidney Int 10: S26, 1976

70. Kuku SF, Zeidler A, Emmanouel DS et al: Heterogeneity of plasma glucagon: patterns in patients with chronic renal failure and diabetes. J Clin Endocrinol Metab 42: 173, 1976

71. Ladefogel J, Winkler K: Hemodynamics in acute renal failure. Scand J Clin Lab Invest 26: 83, 1970

72. Leonard CD, Luke RG, Siegel RR: Parenteral essential amino acids in acute renal failure. Urology 6: 154, 1975

73. Levinsky NG, Alexander EA, Venkatachalam VK: Acute renal failure. p. 1181. In Brenner BM, Rector FC, Jr. (eds): The Kidney, vol. 1. WB Saunders, Philadelphia, 1976

74. Levinsky NG, Bernard DB, Johnson PA: Mannitol and loop diuretics in acute renal failure. In Brenner BM, Lazarus JM (eds): Acute Renal Failure. WB Saunders, Philadelphia, 1983

75. Levy G: Pharmacokinetics in renal disease. Am J Med 62: 461, 1977

76. Llach F, Felsenfeld AJ, Haussler MR: Pathophysiology of altered calcium metabolism in rhabdomyolysis-induced acute renal failure. N Engl J Med 305: 117, 1981

77. Lowenthal DT, Briggs WA, Gibson TP et al: Pharmacokinetcs of oral propranolol in chronic renal disease. Clin Pharmacol Ther 16: 761, 1974

78. McCabe R, Stevens LE, Subramamian A et al: Reduction of acute tubular necrosis (ATN) by furosemide and steriods in cadaveric kidney recovery. Am J Surg 129: 246, 1975

79. McDermott FT, Nayman J, de Boer WGRM: Epithelial cell division in acute renal failure: a radioautographic study in the oesophagus of the mouse. Br J Surg 58: 52, 1971

80. McDermott FT, Nayman J, de Boer WGRM: Effect of acute renal failure upon wound healing: histological and autoradiographic studies in the mouse. Ann Surg 168: 142, 1968

81. McDermot FT, Nayman J, de Boer WGRM: Effect of acute renal failure upon cell division in the jejunum: radioautographic and ultrastructural studies in the mouse. Ann Surg 174: 274, 1971

82. McDonald RH, Jr., Goldberg LI, McNay JL, Tuttle EP, Jr.: Effects of dopamine in man: augmentation of sodium excretion, glomerular filtration rate, and renal plasma flow. J Clin Invest 43: 1116, 1964

83. McNay JL, McDonald RH, Jr., Goldberg LI: Direct renal vasodilatation produced by dopamine in the dog. Circ Res 26: 510, 1965

84. Makoff DL, Da Silva JA, Rosenbaum BJ: On the mechanism of hyperkalemia due to hyperosmotic expansion with saline or mannitol. Clin Sci 41: 383, 1971

85. Massry SG, Arieff AI, Coburn JW et al: Divalent ion metabolism in patients with acute renal failure: studies on the mechanism of hypocalcemia. Kidney Int 5: 437, 1974

86. Matthys E, Patton MK, Osgood RW et al: Alterations in vascular function and morphology in acute ischemic renal failure. Kidney Int 23: 717, 1983

87. Meroney WH, Arney GK, Segar WE et al: The acute calcification of damaged muscle with particular reference to acute post-traumatic renal insufficiency. J Clin Invest 36: 825, 1957

88. Meyers C, Roxe DM, Hano JE: The clinical course of nonoliguric acute renal failure. Cardiovasc Med 669, 1977

89. Mondon CE, Dolkas CB, Reaven GM: The site of insulin resistance in acute uremia. Diabetes 27: 571, 1978

90. Mondon CE, Reaven GM: Evaluation of enhanced glucagon sensitivity as the cause of glu-cose intolerance in acutely uremic rats. Am J Clin Nutr 33: 1456, 1980

91. Murphy GP, Homsy EG, Scott WW: Evaluation of pharmacologically induced renal vasodilatation. J Surg Res 5: 525, 1965

92. Nayman J: Effect of renal failure on wound healing in dogs: response to hemodialysis following uremia induced by uranium nitrate. Ann Surg 164: 227, 1966

93. Novalesi R, Pilo A, Lenzi S, Donato L: Insulin metabolism in chronic uremia and in the anephric state: effect of dialytic treatment. J Clin Endocrinol Metab 40: 70, 1975

94. Olsen NS, Basset JW: Blood levels of urea nitrogen, phenol, guanidine and creatinine in uremia. Am J Med 10: 52, 1951

95. Osswald H, Schmitz HJ, Kemper R: Tissue content of adenosine inosine, and hypoxanthine in the rat kidney after ischemia and postischemic recirculation. Pflugers Arch 371, 45, 1977

96. Paganini EP, Nakamoto S: Continuous slow ultrafiltration in oliguric acute renal failure. Trans Am Soc Artif Intern Organs 26: 201, 1980

97. Parsons FM, Hobson SM, Blagg CR, McCracken BH: Optimum time for dialysis in acute reversible renal failure. Lancet 1: 129, 1961

98. Pelosi G, Proietti R: Acute renal failure: parenteral nutritition with essential and non-essential amino acids. Nutritional Support Services 2: 22, 1982

99. Pfaller W, Gunther R, Silbernagl S: Pathogenesis of HgCl$_2$ and maleate induced acute renal failure. Pflugers Arch 379: R18, 1979

100. Rabkin R, Unterhalter SA, Duckworth WC: Effect of prolonged uremia on insulin metabolism by isolated liver and muscle. Kidney Int 16: 433, 1979

101. Rainford DJ: Nutritional management of acute renal failure. Acta Chir Scand (suppl) 507: 327, 1981

102. Relman AS: Metabolic consequences of acid–base disorders. Kidney Int 1: 347, 1972

103. Renner D, Heintz R: Cell metabolism in uremia. International Congress of Nephrology, Stockholm, 1969

104. Riegel W, Stepinski J, Horl WH, Heidland A: Effect of hormones on hepatocyte gluconeogenesis in different models of acute uraemia. Nephron 32: 67, 1982

105. Rouby JJ, Rottembourg J, Durande JP et al: Plasma volume changes induced by regular hemodialysis and controlled sequential ultrafiltration hemodialysis. Dialysis Transplant 8: 237, 1979

106. Santeusanio F, Faloona GR, Knochel JP, Unger RH: Evidence for a role of endogenous insulin and glucagon in the regulation of potassium homeostasis. J Lab Clin Med 81: 809, 1973

107. Schrier RW: Acute renal failure: pathogenesis, diagnosis and management. Hosp Pract 16: 93, 1981
108. Scribner BH, Magid GJ, Burnell JM: Prophylactic hemodialysis in the management of acute renal failure. Clin Res 8: 136, 1960
109. Selkurt EE: Changes in renal clearance following complete ischemia of the kidney. Am J Physiol 144: 395, 1945
110. Shalhoub RJ, Velasquez MT, Antoniou LD: Reversal of surgical oliguric states by furosemide or ethacrynic acid. The American Society of Nephrology, 60, 1968
111. Siegel NJ, Glazier WB, Chaudry IH et al: Enhanced recovery from acute renal failure by the post-ischemic infusion of adenine nucleotides and magnesium chloride in rats. Kidney Int 17: 338, 1980
112. Siegel NJ, Meade R, Chaudry IH, Kashgarian M: Amelioration of toxic acute renal failure by infusion of ATP-MgCl$_2$. Pediatr Res 14: 625, 1980
113. Smith HW: Principles of Renal Physiology. Oxford University Press, New York, 1956
114. Stahl WM, Stone AM: Prophylactic diuresis with ethacrynic acid for prevention of postoperative renal failure. Ann Surg 172, 1970
115. Stepinski J, Horl WH, Heidland A: The gluconeogenetic ability of hepatocytes in various types of acute uraemia. Nephron 31: 75, 1982
116. Stott RB, Cameron JS, Ogg CS, Bewick M: Why the persistently high mortality in acute renal failure? Lancet 2: 75, 1972
117. Swartz C, Chinitz J, Onesti G et al: Ethacrynic acid in acute renal failure. IVth International Congress of Nephrology, Stockholm, Sweden, 273, 1969
118. Teschan PE, Baxter CR, O'Brien TF et al: Prophylactic hemodialysis in the treatment of acute renal failure. Ann Intern Med 53: 992, 1960
119. Trifillis AL, Kahng MW, Trump BF: Metabolic studies of HgCl$_2$-induced acute renal failure in the rat. Exp Mol Pathol 35: 14, 1981
120. Trump BF, Strum JM, Bulger RE: Studies on the pathogenesis of ischemic cell injury. I. Relation between ion and water shifts and cell ultrastructure in rat kidney slices during swelling at 0–4°C. Virchows Arch [Cell Pathol] 16: 1, 1974
121. Venkatachalam MA, Rennke HG, Sandstrom DJ: The vascular basis for acute renal failure in the rat. Circ Res 38: 267, 1976
122. Vincenti F, Goldberg LI: Combined use of dopamine and prostaglandin A$_1$ in patients with acute renal failure and hepatorenal syndrome. Prostaglandins 15: 463, 1978
123. Wait RB, White G, Davis JH: Beneficial effects of verapamil on postishemic renal failure. Surgery 94: 276, 1983
124. Wallach S, Bellavia JV, Schorr J, Schaffer A: Tissue distribution of electrolytes, ^{47}Ca and ^{28}Mg in experimental hyper- and hypoparathyroidism. Endocrinology 78: 16, 1966
125. Wardle EN, Wright NA: Intravascular coagulation and glycerin hemoglobinuric acute renal failure. Arch Pathol Lab Med 95: 271, 1973
126. Wesson DE, Mitch WE, Wilmore DW: Nutritional considerations in the treatment of acute renal failure. In Brenner BM, Lazarus JM (eds): Acute Renal Failure. WB Saunders, Phildelphia, 1983
127. Whelton A: Post-traumatic acute renal failure in Viet Nam: a milestone in progress. Community Med 38: 7, 1974
128. Whelton A: Antibiotic adjustments in renal failure. Infect Surg 101, 1984
129. Wilkins RG, Faragher EB: Acute renal failure in an intensive care unit: incidence, prediction and outcome. Anesthesia 38: 628, 1983
130. Williams JA, Withrow CD, Woodbury DM: Effects of nephrectomy and KCl on transmembrane potentials, intracellular electrolytes, and cell pH of rat muscle and liver in vivo. J Physiol 212: 117, 1971
131. Wilson DR, Arnold PE, Burke TJ, Schrier RW: Mitochondrial calcium accumulation and respiration in ischemic acute renal failure in the rat. Kidney Int 25: 519, 1984
132. Wright FS: Characteristics of feedback control of glomerular filtration rate. Fed Proc 40: 87, 1981
133. Wright FS, Schnermann J: Interference with feedback control of glomerular filtration rate by furosemide, triflocin and cyanide. J Clin Invest 53: 1695, 1974
134. Wright FS, Thurau K: Renal hemodynamics. Am J Med 36: 698, 1964
135. Zager RA: Glomerular filtration rate and brush border debris excretion after mercuric chloride and ischemic acute renal failure: mannitol versus furosemide diuresis. Nephron 33: 196, 1983
136. Zannad F, Royer RJ, Kessler M et al: Cation transport in erythrocytes of patients with renal failure. Nephron 32: 347, 1982
137. Zech P, Collard M, Guey et al: Renal hemodynamic response to L-dopa during acute renal failure in man. Biomedicine 23: 456, 1975

23

Acute Coagulation Disorders After Trauma

R. Ben Dawson

INTRODUCTION

Hemostasis and coagulation may fail as protective mechanisms in an injured patient as the result of some underlying condition, but more often such acute disorders develop during therapy, such as when large amounts of IV fluids are required. Thus, this chapter will emphasize continuing evaluation (see Table 23-1) for development and prevention, when possible, of an acute coagulation disorder in a patient who was normal with respect to hemostasis and coagulation before the injury or surgery. Acquired or inherited disorders that may predate the injury will also be considered.

Diagnosis of acute coagulation disorders will always involve laboratory confirmation of suspected or observed clinical phenomena. For example, impaired hemostasis due to insufficient platelet activity can often be predicted to occur during massive transfusion or prolonged cardiac surgery, unless provisions are

made for early detection or prevention. Thus, commonly, platelets or soluble plasma coagulation factors need to be supplemented. Rarely, excessive or accelerated consumption of hemostatic platelets and coagulation factors needs to be considered. This will also be discussed.

HEMOSTATIC DISORDERS REPRESENTING IMPAIRED PLATELET ACTIVITY

Pathophysiology

In general, hemostasis refers to maintenance of blood as fluid within the vessels as well as the prevention of excessive blood loss

737

after injury. This function depends on a delicate interplay of three compartments; tissues, blood cells, and plasma. The relative importance of each hemostatic component varies in different species and in humans depends on the size of the blood vessel involved. Upon injury, the vascular wall has the ability to constrict and to contribute a variety of platelet and plasma protein activators. The platelets, by the process of adhesion and cohesion, provide another physical means of arresting blood loss. This second, platelet function, activity is specifically referred to as primary hemostasis. Thus, the injury accompanied by vasoconstriction may expose circulating platelets to native collagen to which platelets adhere. The platelets contribute to their own further utilization by releasing intrinsic substances one of which, adenosine diphosphate (ADP), causes other platelets to cohere, or aggregate, thus forming the definitive hemostatic plug. Thus, the primary hemostasis or formation of the primary hemostatic plug is a function only of the interaction between the platelet and the interrupted vessel wall. But, as such, it will stem bleeding at least temporarily. Coagulation is not involved in primary hemostasis or stopping bleeding but is necessary in structuring the platelet plug and initiating the repair steps. Thus, coagulation is a third phase which is as necessary as the primary hemostatic plug, for without it rebleeding is expected. At the completion of normal coagulation, the fibrin mesh is intertwined with the platelet plug and this undergoes the final action by platelets wherein the clot retracts into a very small, tightly compact, definitive hemostatic plug.

Diagnosis

In patients with mild to moderate aberrations in primary hemostasis, the characteristic is easy bruising and petechial hemorrhages. Nose bleeds and gastrointestinal bleeding, forms of mucous membrane bleeding, occasionally occur. With trauma or surgery, the bleeding is immediate, but if not too severe it usually will respond to local direct measures such as pressure. However, severe disorders

TABLE 23-1. Evaluation Criteria for Bleeding Disorders

Clinical observation
Platelet count and bleeding time
Prothrombin time (PT) (extrinsic)
Partial thromboplastin time (PTT) (intrinsic)
Thrombin time and clot retraction
Fibrinogen and factor assay

of primary hemostasis present a life-threatening situation and must be identified and treated promptly. Inadequate platelet activity is certainly a cause of mortality or morbidity due to exsanguination or trauma, for example, central nervous system hemorrhage, since it represents the failure to form the protective hemostatic plug after which subsequent coagulation and healing events must occur. An understanding of this process requires the grasp of certain broad concepts. Morrison has emphasized that when this information is combined with the knowledge of the proper use of available therapeutic blood components and products, most clinical bleeding problems can be managed satisfactorily.[23]

Early in the management of surgical or trauma patients, the most common reason for failure of primary hemostasis is inadequate platelet numbers due to dilutional thrombocytopenia. The bleeding time (BT) is a specific test of primary hemostasis and its linear correlation with platelet counts will be discussed below. Indeed, the platelet count has the only correlation, an inverse correlation, with numbers of blood units transfused. The platelet count will be higher, as shown in Figure 23-1, than expected from calculations based on blood units given.[2] The other commonly used laboratory screening tests of hemostasis, such as the partial thromboplastin time (PTT), the prothrombin time (PT), and the thrombin time (TT), are characteristically normal in these disorders of primary hemostasis. Even in those extreme situations in which there seems to be coagulation failure due to insufficient plasma factors, perhaps from overtransfusion without supplying these factors, the hoped-for correlation between number of blood units transfused and these tests is not found.

The most useful test that can be performed as a measure of primary hemostasis will be the BT, which, until 15 years ago, was not

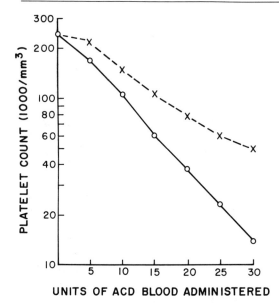

FIG. 23-1. Platelet count as a function of numbers of blood units administered. (X---X) observed; (O—O) calculated.

standardized. Now, the Mielke Template bleeding time is well accepted and has eliminated the two major difficulties: the wide range of normal values between individuals and between sequential determinations in the same individual.[21]

The BT will be abnormally long in the presence of quantitative or qualitative platelet defects. It is not prolonged in the hemophilias or other coagulation deficiencies. Although some vascular abnormalities may be associated with abnormal results, these are inconstant and rarely cause problems in differentiation. However, an acute coagulation disorder in the critically injured patient is usually associated with qualitatively normal platelets. Then, the bleeding time, as mentioned above will be predictive of the platelet count within the clinically relevant range. Indeed, this is the most physiologic relationship we have learned about the meaning of the platelet count in the last two decades. Simply stated, at between 100,000 and 10,000 platelets/μl the bleeding time will vary in an inverse linear manner between 4 and 28 minutes.[15] As shown in Figure 23-2, above 100,000 platelets, the bleeding time will not be any shorter and will be within the broad normal range of 2 to 8 minutes. Below 10,000 platelets, the linear relationship no longer exists; indeed bleeding times greater than 25 to 28 minutes would seem to be infinitely long or indistinguishable from rebleeding. Thus, the expression of such long bleeding time would have no meaning. Finally, the combination of a normal platelet count with a long bleeding time always suggests a qualitative

FIG. 23-2. Bleeding time as a function of platelet count. The Mielke template was used for the bleeding time determinations. Common qualitative platelet defects that greatly prolong the bleeding time in spite of normal platelet numbers (150 to 450 K) are shown. (Adapted from Harker LA, Slichter SJ: The bleeding time as a screening test for evaluation of platelet function. N Engl J Med 287: 155, 1972.)

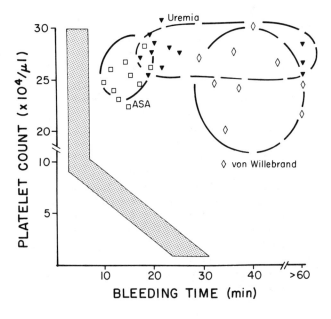

disorder of platelets, the more common kinds of which are indicated in Figure 23-2 and discussed in the last section.

Heparin-induced thrombocytopenia is recognized as the development of a significant thrombocytopenia 8 to 12 days after the initiation of heparin therapy.[1] Its occurrence is independent of the type of heparin used and antibodies directed against the combination of heparin and the platelet membranes seem to cause[6] platelet aggregation and release of platelet factor III. Additional important features of this syndrome are that the bone marrow contains abundant megakaryocytes and, in most studies reported, disseminated intravascular coagulation (DIC) and other such syndromes of accelerated coagulation seem to be ruled out.

Therapeutic Options

Dilutional thrombocytopenia subsequent to the transfusion therapy associated with fluid management in a critically ill patient can be anticipated at certain phases, but should not always be prevented by prophylactic transfusion of platelets. Expectant management is advocated, with the knowledge that at some point near or after the infusion of 1 blood volume, equivalent to 10 red blood cell units or 5 L replacement, the platelet count is likely to go below the lower limit of normal of 150,000/mm[3.]

This decrease in the platelet count is not necessarily a concern since normal hemostasis will still be present as the platelet count reaches 100,000. The platelet count can be allowed to slip down to 60,000 in many patients but not all. Remembering the relationship between platelet count and bleeding time will reassure the anxious that bleeding will stop, although it might take two to as much as six times longer if the platelet count is allowed to reach less than 30,000, which is not advised. Surgical and medical texts have commonly discussed platelet counts of 60,000 and 30,000 as adequate for major and minor surgery, respectively. In the 1980s, platelets are much more readily available and expeditious management of patients bleeding or of potential bleeding

problems warrant the common practice of raising the needed and desired platelet count to 90,000 to provide optimal hemostasis for a critically ill patient.[31]

Platelet transfusions are usually given in multiples of 4 to 6 units at a time to the adult patient who has a defect in hemostasis. This should not be considered a large, but a normal, dose. At best it would represent the platelets in half the circulating volume, and there is some loss during processing and storage. Thus, this 5 unit platelet transfusion will have a volume of 200 to 300 ml and should raise the platelet count by an increment of 25,000 to 40,000. Although granulocytes would be needed very rarely for the transfusion of patients other than those undergoing intensive cancer chemotherapy, some similarities in the need for and dosages of these two cell components make it instructive to discuss them together.

Difficulties in platelet and granulocyte transfusion therapy of the kind that have persisted were first discussed[12] in 1974. At that time hospitals commonly had to draw some of their own blood and frequently prepared platelets for transfusion over weekends. Also, granulocytes were not generally available. Ten years later, preparation of components by blood centers and improvements in blood storage have eliminated these shortages. A major problem, then as now—immune thrombocytopenia (with rapid exponential destruction rates of platelets)—is being effectively treated by infusing[4] 1 to 2 units/hr. This technique is especially useful in patients with idiopathic thrombocytopenic purpura (ITP) who are bleeding, and also occasionally in heavily transfused alloimmunized patients.[4]

However, in general, the failure to produce an increment upon transfusing multiple platelet units from random donors continues to suggest ineffectiveness of therapy. Thus, HLA-matched platelets are indicated from pheresed single donors. The yield of this single donor pheresis platelet product is similar to that of five to seven platelet concentrates from whole blood units. Thus, the dose again approximates that of the platelet activity found in one half a blood volume. Some patients never become alloimmunized even after many weeks of supportive platelet transfusions, but most do after several periods of platelet transfusion support, which necessitates HLA-matched platelet transfusions.

Although a bank of HLA-matched platelets has not been realized yet, platelet freezing[30] with dimethylsulfoxide (DMSO) has been approved by the Food and Drug Administration and is practiced in many cities in the United States and Europe.

Platelets and granulocytes, as well as red cells, are always given through standard 170 μm blood filters. They can be given through microaggregate filters but these expensive and unnecessary special filters have not added to the efficacy of treatment.[33]

Granulocyte transfusion evolved most recently and finally found its limited but important small place in the management of septicemia that is unresponsive to antibiotics in severely granulocytopenic patients. During the late 1950s, the major cause of death in patients with bone marrow failure due to aplastic anemia or hematologic malignancies was hemorrhage, with infection a distant second. However, during the 1960s, as the use of platelet transfusions became commonplace, there was a dramatic decrease in the incidence of hemorrhage as the cause of death in these patients. From 1965 to 1971 infection accounted for about 70 percent of the deaths in such patients, while hemorrhage accounted for only 10 percent. In the 1970s granulocyte transfusions began contributing substantially to the reduction in infections in these patients and also expanded the range of chemotherapeutic agents used.[7]

Granulocytes need to be obtained by pheresis from healthy donors who are stimulated with corticosteroids to release the marginal pool of granulocytes into the circulation.[7] In addition, hydroxyethyl starch is used as a sedimenting agent for red cells during centrifugal separations; this frees the white cells from the red cells so that they can be collected in one of the separation devices. This approximates half or more of the granulocytes normally circulating in a well individual. Arguments have continued about whether HLA and ABO compatibility are necessary for effectiveness of transfusion therapy, but it is agreed that compatibility is desirable. However, an increment in granulocyte count should be achieved after transfusion to predict a clinical response, especially improving the survival of granulocytopenic patients whose septicemia is not responsive to antibiotics alone. Further, the need for a minimum of four consecutive days of therapy with granulocytes continues to require that such patients be treated in specialized hematology, cancer, or transfusion centers. Finally, prophylaxis or prevention of sepsis in granulocytopenic patients by granulocyte transfusion therapy has not been successful in several studies.

COAGULATION FAILURE DUE TO INSUFFICIENT PLASMA FACTORS

Fifteen years ago John Collins reported that transfusion in Vietnam combat casualties was accompanied by dilutional coagulation defects compatible with the level of coagulation factors in stored banked blood. Whereas platelet levels had been known to fall to 100,000/ μl or less during transfusion, the PT, PTT, and fibrinogen levels have been less severely affected. Significant perioperative bleeding was not encountered in conjunction with the mild dilutional coagulation changes seen in those combat casualties. A partial return of the coagulation factors toward normal was accompanied by administration of stored blood to wounded patients who had developed coagulation defects secondary to shock. With the exception of factors VIII and V, all coagulation factors (Figure 23-3) are present in significant amounts in stored whole blood, and whole blood was used in Vietnam. In subsequent combat situations and indeed in most civilian blood banking, whole blood is no longer used. It will no longer be available by the mid 1980s in many areas because of the development of the additive solution blood preservatives; with these, the platelet rich plasma is removed during processing to be replaced by a saline-mannitol based solution. Thus, fresh frozen plasma (FFP) will continue to be the mainstay, and then the only source, of normal biologic activity of all soluble plasma coagulation factors (Fig.

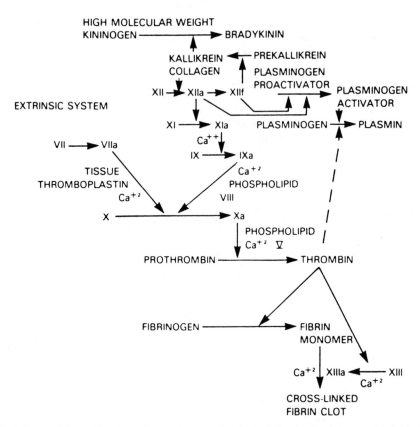

INTRINSIC SYSTEM

FIG. 23-3. A "cascade" amplification scheme of coagulation factors showing the intravascular, intrinsic system starting at the top, and the tissue-activated, extrinsic system starting on the left. Both systems activate factor X, converting it to its activated form, Xa, which completes the cascade by converting prothrombin to thrombin, which converts fibrinogen to fibrin and factor XIII to XIIIa (fibrin-stabilizing factor).

23-3). The minimum concentration of these factors to maintain hemostasis is relatively low, about 30 percent normal for factors VIII, IX, fibrinogen, and prothrombin, and probably 10 percent for factors V, VII, X, XI, XII, and XIII.

As mentioned above, patients with problems following massive transfusion of blood and resuscitative fluids (dilutional effect) who demonstrate thrombocytopenia by count or smear often respond to sufficient platelet concentrates to correct the thrombocytopenia (usually 4 to 8 units). If bleeding persists after platelet therapy, unexpected causes for bleeding must be ruled out: (1) acute hemolytic transfusion reaction, (2) pre-existing heparin or coumadin treatment, or (3) disseminated intravascular coagulation.

The exclusion of these three causes strengthens the case for the bleeding being due to dilution of plasma factors, especially when testing (Fig. 23-4) shows prolonged activated PTT and PT. Therapy then consists of fresh frozen plasma, usually in multiples of 2 units, each unit consisting of 200 ml and capable of raising the level of biologically active factors by about 8 percent. It is noteworthy that platelet concentrates, with their 50+ ml volume, will raise the plasma levels of soluble coagulation factors by 2 percent per unit. Occasionally, cryoprecipitate units are needed as a source

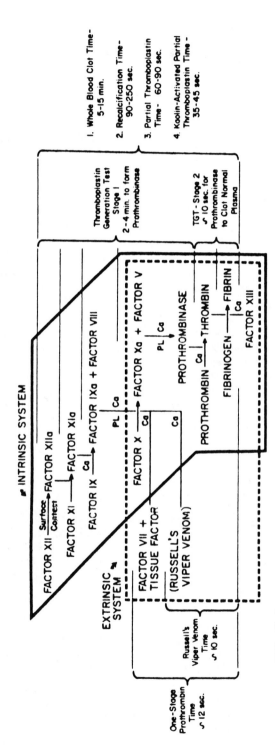

FIG. 23-4. Coagulation tests, showing what factors they measure in the extrinsic, intrinsic, and common systems.

of concentrated factor VIII or fibrinogen, especially if adequate coagulation is not achieved with FFP, and factor VIII or fibrinogen levels are seen to be below the 30 percent or normal levels needed for them to be effective.

Although volume expansion with colloids and crystalloids is discussed in another chapter, infusion volumes in component replacement for blood loss need to be considered together in the context of prolonged surgery or massive volume replacement as in trauma. We and John Collins have used the exchange transfusion models to help us calculate depletion or dilution of plasma factors during massive transfusion.[8,14,20]

After 10 red cell units are transfused with accompanying colloid/crystalloid volumes to maintain vital signs and a hematocrit above 25, the level of coagulation factors remaining, such as fibrinogen, was reduced to 28 percent. At 20 red cell units with accompanying crystalloid/colloid, the depletion was down to 8 percent. Mathematical modeling of a multiple trauma victim with two major sources of blood loss other than several fractured extremities proposed a patient who had lost 50 percent of his blood volume, which had been fully replaced but then the patient continued to bleed and be transfused, maintaining normovolemia. At 10 units, the depletion was to 30 percent of the factors and at 20, 11 percent. These findings are remarkably close to the figures noted above and to the classic exchange transfusion (Fig. 23-5). Thus, bleeding is likely enough at 10 units to warrant expectant preparations and at 20 units to consider unpreparedness a serious and critical threat.[14]

These predictions and comments are based on levels of the soluble coagulation factors that constitute the coagulation cascade. In general, these volume considerations apply to platelet levels and needs as well. However, platelet levels do not fall as low as expected (see Fig. 23-1) due to splenic and other reserves. In the multiple trauma patient of the kind modeled above, bleeding that represents a defect in primary hemostasis frequently occurs at platelet levels less than 100,000 and in all cases after the platelet level falls below 50,000, unless these levels are anticipated.[14] For example, 8 units of platelets per 20 red cell units would be considered a minimum to prevent develop-

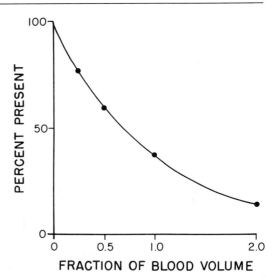

FIG. 23-5. Exchange transfusion: kinetics of depletion. Applied to plasma coagulation factors, the percent present gets below the critical 20 to 30 percent needed between 1 and 2 blood volumes. (Modified from Marsaglia A, Thomas ED: Mathematical consideration of cross circulation and exchange transfusion. Transfusion 11: 216, 1971.)

ment of these levels and the subsequent failure of primary hemostasis.

CONSUMPTION AT AN UNPHYSIOLOGIC RATE OF PLATELETS AND FACTORS, USUALLY BY UNKNOWN MECHANISMS

In the natural or homeostatic form, intravascular coagulation forms thrombin to seal a leaking blood vessel and stop bleeding. Thus, it is a normal local phenomeon. In widespread trauma there is no question that some disseminated intravascular coagulation is a physiologically appropriate mechanism. However, in its extreme or pathologic form, a consumptive disseminated intravascular coagulation is clearly inappropriate and no longer in response to bleeding. It results in decreased blood flow in, either the arterial or venous circulation. The form with thrombosis as the end result is incompletely understood and beyond the scope of this discussion.[36]

Disseminated intravascular coagulation, as opposed to local coagulation, is of concern to us here. It is not commonly appreciated that there are two fairly distinct forms. In the first of these, thrombi form in multiple sites in the body with signs and symptoms resulting from ischemia of the involved organs.[31] The second manifests as generalized bleeding (Fig. 23-6) from disseminated "consumptive coagulation." It has been known for many years that the thrombus formation involves the consumption of various labile coagulation factors, the serine proteases and their substrates that make up the coagulation cascades. These include the major ones commonly tested for, fibrinogen, factors V, VIII, and prothrombin, as well as platelets. Consumption is the result of both the coagulation process itself and various proteases such as plasmin, which increase in amount during coagulation and degrade these coagulation proteins. Several coagulation factors such as factors XIIa and IIa (thrombin) may affect plasminogen activation. Another cause of activation, vascular endothelium plasmogenin activator, is released into the blood when ischemia is present.[28] In recent years attention has been directed to fibrinolysis mediated by cells. It is now apparent that macrophages release fibrinogen activator[37] as well as other enzymes such as elastase,[2] which degrade fibrinogen. Stimulated cells released increased amounts of these enzymes. One such stimulus is fibrin itself, leading to feedback de-

struction of the fibrin.[18] In addition to thromboplastin, leukocytes can also produce elastase and other nonplasmin fibrinolytic enzymes.[25]

The relative in vivo magnitude of these nonclassic fibrinolytic systems is unknown. However, different kinds of fibrinolytic activity are induced by plasmin. These other enzymes probably have additional effects on hemostasis as well. Leukocyte-derived proteases can also degrade[19] factor VIII. These more recently discovered thromboplastic and lytic functions of phagocytes, endothelial cells, and others will occupy a major research focus in the future and no doubt will clarify some current clinical mysteries.

A variety of other coagulation interactions lead to further changes of note. In addition to causing fibrin formation, thrombin first activates (Fig. 23-3) and then degrades[27] factor V and VIII. Other "feedback" mechanisms also exist. Another circulating protein is a vitamin K dependent protein, protein C. Among the variety of newly discovered functions of this material is its ability to inactivate factors V and VIII as well as to stimulate the release of plasminogen activator.[9] Thus, activated protein C can contribute to "consumptive coagulopathy" by increasing the destruction of factor V, VIII, and secondary fibrinolysis. Activation of protein C during intravascular coagulation is likely to contribute also because it is activated by thrombin.

When intravascular coagulation and lytic processes proceed at a pace that outstrips the particular host's ability to synthesize these materials, their levels may be depressed to a point below that necessary for normal hemostasis. Contributing to the hemorrhagic tendency are

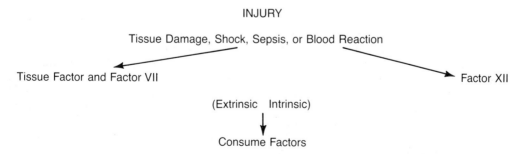

FIG. 23-6. Development of consumptive DIC: proposed steps in tissue injury.

the antihemostatic effects of fibrin/fibrinogen degradation products, which can inhibit both fibrin polymerization[3] and platelet function.[17] Clinical bleeding is the manifestation of these.

Activation of Coagulation

Activation of the coagulation system can occur in several ways, some of which are known. In some instances material may be released from normal or malignant tissue, which affects the coagulation systems. These materials may include tissue thromboplastin as well as various proteases with varying direct and indirect effects on the coagulation and fibrinolytic systems. Malignant tissues, particularly carcinomas, have a propensity for initiating this process. Nonneoplastic tissue does not ordinarily release its contents into the blood stream unless some tissue damage, hypoxia, or trauma has occurred.

The best known associations of normal tissues with DIC are abruptio placenta or pregnancy-related ischemia or dead tissue sources. All of these can cause significant coagulopathies. It is presumed in these cases that tissue thromboplastin released into the maternal circulation is the culprit. Two other complications of pregnancy that can show accompanying DIC by different causative mechanisms are amniotic fluid embolism, which can result in a severe hemorrhage diathesis, and eclampsia. In the former, amniotic fluid has been described as having activity resembling thromboplastic material. However, the active agent would appear to be the particulate material.

In a classic experiment, Steiner demonstrated that filtered amniotic fluid was not effective when injected into animals, whereas unfiltered material was.[35] In eclampsia the degenerative vascular changes are striking pathologic findings, which may cause the coagulopathy in certain patients. There is evidence that the coagulopathy is not the cause of toxemia. Iatrogenically induced DIC due to hypotonic saline used to induce abortion is well known.[34]

Disseminated intravascular coagulation is frequently associated with gram-negative bacteremia, or another source of endotoxin, but has been found with sepsis from a variety of organisms, including viruses, Rickettsia and parasites.[31] The DIC from infection occurs primarily as a result of either direct effects of the microorganisms or their products, such as endotoxin, on the coagulation system or indirect effects, such as endothelial damage, with consequent shock and its sequelae. Endothelial damage is quite characteristic of rickettsial infections and in one of these, Rocky Mountain spotted fever, fulminant DIC occurs commonly.[31]

Platelet aggregation, usually a part of and sometimes an antecedent of DIC, may be induced by a variety of mechanisms. Perhaps the most likely mechanism in vivo would involve changes in the vasculature, either directly due to endothelial injury with exposure of underlying collagen (a powerful platelet aggregator), or indirectly, secondary to changes in levels or concentrations of various prostaglandin metabolites synthesized in the vasculature. Also, dysfunction of platelets is common in massive transfusion.[11,31]

While the degree and causes of activation of the coagulation system are of major importance, of equal significance is the functional capacity of various neutralizing systems. Among these are various circulating enzyme inhibitors, including proteins such as antithrombin III that serves to inhibit thrombin. The other activated serum proteases are α-macroglobulin, α_2 anti-plasmin, α_1 antitrypsin, and others. It is believed that many of these inhibitors, when complexed to the active enzymes, are removed from the circulation in the reticuloendothelial system (RES). Another humoral substance of note is fibronectin, currently thought to be involved in RES clearance, in which circulating fibrin may be involved as a protective mechanism prior to significant thrombus formation.[29] Fibronectin levels decrease both acutely[32] and chronically[24] in DIC.

The second major balance mechanism to control activated coagulation is the RES itself. Here, phagocytic cells can remove circulating enzyme inhibitor complexes, microparticulate fibrin, soluble fibrin, with and without fibronectin, and can synthesize proteolytic enzymes capable of dissolving fibrin. The recently described activity of phagocytic cells to secrete more proteases than do resting cells[37] and documentation that non-plasminogen-dependent fibrinolysis can also occur,[31] add complexity and fine modulation or control.

The third possible mechanism is hepatocellular. This was first studied in the 1960s, when it was shown that certain activated coagulation moieties were removed in the liver by hepatocytes rather than phagocytic cells. The degree to which this system is normally operational is not known and the mechanisms have not been elucidated, although some of the coagulation proteins are glycoproteins, which hepatocytes can clear when sialic acid residues are removed.

Thus, intricate systems play physiologic and pathologic roles in affecting coagulation simply by their various abilities to remove activated products. Although we have attached considerable meaning to such residue as fibrin degradation products and we understand the meaning of critical levels of platelets and fibrinogen, we do not yet have enough clinical experience with such intriguing compounds as antithrombin III and fibronectin to use levels of these in any meaningful way. In addition, individuals under various clinical circumstances vary in their ability to replenish the coagulation factors consumed in an accelerated fashion or when depleted. Finally, another important variable is the intensity and duration of the inciting agent, whether a tissue thromboplastin, vascular damage, or an endotoxin. The balance of these various forces will probably determine whether or not intravascular coagulation will occur in a given clinical situation.

The related area of hypercoagulability is just beginning to be unraveled. This is defined as an altered state of circulating blood that requires a smaller quantity of clot-initiating substance to induce intravascular coagulation than is required to produce comparable thrombosis in a normal subject. However, the slight increased propensity to thrombosis observed in recent decades in people under the influence of premenopausal estrogens may be a harbinger of what this field holds for future exploration. It is worth pondering whether the same group of forces that produce thrombosis in the hypercoagulable state determine whether or not accelerated coagulation will develop.

The role of the endothelium in activated coagulation deserves a mention. Exposure of collagen during endothelial injury and resultant platelet aggregation are well-accepted steps (Fig. 23-7), but the role played by the activation of protein C of the endothelium surface is not so well appreciated.[31] Also, endothelial cells produce prostacyclin, a potent antiaggregant and vasoactive drug, which, at least experimentally, has important anticoagulant effects. A cofactor for antithrombin III with some characteristics of heparin is found on endothelial surfaces.[5] Heparin itself is associated with the endothelium as well as thrombin.

Finally, general influences on the development of DIC would include the observation that DIC is more severe when shock is present, but no additional conclusions are justified. Patients who have had more severe trauma are more apt to be in shock and have DIC, without shock and DIC being otherwise necessarily related. Nonetheless, both experimental and clinical

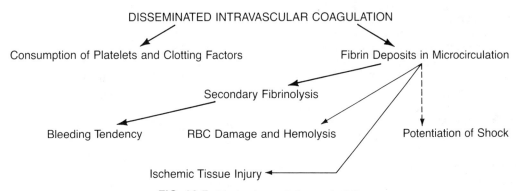

FIG. 23-7. Mechanisms of disease in DIC.

data associating stasis and thrombosis would suggest that a correlation between shock, subsequent acidosis, and the development of DIC is real. The only conclusion or practical lesson must be to place great importance on prompt restoration of normal blood flow in patients with shock or massive transfusion.

Types of DIC

Most episodes of DIC readily divide into acute and chronic types, based largely on the inciting event. Acute DIC, such as that caused by bacterial sepsis, is more apt to be associated with consumptive bleeding than thrombosis. The reverse is true for chronic DIC, although flares in intensity may result in alteration between thrombosis and bleeding. Chronic DIC reflects persistent underlying disease, which is usually more important than the therapeutic decision concerning the DIC. In acute DIC, however, patient management and outcome are often dependent on the successful treatment of this intermediary mechanism. Although removal of the primary cause will lay the cornerstone of success, until that is achieved important management of DIC is sometimes necessary for survival.

The most easily cured acute DIC is that associated with septic shock, and is the best example. Although use of heparin is largely in disfavor, it has its advocates in the literature for patients with septic shock who do not initially respond to antibiotics and antishock measures.[23] Nearly as controversial is the DIC associated with massively transfused patients, whether due to trauma or surgery. In either case, virtually all are massively transfused and have potential sites of bleeding by which a hemostatic insufficiency will be obvious. For this reason, heparin is commonly contraindicated except in a hemolytic transfusion. Also, there is the uncertain therapeutic benefit of heparin in DIC in general. However, in the experience of some individuals and groups, heparin in high enough doses to influence effectively an active acute DIC has been found to be safe if 24 hours or more have passed since the last traumatic or surgical insult.[33]

In these experiences the resultant adequate heparinization has frequently meant a decrease by several times in the need for more than one blood component, such as red cells, platelets, and FFP on a daily basis. Even then fibrinogen concentrations are likely to be low, but the need for platelet concentrates and FFP or cryoprecipitate (cryo) can be greatly reduced by adequate heparinization. Widely accepted diagnostic criteria for the presence of DIC are: abnormalities of platelet count, fibrinogen, and prothrombin time. If only two of these are abnormal, then fibrin split products, euglobulinlysis time, and thrombin time need to be determined to establish a diagnosis (Table 23-2).

Assuming that DIC is accurately diagnosed, then management will necessarily include blood volume replacement or support and appropriate blood component therapy as suggested above. Adequate hemostasis is, of course, the goal. A useful definition of adequate hemostasis in general, and specifically in DIC, includes the following: a platelet count of greater than 100,000, a prothrombin time of less than 1.3 × control, a partial thromboplastin time not greater than 3 seconds over control, and a fibrinogen concentration above 125 mg/dl. Among the exceptions to these will be syndromes with dysfunctional platelets; for example, when a 100,000 platelet count may be inadequate. This is not uncommon in patients who have undergone cardiopulmonary bypass, but is uncommon in severely traumatized patients. The chronic DIC syndromes are not appropriate for discussion in this chapter. However, this author has seen a very rapidly developing DIC in thrombotic thrombocytopenic purpura (TTP) where the three main criteria of Table 23-2 were in evidence, but the PT and PTT remained normal.

Among trauma patients, it is clear from our experience that DIC is more likely in certain groups of injuries than in others. Early DIC, that is, within the first 10 days of the traumatic

TABLE 23-2.   Diagnostic Criteria for DIC

Platelet count less than 100,000/μl
Fibrinogen less than 100 mg/dl
Schistocytes or "helmet" red cell forms on blood smear

If these three are present, high probability of DIC. If only two are present, then additional tests, as suggested in text, are needed.

insult, is more likely to be associated with liver injuries, pelvic fractures, and intracranial injuries. Later development of DIC may occur with these kinds of injuries, but is more commonly associated with the development of infections, with or without septicemia.

The major conclusions about the development of accelerated consumption of coagulation factors that can be drawn from this brief review of physiologic and pathologic mechanisms are that most will be predictable and manageable to some extent, although not explainable. The predictability will be based on the extent or type of the injury or surgery and subsequent events, and the management will consist to a large extent of replacing appropriate consumed coagulation factors such as platelets and plasma factors. Most attention needs to be directed to the planning, to the extent that is practical, based on the nature of the hemostatic defect that may exist, to attribute cause to underlying illness, complications, or errors in treatment. With that background, and an expectation of the known benefits from intervention, most episodes of consumptive coagulopathies can be managed quite satisfactorily. The assistance of a clinical coagulationist or a skilled transfusionist may be necessary.

SUPPRESSION OF PLATELETS OR FACTOR PRODUCTION, ALSO USUALLY BY AN UNKNOWN MECHANISM

This section will discuss the least common group of coagulation disorders found in the critically injured patient. Whereas in the previous section we cited increased consumption of hemostatic platelets and coagulation factors, and in the last section we will consider increased destruction of these as by antibodies and the inherited disorders, here we will elucidate those few fairly well defined defects in production of platelets and coagulation factors.

A large and fairly well understood group of platelet production abnormalities are neoplastic, consisting of leukemias, lymphomas,

and metastatic carcinomas, and aplastic anemia when it involves the platelet precursor, the megakaryocyte. Evidence of adequate megakaryocytes by bone marrow aspiration or biopsy would help to determine whether a known neoplasm is contributing to a thrombocytopenia. Such an examination will help decide whether interference with platelet production is the cause of the thrombocytopenia. Other causes include cancer chemotherapy and radiotherapy as well as a few drugs specific to the megakaryocyte, such as thiazides, estrogens, and ethanol. In addition, folic acid and vitamin B 12 deficiencies can result in a thrombocytopenia with a platelet count as low as 10,000 due to lack of megakaryocytes. Also, iron deficiency in children has been associated with a platelet count as low as 50,000 due to impairment of megakaryocytic maturation. Finally, among acquired causes of megakaryocytic thrombocytopenia the viral diseases that are causative are rubella, rubeola, mononucleosis, the Epstein-Barr virus, influenza viruses, and also the measles vaccine, Thai hemorrhage fever, and dengue fever.

The liver's vitamin K dependent factors[5] are II, VII, IX and X. Factor V is sensitized in the liver and there are suggestions that factors XI and XII may also be.[5] In any case, it is clear that impairment of vitamin K assimilation, as by biliary tract obstruction or poor bile duct drainage, can lead to hemorrhage. Also, there is impaired synthesis of coagulation factors in most patients with liver disease because of hepatic cell failure despite adequate vitamin K stores. The decreased synthetic rate of coagulation proteins in stable liver failure is reflected by a moderately prolonged PT and PTT that is only slightly improved by vitamin K therapy. Also, the liver synthesizes major inhibitors of coagulation, α_2-macroglobulin and antithrombin.[31]

Reduction in inhibitor levels might increase the rate of coagulation reactions, causing some confusion at times in interpreting these tests. Also, liver disease can impair clearance of activated coagulation factors. Further, there may be failure to clear fibrinogen activators secreted in the microcirculation, resulting in increased plasma fibrinolytic activity. Thus, laboratory studies may show a mild increase in plasma fibrinolytic acitivity or a slight elevation in the concentration of fibrin degradation products. However, intense fibrinolysis or overt DIC may occur with sudden prolongation in the PT and PTT as well as a fall in fibrinogen levels, an increase in fibrin degradation products, and a further fall in platelet count. In summary, patients with liver disease have a complex coagulation disorder that may fluctuate so that there is a precarious and limited hemostatic reserve.

Treatment of bleeding and liver disease is complicated. Transfused platelets are sequestered in the spleen if there is increased portal pressure, and the large protein and salt loads that accompany needed infusions of FFP are poorly tolerated. The concentrated vitamin K dependent factors in freeze-dried "prothrombin complex" concentrate that is commercially available are sometimes of significant value, but a limitation is that they cannot adequately replace other needed coagulation factors, such as factors V, VIII, and fibrinogen. These comments are only warnings or precautions, however, as FFP and prothrombin complex concentrates are useful therapy, often with platelets needed as well, in the treatment of bleeding in liver disease. Unfortunately, the prothrombin complex concentrates are the most dangerous blood products available with respect to contamination by hepatitis viruses. In addition, they often contain traces of activated coagulation factors that might trigger inappropriately accelerated coagulation.

PREEXISTING, ACQUIRED, OR INHERITED DISORDERS OF HEMOSTASIS AND COAGULATION

The major problems among these disorders are drug-induced bleeding disorders and the hemophilias. The most common, but fortunately mildest, of these two groups are the aspirin-induced platelet defect and Von Willebrand's disease. However, in injured or surgical patients, an aspirin-induced platelet defect or Von Willebrand's disease can be as serious as complicating disorders, but is not necessarily associated with morbidity or mortality.

On the other hand, drug-induced thrombocytopenia and the hemophilias commonly represent serious bleeding disorders and major complications in surgical management (Table 23-3). In one of the best reviews of drug-induced thrombocytopenia, 50 separate drugs were listed as producing a specific drug–cell–antibody interaction with platelets.[22] Only a fraction of these reported drugs had reactions with leukocytes or red cells, suggesting that thrombocytopenia was the most common of the drug-induced blood dysplasias. Commonly used drugs that were implicated more than once include digoxin, penicillin, quinidine, gold salts, and streptomycin. However, since these are hardly 10 percent of the listed drugs, any question about the possibility of thrombocytopenia being a drug reaction should prompt a call for the assistance of a pharmacist or hematologist. Unfortunately, published reports of drug-induced blood dyscrasias are not commonly found after one or two cases and many commonly used drugs have only a single report associated with them. Examples of these in which the evidence is very strong from the single report for a drug–platelet–antibody causative interaction are hydrochlorothiazide,[13] penicillin,[16] chlorpromazine,[18] and desipramine or imipramine.[26]

The severeness of the drug-induced thrombocytopenia affects the prognosis in a general way. However, since the thrombocytopenia usually resolves within a very few days after use of the drug is stopped, cutaneous bleeding or purpura may be the only consequence. Sometimes, support of platelet count and prevention of further possibly dangerous bleeding

TABLE 23-3. Selected List of Drugs Producing Cytopenias

Drug	Target		
	Platelet	WBC	RBC
Acetazolamide	+	+	+
Acetylsalicylic acid	+		+
PAS	+	+	+
Cephalothin	+		+
Penicillin	+	+	+
Phenylbutazone	+	+	+
Rifampin	+		+
Chlorpromazine	+	+	+
Streptomycin	+	+	+
Sulfas	+	+	
Tetracyclines	+		+
Tolbutamide	+		+

may be necessary with platelet transfusion. With those few drugs that affect platelet function, such as acetylsalicylic acid, hemostatic support, if needed, can be provided by as few as 2 units of platelet concentrates in an adult; the dysfunctional, acetylated platelets will be triggered by the normal transfused platelets.[15]

In the other, mild, common disorder, Von Willebrand's disease, there is also a platelet defect, but the disease is primarily a plasma deficiency of part of the factor VIII complex. Indeed, FFP or cryo, containing concentrated factor VIII, corrects the bleeding disorder and the prolonged bleeding time as well as the abnormal factor VIII/Von Willebrand's factor-dependent platelet test. This latter test, specific for the disease, is characteristically a decreased aggregation of platelets in response to ristocetin. One or two units of either FFP or cryo is usually sufficient to correct the clinical bleeding disorder and the long bleeding time. If not, a repeat dose of 2 units of cryo will suffice.

Finally, the most serious pre-existing disorders in coagulation in a critically injured patient are the hemophilias. Deficient factor VIII or hemophilia A is more serious; factor IX deficiency or hemophilia B less so. High potency, freeze-dried preparations are available with either factor VIII or IX to facilitate the management of these disorders. Coagulation factor assays have traditionally used deficient plasma controls to diagnose the specific factor deficiencies, but the synthetic substrates that react with the serine protease of the coagulation cascade or other activating enzymes greatly improve precision and sensitivity in diagnosing these factor deficiencies in the lab. However, clinical histories continue to be of major importance in realizing that complicating pre-existing disorders of hemostasis or coagulation may be present.

REFERENCES

1. Amsell J, Slepchuk N, Jumar R et al: Heparin-induced thrombocytopenia; a prospective study. Thromb Haemost 43: 61, 1980

2. Banda MJ, Werb Z: The role of macrophage elastase in the proteolysis of fibrinogen, plasminogen, and fibronectin. Med Proc 39: 1756, 1980

3. Bang NU, Fletcher AT, Alkjaersig N et al: Pathogenesis of the coagulation defects of abnormal clot structure by electron microscopy. Clin Invest 41: 935, 1962

4. Bergin JR, Zuck TF: Selected aspects of component therapy. I. Platelets. In Dawson RB (ed): Transfusion Therapy. AABB, Washington, D.C., 1974

5. Busch C, Owen WG: Identification in vitro of endothelial surface cofactor for antithrombin III; parallel studies with isolated, perfused rat hearts and microcarier of bovine endothelium. J Clin Invest 69: 726, 1982

6. Caps CH, Adelstein EH, Rhodes GR et al: Heparin induced thrombocytopenia, thrombosis and hemorrhage. Surgery 86: 148, 1979

7. Cohen E, Dawson RB (eds): Leukopheresis and Granulocyte Transfusions, AABB, Washington, D.C., 1975

8. Collins JA: Massive blood transfusion. Clin Haematol 5: 201, 1976

9. Comp, PC, Emmon CT: Evidence for multiple roles for activator protein C and fibrinolysis. p. 583. In Mann K, Taylor F (eds): The Regulation of Coagulation. Elsevier-North Holland, 1980

10. Comp PC, Nixon RR, Epson CT: Determination of functional levels of protein C, an antithrombotic protein, using thrombin-thrombomodulin complex. Blood 63: 15, 1984

11. Counts RB, Haisch C, Simon TL et al: Hemostasis in massively transfused trauma patients. Ann Surg 190: 91, 1979

12. Dawson RB (ed): Transfusion Therapy. AABB, Washington, D.C., 1974

13. Eisner, EV, Crowell EB: Hydrochlorothiazide-dependent thrombocytopenia due to IgM antibody. JAMA 215: 480, 1971

14. Gill W, Champion HR: Volume resuscitation in critical major trauma. In Dawson RB (ed): Transfusion Therapy. AABB, Washington, D.C., 1974

15. Harker LA, Slichter SJ: The bleeding time as a screening test for evaluation of platelet function. N Engl J Med 287: 155, 1972

16. Hsi YJ, Kuo HY, Ouyang A: Thrombocytopenia following administration of penicillin. Chin Med J (Engl) 85: 249, 1966

17. Jerushal, MAZ, Zucker, MD: Some effects of fibrinogen degradation products (FDP) on blood platelets. Thromb Diath Haem 15: 413, 1966

18. Kautz HD: Blood dysplasia associated with chlorpromazine therapy. JAMA 160: 287, 1956

19. Kopec M, Bykowsa, Lopaciuk S et al: Effects of neutral proteases from human leukocytes on structure and biologic properties of human factor VIII. Thromb Haemost 43: 211, 1980

20. Marsaglia G, Thomas ED: Mathematical consideration of cross circulation and exchange transfusion. Transfusion 11: 216, 1971

21. Mielke CH, Kaneshiro MM, Weiner JM et al: The standardized normal IVY bleeding time and its prolongation by aspirin. Blood 34: 204, 1969

22. Mieschler VA: Drug induced thrombocytopenia. Semin Hematol 19: 311, 1973

23. Morrison FS: Disorders of primary hemostasis and management. In Dawson RB, Morrison FJ (eds): Hemostasis. AABB, Washington, D.C., 1977

24. Mosher DF: Fibronectin concentration is decreased in plasma of severely ill patients with disseminated intravascular coagulation. J Lab Clin Med 91: 729, 1978

25. Plow EF: Leukocyte elastase released during blood coagulation. A potentional mechanism for activation of the alterative fibrinolytic pathway. J Clin Invest 59: 564, 1982

26. Rachmilewitz EA, Dawson RB, Rachmilewitz B: Serum antibodies against desipramine as a possible cause of thrombocytopenia. Blood 32: 528, 1968

27. Rapaport SI, Schiffin S, Patch MJ et al: The importance of activation of anti-hemophilic globulin and proaccelerin of traces of thrombin in the generation of intrinsic prothrombinase activity. Blood 21: 221, 1963

28. Robinson ER, Bandoff M, Nilsson IM: Fibrinolytic capacity in healthy volunteers at different ages as studied by standardized venous occlusions of arms and legs. Acta Med Scand 191: 199, 1972

29. Saba TM, Jaffe E: Plasma fibronectin. Opsonic glycoprotein; its synthesis by vascular endothelial cells and role in cardiopulmonary integrity after trauma related to reticuloendothelial function. Am J Med 63: 577, 1980

30. Schiffer CA, McCready KV: Cell component therapy for patients with cancer. In Dawson RB (ed): Transfusion Therapy. AABB, Washington, D.C., 1974

31. Sherman LA: DIC in massive transfusion. In Collins JA, Murawski K, Shafer WA (eds): Massive Transfusion in Surgery and Trauma. Alan R Liss, New York, 1982

32. Sherman LA, Lee J: Fibronectin. Blood turnover in normal animals during intravascular coagulation. Blood 60: 558, 1982

33. Sohmer PR, Dawson RB: Transfusion therapy. In Spittell JA (ed): Clinical Medicine, vol 5. Harper and Row, Hagerstown, 1984

34. Spivak JL, Sprangler BB, Bell, WE: Defibrination after intraamniotic injection of hypertonic saline. N Engl J Med 287: 321, 1972

35. Steiner ST, Biner PE, Lusbaugh CC: Maternal pulmonary embolism by amniotic fluid as a cause of bstetric shock in unexpected deaths in obstetrics. JAMA 117, 1245, 1981

36. Thomas D: Thrombosis. Br Med Bull 34: 101, 1978

37. Ukeless JC, Gordon S, Reich, E: Secretion of plasminogen activator by stimulated macrophages. J Exp Med 139: 834, 1974

24

Management of Diabetes Mellitus in Surgery and Trauma

Vincent D. Chang
William R. Drucker

INTRODUCTION

A significant by-product of the increased interest of surgeons in "surgical biology" is that the risk of surgery in diabetic patients has decreased substantially in the past few years. This is primarily due to the improved methods of perioperative management and a better understanding by surgeons of the pathophysiology of diabetes. Postoperative morbidity in diabetics has been reduced by increased knowledge of fluid physiology, metabolism, nutrition in surgical patients, improved antibiotic therapy, and by advanced surgical technology.[15,25]

Diabetics undergoing surgery properly are viewed as belonging to a high risk group.[2] This is particularly important when one considers that approximately 50 percent of all diabetics will require surgery during their lifetime.[56] Most patients have a history of the disease but a significant number of them (about 25 percent)

are discovered to have diabetes only preoperatively.[10] While the mortality in diabetics undergoing surgery has been reported to be as low as 3.6 and 3.7 percent, other reports[5,28,71] indicate a mortality rate as high as 13 percent. It is not surprising therefore to find reports of morbidity in the range of 17 percent. The primary causes of morbidity and mortality are cardiac disease and infection. Acute myocardial infarction is the most common cause of death; staphylococcal sepsis is the second most common cause.[13,61] Pulmonary embolism accounts for approximately 10 percent of the deaths. Other potential postoperative complications include infections in the wound or the genitourinary tract, delayed wound healing, phlebitis, hyperglycemia, ketoacidosis, and hypoglycemic shock.

Among the most important contributions to the safety of diabetics undergoing surgery are the recent advances in administering insulin with relative ease and precise monitoring of its effects. These advances have made the

753

perioperative control of diabetes relatively simple and thereby helped to prevent the complications that plagued management in the past. In view of these advances in understanding and technology, the incremental risk of diabetes in a surgical patient today should be very small and the risk of death from previously undetected diabetes should be nearly negligible. The following discussion reviews the advances in knowledge and technology that have contributed to this more optimistic prognosis for diabetics undergoing a surgical procedure; it concludes with a consideration of the management of diabetic patients during the perioperative period.

DIABETES: DIAGNOSIS, CLASSIFICATION, AND PATHOPHYSIOLOGY

Diagnosis and Classification

Although controversy continues over a uniformly acceptable diagnostic criterion for diabetes mellitus, the National Diabetes Data Group has helped to provide guidelines.[47] A strongly positive test for glucose (0.5 percent) in the postprandial urine of a patient with symptoms of diabetes points toward this diagnosis. Measurement of the fasting level of glucose in the blood is still the most reliable and widely accepted test for diabetes. The National Diabetes Data Group recommends that the level of fasting blood glucose exceed 140 ml/dl before a firm diagnosis of diabetes mellitus is established, although other values are quoted by different authors.[38] The glucose tolerance test is the most sensitive means of detecting the disease. In adults with fasting sugar levels greater than 140 mg/dl, the test is superfluous. For those with fasting levels between 115 and 140 mg/dl, performing a glucose tolerance test postoperatively is of no immediate practical value except to determine if a patient has impaired tolerance for glucose or very mild diabetes. In time, however, a diagnosis of dia-

betes should be validated because long-term management supervised by a competent physician is in the best interest of the patient. If the 1 and 2 hour values of blood glucose exceed 200 mg/dl in a well standardized oral glucose tolerance test, the National Diabetes Data Group believe that diabetes is present and treatment warranted.

The syndrome of diabetes mellitus is widely regarded as heterogeneous in origin.[3,33] Most patients can be classified into two groups, type I or type II, on the basis of historical information, clinical findings, and laboratory tests. In a third and smaller group, the cause of disordered metabolism is usually recognizable; these patients manifest either a type I or type II picture of diabetes (Table 24-1).

Type I diabetes is characterized by a rapid onset usually before the age of 30, together with the classic symptoms of polydipsia, polyphagia, polyuria, and weight loss. Symptoms have usually been present for less than 3 months before the disorder is discovered. Plasma insulin levels during fasting are low or absent with minimal response to a challenge with glucose, amino acids, or β-cell stimulants. There is an identifiable structural loss of pancreatic β-cells with consequent insulinopenia.[34] These patients are markedly sensitive to exogenous insulin and may become ketotic when supplementary insulin is withdrawn. The disorder has also been called juvenile-onset or insulin-dependent diabetes mellitus (IDDM).

Type II diabetes, also termed maturity onset diabetes or non-insulin-dependent diabetes mellitus (NIDDM), is seen in patients with altered carbohydrate metabolism often years before the diabetes is diagnosed. These patients are usually over the age of 30 and the diagnosis is often made during an infection or in the perioperative period. Spontaneous ketosis is a rare event; however these patients can develop ketosis if subjected to the stress of infection or surgery. A majority are obese when the diabetes is detected, or they may have a history of obesity or rapid weight gain in the preceding few years. In contrast to the histologically identifiable structural loss of pancreatic β-cells that occurs in type I patients, type II patients have a functional alteration manifested by a variable combination of insulin resistance and relative insulin deficiency. Treatment may be effected by either dietary manipulation or the use of oral hypoglycemic agents.

TABLE 24-1. Classification of Diabetes Mellitus

		Category
Idiopathic Diabetes		
Type I Insulin-dependent diabetes (IDDM)	Thin ketosis without insulin, short history, symptomatic, usually < age 30, female/male 1:1, family history	Insulin deficiency
Type II Non-insulin-dependent diabetes (NIDDM)	Usually obese, ketotic only with stress, long history, symptomatic, usually > age 30, female:male 1:3, family history	Insulin antagonism +/− deficiency
Diabetes Secondary to		
Pancreatic disease	Pancreatectomy, pancreatitis, carcinoma, hemachromatosis, and destructive diseases of the pancreas	Type I
Hormonal excess	Cushing's syndrome, acromegaly, pheochromocytoma, primary aldosteronism, glucagonoma, and other amine precursor uptake and decarboxylation tumors	Type II
Drugs	Diuretics, glucocorticoids, oral contraceptives, phenytoin (Dilantin), phenothiazines, tricyclic antidepressants, and other agents	Either Type I or Type II
Insulin receptor unavailability	With and without circulating antoantibodies	
Genetic syndromes	Hyperlipidemias, myotonic dystrophy, lipoatrophy, leprechaunism, Friedreich's ataxia, Prader-Willi syndrome, and others	Type II or unclear
Gestational diabetes		Type II

(Adapted from Genuth S: Classification and diagnosis of diabetes mellitus. Med Clin North Am 66(6): 1191, 1982. Reprinted with permission from WB Saunders Co., Philadelphia.)

The third group of diabetic patients includes those in whom hyperglycemia is associated with *another* disease process.[33] Most of these patients can be classified as either type I or type II. Patients who have had either significant pancreatic disease or pancreatectomy, or patients on thiazide diuretics may be classified as type I. Those with hormonal excess such as in Cushing's syndrome, pheochromocytoma, or primary glucagonoma, or patients treated with steroids develop a type II diabetic syndrome. Some patients with autoimmune disorders have circulating antibodies directed against insulin receptors that prevent the metabolic actions of insulin and thereby also cause type II diabetes.

Pathophysiology

The diabetic syndrome occurs as a consequence of a deficiency of insulin (type I) or an imbalance between insulin production and release of hormonal or tissue factors that modify the requirements for insulin (type II). In both types, the cardinal manifestations are *hyperglycemia* and *glycosuria*.

It is well recognized that in nondiabetic individuals, normoglycemia is primarily maintained by the coordinated interplay of insulin and glucagon.[65,67] The relative amounts of insulin and glucagon determine not only the glucose concentration but also the net flux of glucose into tissues. This coordination is effected by the intracellular channels between adjacent α-cells (glucagon-secreting) and β-cells (insulin-secreting) known as gap junctions and by a positive/negative feedback between the two hormones. In the normal postprandial state, hyperglycemia is prevented by a burst of insulin secretion. Several signals that originate in the gastrointestinal tract stimulate insulin secretion prior to absorption of carbohydrates (enteroinsulinar axis). These include both vagal signals neurally transmitted to the islet cells, and alimentary hormones such as cholecystokinin, gastric inhibitory peptide, gastrin, secretin, and possibly other factors yet to be identified.

On a cellular level, insulin is the only hormone that has an overall anabolic effect and, as such, has been termed "the banker hormone." Secretion of insulin is stimulated by either carbohydrate, protein feeding, or both via the "enteroinsular axis."[66] Insulin is responsible for the storage of all nutrients, carbohydrates, fats, and amino acids, into stores such as glycogen, triglyceride, and protein, respectively. It drives glucose into metabolically active tissues such as muscle and adipose, while halting lipolysis and proteolysis, thereby sparing other fuels. In the liver, insulin not only promotes lipogenesis and glycogenesis but also inhibits gluconeogenesis in its role as the "banker hormone."

The action of insulin is opposed by glucagon, cortisol, and catecholamines designated as counterregulatory hormones or "stress hormones" due to their increased secretion in response to stress (Table 24-2). Glucagon stimulates gluconeogenesis, glycogenolysis, and ketogenesis when adequate amounts of fatty acids are present. Glucagon also stimulates alanine uptake by the liver. The prime effects of glucagon are on the liver. Cortisol causes a net protein breakdown in extrahepatic tissues. It also stimulates amino acid degradation, gluconeogenesis, and increases the flow of gluconeogenic precursors to the liver. The catecholamines stimulate glycogenolysis and lipolysis, as well as inhibiting the pancreatic release of insulin and the peripheral (muscle) uptake of glucose. Clearly, this group of hormones deserves its designation as counterregulatory due to the combined catabolic influence in opposition to the anabolic role of insulin.

Metabolic homeostasis is dependent on the relative amounts present of insulin and the counterregulatory or catabolic hormones. If there is a significant increase in the concentration of the catabolic hormones, as seen during the early postoperative period, or if there is a relative deficiency of insulin, as in the insulin-deprived juvenile diabetic, the diabetic syndrome develops: the cardinal manifestation being hyperglycemia, frequently associated with glycosuria. While attention to the metabolic alterations of diabetes has been directed traditionally to carbohydrates, it is of paramount importance to recognize that the syndrome involves abnormalities of all three groups of nutrients, fat and protein as well as carbohydrates. The time-honored devotion to alterations of carbohydrate metabolism is readily explicable by the significantly easier measurement of carbohydrates in biologic fluids. It is also due in part to the obvious importance that the carbohydrates exert on the clinically observable signs and symptoms of the syndrome. The advent of improved biochemical techniques for measuring products of protein and fat metabolism has helped us to understand the complex interrelationship of all nutrients in health as well as in diseases such as diabetes.

In the diabetic state, the basic defect is a lack of metabolically effective circulating insulin. This relative or absolute deficiency of insulin causes a decrease in the rate of translocation of glucose from the extracellular fluid into insulin-sensitive cells as well as deficient utilization of glucose in peripheral tissues such as muscle and adipose tissue. Concomitant with the impaired peripheral use of glucose, proteolysis, lipolysis, glycogenolysis, and gluconeogenesis are increased resulting in an increased hepatic output of glucose and a rise in the serum glucose concentration. An excess load of filtered glucose in the urine acts as an osmotic diuretic leading to the loss of large quantities of water, sodium, potassium, and chloride.

When insulin deficiency is marked, ketosis, the result of impaired fat metabolism, compounds the dehydration produced by glycosuria because of further obligatory loss of the

TABLE 24-2. Anabolic and Catabolic Effects of Hormones

	Anabolic effects			Catabolic effects				
	Glyco-genesis	Lipo-genesis	Protein synthesis	Glyco-genolysis	Gluco-neogenesis	Lipo-lysis	Keto-genesis	Proteo-lysis
Insulin	+ +	+ +	+ +	−	− −	− −	− −	− −
Glucagon	−	−	0	+	+ +	(+)	+	0
Cortisol	+/−	+/−	− −	+/−	+	+	(+)	+ +
Catecholamines	−	0	0	+ +	+ +	+ +	+	0
Growth hormone	0	0	+ +	0	+	(+)	(+)	0
Thyroid hormone	0	0	+ ?	0	+	+	(+)	+

+ +, major stimulatory effect; − −, major inhibitory effect; +/−, stimulation if insulin present, inhibitory if insulin absent; (+), important only if insulin absent; + ?, selective stimulatory effect. No attempt has been made to indicate tissues where major actions occur.

See source for further details. (From Alberti KGMM, Thomas DJB: The management of diabetes during surgery. Br J Anaesth 51: 693, 1979.)

positive ions, sodium and potassium, associated with excretion of the cationic ketone bodies. Free fatty acids are released from the adipose tissue, bound to serum albumin, and transported to the liver. Lipogenesis is decreased and lipolysis increased to such an extent that acetyl-coA is produced in excess of the capacity of the Krebs cycle to handle it. This results in the formation of ketone bodies as products of incomplete fat metabolism through the following mechanism: the excess acetyl-coA shunted from the Krebs cycle is metabolized to acetoacetate, which is converted to β-hydroxybutyric acid by hydrogenation and to acetone by decarboxylation. When hepatic production of these ketone bodies exceeds the capacity of peripheral tissue to use them, ketonuria results. The renal loss of sodium and potassium with the ketone bodies therefore compounds the dehydration of glycosuria in diabetes. In time, acidosis develops as a result of two mechanisms: the release of cationic metabolic products from the anaerobic glycolysis induced by hypoperfusion of tissues in dehydrated patients and by the continuing loss of anions (Na and K) with ketones in the urine.

Protein metabolism also contributes to the net catabolic state of diabetics. A negative nitrogen balance results from the combined reduction in protein synthesis and the increased rate of proteolysis, which contributes to the accelerated gluconeogenesis. Protein in muscle is catabolized to amino acids, which are transported to the liver where they are transformed into two and three carbon fragments, and the waste product urea. The urinary excretion of both nitrogen (from proteolysis) and glucose (from gluconeogenesis) contributes additional solutes to the dehydrating osmotic diuresis of uncontrolled diabetes.

METABOLIC RESPONSE IN SURGERY

In his classic series of studies extending over more than four decades, Cuthbertson defined three phases of injury: ebb and flow phases of vitality followed by an anabolic phase.[20] Strictly speaking, convalescence is considered to start directly upon cessation of injury and extend throughout the entire period of recovery, although most studies have been confined to the second, the flow phase, because it has the greatest metabolic variance. Transition between the successive phases, including a fourth and final phase of fat gain, is usually imprecise. Nevertheless, a reasonably uniform sequence of events can be identified to help characterize each phase.[25] The metabolic and physiologic alterations witnessed during these successive phases can be viewed teleologically as serving homeostatic priorities of the organism in defense of a stable internal environment. Defense of circulatory volume is a priority of the first (ebb) phase, followed by defense of energy needs in the second (flow) phase, restoration of protein in the third (anabolic) phase, culminating in storage of energy reserves in the fourth (fat) phase of convalescence. The constellation of these interdependent alterations produced in response to neurohumoral stimuli over the four phases of convalescence constitutes the total biologic response to injury.

Ordinarily, it is during the second or flow phase of convalescence lasting from 1 to 10 days that the greatest threat to control of diabetic patients occurs. But a more complex disruption of metabolism will develop if the initial (ebb) phase is not prevented by careful attention to maintenance of a normal circulatory volume during and following surgery. Under this circumstance the metabolic changes characteristic of hemorrhagic shock will develop and thereby constitute the ebb phase. Nevertheless, even if circulatory volume is not guarded carefully, most patients who are well hydrated and well nourished preoperatively and who do not lose large quantities of blood during surgery will have only a brief and mild ebb phase lasting no more than 24 hours. This reflects the remarkable internal mechanism supportive of circulatory homeostasis.[16,23] If circulatory volume is reduced to the extent that peripheral perfusion is impaired, however, there will be a rapid rise in the level of blood glucose associated with a depressed level of circulating insulin in the well nourished person. These changes are the net result of the increased secretion of the counterregulatory hormones. These hormones foster a marked increase in the hepatic output of glucose due to accelerated gluconeogenesis and rapid glyco-genolysis. Although the peripheral uptake of glucose is increased during the early stage of shock, the level of blood glucose rises due to an even greater output of glucose into the circulation from the liver. If therapy for hypovolemia is delayed, both the hepatic output and peripheral uptake of glucose decline, leading to a progressive fall in the level of blood glucose due to the relatively more rapid fall in hepatic output. As this occurs, mechanisms supportive of the circulation begin to deteriorate.[51,53] Proteolysis and lipolysis support the increased gluconeogenesis that occurs during the initial phase of shock.[44,52] It is noteworthy that the peripheral uptake of glucose is accelerated during the early phase of shock despite the influence of an increased output of epinephrine, which acts to inhibit both pancreatic secretion of insulin and the peripheral uptake of glucose.

Overall, the metabolic changes of the ebb (shock) phase can be viewed as a response to neuroendocrine control that promotes the production of glucose required by hypoxic tissues. Since hypoxic tissues are capable of taking up glucose without the aid of insulin, the relative insulinopenia of this phase may represent a well organized homeostatic device. Unimpeded by insulin the counterregulatory hormones act to increase the hepatic output of glucose, the only exogenous energy substrate that can be used by hypoxic underperfused peripheral tissues. Nevertheless, the peripheral uptake of glucose can be accelerated by insulin in hypovolemic animals.[63] Consequently, the use of insulin as an adjunct to the therapy of hypovolemia remains attractive but very controversial.[6] It is worth re-emphasizing that the metabolic disturbances of the ebb phase can be prevented by careful attention to maintenance of a normal circulatory volume.

In contrast to the ebb phase, the second phase of convalescence cannot be prevented although it can be modified in degree and duration by careful attention to many factors associated with surgery. During this (flow) phase, all patients become "diabetic" as demonstrated by an abnormal glucose tolerance test with glycosuria. This alteration in carbohydrate metabolism may last only 2 to 3 days or as long as 7 to 10 days. Even a relatively minor procedure such as an herniorrhaphy performed under spinal anesthesia with special attention to maintaining an isocaloric intake in the perioperative period causes this alteration in glucose assimilation.[26] In contrast to glucose, fructose is assimilated normally by the postoperative patient because fructose uptake is not dependent on insulin. This suggested that the metabolic response to the stress of surgery is similar to diabetes mellitus, that is, an impaired cellular uptake of glucose.[46] The mechanisms by which the stress of surgery cause metabolic alterations and the significance of the observed changes have been subject to continuing investigative interest over the past quarter of a century.

Surgery is considered to be one of the classic "stress" situations. The postoperative disturbance is characterized by glucose intolerance for an infusion of exogenous glucose, an increased metabolic rate, and an increase in nitrogen loss in the urine. Several factors associated with surgery, such as fasting, hypovolemia (as noted previously), pain, anxiety, tissue damage, and immobilization also contribute to these physiologic and biochemical disturbances. In an uncomplicated elective operation, the basal metabolic rate may increase only by 10 percent and there may be a very small increase in nitrogen excretion. In a more traumatic operation, however, or in the presence of fractures, burns, shock, or sepsis, the metabolic alterations become significantly more extensive.[18,40]

It is now clear that *in contrast to the patient with diabetes,* the postoperative surgical patient with an abnormal tolerance for exogenous glucose is able to oxidize glucose at a normal or even at an increased rate as long as the patient is hemodynamically stable and the blood glucose levels are elevated.[40] An increase in hepatic output of glucose, reflecting enhanced gluconeogenesis and possibly glycogenolysis, occurs despite a rise in the level of blood glucose. The relative nonsuppressibility of gluconeogenesis, a characteristic metabolic alteration of this phase, is more likely to be responsible for the altered tolerance for exogenous glucose than is a decrease in the peripheral uptake of glucose. The hyperglycemia probably reflects an increased flow of glucose with a relatively greater increase in synthesis relative to an increased turnover rate. Under the influence of counterregulatory hormones, gluconeogenic substrates such as pyruvic and lactic acids, amino acids, and glycerol are mobilized from peripheral tissues to promote the increased hepatic output of glucose. This occurs despite the rise in the plasma level of insulin that develops in this second phase of convalescence.[6]

The increase in plasma insulin during the flow phase is in marked contrast to the low level of insulin found in the plasma associated with hyperglycemia in an ebb phase response. While the rise in plasma insulin suggests a plentiful supply of the hormone and an appropriate pancreatic response, the persistence of hyperglycemia with an increase in plasma levels of fatty acids indicates a reduction in the biologic activity of insulin at this time.[35]

Although the cause of the transient insulin resistance during this early postinjury period is unknown, various theories have been postulated. It may be that the conversion of high to low molecular weight insulins results in biologically less active hormone. On the other hand, the insulin may remain biologically normal while changes at the insulin receptor site, distal to it, or in the number of receptors may account for the insulin resistance.[32] Another possibility is development of competitive inhibition at the receptor sites.[72] The degree of influence from the counterregulatory hormones, cortisol, glucagon, epinephrine, and growth hormone cannot be quantitated simply from changes in their concentration in the plasma.

Whatever the mechanism of decreased sensitivity to insulin may be, teleologically this phenomenon can be regarded as useful since it promotes the development of a higher concentration of glucose and fatty acids in the plasma to meet the known increased needs for these energy substrates induced by surgical stress. In time, the decreased sensitivity for insulin becomes progressively less pronounced when convalescence is uninterrupted. This phenomenon is *not* to be confused with the type of insulin resistance that occurs secondary to antibodies directed against insulin or autoantibodies to the insulin receptor.[27] Thus, the alterations found after stress may be phylogenetic adapted features that provide the mobilization of substrates for energy metabolism during this important phase of convalescence from injury. It would be a mistake, therefore, to give patients additional insulin at this time without simultaneously supplying the nutrients required for the wound, acute phase protein synthesis, and other energy-dependent processes.

While the provision of exogenous nutrients does have a significant influence in reducing the degree and duration of metabolic changes that develop during the flow phase, these alterations cannot be prevented completely after a severe stress such as a fracture or multiple system injuries.

Not only the "stress of surgery" causes alterations in intermediary metabolism. Other "nonsurgical" aspects may be involved. For instance, bed rest prolonged for only 3 days will reduce the tolerance for glucose.[21] A reduction in carbohydrate intake while maintaining an isocaloric intake is sufficient to cause a shift to a diabetic type of glucose tolerance after only 3 days.[19] Certain anesthetics and drugs such as morphine have metabolic effects. Hyperglycemia, fatty acid mobilization, and inhibition of insulin secretion occur with both ether and chloroform anesthesia. By contrast, the more modern agents, such as halothane, have only minimal discernible influence on intermediary metabolism. Epidural and spinal anesthetics have the least effects. Failure to distinguish between alterations induced in the normal surgical patient by the acute reduction of caloric intake and other nonsurgical influences from those inherent in the response to surgery has contributed to confusion and controversy about the metabolic changes of convalescence.

In contrast to the nonstressed fasted individual, injury inhibits the adaptation to starvation, thereby allowing hypercatabolism to proceed.[25,40] Prime indices of the catabolic state, characteristic of the flow phase of convalescence, originally identified by Cuthbertson and elaborated by many later studies, include an increase in the excretion of nitrogen in association with sulphur, phosphorus, potassium, magnesium, and creatinine.[20] Since muscle is the primary source of these compounds, their loss can be considered to reflect a reduction in lean body mass. Concomitant with these losses is an increase in the rate of protein turnover, probably tied inextricably to an increase in carbohydrate turnover. Although both synthesis and catabolism of protein are increased, the balance favors catabolism, leading overall to a negative balance in body economy for nitrogen. The enhanced protein synthesis favors tissue repair, formation of acute phase reactant proteins and antibodies, while catabolism mobilizes intracellular material for substrates for the reparative processes. Kinny and his associates have stressed that in the absence of exogenous assistance the protein is more likely used for production of carbohydrate essential for survival than to meet whole body energy requirements.[40] The caloric requirements of this phase are supplied almost entirely by the metabolism of fat excepting only the unique requirements for glucose in neural tissues, erythrocytes, and the wound.

It must be stressed that the alterations in protein metabolism observed during the flow phase are nutritionally dependent. They do not occur after injury in chronically starved or protein-depleted patients. They are significantly less pronounced when a second operation closely follows the initial procedure. Simply staying in bed for 72 hours or an acute reduction in protein intake without surgery induces a negative nitrogen balance similar to that observed after most uncomplicated operations.[21] Continuation of the preoperative quantitative intake of calories and protein into the postoperative period will attentuate greatly the postoperative characteristic metabolic response to surgery as manifested by a negative balance for nitrogen. However, an extensive injury, particularly one associated with sepsis or a fracture, will induce a rapid and sustained loss of nitrogen that cannot be overcome by nutritional intake. Also, the abnormal tolerance for exogenous glucose cannot be prevented by a high protein and caloric intake during the period of injury. Clearly, injury can induce changes distinctly beyond those of starvation.[25,40]

After the initial homeostatic priorities of maintenance of circulatory volume and energy production have been satisfied, the third or anabolic phase begins. Onset of this phase may be abrupt and even quite dramatic in patients who have been through a period of marked catabolism. This metabolic turning point from catabolism to anabolism is characterized by behavior reflecting the restoration of normal physiologic processes. For the diabetic, transition to this phase is particularly important because it signals return of the ability to consume an oral intake. A renewed appetite, the presence of active bowel sounds, and passage of flatus signals transition to the anabolic phase. Unlike the two initial phases, however,

when physician intervention can either obliterate or greatly curtail the metabolic alterations, the phase of anabolism proceeds at its own pace. A gain of lost body weight frequently is slow because the reparative processes must restore the muscle mass lost during catabolism. The rate of restoration of protein is finite and probably cannot exceed 3 to 5 g/70 kg body weight per day. Thus, the total time of the anabolic phase may greatly exceed the brief period of severe catabolism when there seemed to be no absolute restrictions on the quantity of protein that could be lost per day. One can anticipate a weight gain of approximately 1 kg/week at maximum efficiency. Thus, very strict and careful control of the diabetic during this period is important to derive the maximal efficiency from the reparative process.

The final, fat gain, phase starts when the lost protein is restored. It probably reflects more nearly the cultural and emotional needs of the postoperative patient than a response to physiologic priorities for recovery.

All of the energy substrates, protein, fat and carbohydrate, respond to the special requirements induced by injury. The responses vary however as noted in the foregoing sections depending upon the phase of convalescence and the management of the injured patient during these periods. In the uncomplicated patient, the most pronounced metabolic changes occur during the flow phase. The predominance of the catabolic hormone activity over anabolic (insulin) activity may be considered an organized system to channel the appropriate metabolic substrates in defense of the specific energy needs of normal tissues and the wound.

DIABETES IN THE SURGICAL PATIENT

Since the trauma from surgery as well as the complications of surgery such as hemorrhage and infection create significant metabolic derangements, one can anticipate that control of a diabetic patient will become more complicated during the perioperative period. Diabetics are particularly vulnerable to the complications of hyperglycemia such as dehydration, loss of electrolytes, diabetic ketoacidosis, prerenal azotemia, and lactic acidosis. Of particular concern because it may develop incidiously during the early postoperative period is hyperglycemic hyperosmolar nonketotic coma.[1,7,11] Several interrelated factors that may promote development of this syndrome include large exogenous loads of glucose, (both oral and parenteral), medications that induce hyperglycemia, susceptible patient populations (e.g., previously undiagnosed diabetics, uremic patients, and patients with acute or chronic pancreatitis), and dehydration. When diabetic patients develop this acute metabolic disturbance, they are predisposed to infection and vascular thrombosis. Indeed, the increased morbidity and mortality observed among diabetics with hyperglycemic nonketotic coma are primarily due to these additional complications.

Another problem associated with persisting hyperglycemia that the surgical patient encounters is a decrease in the tensile strength and impairment of healing of the surgical wound.[36,57] In part, this reflects the need for adequate replacement of insulin during the early phase of wound healing.[36] Furthermore, impaired polymorphonuclear leukocyte mobilization and function, delayed development of staphylococcal antibodies, and decreased cytotoxic lymphocyte response may increase the susceptibility to infection in the poorly controlled diabetic patient undergoing surgery.[8,9,48] The increased level of circulating free fatty acids as seen in insulin deficiency has been shown to increase myocardial oxygen demand, signaling a decrease in myocardial function.[22,68]

Although not adequately documented, hyperglycemia in the diabetic patient may either exacerbate respiratory insufficiency or even precipitate respiratory failure.[40] This may be the case especially in those patients with underlying obstructive or restrictive pulmonary disease. The mechanism responsible involves an increased demand on respiratory activity in response to the greater production of carbon dioxide and a rise in the respiratory quotient (as seen in carbohydrate loading in parenteral nutrition). Uncontrolled hyperglycemia may be especially hazardous in weaning the surgical patient from a ventilator.

At the other extreme in the control of the diabetic surgical patient is hypoglycemia.[28,65] Although rarely found today, this complication usually results from overzealous control of the level of blood sugar. The symptoms of confusion, lethargy, diaphoresis, tachycardia, and peripheral vasoconstriction subside quickly following intravenous administration of one or two ampules of 50 percent dextrose.

Preoperative Evaluation

The chief goal of the surgeon attempting to control diabetes during an operation is to achieve a smooth and uncomplicated restoration of metabolic homeostasis.[64] In pursuit of this goal, several objectives facilitate preoperative management of the diabetic patient.[12] First is the recognition and evaluation of disorders frequently found in patients with a long history of diabetes such as cardiac and peripheral vascular disease, renal disease, and hypertension. Second is evaluation of fluid and electrolyte status, hematologic status, and control of infection, and, by no means last, the management of the diabetes itself with particular care to avoid the potential iatrogenic complications of ketosis and hypoglycemic reactions.

The heart and peripheral blood vessels can properly be considered the system of primary concern for diabetics faced with the necessity of surgery. The incidence of coronary artery disease in patients with diabetes mellitus is high, as shown by the Framingham study.[31] Not only is there an increased incidence of angina and myocardial infarction in these patients, but they also have an increased risk of cardiovascular mortality in comparison with nondiabetic patients; the latter constitutes the most common cause of death in the diabetic patient. Several intraoperative factors can be expected to stress the cardiovascular system including various vasoactive drugs, volume overload, hypoxia, bleeding with its attendant hypovolemia and hypotension, tachycardia, and/or bradycardia, other arrhythmias produced by the anesthetic agents and, on occasion, the anesthetic agents themselves. In addition, diabetics may have a cardiomyopathy with an increased risk of congestive heart failure. The patient with uncompensated congestive heart failure has a 35 percent chance of developing pulmonary edema, 45 percent chance of exacerbation of the congestive heart failure, and a 25 percent risk of cardiac death.[10] One half of all patients with postoperative myocardial infarctions do not have symptoms of pain; this is particularly true of the diabetic patient who is at increased risk of having a silent infarct because of autonomic neuropathy. Because of the neuropathy, diabetics also may be particularly susceptible to respiratory depression and cardiorespiratory arrest. Both stable and unstable angina occur in patients with coronary artery disease. Whereas stable angina has not been associated with increased risk of surgery, unstable angina has.

Long-standing diabetes is associated with an increased incidence of small vessel disease manifest by thickening of the basement membrane in addition to the aging changes of atherosclerosis in major vessels. The resulting ischemia in peripheral tissues makes the diabetic particularly vulnerable to complications such as claudication, chronic dermal infections with both aerobic and anaerobic organisms, and trophic ulcers.

The kidney also deserves special attention in the preoperative evaluation of diabetic patients. Many patients have chronic renal insufficiency; they therefore require careful fluid and electrolyte management and careful adjustment of medications excreted by the kidneys. Varying degrees of proteinuria may occur. Patients with the nephrotic syndrome have an increased susceptibility to hypotension secondary to a depleted intravascular volume. The peripheral vascular disease often seen in the diabetic patient requires arteriographic evaluation prior to elective vascular surgery. To minimize the risks of the diagnostic studies, diabetics with renal insufficiency should receive a limited amount of intravascular contrast material and must be adequately hydrated prior to the examination. Failure to observe these precautions may lead to exacerbation of the underlying renal insufficiency. Lastly, many diabetics with end-stage renal disease receive chronic dialysis. The dialysis should be performed within 24 hours of operation to prevent major intraoperative fluid and electrolyte perturbations.

Hypertensive disease is commonly observed in the diabetic patient. Uncontrolled hypertension has been shown to be associated with a greater degree of hypotension during anesthesia than that which occurs in the non-hypertensive or well-controlled diabetic patient. Hypotension places an increased stress on the cardiovascular system as does the hypertensive episode that can occur postoperatively when the anesthetic is rapidly reversed. Antihypertensive medications should be continued until the time of surgery. In the postoperative period, hypertension should be controlled with parenteral agents, such as hydralazine, if the patient is unable to take oral medications. In the event of a hypertensive crisis, intravenous nitroprusside may be administered. Oral hypertensive medications should be restarted as early as possible postoperatively.

An essential goal of the preoperative management is adequate hydration and correction of any electrolyte imbalance. Fluid and electrolyte problems are not uncommon preoperatively. Hypokalemia is often seen in diabetic patients who are receiving diuretic agents for either congestive heart failure or essential hypertension. The hypokalemia may be responsible for cardiac arrhythmias during induction of anesthesia. Hyperglycemia may be worsened in the non-insulin-dependent diabetic by either hypokalemia or depletion of total body potassium. A rare entity associated with diabetes is a hyporenin–hypoaldosterone state in which the patient presents with hyponatremia and hyperkalemia. Obviously, this mandates preoperative correction by mineralocorticoid administration. The use of diuretics and the presence of underlying renal disease may contribute to gross fluid and electrolyte imbalance.

It is not unusual to discover anemia preoperatively that may require transfusions of packed red blood cells in preparation for surgery. In the instance of acute massive hemorrhage, transfusion of whole blood is indicated.

Hidden infections (particularly urinary tract infections) are frequently seen in diabetic patients. These are dangerous because they may become fixed chronic infections and are of a particular concern during the perioperative period as a potential source for septic shock. Therefore, any infection must be treated aggressively when discovered in either the pre- or postoperative period.

Obesity is often seen in the non-insulin-dependent (type II) diabetic patient. Ideally this should be controlled prior to elective surgery since obese patients have an increased risk of both pulmonary thromboembolic and anesthetic complications as well as an increased risk of wound infections. Although compliance is low, every sensible effort needs to be directed to bring the weight of a diabetic within a normal range prior to an elective operation.

In addition to the special attention paid to the organs and systems known to be particularly vulnerable to alteration in the diabetic patient, the importance of obtaining a thorough preoperative history and performing a careful physical examination cannot be over-emphasized.[30,49] Important baseline historical data include specific clinical characteristics of diabetes mellitus such as age at onset, the use of insulin or oral hypoglycemic agents, the dietary regimen, an estimation of control (e.g., home urine testing and the frequency and severity of insulin reactions), and problems encountered in previous operations or with previous anesthetics. A history of previous myocardial infarction (especially within the past 6 months), episodes of chest pain (stable vs. unstable angina), or symptoms of congestive heart failure (dyspnea, orthopnea, ankle edema, paroxysmal nocturnal dyspnea, and dyspnea on exertion) provide vital information toward evaluation of the status of the heart. A history of the use of alcohol, tobacco, and other drugs is of obvious importance. The development of autonomic neuropathy may not be apparent until the diabetic patient is questioned frankly and in detail regarding symptoms of postural hypotension, impotence, and diarrhea. A previous history of cerebrovascular events including amaurosis fugaux and transient ischemic attacks (TIAs) may remain hidden, possibly as part of a denial process, until the patient is questioned directly about these harbingers of disastrous complications of vascular disease.

An estimation of control of the metabolic alteration can be obtained by eliciting a history of polydipsia, polyuria, weight loss, episodes of ketoacidosis, and symptoms of hypoglycemia (insulin reaction). Measurement of hemoglobin A_{1c} (HbA$_{1c}$) has been used as a laboratory measure of the adequacy of control of diabetes. Hemoglobin A_{1c} results when normal hemoglobin A is exposed to a high glucose environment, resulting in glycosylation of the amino terminal valine on the β-chain. The normal levels of hemoglobin A_{1c} is 3 to 6 percent of the total hemoglobin. Hyperglycemia in the poorly controlled diabetic results in an increase in this level. Obviously, in an emergency operation, determination of the hemoglobin A_{1c} level is useless; but in elective surgery this can give the clinician additional quantitative data to help assess the control of diabetes.[13]

The essential laboratory data base for these patients will include values for: fasting blood glucose, serum electrolytes, blood urea nitrogen, creatinine, complete blood count with differential, urinalysis, electrocardiogram, and chest radiograph. Since chest pain is often absent in diabetic patients experiencing a myocardial infarction, an electrocardiogram (ECG) is needed preoperatively as a baseline and postoperatively to rule out an intraoperative myocardial infarction.

Use of Insulin and Glucose Monitoring

Before we discuss management of the diabetic patient during surgery, it is necessary to review the time relationship of the two major types of insulin, regular and intermediate acting (Fig. 24-1). Regular insulin, when given subcutaneously, demonstrates activity in about 30 minutes, peaks in 2 to 4 hours, and lasts a total of 6 to 8 hours. The intermediate acting insulin (isophane insulin suspension, NPH, or insulin zinc suspension, Lente) demonstrates metabolic activity in 3 to 4 hours, peaks in 8 to 12 hours, and lasts 18 to 24 hours. To manage hospitalized patients optimally, blood glucose samples should be obtained at both the peaks and troughs of the activity of insulin. Blood glucose levels should therefore be obtained 2 to 3 hours after administration of regular insulin and 8 to 12 hours after intermediate insulin.

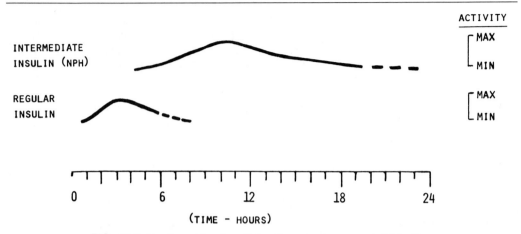

FIG. 24-1 Duration of insulin activity after subcutaneous administration.

When both regular and intermediate insulin are used, the lowest level of activity occurs 18 to 24 hours following their subcutaneous administration.[58]

Insulin has been found to bind to the infusion tubing and bottles thus impairing its accurate delivery to the patient.[70] To avoid this, some of the insulin infusion mixture may be run through the tubing first, but it is no longer necessary to start with a flush of blood.[55]

The former practice of monitoring the diabetic patient through both the operative and postoperative period by urinalysis has been abandoned, having given way to direct measurement of the concentration of glucose in blood. The use of urine for monitoring glucose levels in blood is fraught with many potential problems.[15,58] First, it requires collection of a double voided specimen, which is often difficult to obtain; furthermore, if urinary retention occurs postoperatively, catheterization increases the likelihood of infection. Second, the renal threshold of glucose may be elevated because of renal disease leading to a decrease in the amount of spillage of glucose into the urine and hence a falsely low estimate of the level of blood glucose. Third, many drugs including tetracycline, chloramphenicol, cephalosporin, penicillin G, probenecid, sulfacetamide, salicylates, and ascorbic acid interfere with the estimation of glucose in urine when one uses paper test strips such as Diastix, Clinistix, or Clinitests. Lastly, the use of the urine dip stick in conjunction with an insulin sliding scale delegates full responsibility of insulin administration to the nursing staff and hence may lead to a decreased awareness of the patient's glucose status by the physician.

Blood glucose monitoring is unquestionably the best way to evaluate the diabetic patient.[33] In a modern chemical laboratory, a glucose analyzer can determine the glucose concentration in a drop of blood within an accuracy of 1 to 2 mg/dl in 30 seconds. By using the glucose oxidase enzymatic method, the test is specific for glucose and is not altered by the presence of other reducing substances in the blood (a problem with previous tests).

The relatively new bedside test strips also utilize the glucose oxidase reaction. With a drop of capillary blood obtained by a finger stick, the physician is able to determine a broad range of glucose levels within a few minutes. These tests are reliable and, when read with a portable reflectance meter, are almost as accurate as the analysis performed in the chemistry laboratory. When the blood glucose level is outside the range of 80 to 240 mg/dl, however, a sample of blood should be sent to the laboratory for a more precise determination. The paper test strips are available under the brand names Dextrostix or Reflotest for use with a reflectance meter or under the names Chemstrip BG or Visidex for use with a color chart. There are also highly sophisticated devices that calculate and deliver insulin or glucose based on a continuous analysis of blood glucose concentration. These artificial endocrine pancreases exist primarily within the realm of experimental studies, however, their use has reinforced the desirability and feasibility of controlling blood glucose concentrations with small doses of insulin given intravenously during periods of stress.[4,59]

Preoperative Management

Many diabetes specialists recommend that patients be admitted to the hospital 1 to 2 days prior to elective surgery. Because of the new, easier, and more precise methods of controlling the level of blood sugar, and the shortage of surgical beds in many hospitals, this precaution is no longer necessary for the majority of *stable* diabetic patients. It is best, however, to admit the patient early on the day before surgery for purposes of patient education and assessment of fluid balance, stability of glucose control, and dietary status. If the diabetic goes to surgery with the circulatory volume and electrolytes in order, no special requirements for pre- and postoperative fluid management are imposed.

Among the many regimens for preoperative control of diabetics, the method advocated by Rossini and Hare has the advantage of simplicity with relatively broad boundaries for control.[58] Determinations of the level of blood glucose in the blood are performed optimally at the time when the administered insulin is known to have its maximal activity and at the time when this activity is known to be minimal (Fig. 24-1). A safe "surgical zone" is defined on the basis of the level of the blood sugar falling between 150 and 250 mg/dl. A 10 to 20 percent increase in intermediate insulin is given for levels of blood glucose above the safe zone with the further addition of 10 to 20 units of regular insulin if the glucose level exceeds 350 mg/dl. On the other hand, the intermediate insulin dose is reduced by 10 to 20 percent if blood glucose level falls below 150 mg/dl and glucose is added when the danger of hypoglycemia becomes apparent by a fall in blood glucose below 80 mg/dl.

While opinion is divided regarding the limits of permissible fluctuations of blood glucose during the preoperative period, none will contest that wide fluctuations are not desirable prior to the start of an operative procedure. Ordinarily, the degree of control can be determined readily by careful study during a brief preoperative hospitalization. Appropriate changes in insulin dose and diet can be made according to the rigidity of control desired by the physician. The primary aim is to prevent loss of control to the extent that the feared complications of ketoacidosis, hyperosmotic nonketotic coma, and hypoglycemia might develop during surgery or in the postoperative period. No less important, although less immediate, complications from poor control are infection, impaired wound healing, and cardiovascular problems (stroke, myocardial infarction).

All, nondiabetic as well as diabetic, patients undergoing general anesthesia relinquish control of their perioperative diet to the surgeon. Thus, the surgeon must understand the concepts and techniques of dietary management. The only difference in dietary management of diabetic and nondiabetic patients is the need to monitor the level of blood glucose of the diabetic and to use appropriate mixtures of glucose and insulin to maintain a reasonable concentration of blood glucose. All patients require an adequate intake of calories and a well-balanced preoperative diet to promote glycogenesis. In turn, this will help to conserve protein during the postoperative flow phase. It is desirable, however, to schedule surgery for a time that prevents prolonged fasting, otherwise suitable intravenous alimentation is required to guard against dehydration and depletion of hepatic glycogen.

The classic studies of Gamble during World War II demonstrated clearly that provision of only 100 g glucose daily would prevent the development of ketosis in normal humans.[29] For the diabetic, the need for additional glucose with or without insulin is readily determined by (1) the type of diabetes, including the history of the dietary and insulin regimen followed; (2) the projected magnitude and duration of the surgical procedure; and (3) the estimated time before an oral dietary intake can be resumed. Today, virtually no guess work is involved in making an initial judgment regarding diabetic control and in revising this judgment as necessary due to the availability of the precise and technologically simple methods for monitoring the level of blood glucose at the bedside and in the operating room.

Anesthesiologic Considerations

As noted earlier, various anesthetic agents (e.g., ether, chloroform) will alter carbohydrate metabolism and, in conjunction with the stress of surgery, anesthesia may exacerbate hyperglycemia.[24,37,43] Most modern agents, however, have only minimal effects on metabolism and some, such as halothane, may even reduce the influence of catecholamines.[17,42] Spinal, epidural, and field block anesthesia exert no effect on carbohydrate metabolism nor on the outcome of the surgery with regard to the diabetes. Also, local anesthesia has no effect on carbohydrate metabolism. Therefore, the type of anesthesia and its mode of administration are determined primarily on the basis of the proposed surgical procedure and by the patient's overall medical condition; virtually no anesthetic agent is contraindicated simply by the presence of diabetes.[55]

In the management of the diabetic patient during surgery, the anesthesiologist must address certain predictable problems. Because of the associated autonomic neuropathy, the diabetic patient is especially prone to hypotension during the operation.[54] This common problem mandates close attention to the blood pressure and rate of fluid administration throughout the operative and early postoperative periods.

The anesthesiologist does have the additional task of monitoring and regulating the level of blood glucose throughout the operative procedure. Ordinarily, this is not a challenge because most patients are well controlled before surgery and the duration of most operations is not sufficient to disrupt this control. But procedures lasting over 2 or 3 hours or the development of fluid, respiratory, cardiac, or circulatory problems during the operative procedures signal the need for close supervision of the arterial blood glucose level. Thus, it behooves the anesthesiologist to be fully aware of the preoperative status of diabetic control and of the plan adopted for regulation of glucose metabolism during surgery.

Management During Surgery

Current regimens for the management of diabetes during the surgical procedure are numerous and disparate.[2,69] This undoubtedly reflects the differences in individual experience and stems from the absence of any large scale, properly controlled study comparing the morbidity, mortality, and metabolic alterations of two or more regimens. Nevertheless, guidelines for administration of glucose and insulin during surgery are useful as a point of departure for variations in therapy imposed by the needs of specific patients. The physiological heterogeneity of diabetes is so great that a rigid, all encompassing rule for its management during surgery is neither possible nor desirable. Several alternative regimens have been proposed (Table 24-3).

For the diabetic patient whose condition is controlled by diet only (fasting food glucose levels less than 150 mg/dl) ordinarily, there is no need for insulin therapy perioperatively although a few patients may need insulin temporarily during the early postoperative period.

All type II patients receiving sulfonylureas (chlorpropramide, Diabinese; tolazamide, Tolinase; tolbutamide, Orinase; and acetohexamide, Dymelor) are asked to discontinue use of these oral hypoglycemic agents prior to surgery. Chlorpropamide, which has a longer half-life, should be discontinued 72 hours prior to surgery. Short-acting oral agents or regular insulin are substituted during the immediate preoperative period.[55] For patients receiving insulin, the use of purified pork regular insulin or the newly developed human insulin will reduce the likelihood of insulin resistance, as may occur with beef insulin. Postoperatively, when bowel function returns and the patient is tolerating an oral diet, the oral hypoglycemic agent may be restarted. Occasionally, some patients will continue to require insulin for a short period.

For the insulin-dependent diabetic who is

TABLE 24-3.   Regimens for Administering Glucose and Insulin During Surgery

Type I diabetes (IDDM)	
A: Split normal dose insulin	500 ml with 50 g glucose; 10 mEq KCl; rate = 100 ml/hr
	Give intermediate insulin subcutaneously ($\frac{1}{2}$–$\frac{2}{3}$ total A.M. insulin dose)
	Maintain glucose between 150 and 250 mg/dl; monitor every 4–6 hours
	Sliding scale determines post operative dose regular insulin subcutaneously
B: Continuous IV low dose insulin	500 ml with 50 g glucose; 10 mEq KCl; + 10 u regular insulin; rate = 100 ml/hr
	Maintain glucose between 90 and 150 mg/dl; monitor every 2–4 hours
Type II diabetes (NIDDM)	
C	Monitor; rarely requires insulin
D	Patients using oral hypoglycemic agents switch to regimen A or B during surgery

Preoperative fasting blood glucose should be obtained for all methods.

to undergo elective surgery, the simplest and probably the most commonly used method for administering insulin and glucose on the day of surgery is the "split normal dose" regimen recommended in the 1981 edition of the *American Diabetes Association Handbook for Physicians* [58,55,62] (Table 24-3).

By this method, one half of the usual dose of intermediate-acting insulin (NPN or Lente) plus one half of the usual dose of regular insulin is given subcutaneously as intermediate-acting insulin early on the morning of surgery. If the fasting blood glucose level is more than 200 mg/dl, two thirds of the usual insulin dose is given rather than one half. Postoperatively, short-acting (regular) insulin is administered subcutaneously based on a sliding scale (see Table 24-4), related to measurements of the level of blood glucose made at 4 to 6 hour intervals. The sliding scale, of course, is simply a guide to the amount of supplementary regular insulin to be given based on the level of glucose in the blood. It is a generalization to be modified by the response of individual patients.

An alternative, although a less popular, approach is to start with the sliding scale dose instead of the split normal dose early on the morning of surgery. Some surgeons who start with the split normal dose prefer to give the remaining daily dose after the patient arrives in the recovery room instead of the dose based on the sliding scale. Unless the patient is able to eat supper, however, it is safer and more effective to use the sliding scale dose for subcutaneous regular insulin directly following surgery.

For patients undergoing extensive or prolonged surgery, the level of blood glucose can be determined readily during the operation. The administration of insulin and glucose is adjusted to maintain the blood glucose level in the safe "surgical zone."[58] The intravenous dextrose infusion should provide 50 g glucose for each missed meal with a minimum intake of 150 g in a 24 hour period for all patients.

Because the reduction in activity and total caloric intake is counterbalanced by the adverse effects of stress on insulin sensitivity, it is usually not necessary to administer more

TABLE 24-4.   Determining the Insulin Dosage on the Basis of Blood Glucose Measurements

Subcutaneous insulin (based on a sliding scale of blood glucose determinations at 6-hour intervals)	
Blood Glucose (mg/dl)	*Regular Insulin (units)*
0–60	Notify physician
60–200	0
200–250	2
250–300	4
300–350	6
350–400	8
400	Notify physician

Intravenous Insulin (based on sliding scale of bedside blood glucose determinations at 2- to 4-hour intervals)	
Blood Glucose (mg/dl)	*IV Insulin (units/hr)*
80	$\frac{1}{2}$
80–140	1
140–200	2
200–240	3
240	4+

(From Case SA, Mallory M, Wilcox F, Drucker WR: Diabetes and surgery—how to minimize the risks. Drug Ther 9:29, 1984.)

insulin on the day of surgery than had been received preoperatively. Also, because of the serious consequences of hypoglycemia, a more liberal level of hyperglycemia is tolerated in the immediate postoperative period than would ordinarily be considered acceptable.

A far more rigorous alternative method of insulin administration was adopted on the basis of its successful use in the treatment of diabetic ketoacidosis.[2,45,65] It involves a constant intravenous infusion of low-dose regular insulin coupled with frequent glucose determinations at the bedside (Table 24-3). Given intravenously, regular insulin has a half-life of approximately 4 minutes. The relatively rapid onset and short duration of action of intravenous insulin make the small dose, constant IV infusion method of blood glucose control safer and more concise.

As a detailed example of this regimen, Alberti has proposed a reasonably simple protocol to be used for all insulin-dependent diabetics during surgery. It involves the use of 0.32 units/g of a rapidly acting insulin in conjunction with 10 percent glucose.[2] The insulin infusion regimen is prepared by adding 16 units of a rapid acting insulin and 10 mEq potassium chloride in 500 ml of 10 percent dextrose. After an overnight fast, an infusion of the above is begun at 100 ml/hour. A fasting blood glucose sample is obtained on the morning of operation and the amount of insulin added to subsequent infusions is altered depending on the level of blood glucose measured q 2 h. If the blood glucose is less than 90 mg/dl, the insulin is decreased by 4 units/500 ml; if 90 to 100 mg/dl, continue with 16 units/500 ml; if greater than 180 mg/dl, add 4 units/500 ml. In this regimen, blood glucose is maintained between 90 and 180 mg/dl. The insulin is added directly to the dextrose solution primarily as a safety factor to prevent either being given in excess of the other.

One disadvantage of this method is that an entirely new infusion mixture is required if an alteration in the amount of either glucose or insulin is necessary. Other authors believe that tighter control of metabolism can be obtained when the infusions of glucose and insulin are given in separate bottles.[15] In this method, one infusion can be "piggy-backed"

into the other. In either case, it is important to note that fluids such as blood and crystalloids required for maintenance of volume must be given in an intravenous infusion quite separate from the infusion carrying insulin and glucose. This will allow adjustment of the volume of fluid administration without disrupting the infusions required for control of the blood glucose levels.

The major disadvantage of the low dose constant intravenous infusion technique is the need for more careful observation of the patient during and after surgery. The patient may become hypoglycemic if the glucose infusion stops or if an infiltration at the needle site is not detected. Symptoms of hypoglycemia may not be obvious when the patient is medicated or under anesthesia. In nonspecialized centers, the split-normal dose method therefore may be the safest, although glucose control will not be as tight. Nevertheless, the continuous intravenous infusion of low dose insulin is particularly indicated for the patient undergoing emergency surgery, and for the "brittle" diabetic.

Emergency Surgery

Approximately 1 of 20 diabetics undergoing surgery will be doing so for an acutely emergent situation.[28] The primary needs encountered in this situation are correction of hydration, hyperglycemia, acidosis, and electrolyte disturbances within a short interval. Only under the most urgent circumstances is surgery indicated before dehydration has been corrected. In most instances, treatment of hypovolemia will rectify the acidosis usually associated with it. Control of the glucose under these circumstances is most readily and safely obtained by use of the constant infusion of low dose regular insulin. In the presence of significant hyperglycemia, an intravenous bolus of 10 units of regular insulin can be given immediately before starting a constant infusion of insulin. Even more importantly than in the regimen used for an elective operation, the fluids given to restore adequate circulatory volume must be administered through a separate infusion in patients undergoing an emergency operation. Almost invariably potassium supplementation is indicated because stress, through the action of aldosterone, causes an obligatory loss of potassium in the urine. Also, an intracellular movement of potassium occurs in response to both hydration and the insulin-induced cellular uptake of glucose. In the presence of marked hyperglycemia, the addition of glucose to the insulin infusion is not indicated until the monitored levels of blood glucose decline under the influence of therapy of hypovolemia and acidosis. If hypovolemic or septic shock has been present for some time, the initial levels of blood glucose may be very low. Under this circumstance glucose rather than insulin is the first substance required to bring the diabetes back under control.

Ketoacidosis and the Surgical Emergency

Rarely, the diabetic patient may present with ketoacidosis, nausea, vomiting, and abdominal pain mimicking an acute abdomen. The difficulty for the surgeon in this situation is differentiating an acute surgical abdomen from the abdominal pain of ketoacidosis. In diabetic ketoacidosis, the anorexia, nausea, and vomiting always precede the abdominal pain whereas the opposite occurs in most acute surgical abdomens.[41] If the serum bicarbonate level is greater than 10 mEq/L, it is unlikely that the abdominal pain is due to ketoacidosis alone.[14]

In addition to the difficulty of differentiating between the abdominal pain of an acute surgical emergency and that of ketoacidosis, the surgeon is faced with the potential problem that they will occur together. The increased secretion of counterregulatory hormones in an acute surgical emergency may increase the inhibition of insulin activity to such an extent that, in a diabetic, ketoacidosis is produced. With a careful history, physical examination, and laboratory evaluation, the diagnosis of ketoacidosis can be made and treated by a continuous intravenous infusion of low dose regu-

lar insulin. Most patients will respond to small doses of intravenous insulin infusion ranging from 1.5 to 10.0 units/hr.[39,50,60,64] The importance of simultaneous attention to the needs of these patients for an adequate circulatory volume cannot be overstressed. It is unlikely that control of diabetes will be obtained if restoration of fluids lost consequent to the acute surgical problem is not also achieved.

CONCLUSION

Diabetes mellitus does not constitute a contraindication to surgery. Due to a better understanding of the metabolic alterations that develop following surgery in all patients, coupled with more precise and facile methods for monitoring the level of blood glucose, the surgical mortality of diabetics is approximately on a par with that of age-related cohorts. Nevertheless, the risk of surgery is increased by such complications of diabetes as cardiac, peripheral vascular, and renal disease, and poor control of the metabolic alterations of diabetes. No single regimen is applicable to the management of all diabetics during the perioperative period. Rather, the type of diabetes, the degree of metabolic control, and the planned surgical procedure are the major determinants of the most suitable protocol for care of the diabetic patient undergoing surgery.

ACKNOWLEDGMENTS

This work was supported in part by NIH Grant GM30095. The authors are appreciative of the assistance with the manuscript and illustrations provided by Patricia Semmel, Laurie Stamp, and Frances Wilcox.

REFERENCES

1. Alberti KG, Hockaday TD: Diabetic coma. Clin Endocrinol Metab 6: 421–455, 1977
2. Alberti KGMM, Insulin therapy in diabetic keto-acidosis and surgery. p. 260. In Skyler JS (ed): Insulin Update 1982. Excerpta Medica, Key Biscayne, Florida, 1982
3. Albin J, Rifkin H: Etiologies of diabetes mellitus. Symposium on diabetes mellitus. Med Clin North Am 66: 1209, 1982
4. Albisser AM, Leibel BS, Ewart TG et al: Clinical control of diabetes by the artificial pancreas. Diabetes 22: 115, 1979
5. Alieff A: Das Risiko chirurgischer Eingriffe beim Diabetiker. Zentralbl Chir 94: 857, 1969
6. Allison SP: Effect of insulin on metabolic response to injury. J Parenter Enteral Nutr 4: 175, 1980
7. Ashworth CJ Jr., Sacks Y, William LF Jr., et al: Hyperosmolar hyperglycemic non-acedotic coma: its importance in surgical problems. Ann Surg 167: 556, 1968
8. Bagdade JD: Phagocytic and microbicidal function in diabetes mellitus. Acta Endocrinol (Kbh) 83 (Suppl 205): 27, 1976
9. Bates G, Weiss C: Delayed development of antibody to staphylococcus in diabetic children. Am J Dis Child 62: 346, 1941
10. Beaser SB: Surgical management. p. 746. In Ellenberg M, Rifkin H (eds): Diabetes Mellitus: Theory and Practice. McGraw-Hill, New York, 1983
11. Breuner WI, Lansky A, Engelman RM et al: Hyperosmolar coma in surgical patients: an iatrogenic disease of increasing incidence. Ann Surg 178: 651, 1973
12. Busick EJ: The medical management of diabetic patients during surgery. 8: 22, Diabetes Educator 1982
13. Byyny RL: Management of diabetes during surgery. Postgrad Med 68: 191, 1980
14. Campbell IW, Duncan LJP, Innes JA et al: Abdominal pain in diabetic decompensation: clinical significance. JAMA 233: 166, 1975
15. Case SA, Mallory M, Wilcox F, Drucker WR: Diabetes and surgery—how to minimize the risks. Drug Ther 000: 29–48, 1984
16. Chadwick CDJ, Pearce FJ, Drucker WR: Influences of fasting and water intake on plasma refill during hemorrhagic shock. J Trauma 25:608, 1985
17. Clarke RSJ: The hypoglycemic response to different types of surgery and anesthesia. Br J Anaesth 42: 45, 1970
18. Clowes GHA, O'Donnell TF, Blackburn GL, Maki TN: Energy metabolism and proteolysis in traumatized and septic man. Surg Clin North Am 56: 1169, 1976
19. Craig JW, Miller M, Drucker WR et al: Influence of dietary fructose on glucose tolerance in man. Diabetes 8: 432, 1959
20. Cuthbertson DP: Post-traumatic metabolism: a multi-disciplinary challenge. Surg Clin North Am 58: 1045, 1978
21. Deitrich JE, Whedon GD, Short E: Effects of immobilization upon various metabolic and physiologic functions of normal man. Am J Med 9: 3, 1948
22. DeLeiris J, Opiel H, Lubbe WF: Effects of free fatty acid and enzyme release in experimental glucose on myocardial infarction. Nature 253: 746, 1975
23. Drucker WR, Chadwick CDJ, Gann DS: Transcapillary refill in hemorrhage and shock. Arch Surg 116: 1344, 1981
24. Drucker WR, Costley C, Stults R et al: Studies of carbohydrate metabolism during ether anesthesia. 1. Effect of ether on glucose and fructose metabolism. Metabolism 8: 827, 1959
25. Drucker WR, Gann DS, McCoy S: Response to surgery: neuroendocrine and metabolic changes, convalescence and rehabilitation. p. 3. In Hardy's Textbook of Surgery. JB Lippincott, Philadelphia, 1983
26. Drucker WR, Miller M, Craig J et al: A comparison of the effect of operation on glucose and fructose metabolism. Surg Forum 3: 548, 1952
27. Flier JS: Insulin receptors and insulin resistance. Annu Rev Med 34: 145, 1983
28. Galloway JA, Shuman CR: Diabetes and surgery: a study of 667 cases. Am J Med 34: 177, 1963
29. Gamble JL: Physiological information gained from studies on the life raft ration. Harvey Lect 42: 1946
30. Gastineau CF, Molnar GD: The care of the diabetic patient during emergency surgery. Surg Clinics North Am 49: 1171, 1969
31. Garcia, MJ, McNamara PM, Gordon T et al: Morbidity and mortality in diabetics in the Framingham population. Sixteen year follow-up study. Diabetes 23: 105, 1974
32. Gavin JR, Roth J, Neville DM et al: Insulin-dependent regulation of insulin receptor concentrations: a direct demonstration in cell culture. Proc Natl Acad Sci USA 71: 84, 1974
33. Genuth S: Classification and diagnosis of diabetes mellitus. Med Clin North Am 66(6): p. 1191, 1982
34. Genuth SM: Plasma insulin and glucose profiles in normal, obese and diabetic persons. Ann Intern Med 79: 812, 1983
35. Giddings AEB: The control of plasma glucose in the surgical patient. Br J Surg 61: 787, 1974
36. Goodson WH, Hunt TK: Studies of wound healing in experimental diabetes mellitus. J Surg Res 22: 221, 1977

37. Henneman DH, Vandam LD: The metabolic consequences of epinephrine and insulin administered during ether anesthesia in man. Anesthesiology 19: 104, 1958

38. Ito C, Mito K, Hara H: Review of criteria for diagnosis of diabetes mellitus based on results of follow-up study. Diabetes 32: 343, 1983

39. Kidson W, Casey J, Drayen E et al: Treatment of severe diabetes mellitus by insulin infusion. Br Med J 2: 691, 1974

40. Kinney JM, Felig P: The metabolic response to injury and infection. Endocrinology 3: 1963, 1979

41. Kleeman CR, Liberman B: Diabetic acidosis and coma. In Maxwell MH, Kleeman CR (eds): Clinical Disorders of Fluid and Electrolyte Metabolism. McGraw-Hill, New York, 1972

42. Longnecker DE, McCoy S, Drucker WR: Anesthetic influence on biochemical response to hemorrhage. Circ Shock 6: 55, 1979

43. Marble A, Steinke J: Physiology and pharmacology in diabetes mellitus: guiding the diabetic patient through the surgical period. Anesthesiology 24: 492, 1963

44. McCoy S, Case SA, Swerlick RA et al: Determinants of blood amino acid concentration after hemorrhage. Am Surg 43: 787, 1977

45. Meyer EJ, Lorenzi M, Bohannon NV: Diabetic management by insulin infusion during major surgery. Am J Surg 137: 323, 1979

46. Miller M, Drucker WR, Owens JE et al: Metabolism of intravenous fructose and glucose in normal and diabetic subjects. J Clin Invest 30: 115, 1951

47. National Diabetes Data Group: Classification and diagnosis of diabetes mellitus and other categories of glucose intolerance. Diabetes 28: 1039, 1979

48. Nolan CM, Beaty HN, Bagdade JD: Further characterization of the impaired bactericidal function of granulocytes in patients with poorly controlled diabetes. Diabetes 27: 889, 1978

49. Packovich MJ, Molaar GD, Leonard PF: Management of diabetic patients during surgery. Surg Clinics North Am 45: 975, 1965

50. Page MM, Alberti KGM, Greenwood R et al: Treatment of diabetic coma with continuous low-dose infusion of insulin. Br Med J 2: 687, 1974

51. Pass LJ, Schloerb PR, Chow F et al: Liver adenosine triphosphate (ATP) in hypoxia and hemorrhagic shock. J Trauma 22: 730, 1982

52. Pearce FJ, Weiss PR, Miller JR, Drucker WR: Effect of hemorrhage, anoxia and graded ischemia on hepatic gluconeogenesis. Surg Forum 33: 3, 1982

53. Pearce FJ, Weiss PR, Miller JR, Drucker WR: Effect of hemorrhage and anoxia on hepatic gluconeogenesis and potassium balance in the rat. J Trauma 23: 312, 1983

54. Podolsky S: Clinical Diabetes: Modern Management. Appleton Century-Crofts, New York, 1980

55. Podolsky S: Management of diabetes in the surgical patient. Med Clinics North Am 66: 1361, 1982

56. Root HF: Preoperative care of the diabetic patient. Postgrad Med 40: 439, 1966

57. Rosenthal S, Lerner B, DiBiase F et al: Relation of strength to composition in diabetic wounds. Surg Gynecol Obstet 115: 437, 1962

58. Rossini A, Hare JW: How to control the blood glucose level in the surgical diabetic patient. Arch Surg 3: 945, 1976

59. Schwartz SS, Horowitz DC, Zehfus B et al: Use of glucose-controlled insulin infusion system (artificial beta cell) to control diabetes during surgery. Diabetologia 16: 157, 1979

60. Semple PF, White C, Manderson W: Continuous intravenous infusion of small doses of insulin in treatment of diabetic ketoacidosis. Br Med J 2: 694, 1974

61. Solar NG, Pentecost BL, Bennett MA et al: Coronary care for myocardial infarction in diabetics. Lancet 1: 475, 1974

62. Sussman KE, Kolterman OG: Surgery in the patient with diabetes. p. 225. In Rifkin H, Raskin P (eds): Diabetes mellitus, vol. 5. Robert J. Brady, Maryland, 1981

63. Swerlick RA, Drucker NA, McCoy S, Drucker WR: Insulin effectiveness in hypovolemic dogs. J Trauma 21: 1013, 1981

64. Taitelman U, Reese EA, Bessman AN: Insulin in the management of the diabetic surgical patient—continuous intravenous infusion vs. subcutaneous administration. JAMA 237: 658, 1977

65. Unger RH: Benefits and risks of meticulous control of diabetes. Med Clin North Am 66: 1317, 1982

66. Unger RH, Eisentrant AM: Entero-insular axis. Arch Intern Med 123: 261, 1969

67. Unger RH, Orci L: Glucagon and the A-cell. N Engl J Med 304: 1518, 1981

68. Wahlqvist ML, Kaijser L, Lassers BW et al: Fatty acids as a determinant of myocardial substrate and oxygen metabolism in man at rest and during prolonged exercise. Acta Med Scand 198: 89, 1973

69. Walts LF, Miller J, Davidson MB et al: Perioperative management of diabetes mellitus. Anesthesiology 55: 104, 1981

70. Weisenfeld S, Podolsky S, Goldsmith L et al: Adsorption of insulin to infusion bottles and tubing. Diabetes 17: 766, 1968

71. Wheelock FC Jr., Marble A: Surgery and diabetes. p. 599. In Joslin's Diabetes Mellitus, 11th ed. Lea and Febiger, Philadelphia, 1971

72. Yip CC: Preparation of ^{3}H insulin and its binding to liver plasma membrane. p. 115. In Fritz IB (ed): Insulin Action. Academic Press, London, 1972

25

Endocrine Emergencies in Critical Illness

Glenn W. Geelhoed

INTRODUCTION

Under the stress of critical illness, the body's reserves are mobilized through the integrated actions of at least two reactive systems to maintain homeostasis under duress, the nervous and endocrine systems. The nervous system activates neurogenic impulses, secretes "releasing hormones," and uses peptidergic neurotransmitters to effect shifts in the body economy to facilitate survival. The autonomic nervous system is particularly involved, and the mediators that might normally function as neurotransmitters may even achieve blood levels that circulate as hormones.

The endocrine system is the primary "shock absorber" to adapt to the stress and mobilize energy reserves for repair and extraordinary functions. The global response of the endocrine system is not simply an "all out alert" with hypersecretion of all known hormones in response to nonspecific stress. Rather, the response is modulated and carefully controlled by "feedback loops" so that the "runaway metabolism" does not continue to disrupt the body economy. Only in extraordinary circumstances of exhaustion of some components of the hormonal reserves or in the pathologic process of uncontrolled hypersecretion does a "positive feedback" result, with endocrine disease compounding the original stress. In this chapter, we will examine both the physiologic and pathologic response to stress in critical illness, and determine the measured response that is classified as "critical," that is, a minute-to-minute adaptive response facilitating survival by endocrine coping mechanisms.

HORMONES WITH GENERALLY INCREASED SECRETION IN STRESSFUL ILLNESS

Some, but not all, hormones exhibit an elevated secretion pattern and an increased circulating hormonal activity during the stress of trauma or illness. Table 25-1 lists some of these more characteristic hormone elevations. The anterior and posterior pituitary are stimulated by the releasing factors carried to them by the portal system from the hypophysis. Adrenocorticotropic hormone (ACTH), arginine vasopressin, growth hormone, and prolactin are all increased. As a direct consequence of ACTH stimulation, plasma cortisol can be remarkably elevated to "stress levels" of cortisol secretion rates. Aldosterone is also elevated, but not so much secondary to ACTH elevation as to the remarkable increase in renin secretion and the subsequent rise in angiotensin levels.

Catecholamine output increases remarkably during stress. Ordinarily, epinephrine is the classic adrenergic hormone, and norepinephrine the neurotransmitter, with dopamine being a largely intracellular mediator. In the stress of critical illness, plasma epinephrine levels may increase manyfold, and norepinephrine may increase to the point where it circulates as a hormone rather than functioning as it typically does quite locally as a neurotransmitter.[6] Even dopamine concentrations in plasma rise with stress. The catecholamines have many physiologic actions, but among them are the mobilization of sugar metabolism by the breakdown of glycogen and a shift to readily useable fuels for oxidation. Contributing to this is the increased secretion of glucagon from the pancreatic islets.

Groups of hormones that exist in plasma in such low concentration as to have been undetected before the advent of radioimmunoassay are the neuropeptides. The endorphins and enkephalins are elaborated from pituitary gland and nerve endings and are found to rise in the circulation during stress. A number of behavioral and physiologic effects are attributed to this rise, though the precise role of the endorphins as homeostatic mediators is unclear.

HORMONES WITH GENERALLY DECREASED OR UNALTERED SECRETION DURING STRESSFUL ILLNESS

Table 25-2 lists those hormones with less remarkable changes or actual decreases under the stress of critical illness. Typically thyroxin (T_4) and triiodothyronine (T_3) concentrations are both decreased in shock and other forms of clinical stress. This situation exists despite a normal or unaltered thyroid-stimulating hormone (TSH). Thyroid function, therefore, is decreased despite the stimulating hormone normally responsible for thyroid regulation in a

TABLE 25-1. Hormones with Generally Increased Secretion during Stress

Pituitary
  ACTH
  ADH (vasopressin)
  Growth hormone
  Prolactin
Adrenal
  Aldosterone
  Cortisol
  Catecholamine
Renal
  Renin
Gut
  Glucagon
Neural
  Endorphins (neuropeptides)

TABLE 25-2. Hormones with Decreased or Unaltered Secretion during Stress

TSH
  T_4
  T_3
Insulin
Sex steroids
  FSH-LH and ovarian hormones
  FSH-LH and testicular hormones
  Adrenal androgens

pattern that has come to be known as the "sick-euthyroid" syndrome.

Insulin secretion is not remarkably different under conditions of stress. The insulin effect may differ, particularly under the changes such illnesses as sepsis evokes. Patterns of sugar metabolism certainly change, but the glucagon, growth hormone, and catecholamine concentrations may have more to do with this than any fundamental change in insulin secretion.

The sex steroids from ovarian, testicular, and adrenal origins are not appreciably different under circumstances of stress, and when they are different, they are decreased. This is true despite elevations in ACTH, but levels of follicle-stimulating hormone–luteinizing hormone (FSH–LH) are normal or depressed.

CONSEQUENCES OF ENDOCRINE CHANGES

The metabolic effects of these changes in hormone secretions (Table 25-3) are tissue wasting and weight loss. This comes about from the twin mechanisms of semistarvation, from lack of absorption of foodstuffs, and postinjury catabolism. This breakdown in protein is much greater under the conditions of sepsis, shock, and the withholding of foodstuffs. It is paradoxically much greater in terms of protein loss in young healthy men than in elderly patients. The protein loss and tissue

wasting are also aggravated in patients with some degree of failure of these adaptation mechanisms.

If tissue wasting were the only direct effect of these endocrine changes they would certainly be classified as maladaptive. However, there are direct homeostatic effects of these endocrine changes that tend toward longer-term preservation of the body economy (Table 25-4). The immediate action of the endocrine mediators tends toward salt and water conservation, blood pressure maintenance, and stabilization of the circulation. Furthermore, the tendency of the tissue breakdown is in the direction of supporting oxidative metabolism and ready energy release from fuel stores. Gluconeogenesis and glycolysis serve to shift carbohydrate into its most readily utilizable form and lipolysis breaks down high calorie fat storage into ketones and fatty acids for further substrate supply to fuel aerobic metabolism. These withdrawals from the energy reserve teleologically provide ready energy for the skeletal muscles and myocardium and for the obligate aerobic metabolism of the nervous system. These organ systems are the "effector arms" of the adaptive response.

It would be strategically useful if all the caloric requirement mobilized within the body came from nonfunctional macromolecule sources. However, functional protein is mobilized as part of the consumable fuel as well as the energy storage depots of glycogen and lipid. Initiation of the metabolic response is immediate in all three pathways of caloric fuels (see Fig. 25-1). Carbohydrates are the most

TABLE 25-3. Metabolic Effects of Hormone Changes

Tissue wasting and weight loss
   Postinjury catabolism
   Mimics semistarvation
Disproportionate protein loss in
   Sepsis
   Shock and anoxia
   Failure of adaptation mechanisms
   Withholding of calories and amino acids
   Healthy young men rather than elderly

TABLE 25-4. Homeostatic Effects of Endocrine Stress Adaptation

Circulation
   Salt and water conservation
   Blood pressure maintenance
   Delivery of substrate and oxygen
Fuel
   Gluconeogenesis
   Glycolysis
   Lipolysis
   Mobility of calories
Aerobic energy utilization
   Heart
   Skeletal muscle
   CNS

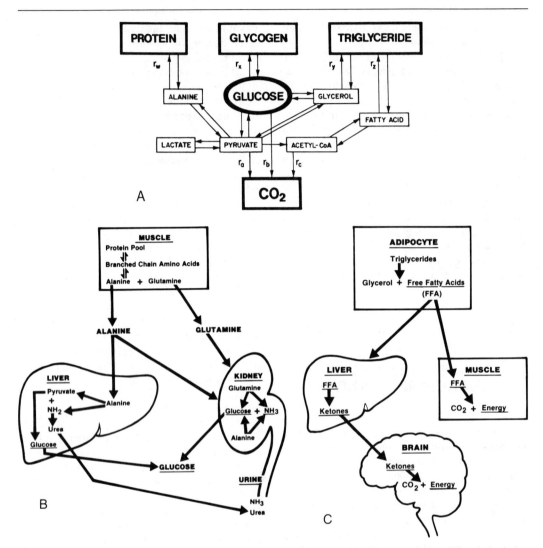

FIG. 25-1 Metabolism is quickened through the effect of these endocrine mediators acting on **(A)** carbohydrate, **(B)** protein, and **(C)** lipid pathways, each converting to mobile calories useful in aerobic metabolism. (Gens D: Nutrition in critical illness. In Geelhoed GW, Chernow B (eds): Endocrine and Metabolic Responses to Critical Illness and Trauma. Churchill Livingstone, New York, 1984.)

readily available substrate for aerobic metabolism, and free glucose is converted out of glycolysis or through the pathways of gluconeogenesis (Fig. 25-1A). However, at the same time, muscle mass and other functioning protein is broken down (see Fig. 25-1B) to serve as a similar ready supply of fuel. The highest energy depot is in lipids, and the lipid pool also serves to contribute substrate, but the endocrine mechanisms of mechanization take longer than the "more expensive" energy reserves in the former two systems that yield only half the calories as a comparable mass of lipid converted to energy[13] (Fig. 25-1C).

SEQUENCE OF PHASES IN RESPONSE TO ILLNESS

In the classic pattern described by Moore,[20] patients responding to the stress of injury go through at least four phases in sequence after their most severe stress. The first, or acute phase, is marked by injury and the response of catabolism. Depending on the degree of the injury, some 48 hours or more later, a "crisis" or critical turning point marks the change from catabolism to a sharp decrease in their nitrogen loss. This period is similar to corticoid withdrawal. As seen in Table 25-5, the third phase is the anabolic period of gain in muscular strength and positive nitrogen balance. Following this recovery phase, in the fourth or final phase, the energy reserves are replenished after nitrogen balance has been achieved. In this final phase positive caloric balance is seen and fat gain occurs. This is the classic pattern seen after isolated injury, but any complication in the patient's course can return the patient from one of the advanced phases back toward an earlier period of catabolism. These effects seen clinically in metabolic balance studies are rational interpretations of the intermediary metabolism effects of the endocrine changes that cause these metabolic shifts.

TABLE 25-5. Phases of Response to Injury as Described by Moore[20]

First: Injury and acute response; catabolism
Second: Turning point; corticoid withdrawal
Third: Muscular strength; anabolism
Fourth: Fat gain; nitrogen balance; but positive energy and calorie balance

(Adapted from Moore FD: Metabolic Care of the Surgical Patient. WB Saunders, Philadelphia, 1959.)

Table 25-6. Only a few of the endogenous hypo- or hyperfunctions in the endocrine system require emergency management, but those that do are critically life-threatening. With respect to the thyroid, hyperfunction is a critical problem requiring much more urgent management than hypothyroidism, although the cardiac and central nervous system effects of thyroid hypofunction make it a highly morbid condition. In infancy, cretinism may result, and we have previously referred to the "sick-euthyroid syndrome" in patients in intensive care units. However, the metabolic disaster of thyroid storm may follow in a thyrotoxic patient after injury or illness and then this endocrine disorder becomes the chief threat to life. It is particularly insidious in the "apathetic hyperthyroidism" that may be seen in some patients, particularly the elderly.

The parathyroid control of calcium homeostasis is a critical problem at both the hypo- and hyperfunction ends of the spectrum. Tet-

HORMONAL FAILURE IN HOMEOSTATIC ADAPTATION

Endogenous endocrine failure would not allow this normal pattern of homeostatic adaptation to occur. With specific endocrine deficiencies, devastating osmolar and electrolyte changes may occur, cardiovascular collapse and mineral or energy deficiencies may also have effects in the nervous system such as seizures. The principal hormone deficiency states that give rise to critical illness are noted in

TABLE 25-6. Endocrine Emergencies that Require Urgent Management for Endogenous Hypo- or Hyperfunction

Hypofunction	Endocrine System	Hyperfunction
Hypothyroidism	Thyroid	Thyrotoxicosis Thyroid storm
Tetany	Parathyroid	Hypercalcemia Coma
Ketoacidosis	Pancreatic islets	Hyperinsulin shock
Addisonian crisis	Adrenal cortex	—
—	Chromaffin system	Pheochromocytoma
Diabetes insipidus	Pituitary	SIADH

(Adapted from Geelhoed GW: Problem Management in Endocrine Surgery. Copyright © 1983 by Year Book Medical Publishers, Inc., Chicago.)

any and interference in respiration may result from hypofunction, and hypercalcemia can lead to coma and seizures as well as systolic arrest from hyperfunction.

The pancreatic islets can give rise to endocrine emergencies particularly with respect to the β-islet cell production of insulin. Failure of insulin production or receptor resistance to its secretion can lead to ketoacidosis. Hyperfunction, however, is also treacherous, since an insulinoma can cause the blood glucose level to drop below levels at which viable central nervous system function can be maintained.

With respect to the adrenal cortex, there are no real emergencies of hyper- or hypofunction of mineralocorticoid or sex steroid, with the possible rare exception of adrenogenital syndrome. Cushing's syndrome is an important diagnosis to make, but it is rarely a crisis requiring emergency management. The principal reason that adrenocortical function is necessary for life is in an adequate supply of cortisol. Either absolutely or relatively, hypocortisolism is a high risk problem termed "addisonian crisis." No real critical problems result from hypofunction of the chromaffin system, but an undiagnosed pheochromocytoma encountered in a patient under circumstances of stress is a critical situation with a high mortality rate. For these critical problems, a pattern of recognition has been described for their management.[10]

These significant deviations from the normal endocrine response to stress and trauma requiring urgent recognition and management are the subjects of this chapter. Exogenous life support may include the use of synthetic hormones or administration of hormone extracts or hormone agonists, or may include receptor blockade or treatment with antagonists, or surgical ablation of the source of excessive hormones. It frequently also entails stabilization of cellular function by ensuring adequate delivery and utilization of nutrients and oxygen. The intensive care physician should understand the use of adrenergic, glucocorticoid, glucose-regulating regimens, and mineral balance metabolism drugs as well as when surgical treatment is indicated in endocrine complications of the critically ill patient.

THYROID DISORDERS IN THE CRITICALLY ILL PATIENT

Hypofunction

Hypothyroidism is a relatively common problem[27] in the general population, occurring with a frequency of 1 to 2 percent. However, critical illness nearly always alters thyroid function, and the measurable thyroid hormones are uniformly decreased, with the exception of the biologically inactive reverse T_3, which is increased.[5] The shift of circulating thyroid hormones from the biologically active T_4 and T_3 forms to reverse T_3 is accounted for by a decrease in thyroid hormone binding to protein and by an inhibition of the enzymatic activity of reverse T_3 degradation. This impairment in thyroid hormone metabolism is uniform in critical illness and the extent of the impairment may correlate with the degree of severity of the hemorrhagic shock as tested in animals and suggested in humans.[29]

Though thyroid metabolism is decreased in acute illness, the measurements of free thyroxin are less reliable precisely when critical illness occurs.[24] Nonthyroidal illness results in disturbances of thyronine-binding proteins, and these alterations change even the free thyroxin index, usually a reliable predictor of thyroid status in patients with thyroid disease alone when uncomplicated by critical illness. The results of one investigation prompted the caveat, "All tests for free T_4 used in this study should be interpreted with caution in severely ill patients."[24]

If seriously ill patients have depressed thyroid hormone levels as a rule, although the measurements become unreliable in the course of the sickness, what effect do these low circulating hormone levels have on the patient? And why not simply administer thyroid hormone to each critically ill patient? This has been tried, but there are some serious questions about its advisability. In the first instance, patients with critical illness do not appear to be other than euthyroid from most clinical measurements except for the thyroid hormone levels. In the second place, T_3 particularly is a catabolic hormone that promotes protein breakdown, oxygen consumption, and a high metabolic demand on the heart. The "sick-euthyroid syndrome" appears to be an adaptive process and may be a quenching mechanism for braking the catabolism of the other hormone excesses, such as catecholamines and corticosteroids. A reciprocal relationship between plasma concentrations of T_3 and catecholamines appears to exist in at least one group of severely injured patients: burn victims. In one study, measurements of the thyroid hormone levels and catecholamines were performed in burn patients and T_3 was administered to half of them; in this study,[1] "treatment with a metabolically active hormone, triiodothyronine, does not alter the level of hypermetabolism accompanying thermal injury." Besides the fact that it does not work, thyroid hormone administration may actually hinder the natural adaptive response.[28]

As already noted in Table 25-2, TSH is one of the hormones not appreciably changed in severe illness. In patients who are not severely ill, if T_4 and T_3 levels were depressed, TSH levels would rise, defining hypothyroidism. As just established, T_4 and T_3 levels are depressed in critical illness, but TSH levels remain the same, so either hypothyroidism is not present or the sick patient is unable to recognize the altered state of thyroid metabolism. To distinguish those patients who are truly hypothyroid from those who are "sick-euthyroid" with similarly depressed thyroid hormone levels in the circulation, a thyrotropin-releasing hormone (TRH) test is performed.

Coincidentally, TRH is one of the neuropeptides of the group to be discussed later, but it usually evokes a two or threefold TSH increase in euthyroid patients and a much greater TSH response in those who are hypothyroid. If one suspected that a patient were both critically ill and hypothyroid, a TRH test would differentiate these on the basis of a very exaggerated TSH response to TRH stimulation.[3]

Those patients who do exhibit a marked TSH response to TRH stimulation (greater than triple the pre-TRH serum TSH level) should be cautiously treated with a maintenance thyroid hormone regimen, even when critically ill. The effects of hypothyroidism include respiratory depression, low cardiac output, and hypothermia. Unexplained hypothermia should alert the clinician to check for evidence of hypothyroidism or hypoadrenocorticism. It is safer to undertreat hypothyroidism than to overtreat and be driving catabolism by thyrotoxicosis.

Hyperfunction

Borderline hyperthyroidism may be present in a patient admitted to the intensive care unit for some other illness, or thyrotoxicosis itself may be the critical illness. Reasonably compensated patients may lose control of their hyperthyroidism under the stress of intercurrent illness or their hyperkinetic activity may lead to an admission for trauma. Patients with evidence of hypermetabolic state, such as hyperdynamic cardiovascular function with high cardiac output, increased temperature, hyperventilation, and increased oxygen consumption, should be thought of as candidates for investigation of possible hyperthyroidism. Many of the symptoms of hyperthyroidism can mimic the hyperreflexic state of the general stress response mediated through other hormones. However, as previously noted, T_4 and T_3 are usually decreased in their circulation, so marked elevations of thyroid hormone in the circulation should be diagnostic in the seriously ill patient. Some part of the critical illness may be attributed to thyroid hyperfunction, particularly with exaggerated response to catecholamines and amplified response to β-adrenergic stimulation.[25]

Some forms of thyrotoxicosis can be readily apparent clinically because of associated findings such as ophthalmologic changes. Graves' disease has distinctive eye findings, but it is not the only type of hyperthyroidism. The eye changes and infiltrative dermopathy are unique characteristics that are not a property of the hypermetabolism of excess thyroid hormone, but concomitants of the thyroid-stimulating immunoglobulins (TSI) including long-acting thyroid-stimulator (LATS).

Graves' disease does share with other forms of hyperthyroidism a common physical finding, an enlargement in the thyroid gland. The goiter in Graves' disease typically shows diffuse hyperplasia, whereas in toxic adenoma, or an autonomous hyperfunction in a multinodular goiter (Plummer's syndrome), the thyroid enlargement may be more discrete or nodular. Each patient in an intensive care unit should have a careful thyroid examination, particularly in retrospect if atypical metabolic responses are noted, or if cardiac arrhythmias or excessive catecholamine sensitivity are noted in combination with the hypermetabolism shared by many patients under severe stress. Measurements of TSH often show the intact thyroid-pituitary axis by TSH suppression, but normal or suppressed TSH findings are also possible with the "sick-euthyroid syndrome." In patients with the latter, levels of TSH as well as the thyroid hormone species are depressed and the patient does not have evidence of hyperadrenergic status.

The hyperthyroid patient, who either coincidentally is victim of a critical illness or injury, or is in the intensive care unit because of thyrotoxicosis, is at risk for several complications. First are the excessive catabolism and nitrogen loss that accompany the hypermetabolic state. The "thermostat" is set too high in such individuals, and both metabolic and behavioral disturbances can result from this overactivity. The "ICU psychosis" is a peculiar, particular risk to these patients since they are stimulated excessively in patterns that do not resemble circadian rhythms. Such patients also are typically administered corticosteroids or are stressed to extraordinary endogenous secretion of these hormones. Their behavioral disturbance and their hyperkinetic reactions to the excess thyroid stimulation often make them difficult nursing challenges. Besides the excessive protein catabolism and its metabolic consequences, cardiac arrhythmias may result, with thyrotoxicosis sensitizing the myocardium to the β-catecholamine effect.

The most dreaded complication of hyperthyroidism in the stressed individual is the runaway hypermetabolism of thyroid storm.[19] Thyroid storm is a diagnosis that should not be used lightly to describe someone with thyrotoxicosis, since the precise application of the term carries with it a very grave prognosis even in the mid-1980s. Thyroid storm is distinguished from hyperthyroidism by the remarkable hyperpyrexia with uncontrollable temperatures rising so high as to cause inactivation of important enzyme systems such as the cytochrome system. Leukocytosis is also the rule. The excessive metabolic demand rapidly exhausts all quickly convertible sources of fuel and a rapid degradation of functional proteins occurs. Management techniques for the control of hyperthyroidism have to be extended for thyroid storm to muscle paralysis of a patient between hypothermia blankets and on ventilator support with full treatment programs of drugs at the level of the thyroid as well as full metabolic support including adrenergic blockade. Surgical treatment may be urgent to control the hyperthyroidism if the hypermetabolic condition can be brought under control to the extent that anesthesia is possible.

The management of hyperthyroidism usually involves drug treatment and may involve radioiodine or surgical therapy. The drugs used for antithyroid treatment are listed in Table 25-7. There are at least three mechanisms by which hyperthyroidism can be reduced in its effect on the critically ill patient. First is through the decrease of thyroid hormone release, and this can be done with iodides or lithium, including those iodides in radiographic contrast material or saturated solutions of potassium iodide. A second technique is by decreasing the production of thyroid hormone

TABLE 25-7. Types of Drug Therapy for Hyperthyroidism

I. Decrease thyroid hormone release
   A. Iodides (Lugol's solution)
   B. Lithium
II. Decrease thyroid hormone production
   A. Thiocynates, perchlorates
   B. Thionamides (PTU)
III. Decrease thyroid hormone response by adrenergic interference
   A. Catecholamine depletion (reserpine, guanethidine)
   B. β-Adrenergic blockade (propranolol)

(Reprinted with permission from Geelhoed GW: Problem Management in Endocrine Surgery. Copyright © 1983 by Year Book Medical Publishers, Inc., Chicago.)

and this happens with thionamides, among which propylthiouracil (PTU) or methimazole (MTZ) are examples. A third drug treatment strategy is to decrease the thyroid hormone response by adrenergic blockade. The most successful of these treatments has been the liberal use of propranolol. The sequence in which these drugs are given varies depending on the elective nature of the thyrotoxic control, but in an intensive care setting propranolol in high dosage would be an effective start to treatment. However, the clinician must be aware of the potential harmful consequences of β-blockade, particularly in a patient who may be dependent on exogenous catecholamine in high output cardiac failure.

Radioiodine is one form of definitive treatment for hyperthyroidism, but is slow in onset and has the unfortunate consequence of producing hypothyroidism if effective in patients who are evaluated long enough. Surgical therapy in the form of subtotal thyroidectomy (see Fig. 25-2) is a nearly ideal treatment for definitive management in the patient who has been rendered euthyroid by appropriate drug treat-

ment. This treatment is used for young candidates because subtotal thyroidectomy is the one form of treatment that may be able to bring the patient back to thyroid–pituitary control with the thyroid hormones and TSH in normal physiologic relationship. Thyroidectomy does carry with it, however, the hazards of injury to the recurrent laryngeal nerves or parathyroid glands, and is a technically challenging procedure.

The control of thyroid abnormalities in the critically ill patient is gratifying. There is reasonable precision in the diagnostic testing, and readily available, cheap, and easily regulated replacement hormone for hypothyroidism, and both acute medical management techniques as well as definitive ablation techniques for hyperthyroidism. The consequences of both hypofunction and hyperfunction are metabolically severe in the patients affected, and the consequences of treatment are very beneficial with acceptable risks. Therefore, thyroid disorders in the clinically ill patient are worth seeking out and appropriate correction of these disorders very quickly pays off in metabolic dividends.

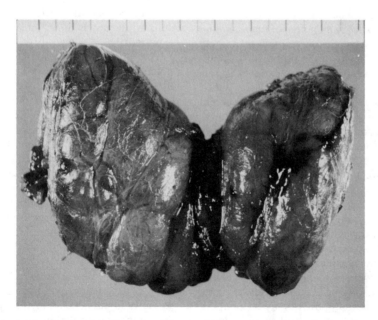

FIG. 25-2 Subtotal thyroidectomy for hyperthyroidism (in this instance, the diffuse hyperplastic goiter of Grave's disease) pays off in immediate metabolic dividends of relief of hypermetabolic stress and has the potential for restoring long-range normal physiologic balance of residual thyroid under pituitary control.

PARATHYROID DISORDERS IN CRITICALLY ILL PATIENTS

Hypofunction

Hypocalcemia is not rare as a finding in critically ill patients, but its interpretation is made difficult unless surgical or traumatic injury to the parathyroid glands was part of the recent history preceding the finding. The parathyroid glands are not the only organs in the body that control calcium homeostasis; many organs are affected in hypofunction when hypocalcemia is the result. For practical purposes, we will limit this discussion to the emergency treatment of hypocalcemic tetany.

The effects of hypocalcemia include cardiovascular manifestations in congestive heart failure, arrhythmia, and hypotension. Neuromuscular manifestations include increased intracranial pressure, the hyperreflexia that is clinically tested in the Chvostek's sign and Trousseau's sign, and the hyperirritability that leads to carpopedal spasm and even seizures. Hematologic consequences include a clotting deficit, since calcium is part of the blood clotting cascade.

Hypocalcemia has extensive interrelationships in the biochemical milieu of the body that determine its severity and response. The only critical compartment of the body calcium that is easily measurable and is accountable for physiologic reactions is the circulating blood calcium. This represents less than 1 percent of the stored inert calcium, principally in bone, and only that component of the circulating calcium in the free ionized state is biologically active at membrane surfaces. Ionized calcium is approximately half or less of the total calcium in the blood. Binding is very important, and the association of calcium with serum proteins, principally albumin, is nearly on the basis of 1 mg of the former per 1 g of the latter. (As a clinical approximation, a change of 1 g in serum albumin equals a change of 0.8 mg in serum calcium.) For example, a serum calcium level that falls outside the lower limits of normal in a normal patient may be compatible with an acceptable ionized serum calcium level if that patient has chronic renal failure and hypoalbuminemia. It is possible to measure the direct component of ionized calcium in the serum, but it is difficult, and a proxy for this determination can be obtained by considering two other factors in the blood: the albumin just alluded to and the pH.

Hydrogen ion concentration changes protein binding of calcium as well as other determinants of the quantity of calcium in free ionized form. This is why hyperventilation in a patient who has the initial symptoms of hypocalcemia makes the problem worse. The serum calcium level does not change during the interval of pH change, but the shift from ionized calcium to the biologically inactive bound calcium occurs with a rise in pH within physiologic range. A patient with critical illness such as anoxia and shock will have little reflection of a low serum calcium level since the pH would reflect a substantial portion of the serum calcium in ionized active form. However, with resuscitation and the nearly universal administration of bicarbonate to restore the pH toward normal or alkalosis levels, hypocalcemic symptoms may emerge. Another binding phenomenon that decreases ionized calcium is the administration of large volumes of blood. This occurs both because of the chelating agents such as citrates in banked blood used as anticoagulants, and because the large volume of blood that is essentially ionized calcium-free would dilute down the calcium circulating in the patient.

Another divalent cation that interacts with ionized calcium metabolism and may also be deficient in critically ill patients is magnesium. Some of the same reasons for decreases in calcium may also cause hypomagnesemia with some similar effects. Hypomagnesemia is often thought to be a consequence of nutritional deficits such as starvation, nasogastric tubes, or gastrointestinal fistulae, medications that interfere with its absorption or promote its excretion, or renal disease that prevents its conservation in the circulation. A low serum magnesium level impairs the release of parathormone (PTH) and competitively inhibits the movement of intracellular or bound calcium back into the ionized form. As a consequence, hypomagnesemia is frequently found accompanying hypocalcemia.

Another factor that has impact on the calcium economy is hypophosphatemia. Hypophosphatemia is a similar consequence of prolonged starvation or "leaking" of phosphates from the body by loss through gastrointestinal or renal failures. Phosphates are part of many metabolic processes, and ATP, creatine phosphokinase, and other components of the "energy currency" systems in the body will be impaired with hypophosphatemia of considerable deficit. Calcium and phosphorus are selectively exchanged in the renal tubules, and a deficit in one will usually be reflected in a deficit in the other, as is seen with hypomagnesemia.

Treatment of hypocalcemia is necessary and critically urgent in the cardiovascular emergencies of cardiac arrest and electromechanical dissociation of myocardial action, and the neuromuscular emergency of tetany. Calcium is available for parenteral injection as the chloride salt or a gluceptate compound. An intravenous injection of 2 g calcium chloride will yield over 100 mg of calcium, and for the average size patient[3] the serum calcium level should rise by 0.5 mg/100 ml. Half of this rise in serum calcium level would remain in the ionized calcium form if the readily dissociable calcium chloride salt is used. For early hypocalcemia or minimal symptoms, the gluceptate variety can be used with a slower release of elemental calcium. The safer technique for administration of calcium is by the enteral route. Calcium wafers can be taken by most patients who are able to eat a regular diet; some forms of antacid preparations in liquid form can be used as calcium suspensions. A more effective form of calcium supplementation is with oral medication that combines calcium and a vitamin D3 congener. Calcitriol is the most potent metabolite of vitamin D, which contributes to the rapid positive calcium balance in these patients. However, antacids that contain magnesium should be avoided while this substance is administered, since hypermagnesemia could result. In patients with renal failure on dialysis, aluminum carbonate or hydroxide gels may be used to control serum phosphate levels. To prevent overdosage of calcium supplementation when vitamin D3 products are used, a rule of thumb is that the serum calcium times the phosphate (Ca × P) product should not exceed 70. This can be helpful in the patient who will require chronic replacement, such as the patient on dialysis treatment or the patient with hypoparathyroidism from an endogenous autoimmune process or surgical excision of the parathyroid glands.

Hyperfunction

Hypercalcemia is a very common finding in hospitalized patients, particularly elderly women. Hypercalcemia as an isolated finding is one of the principal yields of the multiphasic screening biochemical tests run on autoanalyzers. However, hypercalcemia alone does not indicate hyperfunction of the parathyroid glands, but always indicates a problem that must be looked into. The definition of hypercalcemia, like hypocalcemia, depends on the ionized serum calcium level, and is similarly buffered by protein, pH, magnesium, and phosphorus metabolism.

Hypercalcemia has many causes. Some of these are easily fixed, for example, vitamin D excess, milk-alkali syndrome, and the use of certain diuretics or drugs. The presence of hypercalcemia may also indicate a number of benign diseases outside the parathyroid gland such as sarcoidosis, Paget's disease, tuberculosis, thyrotoxicosis, or, most importantly, impaired renal function.

In the older patient, and in the patient with dangerously high serum calcium levels, the leading cause is malignant disease. Other evidence of malignant disease can often be found in the same screening tests if the serum alkaline phosphatase level is also elevated and the phosphorus determination is similarly high. The most likely candidates for cancers causing an elevation in serum calcium are those that produce bony involvement early in their course. Breast cancer, and tumors of thyroid, prostate, renal, lung, and hematologic origins such as multiple myeloma are likely candidates. The presence of bony metastases is not a good prognosis for control of the malignant disease, but the very finding of hypercalcemia is an indication that the patient requires treatment to bring the serum calcium values under control. In the critically ill patient, elevated serum calcium levels are not an "incidental" finding since the metabolic consequences of significant elevations in serum calcium are critical and require immediate management.

Hyperparathyroidism is a very rewarding confirmation in the differential diagnosis of hypercalcemia, since it is relatively easily corrected and has significant long-term injurious consequences in damage to kidneys, vessels, bones, ocular lenses, peptic hyperacidity, pancreatitis, central nervous system malfunction (such as memory loss), and a variety of neuromuscular malfunctions. The symptoms of hyperparathyroidism are protean and they are often unrecognized until they disappear following treatment of the hyperparathyroidism itself.

The differential diagnosis of hyperparathyroidism from the other hypercalcemias may come first from the same SMA-12 and SMA-6 screening tests. Hypophosphatemia commonly occurs in hyperparathyroidism along with hyperchloremia. A general rule of thumb is that the chloride divided by the phosphate should be less than a 30:1 ratio, or hyperparathyroidism is strongly suggested. Serum parathormone levels may be measured by radioimmunoassay, but this is not necessary for the diagnosis of hyperparathyroidism with confidence. The biochemical determinations, particularly if combined with an assay of hypercalciuria, are sufficient in many instances to allow one to schedule surgical therapy. If this set of findings is present in a patient with a consistent history, such as a long history of proven hypercalcemia with mild but persistent elevations off medications and often asymptomatic on first presentation but later found to have had recurrent renal stones, gastric hyperacidity, and a positive family history, the diagnosis and treatment could be carried out without the parathormone determination, which may be inconsistent with the more reliable biochemical pattern.

Serum parathormone levels are usually somewhat delayed in being reported, but may be helpful in those cases that are asymptomatic, particularly if combined with an ionized serum calcium determination. Patients with these findings, however, are not the patients who are typically in intensive care units with severe metabolic disturbance. The recognition of asymptomatic hypercalcemia can occur in an office setting electively. Our current consideration is of emergency management of critical metabolic disturbance, and hyperparathyroidism may also present in such extraordinary distress. One of the most rapid determinations, besides the serum biochemistry, is a radiograph of the skull or hands or other acral extremities showing subperiosteal bone resorption. This radiologic finding coupled with

severe hypercalcemia may be all that is necessary to diagnose the metabolic crisis known by some as "parathyroid poisoning."[31]

The metabolic effects of hypercalcemia do not depend principally on its cause, but the elevated ionized calcium level in the serum from whatever origin has common effects on membrane potentials throughout the body. There are renal causes of hypercalcemia, but there are also certainly renal effects including nephrogenic diabetes insipidus and glycosuria.[8] The presence of hypercalciuria pulls fluid and carbohydrate with it to cause frequent nocturia. Calcium deposition in the kidney may take the form of nephrolithiasis and renal colic may be a complication of this as well as a generalized calcification in nephrocalcinosis. Renal tubular acidosis is also a problem secondary to hypercalcemia. One of the principal reasons for treating the asymptomatic hypercalcemia patient is organ salvage, particularly the kidney.

Serum calcium is a known secretagogue for gastric acid hypersecretion, and peptic ulceration or gastritis may be found in patients with hypercalcemia. This phenomenon is linked inside the multiple endocrine adenopathy syndrome (MEA-I) in which hypercalcemia of hyperparathyroidism coexists with gastric hypersecretion and hypergastrinemia. In the patient with this hereditary form of hyperparathyroidism, the first surgical attack is directed at the source of hyperparathyroidism, since a decrease in the circulating calcium often causes reversion of the gastrin-mediated hyperacidity toward normal.[10] Pancreatitis is a known complication of hyperparathyroidism, and pancreatitis may be one of the presenting symptoms of hyperparathyroidism.

The cardiovascular effects of hypercalcemia may be subtle since calcium is a positive inotrope on the heart. Calcium is necessary for relaxation, and a hypercalcemic cardiovascular death occurs with the patient in systolic arrest. Calcium is linked with other membrane-active agents such as digoxin therapy, and some increase of a depressed calcium levels toward normal is useful for reversing this form of cardiac depression. However, hypercalcemia shows a shortened QT interval on the electrocardiogram (ECG). The peripheral effect of hypercalcemia is a decrease in peripheral vascular resistance, and the combination of an increased inotropic action on the heart and a decrease in resistance leads to a definite increase in cardiac output. In the patient receiving digitalis, increased serum calcium makes the patient susceptible to digitalis toxicity and arrhythmias.

The neuromuscular complications of hypercalcemia are among the most frequent complaints elicited, if not at the time of presentation then often after the patient is relieved of hypercalcemia in retrospect. In the author's experience, headache is one of the most frequent neuromuscular complaints, and the yield from a SMA-12 screening of patients with headaches is much more cost-effective than that done by CT scan of the head. Personality changes and frank behavioral disturbance are frequent, particularly in older patients when it is attributed to senility. A number of patients in the author's experience have been institutionalized in nursing homes for presenile dementia, when other complications have brought their hypercalcemia to light. After correction of their hyperparathyroidism, they have been discharged to independent living. The complaints have ranged from drowsiness and lack of energy to frankly psychotic behavior. In very late central nervous system disease, calcification of the basal ganglia may be seen. Profound muscle weakness and exertional fatigue are frequently reported. Lethargy and musculoskeletal pain and weakness may proceed all the way to coma and death with rapid elevations of the serum calcium. In reversing hypercalcemia, the muscular fatigue may make independent ventilation difficult in the process of weaning from a respirator.

The severity of these metabolic consequences of hypercalcemia mandates treatment, particularly when hypercalcemia is rapidly progressive. Table 25-8 lists the seven steps in the emergency control of hypercalcemia.

Since calcium is excreted in the urine and often pulls with it abundant water, sugar, and salts, restoration of the fluid volume is the first priority and induction of saline diuresis is the important first step. Furosemide natriuresis contributes to this rapid excretion of calcium and oral administration of neutral phosphates such as sodium brushite or binding resins prevents its absorption from the gut. If calcium

absorption can be kept to near zero and a brisk saline and furosemide diuresis can lead to the excretion of nearly 1 g in 24 hours, approximately 1 mg/100 ml reduction in serum calcium can be achieved within the same time.

If the diuresis alone is not sufficient, pharmacologic agents are available to promote calcium elimination further.

A synthetic calcitonin modeled after salmon calcitonin is commercially available and can be given at a dosage of up to 50 units three times daily in combination with corticosteroids. These pharmacologic treatments are a relatively innocuous means of suppressing serum calcium. Another pharmacologic agent, mithramycin, is very effective, but also has considerable marrow toxicity as a highly effective chemotherapeutic agent. For that reason, mithramycin should be employed principally for the treatment of hypercalcemia of metastatic malignant disease rather than for hyperparathyroidism. Hemodialysis against a near-zero calcium bath medium is effective in causing rapid shifts downward in serum calcium levels for patients with renal failure, but must be repeated frequently. Abrupt changes in either direction of serum calcium are dangerous and should be undertaken with caution except in the very extremes of hypocalcemia or hypercalcemia. There is a definite role for urgent surgical parathyroidectomy in the emergency control of hypercalcemia in the extraordinary circumstance of "parathyroid poisoning," in which a large parathyroid adenoma is stimulated to a great deal of parathormone release, often by hemorrhagic infarction. In a series of 10 such patients, the medical management just outlined was truncated as a rapid preoperative preparation, and the hypercalcemia only brought under control by urgent parathyroidectomy.[31] An example of a hemorrhagic parathyroid adenoma is seen in Figure

TABLE 25-8. Seven Steps in Emergency Control of Hypercalcemia

1. Volume restoration with saline infusion
2. Furosemide diuresis
3. Oral neutral phosphates
4. Calcitonin and corticosteroids
5. Mithramycin
6. Dialysis
7. Parathyroidectomy (urgent for parathyroid toxicosis)

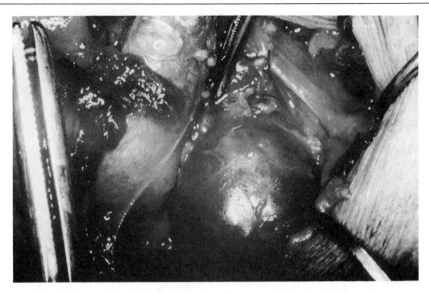

FIG. 25-3 A large parathyroid adenoma that had undergone hemorrhagic degeneration was removed from a patient with "parathyroid poisoning": severe toxicity from rapidly rising hypercalcemia after rapid preoperative preparation with saline diuresis.

25-3, removed from a patient with severe hypercalcemia after an abbreviated preoperative preparation with saline diuresis.

Hyperparathyroidism is probably the most frequent single cause in endocrine surgery for which people are brought to the operating room. Surely more patients with diabetes are found in the operating room, but their operation is not usually designed for the treatment of diabetes, but for its complications. Hypercalcemia is often correctable with an operation that has far less morbidity than does the continuation of the hypercalcemic state. The incidence of hyperparathyroidism in the population at large varies with the sex and age of the population studied, but in women over 60 it may be as high as 1:500 in the population at large.[15] Any number of these individuals can have coincidental critical illness, or the hypercalcemia can abruptly become symptomatic and occasion their severe metabolic derangements.

In following up patients who have had surgical treatment of parathyroid disorders, it is important to be sure that calcium levels in patients who are getting replacement therapy for hypoparathyroidism are maintained within the normal range, and that patients are not gradually becoming hypercalcemic and toxic from iatrogenic sources. It is equally important to check on those patients who have had parathy-

roid adenoma resection to see that they have not had persistent or recurrent hyperparathyroidism. Persistence is defined as hypercalcemia present within 6 months of operation, and recurrence is usually hypercalcemia that follows a period of normal calcium determinations for a period of at least 6 months. It is also important to check in some instances not only the patient but his or her first-order relatives, particularly if the hyperparathyroidism is based in primary hyperplasia of all parathyroid glands, or if the primary hyperparathyroidism occured at a very young age, or if there is other evidence of an MEA pattern in the patient treated for hyperparathyroidism.

PANCREATIC ISLET DISORDERS

Hypofunction

There is an abundant literature on the complications of diabetes in the critically ill patient, particularly when sepsis is a part of the severe illness. Hypofunction of insulin-mediated glucose metabolism is not always a function of decreased insulin secretion from the pancreas, but may also be partly based in insulin resistance at the receptor level on cell membrane surfaces. Since the central nervous system requires minute-to-minute delivery of glucose and oxygen to maintain aerobic metabolism and function, it is not simply the relative deficiency of insulin in stressful illness, but also the "counterregulatory hormones" that assure hyperglycemia for abundant energy substrate by the central nervous system and skeletal muscle effectors.

As seen in Table 25-2, insulin is one of the hormones with generally decreased or unaltered secretion during stress. However, as seen in Table 25-1, each of the counterregulatory hormones in control of blood glucose is increased, and therefore, hyperglycemia is the rule during stressful periods of critical illness.

Glucagon is one of the counterregulatory hormones, and is itself a product of the pancreatic islets. Very rarely, a neoplasm may arise in the pancreatic islets that secretes primarily glucagon in the "glucagonoma" syndrome.[16] These cases are rare, but serve to point out the physiologic function of glucagon in the exaggerated hypersecretion from the islet cell tumor that has been identified. A second counterregulatory hormone is epinephrine, and in severe stress, levels of norepinephrine and the other catecholamines are generally elevated. The catecholamine response of glycolysis promotes immediate conversion to readily usable sugar of those carbohydrate stores in the body, but glycogen is in limited supply in muscle and liver, and is not present in the brain. For that reason a longer-term response is necessary, and comes by way of gluconeogenesis, a potent shift in metabolism largely due to the excess secretion of "glucocorticoids," the third major counterregulatory hormone. Growth hormone is the other counterregulatory hormone and by acting in concert with the others, insulin release is inhibited and ketogenesis is initiated. Counterregulatory hormones all respond to intravascular volume depletion, so the hyperglycemic effect in most severely ill patients is dampened by intravascular fluid restoration.[30]

Treatment of hyperglycemia in the patient with stressful illness involves first the intravenous rehydration just referred to. Insulin ther-

apy is then appropriate also with careful monitoring of the blood sugar, osmolality, and serum potassium. For practical purposes, all critically ill patients require only regular insulin. Long-acting forms or modifications of insulin preparations are not as essential as getting adequate delivery of insulin and glucose for cellular utilization and not having glucose or insulin persist beyond the availability of the other. Unless there are insulin antibodies, one form of insulin is not preferable over another of equal biologic activity except for the additional expense. The critically ill patient with hyperglycemia, whether diabetic or not before the stressful illness, is best managed by continuous low dose insulin infusion by adding insulin to an infusion bottle of fluids with an initial run through the intravenous tubing to saturate the binding sites. Intraoperative glucose management is best achieved by continuous infusion of insulin at low dosage.[32] When highly concentrated sugar solutions such as hyperalimentation fluid are run in simultaneously, and when the patient is under severe stress and has high levels of endogenous counterregulatory hormones or has catecholamines and corticosteroids administered, approximately 10 units/hr of regular insulin may be required for control of hyperglycemia. In the treatment of ketoacidosis without sugar administration, only 10 to 20 percent of this dose will be sufficient to control hyperglycemia. An important factor to recognize is the large shift in potassium that occurs with insulin and glucose infusion, and the correction of acidosis, often with sodium bicarbonate. Often, large quantities of potassium are required for simultaneous infusion as intracellular water is expanded and the extracellular potassium is pumped back in when macromolecular glycogen expands intracellular space and insulin primes the sodium–potassium "pump."

Hyperfunction

Hypoglycemia in many ways is much more dangerous than hyperglycemia because of the dependence of the central nervous system on adequate sugar and oxygen delivery as already mentioned. Hypoglycemia should not be thought of as a problem in diabetes regulation alone, but is a nearly universal finding in the severely stressed patient for a number of reasons. The differential diagnosis of hypoglycemia includes reactive or postabsorptive phenomena such as the "dumping syndrome" after gastrectomy. There may also be deficient glucose production in some patients because of either a failure of reserves of carbohydrate stores (such as alcoholic cirrhosis of the liver with deficient glycogen deposition) or deficiency of the enzymes to convert from protein or lipid metabolism to glucose production (glucocorticoid deficiency, or glucagon or thyroid hormone disturbances). A special case can be made for a particular endocrine surgical problem based on the overutilization of glucose in the fasting state, and the best example of this would be a pancreatic β-cell adenoma (insulinoma).[12] Another potential cause of fasting reactive adult hypoglycemia would be pharmacologic or toxic factors such as factitious insulin shots or oral hypoglycemics or ethyl alcohol.

The effects of hypoglycemia are direct upon the central nervous system from the hypoglycemia itself, and are present as irritability, disorientation, changes in vision, and drowsiness. However, an equal effect of the hypoglycemia is to call forth a surge of catecholamine release, and the autonomic nervous system also gives rise to the characteristic patterns of tachycardia, diaphoresis, and apprehension, mimicking the patient with pheochromocytoma who shares the same catecholamine excess. Hypoglycemia itself calls forth the endocrine consequences of hyperinsulinism. Only in the absence of these counterregulatory hormone balances does a true hypoglycemia result.

The diagnosis of hypoglycemia based on endogenous hyperinsulinism comes from a provocative test such as fasting, which shows the immunoreactive insulin to be high at an inappropriate point when the blood sugar is low (with hypoglycemia arbitrarily defined as 50 mg/100 ml or less of blood glucose). It should be noted that provocative tests are dangerous since they may induce hypoglycemia that would damage the central nervous system that is dependent upon a continuous supply of blood glucose. For that reason, suppression tests are preferred, and administration of intravenous diazoxide depresses insulin release in the hypoglycemic patient, except when the hypoglycemia is due to an autonomous source such as an insulinoma. Radiographic localization is possible by selective pancreatic arteriography. If an insulinoma is identified and localized, surgical treatment is curative in 90 percent of cases. Diazoxide therapy can be used for the management of persistent hypoglycemia as well as an aid in its diagnosis.

Treatment of hypoglycemia in the form of 10 percent glucose solution infusion is often sufficient. If the patient is able to tolerate feedings, protein and other long-lasting nutrient sources are important in supplying a substrate for gluconeogenesis, without further induction of insulin release as would occur with an oral carbohydrate load. If the hypoglycemia is due to exogenous insulin or other hypoglycemic agents such as tolbutamide, these agents should be withheld or the factitial source discovered through the use of insulin antibodies or the absence of C-peptide in equimolar quantities. For those patients with nesidioblastosis[14] or with untreated or untreatable insulinoma that has spread, diazoxide therapy is sometimes useful to prevent dangerous hypoglycemia. A newer method of treatment currently in clinical trial is the administration of an injectable long-acting analog of somatostatin.

ADRENAL CORTEX

Hypofunction

Adrenal insufficiency may be among the most frequent endocrine emergencies encountered in the critically ill patient. Rarely is this due to tuberculous ablation of the adrenal glands, the cause of the problem initially described by Thomas Addison. Only slightly more frequently is it due to replacement of the adrenal glands by metastatic disease, particularly from lung cancer metastases. In some instances of specific types of septicemia, particularly meningiococcemia, the adrenals may undergo hemorrhagic destruction (Waterhouse-Friderichsen syndrome). An autoimmune primary adrenocortical atrophy is responsible for some primary adrenal insufficiencies. Adrenalectomy is carried out more frequently than it had been 50 years ago, often for disease not related to the adrenal glands but for treatment of nonadrenal tumors, such as prostate cancer or breast cancer. It is easy to see why patients who have undergone adrenal ablation are candidates for adrenal insufficiency.

The great majority of cases of adrenal insufficiency encountered today, however, are related to a steroid excess state that has resulted in adrenal suppression when steroids were withdrawn. This "adrenal exhaustion" is a natural consequence of suppression of ACTH stimulation. For practical purposes, the mineralocorticoid (aldosterone, the principal mineralocorticoid in humans) is under the independent regulation of the renin–angiotensin system, and would not be remarkably depressed without ACTH stimulation; the term "adrenal insufficiency" therefore, refers principally to glucocorticoid insufficiency.

Symptoms of acute adrenal insufficiency (an addisonian crisis) include nausea, vomiting, weakness, hypotension, hypothermia, and hypoglycemia. The critically ill patient who cannot seem to mount a stress response is a likely candidate for exogenous steroid treatment under the assumption that at least relative adrenal insufficiency may be present. Measurement of adrenal 17-hydroxy and ketosteroids may be helpful, but is rarely done in the critical care setting, since treatment is often required before such diagnostic delay is possible. Serum cortisol determinations at 8:00 A.M. and 4:00 P.M., and an ACTH stimulation test, are all methods for purists to make diagnoses in the unstressed patient, but the way most adrenal insufficiency is tested for in acutely ill patients is by therapeutic response to exogenous corticosteroids. The preferred method of urgent treatment while still allowing diagnostic testing would be through the use of dexamethasone, which would not be picked up in plasma assays of cortisol or its metabolites in the urine.

As noted in Table 25-9, even under the stress of severe illness, "stress doses" of corticosteroids are all that is necessary for "adrenal replacement." These levels are two to four times the normal 24 hour secretion patterns. "Massive pharmacologic doses" may be given

to the patient in shock or with septicemia for quite different indications than for physiologic replacement of stress level corticosteroids, but steroid treatment of a patient with adrenal insufficiency should not be confused with pharmacologic management of another purpose for which the same drugs may be employed in very different dosages.

The metabolic consequences of deficient cortisol secretion have been alluded to at several points above in our discussion of the severely ill patient's inability to shift to alternative fuels through mechanisms of gluconeogenesis or to maintain stable cardiovascular response to the higher metabolic demand. The detailed outline of subtle features of hypocortisolism has been recently reviewed, and more detailed descriptions of corticosteroid therapy for a variety of illnesses in which the glucocorticoid anti-inflammatory or membrane-stabilizing effects are employed.[22] For purposes of this discussion, corticosteroid treatment will be limited to the emergency replacement of normal steroid secretion of glucocorticoids or their stress levels under the duress of critical illness.

Treatment of glucocorticoid deficiency is possible in many ways using at least 10 differ-

TABLE 25-9. Method of Steroid Replacement after Adrenalectomy

1. Intraoperatively or in crisis situations, the patient still needs no more than stress levels, approximately 100 mg hydrocortisone intravenously, or 300 mg in circadian dosage intervals over 24 hours; do *not* use massive pharmacologic steroid dosage for stress physiologic replacement.
2. Within 48 hours of adrenalectomy, taper dose to 50 mg hydrocortisone intravenously every 8 hours.
3. While the patient is still receiving parenteral steroids, give oral steroids at doses of approximately 35 mg in AM, 15 mg in PM. As patient adjusts to oral intake, discontinue parenteral steroids.
4. In outpatient follow-up, reduce to 20 mg AM, 10 mg PM hydrocortisone and add 0.1 mg fluorocortisone to AM dose.
5. Instruct patient in management of stress, heat tolerance, salt requirements, and use of medical notification bracelet or wallet card.
6. Prepare "stress kit" for 48 hour parenteral supply of hydrocortisone if patient is unable to take in or retain oral feeding.

(Reprinted with permission from Geelhoed GW: Problem Management in Endocrine Surgery. Copyright © 1983 by Year Book Medical Publishers, Inc., Chicago.)

ent steroid preparations. Addisonian crisis is best treated by 100 mg intravenous hydrocortisone. This soluble steroid is rapidly distributed and has some mineralocorticoid activity, which is useful in addisonian crisis. The 100 mg dose offers essentially four times the daily secretion of the equivalent cortisol in a patient in an unstressed state. Yet this steroid preparation results in minimal suppression of the pituitary release of ACTH. By contrast, dexamethasone and methylprednisolone have very little activity in promoting sodium retention, and therefore their utility is high when anti-inflammatory action with minimal mineralocorticoid activity is required. They are also much more potent than cortisol, hydrocortisone, or cortisone; 4 mg of dexamethasone is equivalent to 100 mg of hydrocortisone. Dexamethasone, however, has a long-acting effect and is a potent pituitary suppressing agent, an effect especially utilized in the "dexamethasone suppression test" to differentiate pituitary from adrenal Cushing's syndrome.

Adrenal cortical replacement must be given as long as there is insufficient production of cortisol from the patient's own adrenal glands, which means in perpetuity for the patient with adrenalectomy. As seen in Table 25-9, the patient must be specially prepared for the probability that there will be times when he or she is unable to take a steroid replacement or to retain it. For those occasions, a special "stress kit" for parenteral steroid administration and special wristband or wallet card notification (see Fig. 25-4) is an important part of patient follow-up.

Hyperfunction

Corticosteroid excesses are possible in all three layers of the adrenal cortex with different syndromes produced from hypersecretion. Mineralocorticoid excess is aldosteronism, a syndrome without a phenotypic clinical pattern, but with characteristic biochemical abnormalities. However, the hypertension is not malignant and the hypokalemia is rarely critical. For that reason, treatment of aldosteronism is not generally an emergency, and it is not frequently encountered in critically ill patients.

Glucocorticoid excess is seen in Cushing's syndrome. There is a phenotypic clinical pattern, and these features are of diagnostic importance; however, the blood pressure and blood sugar abnormalities and metabolic disturbances are not usually critical, and emergency treatment for glucocorticoid excess is not necessary.

As outlined in Table 25-2, the levels of adrenal sex steroids are not elevated in critical illness. In fact, there are only very rare instances in which sex steroid excess from the adrenal gland is of critical importance, and it is not the oversecretion of the sex steroid that makes the illness critical, but the deficiency in glucocorticoid in the "adrenogenital syndrome." For all three adrenocortical hypersecretion states, therefore, clinical recognition and management are important, but none require emergency management of crises in the severely ill or injured patient.

THE CHROMAFFIN SYSTEM

Hypofunction

There are abundant nerve endings and postsynaptic ganglia in the chromaffin system for catecholamine production, so there is no genuine catecholamine deficiency state for the normal unblocked patient who is severely ill or injured. This is in marked contrast to the critical metabolic emergencies posed by chromaffin hyperfunction.

Although no deficiency states in catecholamine physiology are of clinical importance, there is widespread utility to the application of catecholamines in critical care medicine. A recent review[4] discusses the endogenous and exogenous catecholamines useful in the critically ill patient, but a deficiency of these catechols does not fit the definition of "endocrine emergency."

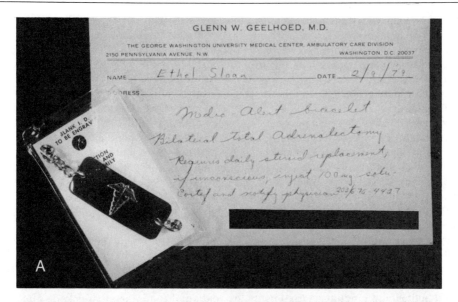

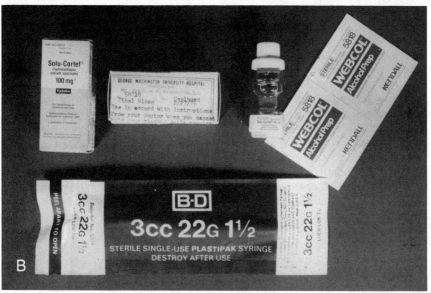

FIG. 25-4 A "stress kit" for parenteral steroid administration is an important follow-up adjunct for the patient who is steroid-dependent for periods of illness when oral steroids cannot be taken in or retained. **(A)** Medical notification of bilateral adrenalectomy is accompanied by **(B)** a parenteral injection kit for a soluble glucocorticoid carried by the patient.

Hyperfunction

The chief endocrine emergency related to the catecholamine system in critically ill patients is the excess secretion of these hormones by pheochromocytoma. Pheochromocytoma is a rare cause of essential hypertension, and occasionally is diagnosed by a very varied clinical pattern. Such patients may be brought to the intensive care unit for control before the correction of their hypertension by removal of the catecholamine source. However, the more serious encounter with an undiagnosed and unsuspected pheochromocytoma may occur in a patient who is acutely stressed or ill, and is found to be reacting bizarrely to this stress. An incidental encounter with an unsuspected pheochromocytoma is more often lethal than not, even in the mid-1980s.[10] The unsuspected "pheo" is termed a "pharmacologic bomb" which may be oncologically benign, but is physiologically malignant. The injection of the enormous quantities of these vasoactive amines into the circulation from such a tumor cannot be withstood by the unprotected cardiovascular system.

The properties of the catecholamines in the endogenous forms (epinephrine, norepinephrine, and dopamine, and their precursors and metabolites) are familiar as treatments to most clinicians dealing with critically ill patients. The inotropic and chronotropic cardiac action and vasoregulatory changes are adaptive responses to critical stresses within physiologic range. In the very much larger quantities in which they may be released from chromaffin neoplasms, these same effects lead to ischemia, arrhythmias, behavioral disturbances, and disorders in other compensatory systems with endocrine responses such as the paradox of "bradykinin shock."[10] Certain anesthetic agents sensitize the myocardium to the arrhythmic potential of catecholamine excess, and sustained circulation of the catecholamines can contribute to an increased "oxygen debt" and myocardial infarction.

An example of a patient presenting for medical treatment with an acute problem (a fractured hip) and a very stormy anesthetic and operative course for the repair of this fractured hip can be described by a reference to Figure 25-5. This patient had an uneventful preoperative evaluation en route to the operating room for pinning of the hip fracture, when, under anesthesia, she developed uncontrollable cardiovascular responses that included extremely high hypertension alternating with cardiac arrest and hypotension. When her condition was finally controlled, it was apparent that she had a very high peripheral resistance and a very sensitive myocardium. Each of these are signs of a catecholamine excess which was proven

by assay of urinary metabolites, metanephrine, and normetanephrine, as well as a documented elevated level of plasma epinephrine. In the intensive care unit, her blood pressure was carefully controlled by phenoxybenzamine at gradually increasing dosages, beginning with 10 mg every 8 hours, and working up to a final 24 hour total of 80 mg incrementally over several days. For acute emergency control, nitroprusside was initiated. This very effective means of controlling the hemodynamic crisis was employed in another patient, also incidentally discovered in the intensive care setting of an unrelated critical illness and described in a previous report.[18]

The contracted plasma volume was gradually restored under the α-adrenergic blockade of phenoxybenzamine, and the arrhythmias were brought under control by the later application of β-adrenergic blockade after α-blockade had been established. Propranolol is a very effective means of blocking the β-stimulation of excess epinephrine. As the contracted plasma volume increased with α-blockade, the hematocrit decreased, and blood transfusion was also possible to compensate for the decrease in vasoconstrictor tone as catecholamine blockade of the reuptake of the released amines into the pheochromocytoma progressed.

The pheochromocytoma was localized by computed tomography (CT) scanning and arteriography under the protection of a pharmacologic blockade. The patient was then taken to the operating room for elective control of this known and localized pheochromocytoma. In contrast to the previous operation (Fig. 25-5) this operation was relatively less stressful (Fig. 25-6). Nitroprusside was used to control the intraoperative blood pressure while the surgical team excised the right adrenal pheochromocytoma. It was of interest that the pulmonary vascular resistance, as reflected in the pulmonary artery pressure, the central venous pressure, and the arterial pressure, stabilized after ligation of the right adrenal vein, thus isolating the source of excess catecholamine from the patient's circulation (Fig. 25-7). With the adrenal vein ligated, the pheochromocytoma was excised without further incident (Fig. 25-8A). Pathologic examination of the specimen revealed a pheochromocytoma originating in the

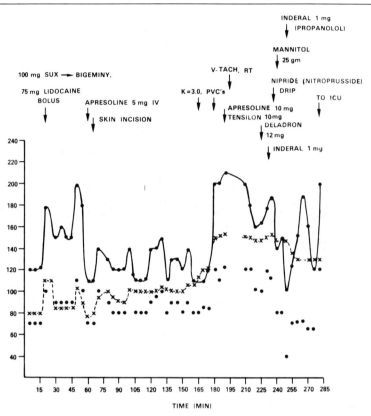

FIG. 25-5 A very stormy operative course observed during a hip pinning operation for a patient later found to have a pheochromocytoma discovered by this cardiovascular reaction to the stress of surgery. (Reprinted with permission from Geelhoed GW: Problem Management in Endocrine Surgery. Copyright © 1983 by Year Book Medical Publishers, Inc., Chicago.)

right adrenal gland that was quite large and showed extremely high levels of tissue catecholamines even after the extensive preoperative preparation and pharmacologic blockade (see Fig. 25-8B).

Many lessons can be learned from the hemodynamic response of this patient and others like her encountered as an endocrine emergency without prior knowledge of her primary endocrinologic pathology until an intercurrent illness forced her into a potentially disastrous complication. Pheochromocytoma should always be on the list of potential abnormalities in anyone who has an unusual cardiovascular response of hypertension, arrhythmias, or myocardial dysfunction that may be due to catecholamine excess. Such a patient should have a screening test for the possibility that the atypical responses are based on catecholamine ex-

cess. The diagnosis can be confirmed by a localization test, only after adequate preparation and pharmacologic blockade with volume expansion. Some of the tests used to localize pheochromocytoma have taken the place of the diagnostic biochemical confirmation, and many of these have resulted in cardiovascular collapse in the patient. For example, glucagon is often used in combination with CT scanning to dilate the gut for orally administered contrast material. Glucagon is one of the most potent provocative stimulators of catecholamine release, and a number of patients have been encountered whose first crushing substernal chest pain attacks with hypertensive crises have occurred either while undergoing a radiographic test such as CT scanning or barium enema, or during endoscopic procedures in which glucagon is used similarly to relax the

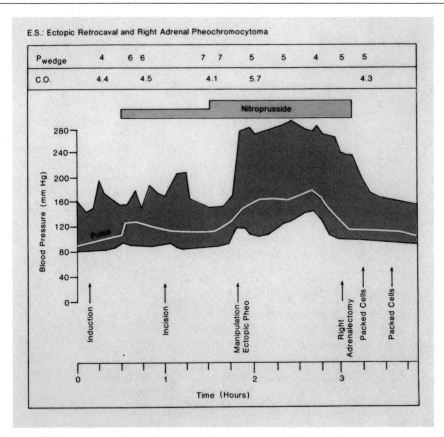

FIG. 25-6 After progressive catecholamine blockade with phenoxybenzamine allowed volume expansion and propranolol protected the myocardium from the arrthymia potentiation of epinephrine, and with nitroprusside protection of acute hypertensive crises, the patient underwent an operation to control the radiographically localized pheochromocytoma.

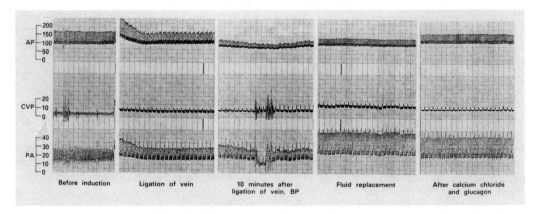

FIG. 25-7 Pulmonary vascular resistance, systemic arterial resistance, and venous pressure normalized after occlusion of the adrenal vein isolated the patient's circulation from the focal source of excess catecholamine.

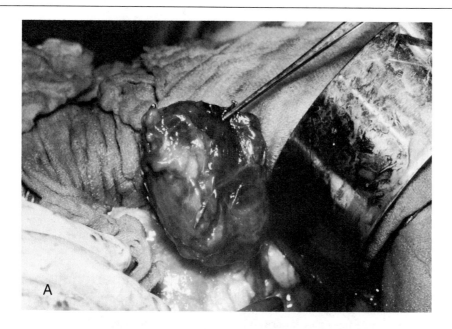

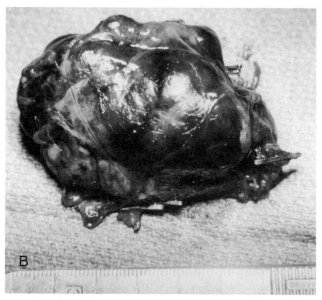

FIG. 25-8 **(A)** After occlusion of the adrenal vein, the pheochromocytoma was excised without further cardiovascular instability. **(B)** Pathologic examination of the tumor showed a large adrenal pheochromocytoma with enormous tissue concentrations of catecholamines.

bowel.[9] Any test to localize a potential pheochromocytoma should be carried out only after diagnostic confirmation by catecholamines in plasma or their metabolites in urine, and any such patient referred for localization of a tumor within the adrenal medulla or the chromaffin chain should be pharmacologically prepared, monitored, and attended. This rule pertains to all tests that are psychologically, physically, or pharmacologically "invasive."

PITUITARY GLAND

Hypofunction

Hypofunction of the anterior pituitary is principally reflected in the deficiencies of the glandular systems that depend upon its trophic hormones. The most important of these is the adrenal cortex and an acute addisonian crisis is the most probable emergency following hypophysectomy. Hypothyroidism is potentially a problem as well. Since each of these endocrine deficiencies are discussed under the glandular systems that secrete these hormones, management of the hypofunction of the pituitary as the "master gland" that controls them is not different than treatment of the hypofunction that results from end-organ failure.

However, there is an emergency endocrine abnormality on both hypo- and hyperfunction extremes with respect to the posterior pituitary.

If the posterior pituitary is missing, as occurs with "stalk section" or some forms of hypophysectomy or loss of function (some related to postpartum complications), disturbances in water balance may occur. The posterior pituitary secretes vasopressin or antidiuretic hormone (ADH). Loss of this hormone leads to an inability to conserve water at the renal tubular reabsorption sites, and diabetes insipidus. When water is lost from the body in excess of the salts normally found in the extracellular water, concentration of the remaining solute and hyperosmolarity occur. Hypernatremia is a frequent finding in patients with excessive water loss, and for a "proxy" measurement, serum sodium levels will in general reflect water balance inversely.

Patients with head trauma or neurosurgical operations are often found to have the condition of excess water loss in diabetes insipidus, reflecting a deficiency of ADH. There are also instances in which osmotic diuretics cause excess water loss, such as in diabetes mellitus with glucosuria or in mannitol diuresis. In addition, there are cases of excess sodium retention such as those seen in aldosteronism or Cushing's syndrome, in which the total body sodium has increased.

The treatment of most forms of water loss, either through osmotic diuresis or excessive perspiration as occurs with fever and increased insensible losses, is to allow free access to water intake by mouth and let thirst control water balance by the delicate mechanisms of the osmoregulators. In cases of hypernatremia, sodium restriction is the rule, or diuretics that work by natriuresis. Simultaneously, the underlying reason for salt retention (such as administration of excess corticosteroids) should be examined.

Hyperfunction

Water intoxication is an endocrine emergency that follows excessive water retention or heavy solute loss, and is usually reflected in hyponatremia and decreased serum osmolality. One of the causes of decreased osmolality is the syndrome of inappropriate antidiuretic hormone (SIADH).

One of the common causes of SIADH is in malignant disease, particularly of amine precursor uptake and decarboxylation (APUD) origin. The APUD neoplasms may secrete peptides closely resembling ADH. However, the SIADH syndrome can also arise from disorders of the central nervous system or secondary to drugs that influence it.

Treatment of water intoxication or SIADH is, most simply and most effectively, water restriction. By not allowing water intake, and with progressive water loss from the insensible routes, gradual increase in osmolality occurs. Untreated, hypo-osmolality and hyponatremia leads to seizures and other neurologic disorders. If such complications are already occurring, an excess solute load in the form of concentrated salt should *not* be administered, since the effect will most likely be to cause further water retention. Rather than giving concentrated salt solutions, an attempt is made to induce a nephrogenic diabetes insipidus through some diuretic or drug that will cause excess free water clearance. One such drug is demeclocycline[7] at dosages of 300 mg four times a day.

OTHER HORMONES AND SPECIAL CONSIDERATIONS FOR EXTRAORDINARY SITUATIONS

Neuropeptides

Endogenous opioid peptides are relatively recent discoveries closely linked to the elaboration of previously discussed hormones such as ACTH and TRH, the latter being an opioid antagonist. No definite hypofunction syndromes are known, although a specific opioid antagonist, naloxone, can cause a mimicking of these deficiency states and can produce narcotic withdrawal. The effects of excess opiates are well known, and these include respiratory suppression and nausea as well as obtundation. No endogenous hyperfunction syndromes are yet known, and most of the experience with excess opiates comes from narcotic abuse or heavy administration to patients with terminal disease. This area of investigation is a "frontier science" at the border between neurophysiology and behavioral science, and may explain a number of phenomena such as addiction, acupuncture, psychotherapy and some psychoses, endurance, shock, hypnosis, and a number of other areas that have remained unexplained in the absence of the appropriate mediators to be monitored.

Renin–Angiotensin

No hypofunction syndromes are known except for those artificially induced by the recently available angiotensin-converting enzyme inhibitor, captopril. Aldosteronopenia is also known as a postoperative phenomenon immediately after the excision of an aldoste-rone-secreting adenoma, but neither of these situations of hypofunction is an endocrine emergency. There is a hyperfunction syndrome in Bartter's syndrome that closely mimics renovascular hypertension. It, also, is not an endocrine emergency, although hypertensive crises can occur in the secondary hypertension syndromes as well as in essential hypertension.

Bradykinin-Kininogens

Some peptides are released from APUDomas such as in the carcinoid syndrome. In some of these, the kinins may be released and cause an endocrine emergency, such as the administration of epinephrine to a patient with one type of carcinoid syndrome that results in "bradykinin shock."[10] In some forms of the carcinoid syndrome, the kinin system is active, and the stimulus to the release of the kinins is epinephrine. Administration of epinephrine to such an individual will paradoxically cause a fall in blood pressure as well as induce bronchoconstriction. One way of inhibiting this emergency is administration of somatostatin,[17] which inhibits the action of the excess of kinin release.

Prostaglandins

Prostaglandins are a family of chemical compounds in the arachidonic acid metabolites that include the compounds known as prostaglandins and leukotrienes. The general term "eicosanoids" describes these molecules and they are active in inflammation and the metabolic pathways of cyclo-oxygenase and lipoxygenase systems. These eicosanoids have been implicated in the changes in metabolism that occur under extraordinary circumstances such as septic shock and myocardial depression. There is an interaction between them and endotoxins and the activation of the complement system. At the present time, there are no clinically apparent hyper- or hypofunction syndromes.

Progesterones

For the total body economy, there is no known excess or deficiency state of progesterone, although this group of steroids is important in maintaining pregnancy. An interesting application of the progesterone compounds, however, is that they seem to have an unusual effect in improving ventilation in patients with sleep apnea or other hypoventilation syndromes.[21]

SPECIAL CONDITIONS

Pregnancy

Pregnant patients are no less likely to develop endocrine emergencies than are nonpregnant women, but the amplified emergency takes into consideration that the disturbance in the mother's circulation is also a crisis for the fetal circulation. A recent review of surgery of the endocrine glands in pregnancy details the hazards of these endocrine crises, best exemplified by pheochromocytoma in pregnancy and thyrotoxicosis.[11] Pregnancy, however, does not protect against many of the other endocrine abnormalities discussed in this chapter, and many are intensified.

Infancy and Childhood

Some considerations of immature endocrine responses in childhood include fixed diabetes insipidus, inadequately developed thermoregulatory mechanisms, and a number of persistent maternal influences through placental transfer or via nursing. The special surgical considerations of metabolic crises in infancy and childhood have been recently reviewed.[23]

Aging

The endocrine responses of the aged are close to those of midlife, with the exception that reserves are limited and the basal metabolic rate is lower. There is a decline in energy utilization in advancing years, and this has both benefit and risk to the aged patient. The caloric requirements are less, but there are fewer reserve nutrient sources or alternative fuels that can be mobilized to meet the stress levels of critical illness.

Burns

A burn victim is a special case of severe critical illness. The caloric demand is extremely high and the endocrine stress is maximal, often leading to unusual complications thought to be unique for burn victims, such as Curling's ulcer and abnormality of the plasma renin secretion.[2] Hypertension may reflect a crisis in burn victims and may be an important negative factor in patients' survival.

Thermoregulation

Disorders of hypothermia and hyperthermia are often endocrine in nature in the absence of external physical loss of heat (convection, radiation or conduction, such as cold water immersion), or infection. Disorders of thermoregulation are often due to the hypothalamic and pituitary axis. Excess temperature means that metabolic rate is increased considerably, and fuels and oxygen are consumed at very high rates. Many of the endocrine enzyme systems are temperature-sensitive, and in such examples as extreme hyperthermia of thyroid storm, some of the endocrine mechanisms are deactivated and can no longer be employed to compensate for the added stress.

Sepsis

Septic shock may be a special case of an endocrine emergency since endotoxin may be a further factor that coexists with or influences endocrine activity for compensatory shifts in metabolism.[26] Many studies seem to indicate that corticosteroid activity at pharmacologic levels is more effective in septic shock than in the comparable magnitude of shock without the endotoxin presence.

SUMMARY

The critically ill patient is mobilizing all neurohumoral compensatory systems to the limit of his or her reserves. Some of these endocrine responses are compensatory, and restore the catabolic metabolism toward normal. Some use an immediate deficit for longer-term benefit, such as the breakdown of functional protein for rapid energy mobilization. Most of the endocrine responses also initiate the self-quenching mechanism of autoregulation. When a pathologic process is initiated that does not result in immediate metabolic dividends to the critically ill patient, decompensation is said to occur and the entire organism spirals into entropic collapse. The alert clinician can recognize these endocrine emergencies and intervene to protect vital function in this period of critical stress.

REFERENCES

1. Becker RA, Vaughan GM, Goodwin CW et al: Plasma norepinephrine, epinephrine and thyroid hormone interactions in severely burned patients. Arch Surg 115: 439, 1980
2. Brizio-Molteni L, Warpeka RL, Angelats J, Lewis N: Endocrine aspects of thermal injuries. Contemp Surg 18: 47, 1981
3. Chernow B: Hormonal and metabolic considerations in critical care medicine. p. 1. In Thompson WL, Shumacher WC (eds): Critical Care: State of the Art. Society of Critical Care Medicine III, Fullerton, California, 1982
4. Chernow B, Rainey TG, Lake CR: The endogenous and exogenous catecholamines in critical care medicine. Crit Care Med 10: 405, 1982
5. Chopra IJ: An assessment of daily production and significance of thyroidal secretion of 3,3'-5' triiodothyronine (reverse T3) in man. J Clin Invest 58: 32, 1976
6. Cryer PH: Physiology and pathophysiology of the human sympathoadrenal neuroendocrine system. N Engl J Med 303: 436, 1980
7. DeTroyer A, Demanet J-C: Correction of antidiuresis by demeclocycline. N Engl J Med 293: 915, 1975
8. Epstein FH: Calcium and the kidney. Am J Med 45: 700, 1963
9. Geelhoed GW: CAT scans and catecholamines. Surgery 87: 719, 1980
10. Geelhoed GW: Problem Management in Endocrine Surgery. Yearbook, Chicago, 1983
11. Geelhoed GW: Surgery of the endocrine glands in pregnancy. In Weingold A (ed): Clinical Obstetrics and Gynecology. Harper & Row, New York, 1983
12. Geelhoed GW: Hypoglycemia in the adult, with special consideration of the management of insulinoma. In Geelhoed GW, Chernow B (eds): Endocrine and Metabolic Response to Critical Illness and Trauma, Clinics in Critical Care Medicine Series. Churchill Livingstone, New York, 1984
13. Gens D: Nutrition in critical illness. In Geelhoed GW, Chernow B (eds): Endocrine and Metabolic Responses to Critical Illness and Trauma. Churchill Livingstone, New York, 1984
14. Harness JK, Geelhoed GW, Thompson NW et al: Nesidioblastosis in adults: a surgical dilemma. Arch Surg 116: 675, 1981
15. Heath H: Incidence of hyperparathyroidism. N Engl J Med 302: 189, 1980
16. Higgins GA, Recant F, Fischman AB: The glucagonoma syndrome: surgically curable diabetes. Am J Surg 13: 142, 1979
17. Klapdor R: Effects of somatostatin in bronchial constriction in a patient with carcinoid syndrome. N Engl J Med 302: 464, 1980
18. Lipson A, Hsu IH, Sherwin B, Geelhoed GW: Nitroprusside in the management of a patient with pheochromocytoma. JAMA 239: 427, 1978

19. Mackin JF, Canary JJ, Pittman CS: Thyroid storm and its management. N Engl J Med 291: 1396, 1974

20. Moore FD: Metabolic Care of the Surgical Patient. WB Saunders, Philadelphia, 1959

21. Orr WC, Imes NK, Martin RJ: Progesterone therapy in obese patients with sleep apnea. Arch Intern Med 139: 109, 1979

22. Passmore J: Adrenal insufficiency and principles of systemic corticosteroid therapy. In Geelhoed GW, Chernow B (eds): Endocrine and Metabolic Response to Critical Illness and Trauma, Clinics in Critical Care Medicine Series. Churchill Livingstone, New York, 1984

23. Pena A: Metabolic considerations in infants and children. In Geelhoed GW, Chernow B (eds): Endocrine and Metabolic Response to Critical Illness and Trauma, Clinics in Critical Care Medicine Series. Churchill Livingstone, New York, 1984

24. Slag MF, Morley JE, Elson MK et al: Free thyroxine levels in critically ill patients: a comparison of currently available assays. JAMA 246: 2702, 1981

25. Sterling K: Thyroid hormone action at the cell level. N Engl J Med 300: 1/3, 1979

26. Trunkey DD: The effects of hormones and toxic factors in shock. Current Concepts, Upjohn Company, 1979

27. Tunbridge WMG: The epidemiology of hypothyroidism. Clin Endocrinol Metab 8: 21, 1979

28. Utiger RD: Decreased extrathyroidal triiodothyronine production in nonthyroidal illness: benefit or harm? Am J Med 69: 807, 1980

29. Vitek V, Shatney CH, Lang DJ, Cowley RA: Thyroid hormone responses in hemorrhagic shock: study in dogs and preliminary findings in humans. Surgery 93: 768, 1983

30. Waldhausl W, Kleinberger G, Korn A et al: Severe hyperglycemia: effects of rehydration on endocrine derangements and blood glucose concentrations. Diabetes 28: 577, 1979

31. Wang C-A, Guyton SW: Hyperparathyroid crisis: clinical and pathologic studies of 14 patients. Ann Surg 190: 782, 1979

32. Woodruff RE, Lewis SB, McLeskey CH, Graney WF: Avoidance of surgical hyperglycemia in diabetic patients. JAMA 244: 166, 1980

SECTION VIII

SELECTED PROBLEMS IN TRAUMA CARE

26

Trauma Protocols for Resuscitation and Evaluation

C. Michael Dunham

INTRODUCTION

External trauma may damage any anatomic structure and cause an immediate threat to life, when injury causes instability in the cardiovascular, pulmonary, or central nervous systems (CNS),[49] or it may affect systems that are usually not life threatening but may cause morbidity by damaging the superficial soft tissues, hollow viscera, or musculoskeletal structures. The trauma patient is managed by a priorities approach to assess and treat pathology rapidly that may result in significant morbidity or mortality. The first priorities are directed toward detecting cardiovascular and respiratory instability and initiating therapy to minimize tissue hypoxia, identifying and treating immediate life-threatening brain injury, and preventing damage to the spinal cord. The second priorities are aimed at detecting cardiovascular, respiratory, or brain pathology that may pose an imminent threat to the patient's life

and identifying potential or actual spinal cord or brain injury that may cause significant morbidity. The purpose of the third priorities is to find indolent pathology that may cause a delayed threat to life and counteract those disruptive processes (Table 26-1). Major injuries are usually easily identified; however, more subtle injuries may not be detected initially. These relatively minor and undetected injuries may lead to later morbidity, however; for example, a perineal laceration may be missed on admission and not become evident until the patient develops sepsis days later. On the other hand, if an obvious peripheral injury, such as a femoral fracture, receives the primary attention, life may be lost due to an undiagnosed thoracic aortic tear or splenic rupture.

Until the general surgeon arrives, it is important that one physician (the general surgeon or the emergency room physician) supervise the multidiscipline care of the trauma patient. The surgeon is best qualified to coordinate management of these patients, since he or she

TABLE 26-1. Protocols for Resuscitation and Evaluation of the Acutely Injured Patient

First priorities
  Protocol
  Respiratory assessment and stabilization
  Cardiovascular assessment and stabilization
  Central nervous system assessment and stabilization

Second priorities
  Protocol
  Neurologic examination
  Spinal injury
  Severe brain injury
  Routine radiographs
  Abdominal injury
    Blunt trauma
    Penetrating trauma
  Miscellaneous considerations

Third priorities
  Protocol
  Systematic physical examination
  Diagnostic modalities
  Elective tracheal intubation
  Pulmonary artery catheterization
  Prophylactic antibiotics
  Tetanus prophylaxis
  Minor brain injuries
  Miscellaneous considerations

has experience in providing physiologic support, possesses invasive skills to counteract life-threatening emergencies, and understands the principles associated with physical injury to all organ systems. Even though the patient may have no general surgical problem, the general surgeon should be in charge until the patient is stable, injuries are clearly delineated, and the patient is assuming a course of recovery.[31]

Trauma protocols based on a priorities concept provide the physician with a structured approach for detecting and managing all injuries relative to their threat to homeostasis. The protocols should be indelibly ingrained in the physician's mind to assist in managing the unstable multiple injured patient. Deviation from the protocols may be clinically appropriate, yet the physician should justify with clear rationale such a waiver. The multiple trauma patient is received by the admitting team and each member has a predesignated duty to maximize efficiency. In many cases, it will be necessary to institute resuscitation measures before a complete diagnostic assessment has been performed. It is imperative that the patient be totally disrobed as rapidly as possible to facilitate assessment and management of all injuries. Since infection is a leading cause of death,[22,63,171] time should be made for adequate skin preparation before invasive procedures except in a few rare situations.

Type and cross-match, hematocrit, white blood cell (WBC) count, sodium, potassium, BUN, creatinine, glucose, coagulation profile, and serum osmolality are routinely obtained in the multiple-injured patient. A toxicology screen is often helpful in identifying substance abuse. The blood for these laboratory determinations is obtained as soon as possible following admission. The blood work may be obtained through a large intravenous catheter, which is subsequently used for volume infusion, by percutaneous needle aspiration or through an arterial catheter.

A supine chest radiograph may be obtained shortly after admission if there is significant respiratory or cardiovascular instability to detect immediately life-threatening intrathoracic injury. The film may also be helpful in the unstable patient to assess quickly the placement of intrathoracic lines, such as central venous catheters, endotracheal tubes, and thoracotomy tubes.

FIRST PRIORITIES

Protocol

1. Upon arrival, rapidly inspect the patient for skin color, chest wall motion, alertness, and extremity movement.
2. Auscultate the chest in each mid-axillary line for the presence and quality of breath sounds.
3. Establish an airway and provide adequate ventilation.
4. Palpate the pulse (slow, rapid, strong, weak).

5. Establish cardiac monitoring.
6. Determine the blood pressure.
7. Establish intravenous catheters and begin volume infusion.
8. Control external hemorrhage.
9. Deflate the MAST garment by section only after volume infusion has been initiated.
10. Note whether the patient follows commands (wiggles fingers and toes).
11. Note the extremity posture in response to noxious sternal compression if the patient is unable to follow commands.
12. Note the size and reactivity of each pupil.
13. Stabilize the neck with a rigid collar and prevent spinal flexion or extension, if movement is necessary.
14. Obtain an arterial blood gas (ABG).
15. Blood is obtained for laboratory assessment as soon as possible.
16. Obtain a supine chest radiograph quickly if there is respiratory or cardiovascular distress.

The objectives of the first priorities are to detect cardiovascular and respiratory instability and initiate therapy to minimize tissue hypoxia, identify and treat immediately life-threatening brain injury, and prevent damage to the spinal cord. As with other life-threatening states, the approach to the severely injured patient is based on the classic ABC concept: *a*irway, *b*reathing, and *c*irculation, cortex, and cord. A great deal of information may be gleaned about the patient regarding circulatory, respiratory, and neurologic function by rapidly inspecting the patient as he or she enters the emergency room and is placed on the receiving bed. The skin color should be noted to be normal, cyanotic, or pallored. The rate and depth of chest wall motion should be evaluated to determine whether the respiratory rate is normal, decreased, or increased and to note asymmetric chest wall motion. Some assessment regarding neurologic function is made by noting whether the patient's eyes are open or closed, thus implying awareness or loss of contact with the environment. Motion of the extremities should be noted to be either rigid or nonrigid. No motion of an extremity may suggest a spinal cord injury, severe peripheral nerve injury, or severe trauma to the musculoskeletal system.

Respiratory Assessment and Stabilization

Hypoxic hypoxia may cause severe cellular damage, especially if there is simultaneous cardiovascular instability. Respiratory insufficiency in the trauma patient may occur secondary to the following:

1. Foreign material in the airway
2. Soft tissue prolapse in the supraglottic region secondary to an impaired level of consciousness or mandibular fracture
3. Laryngeal fracture
4. Tracheal or bronchial laceration
5. Rib fractures with flail chest
6. Aspiration
7. Lung contusion
8. Hemothorax or pneumothorax
9. Pulmonary edema associated with cardiac failure or fluid overload
10. Hypoventilation
    a. Diaphragmatic rupture with abdominal evisceration
    b. Cervical or high thoracic spinal cord deficit
    c. Drug intoxication
    d. Brain injury (structural/metabolic)

The manifestations of respiratory insufficiency may be nonspecific; however, they may clearly reflect the underlying pathology. A foreign body in the airway, soft tissue prolapse into the supraglottic area, a laryngeal fracture or tracheal disruption may present as partial or complete airway obstruction. Manifestations of such pathology may cause stridor, use of accessory respiratory muscles, flaring of the ala nasi, intercostal retractions, noisy respirations, or decreased breath sounds. A bronchial tear may present as a collapsed lung if the disruption is large or as a tension pneumothorax. Multiple rib fractures may manifest as paradoxical chest wall motion during spontaneous breathing. These fractures may cause significant chest wall splinting or an unstable chest wall, especially in the elderly patient, both leading to atelectasis. Patients with significant pulmonary aspiration or lung contusion may present with hypoxia, cyanosis, and tachypnea. A segmental pulmonary infiltrate on chest radiograph commonly represents an aspiration, while a nonsegmental infiltrate is usually associated with a lung contusion. The patient with a lung contusion has bloody bronchial secretions, while the secretions of a patient with aspiration may be bloody or may show oral or gastric contents.

Patients with a lung contusion commonly have rib fractures, though this is not universal. The patient with a large hemothorax or tension pneumothorax usually presents with cardiovascular instability, tachypnea, and a unilateral decrease in the breath sounds. The evisceration of abdominal contents into the thorax from a ruptured diaphragm causes a decrease in breath sounds in the affected hemithorax as well as a mediastinal shift. Patients with a cervical or high thoracic spinal cord deficit have impaired vital capacity manifested as clinical hypoventilation and hypercarbia. Those with suppressant drug intoxication or brain dysfunction secondary to metabolic or structural abnormalities may present with hypoventilation as manifest by decreased breath sounds, decreased chest wall motion, bradypnea, or decreased air exchange from the mouth or nose. Initially, the breath sounds should be auscultated in each mid-axillary line to permit clinical detection of unilateral lung pathology. Auscultation over the central bronchi may be misleading in that a patient may have major lung collapse yet still have good bronchial breath sounds. If the patient has significant cardiovascular or respiratory distress and there is any question regarding the presence of a collapsed lung, a chest tube should be inserted for therapeutic and diagnostic purposes, following needle decompression. If the patient is relatively stable, a supine chest radiograph may be rapidly obtained to detect unilateral or bilateral thoracic injury.

Simple techniques to obtain a patent airway include the jaw thrust technique, removal of foreign material from the pharynx, or insertion of an oral or nasal airway. The most expedient means to control the patient's airway is usually tracheal intubation. Following tracheal intubation, a ventilator is usually necessary to supply adequate ventilation and oxygenation, commonly with the addition of positive end-expiratory pressure (PEEP) to treat or prevent a significant increase in the pulmonary shunt.

Urgent tracheal intubation is indicated for those patients who present with respiratory distress (retractions, tachypnea, or cyanosis), hypoventilation, an inadequate airway, hypoxia, hypercarbia,[170] shock, or impairment in consciousness,[64] in which the patient is nonpurposeful or nonverbal.

Initially, the trauma patient is considered to have a cervical spine injury; the neck should therefore be held in neutral position during urgent tracheal intubation. If the jaws are rigid, an intravenous paralytic agent is administered. One assistant compresses the cricoid ring posteriorly to prevent aspiration of gastric contents while a second assistant holds the head and neck in a neutral position. With visualization of the vocal cords, oral translaryngeal intubation is performed. There is no role for blind nasal translaryngeal intubation in the patient who requires urgent tracheal intubation. If the vocal cords cannot be visualized during oral intubation due to the presence of pharyngeal hemorrhage or for other anatomic reasons, a surgical cricothyroidotomy is performed[93,114] (Fig. 26-1). If a laryngeal fracture or laryngotracheal separation is suspected, a tracheostomy should be performed. For the patient with a laryngeal fracture who is relatively stable and has a thin neck, a standard tracheostomy is performed; however, if the patient's neck is large or there are signs of respiratory embarrassment, a surgical cricothyroidotomy is performed.[93] If the patient presents with an esophageal obturator airway in place, the esophageal obturator airway is not removed until the trachea is intubated and the tracheal cuff is inflated. A chest tube may be necessary to decompress the pleural space in order to obtain lung expansion. If the patient has significant respiratory or cardiovascular instability, or both, and there is any question during physical evaluation regarding the presence of a hemothorax or a pneumothorax, a chest tube should be immediately inserted following needle decompression. Should the patient be relatively stable, a supine chest radiograph is rapidly obtained to determine the need for the insertion of a chest tube. Fluid overload must be prevented[165] and cardiac failure treated with inotropic support to prevent hydrostatic pulmonary edema.[201]

An ABG is obtained as soon after admis-

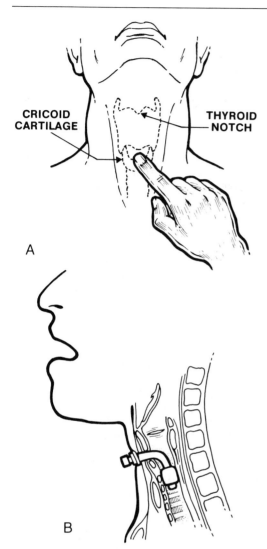

CRICOID
CARTILAGE

THYROID
NOTCH

A

B

FIG. 26-1 Cricothyroidotomy. **(A)** The cricothyroid membrane is located by palpating the thyroid notch with the index finger and moving caudad until the cricoid ring is identified. **(B)** This projection demonstrates the position of a tracheal tube inserted through the cricothyroid membrane.

sion as possible to detect relative or absolute hypoxia, hypercarbia, and acidosis. Virtually all patients with a PaO_2 of less than 60 mmHg on room air have significant respiratory insufficiency. An estimation of the pulmonary shunt is made by calculating the PaO_2/FIO_2 (see ref. 30), which is the partial pressure of oxygen in the arterial blood divided by the inspired oxy-

gen concentration. The normal PaO_2/FIO_2 is 500. For example, a PaO_2 value of 100 on room air, which is 0.2, equals a ratio of 500. A ratio less than or equal to 200 when the patient receives supplemental oxygen implies a pulmonary shunt greater than or equal to 20 percent. A relatively accurate FIO_2 is obtained when the patient is on room air and the FIO_2 is 0.2 or the patient is intubated and the FIO_2 is obtained from the ventilator setting; however, the FIO_2 is not very accurate when the patient is receiving supplemental oxygen by way of nasal prongs or a face mask. If the PaO_2 is less than 60 mmHG on room air or the PaO_2/FIO_2 is less than 200 on supplemental oxygen, tracheal intubation and PEEP or CPAP are virtually always indicated.[54,164] If the arterial CO_2 is greater than 45 and the patient has an acid pH, tracheal intubation is usually necessary to provide adequate alveolar ventilation. A bicarbonate value of less than 26 and a pH of less than 7.35 generally implies significant lactic acidosis, which is primarily managed by adequate restoration of microcirculatory perfusion and the administration of bicarbonate, if the base deficit is severe.

Cardiovascular Assessment and Stabilization

Significant cardiovascular instability creates a deficit in microcirculatory pefusion, which produces cellular hypoxia.[118] Tissue hypoxia leads to a number of metabolic and structural alterations that are reversible initially; however, irreversible destructive changes transpire if the depth or duration reaches a critical magnitude. Since that point of transition is not easily delineated at the bedside, any patient with manifestations of circulatory instability must be aggressively resuscitated in hopes of preventing irreversible cellular damage. Inadequate restoration of microcirculatory perfusion may predispose the patient to multiple physiologic systems dysfunction, which may cause death days to weeks later. Approximately 95 percent of posttraumatic cardiovascular instability is caused by hypovolemia secondary to external or internal blood loss.[118] External hemorrhage is usually readily apparent. However, significant blood loss may occur before the patient's presentation to the hospital; therefore, the medical staff may underestimate the magnitude of the loss. Internal bleeding may occur within the thorax, the peritoneal cavity, or the retroperitoneal space or may be associated with femoral, pelvic, or lumbar spine fractures. An additional cause of cardiovascular instability is mediastinal shock, which is an impairment of central cardiopulmonary circulation. Mediastinal shock may develop secondary to the presence of a tension pneumothorax, cardiac tamponade, or cardiac contusion. Less common causes of cardiovascular instability in the trauma patient are myocardial infarction, quadriplegia, severe, terminal brain injury, or hypothermia. Hypotension, tachycardia, pallor, cool extremities, decreased capillary refill, diaphoresis, cyanosis, or oliguria in any combination are physiologic signs suggestive of cardiovascular instability.

The primary goal of shock resuscitation is to restore adequate tissue oxygen delivery and to treat the underlying pathology to prevent recrudesence of the shock state. Reversal of cardiovascular instability is suggested by normalization of the blood pressure and heart rate, an improvement in color of the mucous membranes and skin, warming of the peripheral extremities, and a urine flow of 30 to 50 ml/hr. Treatment of the blood pressure, heart rate, and other clinical signs and symptoms of hypoperfusion is directed toward restoration of cellular perfusion. Since the primary defect during cardiovascular instability is usually hypovolemia, volume infusion is the primary therapy. Adequate volume loading is initiated after adequate vascular access is obtained, which usually requires the insertion of at least two large-bore venous catheters. Appropriate catheterization may be obtained with a 14- or 16-gauge short line, a pediatric feeding tube, a Swan-Ganz introducer, or a 14-gauge intracath. Catheters may be inserted percutaneously in an arm vein, femoral vein, or saphenous vein at the ankle. If vasoconstriction is significant or the patient is obese and percutaneous venipuncture cannot be performed, peripheral cutdowns or central venipuncture become necessary. Sites at which to perform a peripheral cutdown are the cephalic vein at the wrist, the antecubital fossa, or the saphenous vein at the ankle or groin. Central venipuncture may be used to catheterize the subclavian or jugular vein; however, this technique is commonly associated with an iatrogenic induced pneumothorax in the hypovolemic patient, especially if the operator is inexperienced.[1,179]

Choices of fluid to be infused are colloids, crystalloids, red blood cells (RBCs), fresh-frozen plasma, and platelet packs. Initially, 1,500 to 2,000 ml colloid[37,153,176] is infused and immediately supplemented with RBCs to maintain the oxygen-carrying capacity of the blood, if continued cardiovascular resuscitation is necessary. When possible, type-specific cross-matched blood should be administered; however, if the patient has persistent cardiovascular instability after the infusion of 1,500 to 2,000 ml asanguinous fluids, prior to the availability of type-specific cross-matched blood, type-specific blood or type O RBCs should be administered. Type O-negative packed RBCs with low quantities of antibodies are an ideal replacement if cross-matched blood is not available; however, O-negative RBCs are frequently unavailable. In this situation, O-positive RBCs with low antibody titers are acceptable in males or females except for the Rh-negative female of child-bearing age where there is a risk of sensitization and the subsequent development of erythroblastosis fetalis. If O-positive RBCs are all that are available, the female of child-bearing age who has cardiovascular instability should receive O-positive RBCs and be given Rhogam following the resuscitation. Once cross-matched blood becomes available, it is administered to the patient without anticipating any complications. An alternate plan to the administration of O-positive RBCs is to provide the patient with type-specific uncrossmatched blood until cross-matched blood becomes available.

Coagulability of the blood is maintained by administering adequate quantities of fresh-frozen plasma and platelets. A dilutional coagulopathy may occur in any patient undergoing massive transfusion and may be compounded by disseminated intravascular coagulopathy (DIC) in the blunt-injured patient due to an elaboration of tissue thromboplastins.[27,88,100]

The coagulopathy associated with massive transfusion is usually related to the degree of cardiovascular instability and hemorrhage. To prevent a dilutional coagulopathy, 2 units of fresh-frozen plasma[88] is given for each 5 units of RBCs administered. This ratio should be altered to increase the amount of fresh-frozen plasma depending on the PT, PTT,[100] the degree of hemodynamic instability, and clinical evidence of a coagulopathy.[100] Six to 8 units of platelets[88] is usually administered after the infusion of 8 to 10 units of RBCs; however, the platelet infusion rate may be adjusted according to the platelet count,[29] the degree of hemodynamic instability, or the presence of a coagulopathy.[29] Hypothermia must be aggressively combatted in order to minimize its adverse effect on the clotting mechanism.[88]

In general, the infusion rate for intravascular volume repletion is dictated by the degree of cardiovascular instability and by whether the central venous pressure (CVP) rises significantly with volume infusion. If the CVP rises with volume loading, hemodynamic stability must be obtained by maneuvers other than fluid infusion. With hypovolemia, the CVP is generally low; with depressed myocardial function, the CVP is usually high. If the CVP is less 8 cmH$_2$O and there is persistent hemodynamic instability, more volume infusion and control of the underlying hemorrhagic focus are necessary to stabilize the cardiovascular system. If there is cardiovascular instability and the CVP is greater than 15 cmH$_2$O, there is usually some degree of mediastinal shock secondary to a tension pneumothorax, cardiac tamponade, cardiac contusion, or ventricular dysfunction. If the CVP is not extremely high or low, the change in CVP relative to volume infusion is informative.

When the CVP rises with volume infusion and there is cardiovascular instability, mediastinal shock is present. If the CVP fails to rise with volume infusion and there is persistent cardiovascular instability, active hemorrhage is present. Once some degree of cardiovascular stability has been achieved, an arterial line is inserted to monitor the systemic blood pressure and obtain blood for gas, pH, bicarbonate, hematocrit (HCT), and electrolyte analysis. If the blood pressure is relatively stable, a percutaneous radial or femoral arterial catheter is inserted, but if the pressure is low, a radial arterial cutdown for catheter insertion is performed.

After adequate volume infusion, there may be clinically unrecognizable cardiovascular instability, which can only be detected by pulmonary artery catheter monitoring. Patients likely to fall in this category are those who have a history of cardiac dysfunction, a difficult resuscitation, oliguria, or high-output renal insufficiency or patients who are elderly or on high levels of PEEP.[77,186] Those with hypovolemic shock may incur significant subendocardial ischemia to the point of depressing ventricular contractility, thereby imposing an element of myocardial failure.[7,75] Patients with persistent shock should be monitored with a pulmonary artery catheter to identify the specific abnormalities responsible for the cardiovascular instability. Once hypovolemia has been corrected and the other mechanical causes of cardiovascular instability remedied, dobutamine may markedly improve ventricular performance if the cardiac index (CI) is relatively low and the wedge pressure is elevated.[25,184,217] If the patient is oliguric despite adequate cardiac function, dopamine in the range of 0.5 to 2 μg/kg/min should be administered to improve renal function,[25,36,139] while renovascular and postobstructive uropathy are excluded. It is imperative that adequate oxygenation be maintained during all phases of resuscitation. A patent airway is usually obtained by tracheal intubation, adequate oxygen-carrying capacity is maintained with a hemoglobin (Hb) of 10, and the Hb is optimally saturated with oxygen by providing 100 percent inspired oxygen, PEEP/CPAP when necessary, and adequate alveolar ventilation.

In addition to volume infusion and adequate oxygenation of the patient, specific interventions are usually necessary to treat the underlying pathology that initiated the cardiovascular instability. Sites of external hemorrhage are usually apparent on physical evaluation and are managed by the application of pressure, ligation of bleeding points, or proximal vascular control. A hemothroax is usually identified clinically by the presence of decreased unilateral breath sounds, manifestations of systemic hypoperfusion, and the presence of collapsed veins. Appropriate therapy involves the insertion of a chest tube into the affected pleural space and monitoring of blood flow. A thoracotomy is usually necessary to control the hemorrhage if the flow rate is greater than 500ml over 2 hours after the initial evacuation of blood.[132] A femoral fracture is usually apparent from obvious thigh deformity and is confirmed by x-ray studies. Distal traction is applied to minimize blood loss from the fracture site and soft tissue. Hemorrhage associated with a pelvic fracture may be arrested by the MAST garment in addition to adequate administration of coagulation factors.[48] If there is persistent bleeding and the pelvic ring is clinically unstable, a Hoffman external fixator is rapidly applied to reduce bleeding and produce stability.[128,159] Should bleeding continue, pelvic arteriography is performed to identify points of hemorrhage and embolize those sites other than the common or external iliac artery.[9,48,127,215] If the pelvic ring is stable and bleeding continues despite the use of the MAST garment, an arteriogram is obtained and embolization is performed as indicated.

There may be significant hemorrhage due to the tearing of paraspinous muscles and the perivertebral venous plexus when the lumbar spine is fractured. Low back pain or the presence of paraplegia may be indications of a lumbar spine fracture. The patient may have no local complaints of back pain if there is an alteration in the level of consciousness or the patient has multiple injuries. The diagnosis is confirmed by radiographic examination; the therapy is conservative or surgical immobilization of the spine. Clinical manifestations of a renal injury are hematuria or flank pain, mass, or ecchymoses. The intravenous pyelogram (IVP) may reveal a parenchymal fracture, major dye extravasation, or nonvisualization when there is significant renal damage and associated hemorrhage. If there is significant cardiovascular instability, the patient should be immediately explored to control the hemorrhage. If the patient is relatively stable, better delineation of the pathology is obtained by renal arteriography or computed tomography (CT) scan with administration of a contrast dye. Early surgical intervention to remove, partially resect, or suture the damaged kidney is

indicated only when there is persistent hemodynamic instability.

Intraperitoneal hemorrhage secondary to blunt trauma is detected by diagnostic peritoneal lavage, in which case an RBC count of greater than 50,000 per mm³ in a patient with shock is an indication for surgical intervention; however, an RBC count of less than 100,000 per mm³ is not usually associated with immediately life-threatening hemorrhage. The patient in shock who has a diagnostic peritoneal lavage with an RBC count greater than 100,000 per mm³ or the aspiration of 12 to 15 ml gross blood should undergo emergency celiotomy.[5,6] Abdominal hemorrhage is also inferred if a patient presents with a penetrating abdominal wound and has cardiovascular instability; however, if there are multiple body cavity wounds, each region must be assessed for its contribution to shock. If the patient with cardiovascular instability has been managed with a MAST garment, the trouser should not be deflated until volume repletion has been initiated.[115] The garment should be deflated by section, beginning with the abdominal component and followed by each leg with monitoring of the blood pressure to ensure maintenance of cardiovascular stability.

A tension pneumothorax is usually detected by noting the presence of decreased unilateral breath sounds, minimal chest wall motion of the affected hemithorax, distended neck veins, and manifestations of systemic hypoperfusion. If the patient has relative cardiovascular and respiratory stability, a supine chest radiograph is rapidly obtained to prove or disprove the presence of a pneumothorax. By contrast, if there is severe cardiovascular or respiratory instability, the tube should be inserted immediately following decompression of the pleural space by thoracentesis. The patient should be observed for a large air leak through the chest tube as an indication for bronchoscopy to diagnose a bronchial injury. Patients may have bilateral tension pneumothoraces or a tension pneumothorax on one side and a major hemothorax on the opposite side. Patients with significant cardiovascular instability and a bilateral decrease in breath sounds should receive pleural decompression in each hemithorax.

Cardiac injury and tamponade should be

suspected in any patient sustaining a penetrating wound to the chest or upper abdomen who also has any degree of cardiovascular instability.[41,102] The hemodynamic instability may vary between cardiac arrest to only minimal or transient hypotension. In addition to manifestations of systemic hypoperfusion, the patient may have an increase in CVP or distended neck veins or a paradoxical pulse.[102,202] Occasionally the electrocardiogram (ECG) may reveal evidence of acute cardiac injury.[41] The patient with suspected cardiac injury who has severe cardiovascular instability should be managed by an emergency anterolateral thoracotomy.[178,202] If there is cardiovascular stability after volume resuscitation and a cardiac wound is suspected, a left anterolateral thoracotomy should be performed; however, if the wound is parasternal, a median sternotomy may be elected.[41,196,202] If the patient has had no history of cardiovascular instability, yet a cardiac injury is suspected on the basis of proximity of the wound, a left anterolateral thoracotomy should be performed to evaluate the heart.[196] Serial echocardiograms and CVP monitoring is a conservative method for following such a patient in place of a thoracotomy.

Cardiac tamponade should be considered in any trauma patient who has incurred a blunt traumatic event and who has any degree of cardiovascular instability. The key to diagnosing the injury is to maintain a high index of suspicion for such an entity. The patient may present with systemic hypoperfusion, neck vein distention, increased CVP after volume repletion, facial cyanosis, or pulsus paradoxus. Chest wall fractures and ecchymosis may or may not be present. The patient will commonly respond to volume administration and dopamine infusion. Pericardiocentesis may be performed as a therapeutic and diagnostic procedure; however, there are many false-positive and false-negative results.[202] A small subxiphoid pericardial window (Fig. 26-2) may be performed to detect the presence of a hemopericardium if tamponade is suspected; however, the patient should have relative cardiovascular stability, since this approach will not provide adequate access for repair should a cardiac injury exist.[91] A thoracotomy is performed when the patient has significant hypotension, a cardiac arrest, or a hemopericardium.

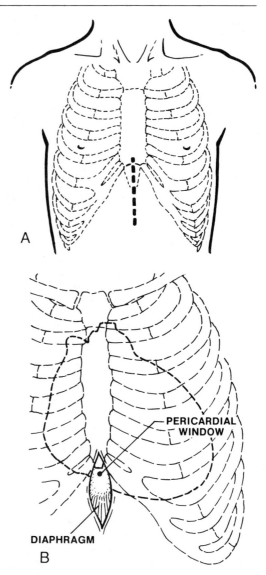

FIG. 26-2 Subxiphoid pericardial window. The xiphoid process **(A)** is removed and dissection performed to expose the pericardium. **(B)** A small aperture is created to detect the hemopericardium.

The diagnosis of cardiac contusion should be entertained if the patient presents with any dysrhythmia, such as a conduction block, tachydysrhythmia, or bradydysrhythmia, or has a ST-T segment abnormality. Other manifestions of cardiac contusion are the presence of systemic hypoperfusion and associated neck vein distention or elevated CVP, friction rub, or heart murmur. Any patient with a lung contusion or chest wall fracture or ecchymosis should be carefully evaluated for the presence of cardiac contusion. There is no diagnostic test specific for cardiac contusion that has a high degree of accuracy.[89,90,95] The ECG may reveal dysrhythmias,[120] ischemia,[89] or acute injury, while CPK[92,95,120] and LDH isoenzymes may be significantly elevated. Radionuclide cardioangiography may show a depression in the ejection fraction or evidence of dyskinesia.[192,200] The cardiac output (CO) may be depressed[200]; however, this is not universal and the two-dimensional echocardiogram may reveal evidence of dyskinesia or intramural hematoma.[90] Cardiac monitoring to detect dysrhythmias is imperative, as is the reversal of hypovolemia, hypoxia or hypokalemia. Any patient suspected of having a cardiac contusion should have a central venous line inserted for pressure monitoring and should be converted to a pulmonary artery catheter if cardiovascular instability develops. If a patient is suspected of having a cardiac contusion and has multiple other injuries or is to undergo an operative procedure, pulmonary artery monitoring is recommended.[192] Inotropic support with dobutamine or the administration of antidysrhythmic agents may be necessary. Rarely, cardiac dysfunction is so severe that the patient may require the insertion of an intra-aortic balloon pump[135,180] or the infusion of afterload reducing agents.

Myocardial infarction should be considered as an etiologic factor in the presence of posttraumatic cardiovascular instability when there is a bradydysrhythmia or tachydysrhythmia, especially in an elderly patient. The ECG will usually reveal evidence of acute cardiac damage. Therapy is directed toward nonspecific management of dysrhythmias and improvement of ventricular contractility with inotropic support or administration of afterload reducing agents, while volume loading is commonly needed to optimize CO.

A quadraplegic patient may present with manifestations of hypoperfusion; however, this patient will usually have an associated bradycardia as opposed to findings in other hypotensive patients. Hypoperfusion in the presence of other signs of cervical spinal cord disruption most commonly directs the physician to suspect a sympathectomy-induced cardiovascular instability. Appropriate therapy consists of judicious fluid administration (500 to 750 ml) and the addition of dopamine as necessary to maintain a systolic blood pressure of approximately 110 and a urinary output greater than or equal to 30 ml/hr. Severe brainstem dysfunction may cause cardiovascular instability in a patient presenting with flaccidity or decerebrate posture and minimal brainstem reflexes. Generally, cardiovascular stability can be gained with the administration of judicious volumes of fluid and dopamine while time is taken to exclude other causes of cardiovascular instability. Hypotension may be caused or exacerbated by the presence of significant hypothermia.[24] The most effective means to diagnose hypothermia is to obtain an accurate core temperature as soon as possible after admission. If the core temperature is less than 32°C, central active rewarming should be instituted, while those patients with a temperature greater than 32°C are managed by passive peripheral rewarming.[123]

Open cardiopulmonary resuscitation may be necessary to obtain adequate cerebral and coronary perfusion. The trauma patient who presents with asystole, ventricular fibrillation, or an idioventricular rhythm usually has an empty heart, in which case closed cariopulmonary resuscitation is generally ineffective.[106,132] The only hope for restoration of an effective sinus rhythm is to restore myocardial perfusion by open cardiopulmonary resuscitation. Commonly the brain has incurred a major hypoxic insult and will be nonfunctional, even though effective spontaneous cardiac function is restored. Open cardiopulmonary resuscitation in a patient who has a cardiac arrest and some signs of life offers the greatest chance to resuscitate the heart and have useful cerebral function.[107,108] Other patients with cardiovascular collapse may benefit from open cardiopulmonary resuscitation short of cardiac arrest. These patients have progressive bradycardia, no obtainable blood pressure, or a systolic blood pressure of less than 90 despite volume infusion, inotropic support, and pericardial or pleural decompression, when appropriate.[105] Once a thoracotomy is indicated, it must be performed immediately in conjunction with tracheal intubation and the application of positive-pressure ventilation, massive volume infusion along with RBCs, compression of the distal thoracic aorta, and administration of appropriate pharmacologic agents such as epinephrine and bicarbonate. As soon as the heart is resuscitated, the underlying pathology causing the arrest must be addressed to prevent recrudescence of the cardiovascular collapse.

Patients with refractory shock are most likely to be hypovolemic and require aggressive volume infusion and control of the bleeding points; however, hypoxia, hypokalemia, hypocalcemia, acidosis, or hypothermia may be contributing factors. Causes of cardiovascular instability other than hypovolemia must be identified and treated appropriately. If the patient has refractory cardiovascular instability the prognosis is poor; however, the administration of dopamine (10 to 20 μg/kg/min), dobutamine, calcium, naloxone, epinephrine (1 to 4 μg/min), Isuprel, glucagon, or corticosteroids may occasionally improve cardiovascular function.[214]

Central Nervous System Assessment and Stabilization

The objective relative to CNS injury during first-priorities management is to identify and initiate treatment for patients needing immediate craniotomy, identify obvious cord dysfunction, and prevent damage to the cord. Cardiovascular and respiratory stabilization is necessary to minimize neurologic tissue damage in any patient with a brain or spinal cord injury.[122] Patients who are unable to follow commands should be suspected of having major intracranial structural pathology. It is important to note that metabolic derangements such as alcohol intoxication are considered the cause of altered neurologic function only after structural brain abnormalities are excluded.[52] If the patient is unable to follow commands, the movement elicited by central noxious stimulation is identified and noted to be a bilateral or unilateral response. There may be flaccidity, minimal movement, or a response described as purposeful, flexion withdrawal, decorticate, or decerebrate. In addition, pupil size and reactivity to light are noted. Unilateral pupillary or extremity dysfunction commonly implies the presence of a focal lesion, which may indicate the need for surgical intervention.

The patient with any degree of brain dysfunction must have adequate oxygenation, ventilation, and cardiovascular stability to minimize neurologic damage.[122] Two types of patients are likely to benefit from emergency craniotomy if the surgery is performed shortly after admission: (1) those who have a witnessed onset of alteration in level of consciousness, that is, who are deteriorating in front of your eyes; or (2) those who present with lateralizing motor dysfunction, marked pupillary inequality, and an altered level of consciousness.[71] These patients are intubated and hyperventilated, administered steroids, and given a bolus of mannitol.[19] A CT scan and neurosurgical consultation are obtained as soon as possible.[71] Medical treatment for intracranial decompression and the minimal time taken to obtain a CT scan for accurate placement of burr holes for formal craniotomy are usually more effective than performing blind burr holes.[19,74] It must be emphasized that cardiovascular and respiratory stability must be maintained at all times for an optimal outcome.[122]

All trauma patients are treated initially as though they have a spinal injury, until proven otherwise. The cervical spine is immobilized in a rigid collar and, if movement of the patient is necessary, spinal column flexion and extension are prevented.[45] Patients who can follow simple commands and who cannot wiggle their fingers or toes should be considered to have a spinal cord injury and treated appropriately. On the other hand, the ability to wiggle the fingers or toes to command does not exclude the possibility of spinal cord or column injury.

SECOND PRIORITIES

Protocol

1. Perform a brief external examination of the head, neck, chest, abdomen, back, pelvis, and extremities.
2. Obtain a pertinent history, if possible.
3. Perform a more complete neurologic examination.
4. Obtain a lateral cervical spine radiograph.

5. Obtain thoracic and lumbar spine radiographs, if indicated.
6. Initiate specific therapy for spinal cord injury.
7. Institute medical treatment for severe brain injury.
8. Obtain an upright chest radiograph if there is no spinal injury.
9. Perform an A-P radiograph of the pelvis.
10. Insert a urinary bladder catheter.
11. Pass an oral gastric tube.
12. Perform diagnostic peritoneal lavage, local wound exploration, or physical examination of the abdomen, as appropriate.
13. Insert an arterial line, when indicated.

The objective of the second priorities is to detect cardiovascular, respiratory, or brain pathology, which is an imminent threat to the patient's life, and identify potential or actual spinal cord or cerebral injury that may cause significant morbidity. A brief external examination from head to toe is performed to identify deformities, lacerations, pulse deficits, penetrating wounds, foreign bodies, areas of ecchymosis, or points of tenderness. At this time, the patient should be cautiously log-rolled onto the side to examine the spine and back carefully for evidence of pathology. The external examination adds further direction to subsequent patient assessment and management. A brief and pertinent history is obtained regarding major symptoms, especially pain or tenderness to palpation of the neck or back, which may represent a spinal injury. Information from the patient, near relative, or observer of the incident relative to the mechanism of injury or past history of allergies, medications, prior surgical procedures, and pre-existing illnesses is often beneficial for optimal patient management.

Neurologic Examination

A more complete neurologic examination is performed to identify those patients with a spinal cord or brain injury that was not apparent on initial examination. The neurologic examination helps assess the magnitude of the neurologic injury as well as the level of the lesion. Amnesia, disorientation, or inability to open the eyes, verbalize words, or follow simple commands are evidence of brain injury. The examination for the corneal reflex, oculovestibular reflex, and pupillary response to light provides an assessment of brainstem function.[19] The deep tendon reflexes may be increased if there is significant brain injury. Spinal cord injury is easy to identify if the patient is able to follow commands and has a complete deficit. A spinal cord injury may be difficult to identify if the patient has an incomplete cord lesion, an altered level of consciousness, or significant instability of the cardiovascular or respiratory systems, which distracts the clinician from performing a careful neurologic examination and obscures the findings. A sensory and motor examination should be undertaken to evaluate each extremity, the chest wall, and the abdominal wall. Hypesthesia, weakness, and poor anal sphincter tone suggest spinal cord injury. The patient should be questioned for evidence of extremity weakness, tingling, or numbness, since these symptoms should suggest the likelihood of a spinal cord injury. Each nerve root should be carefully evaluated, since single nerve root dysfunction may be the only initial indication that a spinal cord injury is present. The deep tendon reflexes are commonly decreased or absent with spinal cord injury.

Spinal Injury

Lateral and A-P spine radiographs are the mainstay of radiographic screening for spinal column injury. Computed tomography of the spine provides the best spatial resolution of the spinal canal, while plain tomography produces a better depiction of the bony pathology relative to plain radiograms. Flexion–extension views of the spine are useful to detect ligamentous and bony instability of the spine when the spinal column appears normal on the plain films. A cross-table lateral radiograph of the cervical spine should be obtained on all patients following blunt trauma and should include all cervical vertebrae.[14,213] Most clinically significant cervical spinal column lesions are obvious on the lateral radiograph[173]; however, a small percentage of lesions may not be identified unless additional views, flexion-extension radiographs, or plain film or CT is performed. Additional views should be obtained if the radiograph of the lateral cervical spine appears normal, yet there is evidence of soft tissue swelling,[213] the patient complains of neck pain,[208] a spinal cord deficit is present, there is a palpable deformity of the neck, or there is a question regarding the possibility of a fracture or abnormal alignment. Additional views consist of an A-P, bilateral oblique, and transoral cervical spine projection. Flexion–extension views are obtained if an alert patient complains of neck pain and has no abnormality on plain films and no spinal cord dysfunction. The patient should voluntarily flex and extend the neck without active assistance from the examiner. Those with persistent focal neck pain and normal cervical spine radiographs should undergo tomography to exclude the presence of an occult fracture.[188,208] A patient with a cervical spinal cord injury, whether or not an abnormal plain radiograph has been obtained, should be considered to have compression of the cord. Spinal cord compression is evaluated by myelography or CT. Thoracic and lumbosacral radiographs should be obtained if the patient has a thoracic or lumbosacral spinal cord deficit, regional back pain, ecchymosis, deformity, or abrasions[140] or is unconscious after sustaining a fall. Appropriate views of the thoracic spine are an A-P and lateral projection, while A-P, lateral, and oblique views are necessary to evaluate the lumbosacral spine. If the patient has no neurologic deficit and has normal lumbosacral radiographs, flexion–extension views should be considered in order to assess stability, if there is a significant complaint of lumbar back pain. For the patient who has normal thoracic and lumbosacral radiographs and a neurologic deficit, spinal cord compression should be evaluated by myelography or CT.

The utilization of corticosteroids is extremely controversial[45,68]; however, these agents may minimize long-term spinal cord dysfunction, especially in the patient who has an incomplete lesion. Relatively high doses of steroids are administered as soon as possible and given for 48 to 72 hours; they are continued if there is neurologic improvement. Fluids should be judiciously administered to maintain a serum osmolality between 290 and 300; however, fluid restriction should not be to such a degree that cardiac preload and output fall. Modest volume expansion and dopamine are administered as necessary to maintain a systolic pressure of 110 to optimize spinal cord perfusion and maintain a urinary output of 30 to 40 ml/hr. Pulmonary artery catheterization for cardiovascular dynamic monitoring is recommended in all quadriparetic patients, in order to optimize cardiovascular performance.

An abnormal spinal column should be immobilized to prevent injury to the spinal cord, while any necessary movement of the patient is performed without flexing or extending the spine. Initially the cervical spine is immobilized in a rigid collar, with the assumption that an injury is present until proved otherwise. The rigid collar is also useful to immobilize patients who have neck pain yet normal radiographs and cord function or those with normal neurologic examination who have a questionable cervical spine fracture. Patients should be placed in cervical spine traction for immobilization if there is a spinal cord deficit, fracture, dislocation, or ligamentous instability. Thoracic or lumbosacral spinal column injuries are best immobilized by placing the patient on a Stryker frame. If the patient has a spinal column dislocation and a neurologic deficit, cord compression is considered to be present; therefore, the spinal abnormality must be reduced as the first step in decompressing the spinal cord. There always exists the possibility that decompression of the spinal cord will result in some return of neurologic function. A dislocation of the cervical spine is commonly reducible by traction; however, open reduction may be necessary if traction fails, while operative reduction of the thoracic or lumbosacral spine is almost always necessary.

Severe Brain Injury

Patients with a severe brain injury are easy to identify, since they are unable to verbalize, unable to follow commands, or are nonpurposeful. Other patients with a lesser degree of neurologic dysfunction must be considered to harbor significant intracranial pathology.[71] Such patients may follow commands, be purposeful, or verbalize but may be agitated, disoriented, or lethargic or have a focal motor deficit. All trauma patients with any neurologic dysfunction are considered to have an intracranial structural lesion, while metabolic cerebral dysfunction (e.g., alcoholic intoxication) is considered a diagnosis of exclusion.[52] The tissue damage following brain trauma is minimized by maintaining cardiovascular and respiratory stability to prevent cerebral hypoperfusion, hypoxia, and hypercarbia, which may markedly increase cerebral blood flow and lead to an increase in intracranial pressure.[19,122] The administration of corticosteroids is quite controversial[19,28,60,81] regarding the ability of these agents to minimize neurologic tissue damage associated with brain injury; however, a single dose of dexamethasone (1 mg/kg) at the time of admission seems reasonable. Intravascular fluids are administered in a judicious fashion to minimize brain edema. Fluids should be given in a manner to maintain a serum osmolality of 290 to 300 mOsm/kg, while acute fluid shifts from excessive dehydration or fluid administration are prevented. Hyperventilation[121] is instituted for the purpose of treating or preventing intracranial hypertension[19,168] in high-risk patients. High risk patients are nonpurposeful or nonverbal, or those who are unable to follow commands and will be under the effects of a general anesthetic.

Most patients who have any neurologic dysfunction should undergo diagnostic imaging to detect intracranial structural pathology.[19] Computed tomography of the brain is the most informative diagnostic study[35,145]; however, carotid/cerebral angiography[19] may be indicated in selected situations. Patients with respiratory and cardiovascular stability can be transported safely to the radiology suite for a CT scan. The CT scan is indicated in those patients who are unable to follow commands, are lethargic, are disoriented, have a skull fracture, or have a focal deficit. Evidence of a focal deficit constitutes the presence of a disturbance in motor, speech, or visual function. Patients who are to undergo a general anesthetic and have any neurologic deficit should undergo a CT scan before being administered the anesthetic agent. Patients with respiratory or cardiovascular instability may be in too tenuous a condition to be transported to the radiologic suite for a CT scan. If such a patient is relatively stable, has a focal deficit, and cannot follow commands, percutaneous carotid angiography is performed; however, if emergency extracranial surgery is mandatory due to marked instability, intracranial pressure monitoring is performed.[19,137] A CT Scan is performed as soon as possible following cardiovascular and respiratory stabilization. If an unstable patient is unable to follow commands and has no focal deficit, intracranial pressure monitoring is performed and a CT scan is obtained as soon as systemically stable.

Patients may be able to follow commands and have evidence of neurologic dysfunction, such as lethargy, disorientation, or amnesia, yet have such a degree of respiratory or cardiovascular instability that transport to the radiology suite for a CT scan is deemed unsafe. If such a patient has a focal deficit and is relatively stable, a percutaneous carotid angiogram is performed in the resuscitation area. If the patient is so unstable that there is no time for a percutaneous carotid arteriogram, intracranial pressure monitoring is performed during surgery. Once the patient is stable, a CT Scan is performed as soon as possible. In the unstable patient who is able to follow commands and in whom the deficit is nonfocal, a CT scan is performed as soon as systemic stability is achieved.

When the CT scan reveals no indication for craniotomy, intracranial pressure monitoring is performed in those patients who cannot follow commands and are going to be under a general anesthetic or in those patients who are nonpurposeful or nonverbal.[101,168] CT scanning and intracranial pressure monitoring to detect brain pathology are more liberally used in patients who will be under the influence of a general anesthetic, since the agent will prevent detection of most episodes of neurologic deterioration.[137] A sustained intracranial pressure greater than 15 mmHg suggests the presence of a mass lesion and should be managed by medical or surgical decompression. Diagnostic imaging should be performed when possible if such has not been recently done.

Adequate oxygenation, hyperventilation, and cardiovascular stability may lower intracranial pressure,[19,168] as may sedation and elevation of the head relative to the thorax. The patient should be evaluated for jugular venous compression, since this may markedly elevate the pressure. If an intraventricular catheter is in place, the pressure may be lowered by aspirating fluid from the system.[19] A mannitol bolus or drip or intravenous lidocaine may also lower the intracranial pressure.[19,168]

Routine Radiographs

If the patient has no spinal injury, an erect chest radiograph should be performed to evaluate the intrathoracic structures. A small pneumothorax or hemothorax is more readily identified on an erect radiograph. A supine radiograph commonly reveals an obscured or widened superior mediastinum; however, the same patient may clearly have a well-delineated aortic knob and a mediastinum of normal dimension on an erect chest radiograph (Fig. 26-3). If the superior mediastinum is wide[69,70] or the aortic knob is obscured,[191] a mediastinal hematoma, which is commonly associated with a rupture of the thoracic aorta or its tributaries, is presumed to be present. The width of the mediastinum depends to some degree on the age of the patient[70]; however, a superior mediastinal width greater than 8 cm is commonly associated with an aortic injury. The clinical impression that a patient has a wide mediastinum has been found to be more reliable than arbitrary dimensions.[20] If a mediastinal hematoma is identified on the chest radiograph, an aortogram is performed to detect the presence and location of an injury to the thoracic aorta

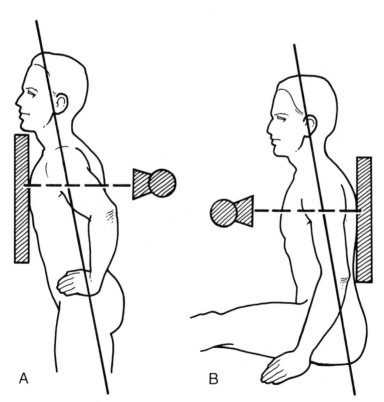

A   B

FIG. 26-3 Chest radiograph. An erect sitting radiograph in the trauma patient provides a nondistorted view of the superior mediastinum and is usually feasible if there is no spine injury. **(A)** True erect P-A chest radiograph. **(B)** True erect A-P chest radiograph.

or its tributaries[70] (Fig. 26-4). Occasionally, the aortic knob may be well delineated on a supine chest radiograph. Patients with spinal injury should have a supine radiographic study of the chest. When the aorta cannot be defined, the x-ray beam is rotated 10 to 15 degrees to visualize the aortic knob posterior to the manubrium; however, if the aortic knob cannot be clearly seen, an aortogram must be performed to exclude the possibility of an arterial injury. There is urgency in making such a diagnosis, since the aorta may rupture and lead to immediate exsanguination. Rarely, a patient with a ruptured thoracic aorta will present with a normal chest radiograph and the aortogram is ordered because the patient had been involved in a major deceleration accident.[69]

The chest radiograph may reveal evidence of a pneumomediastinum, which may be associated with an injury to the esophagus, trachea, or bronchi or may develop secondary to barotrauma. Pneumopericardium is a rare injury that may be detected radiographically, especially if the pericardial space is under tension. Cervical or thoracic wall subcutaneous emphysema may represent injury to the trachea, bronchi, or alveoli. The chest radiograph may reveal a nonsegmental pulmonary infiltrate such as a contusion or a segmental infiltrate representing an aspiration. Occasionally, the patient with a ruptured diaphragm will present with a normal chest radiograph[26,207]; however, the radiograph will commonly reveal at least an obscured hemidiaphragm or an "elevated" diaphragm.[26,38] The radiograph is much more suggestive of a ruptured diaphragm if there are multiple air–fluid levels seen in the hemithorax as a result of abdominal evisceration.[38] Foreign bodies such as bullets or aspirated material such as teeth may be identified on the chest radiograph. Lateral extrapleural hematomas are commonly associated with rib fractures and usually represent injury to intercostal vessels. An apical pleural cap is suggestive of an injury to the thoracic aorta or to one of its tributaries, such as the subclavian artery. Clavicular or spine fractures may be identified on the chest radiograph, as well as rib or scapular fractures, which should alert the clinician to the possible association of abdominal or intra-

thoracic injury. Sternal fractures are not usually identified on an A-P chest radiograph; however, they are usually readily identified on lateral or oblique views of the sternum.

A pelvic radiograph is routinely performed on all patients sustaining blunt trauma, since there may be minimal evidence of such a fracture on clinical examination. Reasons for the paucity of findings on physical evaluation are (1) the fracture may be clinically stable, (2) the patient may have an impaired level of consciousness and not complain of pain, and (3) there is commonly minimal evidence of deformity or ecchymosis. The presence of a pelvic fracture should prompt exclusion of urologic, rectal, or perineal injuries. Should a patient have a pelvic fracture or the question of such a fracture, pelvic inlet and outlet views are obtained for more clear delineation of such pathology. Any question regarding the presence of an acetabular fracture should signal the need for Judet views for further assessment.

Abdominal Injury

Blunt or penetrating abdominal trauma may cause significant hemorrhage, abdominal contamination with bacteria, or organ damage. Following blunt or penetrating trauma, a major goal is to detect the presence of abdominal pathology, which requires therapeutic intervention at the earliest possible point to minimize morbidity and mortality. Physical examination, peritoneal lavage, and diagnostic imaging techniques are useful modalities for evaluating the abdomen.

BLUNT ABDOMINAL TRAUMA: PERITONEAL LAVAGE

Physical evaluation of the abdomen for the detection of visceral injury following blunt trauma has been shown to be accurate in only 50 to 80 percent of large series.[151] Absolute indications for surgery based on physical evaluation are the presence of peritonitis, abdominal

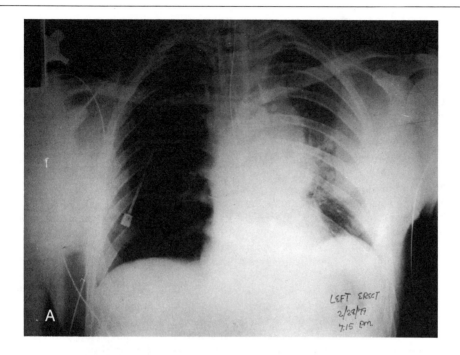

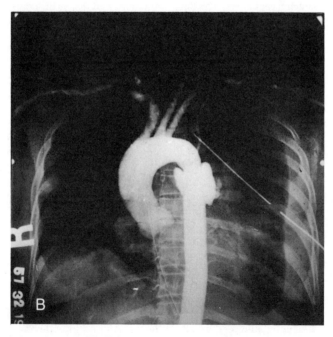

FIG. 26-4 Ruptured thoracic aorta. (A) This erect chest radiograph reveals a widened mediastinum and an obscured aortic knot, implying the presence of a mediastinal hematoma. (B) Aortography reveals the presence of a rupture of the thoracic aorta.

distention with hemodynamic instability, or a disrupted abdominal wall. The diagnostic peritoneal lavage is 98 percent accurate in detecting the presence of significant visceral abdominal pathology[6]; however, the peritoneal lavage may not exclude a retroperitoneal injury such as a pancreatic lesion. A patient with significant abdominal tenderness should be strongly considered for celiotomy to exclude major retroperitoneal injury despite a negative diagnostic peritoneal lavage.[39,58] Indications to perform a diagnostic peritoneal lavage include an altered level of consciousness, spinal cord injury with a nonsensate abdomen,[182] rib or pelvic fractures,[127] abdominal wall tenderness[21,177] or shock. The technique of lavage[32] begins as the anterior abdomen is aseptically prepared and the urinary bladder and stomach are decompressed (Fig. 26-5). The left paraumbilical area is infiltrated with lidocaine (Xylocaine) and a vertical incision is performed through the skin, subcutaneous tissue, and anterior rectus sheath. The rectus muscle is retracted laterally to expose the posterior rectus sheath. The posterior rectus fascia is grasped with a hemostat and a peritoneal dialysis catheter and trocar are gently pushed through the fascia and peritoneum. The catheter is advanced into the pelvis and 1 L saline is infused into the adult, or 15 to 20 ml/kg in a child, by gravity drip. After fluid infusion, the patient is placed alternately in the Trendelenburg and reverse Trendelenburg positions a couple of times, and the fluid is subsequently drained by siphon effect. The result is determined to be positive if greater than 12 to 15 ml of blood is initially aspirated through the catheter, the RBC count on the effluent is greater than 100,000 per mm³, or the WBC count is greater than 500 per mm³.[3,5,6] When the RBC count is greater than 100,000 per mm³, the incidence of significant visceral injury is approximately 85 percent.[151] Most of the time the lavage analysis is considered positive or negative based on the RBC count.[6] The WBC count is rarely helpful since the red cell count is usually elevated when there is significant visceral injury. In addition, the WBC count of the peritoneal cavity usually does not increase for 3 to 6 hours following gastrointestinal (GI) tract disruption, usually long after the diagnostic peritoneal lavage has been performed.[163] An RBC count of 50,000 to 100,000 per mm³ is an indeterminant range in which there is a 25 percent incidence of significant visceral pathology.[5] Because of this relatively low incidence, the surgeon is presented with a dilemma regarding operation versus observation. If the patient is stable, awake, and has minimal other injuries, it is preferable to observe the patient and to follow serial WBC counts, HCT, and physical evaluation and to consider a repeat lavage at a later time. Should the patient have an altered level of consciousness or multiple injuries such that serial evaluation is impossible, a celiotomy is advisable. In other words, the abdomen cannot be repeatedly evaluated, HCT and blood pressure are likely to fall secondary to blood loss associated with extra-abdominal injury or surgical procedures, and signs of peritonitis may not be detected until very late when there is an impaired level of consciousness. Patients without an indication for surgery on the basis of physical examination or diagnostic peritoneal lavage are followed by serial physical examinations and serial HCTs, WBC counts, and serum amylase determinations. The presence of a pancreatic injury should be strongly considered if there is a persistently elevated serum amylase or a rising amylase and the patient has associated abdominal pain.[84,99] Nonoperative candidates are kept NPO and administered minimal pain medications during this evaluation phase. Evidence of subsequent development of an ileus, blood loss, or abdominal tenderness should prompt diagnostic peritoneal lavage or surgery as appropriate. A significant false-negative rate with diagnostic peritoneal lavage is associated with perforations of the GI tract,[14] a ruptured diaphragm,[8,46] and injury to the pancreas, duodenum, or urologic tract.[46] A false-positive RBC count may develop secondary to iatrogenic injury of the mesentery, nonmesenteric vessels, small bowel, colon, urinary bladder, or stomach with the catheter.[151] These injuries are minimized if the urinary bladder and stomach are decompressed before insertion of the catheter and the device is gently advanced into the peritoneal cavity. To prevent a false-positive lavage, patients with a pelvic fracture should have the technique performed in the supraumbilical position and through an opening in the peritoneum, which has a pursestring suture.

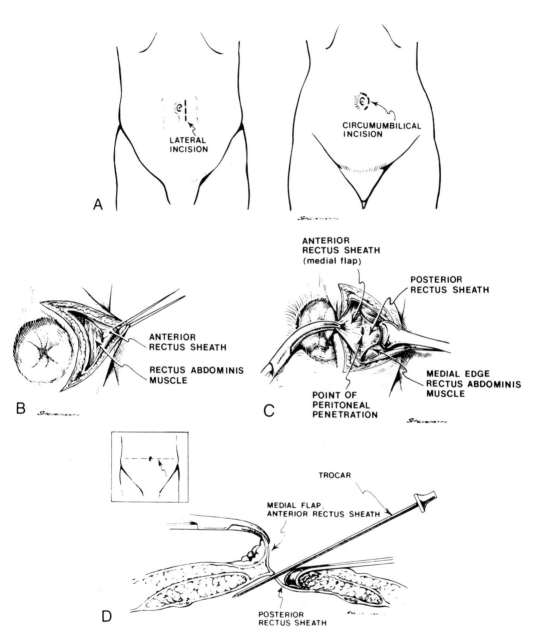

FIG. 26-5 Diagnostic peritoneal lavage. **(A)** The skin incision is performed in the left paraumbilical location. **(B)** An incision through the anterior rectus sheath exposes the rectus abdominus muscle. **(C)** The rectus muscle is retracted to reveal the posterior rectus sheath. **(D)** The trocar punctures the posterior rectus sheath/ peritoneum and is then directed toward the pelvis. (Cox EF, Dunham CM: A safe technique for diagnostic peritoneal lavage. J Trauma 23:152, 1983.)

PENETRATING ABDOMINAL TRAUMA: DIAGNOSTIC LAPOROTOMY VERSUS EXPECTANT TREATMENT

Virtually all medical centers explore patients who have peritoneal penetration as a result of a gunshot wound, since approximately 90 percent of these patients will have significant pathology.[198] About 50 percent of patients with a gunshot wound to the lower chest will have significant abdominal pathology.[198] The determination of peritoneal penetration may be indicated by the entrance and exit wounds or by the entrance wound and the point of implantation, as determined on physical examination or by radiographic evaluation.

Management of an abdominal stab wound depends on the presence or absence of symptoms and on whether the lesion involves the anterior or posterior abdomen, the flank, or the lower chest. Other determinants affecting management depend on whether the patient is alert and cooperative and the availability of an experienced surgical staff to follow such a patient. The major goal in managing patients with an anterior abdominal stab wound is to explore as early as possible all those patients with significant visceral injuries and at the same time to minimize the incidence of unnecessary laparotomies. All clinicians agree that patients with evidence of abdominal hemorrhage or peritoneal irritation should be explored,[134,199] and many operate on the basis of omental evisceration[65]; however, the latter is controversial. The major problem is in deciding which asymptomatic patients should undergo a celiotomy. There are those who strongly support the concept that patients should be explored only after they develop major symptoms.[97,199] Others are highly concerned with the possibility of delayed operative intervention and subsequent increased morbidity and mortality; however, supporters of expectant management state that there is no increase in morbidity and mortality and that the unnecessary laparotomy rate is only 10 to 12 percent.

Patients who are observed and asymptomatic are monitored with serial vital signs, physical evaluation, serial HCT, and WBC counts, are evaluated for hematuria, and have a chest and abdominal radiograph performed.

Local wound exploration has been used to evaluate patients who are asymptomatic or who have equivocal abdominal findings following a stab injury. The advocates of exploration based on peritoneal penetration report a low rate of unnecessary laparotomies,[13] and the opponents find the opposite.[61,199] Peritoneal penetration may be difficult to detect; therefore, diagnostic peritoneal lavage may be used to evaluate those patients who have penetration of the abdominal fascia.[61,134] If the diagnostic peritoneal lavage is positive, a laparotomy is performed, but a primary issue is what indicates a positive lavage. The patient must be observed following a negative diagnostic peritoneal lavage, since the test may yield a false-negative result. The RBC count is the primary determinant for exploration; if the RBC count is too low, the unnecessary laparotomy rate is excessive. If the RBC count is too high, the unnecessary laparotomy rate falls; however, there is an increasing false-negative rate[61] (i.e., a delay in detecting significant visceral injuries). All clinicians agree that an RBC count greater than 100,000 per mm^3 warrants a laparotomy and is associated with a low unnecessary exploration rate.[5,197,198] Currently, the debate is over a range of RBC counts of 1,000 to 100,000 per mm^3.[5,61,134] One report found no patient to have a significant visceral injury if the RBC count was less than 1,000 per mm^3.[134] There are clinicians who circumvent local wound exploration and proceed to diagnostic peritoneal lavage if the patient is asymptomatic or has equivocal findings.[199] However, the debate persists as to what is a positive result.

There is much controversial information in the literature, which usually implies that there is no single way to appropriately manage patients with asymptomatic anterior abdominal stab wounds. The approach to a given patient primarily depends on the availability or lack of availability of an experienced surgical staff to observe the patient; this in turn requires an alert and cooperative patient who can be observed. Patients with signs of abdominal hemorrhage or peritonitis require immediate laparotomy. If an asymptomatic patient is alert and an experienced surgeon is able to follow the patient, one of two plans may be pursued. The first plan may be to observe and operate on the patient only if signs of peritonitis or abdominal hemorrhage develop. The second alternative is to perform local wound exploration and discharge the patient if there is no fascial penetration; if there is fascial penetration, a diagnostic peritoneal lavage is performed. If the RBC count is less than 50,000 per mm³, the patient is observed for 24 hours for the development of abnormal clinical signs. If the RBC count is greater than 50,000 per mm³, a laparotomy is performed. If the patient is not alert or if the patient is alert but repeat examinations cannot be provided by an experienced surgeon, one of two plans is feasible. The first plan is to perform local wound exploration and clear the abdomen if there is no fascial penetration. If there is fascial penetration, a diagnostic peritoneal lavage is performed. If the lavage reveals an RBC count of less than 1,000 per mm³, the patient is observed; if the RBC count is greater than 1,000 per mm³, a laparotomy is performed. The alternative plan is to perform local wound exploration and clear the abdomen if there is no fascial penetration. If there is peritoneal penetration or a likelihood of peritoneal penetration based on anterior or posterior fascial penetration, a laparotomy is performed.

Fifteen percent of stab wounds penetrating the lower chest are associated with abdominal visceral injury.[198] Local wound exploration is not recommended, since the tract is often difficult to follow and more importantly may cause a pneumothorax. A chest tube is inserted if there is a pneumothorax or hemothorax and bleeding is monitored. If a patient with a right-sided wound is alert and cooperative and an experienced surgeon can repeatedly examine the patient, observation is undertaken or a diagnostic peritoneal lavage is performed,[195] with a laparotomy being indicated for an RBC count of greater than 50,000 per mm³. If the patient is not alert or an experienced surgeon cannot follow the patient, a diagnostic peritoneal lavage is performed and a laporotomy is indicated for an RBC count of greater than 1,000 per mm³. Patients with a left-sided lower thoracic wound undergo lavage and are explored if the RBC count is greater than 1,000 per mm³. Celiotomy is performed to close the diaphragmatic rent and to detect visceral injury.

Approximately 10 percent of posterior abdominal stab wounds are associated with significant visceral injury and a reliable physical examination in 90 percent of cases.[198] Diagnostic peritoneal lavage is known to be inaccurate in detecting retroperitoneal injury. The major concern is missing a colon or duodenal injury, which is associated with a 12 to 70 percent infectious morbidity rate. Celiotomy is the safest and most expedient approach to manage deep posterior abdominal stab wounds; however, if the patient is asymptomatic and alert and an experienced surgeon is available, the patient may be observed.[80] There should be some consideration for performing an IVP, upper GI series, barium enema examination, and angiography[80] or CT scan.

Approximately 30 percent of flank stab wounds are associated with visceral injury, and physical evaluation results in a 14 percent false-negative rate.[198] Intraperitoneal or retroperitoneal injury may be present, depending on the trajectory of the blade. The most expeditious and safe route is to explore all patients to detect significant visceral injury.

Miscellaneous Considerations

Critically ill and injured patients often require continuous arterial pressure monitoring and frequent withdrawal of blood samples to follow physiologic parameters. Cannulation of the femoral or radial artery has been shown to be safe and durable.[183] Catheterization is useful in patients with multiple injuries or respiratory insufficiency and in those who are anticipated to have a significant blood loss during surgery. After initial shock resuscitation, continuous arterial pressure monitoring is useful to assess the status of the cardiovascular system.

A transurethral bladder catheter should be inserted in virtually all patients sustaining trauma except for those who are alert and have no evidence of cardiovascular or respiratory instability. The presence of blood at the urethral meatus contraindicates the insertion of a bladder catheter until a urethrogram has been performed to exclude the presence of a urethral laceration. If a pelvic fracture is suspected or proven, a rectal examination should be performed to palpate the prostate. If the prostate is abnormal, a urethrogram should be performed to exclude the presence of a laceration prior to insertion of the bladder catheter. If there is any difficulty in passing a bladder catheter, this procedure should be abandoned until a urethrogram or urologic consult has been obtained.

An orogastric tube should be inserted to empty the gastric contents and to treat or prevent an ileus, as well as minimize the possibility of pulmonary aspiration.[19] An oral tube is recommended as opposed to a nasal tube, since this will decrease the likelihood of developing a paranasal sinusitis or intubation of the skull via a fracture of the cribriform plate.

THIRD PRIORITIES

Protocol

1. Perform a systematic physical examination from head to toe including each orifice.
2. Consider further diagnostic evaluation based on previous findings on physical evaluation and diagnostic studies.
3. Perform emergency surgery and other life-saving interventions after appropriate physical examination and diagnostic evaluation.
4. Consider elective tracheal intubation.
5. Insert a pulmonary artery catheter in high-risk patients.
6. Obtain an accurate core temperature reading.
7. Administer prophylactic antibiotics, when indicated.
8. Consider tetanus prophylaxis in all trauma patients.
9. Obtain specialty consultation as appropriate.
10. Reduce and splint dislocations and fractures.
11. Consider patients with minor brain injury for admission and observation.

The objectives of the third priorities are to detect indolent pathology that may cause a delayed threat to life or subsequent morbidity; initiate therapy to counteract those disruptive processes.

Systematic Physical Examination

A systematic physical examination of each body part is performed to detect abnormalities that subsequently direct diagnostic and therapeutic interventions. Scalp lacerations and hematomas may be detected easily, but small wounds may be hidden within the hair. A laceration or hematoma of the scalp or a skull fracture should alert the physician to the possibility of significant underlying intracranial injury.[53,71] Fractures of the cranial vault may be seen or palpated through scalp or facial lacerations. If the scalp is intact, a fracture may be suspected when there is a scalp hematoma or palpable deformity. A Battles' sign, panda eyes, cerebrospinal fluid (CSF) rhinorrea or otorrhea, epistaxis, hemotympanum, or hemorrhage from the ear may signify the presence of a basilar skull fracture. A facial fracture should be considered whenever a facial laceration or contusion is present and may be identified by palpating the orbital rims, zygomatic arches, mandible, or nose or by grasping the mandibular or maxillary teeth to detect instability. Signs of a jaw fracture are the presence of malocclusion, intraoral ecchymosis, loose teeth, preauricular pain, excessive mobility, and a palpable deformity through a jaw laceration. Signs commonly associated with an orbital fracture are deformity, swelling, ecchymosis, diplopia, and subconjunctival hemorrhage. A zygomatic fracture is suspected if the patient has infraorbital hypesthesia, a subconjunctival hemorrhage, or deformity or ecchymosis in the region of the zygoma. Epistaxis, CSF rhinorrhea, telecanthus, or deformity should suggest the presence of a nasal fracture.

The oral cavity is evaluated for the presence of a laceration, bleeding, or a hematoma. Any laceration of the cheek should be assessed for the possibility of injury to the facial nerve or parotid duct. The presence of a periorbital laceration or swelling or an orbital fracture suggests the possibility of an eye injury. Enophthalmia or dysconjugate gaze may represent extraocular muscle entrapment. When possible, the patient is checked for visual acuity and pupillary response to light. The eye should be carefully observed for the presence of extrusion of intraocular contents. Funduscopic examination is performed to detect the presence of a vitreous hemorrhage or retinal detachment. The eye is examined for the possibility of a corneal abrasion or dislocation of the lens.

The neck is evaluated for hoarseness, airway obstruction, cervical subcutaneous emphysema, and hemoptysis, which commonly reflect injury to the larynx or cervical trachea. Cervical esophageal or pharyngeal injuries may be suggested by the presence of dysphagia, hematemesis, oral bleeding, or subcutaneous emphysema. Injury to carotid or vertebral artery should be suspected if the patient has a pulse deficit, cervical hematoma, impaired level of consciousness, hemiparesis, or bruit. External hemorrhage may represent injury to the carotid or vertebral artery or jugular vein. The entrance wound and exit wound or site of implantation may suggest the possibility of major vascular injury. Cervical soft tissue lacerations are usually apparent and should alert the clinician to the likelihood of an underlying injury to major vascular or visceral structures.

A hemothorax should be suspected if the patient has a diminution in breath sounds and dullness to percussion of the affected hemithorax. A pneumothorax is usually associated with impaired ability to auscultate breath sounds and tympany to percussion. Ecchymosis or abrasions of the chest wall should suggest the possibility of underlying rib fractures and intrathoracic pathology. Paradoxical chest wall motion and crepitus indicate the presence of rib fractures. Rib fractures commonly cause significant chest wall pain which impairs the patient's inspiratory effort. The presence of upper rib fractures should suggest the possibility of intrathoracic injury, while lower rib fractures are commonly associated with intrathoracic or abdominal injuries. The same is true for chest wall abrasions and ecchymosis. Anterior midline crepitus, ecchymosis, abrasions, and paradoxical chest wall motion are commonly associated with sternal fractures. If the patient complains of midline anterior chest pain and has an impaired inspiratory effort, a sternal fracture is likely to be present. A clavicular

fracture is commonly identified on physical examination due to the presence of local tenderness and deformity. A tracheal or bronchial injury is suggested by the presence of progressive massive subcutaneous emphysema, hemoptysis, or tension pneumothorax and should be strongly suspected in a patient who has a transmediastinal penetrating wound.[157] Findings that suggest the possibility of an esophageal injury are the presence of hematemesis, chest pain, transmediastinal penetrating wound,[157] bloody gastric drainage, or cervical subcutaneous emphysema.[193] An injury to the aorta or its tributaries should be considered if the patient has a carotid, brachial, or femoral pulse deficit; interscapular, precordial, or cervical bruit; or impaired level of consciousness. Other findings suggestive of a great vessel injury are the presence of a hemiparesis, hoarseness, transmediastinal penetrating wound,[157] dysphagia, interscapular, or retrosternal pain, or the presence of a cervical or supraclavicular hematoma. Lacerations of the chest wall are usually easily identified and should suggest the possibility of an intrathoracic injury. A rupture of the diaphragm with intrathoracic evisceration is likely in a patient who has a diminution in breath sounds, bowel sounds during auscultation of the chest, tracheal shift, tachypnea, or cyanosis.

The presence of ecchymosis, abrasions, tenderness, laceration, or penetration of the lower thoracic or abdominal wall or pelvis increases the likelihood that the patient has an abdominal or pelvic, vascular, or visceral injury. The presence of abdominal tenderness may represent intra-abdominal visceral injury[21,177] or abdominal wall contusion. Vomiting may reflect a gastric outlet obstruction secondary to an intramural duodenal hematoma, while the aspiration of bloody secretions through a gastric tube may suggest the possibility of a gastric or esophageal wound or swallowed blood. Decreased femoral pulses may occur secondary to an abdominal or thoracic aortic injury. Flank ecchymosis, pain, or hematoma may be associated with a retroperitoneal vascular or renal injury. Hematuria usually signifies an injury to the kidneys, ureter, bladder, or urethra. A urethral injury should be considered present if blood is found at the urethral meatus; if an ill-defined, mobile, or elevated prostate is noted on rectal examination; or if there is a perineal hematoma, pain, or ecchymosis. A uterine injury is suspected if there is bleeding through the cervical os or a pelvic hematoma present on bimanual examination, especially if this is identified in association with penetrating trauma. Vulvar or vaginal lacerations or hematomas are usually identified with appropriate physical examination. Lacerations and hematomas of the penis are easily identified by visual inspection. A rectal injury is suspected if blood is found on rectal examination or the patient has a penetrating wound of the lower abdomen, pelvis, or upper thighs. The presence of a pelvic fracture should always alert the clinician to the possibility of a rectal or anal injury. A pelvic fracture or dislocation should be suspected when pelvic tenderness, iliac wing instability, a pubic symphysis cleft, or perineal ecchymosis, hematoma, or laceration is identified.

Extremity fractures, ligamentous instability, or joint capsule disruption should be suspected when there is local tenderness, crepitus, excessive motion, or impaired motion. Such injury should also be presumed when deformity, ecchymosis, abrasions, or lacerations are identified. To detect arterial or venous injuries, the neck, supraclavicular fossae, groin, and extremities are carefully evaluated. Dislocations should be reduced and fractured extremities pulled out to full length, since vascular insufficiency may disappear after these maneuvers.[15] Decreased or absent pulse is strongly suggestive of an arterial injury, but the presence of a pulse does not exclude such a possibility.[56] Doppler pressures may be useful in identifying those extremities with an embarassment of arterial circulation. External hemorrhage or the presence of a hematoma suggests the likelihood of a vascular injury. Other findings that may indicate the presence of a vascular injury are a bruit, thrill, pallor, impaired capillary refill, cyanosis, paresthesias, hypesthesias, or extremity hypothermia. Soft tissue wounds, fractures, or dislocations should increase the concern for the possibility of an associated vascular injury.

A compartment syndrome should be suspected if the patient has palpable muscular tension and hypesthesia, paresis, or pain with passive motion. Leg edema, cyanosis, and dilated superficial veins are suggestive of the presence of a transected or thrombosed vein or an arteriovenous fistula. A peripheral nerve injury should be suspected when there is a sensory or motor deficit, fracture, dislocation, or laceration. Soft tissue lacerations of the extremity are usually apparent and may or may not be associated with external hemorrhage. Soft tissue injuries are commonly underestimated when the patient has sustained a laceration due to blunt trauma, degloving injury,[94] or gunshot or shotgun wound.[175] Any impairment of extremity motion or the presence of an extremity laceration should suggest the possibility of a tendon injury.

DIAGNOSTIC MODALITIES IN THE STABILIZED PATIENT

Diagnostic imaging, endoscopy, and laboratory tests are supplemental to physical evaluation and useful to guide the surgeon in further therapeutic decision making. The benefit of any diagnostic study must be weighed against the time necessary to perform the test and the potential danger of removing the patient from the resuscitation area. Patients who have severe cardiovascular or respiratory instability should not be transported to a remote diagnostic imaging suite but should remain in the resuscitation area or taken to the operating room as appropriate. Parenchymal anatomic disruption may be further elucidated by CT scan, radionuclide scans, or arteriography. Organ function may be variably delineated by contrast-enhanced CT scan, nuclear scans, or arteriography. Arteriography is the gold standard for imaging trauma-induced arterial pathology.

Head and Face Injuries

Skull radiographs detect significantly depressed fractures, which require surgical intervention, as well as nondepressed skull fractures, which alert the clinician to the possibility of intracranial pathology.[10,47,53,174] Skull radiographs should be obtained if the patient has a penetrating injury or a suspected fracture based on physical examination or has been unconscious for several minutes. For patients who have a normal neurologic examination and a history of brief unconsciousness, a skull radiograph should be obtained before discharge to exclude the possibility of a high-risk fracture, which increases the likelihood that the individual may harbor an extracerebral hematoma. Facial radiographs are indicated when there is clinical suspicion that a fracture is present. A Waters' view, lateral skull, mandibular series, Towne's and submentovertex projections are ordered as appropriate. Better delineation of a nasoethmoid, orbital, zygomatic complex, maxillary, or frontobasilar fracture may be seen on a CT scan. A corneal abrasion may be identified by fluorescein stain, which detects the loss of epithelium. Further diagnostic evaluation by an opthalmologist is indicated when there is an actual or suspected globe injury, an orbital fracture, an abnormality seen on funduscopic examination, a suspected carotid-cavernous fistula, or impaired visual acuity.

Neck and Upper Airway Injuries

For any patient with stridor, hoarseness, cervical subcutaneous emphysema, hemoptysis, or intercostal retractions, a flexible laryngoscopy and tracheoscopy should be performed to exclude injury to the upper airway. Patients with dysphagia, hematemesis, or cervical subcutaneous emphysema should be considered candidates for esophagoscopy, pharyngoscopy, or contrast-enhanced esophagram. A significant false-negative rate is associated with esophagoscopy and esophagram. Barium should be used, since it provides greater mucosal detail; a radioiodinated contrast will cause significant bronchospasm and pulmonary edema if aspirated.

All patients with cardiovascular stability who have a suspected carotid arterial injury should undergo carotid and cerebral angiography.[141,162] The arteriogram will provide an assessment as to proper exposure of the lesion, assist in determining the likelihood of repair versus ligation, and determine the presence of antegrade flow. In addition, the study should evaluate intracranial vessels to elucidate cerebral perfusion, as well as determine external carotid flow should an extracranial–intracranial arterial bypass procedure become a consideration for management. Patients suspected of a carotid arterial injury who have cardiovascular instability should be taken directly to surgery to control the hemorrhage. Cardiovascular stability must be obtained to provide the best cerebral perfusion possible.[98]

Thoracic Injuries

If a patient is suspected of having a sternal fracture, a lateral or oblique sternal radiograph should be obtained. Tracheo-bronchoscopy is performed in patients who present with a pneumomediastinum, a large air leak through a chest tube, a transmediastinal penetrating wound[157] or massive, progressive subcutaneous emphysema. All patients who have incurred a blunt injury and who are suspected of having an aortic injury based on physical examination or chest radiographic findings should have a thoracic aortogram. A patient who has been involved in a high-speed deceleration accident should be considered for aortography even though the chest radiograph may be normal.[69] Patients with cardiovascular stability who have incurred a penetrating injury that has traversed the superior mediastinum[157] or the apex of the hemithorax[132] should undergo aortography to exclude a major vascular injury, even though findings on physical examination or chest radiography may be minimal or absent. The major problem with missing these injuries is that death may ensue after a subsequent bleed into the chest before hemostasis can be obtained by emergency thoracotomy. An esophageal injury following blunt trauma is extremely rare, yet an esophagoscopy and esophagram should be considered in order to diagnose an esophagel injury in any patient who presents with a pneumomediastinum, transmediastinal penetrating wound,[157] or acute hydrothorax.

The diagnosis of a rupture of the diaphragm secondary to blunt trauma may be difficult, since the chest radiograph may reveal only obscuration of the diaphragm or a minimal "elevation of the diaphragm."[26] The differential of an obscured diaphragm includes rupture of the diaphragm with minimal evisceration, hemothorax, or atelectasis, aspiration, or lung contusion of the lower pulmonary lobe.[11] Clarification may be enhanced by performing decubitus chest radiographs, upper or lower GI contrast studies,[26] fluoroscopy of the diaphragm,[209] or thoracoscopy.[38,82] A chest tube in the affected hemithorax may drain peritoneal lavage fluid. In many cases, the only way to make the diagnosis is to perform a celiotomy and evaluate the diaphragm. Patients with rupture of the diaphragm may present with a normal chest radiograph and the diagnosis is made during exploration for a positive diagnostic peritoneal lavage or at a later time, when the patient has a delayed evisceration. Commonly, patients will present with obvious evisceration into the hemithorax, which is well seen on the plain chest radiograph. A 12-lead ECG should be performed on all trauma patients admitted to the hospital.

Abdominal Injuries

In the unstable trauma patient, the abdomen is evaluated by physical examination, diagnostic peritoneal lavage, or celiotomy. Select stable patients may be evaluated by abdominal CT scan, nuclear scans or angiography.[55,85] These patients are alert and have cardiovascular stability and minimal abdominal pain or anemia. The CT scan is useful for identifying splenic and hepatic[124] injuries (Fig. 26-6) and retroperitoneal hemorrhage. Pancreatic injury may be identified on the CT scan, but its reliability is yet to be determined. Nuclear scans of the liver and spleen are helpful in delineating pathology, but the efficacy of those techniques largely depends on the experience of the examiner. Abdominal arteriography may be helpful

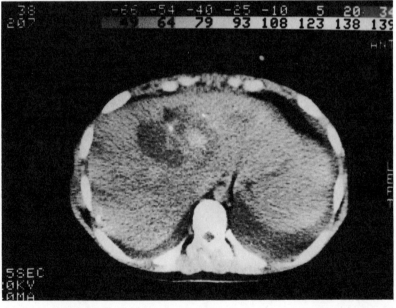

FIG. 26-6 Hepatic hematoma. This intrahepatic hematoma secondary to blunt trauma is readily identified on abdominal computed tomography.

in evaluating solid organs and is indicated if there is another indication for angiography[59] or the CT scan or nuclear scan is equivocal. Abdominal arteriography should be considered in any stable patient who has a femoral pulse deficit following blunt or penetrating trauma. The most definitive diagnostic study for detecting the presence of a duodenal injury following blunt trauma is duodenography.[58] A duodenogram is considered in patients who have epigastric tenderness, vomit, have lower thoracic or upper lumbar spine trauma, or a right renal injury.[206] Proctoscopy is performed to exclude the possibility of a rectal injury in any patient who has sustained a penetrating wound to the pelvis, who has blood on rectal examination, or whose pelvic radiograph reveals a bone fragment projecting into the presacral region.

Renal and Urologic Injuries

The IVP is a useful screening tool to detect significant trauma to the kidneys, ureters, and renal pedicle. Tomographic cuts are ideal, but the transport of the multiple-injured patient to the radiology suite is usually dangerous.[111,142] A nephrogram is commonly poor to absent if there is significant cardiovascular instability. A single bolus of dye and a KUB radiograph 5 minutes after injection will usually provide adequate information about the status of the kidneys and ureters, however, follow up views may be necessary. An IVP should be obtained for virtually all patients with penetrating abdominal trauma, since the absence of hematuria does not exclude the possibility of a ureteral transection.[148] All patients incurring blunt trauma who have gross or large microscopic hematuria should have an IVP, since there is a significant likelihood of renal pathology being present. An IVP is considered in those patients having incurred blunt trauma who present with mild to moderate microscopic hematuria or clear urine if there is a lower rib fracture, flank hematoma, mass, or pain, or lower thoracic or upper lumbar spine fracture.[23,143,144] A normal bilateral nephrogram implies that there is no major renal parenchymal or pedicle injury or

ureteral obstruction. Delayed unilateral filling of the kidney usually suggests a renal contusion. The appearance of only a unilateral nephrogram implies an absent kidney, renal artery occlusion, or a massively injured kidney. Poor visualization of a kidney suggests a contusion or fracture of the kidney. Major perinephric dye extravasation on IVP implies injury to the pelvis or a major parenchymal laceration. A CT scan of the kidney is useful in delineating urinary (dye) extravasation, parenchymal contusion, or lacerations and parenchymal function when contrast is administered, as well as the degree of perinephric hemorrhage.[111] A renal arteriogram is helpful in detecting renal arterial pathology or active renal hemorrhage or in determining the functional status of the parenchyma.[211] Cystography is recommended in all patients who sustain lower abdominal trauma and who have suprapubic pain, hematuria, or a penetrating wound of the pelvis. A urethrogram should be considered in any patient with a pelvic fracture, straddle injury, perineal laceration or ecchymosis, or abnormal prostate on rectal examination; it is mandatory if there is blood at the urethral meatus.

Injuries to the Extremities

A true A-P and lateral plain radiograph should be performed on all extremities with obvious or suspected bone or joint injury. The joint at either end of a long bone fracture must be visualized to exclude injuries to those structures.[166] Special views, stress studies, arthrography, tomography, or examination under anesthesia may be necessary to delineate certain injuries more clearly. Vascular injuries may be identified during exploration of an extremity hematoma or seen on arteriography or venography. Arteriography is useful for patients with apparent arterial injury following blunt trauma to the extremities, since the lesion may not be at the same level as a dislocation or fracture.[190] Patients who have an apparent arterial injury and a shotgun injury or multiple penetrating wounds should undergo arteriography, since it is not certain at which level of soft tissue injury that the vascular injury lies.[203] Similarly, it may not be evident at what point a vessel is traversed when a missile travels parallel to the course of an artery.[203] An arteriogram should be considered when there is a question of an arterial injury and there is no other indication for surgical exploration.[113,117] Angiography for proximal arterial injuries requires catheter insertion under fluoroscopic guidance, usually in the radiology suite. Patient transportation to the radiographic suite is contraindicated if there is cardiovascular or respiratory instability or the patient requires an immediate craniotomy, thoracotomy, or laparotomy. More distal injuries can be evaluated by percutaneous arteriography in the emergency ward. If ischemia is present, the benefit of the arteriogram must be weighed against the fact that ischemic time[190] will be significantly increased.

Emergency Surgery

Ideally, emergency surgery begins after all physiologic systems have been stabilized and all pathology has been identified. Certain life-threatening pathology may require a craniotomy, celiotomy, thoracotomy, or surgical intervention of the neck or extremities to obtain stabilization, thus mandating the need for an operative procedure before the identification of all injuries. Occasionally, life-saving emergency surgery is indicated in more than one body region; therefore, a prioritization as to which is operated first must be made on the basis of which injuries pose the threat of cardiac or cerebral death. Simultaneous surgical procedures may be necessary to prevent cardiac arrest and irreversible brain damage. These scenarios may heavily tax the trauma surgeon's ingenuity to draw from his vast experience.

MAXILLOFACIAL PROCEDURES

Facial fractures should be reduced and stabilized early if the patient's general condition allows. If the patient is unstable, the fractures are accurately reduced and stabilized within 10 to 14 days before the development of fibrous

union.[185] Operative intervention may be necessary shortly after admission to manage certain complications associated with facial fractures. Mandibular and maxillary fractures should be managed initially with at least the application of arch bars, while comminuted jaw fractures must be managed initially by intermaxillary fixation. A nasoethmoid fracture should be reduced if at all possible to minimize subsequent cosmetic impairment, while frontal sinus fractures should at least be drained to prevent the common sequela of sinusitis.[149] Orbital fractures associated with proptosis are reduced to minimize the development of a corneal ulcer. Hemorrhage from facial sinus cavities may present as posterior nasal bleeding and is controlled by the insertion of a nasal pack with an obturator at the posterior choanae. If hemorrhage persists, an external compression dressing of the face may be necessary, while ligation of the internal maxillary, ethmoid, or bilateral external carotid arteries is usually considered as a last resort.

CRANIOTOMY

The primary goals for performing an emergency craniotomy are to remove mass lesions and prevent infection by treating open head injuries. A craniotomy is indicated for penetrating wounds to the skull to debride the brain, remove gross contamination, and close the dura.[71,78] A depressed, closed skull fracture is elevated if there is parenchymal involvement to minimize the occurrence of seizures.[10] An open depressed skull fracture is managed by wound debridement, elevation of the fragment, and closure of the dura.[168] A craniotomy is performed to remove a mass lesion if such is identified on CT scan or carotid angiography and is associated with a significant shift.[168] An immediate craniotomy should be considered to remove a mass lesion if the pupil dilates during extracranial surgery and is unresponsive to medical treatment for intracranial hypertension.[137]

CERVICAL EXPLORATION

Selective operative management of penetrating neck injuries is advocated for patients who have a specific indication for exploration.[116,130,154,189] Pharyngeal or cervical esophageal wounds are surgically repaired and drained; however, if the lesion is large a pharyngostomy or esophagostomy is formed. In patients with a laryngeal fracture, a tracheostomy should be performed and the larynx explored by laryngeal fissure under the guidance of an otolaryngologist.[212] If convenient, a small tracheal wound may be used as a site for a tracheostomy tube, while other tracheal wounds are closed and protected by a tracheostomy tube inferior to the injury.[110,194] The jugular vein should be repaired if possible and at least one vein salvaged, if there is bilateral injury. The patient's head should always remain lower than the heart to diminish the likelihood of developing an air embolism. Patients with a carotid arterial injury and no neurologic deficit or a deficit that is not associated with coma have their artery repaired.[16,96,98,205] If the patient has coma, some clinicians recommend ligation,[96] while others recommend revascularization if possible shortly after the injury.[16,57] Two studies[98,205] found no difference in ligation versus repair for patients with coma. If the lesion cannot be repaired, an extracranial–intracranial bypass should be considered, unless the patient has been comatose for more than 2 hours.[57]

THORACIC PROCEDURES

Thoracic esophageal wounds should be repaired and managed with pleural drainage.[105] Larger wounds are protected with a cervical esophagostomy, ligation of the esophagogastric junction, and a gastrostomy.[40,193] Broad–spectrum antibiotics should be used to prevent mediastinitis. A tracheal or bronchial injury is repaired if the lesion is greater than one-third the circumference of the lumen or if the lung cannot be expanded.[42,66,91,105,110] A thoracotomy is strongly considered if a hemothorax is associated with greater than 500 ml of blood loss within 2 hours after the initial evacuation of blood.[132] The patient should have an exploration of the heart if a hemopericardium is identified by pericardiocentesis or subxiphoid pericardial exploration.[105,132] A thoracotomy is performed in prearrest cases; such situations would include the patient who has a sinus rhythm and is without a detectable blood pressure despite volume infusion or the patient who

has progressive bradycardia with other signs of severe shock.[105] A resuscitative thoracotomy is recommended for the patient who has a witnessed cardiac arrest at admission or an arrest before admission yet has signs of life or a palpable carotid pulse with external cardiopulmonary resuscitation. Injuries of the great vessels of the thorax identified on angiography should be repaired if the patient is deemed salvageable.[105] Any patient suspected of having a penetrating cardiac injury should undergo an exploratory thoracotomy.[41,44] Patients with wounds in close proximity to the heart and no history of cardiac instability may be managed by serial ECGs and central venous monitoring but should preferably undergo a thoracotomy.

INTRA-ABDOMINAL AND RETROPERITONEAL PROCEDURES

There are multiple indications for performing a celiotomy following blunt or penetrating abdominal trauma. Patients with a positive diagnostic peritoneal lavage, peritonitis, free air seen on radiographic evaluation, evisceration, or a penetrating abdominal wound associated with shock should undergo emergency celiotomy. Patients in shock who have gross abdominal distention should undergo an emergency laparotomy; however, gastric dilatation secondary to insufflation must be excluded. Patients with an impaired level of consciousness who have peritoneal penetration identified should undergo a celiotomy. Individuals with significant abdominal pain are likely to have a hollow visceral[21] or pancreatic injury[99] and should be considered for exploration. A CT scan, nuclear scan, angiogram, or duodenogram may reveal significant organ or vascular injury, dictating the need for surgical intervention. An intraperitoneal or major extraperitoneal bladder rupture necessitates closure of the lesion and the insertion of a suprapubic cystostomy or transurethral bladder catheter.[138,210] The initial management of a urethral injury is to perform a suprapubic cystostomy, since urethral exploration may be associated with severe pelvic hemorrhage and a high rate of impotence.[112,150,210] A fracture of the kidney is explored if the patient has significant hemodynamic instability; otherwise, the lesion is managed conservatively.[87,150,211] Major dye extravasation identified on an IVP or CT scan of the kidney with contrast enhancement warrants an exploration, since there is usually damage to the major collecting system.[87,111] A diverting colostomy should be performed for those patients identified as having a rectal injury; repair of the rectal defect, drainage of the perirectal space, removal of stool from the rectum, and administration of broad-spectrum antibiotics should be performed as well.[103,161] A celiotomy is performed to repair a rupture of the diaphragm or to diagnose the injury if it cannot be excluded by other means.

SURGERY OF THE SPINAL COLUMN AND CORD

The goal of acute spinal surgery is to preserve or restore function to the spinal cord and enhance early mobility of the patient when necessary. The persistence of an unreduced bony injury or spinal cord compression is an indication for emergency spinal surgery.[45] Cervical spinal dislocations are commonly reduced by traction; however, surgical reduction may be necessary if traction fails. Dislocations of the thoracic or lumbar spine usually require operative reduction.[92] Following spine reduction, spinal cord decompression is proven by a myelogram or CT scan. Penetrating wounds of the spine are usually stable; however, bone or a foreign body in the canal causing a compression injury should be removed.

SOFT TISSUE REPAIR

The goals of traumatic wound management are to control bleeding, minimize subsequent infection, and consider cosmetic results when appropriate. All soft tissue wounds should be evaluated for associated injury to the nerves, tendons, bone, joint, or vessels. Early removal of foreign bodies and nonviable tissue is mandatory at the earliest possible moment to decrease subsequent wound infection. A high-velocity irrigating system or a jet stream delivered through a 19-gauge needle is necessary to remove small particulate matter, including bacteria. Surgical debridement is an alternate method if viable vital structures are not present. Simple lacerations may be closed after debridement; however, crushing or avulsive wounds[94] commonly contain nonviable tissue

and must be debrided more aggressively. If there is adequate debridement of the wound, it may be closed if there is no tension. When there is any question regarding the adequacy of debridement, delayed closure is performed 3 to 5 days later, to decrease the likelihood of developing an infectious process. If there is significant tissue loss, the wound should be debrided until clean and exposed vital structures such as tendons and vessels are covered with a biologic dressing, such as homograft or heterograft, to decrease the likelihood of dessication. Secondary closure of these wounds are performed by skin grafts or soft tissue flaps.

Administration of antibiotics should be considered in wounds that are likely to be contaminated, such as crush, avulsive, or blast wounds.[62] Antibiotics should also be considered for puncture wounds when the foreign body is suspected to be contaminated. Antibiotics must be given within 3 hours from the time of initial injury to be effective. The greater the lapse of time until wound debridement, the greater the likelihood of tissue invasion with bacteria, hence the greater the need for adequate debridement and delayed closure. Complex wounds of the nose, ears, eyelids, and other facial soft tissue may require the assistance of a skilled plastic surgeon to obtain an acceptable cosmetic result.

PERIPHERAL NERVE INJURIES

When a peripheral nerve injury is associated with a clean laceration, the nerve is repaired shortly after admission.[17] If the soft tissue needs debridement, the nerve is tagged if it can be identified and repaired at a later time.[131] A patient who has a peripheral neural deficit and no soft tissue defect should be observed and the nerve repaired at a later time if necessary.[131]

VASCULAR SURGICAL PROCEDURES

Arterial and major venous injuries of the extremity are usually repaired as soon as possible; however, small peripheral veins may be ligated.[3,72,117] Patients with external hemorrhage or ischemia secondary to vascular injuries should undergo emergency exploration and repair. Individuals with a suspected or proven arterial injury should undergo exploration for repair; however, if there is no ischemia or external hemorrhage and the general status of the patient is poor, repair may be delayed. Life-threatening cranial, thoracic, or abdominal injuries should be addressed before the peripheral arterial injury, or two surgical teams may address the patient concomitantly.

FASCIOTOMY

A fasciotomy may be necessary to prevent muscle or neural damage secondary to a compartment syndrome. A prophylactic fasciotomy should be considered when there has been prolonged limb ischemia,[109,160,218] concomitant arterial and venous injury, or a major venous injury requiring ligation, especially if these are associated with major soft tissue injury.[2,117] A fasciotomy is performed if compartment tension is detected on palpation, and neural or muscular ischemia is present, or if severe compartment hypertension is determined by manometric evaluation. The conventional wisdom is that a therapeutic fasciotomy is generally not indicated if the compartment pressure is less than 50 mmHg.[104] However, our experience with high-velocity blunt trauma is that a compartment pressure greater than 40 mmHg implies the necessity for a fasciotomy. The 30 to 40 mmHg range is a gray zone in which a fasciotomy is not indicated without evidence of neural or muscular ischemia; however, a fasciotomy should be performed if the patient is unconscious and the pressure exceeds 30 mmHg, since clinical examination is inaccurate.

ORTHOPEDIC PROCEDURES

Complete ligamentous disruptions are best treated by early repair before the onset of ligament retraction, which may develop over days to weeks depending on the particular ligament.[119,166] All open joint injuries should be taken to the operating room for exploration, debridement, and thorough irrigation. In the severely injured patient or the patient with severe wound contamination, delayed primary repair or secondary repair is the procedure of choice for a lacerated tendon; otherwise, primary repair is performed. The multiple trauma patient requires frequent turning and chest percussion/postural drainage of all pulmonary segments to prevent the onset of atelectasis and subsequent pneumonia or increase in pulmonary shunt. Management of fractures and dislocations should be directed at early mobilization, when possible.[4,64,158] To obviate some of the problems associated with immobilization by traction, external fixation is an excellent alternative in the multiple injured patient; it is also a superlative mode to manage open fractures associated with extensive soft tissue injury.[4,64] Closed reduction of the hip is usually successful; however, open reduction and stabilization may be necessary, especially if there are bone fragments in the joint or the acetabulum is fractured and unstable. Early reduction is mandatory to prevent avascular necrosis.[155]

Open fractures are managed by intraoperative debridement and jet lavage irrigation as soon as possible to minimize the onset of wound infection and osteomyelitis. When a significant delay in debridement is necessary, the wound should be thoroughly irrigated in the emergency room with the jet lavage irrigator. If a soft tissue defect is present, the fracture is managed by a Hoffman external fixator and the wound is left open to prevent sepsis.[4,12] Displaced fractures of the femoral neck result in traction on the blood supply of the femoral head and are associated with avascular necrosis; they are best managed by early internal fixation.[43] If a fracture or dislocation is associated with a vascular injury, rapid application of a limited external fixator after reduction will provide adequate stability and facilitate the vascular repair.[73,117] Immediate closed intramedullary rodding is the optimal method to manage a femoral shaft fracture.[158] The Neufeld single rope, rolling-traction cast system[18] is an acceptable method for managing femoral fractures in which closed nailing is precluded secondary to excessive comminution of the fracture, the presence of a soft tissue wound, or cases of CNS, respiratory, or cardiovascular instability. A Hoffman external fixator may be necessary to manage complex open fractures. If the patient has bilateral femoral fractures, at least one fracture should be rodded, if at all possible; otherwise, so much distal traction is necessary that the patient cannot be turned and is maintained in the Trendelenburg position, which adversely affects tracheobronchial toiletry.

Central acetabular fractures are commonly managed by traction, which requires combined lateral and distal pull and severely limits the ability to turn the patient in bed. Treatment alternatives are open reduction and internal fixation or triangulation stability by a Hoffman external fixator. Intra-articular fractures are usually best managed by early operative fixation. Clinically unstable pelvic fractures are optimally managed with a Hoffman external fixator early; however, surgical intervention may be necessary to provide adequate stability of the pelvic ring 3 to 5 days after injury.

Limb salvage in the multiple injured patient is one of the most challenging problems facing the trauma surgeon. Every effort should be made to conserve usable structures, especially in the upper extremity. The overall condition and clinical course will dictate to some degree what reconstructive and salvage steps should be taken. By no means should a life be placed in jeopardy in order to salvage a limb. The expected functional return is based on evaluation of the entire extremity, including soft tissue coverage, the skeletal framework, musculotendinous units, motor and sensory nerve supply, and vascularity. Parts should not be salvaged that can neither be restored as useful members nor contribute tissues for overall reconstruction of an extremity. It is possible with microvascular techniques to anastamose one millimeter vessels, thus replantation of digits is possible. Thumb, multiple finger, wrist, transmetacarpal, forearm, arm, and some lower limb amputations should be replanted. Amputated single digits should be replanted only after unusual circumstances.

Elective Tracheal Intubation

Several factors are normally present to optimize respiratory function, such as an alert state of consciousness, mobility, a patent airway, normal chest wall motion, and normal ventilation/perfusion relationships. Commonly, trauma patients have an impairment involving one or more of these factors. Impaired loss of consciousness secondary to brain injury or drug intoxication may lead to the retention of tracheobronchial secretions, to aspiration,

or to an impairment of cough and deep breathing with subsequent formation of atelectasis. The nonmobile patient (e.g., in traction or with impaired level of consciousness) may develop atelectasis with subsequent ventilation/perfusion mismatch or pneumonia. Patients with fractures, hematomas, or edema of the face or neck may have an inadequate airway and sustain subsequent development of acute respiratory insufficiency. Impaired chest wall motion may develop secondary to general depression from drugs, multiple rib fractures,[33,170] or thoracic denervation due to cervical or high thoracic spinal cord injury. Impaired chest wall motion may result in hypoventilation and subsequent hypoxemia or atelectasis with its sequelae, pneumonia, or hypoxia. Pulmonary contusion,[170] aspiration, and heart failure/fluid overload may result in low ventilation/perfusion relationships, leading to a relative or absolute hypoxemia. Each of these adverse components requires individual therapeutic considerations; the more components that are affected, the more invasive and aggressive the treatment must be.[170]

If the patient has multiple factors impairing respiratory function, tracheal intubation and the administration of CPAP or intermittent positive-pressure ventilation (IPPV) with PEEP may be necessary.[33,170] Tracheal intubation permits adequate removal of tracheobronchial secretions and the positive-pressure ventilation helps maintain a normal functional residual capacity.[64,204] Patients should be considered for elective tracheal intubation and positive-pressure ventilation depending on radiographic findings, maximal inspiratory force, vital capacity, ABGs, and level of consciousness. Tracheal intubation and CPAP ventilation is recommended if the chest radiograph reveals new or progressive atelectasis despite the use of maneuvers to maintain bronchial toiletry, maximal inspiratory force is more positive than −30 cm, vital capacity is less than 15 ml/kg, PaO_2/FIO_2 is less than 200, there is respiratory acidosis, or the patient is about to undergo a major surgical procedure. Occasionally, patients are so agitated that intubation and heavy sedation are indicated to prevent injury to the patient or the staff. Patients without a cervical spine injury are intubated by the oral translaryngeal route, while those with cervical spine injury are intubated by an awake blind nasotracheal method or over a flexible bronchoscope.

Pulmonary Artery Catheterization

A pulmonary artery catheter may be necessary to achieve adequate assessment of cardiovascular dynamics. In patients who have had a difficult resuscitation or refractory shock, a pulmonary artery catheter should be inserted for proper evaluation.[77,186] Patients requiring greater than 10 cm PEEP require cardiovascular dynamic monitoring to exclude cardiac insufficiency as a component contributing to the arterial hypoxemia.[152] When undergoing an operative procedure in which major blood loss is anticipated, such as thoracic spine surgery, invasive cardiac monitoring is indicated, if time permits.[147] Certain high-risk patients, such as the elderly, those with a history of cardiac disease, or those suspected of having sustained a cardiac contusion,[89,192,200] who have multiple injuries, or who are to receive general anesthesia should have a pulmonary artery catheter inserted.[147]

Prophylactic Antibiotics

The value of proplylactic antibiotics in the multiple trauma patient has never been adequately studied. Studies from individual disciplines suggest that in certain situations prophylactic antibiotics may be beneficial. An antistaphylococcal drug, such as a cephalosporin or nafcillin, is administered for open fractures as soon as possible following injury.[12,83,129] In addition, open joint injuries are managed with prophylactic antibiotics. Preoperative clindamycin and gentamycin or cefoxitin is given to patients with penetrating abdominal wounds and is continued if an ileal or colonic disruption is identified at laparotomy.[50,76,125,133] Any patient with signs of peritonitis is administered the same preoperative antibiotic regimen. Intravenous penicillin is administered as soon as a maxillary or mandibular fracture that is open into the mouth is identified.[83,216] Because of the high incidence of staphylococcal bacteremia in multiple-injured patients, any patient with a prosthetic heart valve should receive a semisynthetic penicillinase-resistant penicillin for as long as indwelling lines are present. Similarly, any patient with a newly inserted vascular or orthopedic prosthetic device should receive the same therapy.[62] Minimal benefit may be offered to those patients who receive an antistaphylococcal antibiotic soon after sustaining a penetrating chest injury.[67,187] Infection secondary to a cerebrospinal leak or penetrating head injury is relatively uncommon, and prophylactic antibiotics make no difference in the incidence of meningitis. Prophylactic antibiotics alter the patient's flora and are likely to lead to gram-negative colonization; if an infection develops, it will probably be due to a more resistant organism, hence the inadvisability of administering antibiotics in such cases.[34,62,79]

Tetanus Prophylaxis

Tetanus is a risk associated with all traumatic wounds, yet it is generally a preventable disease. Patients with clean minor wounds need no tetanus prophylaxis if a tetanus toxoid booster has been received within the past 10 years. Patients with major wounds should receive absorbed tetanus toxoid if they have had primary vaccinations but have had no booster within the past 5 years or cannot give a history of previous immunization. Tetanus immune globulin is given to all patients with uncertain or no vaccination history and to all patients with major wounds who have had fewer than three previous doses of tetanus toxoid. Patients with no history or an incomplete immunization history should have a full series of tetanus immunization.[51,86]

Minor Brain Injury

It is controversial as to what constitutes appropriate evaluation for patients with minor brain injury and which patients should be hospitalized for observation or sent home. Those with a skull fracture[53] and amnesia for less than 5 minutes[47] as their only neurologic deficit should have a CT scan of the brain and should be discharged if there is no pathology. Hospitalization is recommended if a CT scan cannot be obtained. Most patients with amnesia for more than 5 minutes should have a CT scan and be admitted for observation. Patients who are confused or are unable to answer simple questions should undergo a CT scan within a couple of hours following injury.[71] If there is a history of brief unconsciousness and no clear etiology, the patient should be admitted for evaluation. Patients who are admitted to the hospital should be followed with serial neurologic checks[19] and should undergo urgent CT scan of the brain if deterioration develops.

Miscellaneous Considerations

The patient's temperature is ascertained as soon as possible following admission and should be carefully monitored during the initial phase. Temperature elevation in patients with brain injury predisposes to the formation of cerebral edema. The onset of hypothermia may be associated with cardiovascular instability, life-threatening dysrhythmias, and coagulopathy.

Appropriate specialty medical consultation is dictated by the general status of the patient and by any specific medical or surgical problems. Each consultant's evaluation and recommendation is assessed by the surgical traumatologist in order to develop a coordinated plan for further diagnostic and therapeutic intervention.

Obvious fractures and joint injuries should be splinted as early as possible to reduce pain, bleeding, and tissue damage. Grossly displaced open fractures are splinted as they lie, without attempt at full reduction. Reduction by gentle traction and manipulation are attempted in cases of obvious vascular compromise due to the position of the deformity.[15] Distal traction may be necessary to maintain adequate reduction. Whenever possible, the injured part, once splinted, should be elevated to decrease the formation of tissue edema.

In conclusion, the first priority in managing the multiple injured patient is to diagnose and treat pathology that imposes an immediate threat to life. The second major goal is to diagnose and treat those injuries that may cause morbidity or a late mortality. The surgical traumatologist must supervise all diagnostic and therapeutic interventions and obtain multidiscipline input as deemed appropriate.

REFERENCES

1. Abraham E, Shapiro M, Podolsky S: Central venous catheterization in the emergency setting. Crit Care Med. 11: 515, 1983
2. Adar R, Schramek A, Khodadadi J, et al: Arterial combat injuries of the upper extremity. J Trauma 20: 297, 1980
3. Agarwal N, Shah PM, Clauss RH, et al: Experience with 115 civilian venous injuries. J Trauma 22: 877, 1982
4. Allgower M, Border JR: Management of open fractures in the multiple trauma patient. World J Surg 7:88, 1983
5. Alyono D, Morrow CE, Perry JF: Reappraisal of diagnostic peritoneal lavage criteria for operation in penetrating and blunt trauma. Surgery 92: 751, 1982
6. Alyono D, Perry JF: Value of quantitative cell count and amylase activity of peritoneal lavage fluid. J Trauma 21: 345, 1981
7. Alyono D, Ring WS, Chao RYN, et al: Characteristics of ventricular function in severe hemorrhagic shock. Surgery 94: 250, 1983
8. Aronoff RJ, Reynolds J, Thal ER: Evaluation of diaphragmatic injuries. Am J Surg 144: 671, 1982
9. Athanasoulis CA: Therapeutic applications of angiography. N Engl J Med 302: 1117, 1980
10. Bakay L: Brain injuries in polytrauma. World J Surg 7: 42, 1983
11. Ball T, McCrory R, Smith JO, et al: Traumatic diaphragmatic hernia: Errors in diagnosis. AJR 138: 633, 1982
12. Benson DR, Riggins RS, Lawrence RM, et al: Treatment of open fractures: A prospective study. J Trauma 23: 25, 1983

13. Blaisdell FW: General assessment, resuscitation and exploration of penetrating and blunt abdominal trauma. p. 1. In Blaisdell FW, Trunkey DD (eds): Trauma Management, Abdominal Trauma. Thieme-Stratton, New York, 1982
14. Bresler MJ, Rich GH: Occult cervical spine fracture in an ambulatory patient. Ann Emerg Med 11: 440, 1982
15. Brink BE: Vascular trauma. Surg Clin North Am 57: 189, 1977
16. Brown MF, Graham JM, Feliciano DV, et al: Carotid artery injuries. Am J Surg 144: 748, 1982
17. Brown PW: Factors influencing the success of the surgical repair of peripheral nerves. Surg Clin North Am 52: 1137, 1972
18. Browner BD, Kenzora JE, Edwards CC: The use of modified Neufeld traction in the management of femoral fractures in polytrauma. J Trauma 21: 779, 1981
19. Bruce DA, Gennarelli TA, Langfitt TW: Resuscitation from coma due to head injury. Crit Care Med 6: 254, 1978
20. Burney RE, Gundry SR, Mackenzie JR, et al: Comparison of mediastinal width, mediastinal-thoracic and -cardiac ratios, and "mediastinal widening" in detection of traumatic aortic rupture. Ann Emerg Med 12: 668, 1983
21. Burney RE, Mueller GL, Coon WW, et al: Diagnosis of isolated small bowel injury following blunt abdominal trauma. Ann Emerg Med 12: 71, 1983
22. Caplan ES, Hoyt N: Infection surveillance and control in the severely traumatized patient. Am J Med 70: 638, 1981
23. Cass AS: Immediate radiologic and surgical management of renal injuries. J Trauma 22: 361, 1982
24. Chernow B, Lake CR, Zaritsky A, et al: Sympathetic nervous system "switch off: With severe hypothermia. Crit Care Med 11: 677, 1983
25. Chernow B, Rainey TG, Lake, CR: Endogenous and exogenous catecholamines in critical care medicine. Crit Care Med 10: 409, 1982
26. Christophi C: Diagnosis of traumatic diaphragmatic hernia: Analysis of 63 cases. World J Surg 7: 277, 1983
27. Collins JA: Problems associated with the massive transfusion of stored blood. Surgery 75: 274, 1974
28. Cooper PR, Moody S, Clark WK, et al: Dexamethasone and severe head injury: A prospective double-blind study. J Neurosurg 51: 307, 1979
29. Counts RB, Haisch C, Simon, TL, et al: Hemostasis in massively transfused trauma patients. Ann Surg 190: 91, 1979
30. Covelli HD, Nessan VJ, Tuttle WK: Oxygen derived variables in acute respiratory failure. Crit Care Med 11: 646, 1983
31. Cowley RA, Dunham CM: Shock Trauma/Critical Care Manual. Initial Assessment and Management. University Park Press, Baltimore, 1982
32. Cox EF, Dunham CM: A safe technique for diagnostic peritoneal lavage. J Trauma 23: 152, 1983
33. Cullen P, Modell JH, Kirby RR, et al: Treatment of flail chest: Use of intermittent mandatory ventilation and positive end-expiratory pressure. Arch Surg 110: 1099, 1975
34. Dagi TF, Meyer FB, Poletti CA: The incidence and prevention of meningitis after basilar skull fracture. Am J Emerg Med 1: 295, 1983
35. Danziger A, Price H: The evaluation of head trauma by computed tomography. J Trauma 19: 295, 1979
36. Davis RF, Lappas DG, Kirklin JK, et al: Acute oliguria after cardiopulmonary bypass: Renal functional improvement with low-dose dopamine infusion. Crit Care Med 10: 852, 1982
37. Dawidson I, Eriksson B: Statistical evaluation of plasma substitutes based on 10 variables. Crit Care Med 10: 653, 1982
38. la Rocha AG, Creel RJ, Mulligan GWN, et al: Diaphragmatic rupture due to blunt abdominal trauma. Surg Gynecol Obstet 154: 175, 1982
39. DeMars JJ, Bubrick MP, Hitchcock CR: Duodenal perforation in blunt abdominal trauma. Surgery 86: 632, 1979
40. Defore WW, Mattox KL, Hansen HA, et al: Surgical management of penetrating injuries of the esophagus. Am J Surg 134: 734, 1977
41. Demetriades D, van der Veen BW: Penetrating injuries of the heart: Experience over two years in South Africa. J Trauma 23: 1034, 1983
42. Deslauriers J, Beaulieu M, Archambault G, et al: Diagnosis and long-term follow-up of major bronchial disruptions due to nonpenetrating trauma. Ann Thorac Surg 33: 32, 1982
43. Epps CH: Complications in Orthopaedic Surgery. JB Lippincott, Philadelphia, 1978
44. Ferguson DG, Stevenson HM: A review of 158 gunshot wounds to the chest. Br J Surg 65:845, 1978
45. Feuer H: Management of acute spine and spinal cord injuries, old and new concepts. Arch Surg 111: 638, 1976
46. Fischer RP, Beverlin BC, Engrav LH, et al: Diagnostic peritoneal lavage, Fourteen years and 2,586 patients later. Am J Surg 136: 701, 1978
47. Fischer RP, Carlson J, Perry JF: Postconcussive hospital observation of alert patients in a primary trauma center. J Trauma 21: 920, 1981
48. Flint LM, Brown A, Richardson JD, et al: Definitive control of bleeding from severe pelvic fractures. Ann Surg 189: 709, 1979

49. Foley RW, Harris LS, Pilcher DB: Abdominal injuries in automobile accidents: Review of care of fatally injured patient. J Trauma 17: 611, 1977

50. Fullen WD, Hunt J, Altemeier WA: Prophylactic antibiotics in penetrating wounds of the abdomen. J Trauma 12: 282, 1972

51. Furste W: The Fifth International Conference on Tetanus, Ronneby, Sweden, 1978. J Trauma 20: 101, 1980

52. Galbraith S: Misdiagnosis and delayed diagnosis in traumatic intracranial haematoma. Br J Med 1: 1438, 1976

53. Galbraith S, Smith J: Acute traumatic intracranial haematoma without skull fracture. Lancet 1: 501, 1976

54. Gallagher TJ, Civetta JM, Kirby RR, et al: Post-traumatic pulmonary insufficiency: A treatable disease. South Med 70: 1308, 1977

55. Geis WP, Shulz KA, Giacchino JL, et al: The fate of unruptured intrahepatic hematomas. Surgery 90: 689, 1981

56. Gelberman RH, Menon J, Fronek A: The peripheral pulse following arterial injury. J Trauma 20: 948, 1980

57. Gewertz BL, Samson DS, Ditmore QM, et al: Management of penetrating injuries of the internal carotid artery at the base of the skull utilizing extracranial–intracranial bypass. J Trauma 20: 365, 1980

58. Ghuman SS, Pathak VB, McGovern PJ, et al: Management and complications of duodenal injuries. Am Surg 48: 109, 1982

59. Gilliland MG, Ward RE, Flynn TC, et al: Peritoneal lavage and angiography in the management of patients with pelvic fractures. Am J Surg 140: 744, 1982

60. Gobiet W, Bock WJ, Leisegang J, et al: Treatment of acute cerebral edema with high dose of dexamethasone. p. 231. In Beks JWF, Bosch DA, Brock M (eds): Intracranial Pressure. Vol. III. Springer-Verlag, Berlin, 1976

61. Goldberger JH, Bernstein DM, Rodman GH, et al: Selection of patients with abdominal stab wounds for laparotomy. J Trauma 22: 476, 1982

62. Gorbach SL: Prophylactic antibiotics. J Surg Pract 6: 16, 1977

63. Goris RJA, Draaisma J: Causes of death after blunt trauma. J Trauma 22: 141, 1982

64. Goris RJA, Gimbrere JSF, Van Niekerk JLM, et al: Early osteosynthesis and prophylactic mechanical ventilation in the multitrauma patient. J Trauma 22: 895, 1982

65. Granson MA, Donovan AJ: Abdominal stab wound with omental evisceration. Arch Surg 118: 57, 1983

66. Grover FL, Ellestad BS, Arom KV, et al: Diagnosis and management of major tracheobronchial injuries. Ann Thorac Surg 28: 384, 1979

67. Grover FL, Richardson JD, Fewel JG, et al: Prophylactic antibiotics in the treatment of penetrating chest wounds: A prospective double blind study. J Thorac Cardiovasc Surg 74: 528, 1977

68. Gunby P: Study shows little effect of steroids in spinal injury. JAMA 248: 1035, 1982

69. Gundry SR, Burney RE, MacKenzie JR, et al: Assessment of mediastinal widening associated with traumatic rupture of the aorta. J Trauma 23: 293, 1983

70. Gundry SR, Wiliams S, Burney RE, et al: Indications for aortography in blunt thoracic trauma: A reassessment. J Trauma 22: 664, 1982

71. Gurdjian ES, Gurdjian ES: Acute head injuries. Surg Gynecol Obstet 146: 805, 1978

72. Hardin WD, Adinolfi MF, O'Connell RC, et al: Management of traumatic peripheral vein injuries: Primary repair or vein ligation. Am J Surg 144: 235, 1982

73. Heberer G, Becker HM, Dittmer H, et al: Vascular injuries in polytrauma. World J Surg 7: 68, 1983

74. Hoff J, Spetzler R, Winestock D: Head injury and early signs of tentorial herniation. West J Med 128: 112, 1978

75. Hoffman MJ, Greenfield LJ, Sugerman HJ, et al: Unsuspected right ventricular dysfunction in shock and sepsis. Ann Surg 198: 307, 1983

76. Hofstetter SR, Pachter HL, Bailey AA, et al: A prospective comparison of two regimens of prophylactic antibiotics in abdominal trauma: Cefoxitin versus triple drug. J Trauma 24: 307, 1984

77. Holliday RL, Doris PJ: The critically ill surgical patient. p. 112. In Armstrong PW, Baigrie RS (eds:) Hemodynamic Monitoring in the Critically Ill. Harper & Row, Hagerstown, 1980

78. Hubschmann O, Shapiro K, Baden M, et al: Craniocerebral gunshot injuries in civilian practice—Prognostic criteria and surgical management: Experience with 82 cases. J Trauma 19: 6, 1979

79. Ignelzi R, VanderArk GD: Analysis of the treatment of basilar skull fractures with and without antibiotics. J Neurosurg 44: 721, 1975

80. Jackson GL, Thal ER: Management of stab wounds of the back and flank. J Trauma 19: 660, 1979

81. Jennett B, Teasdale G, Fry, J, et al: Treatment for severe head injury. J Neurol Neurosurg Psychiatry 43: 289, 1980

82. Jones JW, Kitahama A, Watts R, et al: Emergency thoracoscopy: A logical approach to chest trauma management. J Trauma 21: 280, 1981

83. Jones RC: Antibiotics in trauma. J Surg Pract 6: 26, 1977

84. Jones RC: Management of pancreatic trauma. Ann Surg 187: 555, 1978

85. Jones TK, Walsh JW, Maull KI: Diagnostic imaging in blunt trauma of the abdomen. Surg Gynecol Obstet 157: 389, 1983
86. Kalisman M, Millendorf JB, Schiffman E: Clinical tetanus: Prevention and management of an uncommon disease. Infect Surg 3: 291, 1984
87. Karmi SA, Young JD, Soderstrom CA: Classification of renal injuries as a guide to therapy. Surg Gynecol Obstet 148: 161, 1979
88. Kashuk JL, Moore EE, Millikan JS, et al: Major abdominal vascular trauma—A unified approach. J Trauma 22: 672, 1982
89. Katz S, Gimmon Z, Appelbaum A: Cardiac contusion in the patient with multiple injuries. Injury 12: 180, 1980–1981
90. King RM, Mucha P, Seward JB, et. al: Cardiac contusion: A new diagnostic approach utilizing two-dimensional echocardiography. J Trauma 23: 610, 1983
91. Kirsh MM, Sloan H: Blunt Chest Trauma. General Principles of Management. Little, Brown, Boston, 1977
92. Kornberg M, Rechtine GR, Herndon WA, et al: Surgical stabilization of thoracic and lumbar spine fractures: A retrospective study in a military population. J Trauma 24: 140, 1984
93. Kress TD, Balasubramaniam, S: Cricothyroidotomy. Ann Emerg Med 11: 197, 1982
94. Kudsk KA, Sheldon GF, Walton RL: Degloving injuries of the extremities and torso. J Trauma 21: 835, 1981
95. Kumar SA, Puri VK, Mittal VK, et al: Myocardial contusion following nonfatal blunt chest trauma. J Trauma 23: 327, 1983
96. Ledgerwood AM, Mullins RJ, Lucas CE: Primary repair vs ligation for carotid artery injuries. Arch Surg 115: 488, 1980
97. Lee WC, Uddo JF, Nance FC: Surgical judgement in the management of abdominal stab wounds: Utilizing clinical criteria from a 10-year experience. Ann Surg 199: 549, 1984
98. Liekweg WG, Greenfield LJ: Management of penetrating carotid arterial injury. Ann Surg 188: 587, 1978
99. Lucas CE: Diagnosis and treatment of pancreatic and duodenal injury. Surg Clin North Am 57: 49, 1977
100. Lucas CE, Ledgerwood AM: Clinical significance of altered coagulation tests after massive transfusion for trauma. Am Surg 47: 125, 1981
101. Marshall LF, Smith RW, Shapiro HM: The outcome with aggressive treatment in severe head injuries. Part I: The significance of intracranial pressure monitoring. J Neurosurg 50: 20, 1979
102. Marshall WG, Bell JL, Kouchoukos NT: Penetrating cardiac trauma. J Trauma 24: 147, 1984
103. Martinez OV, Lester JL, Arango A, et al: Antibiotic prophylaxis in penetrating colorectal injuries: The comparative effectiveness of clindamycin and cephalothin in combination with an aminoglycoside. Am Surg 45: 378, 1979
104. Matsen FA, Krugmire RB: Compartmental syndromes. Surg Gynecol Obstet 147: 943, 1978
105. Mattox KL: Thoracic injury requiring surgery. World J Surg 7: 49, 1983
106. Mattox KL, Feliciano DV: Role of external cardiac compression in truncal trauma. J Trauma 22: 934, 1982
107. Mattox KL, Beall AC, Jordan GL: Cardiorrhapy in the emergency center. J Thorac Cardiovasc Surg 68: 886, 1974
108. Mattox KL, Espada R, Beall AC: Performing thoracotomy in the emergency center. JACEP 3: 13, 1974
109. Maull KI, Capehart JE, Cardea JA, et al: Limb loss following military anti-shock trousers (MAST) application. J Trauma 21: 60, 1981
110. Mazzei EA, Mulder DG: Closed-chest injuries to the trachea and bronchus. Arch Surg 100: 677, 1970
111. McAninch JW, Carroll PR: Renal trauma: Kidney preservation through improved vascular control—A refined approach. J Trauma 22: 285, 1982
112. McAninch JW, Marshall V: Trauma to the bladder and urethra. Infect Surg 2: 134, 1983
113. McDonald EJ, Goodman PC, Winestock DP: The clinical indications for arteriography in trauma to the extremity. Diagn Radiol 116: 45, 1975
114. McGill J, Clinton JE, Ruiz E: Cricothyrotomy in the emergency department. Ann Emerg Med 11: 361, 1982
115. McSwain NE: Pneumatic trousers and the management of shock. J Trauma 17: 719, 1977
116. Meinke AH, Bivins BA, Sachatello CR: Selective management of gunshot wounds to the neck: Report of a series and review of the literature. Am J Surg 138: 314, 1979
117. Menzoian JO, LoGerfo FW, Doyle JE, et al: Management of vascular injuries to the leg. Am J Surg 144: 231, 1982
118. Messmer KFW: Traumatic shock in polytrauma: Circulatory parameters, biochemistry, and resuscitation. World J Surg 7: 26, 1983
119. Meyers MH, Moore D, Harvey JP: Traumatic dislocation of the knee joint. J Bone Joint Surg 57A: 430, 1975
120. Michelson WB: CPK-MB isoenzyme determinations: Diagnostic and prognostic value in evaluation of blunt chest trauma. Ann Emerg Med 9: 562, 1980
121. Miller JD, Butterworth JF, Gudeman SK, et al: Further experience in the management of severe head injury. J Neurosurg 54: 289, 1981
122. Miller JD, Sweet RC, Narayan R, et al: Early insults to the injured brain. JAMA 240: 439, 1978

123. Miller JW, Danzl DF, Thomas DM: Urban accidental hypothermia; 135 cases. Ann Emerg Med 9: 456, 1980
124. Moon KL, Federle MP: Computed tomography in hepatic trauma. AJR 141: 309, 1983
125. Moore FA, Moore EE, Mill MR: Preoperative antibiotics for abdominal gunshot wounds. A prospective randomized study. Am J Surg 146: 762, 1983
126. Moore JB, Moore EE, Thompson JS: Abdominal injuries associated with penetrating trauma. Am J Surg 140: 724, 1980
127. Murr PC, Moore EE, Lipscomb R, et al: Abdominal trauma associated with pelvic fracture. J Trauma 20: 919, 1980
128. Naam NH, Brown WH, Hurd R, et al: Major pelvic fractures. Arch Surg 118: 610, 1983
129. Newman JH: The prevention of infection in open fractures. J Antimicrob Chemother 11: 391, 1983
130. O'Donnell VA, Atik M, Pick RA: Evaluation and management of penetrating wounds of the neck: The role of emergency angiography. Am J Surg 138: 309, 1979
131. Omer G: Injuries to nerves of the upper extremity. J Bone Joint Surg 56A: 1615, 1974
132. Oparah SS, Mandal AK: Operative management of penetrating wounds of the chest in civilian practice: Review of indications in 125 consecutive patients. J Thorac Cardiovasc Surg 77: 162, 1979
133. Oreskovich MR, Carrico CJ: Complications of penetrating colon injury. Infect Surg 2: 101, 1983
134. Oreskovich MR, Carrico CJ: Stab wounds of the anterior abdomen: Analysis of management plan using local wound exploration and quantitative peritoneal lavage. Ann Surg 198: 411, 1983
135. Orlando R, Drezner D: Intra-aortic balloon counterpulsation in blunt cardiac injury. J Trauma 23: 424, 1983
136. Packman MI, Rackow EC: Optimum left heart filling pressure during fluid resuscitation of patients with hypovolemic and septic shock. Crit Care Med 11: 165, 1983
137. Palmer MA, Perry JF, Fischer RP, et al: Intracranial pressure monitoring in the acute neurologic assessment of multi-injured patients. J Trauma 19: 497, 1979
138. Palomar J, Polanco E, Frentz G: Rupture of the bladder following blunt trauma: A plea for routine peritoneotomy in patients with extraperitoneal rupture. J Trauma 20: 239, 1980
139. Parker S, Carlon GC, Isaacs M, et al: Dopamine administration in oliguria and oliguric renal failure. Crit Care Med 9: 630, 1981
140. Patrick JD, Doris PE, Mills ML, et al: Lumbar spine x-rays: A multihospital study. Ann Emerg Med 12: 84, 1983
141. Perry MO: The management of acute vascular injuries. Williams & Wilkins, Baltimore, 1981
142. Peterson NE: Intermediate-degree blunt renal trauma. J Trauma 17: 425, 1977
143. Peterson NE, Norton L: Injuries associated with renal trauma. J Urol 109: 766, 1973
144. Peterson NE, Kiracofe L: Renal trauma: When to operate. Urology 3: 537, 1974
145. Peyster RG, Hoover ED: CT in head trauma. J Trauma 22: 25, 1982
146. Phillips TF, Brotman S, Cleveland S, et al: Perforating injuries of the small bowel from blunt abdominal trauma. Ann Emerg Med 12: 75, 1983
147. Pietak SP, Teasdale SJ: Anesthesia for the high-risk patient. p. 125. In Armstrong PW, Baigrie RS (eds): Hemodynamic Monitoring in the Critically Ill. Harper & Row, Hagerstown, 1980
148. Pitts JC, and Peterson NE: Penetrating injuries of the ureter. J Trauma 21: 978, 1981
149. Pollack K, Payne EE: Fractures of the frontal sinus. Otolaryngol Clin North Am 9: 517, 1976
150. Pontes JE: Urologic injuries. Surg Clin North Am 57: 77, 1977
151. Powell DC, Bivins BA, Bell RM: Diagnostic peritoneal lavage. Surg Gynecol Obstet 155: 257, 1982
152. Powers SR, Mannal R, Neclerio M, et al: Physiologic consequences of positive end-expiratory pressure (PEEP) ventilation. Ann Surg 178: 265, 1973
153. Rackow EC, Falk JL, Fein IA, et al: Fluid resuscitation in circulatory shock: A comparison of the cardiorespiratory effects of albumin, hetastarch, and saline solutions in patients with hypovolemic and septic shock. Crit Care Med 11: 839, 1983
154. Rao PM, Bhatti FK, Gaudino J, et al: Penetrating injuries of the neck: Criteria for exploration. J Trauma 23: 47, 1983
155. Reigstad A: Traumatic dislocation of the hip. J Trauma 20: 603, 1980
156. Reynolds RR, McDowell HA, Diethelm AG: The surgical treatment of arterial injuries in the civilian population. Ann Surg 189: 700, 1979
157. Richardson JD, Flint LM, Snow NJ, et al: Management of transmediastinal gunshot wounds. Surgery 90: 671, 1981
158. Riska EB, von Bondsorff H, Hakkinen S, et al: Primary operative fixation of long bone fractures in patients with multiple injuries. J Trauma 17: 111, 1977
159. Riska EB, von Bonsdorff H, Hakkinen S, et al: External fixation of unstable pelvic fractures. Int Orthop 3: 183, 1979
160. Robbs JV, Baker LW: Arterial trauma involving the lower limb. J Trauma 18: 324, 1978

161. Robertson HD, Ray JE, Ferrari BT, et al: Management of rectal trauma. Surg Gynecol Obstet 154: 161, 1982

162. Roon AJ, Christensen N: Evaluation and treatment of penetrating cervical injuries. J Trauma 19: 391, 1979

163. Root HD, Keizer PJ, Perry JF: The clinical and experimental aspects of peritoneal response to injury. Arch Surg 95: 531, 1967

164. Roscher R, Bittner R, Stockmann U: Pulmonary contusion. Arch Surg 109: 508, 1974

165. Rutherford RB, Arora S, Fleming PW, et al: Delayed-onset pulmonary insufficiency in primates resuscitated from hemorrhagic shock. J Trauma 19: 422, 1979

166. Ryan JR: Fractures and dislocations encountered by the general surgeon: General principles. Surg Clin North Am 57: 197, 1977

167. Sandor F: Incidence and significance of traumatic mediastinal haematoma. Thorax 22: 43, 1967

168. Saul TG, Ducker TB: Effect of intracranial pressure monitoring and aggressive treatment on mortality in severe head injury. J Neurosurg 56: 498, 1982

169. Saul TG, Ducker TB: Intracranial pressure monitoring in patients with severe head injury. Am Surg 48: 477, 1982

170. Schaal MA, Fischer RP, Perry JF: The unchanged mortality of flail chest injuries. J Trauma 19: 492, 1979

171. Schimpff SC, Miller RM, Polakavetz S, et al: Infection in the severely traumatized patient. Ann Surg 179: 352, 1974

172. Shackford SR, Smith DE, Zarins CK, et al: The management of flail chest: A comparison of ventilatory and nonventilatory treatment. Am J Surg 132: 759, 1976

173. Shaffer MA, Doris PE: Limitation of the cross table lateral view in detecting cervical spine injuries: A retrospective analysis. Ann Emerg Med 10: 508, 1981

174. Shaffer MA, Doris PE: Increasing the diagnostic yield of portable skull films. Ann Emerg Med 11: 303, 1982

175. Shepard GH: High energy, low-velocity close-range shotgun wounds. J Trauma 20: 1065, 1980

176. Shoemaker WC, Hauser CJ: Critique of crystalloid versus colloid therapy in shock and shock lung. Crit Care Med 7: 117, 1979

177. Shuck JM, Lowe RJ: Intestinal disruption due to blunt abdominal trauma. Am J Surg 136: 668, 1978

178. Siemens R, Polk HC, Gray LA, et al: Indications for thoracotomy following penetrating thoracic injury. J Trauma 17: 493, 1977

179. Simpson ET, Aitchison JM: Percutaneous infraclavicular subclavian vein catheterization in shocked patients: A prospective study in 172 patients. J Trauma 22: 781, 1982

180. Snow N, Lucas AE, Richardson JD: Intra-aortic balloon counterpulsation for cardiogenic shock from cardiac contusion. J Trauma 22: 426, 1982

181. Snyder JV, Carroll GC: Tissue oxygenation: A physiologic approach to a clinical problem. p. 652. In Ravitch MM (ed): Current Problems in Surgery. Vol. XIX., Year Book, Chicago, 1982

182. Soderstrom CA, McArdle DQ, Ducker TB, et al: The diagnosis of intra-abdominal injury in patients with cervical cord trauma. J Trauma 23: 1061, 1983

183. Soderstrom CA, Wasserman DH, Dunham CM, et al: Superiority of the femoral artery for monitoring: A prospective study. Am J Surg 144: 309, 1982

184. Sonnenblick EH, Frishman WH, LeJemtel TH: Dobutamine: A new synthetic cardioactive sympathetic amine. N Engl J Med 300: 17, 1979

185. Spiessl B: Maxillofacial injuries in polytrauma. World J Surg 7: 96, 1983

186. Sprung CL, Jacobs LJ: Indications for pulmonary artery catheterization. p. 7. In Sprung CL (ed): The Pulmonary Artery Catheter. Methodology and Clinical Applications. University Park Press, Baltimore, 1983

187. Stone HH, Symbas PN, Hooper CA: Cefamandole for prophylaxis against infection in closed tube thoracostomy. J Trauma 21: 975, 1981

188. Streitwieser DR, Knopp R, Wales LR, et al: Accuracy of standard radiographic views in detecting cervical spine fractures. Ann Emerg Med 12: 538, 1983

189. Stroud WH, Yarbrough DR: Penetrating neck wounds. Am J Surg 140: 323, 1980.

190. Sturm JT, Bodily KC, Rothenberger DA, et al: Arterial injuries of the extremities following blunt trauma. J Trauma 20: 933, 1980

191. Sturm JT, Marsh DG, Bodily KC: Ruptured thoracic aorta: Evolving radiological concept. Surgery 85: 363, 1979

192. Sutherland GR, Calvin JE, Driedger AA, et al: Anatomic and cardiopulmonary responses to trauma with associated blunt chest injury. J Trauma 21: 1, 1981

193. Symbas PN, Hatcher CR, Vlasis SE: Esophageal gunshot injuries. Ann Surg 191: 703, 1980

194. Symbas PN, Hatcher CR, Vlasis SE: Bullet wounds of the trachea. J Thorac Cardiovasc Surg 83: 235, 1982

195. Talbert J, Gruenberg JC, Sy G, et al: Peritoneal lavage in penetrating thoracic trauma. J Trauma 20: 979, 1980

196. Tate JS, Horan DP: Penetrating injuries of the heart. Surg Gynecol Obstet 157: 57, 1983

197. Thal ER: Evaluation of peritoneal lavage and local exploration in lower chest and abdominal stab wounds. J Trauma 17: 642, 1977

198. Thompson JS, Moore EE: Peritoneal lavage in the evaluation of penetrating abdominal trauma. Surg Gynecol Obstet 153: 861, 1981

199. Thompson JS, Moore EE, Van Duzer-Moore S, et al: The evolution of abdominal stab wound management. J Trauma 20: 478, 1980

200. Torres-Mirabal P, Gruenberg JC, Brown RS, et al: Spectrum of myocardial contusion. Am Surg 48: 383, 1982

201. Tranbaugh RF, Elings VB, Christensen J, et al: Determinants of pulmonary interstitial fluid accumulation after trauma. J Trauma 22: 820, 1982

202. Trinkle JK, Toon RS, Franz JL, et al: Affairs of the wounded heart: Penetrating cardiac wounds. J Trauma 19: 467, 1979

203. Turcotte JK, Towne JB, Bernhard VM: Is arteriography necessary in the management of vascular trauma of the extremities? Surgery 84: 557, 1978

204. Tyler DC: Positive end-expiratory pressure: A review. Crit Care Med 11: 300, 1983

205. Unger SW, Tucker WS, Mrdeza MA, et al: Carotid arterial trauma. Surgery 87: 477, 1980

206. Vukich DJ, Moore EE, O'Connor ME, et al: Duodenal hematoma. Ann Emerg Med 11: 36, 1982

207. Waldschmidt ML, Laws HL: Injuries of the diaphragm. J Trauma 20: 587, 1980

208. Wales LR, Knopp RK, Morishima MS: Recommendations for evaluation of the acutely injured cervical spine: A clinical radiologic algorithm. Ann Emerg Med 9: 422, 1980

209. Ward RE, Flynn TC, Clark WP: Diaphragmatic disruption secondary to blunt abdominal trauma. J Trauma 21: 35, 1981

210. Weems WL: Management of genitourinary injuries in patients with pelvic fractures. Ann Surg 189: 717, 1979

211. Wein AJ, Arger PH, Murphy JJ: Controversial aspects of blunt renal trauma. J Trauma 17: 662, 1977

212. Whited RE: Laryngeal fracture in the multiple trauma patient. Am J Surg 136: 354, 1978

213. Williams CF, Bernstein TW, Jelenko C: Essentiality of the lateral cervical spine radiograph. Ann Emerg Med 10: 198, 1981

214. Wilson RF, Wilson JA, Gibson D, et al: Shock in the emergency department. JACEP 5: 678, 1976

215. Yellin AE, Lundell CJ, Finck EJ: Diagnosis and control of posttraumatic pelvic hemorrhage: Transcatheter angiographic embolization techniques. Arch Surg 118: 1378, 1983

216. Zallen RD, Curry JT: A study of antibiotic usage in compound mandibular fractures. J Oral Surg 33: 431, 1975

217. Zimpfer M, Khosropour R, Lackner F: Effect of dobutamine on cardiac function in man: Reciprocal roles of heart rate and ventricular stroke volume. Crit Care Med 10: 367, 1982

218. Zweifach SS, Hargens AR, Evans KL, et al: Skeletal muscle necrosis in pressurized compartments associated with hemorrhagic hypotension. J Trauma 20: 941, 1980

27

Anesthesia for the Critically Ill Trauma Patient

John K. Stene

GENERAL DEMOGRAPHIC CONSIDERATIONS

Professional anesthesia care is an indespensible part of the care of the trauma patient. Modern surgical care of the trauma patient requires rapid diagnosis concurrently with resuscitation and operation. Highly skilled anesthesia practice is required to provide intraoperative critical care for these patients to ensure prompt definitive surgical treatment. As infectious diseases and chronic diseases are controlled by good preventive care and medical management, traumatic disease assumes a larger share of our national mortality rates, hospital utilization, and health care expenditures.[5] Currently traumatic disease accounts for the largest utilization of hospitalization in United States in terms of hospital days per disease per year.[54] The high cost of trauma care includes a high rehabilitative cost for young patients with long life expectancies after their initial injury. These patients require both extensive rehabilitative care as well as expensive custodial care for long periods of time. Also added to this cost is the loss of productivity of young members of our population. Since the effects anesthesia care are manifested long beyond the end of the operation, appropriate anesthesia management in the initial phases of trauma will help reduce the morbidity, mortality, and therefore the cost of trauma.[16]

Any demographic discussion of trauma must include different mechanisms of injury. From 1960 to 1980, the relative distribution of injuries in society changed.[54] Assaults and motor vehicle accidents have assumed a greater proportion of traumatic injuries in the United States. Certain types of trauma, such as home injuries (falls) have decreased over that period of time. Assaults frequently involve penetrating trauma, secondary to knife and bullet wounds. Motor vehicle accidents usually involve blunt trauma. The type of surgical care differs depending on the type of trauma. The

843

anesthesiologist needs to be aware of the types of injury the patient may have in order to prepare properly for intraoperative management.

Appropriate anticipation of the expected injuries that occur with different types of trauma will direct the anesthesiologist's attention toward appropriate care for these patients. For example, a patient with a gunshot wound to the chest might reasonably be expected to require a chest tube to drain the intrapleural hemorrhage and no further surgical care.[43] By contrast, a person involved in a high-speed automobile accident with blunt chest trauma, secondary to hitting the steering wheel, could have several serious injuries, including pulmonary or myocardial contusions, a possible ruptured aorta or bronchus, as well as multiple broken ribs with a flail chest.[43] The anesthesiologist should anticipate the need for early intubation and mechanical ventilation in such a patient. Mechanical ventilation stabilizes broken ribs, maintains contused lung at optimum volume for healing, and prevents splinting from pleuritic pain. Also, anesthesiologists must be aware of certain types of organ damage that cluster together from certain injuries. Such knowledge will help direct the appropriate critical care to the anesthetized patient.

Patients with chronic disease become victims of trauma and challenge the anesthesiologist by presenting with both chronic and acute disease. Since most trauma victims are young, they exhibit few of the chronic diseases often associated with the general surgical population.[39] One exception is juvenile-onset diabetes mellitus in the young patient. Patients with diabetes who sustain fractures and vascular injuries to the limbs often have poor healing of their extremities and may eventually require amputation. Diabetics frequently develop ketoacidosis following trauma. The anesthesiologist will have to treat intraoperative ketoacidosis with insulin and K^+.[25] Some older patients with coronary artery disease may sustain a myocardial infarction while driving and thus may be involved in a motor vehicle accident. The anesthesiologist needs to be prepared to treat such a patient like any other surgical patient with a high cardiac risk.[19] The additive effect of an acute traumatic insult on an elderly patient weakened by chronic disease is one reason that overall mortality rates from trauma increase with age.[5] Successful treatment of the elderly trauma victim requires treatment of both acute and chronic disease.

A common preoperative problem is the association of drug use and trauma in the young patient population. Many patients come to the hospital because they are injured while under the influence of alcohol or other central nervous system intoxicants.[55] A knowledge of the prevaling drug use in the community will help the anesthesiologist anticipate potential drug interactions before a drug screen is completed.[53]

The distribution of traumatic deaths following time of injury is trimodal: immediate deaths, early deaths, and late deaths.[54] Immediate deaths occur within minutes of the injury; they are usually due to major vascular laceration with a rapid fatal hemorrhage or a devastating brain injury resulting in immediate brain death. Early death occurs within a few hours of the trauma; these are usually secondary to slow but uncontrolled hemorrhage or prolonged inadequate gas exchange leading to hypoxic death. This group of patients is amenable to life-saving hospital emergency room therapy and includes most of the "preventable trauma deaths." Most will require surgical treatment and the services of the anesthesiologist. Late deaths occur with a peak of about 3 weeks following injury. These deaths are usually due to sepsis and multiorgan failure. This is the human manifestation of "irreversible shock" described by physiologists in laboratory animals.[23] Prolonged low blood flow to vital organs causes cell necrosis and organ death, resulting in death from multiorgan failure.[7] The immune system fails along with other organs; these patients become susceptible to bacterial infections. An overwhelming bacterial infection with sepsis accounts for most deaths in this group. If shock is recognized early and patients are aggressively treated in the emergency room and the operating room, many late trauma deaths may be prevented. Time is of the essence in resuscitating trauma patients to prevent many deaths due to early and late trauma.

In summary, the anesthesiologist must be aware of patterns of trauma in the community in order to anticipate the types of patients who will require anesthesia management for surgical treatment of their injuries. Since emergency surgical treatment of trauma rarely allows the anesthesiologist time for extensive preoperative evaluation of the patient, a knowledge of diseases to expect in the patient's age group, of predisposing factors that could lead to trauma, and of how the mechanism of injury can lead to multiple organ systems involvement is important. The anesthesiologist armed with this kind of knowledge can make appropriate preoperative judgements to provide the best possible anesthesia management, and anticipate possible complications that may arise. Such high-quality anesthesia care will reduce postoperative morbidity and mortality in trauma patients.

PREOPERATIVE ASSESSMENT

History

For patients who come to the operating room or emergency room directly from the scene of the accident, preoperative history is often limited to knowledge of the type of accident that occured and a brief description of the patient's course following the arrival of emergency medical personnel. The need to provide resuscitation treatment simultaneously with diagnosis further reduces the preoperative history. The anesthesiologist needs to be most attentive to such history of the present illness as trends in the patient's level of consciousness, patient's total fluid intake and output balance, the type of accident the patient suffered, and injuries received. The anesthesiologist and surgeon need to confer on the proposed surgical correction for those injuries. It is obvious that the patient who has suffered penetrating trauma to one body region will have a different type of surgical approach and a different anesthesia problem than a patient who has suffered blunt trauma to several body regions. The anesthesiologist must be cognizant of anticipated surgery to be done on the patient to be prepared for all problems. This communication

between anesthesiologists and surgeons is especially important for patients whose surgery is part of resuscitation.

There is a tendency for anesthesiologists to underestimate the "disease" effect of trauma on a patient. Many anesthesia complications in trauma surgery occur because anesthesiologists consider a young robust person with major trauma to be an ASA class I anesthetic risk. The goal of the preoperative anesthetic assessment is to document the extent of acute disease (how many systems involved) that changes the patient's ASA risk classification to II, III, IV, or even V. Experience in caring for trauma patients will allow the anesthesiologist to estimate the severity of the patients illness.

Many critically ill trauma patients will come to the operating room from the intensive care unit (ICU). These critically ill patients are just as demanding anesthetically as are patients who arrive in the emergency room directly from the scene of the accident. Important historical points to record in ICU patients are total fluid intake and output, laboratory changes that have occurred during the intensive care course, and any cardiorespiratory complications and treatments. It is especially useful to ascertain treatments that have worked for cardiorespiratory complications, as these same treatments are likely to work in the operating room. A general review of systems completes the preoperative history with information on the hepatic, renal, coagulation, hematologic, and neurologic systems.

A careful analysis of these historical data will prepare the anesthesiologist for most occurrences in the operating room. The patient's response to the stress of surgery will be similar to the response to the stress of the illness in the ICU. The types of therapy that have worked in the ICU will probably work as well in the operating room. This is why it is extremely important for the anesthesiologist to analyze the preoperative intensive care course carefully. Patients who have been in the ICU for some time before transfer to the operating room will also have accumulated a more complete medical history. Family members can be questioned about drug allergies, pre-existing medical problems, smoking,[37] drinking,[11] and medication history. Also, the patient's primary physician should be known by this time and can be questioned about any previous medical history.

Physical Examination

Since many trauma patients have reduced levels of consciousness, much of the anesthesiologist's preoperative preparation involves the physical examination. The most important preoperative examination of the critically ill trauma patient concerns respiratory and cardiovascular systems. The anesthesiologist examines the patient's respiratory status by recording the type of airway, ventilatory support, and FIO_2 (fraction of inspired oxygen) required for adequate oxygenation. The anesthesiologist also auscultates the lungs for evidence of excessive secretions, pulmonary edema, or atelectasis.

The cardiovascular examination consists of (1) inspecting the patient for signs of cardiac insufficiency, such as edema, pallor, and cyanosis, (2) palpating peripheral pulses, and (3) auscultation of heart sounds, although noisy ICU and emergency room (ER) environments make ascultation difficult. Evaluation of electrocardiograms (ECGs), pulse waveforms measured by indwelling catheters (arterial, pulmonary artery), and availability of intravenous catheters for fluid management completes the preoperative cardiovascular examination. The anesthesiologist should use this information to prescribe appropriate cardiovascular monitoring and therapy for intraoperative care.

It is important to include the neurologic system in the preanesthetic physical examination. The anesthesiologist needs to know the patient's baseline neurologic status preoperatively to organize the anesthetic management to avoid neurologic damage. The neurologic examination (Table 27-1) begins with a level of consciousness evaluation. The Glasgow coma scale is a reliable simple method for recording the level of consciousness[26]; however, patients who are intubated and who cannot speak cannot be adequately evaluated on the verbal section. Next, cranial nerve functions are examined. The size and reactivity of the pupils, the extra ocular muscle movement and facial muscle function are usually the only cranial nerve examination possible. (Frequently, the neurologic examination is limited because the therapeutic devices attached to the patient interfere.) Evaluation of the patient's ability to perform motor movements, discern peripheral sensory stimuli, and respond reflexively completes the neurologic physical examination.

If the patient is not intubated preoperatively, the anesthesiologist must evaluate the teeth and airway as for any surgical patient. If the patient has not had a cervical spinal fracture ruled out, the neck must remain in some type of fixation device to protect the cervical spinal cord. Additional intravenous catheters needed to replace the anticipated blood and fluid losses during surgery need to be placed before the patient is draped for surgery.

Laboratory Data

Useful laboratory data to prepare a critically ill trauma patient for the operating room (OR) includes the ECG and the chest radio-

TABLE 27-1. Preoperative Neurologic Examination

Glasgow Coma Scale[a,b]		
Eye opening	Spontaneous	E4
	To speech	3
	To pain	2
	None	1
Best motor response	Obeys commands	M6
	Localizes	5
	Withdraws	4
	Abnormal flexion	3
	Extension	2
	None	1
Verbal responses	Orientated	V5
	Confused conversation	4
	Inappropriate words	3
	Incomprehensible sounds	2
	None	1

Reactivity and size of pupils
  May be affected by drugs or trauma to eye or cranial nerves

Eye position and movements

Other cranial nerves

Spinal cord function
  Level of paralysis
  Level of sensory deficit

Level of reflexes

[a] From Jennett B, Teasdale G: Aspects of coma after severe head injury. Lancet 1:879, 1977.

[b] Add E, M, and V; 15 is normal; <7 after 6 hours indicates severe head injury.

graphs. Chest radiographs rarely yield information on healthy adults without respiratory symptoms who are scheduled for general elective surgery.[41] However, following trauma the chest radiograph is an indispensible diagnostic tool, illustrating intrapulmonary, chest wall, and diaphragmatic pathology as well as dwelling line placements.[3] The ECG is used to diagnose cardiac disease such as myocardial ischemia, contusion, and cardiac dysrhythmias. Further laboratory data of special interest are the arterial and mixed venous blood gases. Cardiac output (CO) measurements, serum electrolytes, osmolality, glucose, BUN, creatinine, and creatinine clearance (very important, since renal failure is quite common in patients who suffer hemorrhagic shock and aggressive treatment of prerenal azotemia prevents serious prolonged renal failure)[14,42] are essential to the preoperative preparation. The hemoglobin (Hb) and hematocrit (Hct) are measured to assess the adequacy of red blood cell (RBC) oxygen-carrying capacity. Also, Hct changes that occur during fluid resuscitation (which increases the rapidity of hemodilution) provide a reliable estimate of the amount of blood loss the patient suffered prior to operation.[35] The percentage change in RBC volume calculated from Hct changes before and after fluid replacement has restored normal blood volume will provide an estimate of the total volume of RBCs lost. The volume of blood loss can be calculated by dividing the volume of red cells lost by the initial Hct. Many trauma patients develop dilutional coagulopathy; therefore, coagulation studies, including platelet count, partial thromboplastin time (PTT), and the prothrombin time (PT), need to be evaluated[33] preoperatively and followed intraoperatively.

brain trauma anatomically. Some critically ill patients transferred from the ICU to the operating room may have had radionuclide myocardial contractility studies. Knowledge of the left and right heart ejection fractions and wall motion is an invaluable addition to the cardiovascular data base used to prescribe appropriate anesthetic and cardiovascular monitoring.[4] Two further tests that are most helpful for evaluating a patient's response to trauma and resuscitative measures are oxygen consumption as a function of CO and ventricular function (Starling) curves in response to fluid challenges.[6] Oxygen consumption can be measured either as the oxygen uptake by the lung or as the arteriovenous oxygen content difference ($Ca-\bar{v}O_2$) multiplied by the CO. Mass spectrometer systems are commercially available to measure pulmonary oxygen uptake reliably, but caution should be applied to interpreting results unless averaged over a long enough period of time to reflect whole-body cellular oxygen consumption. Oxygen consumption appears to be an important predictive variable for ultimate survival following posttraumatic resuscitation.[50] (see Chapter 9). The anesthetic care of the trauma patient is directed toward maximizing oxygen consumption of the whole patient as well as optimizing individual organ oxygen comsumption. The preoperative evaluation of the patient should prepare the anesthesiologist to give special attention to the heart, lung, brain, and kidneys.

Special Studies

Many trauma patients undergo angiography for surgical diagnosis. Such patients may have received a large volume of intravenous contrast material and require an elevated high urine output to minimize renal toxicity from the contrast material.[18,49] Cranial computed tomography (CT) scan with and without contrast material is often done preoperatively to outline

PREOPERATIVE MANAGEMENT

Airway Control

Ideally the anesthesiologist caring for trauma patients will be available in the ER to evaluate the patient upon admission. Evaluation and treatment of the patient's airway status must proceed simultaneously. If the patients airway status is adequate, treatment may simply consist of increased oxygen delivery.

If the airway is compromised or the patient needs ventilatory support, a secure intratracheal airway is needed. Such airways can be an orotracheal, nasotracheal, or tracheostomy tube (Fig. 27-1).

Many trauma patients are rendered unconscious by their injury or require drugs that decrease the level of consciousness in order to tolerate diagnostic and therapeutic surgical procedures. The care of the unconscious patient requires maintenance of a secure airway by a cuffed tube in the trachea. Such a tube provides a patent route for respiratory gas exchange by positive-pressure devices. The cuffed tube in the trachea also isolates the lungs from fluids, either blood or gastric juice,

that may enter the mouth and prevents pulmonary damage secondary to aspiration. An artificial tracheal tube also provides a sure route for tracheal suction.

The anesthesiologist can intubate the trachea either through the larynx through a tracheostomy incision.[40] In an unconscious patient with an artificial airway, the medical personnel caring for the patient must pay strict attention to an adequate respiratory gas source. An adequate respiratory gas source includes proper oxygen concentration, proper pressure of gas, as well as proper humidification. Bypassing the patients nose and upper airway removes the patient's ability to humidify the gases and the patient's ability to

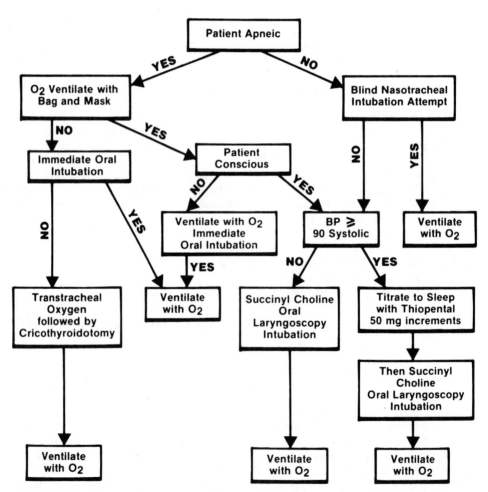

FIG. 27-1 Decision tree for emergency airway control in trauma patients. Intubation technique.

keep his own airway clear, so the medical personnel also must pay strict attention to keeping the artificial airway clear and free of debris. Airway obstruction in the hospitalized intubated patient is an unexcusable iatrogenic complication.

Blunt head and facial trauma is associated with a 5 to 10 percent incidence of cervical spine fractures.[12,31] The dire consequences of excessive movement of a fractured cervical spine should cause the anesthesiologist to be extremely careful when intubating a blunt trauma victim. Intubation can be difficult in the best of circumstances in a patient with in-line cervical traction with Gardner-Wells tongs. In such a patient, preparations need to be made for topical anesthesia to the larynx followed by an awake intubation, either blindly or guided over a fiberoptic bronchoscope. Such intubations can use either the nasal or oral route.

The route of choice for securing the airway depends on several factors. Blunt trauma patients should be assumed to have a cervical spine fracture until it is absolutely proven otherwise. Therefore, manipulation of the neck is strictly contraindicated. There are those who advocate blind nasal tracheal intubation in such patients using the patient's own respiratory efforts to aspirate the endotracheal tube into the trachea. However, patients who have poor respiratory exchange may not generate enough air movement through the vocal cords to guide intubation blindly. Nasal tracheal intubation is also frought with certain long-term hazards, passing a large tube through a narrow nasal passage can lead to excessive hemorrhage as well as delayed appearance of sinusitis secondary to obstructed sinuses. Oral tracheal intubation avoids the complications of nose bleeds and sinusitis; however, many practitioners believe that direct laryngoscopy involves the hazard of neck manipulation. We have found that patients who are lying on a long spine board with an assistant holding their occiput on the board can undergo laryngoscopy with minimal changes in the position of the cervical vertabrae (Fig. 27-2). Although optimum exposure of the larynx is often unachievable under such conditions, most experienced anesthesiologists can intubate patients without seeing the vocal cords. A sharply bent stylet curves the endotracheal tube (hockey stick) to pass behind the tongue and through the glottis. Cricoid pressure provided by an assistant is absolutely essential to protect the patient from aspirating gastric contents.[46] Tracheostomy is reserved for patients who cannot be intubated either nasally or orally. Frequently there are patients with massive facial trauma that distorts the pharyngeal anatomy to the point that the glottic opening is unrecognizable (see Fig. 27-1). Emergency tracheostomy can be performed through the cricothyroid membrane with a small midline incision and a small tracheostomy tube placed through the cricothyroid membrane. Alternatively, oxygenation can be supported by a cricothyroidotomy with needle jet ventilation while the patient is having a formal tracheostomy. Bleeding is usually minimal with a cricothyroidotomy. All anesthesia practitioners should be familiar with the technique of emergency tracheostomy through the cricothyroid membrane, as there are times when this is the only way of establishing an airway. It is controversial as to whether the tracheostomy tube should remain in the cricothyroid membrane or be converted to a more formal tracheostomy within the first 24 hours.

Many patients who have fractures of the maxilla and mandible have their fractures reduced and fixated by intramaxillary fixation (IMF) over arch bars placed along the teeth. Such patients who then return to the OR for other procedures present a special airway problem to the anesthesiologist. Patients with a reduced level of consciousness who require IMF should have a tracheostomy performed during the original surgery. This will assure a continuously patent airway for ventilation of the patient; a cuffed tracheostomy tube can protect the airway from foreign material aspiration. If the tracheostomy tube becomes dislodged, it can be easily replaced. A dislodged oral or nasal tracheal tube is extremely difficult to replace unless the IMF is disrupted. However, patients with a normal level of consciousness can be extubated as soon as they recover from the anesthesia enough to protect their own airway. However, when these patients return to the operating room, spontaneous respirations will be compromised if they have been heavily sedated. It is also difficult for the patient in IMF to handle oral secretions easily

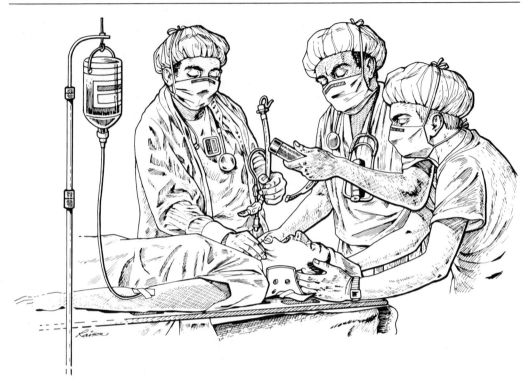

FIG. 27-2 Technique for oral intubation. Patient is supine on long spine board with semirigid (Philadelphia) collar in place. Drugs are given as needed to provide patient cooperation and good intubating conditions. Before paralyzing the patient, the anterior half of the collar is removed and cricoid pressure applied as another assistant holds head in neutral position on the spine board. Positive-pressure ventilation should be applied with bag and mask to assure ability to ventilate patient before neuromuscular paralysis. Cricoid pressure will keep gas out of the stomach. A rapid-acting neuromuscular blocking drug is given and ventilation continued to optimize alveolar gas tensions. When the patient is relaxed, oral intubation with laryngoscope and the tube is performed, while assistant prevents occiput from moving off the board. Cricoid pressure is maintained until the cuff on the endotracheal tube is inflated. Tube position is confirmed by listening for bilaterally equal breath sounds (both axilla) and absence of air entry into stomach. The cervical collar is reapplied, tube tapped, and the patient is connected to ventilator.

when lying supine and sedated. Therefore, these patients should receive minimal sedation until they are in the OR, where the airway can be easily controlled.

There is a great temptation to provide regional anesthesia for patients with IMF. However, spinal and epidural anesthesia have to be carefully evaluated. If a high spinal anesthetic level is required for surgery, the anesthesiologist has to be prepared to support the patient's ventilation if the spinal anesthetic paralyzes the respiratory muscles. Patients in IMF cannot be ventilated well with a mask due to facial fractures and also cannot be rapidly intubated due to the IMF rubber bands or wires

holding the teeth tightly shut. Even without a high spinal block, if some of the accessory muscles of respiration are paralyzed and the patient is forced to lie supine, breathing may be difficult because the patient cannot open the mouth and keep the tongue forward out of the glottis. Many of these patients are best managed with an awake "elective intubation," followed by general anesthesia in order to maintain a secure airway.

Patients with suspected laryngeal fractures should be approached with caution when establishing on emergency airway. Laryngoscopy should be performed while the patient is breathing spontaneously. If there is cartilaginous disruption and exposure in the larynx, the patient requires tracheostomy and an emergency ENT consultation. Tracheostomy should be performed with local anesthesia. If there is no exposed cartilage in the larynx, intubation with a small endotracheal tube can be performed before tracheostomy. Such an intubation should obviously be done in the most gentle manner possible. This endotracheal tube should be used to maintain an airway while a formal tracheostomy is done.

The critically ill injured patient who is to have surgery on either the aorta or the tracheal bronchial tree in the lateral position will benefit from the use of a double-lumen endobronchial tube to collapse one lung or to permit the use of synchronous independent lung ventilation to balance ventilation and perfusion to the dependent lung. Endobronchial tubes can be extremely difficult to place in the patient whose neck is either in traction or stabilized with a hard cervical collar. This technique may have to be abandoned in these patients.

To secure the airway by either the oral or nasotracheal route in patients with responsive airway reflexes, the patient usually requires induction of general anesthesia. Anesthetic drugs, both muscle relaxants and sedative/hypnotics, reduce the chance of the patient's "fighting" the ventilator as well as providing easier intubation (Table 27-2).

Choice of Anesthetic

Anesthesiologists caring for critically ill trauma patients must learn to adjust the doses of anesthetics they administer, to avoid compromising the safety of the patient. Drugs such as opiates and barbiturates should be administered in smaller doses to avoid profound cardiovascular depression. Other drugs such as ketamine and halogenated hydrocarbons elevate intracranial pressure and are contraindicated in head trauma. Drugs such as ketamine, nalbuphine, and naloxone are especially useful to stabilize the cardiovascular pathology associated with hemorrhagic shock and trauma. Patients who are in profound hemorrhagic shock and admitted to the operating room for life-saving surgery often are treated with 100 percent oxygen and a muscle relaxant to facilitate surgical exposure.[9] Pancuronium bromide (Pavulon) is the preferred muscle relaxant, as its side effects include vagal blockade but not sympathetic blockade at clinically useful doses.[44] Unfortunately, approximately 40 percent of patients treated with oxygen and pancuronium for trauma anesthesia recalled their surgery as the worst experience they had during their hospital course.[8,9] A control group that received general anesthesia had about a 10 percent incidence of recall.[9] Judicious use of thiopental and/or opiates used in doses low enough to not aggravate hypotension may reduce some of this recall. Thiopental should be titrated in 50-mg increments and fentanyl in 50-μg increments until the desired effect is achieved without compromising blood pressure. The opiate agonist/antagonist, nalbuphine, has cardiovascular properties similar to that of naloxone and is useful in providing analgesia for trauma patients while not aggravating hypotension and shock (J. K. Stene, unpublished data). Nalbuphine has demonstrated marked cardiovascular stability in normal patients.[27] An initial nalbuphine dose of 1.0 mg/kg IV with an 0.25-mg/kg hourly dose of nalbuphine provides surgical analgesia as a component of balanced anesthesia.[32] Nalbuphine will not provide total anesthesia and must be supplemented with inhalation or intravenous drugs.

Muscle relaxants to facilitate intubation include succinylcholine, pancuronium, and

TABLE 27-2. Drugs for Anesthesia Induction

Muscle relaxants
  Succinylcholine, 1.0 mg/kg IV push
  Pancuronium, 0.1–0.2 mg/kg IV push

Sedatives/Hypnotics (use for noncomatose patients)
  Thiopental, titrate 50-mg IV doses until patient closes eyes
  Ketamine, 1.0–2.0 mg/kg IV push
  Etomidate

Analgesics
  Fentanyl, titrate 50 μg IV for analgesia; stop if BP decreases $\geq$ 10 mmHg
  Butorphanol, 0.1 mg/kg slow IV push; stop infusion if BP decreases $\geq$ 10 mmHg
  Nalbuphine, 1.0 mg/g slow IV push; full dose useful in hypovolemic patients

vecuronium. These agents are safe to use as adjuncts to anesthesia in patients with hemorrhagic shock to facilitate intubation. Succinylcholine will elevate plasma potassium levels in patients with spinal cord injuries and burns more than 24 hours postinjury.[14] In practice we have not seen large increases in plasma potassium in patients with other types of injuries. Many head-injured patients have trismus and will not open their mouths to admit a laryngoscope or an endotracheal tube; because of this, muscle relaxants are needed. Intubating doses are as follows: succinylcholine, 1.0 mg/kg; pancuronium, 0.1 to 0.2 mg/kg; and vecuronium, 0.1 to 0.2 mg/kg (more clinical experience is needed to refine this dose). Thiopental should be administered before giving muscle relaxants to patients who are alert or who have a systolic blood pressure of $\geq$ 90 mmHg. Ketamine is a popular alternative to thiopental because it elevates blood pressure and heart rate.[57,58] However, ketamine also elevates intracranial pressure, which is undesirable in patients with head trauma.[48] Patients with head trauma need an anesthetic that will reduce intracranial pressure. Thiopental and opiates as part of a balanced anesthetic are the drugs of choice for head-injured patients.[47] The use of isoflurane or other halogenated inhalational drugs has to be accompanied by hyperventilation to lower the $PaCO_2$ to keep the intracranial pressure low (Table 27-3).

The anesthesiologist must remember that the patient with reduced blood volume, in whom primarily the brain and heart, is perfused, will have a reduced volume of distribution for anesthetic drugs. The anesthesiologist must be aware of the altered pharmokinetics and adjust the drug doses downward. These patients will receive a much higher drug concentration in the bloodstream than do normovolemic patients at any given drug dose.[24,56] This is especially important for highly lipophilic drugs, such as fentanyl and thiopental, for which a very small dose will render the hypovolemic patient unconscious because most of the intravenous bolus will directly cross the blood-brain barrier.[20] In a patient with normal blood volume and a larger volume of distribution, a smaller fraction of the injected intravenous dose will be delivered directly to the brain.

Pre-existing, self-administered drugs that interact with anesthetics are a common problem in trauma patients. Alcohol is commonly associated with traumatic injury in the patients treated at Maryland Institute for Emergency Medical Services Systems. Alcohol was involved in 50 percent of the motor vehicle accident victims between the ages 15 and 40 years. Serum osmolality, sodium, and glucose levels will give the anesthesiologist an estimate of the blood alcohol level in the acutely intoxicated patient (Fig. 27-3). Serum osmolality is most dependent on small osmotically active particles such as sodium, glucose, and alcohol. If the osmolality is much higher than can be accounted for by calculating

$$\text{Sodium concentration} \times 2 + (\text{glucose} \div 18)$$

the unaccounted osmotic load is most likely to be from ethanol. Knowledge of the precise blood alcohol level is unnecessary to anesthetize these patients. However, it is useful to know the magnitude of the ethanol level, since ethanol will enhance the effects of anesthetic and sedative drugs and will reduce the minimum alveolar concentration (MAC) required for general anesthetics.[11] The depth of anesthesia should be carefully monitored in these patients, since the blood alcohol concentration will be decreasing throughout a prolonged surgery. The patient will have far less effect from the alcohol at the end of the operation then at the beginning of the operation and may need an increased depth of inhalation anesthetics as time proceeds. Also, patients with acute and chronic ethanol toxicity may develop severe

TABLE 27-3. Drug Contraindications for Trauma Patients

Head-Injured Patients
  Ketamine: increases intracranial pressure
  Halothane/enflurane: increases intracranial pressure
  Relative contraindication: isoflurane use with hyperventilation; least increase in intracranial pressure of all halogenated anesthetics
Burn and spinal cord-injured patients
  Succinylcholine: safe during first 24 hours; after 24 hours until healing complete, potential lethal hyperkalemia
Open eye injuries
  Succinylcholine: relative contraindication, as it raises intraocular pressure

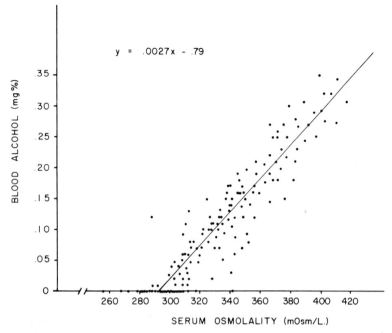

$$y = .0027x - .79$$

FIG. 27-3 Relationship between serum osmolality and blood alcohol in acutely injured patients. Data collected on admission to Maryland Institute for Emergency Medical Services Systems.

alcohol withdrawal symptoms during the post-operative period.

Other drugs that can cause problems range from self-administered opiates to phencyclidine (PCP).[53] Patients addicted to opiates will develop withdrawal if a source of opiate is not available within a few hours. Furthermore, the use of narcotic antagonists for these patients will precipitate an abstinence syndrome. PCP is an incidious problem, as the drug is very slowly metabolized. Intensive periods of hypertension, tachycardia, and rage reaction can occur in PCP users. Treatment consists of acidifying the urine, administering gastric charcoal, and drugs for sedation (diazepam, droperidol), of controlling autonomic reflexes (propranolol), and of increasing output of acidic urine (intravenous fluids, furosemide, and ascorbic acid). Treatment may also require endotracheal intubation, ventilation, and management of hyperthermia. Other drugs commonly associated with trauma are cocaine and marijuana, both of which have sympathomimetic effects. Cocaine stimulates the adrenergic responses causing vasoconstriction and hypertension. By contrast, marijuana is a adrenergic agonist causing tachycardia and vasodilation. Intravenous propranolol in small doses will reduce cocaine toxicity due to inhibition of catecholamine uptake. Marijuana poisoning is probably not lethal and can be treated by supportive care.[53]

The choice of drugs for anesthesia must be carefully selected on the basis of the preoperative assessment in order to optimize the anesthetic management and provide for an uneventful recovery from anesthesia.

Monitoring

Monitoring of the trauma patient in the OR includes not only the use of devices to measure directly the patient's hemodynamic activity but also includes frequent laboratory measurements and computations of derived variables. These derived variables help the anesthesiologist interpret changes that occur in the patient's condition. The goal of monitoring is to ascertain accurately the patient's physiologic state so that the anesthesiologist can modify therapy as needed to improve the patient's physical status and prognosis. Theories of the pathophysiologic changes during anesthesia have been determined by the availability of monitoring. The dependence of anesthesia theories on monitoring is a manifestation of the principle that you won't discover anything unless you look for it. Patients will suffer extreme pathophysiologic changes that will be unexpected unless the clinician monitors the patient thoroughly and corrects potentially deleterious changes. Therefore, when dealing with critically ill patients, the anesthesiologist must use extensive monitoring.

Monitoring systems start with simple vital sign measurements which include pulse rate, arterial blood pressure, respiratory rate, and temperature. More extensive monitoring includes the electroencephlagram (EEG) to assess cerebral perfusion and function, measurements of inspired and expired gas tensions (both the respiratory gases and anesthetic gases), intravascular measurement of arterial pressure, CVP, and pulmonary artery pressure as well as CO (Table 27-4). Monitoring of renal function includes urine output and composition as well as serum BUN and creatinine. Complete monitoring includes measurements of serum electrolytes, glucose, Hb, Hct, and the coagulation profile. The critically ill or injured patient

TABLE 27-4. Cardiovascular Monitoring of Patients

ECG: precordial electrode for ischemic heart disease
Arterial blood pressure: use intra-arterial catheter to follow pressures and waveforms in patients with heart disease or large volume shifts
Urine output: adequacy of renal perfusion
Cardiac filling pressures: central venous catheter for one system trauma, healthy heart, prior to pulmonary artery catheterization
Pulmonary artery catheter: thermodilution cardiac output
  Multiple systems injury with large volume loss
  Ischemic heart disease
  Cardiac output and oxygen consumption monitored for critically ill patients.
  Head and spinal cord injury use to optimize fluid management
Transcutaneous oxygen tension: adequacy of skin perfusion

in the operating room needs to be treated as if he or she were in an ICU environment in order to have the best chance of surviving the operation.

INTRAOPERATIVE COURSE

Drugs

Anesthetic management of the trauma patient requires the choice of drugs that will render the patient senseless to the pain of surgery and trauma but maintain optimum oxygen consumption for the whole body as well as individual organs. Pain from trauma or surgery can trigger reflex release of vasoactive humoral agents that interfere with homeostasis and healing. Therefore, the goal of controlling pain is to make the patient psychologically comfortable and to reduce stress-hormonal release. General anesthesia reduces oxygen consumption to basal levels, although isolated tissue preparations show a further reduction of oxygen uptake under the influence of anesthesia.[15,52] The following discussion of anesthetic and vasoactive drugs weighs the need to reduce pain perception and stress-hormonal responses against the need to preserve CO, systemic blood pressure, and oxygen consumption.

The use of oxygen and muscle relaxants has already been mentioned as a compromise to prevent further depression of CO and blood pressure. Pancuronium bromide has been particularly useful for this purpose, since it has rapid onset in large doses (0.1 to 0.2 mg/kg IV) and vagolytic cardiovascular side effects. Very high doses of pancuronium are needed to develop ganglionic sympathetic blockade. Pancuronium also has minimal histamine release. The drawbacks of pancuronium are its long duration of action in high doses and the need for renal clearance of the drug.

Other useful muscle relaxants are metocurine iodide, vecuronium bromide, and atracurium besylate. These drugs have minimal cardiovascular side effects in doses used for maintenance of relaxation, but metocurine and atracurium will trigger histamine release in large doses. Atracurium is interesting, as it undergoes Hoffman degradation in the plasma and thus requires neither renal or hepatic function for excretion. Combinations of these drugs with pancuronium may be useful to potentiate onset of blockade at doses that are easily reversed.[28]

The inhalational anesthetics (halothane, enflurane, and isoflurane) are useful for patients requiring trauma surgery; however, they cause profound cardiovacular depression when the alveolar concentration exceeds $1.5 \times MAC$. However, these drugs can be safely used in low concentrations supplemented by intravenous sedations, narcotics, and muscle relaxants. The combination of nitrous oxide with these drugs needs to be examined with caution. Nitrous oxide has a predilection to accumulate in closed air spaces (pleural, cerebral, or intrabowel). Thus, it may aggravate pneumothoraces, pneumocephalus, and bowel obstruction. There is some evidence that nitrous oxide may impair left ventricle contractility; thus it may lead to left ventricular failure in patients recovering from shock.[17,29,45]

Fluid Management

Fluid management of the trauma patient involves not only maintenance fluid replacement typically required by all surgical patients but replacement of hemorrhaged blood as well. There are many useful formulas for estimating the maintenance fluid requirements in surgical patients.[14] Consideration must be given to the soft tissue injury, which causes third-space loss of water and electrolytes.[30] Such third-space losses need to be replaced. The amount to be replaced can be estimated from knowledge of third-space losses with elective surgery. The anesthesiologist needs to monitor serum and urine volume, osmolality, and electrolytes to fine-tune the fluid replacement of third-space losses. Burn patients require accurate fluid replacement to prevent complications of hypovolemia, as they have a large exposed surface area to evaporate water. Many formulas, such as that from Brook Army Hospital, can be useful in calculating the amount of fluid required by the burn patient.[34] Head injury patients require less fluids than do other patients in order to minimize cerebral edema by maximizing oncotic forces that will transfer water from the brain to the bloodstream. Sophisticated management of these patients requires measurement of intracardiac filling pressures, CO, and intracranial pressure, instead of empirically dehydrating the patient. Such a sophisticated approach should optimize cerebral blood flow and oxygen delivery to help the injured brain heal.[10]

The most common problem encountered by the trauma anesthesiologist is that of optimizing blood volume replacement. Some injuries, such as large liver lacerations and disruptions of the aorta or vena cava, cause the patient to lose massive amounts of blood very rapidly. If the patient is to survive until a surgical correction can be made, large amounts of blood need to be transfused rapidly. The major goal of the anesthesiologist is to have enough large bore intravenous catheters so that massive blood replacement can be accomplished. Large bore intravenous tubing with filters capable of high blood flow will maximize the effect of the intravenous catheters. Mechanical pumps may be used to force large volumes of fluid into the patient, but the expense and complications of mechanical pumps encourage most anesthesiologists to rely on pressure bags to force fluids. Dilutional coagulopathy occurs from replacing shed blood with blood bank blood especially during massive volume replacement. Preoperative preparation of an autotransfusion system will help replace some of the shed clotting factors as well as reduce the amount of blood needed from the blood bank.

Replacement of hemorrhagic loses requires accurate estimates of the amount of hemorrhage. The American College of Surgeons has developed a classification of hemorrhage that allows such estimation of the blood loss on admission from changes in vital signs (Table 27-5). It is important for the anesthesiologist to be familiar with these methods of quan-

TABLE 27-5. Estimated Fluid and Blood Requirements[a-c]

	Class I	Class II	Class III	Class IV
Blood loss (ml)	up to 750	750–1,500	1,500–2,000	2,000 or more
Blood loss (%BV)	up to 15	15–30	30–40	40 or more
Pulse rate	< 100	> 100	> 120	140 or higher
Blood pressure	Normal	Normal	Decreased	Decreased
Pulse pressure (mmHg)	Normal or increased	Decreased	Decreased	Decreased
Capillary blanch test	Normal	Positive	Positive	Positive
Respiratory rate	14–20	20–30	30–40	> 35
Urine output (ml/hr)	30 or more	20–30	5–15	Negligible
CNS-mental status	Slightly anxious	Mildly anxious	Anxious and confused	Confused– lethargic
Fluid replacement (3:1 rule)	Crystalloid	Crystalloid	Crystalloid + blood	Crystalloid + blood

[a] Based on patient's initial presentation.
[b] For a 70-kg male.
[c] Committee on Trauma (ATLS): Advanced trauma life support course. American College of Surgeons, Chicago, 1984, p. 185.

tifying hemorrhage in the trauma patient, since most trauma patients will have lost blood before arriving at the hospital. Such blood loss cannot be visually ascertained. Also, following blunt trauma, patients will collect blood in body cavities or spaces where it is unavailable to the circulation. Assessment of the amount of blood in such hematomas is vital for devising accurate replacement schemes. Obviously, blood loss can be assessed by visually quantifying loss from chest tubes, wounds, suction bottles, on the bed, and on the floor. It is desirable to replace shed blood with equal volumes of transfused blood once the hemorrhage continues beyond the 2 units. It should be understood, however, that applied blindly, the guidelines given in Table 27-5 can result in excessive or inadequate fluid administration. For example, a patient with a crash injury to the extremity will have hypotension out of proportion to blood loss and will require fluids in excess of the 3:1 guidelines. By contrast, a patient whose ongoing blood loss is being replaced will require less than 3:1. The use of bolus therapy with careful monitoring of the patient's response can moderate these extremes.

Since accurate blood replacement in the trauma victim who has ongoing hemorrhage is desirable, the anesthesiologist must monitor the patient to assess the degree of intravascular volume continually. Such monitoring is discussed in another section but includes measurement of pulse rate, as well as ECG waveforms, and blood pressure, including intra-arterial, right atrial (CVP), and pulmonary

arterial. Also, CO and urinary output measurements are required to assess ongoing volume losses and replacements. Accuracy is important in blood volume replacement. Excessive volume replacement can lead to cerebral and pulmonary edema and increased morbidity. Inadequate replacement of lost volume can lead to tissue ischemia in vital organs, as well as marked morbidity.

Use of blood component therapy to replace blood loss generates a dilutional coagulopathy. Hemorrhaged blood contains RBCs, plasma proteins, and platelets. Plasma proteins and platelets are involved in propagating blood clots for hemostasis. Therefore, replacement of hemorrhaged blood should include replacement of platelets and coagulation proteins, as well as RBCs. It is our policy to give 4 units of fresh-frozen plasma for the first 10 units of packed RBC replacement and 1 unit of fresh-frozen plasma for each unit of packed RBCs for further volume replacement. Platelets are given on an empirical basis when the platelet count falls below 50,000 platelets/mm^3 of blood. Aggressive replacement of coagulation factors helps prevent profound drops in platelet count. During replacement of large volumes of shed blood with blood bank products, citrate accumulates in plasma and chelates calcium. Thus, patients who receive large quantities of blood bank products will need calcium replacement to maintain proper levels of ionized calcium. Decreases in ionized calcium leads to hypotension and left ventricular depression. $CaCl_2$ is the most rapid method of increasing plasma ionized Ca^{++} levels. We give by slow intravenous injection 1 g $CaCl_2$ for every 10 units of blood replacement.

Intracranial Pressure Management

Elevated intracranial pressure is a major problem with patients who have head injuries.[10] Elevated intracranial pressure is caused by brain, CSF, and blood overfilling the rigid cranial vault. Such overfilling of the cranial vault compresses cerebral blood vessels and reduces blood flow to healthy as well as injured brain tissue. Thus, elevated intracranial pressure tends to reduce the amount of oxygen and nutrients delivered to the uninjured brain. The goal for treatment of patients with head injury is to preserve as much uninjured brain tissue as possible. One needs to be aware of all causes of elevated intracranial pressure. All etiologies of intracranial hypertension produce an increase in (1) brain tissue volume, (2) blood volume, (3) and cerebrospinal fluid (CSF) volume with the cranial vault.[36]

The increase in brain tissue volume occurs secondary to either intracerebral hemorrhage or intracerebral swelling (extracellular and cellular edema). Reducing the body water and providing an osmotic gradient for water flow from the brain cells and interstitium to blood and then to urine will reduce intracerebral water and swelling. This can be achieved with diuretics and with hyperosmolar agents such as mannitol and urea. Unfortunately, the hyperosmotic agents tend to be distributed through injured capillaries into the brain tissue intially, causing an early rise in intracranial pressure before a diuresis reduces the body and brain water and decreased intracranial pressure. Diuretics such as furosimide and ethacrynic acid not only increase water excretion at the kidney but also reduce intracellular and extra cellular brain water.[36]

The amount of CSF generated is probably not under the control of the anesthesiologist; however, CSF removal may be under his or her control. Halothane causes a progressive increase in resistance to CSF reabsorption, while fentanyl causes a decrease in resistance to CSF reabsorption.[2] Other halogenated hydrocarbons may also decrease the uptake of CSF from the brain; thus they would be contraindicated in head-injured patients.[1] This increased resistance to reabsorption of CSF from the brain could cause a prolonged increase in the cerebral CSF. Since fentanyl actually decreases the resistance of the CSF flow out of the brain, it may help relieve the brain from excess CSF.

The amount of blood volume in the brain can be controlled by the anesthesiologist, since blood volume is proportional to cerebral blood flow and cerebral blood flow is inversely proportional to the partial pressure of carbon dioxide in the arterial blood. The most rapid and effective means of lowering the intracranial pressure is to hyperventilate the patient to a low $paCO_2$, thereby reducing cerebral blood flow, hence cerebral blood volume.[48] Also the degree of interstitial edema at any given level of brain capillary permeability and cerebral blood flow is a function of the jugular venous and right atrial venous pressure. Therefore, mechanical elevation of the brain venous outflow above the level of the right atrium and the use of cardiac inotropic agents to reduce right-sided filling pressure will markedly help in lowering the level of brain edema.

Besides diuresis and hyperventilation, drug therapy can manage intracranial pressure. Thiopental decreases intracranial pressure and cerebral metabolic rate. Thus, thiopental is the main anesthetic drug for patients with head injuries. Intravenous lidocaine has been used to drop intracranial pressures acutely, especially to prevent the rise in intracranial pressure associated with coughing and airway suction maneuvers. Narcotics are indicated for neuroanesthesia to supplement thiopental because they tend to cause either no change or a decrease in cerebral metabolic rate and no change or decrease in cerebral blood flow[47] (Table 27-6).

Temperature Regulation

Prevention of hypothermia is of upmost importance in the trauma patient who requires a prolonged operation in a cold operating room. There are many maneuvers the anesthesiolo-

TABLE 27-6. Trauma Management of the Head-Injured Patient

ICP monitoring: on all head-injured patients, regardless of type of operation
Drugs that lower ICP
  Barbiturates: thiopental, 2.5–4.0 mg/kg IV, repeated every hour
  Lidocaine: 1.5 mg/kg IV
  Diuretics
Drugs that do not affect ICP (usual anesthetic doses)
  Narcotics
  Benzodiazipines
  Butyrophenones
  PEEP, to optimize oxygenation
Monitoring cardiac output and cardiac filling pressures to optimize fluid therapy
  High normal cardiac output with low filling pressures
Monitoring urine output: polyuria with low specific gravity caused by diabetes insipidus treat with vasopressin 5 units IV initially, with subsequent doses adjusted to urine output

gist can attempt to prevent the development of profound hypothermia. Keeping the patient covered as much as possible in the cold OR will prevent radiant heat loss from the skin. Keeping patients dry will prevent rapid evaporative cooling of wet skin. Keeping the OR warm will prevent rapid heat loss from large exposed surfaces, such as burned skin or exposed peritoneal contents. Other techniques that prevent the patient from rapid cooling are ventilation through a heated humidifier set to deliver inspired gas at 100 percent relative humidity above body temperatures.[51] The condensation of water vapor in the lung will transfer heat to the blood across the large alveolar-capillary membrane area. A heated humidifier also prevents evaporative water loss from the lung, preventing evaporative cooling of the patient. In extreme situations, all intravenous fluids can be warmed through warmers. Warmers are somewhat limited in their ability to provide heat input into the body, since the amount of intravenous fluid going into the patient during any particular period of time is a small fraction of the patients total weight. Therefore, the amount of heat available from the intravenous fluid will be rapidly dissipated in the whole patient. However, cardiac dysrhythmias will be less common if the venous blood bathing the sinoatrial (SA mode is not profoundly cold. The abdominal cavity should be irrigated with warm saline following a laporatomy. Warm fluids can be instilled in the bladder or the stomach in order to help warm the patient. In

selected cases, the use of partial extracorporeal circulation with a heat exchange may be indicated, if the patient can tolerate a brief period of heparinization.

Profound hypothermia in the trauma patient following severe hemorrhagic shock may be untreatable and diagnostic of massive cell death. If the patient's oxygen consumption has been severely reduced by cell necrosis, body heat production will be severely compromised and hypothermia may be the first sign of death.

Hyperthermia is another temperature regulation problem that effects the trauma patient. This occurs especially following maxillofacial trauma. These patients are well covered in the OR except for the face. They can also rapidly develop bacteremia from multiple fractures through the perinasal sinuses. Hyperthermic patients need to be evaluated on the basis of ABGs to rule out malignant hyperthermia. Cooling attempts include reducing heated humidifiers to below body temperature (about 35°C), running intravenous fluids at room temperature, and exposing more of the patients skin. Also, appropriate antibiotic therapy should be initiated or continued.

Some patients will develop the syndrome of malignant hyperthermia with total uncontrolled temperature regulation.[22] These patients need to be treated with ice cold intravenous solutions and removal of triggering anesthetic drugs to stop the malignant hyperthermia process, intravenous dantrolene to restore cellular homeostasis, and, in extreme cases, packing in ice or cooling by attaching to cardiopulmonary bypass pump with a cold heat exchanger. Classically malignant hyperthermia is distinguished from other etiologies of fever and tachycardia by the presence of metabolic and respiratory acidosis. An extremely high oxygen consumption and carbon dioxide production associated with uncoupled mitochondrial oxidation causes the acid–base disturbance and the fever. Treatment is outlined in Table 27-7.

Prolonged Anesthesia

Patients who suffer severe blunt multiple trauma become a real physiologic management problem for the anesthesiologist not only be-

TABLE 27-7. Malignant Hyperthermia

Diagnosis of malignant hyperthermia
  Tachycardia: > 120/min precedes temperature rise
  Hyperthermia: rapid rise $\geq 40°C$
  Metabolic/respiratory acidosis: $PaCO_2 \geq 50$
    mmHg + BE $\leq$ −3 mEq/L
Treatment
  All anesthetics turned off; machine changed to avoid
    trace contamination of anesthetics
  Infusion of cold intravenous normal saline at a rate
    to maintain urine output $\geq$ 1 ml/kg/hr
  Dantrolene 3 mg/kg IV, repeated if necessary q 30
    min to total dose of 10 mg/kg/IV
  Patient transferred to ICU for monitoring cardiovascu-
    lar and temperature
  Maintenance dantrolene 3 mg/kg IV q6h
Prophylaxis
  Administration of safe drugs (e.g., droperidol, fenta-
    nyl, morphine, nalbuphine, pancuronium, O_2 and
    N_2O) as needed to provide general anesthesia
  Pretreatment with dantrolene 3 mg/kg IV

cause they are "sick," having suffered major disruption of many organs systems and therefore require a large degree of monitoring and therapy, but also because they are a challenge to anesthetize safely. The patient's best chance of survival postoperatively occurs if all injuries are treated during the first operation. This is especially true with multiple fractures. If most of the fractures are internally fixated, the patient can be mobilized in bed and turned to provide good pulmonary care and can receive adequate chest physical therapy in bed. These patients can also be mobilized out of bed early, thereby reducing pulmonary complications. If the multiple fractures are casted or put in traction so that the patient cannot be fully mobilized, the postoperative complications and the mortality are increased.[21]

It is advantageous to treat all injuries at the initial surgery immediately after stabilization following admission. Such operations may be extremely long. This presents a new challenge to the anesthesiologist, who now has to provide continuous intensive care under anesthesia for a very sick patient for an extended period. Such prolonged intraoperative critical care requires a teamwork approach to anesthesia. More than one anesthesia provider is required to keep up the intense therapy over a long period.

There are very few reports in the literature concerning the problems of extended anesthesia.[13] One of the problems with inhalation anesthetics is the anesthetic saturation of body tissues after a prolonged period, which will necessitate corresponding a prolonged period of washout of inhaled anesthetic.[13] The patient is usually lying in an unchanging position on the operating table for a very long period of time, which can lead to blood pooling in the dependent regions. This may also result in skin necrosis and decubitus ulcers at points of pressure. The same considerations hold true for the lungs because V/Q distribution will be affected by prolonged lying in one position.[38] Increased V/Q ratios in the nondependent part of the lung and decreased ratios and localized regions of pulmonary interstitual edema in the dependent part of the lung need to be treated with periodic sighs. Failure to provide adequate tidal volumes to the lungs will lead to alveolar collapse and atelectasis. There does not seem to be any particular cardiovascular toxicity associated with prolonged anesthesia; however, prolonged surgery may expose a patient to a long period of surgical hemorrhage and blood replacement. Transfusion requirements will mount up in long periods of surgery. All the problems associated with massive transfusion requirements that conspire to produce the posttraumatic acute respiratory distress syndrome (ARDS) are seen in the patient requiring prolonged surgery. These patients need to be monitored very carefully so that the anesthesia care team can provide an ICU environment. Excellent intraoperative critical care will help these patients survive after a prolonged operation.

Transportation

The critically ill trauma patient needs special attention during transportation. These patients require transportation from the ER to the OR and the x-ray suites. Since these transportations often involve long distances and elevator rides, patients need to be monitored during transportation just as seriously as they do in the OR. The unmonitored patient can suffer a cardiac arrest or have a severe hypotensive episode during transport that will compromise the overall outcome. During transportation, a portable battery-powered monitor is used to monitor the ECG and intra-arterial pressure if the patient has an arterial line. Many of these portable monitors will also monitor a second pressure source, which could be the intracranial pressure or the pulmonary artery pressure.

The patient's intravenous solutions need to be hung on the transporting bed in such a way that they will continue to function during transportation. All medications infused through a pump need to be continued during transportation. Failure to continue intravenous fluids and drugs during transport will jeopardize the patient's care.

Hypovolemic patients who have vasoconstricted to maintain blood pressure may develop profound hypotension following a sudden change in body position. This occurs when the stretcher goes over a bump or around a corner too fast, or when the patient is transferred from the transport cart to the x-ray table or OR table. This hypotension occurs secondary to gravitational redistribution of blood volume within the body, decreasing venous return. Therefore, the patient's volume status must be appropriately adjusted before transport and the patient should not be moved too roughly. A secure airway and source of enriched oxygen needs to be obtained before transportation and arrangements are made for ventilatory equipment to be ready at the site and sometimes during transport as well (Table 27-8).

Transportation also involves intrahospital transportation. The major problem with transporting the critically ill patient between hospitals is to provide appropriate ventilatory support. Human fatigue often sets in when patient ventilation is provided by prolonged manual bag squeezing. After long periods of hand ven-

TABLE 27-8. Transportation of the Traumatized Patient [a]

*A*irway: Intubate comatose patients or patients with respiratory distress before transporting.
*B*reathing: Portable ventilator may be needed; maintain PEEP during transport.
*C*ardiovascular monitoring: Battery-powered ECG, pressure monitor.
*S*upportive systems: Maintain all necessary intravenous infusions, use battery-powered pumps; portable defibrillator.

[a] Given technologic advances, even the severely injured patient can be moved provided the appropriate equipment and personnel are available. Do not forget to recharge the batteries after use.

tilation, the ventilating person's hand tires and the tidal volume that is delivered decreases. Various kinds of transport ventilators have been developed to reduce danger to the patient during transport and should be utilized during intrahospital transportation.

In summary, the anesthesiologist caring for trauma patients faces many challenges. These include limited preoperative history, devastating injuries that necessitate many surgical procedures to save the patient, hypovolemic shock requiring massive volume replacement, potential interactions of anesthetic drugs with the patient's altered pathophysiology, requirements for extensive intraoperative monitoring to provide critical care in the OR, and responsibility for safe transportation of these patients. Skillful delivery of anesthetic care to trauma patients will help decrease the morbidity and mortality associated with trauma.

REFERENCES

1. Artru AA: Effects of enflurane and isoflurane on resistance to reabsorption of cerebrospinal fluid in dogs. Anesthesiology 61: 329, 1984
2. Artu AA: Effects of halothane and fentanyl anesthesia on resistance to reabsorption of CSF. J Neurosurg 60: 252, 1984
3. Ayella RJ: Radiologic Management of the Massively Traumatized Patient. Williams & Wilkins, Baltimore, 1978
4. Ayres SM: Ventricular function. I(C)1. In Shoemaker WC, Thompson WL (eds): Critical Care State of the Art. Vol. 1. Society of Critical Care Medicine. Fullerton, CA, 1980
5. Baker SP, O'Neill B, Karpf RS: The Injury Fact Book. Lexington Books, Lexington, MA, 1984
6. Barash PG, Chen Y, Kitahata LM, Kopriva CJ: The hemodynamic tracking system: A method of data management and guide for cardiovascular therapy. Anesth Analg 59: 169, 1980
7. Berk JL: Multiple organ failure. p. 3. In Berk JL, Sampliner JE (eds): Handbook of Critical Care. 2nd ed. Little, Brown, Boston, 1982
8. Blacher RS: Awareness during surgery. Anesthesiology 61:1, 1984
9. Bogetz MS, Katz JA: Recall of surgery for major trauma. Anesthesiology 61: 6, 1984

10. Bruce DA, Matjasko J, McKay RD: Head trauma. p. 283. In Newfield P, Cottrell JE (eds): Handbook of Neuro Anesthesia: Clinical and Physiological Essentials. Little, Brown, Boston, 1983
11. Bruce DL: Alcoholism and anesthesia. Anesth Analg 62: 84, 1983
12. Byrnes D: Management of the head-injured patient. p. 107. In Salcman M (ed): Neurologic Emergencies Recognition and Management. Raven Press, New York, 1980
13. Caplan RA, Long MC: Prolonged anesthesia management and sequelae of a two-day general anesthetic. Anesth Analg 63:353, 1984
14. Catron DG: The Anesthesiologist's Handbook. 3rd ed. University Park Press, Baltimore, 1983
15. Cohen PJ: Effect of anesthetics on mitochondrial function. Anesthesiology 39: 153, 1973
16. Dripps RD, Eckerhoff JE, Vardam JD: Introduction to Anesthesia, The Principles of Safe Practice. 6th ed. WB Saunders, Philadelphia, 1982
17. Eisele JH: Cardiovascular effects of nitrous oxide. p. 125. In Eger EI (ed): Nitrous Oxide/N_2O. Elsevier, New York, 1985
18. Goldberg M: Systemic reactions to intravascular contrast media. Anesthesiology 57: 9, 1982
19. Goldman L, Wolf MA: The heart and circulation. p. 1. In Vandam LD (ed): To Make the Patient Ready for Anesthesia Medical Care of the Surgical Patient. Addison-Wesley, Menlo Park, CA, 1980
20. Goldstein A, Aronow L, Kalman SM: Principles of Drug Action: The Basis of Pharmacology. 2nd ed. Wiley, New York, 1974
21. Gori RJA, Gimberse JSF, Van Nieberk JLM, et al: Early osteosynthesis and prophylactic mechanical ventilation in the multitrauma patient. J Trauma 22: 895, 1982
22. Gronert G: Malignant hyperthermia. Anesthesiology 53: 395, 1980
23. Guyton AG, Jones CE, Coleman TG: Circulatory Physiology: Cardiac Output and Its Regulation. WB Saunders, Philadelphia, 1973
24. Hug CC: Pharmacokinetics of drugs administered intravenously. Anesth Analag 57: 704, 1978
25. Izenstein BZ, Dluhy RG, Williams GH: Endocrinology. p. 112. In Vandam LD (ed): To Make the Patient Ready for Anesthesia Medical Care of the Surgical Patient. Addison-Wesley, Menlo Park, CA, 1980
26. Jennett B, Teasdale G: Aspects of coma after severe head injury. Lancet 1: 879, 1977
27. Lake C, Duckworth EN, DiFazio CA, et al: Cardiovascular effects of nalbuphine in patients with coronary or vascular heart disease. Anesthesiology 57: 498, 1982
28. Lebowitz PW, Ramsey FM, Savarese JJ, et al: Combination of pancuronium and metocurine, neuromuscular and hemodynamic advantages over pancuronium alone. Anesth Analg 60: 12, 1981
29. Lilleaasen P, Semb B, Linberg H, et al: Hemodynamic changes with administration of nitrous oxide during coronary artery surgery. Acta Anaesthesiol Scan 25: 533, 1981
30. Lowery BD, Cloutier CT, Carey LC: Electrolyte solutions in resuscitation in human hemorrhagic shock. Surg Gynecol Obster 133: 273, 1971
31. McCabe JB, Angelos MG: Injury to the head and face in patients with cervical spine injury. Am J Emerg Med 2: 333, 1984
32. McGruder MR, Cristofforetti R, Difazio CA: Balanced anesthesia with nalbuphine hydrochloride. Anesthesiol Rev 7: 25, 1980
33. MIller RD: Coagulation defects associated with massive blood transfusion Ann Surg 174: 794, 1971
34. Moncrief JA: Burns. N Engl J Med 288: 445, 1973
35. Moore FD: Effects of hemorrhage on body composition. N Engl J Med 273: 567, 1965
36. Newfield J, Cottrell JE: Handbook of Neuro Anesthesia: Clinical and Physiological Essentials. Little, Brown, Boston, 1983
37. Pearce AC, Jones RM: Smoking and anesthesia: Preoperative abstinence and perioperative morbidity. Anesthesiology 61: 576, 1984
38. Rehder K, Knopp TJ, Sessler AD, Didier EP: Ventilation–perfusion relationships in young healthy awake and anesthetized-paralyzed man. J Appl Phys 47: 745, 1979
39. Rembert FC: State of health at time of injury. p. 17. In Geiseche AH (ed): Anesthesia for the Surgery of Trauma. FA Davis, Philadelphia, 1976
40. Roberts J: Fundamentals of Tracheal Intubation. Grune & Stratton, New York, 1982
41. Roizen MD: Routine preoperative evaluation. p. 3. In Miller RD (ed): Anesthesia. Vol. 1. Churchill Livingstone, New York, 1981
42. Rosen SM: Renal failure during and after shock. Int Anesthesiol Clin 7: 861, 1969
43. Rutherford RB: Thoracic injuries. p. 371. In Zuidema GD, Rutherford RB, Bollinger WF (eds): The Management of Trauma. WB Saunders, Philadelphia, 1979
44. Savarese JJ, Kitz RJ: Pharmacology of relaxants. p. 153. In Hershey SG (ed): ASA Refresher Courses in Anesthesiology. JB Lippincott, Philadelphia, 1975
45. Schulte-Sasse U, Hess W, Tarnow J: Pulmonary vascular response to nitrous oxide in patients with normal and high pulmonary vascular resistance. Anesthesiology 57: 9, 1982
46. Sellick BA: Cricoid pressure to control regurgitation of stomach contents during induction of anesthesia. Lancet 2, 404, 1961

47. Shapiro HM: Intracranial hypertension: Therapeutic and anesthetic considerations. Anesthesiology 43: 445, 1975

48. Shapiro HM, Wyte SR, Harris AB: Ketamine anaesthesia in patients with intracranial pathology. Br. J Anaesth 44: 1200, 1972

49. Shehadi WH: Problems and toxicity of contrast agents. AJR 97: 762, 1966

50. Shoemaker WC, Pierchala C, Chang P, State D: Prediction of outcome and severity of illness by analysis of the frequency distributions of cardiorespiratory variables. Crit Care Med 5: 82, 1977

51. Stone DR, Downs JB, Paul WL, Perkins HM: Adult body temperature and heated humidification of anesthetic gases during general anesthesia. Anesth Analg 60: 736, 1981

52. Theye RA, Michenfelder JD: Whole-body and organ VO_2 changes with enflurane, isoflurane and halothane. Br J Anaesth 47: 813, 1975

53. Thompson WL: Poisoning: The twentieth-century black death. I(N)1. In Shoemaker WC, Thompson WL (eds): Critical Care State of the Art. Society of Critical Care Medicine, Fullerton, CA, 1980

54. Trunkey DD: Trauma. Sci 249(2): 28, 1983

55. Watson TD, Lee JF: Intoxication and trauma. p. 31. In Giesecke AH Jr (ed): Anesthesia for the Surgery of Trauma. FA Davis, Philadelphia, 1976

56. Wilkenson GR: Pharmacokinetics in disease states modifying body perfusion. p. 13. In Benet LZ (ed): The Effect of Disease States on Drug Pharmacokinetics. American Pharmaceutical Association, Washington, DC, 1976

57. Zimmerman BL: Uncommon problems in acute trauma. p. 635. In Katz J, Benumof J, Kadis LB (eds): Anesthesia and Uncommon Diseases. WB Saunders, Philadelphia, 1981

58. Zsigmond EK, Domino EF: Ketamine clinical pharmacology, pharmacokinetics and current clinical uses. Anesthesiol Rev 7(4): 13, 1980

28

Acute Thoracic Injuries

Marvin M. Kirsh

The combination of technologic advances and man's fascination with high-speed propulsion has produced a steady increase in disasters on our streets and highways. Every year more than 200,000 people are killed in road accidents around the world. Approximately 25 percent of these traumatic civilian fatalities are due entirely to thoracic injuries, while in another 25 to 50 percent, injury of the thorax is a major contributing factor. Twenty-five years ago the mortality from isolated chest injuries approached 50 percent. However, improvement in ambulance transport systems and in prehospital care has not only increased the number of potentially salvagable patients but has lowered the mortality to less than 15 percent as well. It is hoped that earlier recognition, better understanding of the pathophysiology, and improvement in management will even further reduce the number of deaths due to thoracic injuries.

GENERAL PRINCIPLES OF MANAGEMENT

The condition on arrival in the emergency room of the person who has sustained blunt trauma to the chest varies greatly. Most patients are first seen in a critical condition with obvious chest injuries and require immediate treatment. It is also important to recognize that serious intrathoracic injury can occur without obvious external chest injuries or rib fractures. The semirigid chest wall of the elderly absorbs energy in the process of fracturing ribs that would otherwise be transmitted to the lung parenchyma and great vessels. However, the flexible chest wall of the young patient will transmit essentially all the kinetic energy to the thoracic contents. Thus the absence of rib fractures does not rule out the possibility of life-threatening injuries. If the injury is not recognized early, death frequently results. The physician caring for patients who are suffering from blunt chest trauma must not be deceived by an initially good condition and must always be alert for the likelihood of later clinical deterioration. Careful and frequent observation of any patient with a blunt chest injury is as important as the initial evaluation.

Patients with severe thoracic injuries frequently sustain multiple extrathoracic injuries. The physician's attention must not be diverted from thoracic injuries by obvious extrathoracic injuries, such as abdominal or central nervous system (CNS) injuries. After any immediate life-threatening emergencies have been treated, the physician should undertake a careful history, if possible, and should methodically examine all systems in the injured patient. Knowledge of the patient's past medical history, allergies, and medications may influence subsequent therapy. Guidelines to the likely injuries may be gained from the knowledge of the circumstances under which the injury occurred.

Arterial blood gas (ABG) determinations are a means of indirectly measuring and following the functional impairment caused by pulmonary injury. Often the first sign of impending respiratory failure may be the marked hypoxia exhibited. Serial ABG determinations compared with baseline data obtained on room air may be useful in predicting trends in respiratory function. Using a FIO_2 0.21 permits consistent serial comparisons and gives a more accurate estimation of the severity of the respiratory impairment. Patients should be followed initially every 4 hours for 48 hours with ABG determinations to detect subtle changes that prompt modification of treatment.

PULMONARY CONTUSION

Pulmonary contusion is defined as damage to the lung parenchyma that results in edema and hemorrhage without accompanying pulmo-

nary laceration. Although often mild and frequently masked by other more dramatic injuries, pulmonary contusion deserves careful consideration in the management of any patient with blunt chest trauma because it is now well recognized that left untreated, it is frequently progressive and may be fatal because of respiratory insufficiency.

Pathogenesis

Pulmonary contusion usually results from a compression—decompression injury to the chest wall. Most of the victims of automobile accidents sustain pulmonary injury when their chest strikes the steering wheel during deceleration. The precise pathogenesis of pulmonary injury in these patients is unknown, but most believe it is analogous to the mechanism thought to operate in a blast injury—a forceful high-pressure wave that compresses the thoracic cavity. The force is also transmitted to the lung by virtue of its continuity with the tissues of the chest wall. The increase in intrathoracic pressure compresses the lung by diminishing the size of the thorax and results in parenchymal hemorrhage and edema. When the force of compression is removed, decompression occurs and the distorted thorax springs back creating an instant of negative intrathoracic pressure that leads to additional injury in the areas ruptured during compression. Among the factors that influence the severity of the lesions produced are the amount of padding on the thoracic wall and the flexibility of the chest wall. Zuckerman[19] was able to prevent animals from developing lung injury by protecting the chest with a sponge jacket when the animals were subjected to blast explosions. His finding is supported by our clinical observations that obese patients do not sustain as severe pulmonary contusions as asthenic patients. If the ribs are sufficiently elastic, severe compression of the lung can occur without a break in the costal cage. Some of the most severe pulmonary contusions we have seen have occurred in patients who exhibited no rib fractures or discontinuity in the chest cage. In the past, it was conjectured that fractures of the ribs served as a protective mechanism by breaking the force of trauma before severe compression of the chest occurred, thus preventing or reducing the severity of the injury. This belief is no longer considered valid by some since flail chest is frequently complicated by pulmonary contusion.

Pathophysiology

Pulmonary contusion is frequently associated with multiple injuries and the injured lung is often subjected to incidental resuscitative measures that ultimately prove harmful, namely, the administration of large volumes of fluid that are directed at the other injuries. The adverse effects of rapid administration of large volumes of fluid in animals with pulmonary contusion have been shown by several investigators. Fulton and Peter[4] studied the physiologic and histologic effects of rapid infusion of saline solution into animals with pulmonary contusion. These workers found damage not only to the injured lung but to the noninjured lung as well. After the pulmonary contusion, the pulmonary blood flow through the damaged lung decreased in association with an increase in pulmonary vascular resistance. The pulmonary blood flow increased through the uninjured lung with a decrease in pulmonary vascular resistance. Rapid infusion of saline solution produced an increase in pulmonary artery pressure and blood flow, particularly in the uninjured lung. The fall in pulmonary vascular resistance in the normal lung allowed the pressure to reach the capillaries. The increased capillary pressure forced blood and fluid out of capillaries into the interstitium and alveoli with resultant pulmonary congestion. As congestion develops in one part of the lung, the pulmonary blood flow shifts into another portion of the lung with lowered resistance and the same results. Thus, the process is self-perpetuating.

The animals in this study demonstrated more intrapulmonary shunting and resultant systemic hypoxemia than did the group with pulmonary contusion that did not receive rapid infusion of saline solution. Administration of large volumes of fluid (greater than 30 ml/kg of body weight) produced alterations in osmotic pressure. Since the lung has a greater propensity to leak fluid into interstitial spaces than other organs do, the decrease in colloid osmotic pressure tends to accentuate transcapillary fluid movement resulting in interstitial pulmonary edema. The percentage of water increased in both the normal and the contused lungs of the experimental animals. The results of the studies suggest that some of the progression of pulmonary contusion as seen clinically and radiographically is due to damage in both the normal and the injured lung. Similar conclusions have been reached by Trinkle and associates,[15] who demonstrated that the contused lung was damaged by noncolloid fluid administration. These investigators also found that

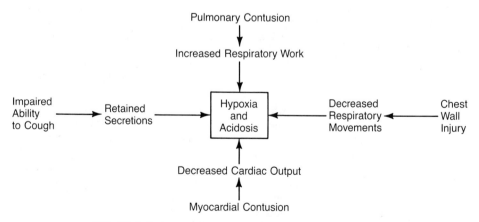

FIG. 28-1 Pathophysiology of untreated pulmonary contusion.

when plasma was used, even in large volumes, there was a minimum increase in the weight of the injured lung or its water content. By maintaining a normal colloid osmotic pressure, plasma prevented local water loss into the injured lung.

The pathologic changes found in pulmonary contusion are the result of alveolar capillary damage with interstitial and intra-alveolar extravasation of blood as well as interstitial edema. The injury as a rule does not produce much more than intra-alveolar hemorrhage initially. Edema then begins to accumulate in the interstices of the lung and enters the interstitium and the alveoli. After the influx of edema, the cellular response to injury occurs.

The combination of blood, fluid, and cellular debris leads to atelectasis by obstruction of the bronchioles and alveoli (Fig. 28-1). Trauma to the lung stimulates the tracheobronchial mucosa, and there is an increase in mucus production. The patient is unable to rid himself or herself of the pulmonary secretions because pain makes the cough ineffective and there is reduced motion of the chest wall from soft tissue injury. Further atelectasis results, and a vicious cycle occurs with the production of more secretions. The resultant atelectasis removes these areas as effective units of ventilation and produces alterations in ventilation/perfusion ratios with systemic hypoxia. Intrapulmonary shunting may be increased in these patients if they receive rapid infusion of large volumes of crystalloid solutions or massive blood transfusions without the use of fine-screen infiltration. Resistance to air flow is markedly increased. The elasticity of the lungs is reduced and more respiratory work is needed to move air in and out of the lungs. The oxygen demand for the increased work of respiration cannot be met and an oxygen deficit occurs with additional hypoxia and respiratory acidosis. Another vicious circle occurs, with hypoxia begetting hypoxia. Circulatory adaptations occur in an effort to maintain oxygen delivery, namely, an increase in the pulse rate and cardiac output (CO). If the patient's CO does not increase above normal levels to satisfy the increased demands for oxygen delivery to the tissues, myocardial decompensation occurs. Similarly, myocardial failure occurs if it becomes necessary for the patient

to maintain an increased CO for a prolonged period of time. Myocardial decompensation results in inadequate tissue perfusion with accumulation of lactic acid. Thus the resultant metabolic acidosis is superimposed on the already established respiratory acidosis. Additional myocardial decompensation may result from a myocardial contusion in 15 to 25 percent of these patients. Unless it can be corrected, the combination of metabolic and respiratory acidosis may prove fatal.

Roentgenographic Findings

The roentgenographic findings depend on the severity of the pulmonary contusion and may vary widely in both distribution and appearance. In 70 percent of patients, roentgenographic changes occur within 1 hour after injury. In the remaining 30 percent there may be a time lag of 4 to 6 hours between the time of injury and the appearance of radiographic abnormalities.

Two basic roentgenographic patterns have been described for this lesion. The most frequent finding is a pulmonary infiltrate characterized by patchy, ill-defined areas of increased parenchymal density. The degree of involvement may range from small localized areas (nodular densities) to extensive hemogeneous opacification in one or both lungs that is caused by intra-alveolar hemorrhage. The lung that is extensively affected by pulmonary contusion is larger in size than the uninvolved lung. In addition, the diaphragm on the side of the injured lung is pushed down by the increased weight of the lung. The less frequent pattern is a linear irregular infiltrate with a peribronchial distribution produced by peribronchiolar or perivascular hemorrhage.

After treatment is instituted, signs of resolution usually begin within 48 to 72 hours, but it may take as long as 14 to 21 days for complete clearing to occur. If resolution does not begin to occur or if there is progression of the lesion despite appropriate treatment, a superimposed complication such as a fat embolism, pneumonia, or a pulmonary embolism should be suspected and aggressively sought.

Management

It is important to remember that regardless of the severity of the injury to the lung there may be a delay in the onset of symptoms as seen in the roentgenographic findings. In addition, the clinical signs of hypoxia may be difficult to recognize, especially in patients with multiple injuries. Arterial blood gas measurement is the only effective way to accurately evaluate the efficiency of gas exchange. An arterial oxygen tension (PaO_2) of less than 60 mmHg with the patient breathing room air or a PaO_2 of less than 300 mmHg with the patient breathing 100 percent oxygen is indicative of significant pulmonary dysfunction. The presence of an elevated arterial $PaCO_2$ (40 mmHg), along with hypoxemia is an even more ominous finding. Normally, the patient with hypoxemia hyperventilates and thus any elevation of $PaCO_2$ is evidence of marked reduction in pulmonary function and indicates the need for respirator support. These determinations will help to prevent delays in instituting treatment.

It should be emphasized that the keys to successful management of patients with pulmonary contusion are as follows: (1) early and vigorous therapy, as the first 24 hours of treatment are by far the most important; (2) restoration and maintenance of oxygenation while avoiding resuscitative measures that might aggravate the pulmonary contusion; (3) good tracheobronchial care, including intratracheal suction and physical therapy. The following steps should be taken in the treatment of pulmonary contusion:

1. Insert a percutaneous radial artery catheter for frequent blood gas determination and a Swan-Ganz catheter to monitor filling pressures and CO.
2. Restrict crystalloid solution to 1,000 to 1,500 during resuscitation and 50 ml/hr thereafter.
3. To decrease excess fluid within the lung, administer 40 mg furosemide immediately and 20 mg every 6 to 12 hours until no longer needed.
4. Maintain serum pressure by infusing albumin (25 g/L fluid) at 50 ml/hr for 48 to 72 hours.

5. Since large doses of steroids have been shown to reduce the size of experimentally induced pulmonary contusion by lysosomal stabilization of the cell wall and decreasing capillary permeability, administer methylprednisolone (30 mg/kg body weight) immediately and in divided doses thereafter for 2 to 4 days.
6. Insert a nasogastric tube and connect to low suction.
7. Obtain adequate relief of pain by the use of small, frequent doses of narcotics or intercostal nerve blocks.
8. Since the damaged lung is susceptible to infection, broad-spectrum antibodies should be administered. Cultures of the sputum should be obtained periodically and antibiotics altered accordingly.
9. If the patients are not intubated, maintain PaO_2 above 60 mmHg by administering oxygen by mask or nasal cannula. Sterile techniques must be employed during endotracheal suctioning. Ultrasonic nebulization by mist or intermittent positive-pressure ventilation (IPPV) with bronchodilators such as aminophylline should be used when there is evidence of bronchospasm.
10. Indications for ventilator support through an endotracheal tube are listed in Table 28-1. The lowest FIO_2 should be used to maintain PaO_2 at 60 mmHg. Use PEEP if unable to maintain PaO_2 of at least 60 mmHg on an FIO_2 of 0.6. Indications for weaning are listed in Table 28-2.
11. Maintain HCT between 40 and 45 percent

TABLE 28-1. Indications for Respirator Support

Function	Value
Mechanics	
Respiratory rate (per min)	> 35
Vital capacity (ml/kg body weight)	< 15
FEV_1 (ml/kg body weight)	< 10
Inspiratory force (cmH_2O)	<−25
Oxygenation	
PaO_2 (mmHg)	< 60 (suppl. O_2)
A–aDO_2 (mmHg)	>450 (on 100% O_2)
Ventilation	
$PaCO_2$ (mmHg)	> 55
V_D/V_T	> 0.60

TABLE 28-2. Indications for Weaning from Respirator

Function	Value
Mechanics	
Respiratory rate (per min)	< 30
Vital capacity (ml/kg body weight)	> 15
FEV$_1$ (ml/kg body weight)	> 15
Inspiratory force (cm H$_2$O)	>−20
Oxygenation	
PaO$_2$ (mmHg)	> 60 (suppl. O$_2$)
A–aDO$_2$ (mmHg)	< 300 (on 100% O$_2$)
Ventilation	
PaCO$_2$ (mmHg)	< 40
V$_D$/V$_T$	< 0.60

by transfusions of whole blood or packed red blood cells (RBCs). Bank blood contains a reduced amount of 2,3-diphosphoglycerate; consequently, the ability of Hb to release oxygen is decreased. Therefore, freshly drawn blood or packed RBCs should be used to increase the oxygen carrying capacity of blood.

12. Maintain pH between 7.35 and 7.45, since an alkaline pH may shift the oxygen dissociation curve to the left and reduce the ability of Hb to release oxygen.

13. A significant contribution to the demise of many severely injured patients today is inadequate nutritional support. In patients with significant chest injury, the impairment of host defenses secondary to malnutrition with subsequent sepsis and death becomes a major concern. These patients often have associated injuries that limit mobilization, create increased metabolic demands, and compromise the mode of enteral alimentation. Combinations of alimentation utilizing peripheral, enteral, and central routes are all employed early to stop catabolism. Immediately after these patients are resuscitated attention must be directed to providing nutrition support to avoid the complications of sepsis and multisystem failure.

Outcome

The course of illness in most patients is determined by the severity of the initial injury. In those patients with mild pulmonary contu-

sion and who do not require ventilatory support, the course of the illness is characterized by rapid resolution of the parenchymal abnormality (in 72 to 96 hours) and return of ABGs to normal. In those patients who require ventilatory support there is a gradual resolution of the parenchymal abnormalities in association with improvement in clinical condition and ABGs by 10 to 14 days. Patients can be successfully weaned from the ventilator at that time (Table 28-2). In any patient with a pulmonary contusion in whom there is a delay in the radiographic improvement, one should suspect a superimposed complication such as pneumonia, fat embolism, or pulmonary embolism. Early detection of these complications is possible by serial determinations of the alveolar–arterial oxygen gradient. The value of serial determinations of alveolar–arterial gradients in patients with chest trauma in evaluating the efficacy of respirator support and the progress of the pulmonary abnormalities has been emphasized by Wise et al.[17] In patients with pulmonary contusion who survive and who do not develop superimposed pulmonary complications, the alveolar–arterial gradient will rise to a maximum on the third or fourth day but fall to initial levels or below by the fifth or sixth day. Patients in whom pulmonary complications develop have progressively wider alveolar–arterial oxygen gradients that may remain elevated. At times, these changes in gradients occur even before the decline in pulmonary function becomes apparent either clinically or radiographically. Despite optimum therapy, approximately 15 percent of the patients die from progressive respiratory insufficiency.

CHEST WALL FRACTURES

First Rib Fractures

The first rib in its protected position low in the neck is short, broad, flat, and relatively thick. Consequently, it requires an extremely violent force to become fractured. The mechanism of these isolated first rib fractures is a sudden forward movement of the head and neck. In motor vehicle accidents the movement of the torso or head is stopped quickly by a seat belt, dashboard, steering wheel, or windshield. The net vector of force causes a bending strain on the first rib and results in a fracture usually just behind the scalene medius since the first rib has two major points of fixation—anteriorly at the clavicle and manubrium and posteriorly at the transverse process of the first thoracic vertebra. Major chest, abdominal, and cardiac injuries are infrequent, since the force needed to fracture the first rib is confined. However, there is a high incidence of serious maxillofacial or neurologic injuries.[14] Injury to the subclavian artery and neck has been reported to occur in 5 to 15 percent of patients with first rib fracture. The indications for arteriography in first rib fractures whether isolated or not should include patients with (1) absent or decreased upper extremity pulse, (2) evidence of brachial plexis injury, (3) marked displacement of fragments especially if posterior, (4) altered serial chest roentgenograms (increased pleural cap or hemothorax), and (5) subclavian groove fracture (anteriorly). There is no specific therapy for the treatment of first rib fracture. Their only significance is to alert the physician to the possibility of associated intrathoracic and extrathoracic injuries.[16]

because of its protected position between the flare of the costal margins bilaterally.

Severe trauma is usually necessary to produce a sternal fracture; this explains the high incidence of serious associated injuries (Table 28-3). The actual presence of the sternal fracture suggests that severe associated injuries might be present.

The diagnosis is confirmed by visualization of the fracture site on only a lateral or oblique chest roentgenogram. All patients with sternal fractures should be investigated for associated cardiac or other intrathoracic injuries. Surgical treatment of the sternal fracture should be delayed until evaluation and possible treatment of the associated injuries have been completed. Treatment of the sternal fractures is dependent on its severity and in undisplaced fractures, treatment should be directed toward the relief of pain. Analgesics will usually suffice, but on occasion the injection of lidocaine or related compounds into and around the fracture site are needed for relief of pain. If pain cannot be relieved by these measures, operative stabilization should be performed. Open reduction and stabilization should be carried out on all patients with severely displaced fractures, especially those who also exhibit paradoxical motion. The mortality associated with sternal fractures is directly attributable to the associated injuries and not to the fracture itself.

Fractured Sternum

Fractures of the sternum most often occur following direct injury to the front of the chest (e.g., from a steering wheel or a forceful blow), but they can also occur following any crushing or hyperflexion injury. The sternum is seldom fractured in children and young adults because of the elasticity of the ribs and anterior costal cartilage. Most sternal fractures occur in the body of the sternum near its junction with the manubrium. Because of fixation to the manubrium sterni, there is usually anterior displacement and overriding of the distal fragment. Despite this overriding, the periosteum on the posterior surface of the sternum remains intact. Fractures of the xiphoid process rarely occur

Rib Fractures

Fractures of the ribs are more common in adults than in children because the cartilage in children is more resilient and can absorb the impact without breaking. On the other hand, the ribs of elderly persons are brittle and can be broken even by minor degrees of trauma. The ribs usually break at the point of impact or at the posterior angle, which structurally is the weakest point. The fifth through ninth ribs are the ones most commonly broken. The lower two ribs are mobile and yielding and therefore fracture least often. Because of the location, lower rib fractures are often associated with injuries to the liver, spleen, and kidney.

**TABLE 28-3.
Associated Injuries with
Fractured Sternum**

Flail chest
Pulmonary contusion
Ruptured bronchus
Hemothorax or pneumothorax
Hemopericardium
Lacerated pericardium
Myocardial contusion
Valvular cardiac injuries
Cardiac rupture
Ruptured thoracic aorta
Abdominal visceral injuries
Spinal injuries

The number of ribs fractured and the degree of displacement of rib fragments and injury to the underlying lung are dependent on the force and direction of the impact and the area of its distribution. If the injuring force is applied over a wide area, especially in the anteroposterior projection, the ribs buckle outward and thus break in the mid-shaft position without injuring the pulmonary parenchyma. A direct injury tends to drive the rib fragments inward over a limited area and can cause lacerations of the pleura, pulmonary parenchyma, and intercostal vessels producing pneumothorax, hemothorax, or both, which may be life threatening when pneumothorax or massive intrathoracic bleeding occurs.

A delayed complication that is apt to occur in elderly patients or in patients with preexisting chronic lung disease is pneumonia and possibly respiratory failure. Rib fractures are invariably accompanied by pain. To reduce the pain to tolerable levels, the patient both consciously and unconsciously restricts excursion of the chest wall by shallow breathing. Such shallow breathing results in fewer alveoli being ventilated. The unaerated alveoli collapse, secretions accummulate, and atelectasis develops. Because coughing causes pain, the patient consciously reduces coughing and thus becomes less efficient in removing secretions. As a result, additional atelectasis develops thereby setting up a vicious cycle, which if uninterrupted could lead to death. It is during the first few days after injury that the pain is most severe and the patient is at the greatest risk from respiratory complications. While this sequence of events is unlikely to occur in young, healthy patients, it is imperative that rib fractures never be considered insignificant until proven so.

Almost all conscious and alert patients with rib fractures experience a pleuritic type of chest pain that is usually localized to the site of fracture. The pain is localized when one rib is fractured, but it may occur over a wide area when a number of ribs are fractured. The pain is aggravated by coughing, deep breathing, and motion. On physical examination, there is tenderness to palpation and if displacement is present, bone crepitus may be felt.

The diagnosis is suggested by the history of trauma and the eliciting of pain on palpation and is confirmed by visualization of the fracture site on chest roentgenogram. Since anterior or lateral rib fractures may not be seen on a posteroanterior chest roentgenogram, it is best to obtain left anterior oblique and right anterior oblique views as well so that all regions of the ribs may be visualized. In obese or thick-muscled patients, the Bucky technique may be necessary for adequate visualization. Serial chest roentgenograms should be obtained in all patients with rib fractures since delayed pneumothorax or hemothorax may develop late after the initial injury because of trauma to the lung, parenchyma, or intercostal vessels by rib fragments.

When rib fractures are complicated by pneumothorax or hemothorax, these complications must be treated promptly and before treatment of the rib fractures. Treatment of rib fractures is dependent on the severity of the injury, age of the patient, the presence of preexisting lung disease, and the pain threshold of the patient. In the elderly patient, a rib fracture is a serious injury; these patients should be hospitalized regardless of initial appearance. Likewise, patients with poor cardiovascular reserve or underlying chronic lung disease should be admitted, since the additional insult of the rib fracture may result in pulmonary or cardiac decompensation. In these elderly patients or in patients with pre-existing lung or cardiac disease, therapy should be instituted early and aggressively in order to prevent pulmonary complications. Narcotics should be given immediately to control pain; they may be repeated as often as necessary.

Large doses should be avoided because of the respiratory depressant effect. Intercostal nerve block that includes two nerves above and two below the fracture sites will relieve pain and permit the patient to ventilate and cough.

With adequate relief of pain, the patient can be made to cough and breathe deeply, and bronchial secretions can be effectively expelled, thereby minimizing the danger of developing atelectasis and pneumonia. Other helpful measures include intratracheal suctioning, ultrasonic nebulization by mist or by intermittent positive-pressure breathing (IPPV), and chest physiotherapy. Since adhesive chest strapping decreases respiratory excursion bilaterally, it is indicated only in the simplest of injuries and in the healthiest of patients.

On occasion patients with rib fractures have an associated small pleural effusion on the initial chest roentgenogram. A follow-up chest roentgenogram should be obtained within several days to assure that a large effusion has not developed.

FLAIL CHEST

Flail chest usually results when there are multiple fractures in several ribs with or without separation of the costochondral junction or when rib fractures are associated with fracture of the sternum. As a result of the multiple fractures, the injured or damaged segment of the chest wall no longer maintains its continuity with the remainder of the chest wall and becomes flail. The flail portion of the chest wall is then subject to changes in intrathoracic pressure and begins to move independently of and in an opposite direction to the intact portion of the chest wall. The flail segment may occur in the lateral, anterior, or posterior portion of the chest. The lateral type of flail chest is the most frequent and is characterized by multiple fractures of two or more adjacent ribs in the anterolateral or posterolateral regions of the chest. The anterior type of flail chest occurs when the ribs become separated at their costo-

chondral junction with or without an associated fracture of the sternum. The posterior type results when the ribs in the back of the chest are fractured; the unstable segment lies posteriorly. The paradoxical motion is usually slight because of the support supplied by the scapula and muscles in this region and because the excursion of the posterior rib is normally less than that of the anterior portion.

Because a great force is required to produce a crushing injury of the chest, associated intrathoracic and extrathoracic injuries are common. In Brewer's series, extremity fractures occurred in 17 percent of patients, abdominal injuries occurred in 21 percent of patients, and neurologic injuries occurred in 21 percent of patients.[3] A similar incidence of associated injuries has been reported by other investigators.[9] More important are the associated intrathoracic injuries: pulmonary contusion, pneumothorax, hemothorax, and hemopneumothorax. In Brewer's series of patients with crushing chest injuries, pulmonary contusion, hemothorax, and pneumothorax occurred in 68, 49, and 33 percent of patients, respectively.[3] These associated injuries may make diagnosis and treatment more difficult and may increase the mortality as well.

Pathophysiology

The physiologic alterations that occur with flail chest result not only from the disruption in chest wall mechanics but from the associated pulmonary injury as well. As a result of the chest wall injury, the bellows action of the muscles of the chest wall is reduced. During inspiration, the intact portion of the rib cage expands drawing air into the lungs. However, the flail portion does not expand, since it is no longer in continuity with the normally expanded portion. Atmospheric pressure is exerted on the unstable segment, forcing it inward. This inward motion is enhanced by the gradient produced by the negative intrapleural pressure. A reverse relationship develops on expiration in that the intrathoracic pressure exceeds atmospheric pressure and the flail segment is pushed outward, while the remainder of the thorax contracts normally. Thus, the loss of the structural integrity of the thoracic cage does not permit sufficient negative intrapleural pressure to develop. As a result, the patient lacks the mechanical ability to produce adequate pulmonary ventilation. In fact, the larger the flail segment, the more diminished is the mechanical ability to ventilate. As a result of decreased alveolar ventilation in the presence of continued perfusion, ventilation/perfusion abnormalities occur and lead to hypoxia. The paradoxical motion limits the patient's ability to cough effectively, which in turn leads to accumulation of secretions. In addition, the inadequate ventilation also tends to cause both atelectasis and accumulation of secretions, which lead to increased airway resistance. An additional increase in airway resistance develops as a result of alterations in the intrapleural pressure dynamics and in an attempt to overcome these abnormalities, respiratory work increases.

The associated pulmonary parenchymal injury produces additional physiologic derangements. As a result of the lung damage (contusion, atelectasis), there is a marked reduction in lung compliance, an increase in airway resistance, decrease in pulmonary diffusion and alterations in ventilation/perfusion ratios. These changes lead to even further increases in respiratory work. In a study of patients with crushing chest injuries, Garzon et al.[6] found that the compliance was decreased to approximately one fourth of normal and the airway resistance was increased twofold. In addition, they found that the work of breathing was three times that of normal and the total respiratory work per unit of time (actual respiratory work performed) was five times that of normal. The oxygen demands of the increased work of respiration cannot be met, and the net result is a reduced arterial oxygen tension (PaO_2). Garzon and co-workers also found arterial oxygen desaturation in all patients with crushing chest injuries. In some of their patients, the desaturation was difficult to correct in spite of the use of a high concentration of inspired oxygen and mechanical ventilation. Garzon attributed the oxygen desaturation to pulmonary arteriovenous shunting.

On the other hand, Trinkle et al.[16] consider the paradoxical motion of the chest wall a relatively minor part of the total defect but the respiratory distress to be primarily due to the underlying pulmonary contusion. They also believe that if the underlying pulmonary contusion is treated appropriately and aggressively, the paradoxical motion of the chest wall could be ignored; thereby eliminating the need for mechanical ventilation or even surgical stabilization of the chest wall.

Diagnosis

Careful observation of the chest wall excursion will demonstrate the presence of paradoxical respiration. Excursions of the chest wall are best observed standing by the patient's side. At times, paradoxical respiration can be demonstrated only by having the patient breathe deeply or cough.

In patients with the anterior type of crushing chest injury, the resultant breathing pattern is of the seesaw type; that is, when the chest wall sinks in the abdominal wall goes up and vice-versa. The paradoxical motion of the chest wall may not be seen initially, since the tissue swelling and chest wall hematoma may obscure visualization of its movement. Also, paradoxical motion of the chest wall will not be seen if the patient does not breathe deeply enough to create an intrapleural atmospheric pressure gradient.

Paradoxical motion of the chest wall is most severe and leads to the worst physiologic consequences when multiple fractures occur anteriorly, especially with bilateral costochondral separations or fractures of the sternum. Posterior fractures produce less extensive paradoxical motion and rarely lead to serious physiologic consequences.

The chest roentgenogram is of limited value in establishing the presence of paradoxical respiration, but it is useful in demonstrating the presence of chest wall fractures, pulmonary contusion, atelectasis, hemothorax, or pneumothorax.

Arterial blood gas measurements are of value in estimating the severity of the patient's condition on admission, even in the absence of obvious symptoms. The measurements are also helpful in following the clinical course of the patient once therapy is instituted. As a general rule, most patients with a flail chest will have a low PaO_2 on admission (less than 80 mmHg while breathing room air). A pH value in the range of 7.40 to 7.49 and a $PaCO_2$ greater than 40 mmHg indicate the presence of a more serious degree of hypoxia. Since hypoxia will stimulate compensatory hyperventilation, patients with serious degrees of hypoxia may have arterial blood gases that show an alkalotic pH (7.50) and a low $PaCO_2$ (less than 20 mmHg) in addition to a low PaO_2 (less than 60 mmHg).

Treatment

Treatment of flail chest depends on the severity of the chest wall injury, the condition of the underlying lungs, and the degree of hypoxia. In patients with unilateral paradoxical motion, those with a small volume of chest wall paradox, mild to moderate pulmonary contusion, and a PaO_2 greater than 60 mmHg while breathing room air, or greater than 80 mmHg while breathing supplemental oxygen, or with a tidal volume greater than 10 to 15 ml/kg of body weight can be treated without mechanical ventilation of the chest wall. Instead, the treatment regimen is the same as that discussed earlier for pulmonary contusion. Patients undergoing treatment in this manner should be observed carefully and followed with frequent measurements of arterial blood gases. If signs of ventilatory insufficiency develop, intubation with an endotracheal tube must be promptly carried out and mechanical support of ventilation instituted.

Patients who initially present with evidence of pulmonary insufficiency (a PaO_2 less than 60 mmHg while breathing room air or less than 75 mmHg while breathing supplemental oxygen and a tidal volume less than 10 ml/kg) as well as severe bilateral paradoxical respiration, should be initially treated by endotracheal intubation and mechanical ventilatory support. Mechanical ventilation not only improves ventilation but also reduces the work of breathing, thereby relieving hypoxia and decreasing oxygen consumption and need.

According to Avery et al.,[2] during mechanical respiration the air is distributed into the lungs under a pressure that exerts a gentle, evenly distributed outward push on all the damaged parts, holding them in the normal position during passive expiration, while the intrathoracic pressure drops toward atmospheric levels so that the inside push gradually diminishes. In this way, the ribs move within their normal arcs as they passively ride on the cushion of air caused by the expansion and contraction of the lungs. All paradoxical motion of the rib cage is stopped by this "internal pneumatic stabilization."

Operative Management

Numerous devices and techniques of external traction to elevate and stabilize the flail segment in an outward position (e.g., towel-clip traction, soft tissue traction, or skeletal traction) have been used. But since these traction devices have been associated with a number of complications including necrosis of bony and soft tissues, infection, inadequate stabilization of the flail segment, limited patient mobility, interference with tracheobronchial hygiene, and bone deformity, they are no longer used. If temporary chest wall stabilization is needed, the simplest and quickest way to achieve this is either by turning the patient on the affected side and placing a sandbag against the involved segment or simply by firmly pressing the hand against the paradoxical portion of the chest wall.

On the other hand, direct operative stabilization of the paradoxical segments of the chest wall is a very effective method of treatment. According to Moore,[12] this approach is indicated when (1) the patient is prevented from ventilating adequately because of paradoxical motion and pain; and (2) the injuries are such that they will inevitably result in deterioration of ventilation and the ability of the patient to cough if stabilization is not achieved. The major advantage of operative stabilization is that it avoids endotracheal intubation and mechanical ventilation or reduces its duration. It also allows for direct inspection and correction of associated intrathoracic injuries and restores the anatomic integrity of the chest wall. Operative stabilization can be carried out immediately after admission or as late as 72 to 96 hours following injury. Before operative stabilization is carried out, one should rule out the presence of associated severe injuries that might be adversely affected by general anesthesia.

The mortality for crushing chest injuries varies from 15 to 89 percent in the literature. The mortality is directly related to the age of the patient, the severity of the injury, and the number of associated injuries. The mortality for patients under 30 years of age or for those whose sole injury is the flail chest is less than 3 percent, whereas it approaches 50 to 60 percent for those 60 years and older and for those with multiple injuries. The mortality is higher in those with head injuries (40 percent) than in those without head injuries (16 percent); higher in those who are in shock on admission (61 percent) than in those who are normotensive on admission (17 percent); and higher in those with seven or more rib fractures (33 percent) than in those with fewer fractures (16 percent).[9]

RUPTURE OF THE INTRATHORACIC TRACHEA AND BRONCHI

Although every level of the trachea and almost all the major bronchi have been involved, more than 80 percent of the injuries are within 2.5 cm of the carina. Intrathoracic tracheal lacerations usually occur at the junction of the membraneous and cartilaginous trachea. They are usually vertical lesions and occur posteriorly where the cartilage is deficient. The most common site of bronchial injuries involve the main stem bronchus within 2.5 cm of the carina. Tears in the bronchi are usually transverse. Serious concomitant intrathoracic and extrathoracic injuries are infrequent.

Pathogenesis

The precise mechanism of tracheobronchial disruption is unknown, but several theories have been proposed. The first theory states that the type of injury associated with tracheobronchial disruption is usually one of sudden forceful compression of the thoracic cage. A decrease in the anteroposterior diameter of the thorax occurs with widening of the transverse diameter. The lung remains in contact with the chest wall as a result of the negative intrapleural pressure and the surface tension that exists between the visceral and parietal pleura. The lateral motion pulls the two lungs apart, producing traction on the trachea at the carina. If this force exceeds the elasticity of the tracheobronchial tree, rupture occurs.

A second theory proposes that the glottis is closed at the moment of impact. If during this time the trachea and major bronchi are crushed between the sternum and vertebral column, an acute increase in intrabronchial pressure is produced by compression of the air within the tracheobronchial tree. The greatest tension develops in the larger bronchi. When the elasticity of the tracheobronchial tree is exceeded, rupture occurs.

A third theory states that the effect of rapid deceleration on the lung, which is fixed at the cricoid cartilage and carina, produces shearing forces that disrupt the lung and bronchi.

Clinical Manifestations

There are two distinct clinical patterns depending on whether there is free communication between the site of the disruption and the pleura. In pattern one the bronchus opens into the pleural cavity and as a result there is a large pneumothorax. Insertion of an intercostal tube results in continuous bubbling of air in the underwater-seal drainage bottle. As a rule, suction fails to re-expand the lung. The usual signs of tracheobronchial disruption in this group of patients are dyspnea, hemoptysis, and subcutaneous and mediastinal emphysema. Tension pneumothorax is uncommon, since the intrapleural air decompresses itself through the mediastinal pleural rent into the mediastinum.

In pattern two, although the transection is complete, there is little or no communication between it and the pleural cavity. As a rule, there is no pneumothorax or, if present, it tends to be small. If an intercostal tube is inserted, the lung re-expands. After the tube is removed, there is usually no recurrence of the pneumothorax. Initially, the peribronchial tissues are firm enough to maintain an airway and ventilation of the lung continues. If the transection is complete, the proximal and distal ends heal by granulation and epithelialization. However, at some time between the end of the first and third weeks after injury, granulation tissue obstructs the airway or bronchus and lung with the development of delayed atelectasis. If transection is incomplete, granulation tissue forms in an attempt to bridge the gap. When the granulation tissue epithelializes, a fibrous stricture develops producing a partial bronchial obstruction. The retention of secretions distal to the obstruction often results in pulmonary suppuration and eventual irreversible destruction of pulmonary parenchyma.

Several radiographic findings are highly suggestive of bronchial rupture: pneumomediastinum, deep cervical emphysema, subcutaneous emphysema, pneumothorax, air surrounding the bronchus, and obstruction in the course of an air-filled bronchus. It should be emphasized that these findings are not diagnostic but indicate the need for a more definitive diagnostic procedure. Bronchoscopy is the most reliable means of establishing the site, nature, and extent of bronchial disruption and should be done when the diagnosis is suspected. The bronchoscopy should be performed under operating room conditions with facilities readied for immediate thoracotomy in case it becomes necessary.

to this is if bronchoscopy shows the bronchial tear to involve less than one third of the circumference of the bronchus and if the intercostal underwater-seal drainage results in complete persistent re-expansion of the lung with an early cessation of the air leak as well. Early surgical intervention is advantageous because it permits primary reconstruction of the tracheobronchial tree before infection or extensive scarring complicates the injury.[7]

A double-lumen tube (or a long-cuffed endotracheal tube) can be inserted beyond the area of tracheal transection or into the opposite bronchus for adequate ventilation during operation. Additional sterile endotracheal tubes should be present in the surgical field for ventilation of a transected trachea or bronchus if ventilation becomes necessary. Tears of the thoracic trachea or right bronchus are best approached through a right posterolateral thoracotomy by the way of the fourth intercostal space. When the left bronchus is transected, a left thoracotomy is required. The preferred method of repair is debridement of the divided tracheal or bronchial edges and primary anastomosis with interrupted 4–0 polyglycolic acid sutures carefully approximating mucosa to mucosa. The suture line should be reinforced with a pericardial or pleural flap.

At times it is inadvisable to perform a thoracotomy because of the condition of the patient. Under these circumstances an endotracheal tube should be inserted beyond the area of tracheal transection or into the opposite bronchus to establish satisfactory ventilation to allow for aspiration of secretions and to minimize the effects of tracheobronchial rupture. Repair should be carried out when the condition of the patient improves to the point that a thoracotomy can be safely tolerated.[11]

Treatment

When the diagnosis of tracheobronchial disruption is established, thoracotomy should be performed as soon as the patient's condition permits such a procedure. The only exception

RUPTURE OF THE AORTA

That anyone survives traumatic rupture of the aorta is almost unbelievable. However, 10 to 20 percent of persons who have sustained traumatic rupture of the aorta reach the hospital alive because the aortic blood is contained temporarily by the adventitia or mediastinal pleura.[10] Left untreated, this thin-walled false aneurysm follows an unpredictable course but usually ruptures within 3 weeks after the injury. In order to prevent this catastrophic outcome, it is imperative that the diagnosis be established quickly so that appropriate therapy can be carried out.

Mechanism of Injury

Traumatic rupture of the thoracic aorta can be caused by one of the following mechanisms:

1. Horizontal deceleration with or without chest compression, such as occurs in motorcycle or automobile collisions
2. Marked compression of the chest, such as occurs when a person is run over by a car or kicked in the chest by an animal
3. Vertical deceleration, such as occurs when a person falls from a great height or is struck by a car
4. Crushing injuries that involve some flexion to the spine

The factors responsible for traumatic rupture of the thoracic aorta have not been clearly defined, but they are believed to be different for each rupture location. The most widely accepted explanation concerning aortic rupture at the isthmus is that it is caused by unequal rates of horizontal deceleration of different portions of the aorta, especially at points of fixation. The three mechanical factors thought to contribute to rupture of the descending aorta at the isthmus are shearing stress, bending stress, and torsion stress. The difference in deceleration between the mobile aortic arch and the relatively immobile descending aorta exposes the aortic isthmus to tension and leads to rupture opposite the site of fixation (shearing stress). With bending stress, the heart exerts traction on the aortic arch, resulting in hyperflexion of the blood filled aortic arch on the "transverse mechanical bar and fulcrum" cre-

ated by the hilar structures of the left lung. Torsion stress occurs when there is anteroposterior compression of the chest with displacement of the heart to the left, which produces a pressure wave of blood transmitted through the aorta. The maximum internal pressure is produced at the point of greatest fixation of the aorta (the ligamentum arteriosum). These three forces combine to produce maximum stress at the inner surface of the aorta and the tears lead from the intima toward the adventitia. The adventitia, which has the lowest elastic limit, often withstands the stress.

The hypotheses just described are supported by the observation that 80 to 90 percent of the descending aortic tears from blunt trauma occur within the vicinity of the aortic isthmus and by the fact that most aortic tears are linear and invoke partial or complete transection. Another hypothesis suggests that the sudden increase in intraluminal pressure ruptures the aorta in an accident. Oppenheimer calculated the bursting pressure of a healthy adult human aorta and found it to range from 580 to 2,500 mmHg. Most observers believe that the bursting pressure is unlikely to be exceeded in vehicular accidents. However, the fact that multiple ruptures can occur lends some credence to the hypothesis that the suddenness of the rise in intra-aortic pressure is the primary force in producing aortic rupture.

Vertical deceleration injuries usually cause rupture of the ascending aorta. The vertical deceleration produces acute lengthening of the aorta, with resultant development of a pressure wave in the aortic blood column. This pressure wave produces a water-hammer effect (a pulse characterized by a rapid forceful ascent or upstroke) that is greatest in the ascending aorta and is believed to cause, or at least contribute greatly to, rupture in that location.

The mechanism of rupture of the innominate artery and left subclavian artery results from the interaction of two forces. One is a compression force that displaces the heart into the left chest and places the brachiocephalic vessels under tension at their attachment to the aortic arch. The other force occurs when hyperextension of the neck and rotation of the head to one side place the opposing brachiocephalic vessel under additional tension. The tension leads to the development of maximum shearing stress at the origin of these vessels with resultant rupture.

The fact that the overwhelming majority of brachiocephalic injuries involve the origin of the innominate or subclavian artery suggests that a major stress occurs along these vessels rather than along the carotid arteries.

The more frequent sites of rupture of the thoracic aorta are (1) the descending aorta just distal to the origin of the left subclavian artery (aortic isthmus); (2) the ascending aorta proximal to the origin of the innominate artery; and (3) the origin of the innominate artery from the aortic arch. Other sites of involvement include the distal descending aorta at the aortic hiatus in the diaphragm, the mid-portion of the descending aorta, and the left subclavian artery.

INJURIES OF THE DESCENDING AORTA

The single most important factor in establishing the diagnosis of acute traumatic aortic rupture is maintenance of a high index of suspicion and a constant awareness of the likelihood of this lesion in anyone who has sustained an accident characterized by sudden deceleration regardless of whether or not there is external evidence of chest injuries. One third of our patients had no external evidence of thoracic injury at the time of initial physical examination.[10] Despite the severe nature of the injury, the clinical findings are usually deceptively meager. Clinical findings of importance are the acute onset of upper extremity hypertension, especially if coupled with evidence of massive blood loss, the presence of a harsh systolic murmur heard over the precordium or posterior interscapular area, and a difference in blood pressure between the upper and lower extremities. These findings either alone or in combination occur in only one-third of patients with aortic rupture.

Radiographic Findings

Radiography of the chest is invaluable in arousing suspicion of aortic rupture. It is important to emphasize that careful evaluation of the chest roentgenogram is mandatory in victims of blunt chest trauma since many patients have died because the presence and significance of radiographic abnormalities were not appreciated. Radiographic features of importance are as follows: (1) widening of the superior mediastinum, especially if greater than 8 cm in width; (2) obscuration of the aortic knob shadow; (3) loss of sharpness of the aortic outline; (4) deviation of the trachea to the right; (5) depression of the left main stem bronchus; (6) deviation of the nasogastric tube; and (7) obliteration of the paraspinous stripe.[8] Although these findings are highly suggestive of aortic rupture, they are not diagnostic because they can occur without aortic rupture. Conversely, aortic rupture may exist without these radiographic findings being present. This is true even when they are associated with upper extremity hypertension and a systolic murmur.

The standard upright posteroanterior chest roentgenogram is often recommended in the evaluation of acute aortic rupture. Even if it could be obtained easily, it adds no useful information that is not already present on the supine film. Serial chest roentgenograms might solve the diagnostic problem, but it is our belief that they are contraindicated if exsanguination from secondary rupture is to be avoided. Traumatic aortic rupture has occurred in some of our patients with a normal chest roentgenogram (Figs. 28-2 A and 28-2 B). Since a widened mediastinum is not always caused by aortic rupture and since rupture of the aorta is not always associated with a widened mediastinum, a definitive diagnostic procedure is necessary. In addition, the location of the aortic rupture cannot be determined by the plain chest roentgenographic findings.

Aortography is the only definitive means for establishing the diagnosis of acute aortic rupture. It should be performed on any patient who has sustained a high-speed deceleration injury or blunt trauma to the chest whether or not there is external or radiographic evi-

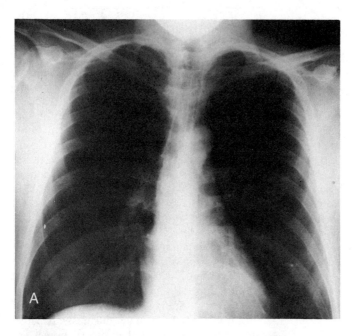

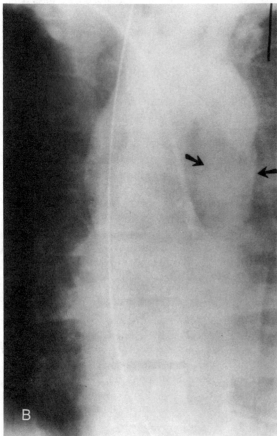

FIG. 28-2 (A) Normal chest roentgenogram in a 24-year-old man with high-speed decelerating injury. **(B)** Aortogram demonstrating pseudoaneurysm of aortic rupture.

dence of thoracic wall injuries, whether or not there are clinical findings suggesting aortic rupture, and whether or not there are changes in the serial chest roentgenograms. The following list summarizes the indications for aortography in victims of blunt chest trauma:

1. History of deceleration injury
2. Any of the following chest roentgenographic findings
   a. Superior mediastinal widening
   b. Obscuration aortic knob shadow
   c. Obliteration of aortic outline
3. Massive hemothorax
4. Pulse deficits
5. Upper extremity hypertension
6. Systolic murmur
7. Unexplained hypotension

Although the transaxillary approach theoretically offers certain advantages because the catheter does not pass through the area of transection, the preferred method is by retrograde catheterization (right femoral arteriography using a long, soft, J-shaped catheter passed under fluoroscopic control). Retrograde catheterization is technically easier, can be performed in the severely injured or uncooperative patient, and allows important angiographic evaluation of other areas of suspected injury. Characteristically, the aortogram in acute aortic rupture demonstrates the presence of a pseudoaneurysm at or near the ligamentum arteriosum without extravasation of contrast medium. In those instances in which the intimal flap acts as a ball valve, complete interruption of the aorta at the site of transection will be seen without distal filling of the aorta beyond the transection. The intimal tears are usually visualized as irregular filling defects within the lumen of the aorta. Since the rupture can be complicated by medial dissection, this complication should be carefully searched for when evaluating the aortogram. At times, the angiographic appearance of a ductus diverticulum may be misinterpreted as a pseudoaneurysm. This can be avoided if one remembers that the ductus diverticulum is characterized by an area of bulging limited to the inferomedial aspect of the aorta without any intimal tears, and most importantly by a smooth interface with the aorta.

Treatment

Because lethal secondary rupture of the false aneurysm is likely, immediate surgical repair should be carried out as soon as the diagnosis is established and the site of rupture localized. Aortography should always precede thoracotomy unless contraindicated by rapid deterioration of the patient's condition. In patients with multiple injuries, a brief delay to establish management priorities is advisable. The decision whether first to treat the major associated injuries (celiotomy) or to repair the aortic rupture must fit the circumstances. Initially in our experience, treatment of the coexisting abdominal injuries was carried out prior to thoracotomy in six patients, five of whom exsanguinated before thoracotomy could be performed. In addition, six other patients died because repair of the aortic rupture was delayed for various reasons. This experience, as well as the fact that the untreated aortic rupture follows such an unpredictable course, has led us to recommend that aside from rapidly progressing craniocerebral injuries such as epidural hemorrhage or massive intra-abdominal bleeding, traumatic rupture of the aorta deserves the highest priority and that its repair be carried out first. Since repair of the aorta can be performed with a shunt that does not require systemic heparinization, intra-abdominal bleeding will not, as a rule, increase during thoracotomy. If it does, exploration of the abdomen can be carried out by converting the incision into a thoracoabdominal one. Before doing this, proximal and distal control of the aorta should be obtained.

In circumstances in which repair of the aortic rupture must be delayed because another operation is needed or because the condition of the patient (severe closed head injury) makes thoracotomy inadvisable, these patients should be managed in the manner in which patients with spontaneous aortic dissection are treated. The systolic blood should be maintained below 120 mmHg with Guanethidine and reserpine, in conjunction with Propranolol. These drugs lower the blood pressure and decrease the force of contraction of the heart which decreases the "shearing jet effect" of the pulse and decrease the possibility of aortic rupture.

Operative Management

A useful adjunct during the operative management of these patients is the use of a double-lumen endotracheal tube in conjunction with high-concentration oxygen ventilation. Selective collapsing of the left lung facilitates exposure and dissection of the aorta. This makes retraction of the left lung unnecessary and minimizes the amount of damage that normally occurs with retraction.

The patient should be positioned on the operating room table in the right lateral decubitus position with the pelvis rotated 45 degrees backward and the left hip fully extended. A standard posterolateral thoacotomy incision through the bed of the fourth intercostal space provides optimum exposure.

The hematoma surrounding the transection often covers most of the descending thoracic aorta and extends over the transverse arch as well. The pericardium is opened anterior to the phrenic nerve and by beginning the dissection from within the pericardium, one may encircle the aorta proximal to the left subclavian artery without entering the mediastinal hematoma and possibly releasing its tamponading effect. Distal aortic control should also be obtained well outside the area of mediastinal hematoma.

While performing aortic repair, ischemic injury to the spinal cord and kidneys must be avoided, the cerebral vessels spared from hypertension, and acute left heart failure prevented. The techniques most widely used to accomplish these goals are left heart bypass or femoral vein–femoral artery partial bypass. During the bypass, systolic pressures in the right radial artery should be continuously recorded and kept at acceptable levels (100 to 130 mmHg) by maintaining the flow rates between 60 and 100 ml/kg of body weight/min. Despite continuous left atrial pressure monitoring and careful control of the left atrial pressures with these techniques, left atrial hypertension and pulmonary edema have occasionally developed either alone or in combination. A more common problem associated with the necessary total body heparinization has been excessive bleeding from the dissection necessary to isolate the aorta. Heparinization may also increase intra-abdominal or intracerebral bleeding. The latter occurred in three of our patients and the resultant brain damage was responsible for the death of two of them. Postoperative hemorrhagic diathesis resulting from alteration in coagulation factors during extracorporeal circulation with its attendant complications also occurs.

To avoid these problems during aortic cross-clamping and to achieve the goals previously discussed, we prefer to use an external shunt composed of a plastic arterial cannula connected to Tygon tubing that does not require systemic heparinization. Two sizes of cannula have been used: a 7.5-mm cannula connected with a 8-mm tubing and 9-mm cannula connected with 12-mm tubing. The tubing is filled with 50 ml saline solution containing 1,000 units of heparin to prevent clotting when there is no flow through the shunt. To ensure adequate flow through the shunt, the clamps on the shunt must not be released until the aorta proximal and distal to the rupture is clamped. The left subclavian artery should not be used for proximal cannulation because of the severe neurologic sequelae (e.g., paraplegia, brain stem injury) that have been associated with its use. If the aortic rupture is complicated by proximal medial dissection or if technical difficulties are encountered in cannulating the ascending aorta, a left ventriculoaortic bypass shunt is a reasonable alternative technique. The technique of shunt insertion into the left ventricle is exactly the same as that used in decompression of the left ventricle during cardiac surgery. To avoid air embolism, the shunt must be filled with heparinized saline solution before it is inserted into the left ventricle. Since diastolic return to the ventricle through the shunt represents a small percentage (less than 15 percent of the forward flow), a directional flow valve within the shunt is not needed.

Appelbaum et al.[1] repaired ruptured thoracic aortas without a shunt or without partial cardiopulmonary bypass. None of the patients in their series treated in this manner developed paraplegia. Since the period of time that the aorta can be clamped with this technique cannot exceed 30 minutes, it should be used only by experienced and fast-working surgeons.

Although primary end-to-end anastomosis has been successfully accomplished by ourselves and others, the overwhelming majority of repairs have been accomplished with the use of woven prosthetic grafts. In fact, woven prosthetic grafts were used to reconstruct the aorta in all but five of our patients undergoing operation.[13] The marked friability of the aortic wall, the retraction of the two ends, and mediastinal hemorrhage and its surrounding reaction prevent adequate end-to-end anastomosis, thereby necessitating the use of a prosthetic graft.

INNOMINATE ARTERY INJURY

In cases in which the patient survives long enough for diagnosis and repair, avulsion of the innominate artery from the aortic arch is second in frequency only to rupture of the aorta at the aortic isthmus. Associated injuries such as rib fractures, flail chest, hemopneumothorax, fractured extremities, head injuries, facial fractures, and abdominal injuries occur alone or in combination in more than 75 percent of patients.

The diagnosis may be difficult, since there are no characteristic physical findings. Although there is diminution of the radial or brachial pulse in about 50 percent of these patients with innominate artery avulsion, a decreased pulse and blood pressure may be the only clues to the diagnosis. Signs and symptoms of distal ischemia are uncommon and cannot be relied on to draw attention to the injury.

The chest roentgenographic findings are usually no different from those in aortic isthmus rupture (i.e., a widened mediastinum with obscuration of the aortic knob shadow). However, the outline of the descending aorta may be preserved. Aortography must be performed for the diagnosis to be established. The right posterior oblique position is best for visualization of the proximal aorta and origin of the brachiocephalic vessels. Avulsion of the innominate artery typically shows bulbous dilatation of the vessel just distal to its origin.

Because of the ever-present danger of sudden cataclysmic hemorrhage from secondary rupture of the pseudoaneurysm, the treatment is immediate surgical repair. The best approach is through a median sternotomy incision with extension of the incision into the soft tissues of the right side of the neck. Cerebral ischemia must be prevented during the period of arterial occlusion since the incidence of paralysis following occlusion of the carotid artery is 25 percent. This is best avoided by placing an external or internal bypass shunt from the ascending aorta to the distal carotid artery. Cardiopulmonary bypass should be available for all patients in the event that extension of the tear or unrecognized associated aortic injuries are found during thoracotomy. Our preference is for the use of an external bypass shunt. The advantage of this technique is that it avoids heparinization and its attendant risks. Reconstruction is usually carried out with a prosthetic graft or a reversed autogenous saphenous graft but an end-to-end anastomosis should be performed if possible.

SUBCLAVIAN ARTERY INJURY

Although most subclavian ruptures result from deceleration types of injuries, an occasional rupture has occurred from impingement of a fractured first rib or clavicle on the vessel. Clinically, the cardinal sign is absence of a radial pulse in association with signs and symptoms of distal ischemia. However, this sign is present only in patients with associated thrombotic occlusion of the artery. In patients with partial lacerations and without thrombotic occlusion, the radial pulse will be palpable because of continuous flow through the injured vessel. The chest roentgenogram shows the presence of a widened superior mediastinum without obscuration of the aortic knob shadow. Accurate diagnosis of the injury requires aortography through the retrograde femoral technique and with the patient in the right posterior oblique position. The aortogram characteristically demonstrates the presence of occlusion in the subclavian artery at its site of injury.

Treatment of acute subclavian rupture is immediate surgical repair. For injuries to the left subclavian artery, an anterolateral fourth intercostal incision is made. If additional exposure of the vessel is needed, a separate supraclavicular incision can be made. Reconstruction should be by means of a prosthetic graft or reversed saphenous bypass graft.

ASCENDING AORTIC INJURIES

Few patients with ascending aortic ruptures have survived long enough for the diagnosis to be established and the repair to be carried out. The high mortality is explained by the frequent association of ascending aortic injuries with severe cardiac injuries and by the fact that most ascending aortic tears occur within the pericardium, leading to the early development of pericardial tamponade. There are no characteristic physical findings to suggest that ascending aortic rupture has occurred. The chest roentgenographic findings are the same as those of aortic rupture in the other locations: a widened superior mediastinum with or without obscuration of the aortic knob shadow. Aortography must be performed for the diagnosis to be established. The aortogram will show a pseudoaneurysm, and the intimal tear will be seen as an irregular filling defect within the lumen of the aorta. If there is associated aortic valvular injury, aortic insufficiency of varying magnitude will be seen. For obvious reasons, the treatment is immediate surgical repair with the use of cardiopulmonary bypass. Depending on the nature of the injury, either direct end-to-end anastomosis or graft interposition should be used for reconstruction of the aorta.

REFERENCES

1. Appelbaum A, Karp RB, Kirklin JW: Surgical treatment for closed thoracic aortic injuries. J Thorac Cardiovasc Surg 71: 458, 1976
2. Avery EE, Morch ET, Benson DW: Critically crushed chests: A new method of treatment with continuous mechanical hyperventilation to produce alkalotic apnea and internal pneumatic stabilization. J Thorac Surg 32: 291, 1956
3. Brewer L, Steiner L: The management of crushing injuries of the chest. Surg Clin North Am 48: 1279, 1968
4. Fulton R, Peter E: Physiologic effects of fluid therapy after pulmonary contusion. Am J Surg 126: 773, 1973
5. Franz J, Richardson JD, Grover FL, Trinkle JK: Effect of methylprednisolone sodium succinate on experimental pulmonary contusion. J Thorac Cardiovasc Surg 68: 842, 1974
6. Garzon A, Seltzer B, Karlson E: Pathophysiology of crushed chest injuries. Ann Surg 168: 128, 1968
7. Grover FL, Ellestad C, Arom K et al: Diagnosis and management of major tracheobronchial injuries. Ann Thorac Surg 28: 384, 1979
8. Gundry SR, Wilton G, Burney R et al: Double-blind assessment of mediastinal widening and its role in predicting aortic rupture in trauma patients. J Trauma 23: 293, 1983
9. Hankins JR, Shen B, McAslan T et al: Management of flail chest: An analysis of 99 cases. Am Surg 45: 176, 1979
10. Kirsh MM, Behrendt DB, Orringer MB et al: The treatment of acute traumatic rupture of the aorta—ten year experience. Ann Surg 184: 308, 1976
11. Kirsh MM, Orringer MB, Behrendt DB, Sloan H: Management of tracheobronchial disruption secondary to non-penetrating trauma. Ann Thorac Surg 22: 93, 1976
12. Moore BP: Operative stabilization of non-penetrating chest injuries. J Thorac Cardiovasc Surg 70: 619, 1975
13. Orringer MB, Kirsh MM: Primary repair of acute traumatic aortic disruption. Ann Thorac Surg 35: 672, 1983
14. Phillips EH, Rogers WF, Gaspar MR: First rib fracture: Incidence of vascular injury and indications for angiography. Surgery 89: 42, 1981
15. Trinkle J, Furman RW, Hinshaw M et al: Pulmonary contusion—Pathogenesis and effect of various resuscitative measures. Ann Thorac Surg 16: 568, 1973
16. Trinkle JK, Richardson J, Franz JL et al: Management of flail chest without mechanical ventilation. Ann Thorac Surg 19: 355, 1975
17. Wise A, Topuzlu C, Mills E, Page HG: The importance of serial blood gas determinations in blunt chest trauma. J Thorac Cardiovasc Surg 56: 520, 1968
18. Yee ES, Thomas AN, Goodman PC: Isolated first rib fracture: Clinical significance after blunt chest trauma. Ann Thorac Surg 32: 278, 1981
19. Zuckerman S: Experimental study of blunt injuries to the lung. Lancet 2: 219, 1940

29

Blunt Trauma to the Abdomen

Everard F. Cox
John H. Siegel

INTRODUCTION

Etymologists tell us that the word abdomen is derived from the latin *abdere,* meaning to hide, and indeed, in blunt abdominal trauma the consequences of the forces delivered to the torso are often hidden—for a time. While injuries to organs within the abdomen have been described from the beginnings of medical science, the advent of the modern engines of conveyance, the motor car, the motorcycle, the railway, and the airplane and the explosive growth of the industrial age and its accidents have projected this form of trauma into the forefront of injury.

The forces dissipated on the human body as a result of the modern mechanisms of blunt trauma can be of enormous magnitude, since the force exerted on impact equals the mass times its velocity divided by the time to decelerate to zero velocity. The pressure equals this force divided by the fraction of the body sur-

face area that receives the impact. For example, the torso of a 100-kg (220-lb) motorcyclist of 2.0 m² body surface area (BSA) who leaves his machine at 30 miles per hour (44 ft/sec) and decelerates in 0.01 seconds on impact with a telephone pole or road abutment receives 30,108 lb of force. If this is exerted on an area of his right lower chest and upper abdomen of 310 square inches (equivalent to 5 percent of BSA) he has a pressure delivered of 97 lb/sq inch. Similarly a 220-lb construction worker who falls 33 feet from a scaffold will achieve a velocity of 45.3 ft/sec on impact with the ground. If he also decelerates in 0.01 seconds and lands on the same area of thorax and upper abdomen he will receive a force on impact of 30,998 lb or 100 lb/square inch. In contrast, a pedestrian crushed against the side of a building by a 3000 lb automobile braking to only 15 miles per hour (22 ft/sec) which also decelerates over 0.01 seconds on impact with 5 percent of BSA at the lateral pelvis and flank receives 205,288 lb of force, or a pressure of 662 lb/sq inch. Even if this is equally dissipated over two additional 5 percent BSA areas of femur, and face and head, this could mean a pressure of 220 lb/sq inch to each body part. If this full decelerating impact is concentrated over a much smaller area (1 percent of BSA), such as a bumper injury to the tibia, the pressure on impact could rise as high as 3311 lb/sq inch. To put these forces and pressures in perspective, consider that a man using a 9-lb sledge hammer to hit a brick wall at a velocity of 10 ft/sec exerts a pressure on the order of 67 lb/sq inch, but administers a total force of only 268 lb per impact.

The result of these very large forces transmitted through the viscous semisolid medium of the chest, abdominal, or pelvic viscera, or the brain, is to create shearing, compression, or bursting injuries of a formidible magnitude. By its nature blunt trauma, as opposed to single penetrating injuries, usually has several points of impact. The consequence of this force transmission is to produce a pattern of multiple organ and skeletal injuries with devitalization of tissues and impairment of complex host defense mechanisms that compound the trauma itself and predispose to septic complications. Even the specific injuries have characteristic features that are often lacking in simpler accidents. Applied to the long bones or pelvis, forces of this magnitude produce shattering, comminuted injuries with massive soft tissue damage, or loss, and frequently there are torsion rotational tears of the internal linings of limb vessels. When the head is the point of impact, crushing injuries of the face and skull occur, combined with major contusions of the brain, or shearing forces on the subarachnoid or dural vessels. Applied to the chest, they can cause contusion or rupture of lung parenchyma and bronchi, myocardial contusion, and shearing of the descending aorta at points of vascular fixation to tethering vessels.

Impacting forces of this magnitude on the abdomen or lower thorax produce deep lacerating or fracturing injuries of the liver or spleen, bursting perforations of the bowel or bladder, shearing devascularizations of the bowel mesentery, and explosive tearing perforations of the diaphram with acute herniation of abdominal contents into the thoracic space. In severe multiple trauma produced by blunt forces of these magnitudes some, if not all, of these injuries may occur together. Thus, the common clinical features of abdominal visceral injury may be hidden behind the signs and symptom complex produced by brain contusion and/or hemorrhagic shock resulting from major extremity fractures. Indeed 50 percent of our patients with blunt intra-abdominal injury had at least one other major system injury and nearly 40 percent had two additional systems traumatized.

To place this type of trauma in perspective in the context of this book it is of help to review the recent experience of the Maryland Institute for Emergency Medical Services Systems (MIEMSS) whose trauma demographs were described in Chapter 1.

Over a 5-year period (1978 to 1982) at MIEMSS, injury to the abdomen requiring investigative celiotomy was seen in 12.9 percent of 6,745 patients admitted following blunt trauma from whatever cause.[8] Injury by vehicular accident was responsible for 90.4 percent of blunt abdominal trauma. The great majority of patients arrived by helicopter from the scene of the accident where an effective emergency medical system had already instituted early resuscitation. At the trauma center, a full-time traumatologist continued the resuscitation started in the field, and began diagnostic evaluation. Of the 870 patients who had celiotomy, the average age was 29.8 years with a 2.7:1 male to female ratio. The ingestion of intoxicating beverages played a major role as a predisposing factor to the injury. Blood alcohol values above 100 mg/dl were observed in 22.9 percent of the patients. An additional 6.7 percent of the patients had detectable blood alcohol levels less than 100 mg/dl. Automobile accidents accounted for 69.4 percent of the victims and motorcycles for 11.7 percent, and 9.3 percent were pedestrians. Industrial accidents accounted for 3.1 percent and domestic home and farm accidents for 4.1 percent, and 2.7 percent had unrecorded injuries (Table 29-1).

Of the 870 patients with blunt abdominal trauma, 50.5 percent (493 patients) had an associated injury (Table 29-2) and 38.2 percent had two or more associated injuries. There were 301 patients (34.6 percent) with extremity or axial skeleton injuries, 32.6 percent with facial injuries, 18.5 percent had central nervous sys-

TABLE 29-1. Profile of Patients with Blunt Abdominal Trauma (BAT)

	No.	% of BAT
Total trauma admissions (1978–1982)	6745	
BAT patients requiring celiotomy	870	12.9
Average age (years)	29.8	
Male	637	73.3
Female	232	26.7
Positive blood alcohol (BAL)	257	29.5
BAL ≥ 100 mg/dl	199	22.9
Cause of trauma		
Automobile	600	69.4
Motorcycle	102	11.7
Pedestrian	81	9.3
Industrial	27	3.1
Home and farm	36	4.1
Unrecorded	24	2.7

(Data from Cox EF: Blunt abdominal trauma: a 5-year analysis of 870 patients requiring celiotomy. Ann Surg 199:467, 1984.)

TABLE 29-2. Associated Injury Requiring Surgical Intervention in 870 Patients Undergoing Celiotomy for Blunt Abdominal Trauma

Number of Patients	%	Associated Injuries
439	50.5	One associated injury
332	38.2	Two or more injuries
301	34.6	Extremities and axial skeleton
284	32.6	Facial
161[a]	18.5	Head and central nervous system
65	7.4	Mandible and maxillary alveolus (dental)
50	5.7	Thorax (aorta 16/50 = 32%)

[a] Intraventricular pressure monitoring or craniotomy required.

(Data from Cox EF: Blunt abdominal trauma: a 5 year analysis of 870 patients requiring celiotomy. Ann Surg 199:467, 1984.)

tem injuries, 7.4 percent had mandible or maxillary injuries, and 5.7 percent had injury to the thorax (Table 29-2). In all cases the diagnosis of organ injury within the abdomen was confirmed at the time of celiotomy.

PERITONEAL LAVAGE

Role

Since these patients were critically injured, the indication for celiotomy was based on clinical criteria such as a rapidly distending abdomen and shock, or on the use of diagnostic peritoneal lavage as described by Root and associates[29] in 1965. This has subsequently been accepted by most traumatologists as a valid basis for making the diagnosis of intra-abdominal organ injury. While the initial experience with the use of computer tomography (CT) as a diagnostic modality for the detection of intra-abdominal organ injury seems promising,[15] the full range of capability of this new methodology needs to be evaluated with regard to its potential for false-negative diagnoses as well as in its value in avoiding an unnecessary laparotomy. However, the use of alternative diagnostic modalities for the detection of visceral trauma has not been a major factor at MIEMSS since such a large percent of these patients have a serious associated injury, frequently involving the brain or spinal cord. The priorities in diagnostic evaluation of abdominal injuries in these patients are often dependent upon whether patients are going to need other emergency surgical procedures that require alteration of the normal sequence of diagnostic evaluations and reduce the time available for such examination. Under these circumstances diagnostic peritoneal lavage in patients sustaining suspected blunt abdominal trauma appears to be a rapid, inexpensive, and reliable means of diagnosis. We have relied on peritoneal lavage with great confidence, and we believe it to be an effective safeguard against complications resulting from missed organ injuries.[8,9]

Early experience with peritoneal lavage in many centers resulted in a high percentage of inappropriate or negative celiotomies.[8] As experience has been gained, a more specific set of criteria for performing this study has been established and a highly reliable technique of peritoneal lavage has been developed.[9] At present, in our institution the number of completely negative explorations has fallen to 2 percent. There is a current incidence of less than 1 percent false-negative results, mainly due to retroperitoneal injuries diagnosed by radiologic means because of a high index of suspicion on clinical grounds. However, a low incidence of negative explorations is considered good medical practice, since occult injuries such as a ruptured diaphragm, or a localized bowel perforation, can occur without meeting the criteria for a diagnostically positive peritoneal lavage. If these borderline cases are excluded from celiotomy, there will be serious clinical problems in a later phase of the patient's recovery.

Technique

No single set of indications can cover all clinical situations and good clinical judgment should prevail in determining who should undergo diagnostic peritoneal lavage. Our present technique of peritoneal lavage takes advantage of the anatomic constancy of the posterior sheath of the rectus abdominus muscle (Fig.

29-1). The peritoneum is adherent to the rectus sheath and there is little or no fat between the rectus sheath and the peritoneum. The surgical approach is based on a belief in the superiority of control and the increased safety of the open, or semiopen, technique compared to a closed technique.

The incision for peritoneal lavage is made lateral to either side of the umbilicus (Fig. 29-2). If cosmetic appearance is considered important, a circumumbilical incision, though slightly more tedious, allows unencumbered access to the anterior rectus sheath (Fig. 29-3). The anterior rectus sheath is incised longitudinally about 1 cm lateral to the lateral border of the linea alba for 2 to 3 cm. The medial flap of the incised rectus sheath is lifted and the medial fibers of the rectus muscle are gently retracted laterally, exposing the posterior rectus sheath (Fig. 29-4). The posterior rectus sheath may be opened for direct visualization of abdominal viscera before placing the catheter, or, as we prefer, by depressing the hand laterally, the trocar is pushed in an almost horizontal plane through the lifted rectus sheath (Fig. 29-5). As the trocar sheathed by the cath-

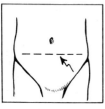

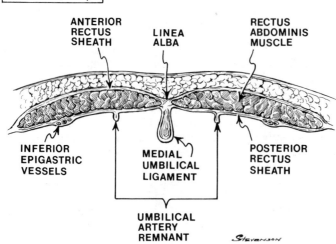

ANTERIOR RECTUS SHEATH   LINEA ALBA   RECTUS ABDOMINIS MUSCLE

INFERIOR EPIGASTRIC VESSELS   MEDIAL UMBILICAL LIGAMENT   POSTERIOR RECTUS SHEATH

UMBILICAL ARTERY REMNANT

FIG. 29-1 Anatomic relations of the posterior sheath of the rectus abdominus muscle. (Cox EF, Dunham CM: A safe technique for diagnostic peritoneal lavage. J Trauma 23: 152, 1983.)

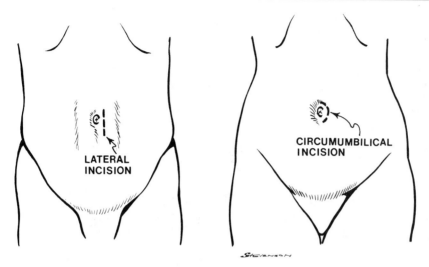

FIG. 29-2 Periumbilical incisions for peritoneal lavage. (Cox EF, Dunham CM: A safe technique for diagnostic peritoneal lavage. J Trauma 23: 152, 1983.)

FIG. 29-3 Exposure of anterior rectus sheath and rectus abdominus muscle. (Cox EF, Dunham CM: A safe technique for diagnostic peritoneal lavage. J Trauma 23: 152, 1983.)

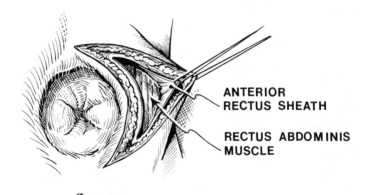

FIG. 29-4 Exposure of posterior rectus sheath. (Cox EF, Dunham CM: A safe technique for diagnostic peritoneal lavage. J Trauma 23: 152, 1983.)

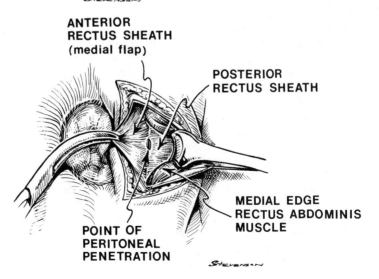

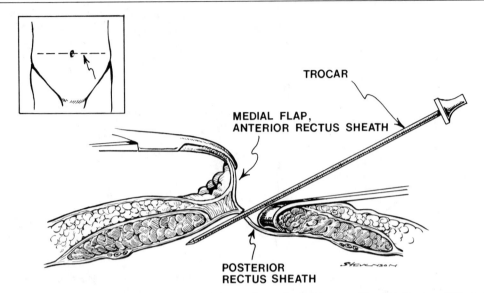

FIG. 29-5 Technique of trocar insertion into abdomen for peritoneal lavage. (Cox EF, Dunham CM: A safe technique for diagnostic peritoneal lavage. J Trauma 23: 152, 1983.)

eter enters the abdomen, a distinct "give" in the exerted pressure is felt; the trocar is then removed and the catheter is redirected toward the pelvis. One or two sutures are placed in the incised anterior rectus sheath and the sutures in the skin are completed as the perfusate of normal saline is run into the peritoneal cavity. The catheter is easily withdrawn through the closed incision.

If the patient strains during the procedure, it is interesting to observe that the rectus muscle, as it contracts, closes the incision, reducing the likelihood of evisceration of the bowel. This procedure of peritoneal lavage is easily done under local anesthesia. It has proven to be very safe and is accomplished with little discomfort or danger to the patient.

The criteria for surgical exploration based on the effluence of the peritoneal lavage is generally considered to be standardized at 50,000 red blood cells/ml fluid.[9,29] Using this criterion, in some of the celiotomies the surgeon may find that the injury is limited to minor tears in the mesentery or bowel, serosa, or to minor hepatic lacerations of other injuries that are not clinically significant. However, in the overall management of multiply injured patients with severe blunt trauma, the complications associated with negative exploration of the ab-

domen are few compared to the consequences of overlooking a devascularized or perforated intestine or a diaphragmatic laceration.

CHOICE OF INCISION FOR CELIOTOMY

If patients with pelvic fracture (where urinary bladder ruptures are common) are excluded, as demonstrated in this series, the majority of injuries are in the upper half of the abdomen. Palomar and associates, in a study of 34 patients with bladder rupture following blunt trauma noted that 74 percent had pelvic fractures.[26] In this MIEMSS study as well, all patients who had ruptured bladders, except one, had associated pelvic fractures. In view of these data, rigid adherence to the vertical midabdominal incision, which is used by preference in many institutions, does not seem warranted in all occasions. A midepigastric transverse incision gives superior exposure to the spleen and to the liver. In patients who are resuscitated, physiologically stable, and carefully evaluated for other injuries, the presumed advantage of more rapid access to the abdominal cavity through the midline incision in blunt trauma does not outweigh the disadvantages of compromised exposure to the lateral flanks of the upper abdomen. This is especially true in major splenic injuries requiring emergency splenectomy where iatrogenic injury to the colon, stomach, or pancreas, often followed by abscess formation, can be a consequence of a poor exposure through a vertical incision. It is estimated that approximately 2 percent of the splenic injuries in this series were iatrogenic and eight pancreatic complications occurred as a result of splenectomy for trauma where exposure was not ideal. If access to the dome of the liver is needed, the transverse incision can be converted to an extra pleural thoracotomy by extension through the eleventh rib interspace. If entrance into the chest becomes necessary because of cases of severe hepatic lacerations or fracture that require caval control, a vertical limb can be extended up the midline as a median sternotomy, or a transection through the ninth rib interspace on the right can be used to gain access to the diaphragmatic surface of the liver. However, incisions that enter the thoracic cavity should be avoided unless deemed necessary for control of major hemorrhage, since they lead to severe morbidity following operative procedures in the abdomen.

INCIDENCE OF VISCERAL ORGAN INJURY

Table 29-3 shows the incidence of the blunt abdominal visceral injuries found on celiotomy. In the MIEMSS series, as in most others considering blunt trauma to the abdomen, splenic trauma was the most frequent injury.[8] It occurred in 42.2 percent of the patients, but in this group of multiply injured patients in only

TABLE 29-3. Incidence of Abdominal Organ Injury Due to Blunt Trauma in 870 Patients Requiring Operative Intervention (1978–1982)

Organ Injured	Number of Patients	% of Total with Injury
Spleen	367	42.2
Liver	310	35.6
Retroperitoneal hematoma	127[a]	14.6
Serosa and mesentery of bowel	113[b]	13.0
Diaphram	44	5.1
Bowel wall rupture	41	4.7
Small bowel	30	3.4
Colon	11	1.3
Bladder	28[c]	3.2
Kidney	23	2.6
Mesenteric vascular (SMA or SMV)	17	2.0
Vena cava or iliac vein	9	1.0
Ovarian cyst rupture	9	1.0
Stomach	2	<0.1
Pancreas	2[d]	<0.1
Duodenum	1[e]	<0.1
Aorta	1	<0.1

[a] Not associated with major retroperitoneal organ injury.
[b] Injuries requiring repair or bowel resection.
[c] All but one associated with pelvic fracture.
[d] Eight additional injuries in association with splenectomy.
[e] Six paraduodenal hematomas.
(Data from Cox EF: Blunt abdominal trauma: a 5-year analysis of 870 patients requiring celiotomy. Ann Surg 199:467, 1984.)

8 percent was splenic trauma the sole injury.

Of the 870 with blunt abdominal trauma, 310 (35.6 percent) sustained injuries to the liver. These ranged from minor capsular tears to major fractures involving the retrohepatic vena cava. As in other reports,[1,24,34] severe liver injury was the leading cause of intraoperative death. In this series of unselected blunt abdominal trauma 29 (9.4 percent) patients with major hepatic injury died intraoperatively.[8]

In the MIEMSS experience with multiply injured patients, clinically insignificant injuries to the bowel serosa and/or mesentery secondary to blunt trauma were the most common type of insult sustained in the abdomen. This type of trauma was the most frequent cause of the false-positive diagnostic peritoneal lavage. Serosal injury to the mesentery that, in the opinion of the surgeon, required repair was discovered in 13 percent of patients. The bowel repair most often carried out consisted of control of small vessel mesentery bleeding and closure of rents in the small bowel mesentery. A bowel injury due to blunt trauma requiring resection because of perforation occurred in 41 patients (4.7 percent) of the patients with abdominal trauma; 30 of these were in small bowel and 11 were in colon. There was no apparent site of predilection in the small bowel injuries. One gastric and one prepyloric rupture of the stomach was seen, and one duodenal rupture occurred and was repaired without resection. Paraduodenal hematomas were encountered in six other patients, but no specific surgical intervention was necessary. In one patient a fractured pancreas was initially missed on the basis of peritoneal lavage, but was discovered using computed tomography and managed with resection of the distal pancreas with eventual recovery. Though blunt traumatic injuries to the extrahepatic biliary duct system are seen, they are uncommon[22,24] and none occurred in this group of patients. The diaphragm was ruptured in 44 patients, for an incidence of 5.1 percent of abdominal injuries.

Nearly 15 percent (14.6) of all patients with intra-abdominal trauma had retroperitoneal hematomas and there were 27 patients (3.1 percent) with major vascular injuries within the abdominal confines. Of the vascular injuries encountered due to blunt trauma, the abdominal aorta was ruptured in the one patient and there were no injuries to the iliac artery. The vena cava was ruptured on eight occasions, the iliac vein injured in one patient, and there was vascular disruption at the root of the small bowel mesentery in 17 patients. This injury carries a high mortality in most series.[3,11,35] The kidney was fractured, or severely contused, requiring opening of Gerota's fascia in 23 patients, resulting in 9 nephrectomies. The urinary bladder was ruptured 28 times and in all but 1 case there were associated pelvic fractures. Nine women had ruptured ovarian graafian follicles as an incidental finding at celiotomy.

MANAGEMENT OF SPECIFIC ORGAN INJURIES

Spleen

The management of splenic trauma has undergone a major revision in approach during the past 20 years. As was indicated earlier, access to spleen is best achieved through an epigastric transverse incision, although good exposure can usually be obtained through a midline approach. Until the early 1960s, splenectomy was considered to be the only acceptable treatment for all splenic injuries. This concept was based on a lack of appreciation of splenic function, as well as the belief that the splenic capsule was too thin to hold sutures and was therefore not amenable to repair. In 1962, Christo[6] in Brazil successfully performed segmental splenic resection in eight traumatized patients. Following this, Boda and Verzosa[2] described the use of absorbable gelatin sponges (GelFoam) in the repair of incidental splenic capsular tears. Since King and Schumacher[17] first described overwhelming postsplenectomy sepsis in 1962, the management of splenic injury has undergone continued re-evaluation. Initially, it was believed that this entity occurred only in children with hematologic disorders, until Singer[31] in 1973, on review of the literature, reported a 1.45 percent incidence of postsplenectomy sepsis after trauma. In children with splenectomy there was a mortality rate 60 times greater than normal children, regardless of the reason for splenectomy. It is now generally accepted that there is an increased susceptibility to infection in asplenic children and there is also evidence that this can occur in adults, although the incidence appears to be much less.

Successful splenorrhaphy in adults is now a well accepted procedure. However, the techniques to accomplish splenic repair are compromised by not gaining complete access to the spleen. To allow one to assess the extent of splenic injury accurately, the spleen must be completely mobilized into the incision by dividing all the lateral peritoneal attachments, as well as the lienophrenic, lienocolic, and lienorenal ligaments. In exposing the spleen for examination, one should avoid pulling down the omentum or depressing the stomach lest the vascular pedicle be avulsed. Where necessary, the short gastric vessels must be divided so that the spleen can be gently manipulated from its fossa in the left upper quadrant to the middle of the wound. Only through this type of exposure can adequate assessment of the injury to the spleen be accomplished and injury to the tail of the pancreas avoided. A common mistake is to try to assess the injury to the spleen before these mobilization maneuvers are completed.

One should be guided as to the nature of the definitive management of the splenic injury by an overall assessment of the patient's condition, which includes an evaluation of hemodynamic instability, the presence of dilutional or consumptive coagulopathy, or a splenic injury that is not amenable to repair. In addition, severe fecal contamination in the left upper quadrant, or multiple associated injuries, are usually contraindications to splenorrhaphy.

At the present time, when these criteria for splenorrhaphy are used, approximately 50 percent of MIEMSS patients with injured spleens are able to have surgery that conserves the spleen. The question as to whether splenorrhaphy can be successfully done has been answered affirmatively. It is a feasible procedure and it should be considered when possible and if the clinical circumstances are right. There is statistical evidence in our study that the requirements of time and blood replacement are slightly increased with splenorrhaphy. However, in our experience in the multiply injured patient there does not appear to be a significant increase in mortality or serious morbidity if one chooses to do this procedure based on the above exclusion criteria.

However, when the spleen must be removed, drainage of the splenic fossa is not a necessary part of the splenectomy, unless there is concomitant injury to the tail of the pancreas, or if there is an associated perforation of the stomach or the colon due to the original injury, or secondary to iatrogenic injury.

Liver

Liver injury occurred in 35.6 percent of trauma patients who sustained blunt injury to the abdomen.[8] When very severe, liver injury can be the most difficult injury to manage in blunt abdominal trauma. J.H. Pringle[27] in 1908 noted that "rupture of the liver is fortunately an accident not often met with, but one which when it is seen, may be associated with a condition of a patient as serious as anyone can meet in surgical practice." Small lacerations of the liver substance may stop bleeding spontaneously and permit recovery without surgical interference. However, if the laceration is extensive causing intrahepatic vessels of any magnitude to be torn, hemorrhage will continue owing to the structural arrangement of the liver. Since up to 20 percent of the normal cardiac output perfuses the liver by the time such a patient comes under the care of a surgeon, the physiologic state is almost invariably bound to be extremely grave from the combination of hemorrhage and circulatory shock. As also noted by Pringle, this sequence of events is of particular consequence in those hepatic injuries "due to contusing violence in which there is often gross injury inflicted on parts other than the liver, and where shock is liable to be more severe than in localized injury caused by sharp instruments."[27]

In the years since Pringle's notes on hepatic trauma, the surgeon's frustration in managing serious blunt injury to the liver remains and the mortality associated with it is virtually unchanged.[19,22,24,25,32,34] Our experience over a 6-year period with 281 patients with blunt traumatic liver injury is depicted in Tables 29-4 through 29-6. Of these patients, 42.7 percent had minor hepatic injuries with no mortality, 21.4 percent had moderate hepatic injuries also with no mortality, and 35.9 percent had severe hepatic injuries with a 58.4 percent mortality. Overall, 20.9 percent of patients with blunt liver injuries died. An additional 42 patients with minor or insignificant liver injuries died of causes unrelated to their hepatic trauma such as severe closed head injury, ruptured aorta, and others.

The surgical treatment of minor or moderate blunt hepatic injuries should give excellent results with few complications. As shown in Table 29-4, there was no mortality for hepatic injury in 180 patients with these injuries. No therapy was required in minor injuries and 83.3 percent of moderate injuries were repaired by simple suture alone. There was a 10 percent complication rate, mostly of a septic nature, which was related in part to the presence of other injuries. However, controlling bleeding from the liver severely injured by blunt trauma is a challenging and difficult problem.

In the 101 patients with severe blunt hepatic injury (Tables 29-5, 29-6), there was a 58 percent mortality. Of those patients with fatal outcomes, 71 percent died during the intra- or perioperative period because of massive hemorrhage compounded by coagulopathy, or other major nonhepatic injuries.

The high mortality in this group of severe

TABLE 29-4. Liver Injury Due to Blunt Trauma

	Minor Injury (No Therapy Required)		Moderate Injury (Surgical Therapy Required)	
	Number (n = 120)	% of Group	Number (n = 60)	% of Group
Vital signs				
Stable	97	80.8	45	75.0
Unstable	23[a]	19.2	15	25.0
Surgical therapy				
None required	120	100.0	—	—
Suture only	—		50	83.3
Cautery only	—		3	5.0
Packing with removal prior to closure	—		2	3.3
Hemostatic agent alone or in combination with above	—		10	16.6
Blood given (mean units)[a]				
Admission and OR	2.98		5.92	
Abdominal complications				
No drains, no complication	66	55.0	37	61.7
Drained, no complication	44	36.7	15	25.0
Drained with complication[b]	8	6.7	6[b]	10.0
No drains with complication[c]	2	1.6	2[c]	3.3
Total abdominal complications	10	8.3	8	13.3
Length of stay (LOS; mean days)[d]	15.2[d]		15.9[d]	
Mortality	0		0	

[a] Stability of vital signs and blood replacement in minor hepatic injury related to extrahepatic and nonabdominal trauma.

[b] Complications included wound infections, wound dehiscence, subphrenic abcesses, and bleeding requiring reoperation (1 case) in moderate injury group.

[c] Complications included wound infections, wound dehiscence, and one case of pancreatitis in minor injury group.

[d] LOS does not include patients with associated head injury or complicated orthopedic injuries.

blunt trauma injuries is similar to that reported in other series for patients with major blunt hepatic injuries.[24,34] As shown in Table 29-5 the perioperative (OP) deaths occurred in patients with multiple hepatic injuries. The OP deaths averaged more than 1.6 major liver injuries per case, including multiple bilobular parenchymal fractures, and were more likely in those with major stellate fractures and avulsions of the hepatic veins or tears into the hepatic vena cava. Although occasionally patients survive with those latter types of injuries, there were no survivors in this series. Also, the fatal cases of severe hepatic injury had a much higher incidence of other abdominal visceral or extra-abdominal injuries. Using the ratio of the incidence of deaths to survivors (ratio D/S) as a guide, the most important among the

associated abdominal organ injuries were those to the bowel (D/S = 6.0:1), diaphragm (D/S = 2.5:1), and spleen (D/S = 1.6:1), perhaps because those types of injury predisposed to shock or infection (Table 29-5). The most important extra-abdominal associated injuries predisposing to an early or late fatal outcome were a severe closed head injury (D/S = 2.4:1) or associated chest and lung trauma (D/S = 1.5:1).

The remaining deaths (29 percent occurred in the late postoperative period and were mainly due to sepsis and its late complications of ARDS, hepatic failure with coagulopathy, renal, or multiple organ failures (Table 29-6). In this regard, it is of significance to note that the incidence of major septic complications was three times as high in those patients who

TABLE 29-5. Severe Liver Injuries Due to Blunt Trauma

	Survivors N (%)	OP Deaths N (%)	Late Deaths N (%)	Total Deaths (%) N (%)	Total Patients (101)
	42 (41.5)	42 (41.5)	17 (16.8)	59 (58.4)	Ratio D/S[c]
Hepatic Injury					
Laceration R Lobe	29	32	9	41	**1.4:1**
Laceration L Lobe	9	10	5	15	**1.6:1**
Laceration Bilaterial	5	4	3	7	**1.4:1**
Stellate fracture	2	5	3	8	**4.0:1**
Caudate Laceration			1	1	1:0
Hepatic vein		8		8	**8:0**
Vena cava		9		9	**9:0**
Total	45 (1.1)[a]	68 (1.6)[a]	18 (1.1)[a]	89 (1.5)[a]	
Associated Abdominal Injury					
None	20	19	7	26	1.3:1
Gallbladder[b]	7	1	2	3	1.4:1
Spleen	13	12	9	21	**1.6:1**
Diaphram	2	3		5	**2.5:1**
Bowel	1	5	1	6	**6.0:1**
Kidney	1	2		2	2.0:1
Vascular	1	1		1	1.0:1
Pancreas	2				
Stomach	2				
Retroperitoneal	4	5	1	6	1.5:1
Associated Extra-abdominal Injuries					
None	9	5	5	10	1.1:1
Closed head injury	8	13	6	19	**2.4:1**
Face	10	5	4	9	0.9:1
Chest	17	22	3	25	**1.5:1**
Skeleton	16	11	9	20	1.3:1
Thoracic aorta	1		1	1	1.0:1

[a] Mean number of separate hepatic injuries per case.
[b] All gallbladder injuries were extensions of hepatic injury.
[c] Bold indicates death/survival ratios for the most important injuries.

TABLE 29-6. Severe Liver Injuries Due to Blunt Trauma

	Survivors		OP Deaths		Late Deaths		Total Deaths		Total Patients (101)
	N	%	N	%	N	%	N	%	
	42	(41.5)	42	(41.5)	17	(16.8)	59	(58.4)	Ratio D/S[b]
Surgical Intervention									
Suture	26		12		8		20		0.8:1
Resection debride	14		3		2		5		0.4:1
Anatomic lobectomy			6		2		8		**8:0**
Partial lobectomy	3		3		2		5		**1.6:1**
Packing	3		10		3		13		**4.3:1**
Hepatic artery ligation	3		4		7		11		**3.7:1**
IVC shunt			7				7		**7:0**
Omental pack	1								**0:1**
Death before Sx			7				7		**7:1**
Complications									
None	30								0:30
Wound infection	3								0:3
Sepsis or abscess	5				15		15		**3:1**
Rebleed	3				3		3		1:1
Pulmonary embolus	1								0:1
Renal failure					5		5		**5:0**
Coagulopathy					5		5		**5:0**
MI					1		1		1:0
Pulmonary failure					3		3		**3:0**
MOFS					5		5		**5:0**
LOS (days)	26.0				13.5[a]				

[a] Days till death.
[b] Bold indicates death/survival ratios for surgical procedures and complications in the most important injuries.

had a late fatal outcome as in the patients who survived. Also, while all patients with major hepatic trauma show some degree of hepatic dysfunction on a transient basis, the associated isolated organ failures as well as the multiple organ failure syndrome (MOFS) occurred almost exclusively in the nonsurviving group in this series. While ARDS and MOFS do occur in some surviving patients with major sepsis complicating hepatic trauma (Chap. 15), these complications represent an extremely high risk event that requires the full armamentarium of cardiorespiratory and metabolic support therapies if the patient is to survive. The successful management of this type of liver injury requires optimal planning and preoperative resuscitation, surgical expertise and judgement, and a sophisticated critical care capability. Controlling the bleeding from the liver severely injured by blunt trauma is a particularly challenging and difficult problem in the operating room.

Respected investigators from good institutions worldwide have proposed many measures for the emergency treatment of these injuries.[1,14,19,23-25,27,30,32-34] No dominant surgical technique has emerged to be used in every patient. An important finding with blunt trauma, as seen here, is that 81.2 percent *of all patients with major hepatic injury had severe associated extra-abdominal trauma* and 54.5 percent had another intra-abdominal organ injury complicating the severe condition of the liver and compromising all of the possible technical approaches to control bleeding from the liver.

Surgical Approaches to Liver Injury

SUTURING

Though suturing of the liver has been condemned by Mays,[22] Trunkey and co-workers,[34] reporting on a large series of patients, noted that 20.4 percent of their patients with extensive lacerations to the liver were treated using 0 to 1 chromic catgut with interlocking horizontal mattress sutures. As a result of their experience they advocated that bleeding points be managed by direct suture. It was thought that this technique reduced the chance of hepatic necrosis and hemobilia. However, only 21.3 percent of the 811 patients they reported were victims of blunt trauma and their data do not make clear whether these complications occurred to the same extent in this group as in the patients with penetrating trauma. In our experience, suturing of the liver as described above, with variations according to the operator's preference, was the most often used technique (Table 29-6). This technique was successfully used in all of the 60 patients with moderate injuries, and in 46 of 101 (45.5 percent) of the patients with severe hepatic injury, where it was successful in controlling hemorrhage in 74 percent of the injuries in which it was tried. In blunt trauma where there are multiple planes of fracture and where point ligation of bleeding vessels would require technical maneuvering that adds to the existing trauma, this simple, quick, traditional method of primary suture has been very effective in limiting blood loss. However major, or persistent, bleeding vessels should be individually suture ligated after the small vessel bleeding is controlled by suture of the hepatic substance. Lucas and Ledgerwood[19] have claimed that liver suture will cause hepatic ischemia. However, only 9 percent of Lucas and Ledgerwood's group of 637 patients had experienced blunt injury. We experienced none of the complications often alluded to (hemobilia and liver necrosis) in this group. Among the patients with severe hepatic injuries who died intraoperatively, the use of the suturing technique failed to result in survival in only 12 of the 42 patients (28.6 percent), but 5 of these patients who died had no detectable blood pressure on admission. No patient died specifically because the hepatic suture technique did not control bleeding.

RESECTION

Successful liver resectional debridement, completion resection, or partial lobectomy (segmentectomy) resection was performed in 27 patients (Table 29-6). These techniques were usually limited to removal of the injured frag-

ment peripheral to the normal blood flow and distal to the fracture line of the liver. Two patients required reoperation for bleeding that had been previously treated with ligation of the right hepatic artery. One patient's subsequent bleeding was controlled by suture of the offending vessel.

Major resection along anatomic planes was attempted eight times and was never successfully accomplished with a surviving patient. Mays,[22] in his monograph on hepatic trauma, in referring to anatomic lobectomy in acute injuries of the liver, states: "The mortality rate forbids it." Pachter and Spencer[24] in New York noted a mortality above 50 percent and commented that "though the techniques of hepatic resection have been well defined, there is a declining frequency in its [anatomic lobectomy] use." The experience in our institution substantiates the warnings of these investigators. However, when resectional debridement or limited resection is carried out, the finger-fracture technique advocated by Pachter et al.[25] appears to be very satisfactory.

INTRACAVAL SHUNTING

In 1968, Schrock and associates[30] described the use of intracaval shunting in a victim of a fall with avulsion of the hepatic veins and a lacerated inferior vena cava. Since that report, refinements of this technique have been added in search for a reliable approach to controlling bleeding when the injury to the liver includes the retrohepatic vena cava or the hepatic veins. In general, the results of intracaval shunting have been poor, but it is usually attempted in desperate situations. Yellin and associates[38] advocate venous isolation with occlusion of the inflow to the liver. Balasegaram,[1] reporting from Malaysia on 12 patients with "juxtahepatic venous" injury, had 8 survivors when venous isolation was used. He contends that sternotomy to gain supradiaphragmatic caval or right atrial exposure takes too much time in these desperate circumstances. He used intracaval shunting in seven patients without a survivor. All three approaches usually described, sternotomy or thoracoabdominal incision for the right atrial approach, or use of the suprarenal inferior vena cava for the insertion of this shunt, have been attempted.[1,22,24,30,34,38] Unfortunately, patients with these injuries generally die of exsanguination in spite of isolated reports of successful use of any of these shunting methods. This has led to a resumption of interest in packing for control of initial hemorrhage with later re-exploration, when coagulation factors are normal, for planned definitive therapy as necessary.

LIGATION OF ARTERIAL INFLOW

In 1933, Graham and Cannell[16] postulated that operative interference with the hepatic artery could be successfully done without hepatic necrosis. Hepatic artery ligation enjoyed a brief vogue in the treatment of cirrhosis when introduced by Rienhoff[28] in 1951. Mays[21] suggested that hepatic artery ligation be used in some cases of liver injury. More recently, Mays[23] has promulgated lobar dearterialization of the liver in selected patients for severe liver injury with certain limits. However, when the right hepatic artery is ligated the gallbladder must be removed to avoid necrosis. While some surgeons see a place for the use of this technique, others see it as an unnecessary hazard for the patient.[36] In our experience, two patients with right hepatic artery ligation and one patient with ligation of the proper hepatic artery survived. These were the only survivors of 14 patients who had emergency hepatic artery ligation. Of these three patients, the two survivors of the right hepatic artery ligation required reoperation for continued bleeding. The third survivor with ligation of the proper hepatic artery had an uncomplicated recovery, and he was discharged in 21 days. Therefore, the record for hepatic artery ligation in our study shows one unqualified success in 14 patients.

OMENTAL PACKING OF THE LACERATION

Stone and Lamb[33] in 1975 described the use of an isolated omental pedicle placed into the fracture defect and held in place by sutures. An updated experience by Fabian and Stone[14] in 1980 described their experience with 115 pa-

tients in which this method of packing was used to gain successful hemostatic control 90 percent of the time. However, most of their patients had penetrating hepatic trauma and their experience with the study of omental packing was limited to patients without severe arterial bleeding. In the experience in our institute, there has been one successful use of this technique for major hepatic fractures in the manner proposed by Stone and his colleagues. Pachter and colleagues[25] also advocated the use of an omental pack with good success, but only after resectional debridement. This latter approach has appeared to be a more effective use of the omental pack in our clinical experience with major hepatic injuries.

PACKING WITH GAUZE

Long considered a last, desperate measure to control bleeding from the liver, packing with gauze rolls or laparotomy pads under conditions where a major hepatic contusion with possible hepatic vein injury is associated with evidence of coagulopathy has been advocated as a deliberate planned first approach with reoperation 48 to 72 hours after coagulation parameters have returned to normal. Packing with laparotomy pads, with radiopaque identifiers, was used on 16 occasions (Table 29-6) in the MIEMSS 1978 to 1982 experience: 10 times as a late desperate measure in severe coagulopathy without success, 3 times without complication, and 3 times as a successful measure for hemorrhage, but where the patient developed severe intra-abdominal infection and sepsis with an eventually fatal outcome. Our more recent clinical results using this technique as a primary procedure early in the operation when major coagulopathy is present, have confirmed these initial findings: while hemorrhage generally can be well controlled, the risk of infection is high, and secondary and tertiary procedures for debridement and drainage of septic collections are the rule rather than the exception. These data would suggest that packing is a valid emergency measure for uncontrollable hemorrhage, but that one can expect serious septic complications as a consequence.

DRAINS AND COMPLICATIONS

The use of drainage following repair of hepatic injury is a controversial issue, with strong advocates on either side of the question. In the MIEMSS series when the patients who died early from associated injuries or intraoperatively were excluded (because drainage of the liver could not have been a complicating factor in their deaths), 239 patients could be evaluated with regard to the use of drains on outcome. Of these patients, 51.8 percent were closed without drains and 48.1 percent were closed with drains. However, when these cases of hepatic trauma are subdivided into a group with minor or moderate injury and compared to the severe trauma group who survived the initial posttrauma period (Table 29-7), a striking difference can be seen. In the 180 less severe cases, drainage was carried out in 73 patients (40.6 percent) and was associated with a 19.2 percent complication rate, primarily of a septic nature. This compared to only a 3.7 percent complication rate in the 107 (59.4 percent) undrained patients. Neither the drained nor the undrained patients with minor or moderate hepatic injuries died as a result of those complications. In contrast, in the 59 severe hepatic trauma patients, drainage was carried out in 42 (71.2 percent) and only 17 (28.8 percent) were not drained. The complication rate was somewhat higher in the drained group (35.7 percent) than the undrained patients (23.5 percent), but in those who subsequently died sepsis or a septic complication was the cause of

death in all of those not drained and in 64 percent of those drained. No patient in this series of 239 patients had bile peritonitis although some of the septic collections subsequently drained were bile-stained. No T-tube drainage of the common duct was used.

These data are consistent with the view that routine drainage is not advisable in minor or moderate hepatic trauma. However, the high septic complication rate in severe hepatic trauma would support the use of closed system drainage in major hepatic trauma and the use of wide drainage in those circumstances where a septic complication can be anticipated, for instance, where bowel contamination is associated with a severe liver injury.

As a final thought in this matter, no drains should be used at the initial procedure in patients in whom abdominal packing is used to control massive intraoperative hemorrhage. However, at the time of reoperation to remove the pack, the intra-abdominal blood clots should be removed by irrigation and any obviously necrotic liver should be debrided. An adequate number of drains, preferably of the closed-system type, should be placed in the area of major hepatic injury, or, alternatively, planned reoperation should be scheduled 48 to 72 hours after pack removal to debride any remaining necrotic liver again. Since sepsis is the major late complication leading to death in this group of patients, an effort should be made to remove all potential collections of blood or dead tissue that can serve as a nidus for infection and abscess formation.

TABLE 29-7. Use of Drains in Multiply Injured Patients with Hepatic Trauma (n = 239)[a]

Minor or moderate trauma			Complication rate[b] (%)
Not drained	107	(59.4%)	3.7
Drained	73	(40.6%)	19.2
Total	180		
Severe trauma			Complication rate[b] (%)
Not drained	17	(28.8%)	23.5
Drained	42	(71.2%)	35.7
Total	59		

[a] Perioperative deaths and early deaths from associated injuries with minor hepatic trauma are excluded.

[b] All septic in nature except one rebleed and one pancreatitis case in the minor and moderate group.

CONCLUSIONS REGARDING BLUNT LIVER INJURY

In patients with blunt traumatic injuries, the frequency and severity of the associated injuries, both abdominal and extra-abdominal, creates a disease entity distinct from that seen with most penetrating hepatic trauma. Such injuries require special considerations in judgment and management. Our experience confirms that of other students of this disease,[24,25] that a more conservative approach to major hepatic injury may be justified. While some surgeons still advocate extensive surgical procedures to deal with the consequences of major liver trauma, most experienced trauma surgeons are less inclined to attempt formal anatomic resections and prefer resectional debridement instead. Hepatic artery ligation does not appear to be of great value in arresting uncontrollable hepatic bleeding, and there are only a few instances in which intracaval shunting has been successful in treating major hepatic trauma complicated by hepatic vein or vena caval lacerations. Though the use of these devices has been successful in some cases, we believe that the contention that these procedures can be carried out with good success in all instances of severe trauma is misleading. In many instances the inappropriate use of these measures in desperation may have contributed to some less than favorable outcomes, where hepatic packing and later re-exploration might have achieved a successful result.

The mortality from liver trauma bears a direct relationship to the severity of the injury, and an inverse relationship to the judgment and skill of the team caring for the patients. Since the best results reported seem to come from institutions where a one-person, or one-team, approach is used, it may be well to consider means of stabilizing the patient until the "liver team" can be assembled.

On admission, most of the patients with severe liver injury have obvious abdominal distention, or gross blood return on diagnostic peritoneal lavage. They will usually be hemodynamically unstable. Since control of the bleeding is the ultimate goal, as soon as there is any suspicion of major liver trauma resuscitation with reconstituted fresh frozen plasma or warm whole blood should be started to reduce the high incidence of coagulopathy that develops with the use of red cell component transfusion only. Also, the infused blood and all other fluids should be warmed, from the very beginning of therapy, since hypothermia contributes to the coagulopathy and myocardial depression that often cause death, even when major bleeding has been controlled.

At operation, minor hepatic injuries that are not bleeding need little or no treatment. In more severe injuries, graded towards those with retrohepatic vena cava injury or hepatic vein involvement, the major goal should be to control bleeding. From these data the great majority of hepatic bleeders will be controlled with simple sutures placed 2 to 3 cm from the edge of the laceration or fracture. Absorbable suture material is used on a blunt-point needle with a large arc, and sutures are placed in the liver in an interlocking fashion so as to buttress each other. Larger bleeding vessels may need to be controlled with direct suture using nonabsorbable suture ligatures. However, concern over the later development of intrahepatic hematomas, hemobilia, liver necrosis along the suture line, bile collections, or biliary fistulas appears largely unwarranted, since these are very infrequent complications. The more peripheral the hepatic injury, the better the simple suture method works. If done with a minimum of meddling, this will save blood, time, and lives.

Deeper, more centrally placed, injuries may require more complicated surgical interventions. Often there is a blood clot in the fracture fissure. Before succumbing to one's curiosity to probe the depths of the wound, it is well to dry up the area and ascertain the degree of bleeding. Major arterial or portal vein branches should be suture ligated if they are actively bleeding, but if only capillary oozing is present this may be an instance where an omental pack is justified. Devitalized fragments should be conservatively debrided after placement of proximal liver sutures to control hemorrhage. If there is major deep hemorrhage, and especially if a coagulopathy is present, one option gaining favor is that of packing with laparotomy pads carefully placed between the liver and the diaphragm. These are stabilized with several additional pads in the subhepatic space. Empirically, some individuals advocate that the pads be dampened with an antibiotic solution, but there is no conclusive evidence to support this use of topical antibiotics. When tamponade packing is utilized no drains are used, and after 48 to 72 hours, when coagulation factors have been returned to normal, the patient is operated on again, the pads removed, and blood clots gently irrigated away and obviously devitalized tissue removed.

In some of these deeper injuries to the liver, the bleeding is too great to ignore and cannot be controlled by simple measures. These cases lend themselves to point ligation of the bleeding by widening the "hepatotomy." Though our direct experience with omental packing is limited, it has been strongly advocated for use in these situations by Stone[33] and by Pachter et al.[25]

In the management of the severe fragmented fracture of the liver, where the viability of the distal segment is questionable, completion resectional debridement with bleeding points controlled by suture ligation is preferable to the use of electrocautery or hemoclips, since the repeated "mopping" with gauze pads tends to pull off the clips and the eschar. These procedures can be tedious and time-consuming. The infrared laser has been used for this type of case in Europe, but is not generally available in this country at the present time. Impatience or persistence in operating in the face of uncontrolled bleeding is not often rewarded by successful outcome. The patient must be hemodynamically stable, if possible, before complicated technical maneuvers are undertaken. The Pringle maneuver (compression of the porta hepatis including the hepatic artery and the portal vein, plus compression of the liver, while waiting for replacement of blood) often can control the bleeding from smaller vessels, making identification of major hepatic vessels possible. This approach seems easy to do, but it is often ignored.

There is a critical point in massive hepatic hemorrhage at which the clotting factors become depleted and the patient's clotting time becomes greatly extended. When this point is recognized, if major arterial bleeding is controlled the better part of valor is to pack the hepatic injury and close the abdomen. One can then hope to try another day after the bleeding is brought under control by the use of fresh frozen clotting factors and/or fresh warm whole blood. In the intraoperative volume replacement of patients with major hepatic trauma, fresh frozen plasma and platelet transfusions must be used as early as is possible, and continued through the postoperative period (see Chap. 23). The liver is the origin of many clotting factors and it is reasonable to assume that it has been functionally impaired by the injury, the associated hypovolemic shock, and the transfusion-related hypothermia.

Measures to deal with injuries to the liver that involve the retrohepatic vena cava and hepatic veins using intracaval shunts have been described.[1,30,38] Our experience is the same as that described by Walt[36]: only when such massive injuries are anticipated and suspected in advance, and if the patient's condition allows time for deliberate planning of the surgical approach to the vena cava, do the shunting and inflow procedures advocated stand a reasonable chance of success. Until some new technical advance allows controlled access to these injuries in a dry operating field, the mortality for these types of injuries will continue to be forbidding.

Since the original techniques proposed by Pringle,[27] there have been constant advances in the intensive care of critically injured hepatic trauma patients, especially in the areas of treatment of hypovolemic shock (Chap. 9), control of sepsis and hepatic failure (Chaps. 15 and 16), support of respiratory function care (Chap. 19), and nutrition (Chap. 17). The concept of a liver trauma team of experienced trauma surgeons alluded to by Spencer[32] should be considered for general use as more trauma centers evolve to improve the care of civilian trauma.

Intestine

Intestinal injury, if not diagnosed on initial evaluation, has a greater chance of producing late septic complications and death than almost any other abdominal injury. Blunt trauma to the abdomen can result in perforation or devascularization of the intestine. The relative infrequency of this event, the mechanisms of bowel injury, and the location of these injuries and the difficulty in their diagnosis have been the theme of many reports.[3,7,11,35] In 1899 Geill, as noted by Vance,[35] reported an 11 percent incidence of major intestinal injury among patients sustaining blunt abdominal trauma. This figure is consistent with the 5 to 15 percent incidence reported in modern series of blunt trauma, making the intestinal tract the third most commonly injured organ in the abdomen. In spite of this, the overall occurrence of blunt intestinal injury is low. Bosworth's[3] study in 1948 calculated an incidence of only 1:10,000 to 20,000 admissions for the general surgical services in six major hospitals in New York City during a 10-year period. Although more common today due to an increased number of high speed motor vehicle accidents, these injuries are still relatively infrequent. Many theories have been introduced to explain why these injuries occur. Vance[35] credits Moty with postulating the three most popular mechanisms: (1) crush injury between the vertebrae and anterior abdominal wall, (2) a sudden increase of intraluminal pressure of the bowel, and (3) tangential tears at a relatively fixed point along the bowel. Others think that such factors as age and the degree of intoxication may positively influence the incidence of these injuries because of their lessening of the protective role of the musculature of the abdominal wall.

In 1935, Counseller and McCormack[7] gave evidence to support the fixed point theory of traumatic bowel injury in a review of the world literature on the subject. They analyzed over 1,000 cases and reported that the majority of small bowel injuries occurred in the proximal jejunum or distal ileum. They reported a high mortality: 73 percent. In most centers the advent and use of the diagnostic peritoneal lavage have lessened the chance of missing these injuries due to delayed diagnosis. Dauterive and colleagues[11] reviewed all patients sustaining major intestinal injuries at MIEMSS during the 5-year period 1978 to 1982. Sixty patients sustained major intestinal injuries. The average age was 33.2 years and the male to female ratio was 7.5:1. Automobile accidents accounted for 77 percent of the patients, motorcycle accidents claimed 13 percent, and the re-

mainder were the results of miscellaneous accidents, such as falls or crush injuries.

The incidence[8] of major bowel injury in the 870 MIEMSS blunt trauma patients who had abdominal trauma proven by celiotomy was 6.9 percent. In all instances, the diagnosis of intestinal trauma was made at the time of celiotomy. This is consistent with the descriptions of intestinal injury reported in the various studies made in the past.[3,7,11,35] There were 83 major injuries among the 60 patients reported (Table 29-8). As shown in Figure 29-6, 30 perforating or transecting small bowel injuries occurred between the ligament of Treitz and the ileocecal valve without any preference for specific location. There were only two perforations of the duodenum, and seven bowel perforations or transections were distributed throughout the colon.

The operative findings in this group of injuries showed that of the 30 patients with perforations of the small bowel, 50 percent underwent debridement and primary closure while 43 percent required resection with anastomosis. One patient had two perforations treated with one resection and another patient died intraoperatively of other causes before the small bowel perforation was treated.

Major mesenteric injuries (Fig. 29-7) accounted for 41 of the lesions in this series of cases. There were 24 involving the small bowel with a predilection for the distal ileum. The colonic mesentery was disrupted seven times, six in the right colon. Twenty-two of these patients underwent resection with primary anastomosis, while two died intraoperatively of other major injuries before treatment of the bowel injury could be undertaken.

In this group of intestinal blunt trauma patients, there were 17 with large bowel injuries

TABLE 29-8. Site of Major Intestinal Injuries in 60 Patients with Blunt Abdominal Trauma

	Small Bowel	Colon
Perforation/transection	30	7
Devascularization	34[a]	7
Severe contusion	0	5

[a] Includes 10 injuries to the root of the mesentery.
(Dauterive AH, Flancbaum L, Cox EF: Blunt intestinal trauma: a modern day review. Ann Surg 201:198, 1985.)

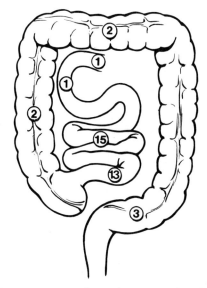

FIG. 29-6 Sites of bowel perforations or transections. (Dauterive AH, Flancbaum L, Cox EF: Blunt intestinal trauma: a modern day review. Ann Surg 201: 198, 1985.)

(Figs. 29-6, 29-7). Seven had perforations of the colon, five sustained ischemic injuries resulting from mesenteric devascularizing trauma, and five patients had local serosal tears or contusions of the colonic wall. Four of these seromuscular tears were located in the sigmoid colon and one was in the transverse colon. With the exception of two patients with minimal perforations that could safely be closed primarily with good serosal approximation, and two patients who died intraoperatively of other massive injuries, the rest were all treated by surgical procedures to remove the injured bowel from the peritoneal cavity. Ten patients had resection of the injured colon with either colostomy or cecostomy (for cecal and ascending colon injuries), and three patients with sigmoid colon serosal tears or other significant local damage had primary repair and exteriorization of the injury. The danger of anastomotic or suture line breakdown in unprepared large bowel is very great, with the inevitable consequences of peritonitis or abscess formation, which are poorly tolerated by the multiply injured patient. Therefore, resection of the injured area with colostomy is the safest choice for surgical repair of blunt traumatic injuries of the colon.

In favorable instances where only a limited antimesenteric laceration or perforation is present, primary repair with exteriorization of the traumatized area can be an alternative to colostomy, with the knowledge that at least 50 percent of exteriorization repairs will fail and need to be converted to a colostomy.

Ten patients had injuries to the root of the mesentery with lacerations of the superior mesenteric vein, three with simultaneous avulsion tears of the mesenteric artery and all of whom died. Suture repair of the superior mesenteric vein was performed in six patients with 100 percent survival. The seventh patient, whose injury extended into the portal vein, died intraoperatively.

The overall mortality in this group of 60 patients with intestinal injuries was 26 percent. However, five of these deaths were the result of serious head injuries and four other patients had vascular injuries at the root of the mesentery that resulted in death. One patient who was transferred from another hospital with a missed colon injury on initial lavage suffered sudden death postoperatively from myocardial

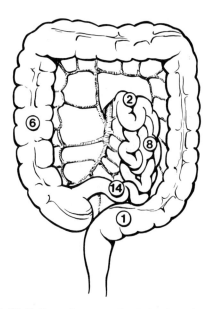

FIG. 29-7 Sites of mesenteric injuries throughout the intestines, excluding disruptions of superior mesenteric vessels at the root of the mesentery. (From Dauterive AH, Flancbaum L, Cox EF: Blunt intestinal trauma: a modern day review. Ann Surg 201: 198, 1985.)

TABLE 29-9. Mortality Directly Related to Complications of Bowel Injury

No.	Age/Sex	Mode of Injury	Bowel Injury	Other Injury	Complication	Time from Accident to Death
1	50 M	Auto	Avulsion of distal ileum	Ruptured spleen Fracture pelvis	Pelvic abscess → multiple organ failure	22 days
2	50 M	Auto	Perforation of distal ileum/devascularization of segment of ileum and right colon	None	Iatrogenic disruption of anastamosis at reoperation for GI bleed → sepsis	18 days
3	15 F	Auto	Perforation of distal ileum	Pelvic fracture Bilateral femur fracture Radius fracture Ruptured spleen Ruptured bladder	Pelvic abscess with probable infected retroperitoneal hematoma	30 days
4	37 M	Auto	Perforation of midjejunum Mesenteric hematoma	T_9 fracture and paraplegia Multiple rib fractures	Intra-abdominal abscess/sepsis/renal failure	19 days
5[a]	35 M	Auto	Perforation of mid small bowel and sigmoid colon	Fractured humerus Fractured tibia–fibula	Missed jejunal injury → sepsis → multiple organ failure	20 days
6	55 M	Airplane	Mesenteric injury to distal ileum	Laforte III Ruptured spleen Bilateral femur fractures	Intra-abdominal abscess/gangrenous cholecystitis	60 days

[a] Transferred to MIEMSS Shock Trauma unit after laparotomy.
(Dauterive AH, Flancbaum L, Cox EF: Blunt intestinal trauma: a modern day review. Ann Surg 201:198, 1985.)

infarction. He had a previous history of angina pectoris and hypertension. The remaining six patients (Table 29-9) all had late septic complications as a direct result of their bowel injury that contributed at least in part to their death.

Most publications dealing with blunt intestinal trauma are based on a few cases collected over many years. Over extended periods of time, changes in the mode of injury, methods of diagnosis, and method of treatments can affect these results and conclusions. Whatever the mechanism, the early recognition of bowel injury lesions can be difficult. The patients in this report were identified by a similar diagnostic protocol during a relatively short period of time and with one exception, a late transfer, were treated early in their clinical course. An overlooked bowel injury is perhaps the most dangerous of all abdominal injuries because of the great potential for infection. Repeated studies have shown that an increased mortality is directly related to the delay in diagnosis. Peritoneal lavage has proven to be extremely useful in the early detection of intraperitoneal injuries. It was diagnostic in 33 of 34 patients (97 percent) with isolated bowel injuries reported here and was probably improperly performed in the one missed case.

In patients injured by blunt trauma, the danger of failing to recognize a perforation of the intestine cannot be overstated. It has been estimated that if hemodynamically stable, at least 50 percent of the patients with blunt abdominal trauma would not require celiotomy, even with a positive peritoneal lavage, except that the risk of leaving perforated intestine dictates early exploratory celiotomy. If some means of ruling out perforated intestine in stable patients were possible, it would be a significant advance in the management of the abdomen in the acutely injured patient with nonpenetrating trauma. In investigating a solution to this problem Cox and Uddo[10] did a series of experiments on dogs, in which the bowel was perforated by insertion of a trocar through the anal canal. Using nitrogen gas insufflated through a needle into the peritoneal cavity, evacuated in 5 minutes and analyzed by gas chromatography, they were able to identify methane, hydrogen sulfide, and other gases from the bowel. Future clinical studies with this technique may make it possible to exclude

from celiotomy stable blunt trauma patients without perforated intestines.

Retroperitoneal Bowel

Retroperitoneal injuries of bowel resulting from trauma are often very difficult to diagnose since peritoneal lavage may be negative or equivocal unless there is also a free intraperitoneal perforation component to the injury. This is especially true of duodenal injuries. When injuries of this sort are suspected based on the history or physical findings on abdominal flat film x-ray, a CT scan of the abdomen looking for retroperitoneal gas or fluid is essential. However, regardless of the findings, if the index of suspicion is high exploration is justified, in view of the poor prognosis following delayed treatment of these injuries.

In the MIEMSS experience from 1978 to 1982 only two blunt perforations of the duodenum were seen, and by the 1983 to 1984 year this had risen to six cases. Coincidentally, only three major pancreatic injuries and one stomach perforation from blunt trauma were seen. These injuries usually occur by direct blows from objects such as the steering wheel or gear shift of an automobile. However, they are more prone to follow insults from well-localized blows from fist, feet, bicycle handlebars, and small weapons.

Unless there is some index of suspicion from radiographic studies, the duodenum is not routinely mobilized in the absence of bile staining or localized retroperitoneal bleeding. This maneuver, although simple, prolongs the operation and may result in iatrogenic injuries. Yet of the injuries to the small intestine, injury to the duodenum is the most difficult to diagnose. In our environment where, due to the urgency of the situation, the nature of the intra-abdominal injury is diagnosed largely on the basis of celiotomy, careful examination of the duodenum has generally established the presence of this problem. Whenever a paraduodenal hematoma is noted, there must be a thorough exploration of the first, second, third, and fourth portions of the duodenum to rule out rupture of this viscus. This is best done by employing the

Kocher maneuver: incising the peritoneum at the outer or convex margin of the duodenum, mobilizing the hepatic flexure and right transverse colon, and lifting the duodenum to explore all surfaces of the first, second, and proximal third portion of the duodenum. The remaining portions of the duodenum can be examined by turning to the root of the mesentery and incising the ligament of Treitz if necessary. Using these maneuvers, the integrity of the superior mesenteric artery and vein can also be established.

When small perforations of the duodenum are discovered that do not have extensive associated contusion, they can be treated by simple closure of the perforation, which can be reinforced, if necessary, by bringing up a loop of proximal jejunum as a serosal patch. More difficult or more extensive duodenal injuries can be treated by converting the injury to a side-to-side jejunoduodenostomy, or in some instances, a Roux-en-Y jejunal loop can be brought to the injured portion of the duodenum. Under special circumstances where no other alternatives exist, a duodenal diverticulum can be established and a gastrojejunostomy used to divert the gastric contents from the duodenum.

Pancreas

The pancreas presents a special problem in blunt abdominal trauma because of its retroperitoneal location, and its position posterior to the lesser omental bursa, which may produce a false-negative peritoneal lavage. In this study, one instance of ruptured pancreas was missed by peritoneal lavage. However, the use of CT in patients with potential pancreatic injury can permit a diagnosis to be made. In general, pancreatic lesions are seldom, if ever, isolated injuries and although they can be missed by peritoneal lavage, this will usually be a rare circumstance. Any evidence of contusion of the gastrocolic megacolon or other evidence of injury to the stomach, transverse colon, or mesenteric root dictates that the omental bursa be opened and the pancreas carefully examined. Unless there is bleeding that is not easily

controlled, conservative measures such as sump, or a closed system drainage to the injury site, is the best method of management for these types of injuries, even if the head of the pancreas is severely contused. However, if there is any suspicion of a major ductal injury, which usually occurs in the body of the pancreas where it overlies the spine, the duct should be visualized by pancreatography if the patient's condition permits. A major duct or pancreatic gland transection should be treated by distal resection, with closure of the pancreatic stump rather than by internal drainage by a Roux-en-Y loop. This is because the traumatized normal gland holds sutures poorly and opening an otherwise intact bowel merely converts a traumatic pancreatic injury into an infected pancreatic injury with a great potential for sepsis and abscess formation.

Dramatic procedures such as a pancreatoduodenectomy are not warranted unless a massive injury has destroyed both organs or uncontrollable pancreatic bleeding is present. Adequate drainage of all pancreatic injuries is essential. Both sump and passive drains should be led out of the flanks over the top of Gerota's fascia to ensure good dependent drainage of the patient lying in the supine position, since the enzymatic action of the pancreas on tissues in the abdomen can cause serious peritonitis or retroperitoneal necrosis and erosion of vessels with major hemorrhage.

Diaphragm

Diaphragmatic rupture was first recognized, as early as 1541 and its documentation is credited to Sennertus. In 1578 during a postmortem examination, Ambroise Paré discovered loops of bowel herniated through the left diaphragm of a French army captain who had sustained an abdominal gunshot wound months before. The first premortem diagnosis of traumatic diaphragmatic hernia was reported by Bowditch[4] in 1853, when he described a 17-year-old boy with this injury, and reviewed the world literature. Since that time, numerous articles dealing with blunt and penetrating injuries to the diaphragm have appeared. Because of its relative infrequency, large series of patients with blunt diaphragmatic injury have only been accrued over long periods of time.[13] Over a 5-year period (1978 to 1982), 44 patients who had ruptures of the diaphragm were seen at MIEMSS. Thirty-three of the ruptures were left-sided (75 percent), eight were right-sided (18 percent), two were ruptured through the central tendon and pericardium, and one was bilateral. The mean age was 34 years of age, and there were 33 male and 11 female patients. Motor vehicle accidents accounted for all but one of the injuries.

On physical examination, evidence suggestive of diaphragmatic injury was nonspecific and seldom unequivocal. Chest and abdominal wall contusions were the most common finding, but were present in only seven patients, and were not helpful in establishing the diagnosis. Hypotension, less than 90 mmHg, as an indication of severe trauma was seen in 15 patients (34 percent). Chest radiographs were obtained in 42 patients at the time of admission and abnormalities were noted in 34 of 37 patients (92 percent) whose chest radiographs were available for retrospective reviews (Table 29-10). The majority of abnormal findings were rib fractures, pneumothorax, hemothorax, and pulmonary contusion and were present as nonspecific findings in only 14 patients (32 percent), when the initial chest radiograph demonstrated diaphragmatic rupture. The findings thought to be diagnostic were a markedly elevated left hemidiaphragm, the presence of a herniated abdominal viscus into the chest, a double shadow overlying the diaphragm, and the presence of a nasogastric tube in the chest. However, 8 percent of the patients with a documented diaphragmatic hernia had radiographs interpreted as normal.

Diagnostic peritoneal lavage was positive in only 22 patients (50 percent), but was the most common indication for operation. Six patients (21 percent) had false-negative peritoneal lavages, and were operated on for specific radiographic evidence of a ruptured diaphragm. Overall, in 41 of the 44 patients (93 percent) a diagnosis of ruptured diaphragm was established within 6 hours of admission. Nineteen patients operated on acutely had a preoperative diagnosis of diaphragmatic rupture, while in 17 patients the ruptured diaphragm was an incidental finding during celiotomy (Table 29-11). Five patients had the diagnosis made during thoracotomy for associated injuries, and five had the diagnosis established by visualization of intraperitoneal fluid or omentum extruded through a thoracostomy tube placed as an emergency procedure to relieve an acute pneumo- or hemopneumothorax. The remaining three patients (7 percent) had delayed diagnosis, two confirmed by upper gastrointestinal contrast studies and one by CT scan, 3 to 5 days following admission.

The operative findings on all 44 patients with ruptured diaphragms due to blunt trauma are summarized in Table 29-12. All patients with right-sided diaphragmatic or central diaphragmatic rupture had associated intra-abdominal injuries, as did 20 patients (61 percent) with left-sided injuries. Only nineteen patients (43 percent) had a sustained herniation of abdominal viscera into the chest. The operative approach was transabdominal in 18 of these 19 patients, and in only one case was extension from the abdomen into the left chest required

TABLE 29-10. Radiographic Findings at Admission in Acute Posttraumatic Diaphragmatic Herniation

Findings	Number of Patients
Rib fractures	16
Pneumothorax	11
Hemothorax	9
Pulmonary contusion/infiltrate	7
Herniated viscus into chest	7
Elevated left hemidiaphragm	6
Nasogastric tube in left chest	1
Normal	3

TABLE 29-11. Method of Diagnosis of Acute Posttraumatic Diaphragmatic Herniation

	Number of Patients
Early	
Chest radiograph	14
Egress of fluid via chest tube	5
Incidental finding at thoracotomy	5
Incidental finding at celiotomy	17
Late	
UGI contrast studies	2
Computed tomography	1

TABLE 29-12. Operative Findings in Acute Posttraumatic Diaphragmatic Herniation

Findings	Left	Right	Central Tendon
Splenic injury	10	3	—
Liver injury	4	3	3
Hollow viscus injury	2	3	2
Retroperitoneal hematoma	2	—	1
Ruptured bladder	2	—	—
Fractured kidney	2	—	—
Stomach in chest	13	—	—
Spleen in chest	11	—	—
Small bowel in chest	3	—	—
Omentum in chest	4	—	—
Colon in chest	1	—	—
Liver in chest	—	2	—
Pericardial rupture	2	1	2

to complete the diaphragmatic repair. Two patients had emergency thoracotomy following cardiac arrest and the diaphragmatic injury was repaired by that incision. Two patients had elective right thoracotomy, one for persistent bleeding through a chest tube, and one after delayed diagnosis of a right-sided diaphragm injury. One patient had an open left chest wound explored for bleeding. Complications developed in 26 (59 percent) of all patients with diaphragmatic rupture. These were largely related to pulmonary complications, atelectasis, lung abscess, empyema, and persistent pneumothorax. There were no deaths directly attributable to the diaphragmatic injury per se. However, death due to associated organ injuries or sepsis occurred in 20.5 percent of all cases.

Operative management of these injuries was predominantly through the abdomen for both left- and right-sided diaphragmatic injuries. There is a continuing controversy concerning the operative approach for right-sided injuries. Seven of the eight patients with this injury were operated on acutely, and the injury was repaired *without* extension into the right chest. In the acute situation, where associated intraabdominal injuries are likely, the transabdominal approach should be utilized primarily and, if necessary, a second thoracotomy incision performed to reduce the hernia. As demonstrated 17 times (39 percent) in the 44 cases in this study, it is still vitally important that the surgeon operating on the abdomen following blunt trauma *feel carefully along the entire diaphragmatic surface* to avoid missing an unsuspected rupture.

Although signs of thoracic injury were commonly present (rib fractures, hemothorax, pneumothorax) the evidence accumulated from these patients indicated that this injury occurred secondary to impact of the abdomen. It is of interest in this regard that six of these patients who were personally questioned after postoperative recovery by Cox. They each claimed to be aware of the pending crash, were conscious at the time, and recalled bracing themselves for the impact while holding their breath. With the victim in a Valsalva position and with the tightened anterior abdominal wall, the diaphragm offers the weakest point for the release of the increased pressure created by the impinging steering wheel, dashboard, or other hard surface. This is consistent with postulated mechanisms discussed by Desforges[12] and Wise.[37] In contrast with these findings, Ebert[13] has suggested that diaphragmatic ruptures occur more frequently in thoracic trauma.

In conclusion, in diaphragmatic ruptures due to blunt trauma overt evidence of a ruptured diaphragm is present in only about half of the cases. These are patients in whom peritoneal lavage fluid, or omentum passes through a previously placed chest tube, or where unequivocal radiograph evidence demonstrates the abnormality. In the remaining patients with this entity the diagnosis will be made incidentally, during thoracotomy or celiotomy for associated injuries. This is also confirmed by previous reports[12,13,37] that describe the lack of specificity of physical examination and chest roentgenography in diagnosing this entity. This degree of uncertainty in preoperative diagnosis makes it imperative that a careful exploration of all portions of the intra-abdominal diaphragmatic surface be carried out during surgery in every patient with blunt abdominal trauma who requires exploration for any other cause. Also, the incidence of delayed discovery of diaphragmatic rupture, although small (7 percent in this series), suggests that a minimal injury may enlarge over time to produce a diaphragmatic herniation. It also implies the need for careful follow-up radiographic examination in all patients with severe blunt abdominal trauma who do not require emergency surgical exploration.

Retroperitoneum

Trauma causing bleeding into the retroperitoneal space that does not involve major retroperitoneal organs was noted in 15 percent of blunt trauma patients in the MIEMSS series. Retroperitoneal hematomas not suspected of involving specific organs are seldom opened since the bleeding is difficult to control once the tamponade of the peritoneal tissues is relieved. In general, retroperitoneal bleeding here serves to alert the surgeon to the fact that the patient has sustained severe injury and that continuing volume infusion and observation of blood coagulation factors are essential.

Kidney, Bladder and Ovary

Although the kidneys and the bladder are not truly abdominal organs, they are included in this series because the preferred surgical access is through the abdominal wall in the usual trauma setting. The kidney was fractured, or severely contused, requiring opening of Gerota's fascia in 23 patients (2.7 percent) of the 870 blunt trauma patients with intra-abdominal injuries. Surgical exploration of the kidneys resulted in nine nephrectomies. The urinary bladder was ruptured 28 times (3.3 percent) and in all but one case there were associated pelvic fractures. The incidence of these injuries makes a thorough radiographic study of the urinary tract mandatory in any case of blunt trauma in which hematuria is present. If emergency surgery is required for other life-threatening injury, a cystourethrogram as well as a one-shot (intravenous pyelogram) (IVP) can be done in the emergency admitting area using portable equipment. Both a distended view and a postevacuation view of the contrast-filled bladder are essential if retroperitoneal as well as intraperitoneal bladder ruptures are to be diagnosed. If time permits, or if an abdominal or head CT examination is required for another cause, the preferred visualization of the extent of renal injury is by this modality and a more rational decision regarding renal exploration can be made. Unless the kidney does not take up contrast, or shows major disruption with extravasation of urine into the retroperitoneal space, conservative management is indicated, since the incidence of nephrectomy increases if the Gerota's fascia is opened. In cases where nonvisualization of the kidney occurs and is confirmed by repeat radiographic or CT study, immediate renal arteriography should be done unless other more life-threatening injuries mandate immediate surgery, since the incidence of renal arterial intimal tears with arterial thrombosis is high in these cases. Repair or bypass of such lesions within 4 to 6 hours after injury is the only therapy with a reasonable chance of salvaging the kidney.

Another retroperitoneal organ that can produce positive findings on peritoneal lavage is the ovary. Nine women in the MIEMSS series had ruptured ovarian graafian follicles as the sole finding on celiotomy that had produced abdominal signs or positive peritoneal lavage. The treatment of injuries to the uterus during pregnancy is discussed in Chapter 35.

Aorta and Vena Cava

Of the vascular injuries encountered in the retroperitoneal space, the abdominal artery was ruptured in one patient and there were no injuries to iliac arteries. Blunt traumatic injuries to the aorta are extremely rare, usually infrarenal in location, and are most commonly associated with steering wheel injuries.[18] Their most common presentation is as thrombosis secondary to intimal disruption 2 weeks to 1 year after injury. However, disruption of the aorta with pseudoaneurysm can occur, usually presenting as an acute abdomen with pain, mass, and an abdominal bruit. Prompt aortography and graft replacement should be done unless there is contamination of the abdomen by bowel disruption. In this case, closure of the proximal and distal aorta should be done with resection of the damaged segment and extraanatomic bypass using axillobifemoral or bilateral axillofemoral Dacron or Gortex grafts. Later, when all intra-abdominal injuries have healed and no evidence of infection is present, anatomic graft anastomosis of proximal and distal segments can be done if necessary.

The vena cava, the most commonly injured great vessel, was ruptured on eight occasions. There were 17 vascular disruptions at the root of the mesentery as described in the small bowel section. This is a serious injury and was associated with high mortality. Such injuries required an aggressive approach to management, as discussed more thoroughly in Chapter 30. Recently, Maddox[20] has described a retroperitoneal approach to these lesions by mobilizing all the left-sided viscera, which may improve the chances of satisfactory repairs. However, in all cases of major injury to the superior mesenteric artery or vein with repair of these vascular structures, it is essential to plan a *second-look* procedure within 24 to 48 hours to check for the presence of nonviable bowel. If this is present, resection with anastomosis of viable small bowel, or ileostomy or colostomy for right- or left-sided colon lesions, respectively, is usually necessary if the patient is to survive. Major advances have occurred in chronic intravenous hyperalimentation and the development of nutritional fuels (Chap. 17) that can be absorbed from short segments of proximal bowel. The surgeon confronted with major portions of nonviable bowel in a young or otherwise previously healthy person should therefore not hesitate to resect widely and perform any possible anastomosis between viable structures, or even to produce a temporary high small bowel ostomy, since these patients can often be salvaged by aggressive nutritional support.

COMPLICATIONS AND MORTALITY

Due to the complexity of injuries in blunt trauma patients who require celiotomy for major intra-abdominal organ trauma, it is not warranted to ascribe all mortality to the injuries found in the abdomen. As discussed in Chapter 1, in this type of multiply injured patient treated at MIEMSS the incidence of severe head injuries has remained a fairly constant 13 to 15 percent of all admissions, with some form of head trauma present in 34 percent of the trauma patients. There is also a small, but significant, incidence of nonsurvivable cardiac, aortic, and open pelvic fracture injuries. However, the intraoperative mortality from all causes from 1978 to 1982 was 2.1 percent, with that from all intra-abdominal procedures representing 55 percent of the total, due largely to the mortality from severe hepatic injuries.[8] Improved resuscitation techniques and physiologic monitoring have caused this intraoperative death rate to continue to decrease, as discussed in Chapter 1. However, certain types of injuries were fatal regardless of use of the most sophisticated intervention. The late deaths were usually associated with sepsis or with deterioration of brain function in patients with an associated severe head injury. Caplan and Hoyt[5] (see Chap. 16) have studied MIEMSS infections and concluded that the nature of the organ injury and the invasive procedures required for management of these patients are the major causes of infection. However, as discussed in Chapter 14, major trauma compromises the host defense mechanisms. Multiorgan and/or pulmonary failure was present in all but a few of those who died late.

As also shown in Chapter 1, there has been an encouraging year-to-year improvement observed in the mortality rate. The most significant factor would appear to be the development of established protocols for resuscitation and care (Chap. 26) and the combined increase in experience of a young, stable staff of dedicated trauma surgeons. There has also been a general increase knowledge in techniques of physiologically based pre- and postoperative support (Chaps. 9 and 15) and respiratory (Chap. 19) and nutritional adjuncts (Chaps. 15 and 17), and infection control (Chap. 16). It is possible that the severity of injuries has decreased since the energy crisis of the late 1970s. This seems unlikely, in view of the data presented in Chapter 1 that the injury severity scores of patients admitted to MIEMSS have remained stable or increased. While the increasing national outrage against the drunk driver has stimulated legislative action to control this hazard, the incidence of alcohol-related accident victims admitted to MIEMSS has remained relatively constant. Public pressure on auto manufacturers, increased highway policing, and constant media awareness of safety devices (seat belts, air bags) will, we hope, combine to make motor vehicle travel safer in the future and lessen the incidence of intra-abdominal injuries. However, the preponderance of data suggests that the major factor that will improve the survival of those who are injured is a well-organized trauma center made available to the public by a coordinated system of trauma field triage and rapid transport of the trauma victim.

REFERENCES

1. Balasegaram DM: Hepatic resection in trauma. Adv Surg 17: 129, 1984
2. Boda GR, Verzosa ES: Incidental splenic injury: is splenectomy always necessary? Am J Surg 113: 303, 1967
3. Bosworth BM: Perforation of the small intestine from nonpenetrating abdominal trauma. Am J Surg 76: 472, 1984
4. Bowditch HI: Diaphragmatic hernia. Buffalo Med J 9: 1, 65, 1853
5. Caplan ES, Hoyt N: Infection surveillance and control in the severely traumatized patient. Am J Med 70: 638, 1981
6. Christo MC: Segmental resections of the spleen: report on the first eight cases operated on. Hospital (Rio de Janeiro) 62: 575, 1962
7. Counseller VS, McCormack CJ: Subcutaneous perforation of the jejunum. Ann Surg 102: 365, 1935
8. Cox EF: Blunt abdominal trauma: a 5 year analysis of 870 patients requiring celiotomy. Ann Surg 199: 467, 1984
9. Cox EF, Dunham CM: A safe technique for diagnostic peritoneal lavage. J Trauma 23: 152, 1983
10. Cox EF, Uddo, J: Work in progress.
11. Dauterive AH, Flancbaum L, Cox EF: Blunt intestinal trauma: a modern day review. Ann Surg 201: 198, 1985
12. Desforges G, Strieder JW, Lynch et al: Traumatic rupture of the diaphragm: clinical manifestations and surgical treatment. J Thorac Surg 14: 779, 1957
13. Ebert PA, Gaertner RA, Zuidema GD: Traumatic diaphragmatic hernia. Surg Gynecol Obstet 125: 59, 1967
14. Fabian TC, Stone HH: Arrest of severe liver hemorrhage by an omentum pack. South Med J 73: 1487, 1980
15. Federle MP, Crass RA, Jeffrey B et al: Computed tomography in blunt abdominal trauma. Arch Surg 117: 645, 1982
16. Graham EW, Cannell D: Accidental ligation of the hepatic artery. Br J Surg 20: 566, 1933
17. King H, Schumacher HB: Splenic studies. 1. Susceptibility to infection after splenectomy performed in infancy. Ann Surg 135: 239, 1952
18. Lassonde J, Lawrendeau F: Blunt injury of the abdominal aorta. Ann Surg 194: 745, 1981
19. Lucas CE, Ledgerwood AM: Prospective evaluation of hemostatic techniques for liver injuries. J Trauma 16: 442, 1976
20. Maddox KL, McCollum WB, Jordon GL et al: Management of upper abdominal vascular trauma. Am J Surg 128: 823, 1974
21. Mays ET: The hepatic artery. Surg Gynecol Obstet 139: 595, 1974
22. Mays ET: Hepatic trauma. Curr Probl Surg 11: 47, 1976
23. Mays ET: Lobar de-arterialization for exasanguinating wounds of the liver. J Trauma 12: 397, 1972
24. Pachter HL, Spencer FC: Recent concepts in the treatment of hepatic trauma. Ann Surg 190: 423, 1979
25. Pachter HL, Spencer FC, Hofstetter SR, Coppa GF: Experience with the finger fracture technique to achieve intra-hepatic hemostasis in 75 patients with severe injuries of the liver. Ann Surg 197: 771, 1983
26. Palomar J, Polanco E, Trentz G: Rupture of the bladder following blunt trauma. A plea for routine peritoneotomy in patients with extraperitoneal rupture. J Trauma 20: 239, 1980
27. Pringle JH: Notes on the arrest of hepatic hemorrhage due to trauma. Ann Surg 48: 541, 1908
28. Rienhoff WF, Jr.: Ligation of hepatic and splenic arteries in the treatment of portal hypotension with a report of 6 cases. Bull John Hopkins Hosp 88: 365, 1951
29. Root HD, Hauser CW, McKinley CR et al: Diagnostic peritoneal lavage. Surgery 57: 633, 1965
30. Schrock T, Blaisdell FW, Mathewson C, Jr.: Management of blunt trauma to the liver and hepatic veins. Arch Surg 96: 698, 1968
31. Singer DB: Post-Splenectomy Sepsis: Perspectives in Pediatric Pathology. Year Book, Chicago 1973
32. Spencer FC: Discussion: recent concepts in the treatment of hepatic trauma. Ann Surg 190: 423, 1979
33. Stone HH, Lamb JM: Use of pedicle omentum as an autogenous pack for control of hemorrhage in major injuries of the liver. Surg Gynecol Obstet 141: 92, 1975
34. Trunkey DD, Shires GT, McClelland R: Manage-

ment of Liver Trauma in 811 consecutive patients. Ann Surg 179: 722, 1974

35. Vance BM: Traumatic lesions of the intestine caused by nonpenetrating blunt force. Arch Surg 7: 197, 1923

36. Walt AJ: Questions and answers: hepatic artery ligation. JAMA 248(15): 1900, 1982

37. Wise L, Connors J, Hwang Y et al: Traumatic injuries to the diaphragm. J Trauma 13: 946, 1973

38. Yellin AE, Chaffer CB, Donovan AJ: Vascular isolation in treatment of juxtahepatic venous injuries. Arch Surg 102: 566, 1971

30

Major Intra-Abdominal Vascular Trauma

H. Harlan Stone

INTRODUCTION

Probably the severest test of clinical experience, technical skills, knowledge of anatomy, and emotional composure for any trauma surgeon is an exsanguinating injury to one of the major intra-abdominal vascular structures. Immediate laparotomy is essential. Hemorrhage must first be controlled, followed by appropriate repair of damaged vessels as well as all other injuries to associated intra-abdominal viscera. Finally, because of the attendant shock, requirments for massive transfusion, and frequent occurrence of peritoneal contamination by enteric contents, postoperative care uniformly demands the moment-to-moment monitoring and expert organ system support readily available only in an intensive care unit.

INITIAL MEASURES

Patients who have sustained major intra-abdominal vascular trauma almost uniformly present with obvious blood loss into the peritoneal cavity. The resultant hypovolemic shock either fails to respond even partially to massive fluid therapy with a crystalloid solution (such as 2 or 3 L of Ringer's lactate rapidly infused through a large-bore intravenous line over a 5 to 10 minute interval) or shock promptly recurs after a favorable initial response to energetic fluid therapy. Usually there is insufficient time for a completed cross-match of blood, so that the most immediately available volume expander (a buffered salt solution containing 5 percent glucose) should be used. Dextran and other agents that may complicate future crossmatches or that may favor a coagulopathy should be avoided. Once cross-matched blood is available, it is administered as rapidly as possible. If more than 8 or 10 units of transfused blood are required, then type-specific blood should be given as there is no longer additional safety gained by a cross-match.

Once the diagnosis of a major intra-abdominal vascular injury has been made, all additional resuscitative efforts should be made on the operating table during the induction of anesthesia and the exploratory laparotomy that follows.[3,9] Waiting for the blood pressure eventually to respond to additional boluses of intravenous fluid only compounds the problem. Shock is unnessarily prolonged and total transfusion requirements are increased. On the other hand, the abdomen should never be opened in an emergency room; the available facilities are woefully inadequate for a formal laparotomy, experienced assistance (both medical and nursing) is seldom present, and results obtained even under the best of circumstances have been dismal. It has consistently been found that any delay in transferring the patient from the emergency receiving area to the operating room generally precludes any real chance for survival.[3]

When the patient reaches the operating room, anesthesia is immediately induced despite the patient's shock-like state. An airway is established during the initial stages of general anesthesia or after the intravenous administration of a narcotic. Agents for muscle relaxation become the mainstay of anesthesia from this point on. Since occulsion of the inferior vena cava, and thus interruption of adequate blood return to the heart, may be necessary, lines for massive fluid infusion should be placed in the arms or neck.

The abdomen is prepped and draped from the clavicles to the midthighs. There must always be preparations for entering the chest through a sternal split or an intercostal incision; control and repair of vessels as they enter and exit the abdomen may otherwise be impossible. The abdomen is opened as rapidly as possible; most trauma surgeons use a vertical midline incision. Speed is crucial, for the ab-

dominal tamponade has retarded the rate of hemorrhage. Once the tamponade has been released, bleeding resumes its massive proportions. The aortic compressor (Fig. 30-1 A) is placed over the aorta as it passes through the diaphragmatic hiatus (Fig. 30-1 B),[2] compressing the aorta between the instrument foot-plate and the vertebral body below until an aortic vascular clamp can be applied (Fig. 3-1 C, D). This maneuver immediately increases peripheral resistance below the diaphragm and thereby improves both coronary and cerebral perfusion. The abdomen is then cleared of blood, preferably with a sterile bath towel. Wounds responsible for the hemorrhagic shock can then be sufficiently identified to permit at least partial control of the massive bleed: a finger or thumb is pressed over the hole in a major artery or a laparotomy pad can be used to compress the injured vein. Care must be taken not to make the vascular wound larger, so composure on the part of the surgeon is equally important. Generally, hemorrhage from a a solid viscus can best be stemmed by hand compression of the organ. Clamps are used only when the bleeding vessel can be easily and quickly exposed, such as with wounds of the bowel mesentery.

Once the rate of blood loss from the vascular tree has been significantly reduced, the volume of infused fluid will remain within the vascular compartment and can thereby correct those derangements due to hypovolemic shock. There is no great urgency in repairing the vessels. It is best to wait until the blood volume has been fully expanded. Whole blood and fresh frozen plasma are administered as soon as available; the latter is particularly critical to avoid subsequent coagulopathies. While you await the arrival of additional surgical assistance, the incision is extended, and bleeding vessels that had been ignored during the rapid abdominal entry are controlled. Never attempt to perform definitive repair of any major vessel until the patient has a stable cardiovascular system, appropriate exposure has been achieved, and all of the necessary instruments and lighting are available.

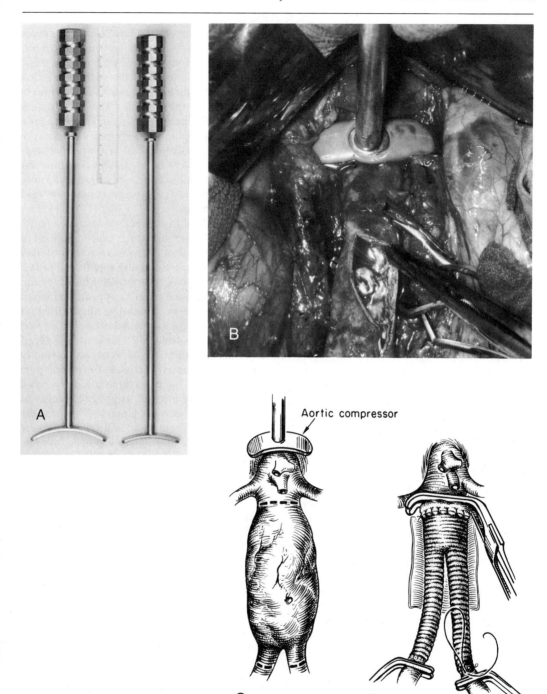

Fig. 30-1 To control massive bleeding, the aortic compressor (**A**) is placed over the aorta as it passes through the diaphragmatic hiatus (**B,C**), compressing the aorta between the instrument foot-plate and the vertebral body below until an ortic vascular clamp can be applied (**D**). (Figures 30-1 A, C and D from Conn J Jr, Trippel OH, Bergan JJ: A new atraumatic aortic occluder. Surgery 64: 1158, 1968.)

TREATMENT OF SPECIFIC INJURIES

Aorta

It is imperative that both proximal and distal control of the responsible vessel be obtained before an attempt is made to repair the injury. For the suprapancreatic aorta, the sternum should be split up to the sternal angle. To reach the retropancreatic aorta, the neck of the pancreas is divided so as to give direct access to site of the injury.[9] (After aortic repair, the distal pancreas is resected, leaving the spleen intact; the remaining stump of pancreas is oversewn, an omental apron is placed between the stump of the pancreas and the aortic suture line, and the stump of the pancreas is drained with a sump.) That part of the aorta immediately below the pancreas is easily exposed by merely reflecting the base of the small bowel mesentery. The iliac vessels are likewise reached without difficulty.

The aorta is repaired with a running suture of a synthetic monofilament. However, if there is consequent narrowing to less than 30 percent of normal diameter, a synthetic bypass graft is inserted by end-to-end anastomosis proximally and end-to-side far distally. The distal stump of the aorta is oversewn. Recently, an aortic graft insert has become available.[4] This permits easy and rapid insertion of a synthetic graft into both lumens of the divided aorta. The graft is fixed by ligation of the ends of the aorta over terminal rings in the graft. Flow can be re-established in this way within a matter of only a few minutes. Occasionally, a through-and-through wound lends itself to repair by enlargement of the anterior wound into a formal longitudinal aortotomy and then repair of the posterior wound through the lumen of the open aorta. The anterior wound is then isolated by a partial occlusion clamp, thereby permitting aortic flow while the anterior wound is being sutured.

Vena Cava

Wounds of the inferior vena cava below the level of the renal veins are repaired with a tangential suture line unless there has been total destruction of the vessel.[6] In this instance, the vena cava is ligated just below a major confluence, proximally as well as just distal to the wound. Injuries of the vena cava below the liver, yet above the renal veins, should be repaired if at all possible. This may require insertion of a patch of saphenous vein. However, should ligation be required, a side-to-side shunt with a Gortex graft is placed between inferior vena cava below the level of the renal veins to the side of the superior mesenteric vein just below its passage behind the neck of the pancreas.

Wounds of the inferior vena cava situated behind the liver are particularly difficult to manage.[5] Occlusion of the cava at the proximal level (just above the liver) significantly interferes with venous return to the heart. Within a few minutes, arrhythmias appear, and within another minute or so fatal cardiac arrest occurs. If at all possible, it is best not to explore the suspected retrohepatic caval wound. Bleeding anteriorly through the liver can instead be controlled by insertion of an apron of omentum, mobilized from the transverse colon and based upon one or the other of its gastroepiploic vascular pedicles, into the wound.[8] This provides a viable pack of autogenous tissue that almost always controls bleeding of venous origin. The same can be done for wounds of the immediate retroperitoneal area, yet the results are somewhat less reliable.

If, however, the retrohepatic cava must be inspected, the cava should be isolated with umbilical tapes above (generally best done via the pericardium through a sternal split or intercostal extension of the incision) as well as below the liver. The aorta at its diaphragmatic hiatus is then identified, by splitting its anterior crus from below. The porta hepatis is also isolated. Not until all structures are accessible, however, is the cava occluded. Instead, first the porta hepatis and then aorta are clamped with vascular instruments. Then the cava can be occluded both above and below, the right lobe of the liver is mobilized and rolled medially, and at last the retrohepatic cava can be exposed. If possible, a partial occlusion clamp is used to allow loosening of the occluding umbilical tapes around the cava and thus re-establishing better venous return to the heart from below. A running suture line up and then back down is placed; the needle end of the suture should be tied to its original loose end at the initial knot. Wounds of the hepatic veins can almost never be sewn or ligated. They are best managed by insertion of autogenous tissue plugs of free omentum or rectus muscle.

Experience with the caval shunt has not been as successful as reports in the literature might suggest.[5] It has been found more practical to leave the retrohepatic cava undisturbed if bleeding from its overlying liver or somewhat adjacent peritoneal defects can be controlled with tissue packs. Nevertheless, if the retrohepatic cava must be exposed, aortic cross-clamping is imperative throughout the period of caval occlusion.

Hepatic Veins

Although not readily identified as a single vascular injury, bleeding from the liver can be massive and cause death within a short time from exsanguination. In blunt trauma, the liver has usually been disrupted along planes between the respective lobes, segments, and subsegments where there is no supporting framework of artery, duct, and portal vein—the so-called triad structures. Such bleeding almost always emanates from large tears in the draining hepatic veins whose course passes within these spaces.[8] Immediate control is relatively easy: simply compress the liver together to close the veins located beneath.

Once shock has been reversed by fluid repletion, the hepatic wound can safely be inspected. Occasionally a small artery has also been divided, so the depths of the crevice within liver must be exposed. To do so, however, before venous pressure has been restored predisposes the patient to air entry through the open vein and subsequent air embolism.

Bleeding arteries are ligated with sutures and the liver wound is once again compressed between both hands. A viable omental pack is then inserted into the defect within the liver. As mentioned above, the omentum has been mobilized from the colon and is based upon one or the other gastroepiploic vessels. To maintain the viable pack in place, the liver surface is oversewn with a running suture of large-caliber Prolene. During this suturing, the liver is compressed so that when the stitch has been tied, release of the pressure will allow the entire liver to swell as it refills with blood and in this way put tension on all suture bites equally. To buttress the suture and thereby avoid tearing of liver capsule, the falciform ligament can be turned down or a strip of Prolene mesh can be applied.

For penetrating wounds, only the artery need be repaired. Wounds of the hepatic and portal veins are managed by the pack–tamponade procedure described above.[8] If the specific artery cannot be reached easily through the liver wound, then the feeding right or left hepatic artery is ligated. One can confirm which artery should be ligated by applying a vascular clamp to the individual artery, since approximately 10 percent of patients will have a major contribution to hepatic arterial supply by an aberrant branch from the superior mesenteric artery.

Portal Vein

Wounds of the portal and superior mesenteric veins should be repaired by a longitudinal suture line whenever possible.[7] If this is not practical, either vein can be ligated without fear that the patient will die.[1] However, when there is interruption to returning flow of blood from the splanchnic circulation, the patient will rapidly sequester large volumes of blood into the portal venous system. This will require significant overtransfusion, often to a volume equal to the patient's own normal blood volume (as dictated by carefully filling pressures of the heart, that is, central venous pressure or pulmonary artery pressure).[1,7] Creation of a portocaval shunt should be avoided.

If both the portal vein and hepatic artery have been destroyed, it is absolutely crucial to repair one or the other so as to provide oxygenated blood to the liver. Generally, it has been found easier to ligate the artery and replace the vein with a shunt between the stump of the portal vein superiorly and side of the superior mesenteric vein below, the inferior stump of the portal vein having been ligated.[7]

A reversed saphenous vein or Gortex graft serves this purpose equally well.

Hypogastric Vessels

Fractures of the pelvis due to blunt trauma seldom cause massive bleeding unless there has been fracture–dislocation through the sacroiliac joint with a corresponding break in the anterior pelvic ring. This leads to ipsilateral disruption of the hypogastric artery or one or more of its major branches. The resultant hematoma should never be opened, no matter how tempting even at the time of abdominal exploration. The associated vein disruptions are extensive and exceedingly difficult to control once the tamponading peritoneum has been removed. Instead, the patient should be carried immediately to the angiography suite for direct embolization of both hypogastric arteries. Embolization of a single side is inadequate, since there is excellent collateral circulation between the right and left hypogastric vessels.

Penetrating injuries to the pelvic vessels, on the other hand, always warrant exploration. Proximal control, regardless of whether the wound is to an iliac artery or vein, always requires cross-clamping of the terminal aorta. The arterial collateral circulation is so extensive that occlusion of the involved iliac artery only partially reduces the brisk retrograde flow from the distal vessel end. Similarly, the venous flow from below is exceedingly heavy whenever the proximal vein or cava has been occluded; this can only be diminished by clamping the terminal aorta. Wounds of the common and external iliac arteries are appropriately repaired. If extra length is needed, the ipsilateral hypogastric artery can be ligated to make the vessel course more direct, thereby gaining an extra 3 or 4 cm in length. The injured hypogastric artery is routinely ligated. If there is difficulty in maintaining good control of the distal vessel end, ligation of the contralateral hypogastric artery will significantly reduce the rate of back-bleeding.

Common and external iliac veins should be repaired to maintain venous return and avoid later problems with various manifestations of thrombophlebitis. Hypogastric vessels are oversewn. If bleeding from the extensive venous network in the pelvis cannot be controlled, the pelvic space should be packed with laparotomy pads, the abdomen closed, and the patient re-explored in 2 or 3 days. By that time, only large venous channels are still open. They can then be easily identified and more definitively closed.

Finally, it must be remembered that many patients present in profound shock because of bleeding of multiple small intra-abdominal vessels, rather than from a single large vascular structure. The resultant mortality rate is identical unless the same basic principles of immediate exploration and concomitant energetic fluid resuscitation are applied.

Coagulopathy

After 12 to 15 units of blood have been transfused, coagulopathies begin to appear. Part of the problem is dilutional because of the massive infusion of crystalloid solutions as well as various blood products. However, platelet depletion and malfunction, low fibrinogen levels, and a multitude of other clotting element deficiencies occur. In addition, there is usually some degree of passive transfusion reaction between the various donor units. At the operating table, an ooze of blood from most raw surfaces is noted, and a failure of blood shed into the abdomen to clot.[10]

At this juncture, continuing with operation only allows for further loss of blood with its resultant demand for more transfusion and thus a greater compounding of the coagulopathy. The surgical procedure must be terminated as soon as possible to reduce this extra transfusion load. Only critical vessels are repaired; all others are ligated. Expendable solid viscera whose wounds still bleed are rapidly extirpated. Bowel ends are ligated, as are open ureters. Lateral wounds to hollow viscera are closed with a single purse-string. No extraordinary attempt is made to close holes in any hollow structure other than the alimentary tract. Leaks of urine, bowel, and pancreatic juice are ignored.

The abdomen is then packed with laparotomy pads, operating gowns, towels, or other sterile space-filling items.[10] There must be no intestinal or other vents or any drain tracts whatsoever. Once tightly packed, the abdomen is closed with large running sutures for fascia as one layer and skin as a second. Blood product repletion is then provided as indicated by platelet count and measurements of fibrinogen levels. Tests for the adequacy of other clotting elements are usually unreliable. Fresh frozen plasma is then given as the main volume expander beyond the need for red cell mass. Once the blood will clot in a test tube (Lee-White clotting time of 6 minutes or less), it is safe to re-explore the abdomen and complete the initial operation. This may take as long as 36 hours, yet operation must be put off until the coagulopathy has been corrected.

In the interval between abdominal pack closure and re-exploration, the patient requires continued support in an intensive care unit. Because of the abdominal tamponade, diaphragms have been significantly elevated and thus continous airway pressure must be maintained, often to as high as 30 cmH$_2$O, if ventilation is to be adequate. Likewise, there is considerable increase in venous back pressure on the kidney. The resultant oliguria must be accepted, yet administration of an osmotic diuretic such as mannitol will evoke at least a small increase in urine production. These attendant setbacks must be taken as representing only a temporary state, and will soon revert toward normal once the abdominal tamponade has been released.

At the time of re-exploration, a thorough peritoneal toilet is required to remove all packing material, blood, and spill from hollow viscera. Wounds of solid organs are appropriately sutured and/or drained, the urinary tract is repaired as needed, the extrahepatic bile ducts are sutured and drained when indicated, and bowel anastomoses are performed. If there are wounds of the stomach and duodenum, these ogans should be decompressed by tubes as well as repaired. For small and large bowel injuries, the most proximal wound should be exteriorized as a Mikulica double-barrel enterostomy. The distal wounds, now protected by a proximal diversion, can be closed or primarily resected almost with impunity.

CONCLUSION

Patients with wounds of major intra-abdominal vascular structures almost always present in severe to profound hypovolemic shock. Implementation of an algorithm for resuscitation, exploration, and injury management individualized for the vessel involved is crucial. A successful outcome is far more likely to follow if personnel in attendance have acquired the necessary experience, either by actual encounter with such wounds before or by mental dress rehersal.

REFERENCES

1. Boswick J. III, Stone HH: Trauma to the portal venous system. South Med J 68: 1369, 1975
2. Conn J, Jr., Trippel OH, Bergan JJ: A new atraumatic aortic occluder. Surgery 64: 1158, 1968
3. Ekbom GA, Towne JB, Majewski JR, Woods JH: Intra-abdominal vascular trauma—a need for prompt operation. J Trauma 21 (12): 1040, 1981
4. Krause AH, Chapman RD, Bigelow, JC, et al: Early experience with the intraluminal graft prosthesis. Am J Sur 45: 619, 1983
5. Schrock T, Blaisdell FW, Mathewson C., Jr.: Management of blunt trauma to the liver and hepatic veins. Arch Surg 96: 698, 1968
6. Stewart MT, Stone HH: Injuries of the inferior vena cava. Am Surg 52: 9, 1986
7. Stone HH, Fabian TC, Turkleson ML: Wounds of the portal venous system. World J Surg 6: 335, 1982
8. Stone HH, Lamb JM: Use of pedicled omentum as an autogenous pack for control of hemorrhage in motor injuries of the liver. Surg Gynecol Obstet 141: 92, 1975
9. Stone HH, Oxford WM, Austin JT: Penetrating wounds of the abdominal aorta. South Med J 66: 1351, 1973
10. Stone HH, Strom PR, Mullins RJ: Management of the major coagulopathy with onset during laparotomy. Ann Surg 197: 532, 1983

31

The Head Injury Patient

Fred H. Geisler
Michael Salcman

INTRODUCTION

Head trauma represents an enormous medical problem because of its high incidence in the United States and the frequent long-term sequelae of the initial injury. An estimate of the annual incidence of head injury requiring medical attention is 200:100,000 population.[61] Thus, approximately 500,000 Americans each year suffer cerebral lesions including cerebral concussion, cerebral contusion, diffuse axonal injury, cerebral laceration, skull fracture, epidural hematoma, subdural hematoma, intracerebral hematoma, and cerebrospinal fluid leak.

Head injury has a peak incidence in persons aged 15 to 24 years.[30,65] Trauma is the leading cause of death in males under 35 years of age and brain injury is present in 75 percent of patients who die from motor vehicle accidents.[11,24,43] Although most patients require only close observation for 1 to 3 days, 2 percent of all head injury patients have intracranial

hematomas and 3 percent die.[65] The most severely injured patients, those that are posturing and have intracranial hematomas, experience a mortality of 60 to 70 percent.[9,57,62] Approximately 8 percent of head-injured patients are in a coma during the first days postinjury and have a mortality of 30 to 50 percent.[27]

In a large percentage of the survivors of head injury, major cognitive deficits persist and limit patients' ability to maintain their former employment or level of interaction with family and friends. Head injury patients have physical and emotional symptoms that extend far beyond the period of initial intensive medical and/or surgical care. Many head-injured patients require physical or cognitive rehabilitation to achieve the highest degree of motor and cognitive recovery. Such rehabilitation often requires support for the family unit as well as for the patient. The physical and cognitive recovery of the severely injured patient requires inpatient rehabilitation for several months. The ultimate neurologic level of performance is not

919

obtained for 12 to 24 months following the injury. Similar rehabilitative efforts are often helpful in the cognitive retraining of the moderately injured patient and greatly aid in reintegrating the patient into society.[9,71]

Patients with minor head injury have a high incidence of persistent headaches, memory disturbances, gait disturbances, and psychogenic symptoms at 3 months following the injury. In many patients these symptoms are severe enough to limit their employment and interfere with their personal goals.[81,102,103]

Extensive community-based medical services are required to complete the rehabilitation of head-injured patients and to provide long-term support. Motor and cognitive rehabilitation/retraining is a crucial aspect in the total care of any head injury since permanent neurologic disability that prevents the patient from living a meaningful life is often as disastrous an outcome for the individual, family, and society as the death of the patient.

PRIMARY AND SECONDARY INJURY

The pathophysiology of head injury can be divided into two distinct phases in which the brain tissue is damaged by different pathologic processes. An understanding of the two phases provides insight into the rationale for medical therapy and sets limits on the ultimate neurologic outcome.[27,41,77,83,84,97]

In the first phase, primary brain injury is caused "directly" by the impact and continues at the scene of the accident before medical treatment is begun. During this period, direct biomechanical damage to the neurons, dendrites, axons, myelin sheaths, and blood vessels occurs. Gross disruption of neural tissue may additionally occur from the acceleration–deceleration forces of the injury. For the present, these primary effects of head injury have no known treatment.

In addition, once the force-related damage has occurred, a cascade of events leads to further injury at the scene. Among the early pathophysiologic responses to trauma that increase "direct" brain injury are systemic hypotension, hypoxia, and hypercarbia. Hypoxia and hypercarbia can be caused by apnea related to the primary brain injury itself or may result from other systemic injuries. For example, brain injury can be complicated by traumatic injury to the chest with respiratory failure or aspiration. Hypotension is commonly a result of internal or external bleeding from other injuries such as a ruptured spleen, fractured pelvis, or lacerated artery. These injuries can impair oxygen delivery to the brain and cause subsequent anoxic brain damage.

Other initial complications of some head injuries include direct penetration of the cranial cavity by fractured bone, foreign objects, or gunshot wounds with resultant dural penetration, brain disruption, intracranial hematoma, and/or contusion. Implantation and dural penetration of potentially infected foreign material or tissues (e.g., nasal sinus mucosa) also can occur with disastrous consequences including meningitis, cerebritis, and brain abcess.

In the second phase of head injury, other pathologic processes cause additional brain tissue to infarct or otherwise become dysfunctional hours or days after the initial damage. The secondary mechanisms include intracranial hypertension, low cerebral compliance, cerebral infection, and seizure disorders.[3] These secondary causes of brain damage are a direct result of the pathophysiologic evolution of injured brain tissue over time and are usually limited to the first few days or weeks after the head injury.

The intensive care management of head injury patients is designed to minimize or eliminate the secondary effects of head injury by intensive monitoring of cerebral perfusion and neurologic function. Aggressive surgical and intensive medical therapies can prevent or lessen the effects of secondary brain damage, especially when it is detected early. The management goals of adequate cerebral perfusion, oxygenation, and nutrition provide the optimal environment for the electrically dysfunctioning neurons to undergo metabolic recovery and return to preinjury function. The resumption of normal electrical activity is believed to be an important aspect of neurologic recovery and corresponds clinically to the patient regaining consciousness and higher cortical function. The physical integrity of the neuron and its continued electrical activity are known to depend on a critical level of cerebral blood flow (18 ml/100 g tissue/min).[1]

The secondary pathologic effects of head injury can appear in a cascade fashion, such that a small deterioration in the value of a single physiologic parameter may cause a disproportionate deterioration in many other physiologic parameters and result in massive brain injury. If the cascade is left unchecked, cerebral herniation and death will occur. The cascade of secondary brain damage that represents the pathophysiologic response to head injury is shown in Figure 31-1. The objective of the medical and surgical therapy of head injury is to break or eliminate the cascade and prevent the secondary damage.[26]

CONCUSSION, CONTUSION, AND DIFFUSE AXONAL INJURY

An impaired level of consciousness is the clinical hallmark of a serious head injury.[21] When an accident occurs the patient may lose consciousness or have a clouding in mental processes as a direct result of the impact energy transmitted to both hemispheres or the brain stem.

Cerebral concussion represents the mildest form of head injury. The prototype of a cerebral concussion is a knockout in boxing. The boxer receives an acceleration–deceleration impact usually associated with a significant amount of angular acceleration-deceleration of the head and this results in a loss of consciousness for a brief period of time. During the period of unconsciousness the boxer has no spontaneous motion and is unresponsive to verbal and painful stimuli. The boxer then awakens and is initially mentally cloudy and unsteady of gait. These neurologic signs are caused by dysfunction of the interconnecting cortical white matter tracts in both the motor coordination and cognitive neuronal circuits of the brain. These gross neurologic abnormalities gradually clear over a variable length of time, usually minutes to hours, and sometimes days in the severest cases. The computed tomographic (CT) scan is either normal or demonstrates minimal global edema or swelling.

Although cerebral concussion of this type was once viewed as benign with no demonstrable pathologic lesions, evidence has been presented that concussion, especially on the repetitive basis seen in boxing, causes significant permanent injury to the brain as measured by both the electroencephalogram (EEG) and neuropsychometric testing.[20,106]

Head-injured patients with cerebral contusion have experienced a larger insult to the brain than those with cerebral concussion. Cerebral contusions are microhemorrhages into the brain substance resulting from cortical tissue damage produced by the absorbed energy of the impact. The CT scan initially demonstrates a region of mixed localized high density (blood) with interspersed and surrounding low density (edema) at the site of the damage. Figure 31-2 shows an example of massive bilateral cerebral contusions and demonstrates the mixed-density appearance of the lesions. The initially small area of perilesional edema evolves to a larger layer of low density surrounding the contusion. This swelling can be sizable and peaks in volume at 48 to 72 hours following brain trauma. Contusions of the brain occur in all lobes and the basal ganglia. However, the bony configuration of the skull base and the typical rotation acceleration–deceleration forces in head injury commonly produce contusions in the temporal tips and the inferior frontal lobes.[77,94] These contusions are caused by the relative motion of the skull and the brain at the time of impact. A history of unconsciousness at the accident scene can be obtained in almost all patients with cerebral contusions. Patients with cerebral contusions vary widely in their clinical presentation in the emergency room. They may be awake and conversive with the examiner or possess major motor, speech, or cognitive deficits, or may even present in coma.

Hemispheric contusions as seen on CT scan are usually not responsbile for the uncon-

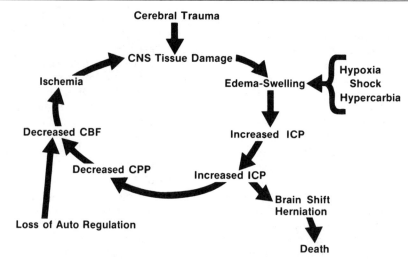

Fig. 31-1 Cascade of secondary brain damage following head injury. This represents the cascade of secondary brain damage that may result as the pathophysiologic response to head injury. Damaged central nervous system tissue leads to a variable amount of edema and swelling, accentuated by hypoxia, shock, and hypercarbia. The edema and swelling result in an increased intracranial volume and increased intracranial pressure. This high pressure leads to brain anoxia, midline shift, herniation, and a decrease in cerebral perfusion pressure. Cerebral autoregulation is typically impaired; this results in a decrease in the cerebral blood flow. The decreased cerebral blood flow produces local ischemia that may produce more tissue damage, thus completing the cycle. The object of medical and surgical management of head injury is to halt or eliminate this cascade.

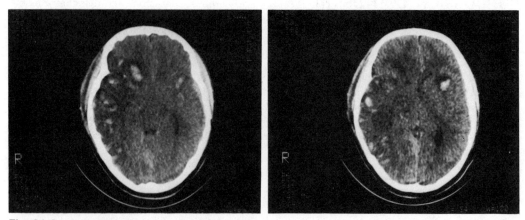

Fig. 31-2 Massive bilateral cerebral contusions. The CT scan demonstrates massive bilateral cerebral contusions with a characteristic mixed-density appearance. The basal cisterns and the ventricular system are compressed by the cerebral swelling. The whiter or higher-density areas in the CT scan represent blood within the brain parenchyma and the lower-density areas represent edema in the surrounding brain. No significant midline shift is present because the damage is bilateral.

scious and unresponsive clinical state since they are focal cortical lesions and should only produce focal neurologic deficit. The unconscious state can only result from cerebral contusion when massive bilateral hemispheric damage occurs or when subsequent swelling and raised intracranial pressure cause midbrain compression. The prolonged unconscious state seen in some patients with cerebral contusion results from a diffuse axonal injury affecting deep midline structures including the reticular activating system.[21]

In 1 to 2 months the CT scan image of a hyperdense or mixed cerebral contusion may completely resolve or develop into focal encephalomalacia at the site of the initially visualized contusion. On occasion, some contusions coalesce into a hematoma and require surgical removal in the first few days after injury. Coagulation defects are common in these patients. The size of the zone of edema surrounding the cerebral contusion is a function of both the state of hydration of the body and the initial brain damage. This zone of edema can expand greatly in an overhydrated patient and can act as a secondary mass lesion that greatly accentuates the effect of the contusion itself. Intensive medical management of fluid therapy is used to achieve a state of mild dehydration with a concomitant elevation in the serum osmolality. This may diminish the effective size of the edema surrounding the contusion. In this way, one may achieve successful nonsurgical management of the majority of cerebral contusions.[2,10,74,86]

Diffuse axonal injury describes damage in multiple areas of the white matter of the cerebral hemispheres, corpus callosum, periventricular area, dorsal midbrain, and pons. This damage is especially prevalent in head injuries when the impact involves large acceleration–deceleration forces. Direct damage to the midbrain, pons, or reticular activating system may cause some patients to have decerebrate posturing and to be in unresponsive coma for a prolonged period of time or indefinitely. Furthermore, in patients who do wake up from prolonged coma, the damage to the deep interconnecting tracts of the cerebral white matter produces most of the major motor and cognitive residual deficits.[40,77]

Damage to the interconnecting white fiber tracts of the cerebral hemispheres can be documented by mathematical analysis of a 20-lead EEG using signal processing techniques such as the calculation of power spectrum and coherence in the neurometrics test. Most patients wake up from coma but have a major cognitive deficit in some or all areas of memory, speech, personality, judgment, or intellect. A significant recovery in cognitive function is possible with retraining over 6 to 24 months, especially in young patients. Although CT scanning of the head sometimes discloses the diffuse axonal injuries in the brain substance as small contusions in the brain stem (Fig. 31-3) or white matter, they are usually not visualized.[41] Diffuse axonal injury may be diagnosed with a higher sensitivity and specificity with high-resolution magnetic imaging techniques.[48]

PATHOPHYSIOLOGY OF INTRACRANIAL MASS LESIONS AND CEREBRAL BLOOD FLOW

Any intracranial mass lesion can cause neurologic dysfunction. The mass lesion can be a hematoma within the brain substance, subdural space, or epidural space; it can be a localized swelling of the brain itself or even ventricular enlargement. All expanding intracranial mass lesions can have potentially disastrous effects on the cerebral hemispheres and brain stem. The effects of an expanding lesion are accentuated by the unique anatomic position the brain occupies within the body. The brain is enclosed in a rigid bony cavity, the skull, and if the brain swells or another mass lesion is placed in the skull, a massive elevation in intracranial pressure can occur with physical displacement and distortion of the brain substance.[1,99]

The normal cranial vault contains 500 to 700 ml of neurons, 700 to 900 ml of glia, 100 to 150 ml of blood, and 100 to 150 ml of cerebrospinal fluid (CSF). These fluid compartments form a dynamic physiologic system in which an increase in the volume of one com-

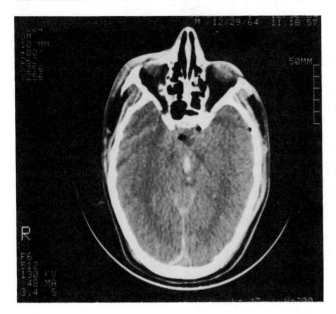

Fig. 31-3 Traumatic hemorrhagic brain stem contusion. The CT scan demonstrates a high-density hemorrhagic lesion in the dorsal region of the midbrain. Intracranial air is visualized in the collapsed basal cistern and gained access to the subarachnoid space by a basal skull fracture. The perimesencephalic and quadrigeminal cisterns are obliterated by diffuse cerebral swelling visualized on higher cuts of the CT scan.

partment is compensated by a decrease in the volume of another. For example an increase in the volume of the brain by 50 ml of brain swelling might be compensated by a 50 ml decrease in the volume of the CSF. This reciprocal shift of fluid maintains constancy of the intracranial volume. Fluctuations in the intracranial blood volume and the volume of CSF normally occur with each change in pulse, respiration, or posture.[78]

The major component of all intracranial compartments is water, which is essentially incompressible. When an expanding mass lesion is small, the brain can accommodate it by shifting fluid of the same volume from the vascular or CSF compartments. About 75 to 100 ml of pathologic tissue or fluid can be managed intracranially without a significant rise in the intracranial pressure (ICP). As the size of the intracranial mass lesion increases further, an elevation in the ICP is an unavoidable consequence of increasing the volume of incompressible materials in a fixed space. Once all physiologic compensatory mechanisms are exhausted, changes as small as 1 ml in the size of the mass lesion can result in severe elevations in the ICP with tentorial herniation or lethal reductions in cerebral perfusion.[101] The precise nature of the pressure–volume interac-

tion can be inferred from cerebral compliance measurements. The compliance is directly measured by observing the time of response of the intracranial pressure to either small injections or withdrawals of small volumes of CSF from the lateral ventricles.[75]

In the normal brain, cerebral blood flow is autoregulated to provide constant blood flow over a broad range of systemic arterial pressures. In normotensive individuals the autoregulation range extends from a mean pressure of 55 mmHg to a mean of 150 mmHg. The average cerebral blood flow for the cerebral hemispheres is 50 ml/100 g tissue/min with white and gray matter flows of 20 ml/100 g tissue/min and 80 ml/100 g tissue/min, respectively. Autoregulation is controlled by myogenic, neurogenic, and local metabolic factors. The vascular smooth muscle in the arterioles can constrict or dilate, based on the transluminal pressure. The cerebral vasculature has both sympathetic and parasympathetic innervation. Regional cerebral blood flow (CBF) is inversely related to the local tissue pH; the CBF falls as pH rises and rises with acidosis. Local metabolites such as lactic acid, systemic vasoactive substances, and extracellular potassium also influence the cerebral blood flow by modulating the tone of the arterioles.[30,69,76] The cerebral blood flow is accurately balanced to the cerebral metabolic rate for oxygen consumption (CMRO$_2$) by these mechanisms.[109]

Cerebral blood flow in injured brain manifests a variety of abnormalities not present in normal brain. The cerebral blood flow after acute severe head injury varies over a wide range.[18,76] The CMRO$_2$ in coma is depressed greater with deeper levels of coma.[93] Dissociation of CBF and metabolism is referred to as luxury perfusion. The relative cerebral hyperemia is due to defective autoregulation resulting from the trauma. Defects in the blood–brain barrier either resulting from, or concomitant with, the autoregulation derangement can lead to formation of edema. The cerebral blood vessels in many patients with severe head injury patients behave as if they are in vasomotor paralysis, with the CBF passively following the systemic blood pressure; this is the hallmark of defective autoregulation. Direct transmission of the arterial pulse to the capillaries results in transudation of edema fluid. The decrease in vascular tone produces an increase in the cerebral vascular volume and this also can cause an increase in the ICP.[68]

Systemic arterial hypertension aggravates the management of patients with significant vasomotor paralysis by exposing the arteriolar and capillary lumens to a higher hydrostatic pressure and hence there is a greater propensity to produce edema.[74] The vasomotor defect appears to be selective since the vessels remain responsive to changes in the arterial carbon dioxide concentration.[96]

The hyperemia following severe head trauma has a duration of 1 to 8 days and is present in 55 percent of patients. The remaining 45 percent of the patients have a consistent depression in cerebral blood flow. Although the hyperemia usually occurs in the initial phase of head injury, it may be delayed for 1 to 2 days. Metabolic acidosis in the brain can be inferred from lactic acidosis in the cerebrospinal fluid and is theorized to cause the hyperemia. The hyperemic phase is associated with an elevation in the ICP. Two distinct groups of patients can be defined by the relationship of the cerebral arterial–venous difference in oxygen content to the CBF. One group has decoupling of flow and metabolism and is hyperemic; the other group has coupling of flow and metabolism with both at a low level. In the latter case, the brain is not made ischemic by the reduced flow but responds by correctly autoregulating the flow necessary for the level of metabolic demand. The increased CBF and the resultant hyperemia have important clinical implications. The most potent and useful means of reducing intracranial pressure is a reduction in the arterial carbon dioxide concentration. The resultant vasoconstriction reduces both the CBF and cerebral blood volume. When the patient is in the hyperemic phase of head injury, a reduction in cerebral blood produced by a decrease in the arterial carbon dioxide tension can still provide sufficient flow for the metabolic demands of the brain. However, if the brain is in a low-flow state, a similar reduction in blood volume may produce ischemia and possibly infarction. Thus, hyperventilation therapy should optimally be employed, with consideration of the known interactions of CBF, cerebral metabolic rate, systemic hemodynamics, and intracranial pressure.[93]

The calculated cerebral perfusion pressure (CPP) is a useful clinical management tool. It is defined as the difference between the mean cerebral arterial and mean cerebral venous sinus pressures. The CPP is approximated by the difference between the mean systemic arterial pressure (SAP) and the mean ICP. The CBF can be defined as the ratio of the CPP to the cerebrovascular resistance (CVR):

$$CBF = \frac{CPP}{CVR} = \frac{SAP - ICP}{CVR}$$

If an untreated mass lesion expands beyond a critical volume, the ICP rises abruptly and may approximate the mean arterial pressure. When this occurs, the blood flow to the cerebral hemispheres drops to zero because there is no pressure differential between the extracranial arterial pressure and the intracranial pressure, that is, no driving force exists to provide CBF. Ischemic infarction of both cerebral hemispheres and brain death will occur without prompt reinstitution of CBF. Current head injury therapy is directed toward preventing any abnormal elevation in the ICP and thereby stopping the cascade of events leading to brain herniation or cerebral death. The clinical signs of cerebral herniation depend on the site of the expanding mass lesion.[99]

The most important step in the control of intracranial hypertension is the surgical removal of any mass lesion causing an abnormal elevation in ICP. Mass lesions are also removed before ICP is elevated if there is a deterioration in the patient's clinical status. Hematomas and a few large contusions are removed surgically, whereas the majority of contusions are treated by hyperventilation, dehydration, and hyperosmolar therapy. This management scheme has developed because hematomas as a group tend to expand in size unless bleeding is controlled surgically, and intensive medical therapy for contusion has been successful when carefully adhered to. The monitoring of ICP allows continuous assessment of the cerebral perfusion status and provides early warning of most expanding intracranial mass lesions.

The different time course of some expanding lesions and simple concussion allows clinical differentiation in some cases. Hematomas, whether epidural, subdural, or intracerebral, are either absent or small at the time of impact and then expand as bleeding continues. Thus, the mass effect can be delayed in slow continuous bleeding. At the instant of impact the patient is rendered unconscious by the concussion and then may regain consciousness after a variable length of time. Patients who regain consciousness and talk, only to return to unconsciousness as the hematoma expands to cause delayed mass effect, can be described as having a lucid interval. If the patient does not regain consciousness from the concussion before the onset of mass effect, then the evolution of the hematoma can only be detected by CT scan or by an increase in ICP. Hence the imaging of every unconscious head injury patient by emergency CT and the continuous measurement of ICP are essential.

Head injuries commonly result in a mixture of several pathologic brain insults discussed above. For instance, a rotational acceleration–deceleration injury to the brain may cause concussion with loss of consciousness, contusion as the temporal tips impact on the sphenoid ridge, diffuse axonal injury from energy absorbed in the deep white matter, and anoxic brain damage from apnea following the injury. The patient may also harbor an expanding mass lesion in the early stage, the removal of which will prevent permanent disability or death. It is the task of the physician caring for patients with head injury to differentiate these various processes while deciding on treatment and prognosis. A major advance was made in the treatment of head injury a decade ago with the development and wide deployment of CT scanning of the brain. This method identifies all mass lesions, midline shifts, and ventricular enlargements that require operative treatment. The CT also identifies the location of major cerebral contusions. The size of the basilar cisterns and lateral ventricles on CT can be used as an indicator of brain stem compression due to global edema; this feature provides prognostic information.[113] More recently, use of evoked potentials and computerized EEG analysis has aided in the determination of the type, site, and severity of brain injury. Serial examination with this technique can accurately predict recovery.[44,49,63,64]

INITIAL NEUROLOGIC EXAMINATION

The initial examination of the head-injured patient provides an estimate of the severity of the head injury, determines the initial clinical management, and makes an estimate of the prognosis for both survival and neurologic outcome.[106a] Although an ideal scheme for the initial assessment of all head injuries has yet to be developed, the Glasgow coma score is useful for all of these goals. This scale uses three readily obtainable clinical parameters: eye opening, verbal response, and best motor response.[111] Many centers in Europe and the United States have reported a correlation between the Glasgow coma score and mortality and neurologic outcome.[68] The Glasgow coma scale is reproduced in Table 31-1. The total score is the sum of the three components and varies from 3 to 15, with 3 corresponding to unresponsive coma.

In the range of 3 to 7, the Glasgow coma score uses only the motor examination to separate different levels of coma. The motor exam

TABLE 31-1. The Glasgow Coma Scale[a]

Sign	Evaluation	Score[a]
Eye Opening	Spontaneous	4
	To Speech	3
	To Pain	2
	None	1
Best Verbal Response	Oriented	5
	Confused	4
	Inappropriate	3
	Incomprehensible	2
	None	1
Best Motor Response	Obeying	6
	Localizing	5
	Normal Flexion	4
	Abnormal Flexion	3
	Extending	2
	None	1

[a] Individual points are given for each of the categories; the total score (3 to 15) is the sum of the three categories.
(Teasdale G, Jennett B: Assessment of coma and impaired consciousness. A practical scale. Lancet 2: 81, 1974.)

assesses the highest level of function in the neural axis of patients who are unable to speak, open their eyes, or follow commands. Holding up two fingers to answer verbal command demonstrates that large areas of the cortex are functionally connected, integrating information, and programming motor tasks correctly. The Glasgow motor examination score is 6 in such patients. Continuity of the projection of motor control through the brain stem is also demonstrated.

The ability to localize a painful pinch on the chest indicates that the sensory and motor cortex are functioning as a local neuronal circuit to localize accurately the site of pinch and program the correct defensive motor response. The motor and sensory cortex are located adjacent to one another on the hemisphere and hence only a local cerebral communication is clinically demonstrated. These patients have a localizing motor response and a Glasgow motor index of 5.

When localization fails, a flexor response is manifested due to partial disconnection of the hemispheres and the brain stem. These patients have a flexor withdrawal response and a Glasgow motor score of 4.

A decorticate response with a Glasgow motor score of 3 results when the cerebral hemispheres are not providing inhibitory input

to the diencephalon and brain stem. The decerebrate response is a brain stem reflex that may occur with damage in the midbrain and upper pontine area. A Glasgow motor score of 1 corresponds to flaccid extremities and indicates dysfunction to the lower pontomedullary area of the brain stem.

Patients are not considered in coma when they are able to follow commands, open their eyes, or make sounds. Glasgow coma scores between 8 and 14 correspond to levels of consciousness between coma and full alertness. Scores in this region of the scale are more prone to interobserver variability and the effects of drugs than are scores at the low end of the Glasgow coma scale.[54]

Patients with a Glasgow coma score of 13 or 14 or a history of unconsciousness have mild head injuries, and good neurologic recovery is the rule. However, the superficial appearance of neurologic normality in these patients can be misleading. Detailed neuropsychological examination of these patients often reveals persistent personality, cognitive, or memory deficits. Clinical management involves serial neurologic examinations and careful observation for late neurologic deterioration.

Moderate head injury describes those patients with a Glasgow coma score of between 9 and 12. Deaths are relatively uncommon in this group, but major deficits of memory, speech, personality, or judgment are common in long term follow-up. Clinical management utilizes serial CT scans of the head along with serial neurologic examinations.

Patients with Glasgow coma scores of between 3 and 8 form the severe head injury group. These patients are treated with ICP monitoring, intubation, and hemodynamic monitoring. Deaths are common in this group, especially in those with Glasgow coma scores of 3 and 4. The majority of surviving patients eventually wake up but severe or moderate neurologic disability is common. A few patients who survive never wake up and remain in a persistent vegetative state.[99]

Although the Glasgow coma scale remains the standard by which all other coma scales are measured, it contains many major deficiencies and is not a replacement for a detailed serial neurologic examination. The major criticisms of the Glasgow coma scale include the

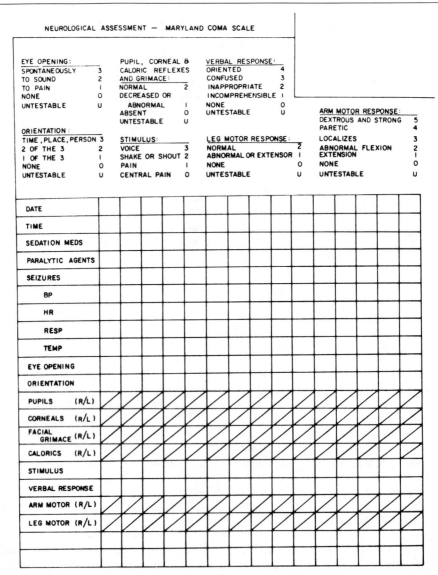

NEUROLOGICAL ASSESSMENT — MARYLAND COMA SCALE

EYE OPENING:
SPONTANEOUSLY	3
TO SOUND	2
TO PAIN	I
NONE	O
UNTESTABLE	U

ORIENTATION:
TIME, PLACE, PERSON	3
2 OF THE 3	2
I OF THE 3	I
NONE	O
UNTESTABLE	U

PUPIL, CORNEAL & CALORIC REFLEXES AND GRIMACE:
NORMAL	2
DECREASED OR ABNORMAL	I
ABSENT	O
UNTESTABLE	U

STIMULUS:
VOICE	3
SHAKE OR SHOUT	2
PAIN	I
CENTRAL PAIN	O

VERBAL RESPONSE:
ORIENTED	4
CONFUSED	3
INAPPROPRIATE	2
INCOMPREHENSIBLE	I
NONE	O
UNTESTABLE	U

LEG MOTOR RESPONSE:
NORMAL	2
ABNORMAL OR EXTENSOR	I
NONE	O
UNTESTABLE	U

ARM MOTOR RESPONSE:
DEXTROUS AND STRONG	5
PARETIC	4
LOCALIZES	3
ABNORMAL FLEXION	2
EXTENSION	I
NONE	O
UNTESTABLE	U

DATE	
TIME	
SEDATION MEDS	
PARALYTIC AGENTS	
SEIZURES	
BP	
HR	
RESP	
TEMP	
EYE OPENING	
ORIENTATION	
PUPILS (R/L)	
CORNEALS (R/L)	
FACIAL GRIMACE (R/L)	
CALORICS (R/L)	
STIMULUS	
VERBAL RESPONSE	
ARM MOTOR (R/L)	
LEG MOTOR (R/L)	

Fig. 31-4 Flow chart of the Maryland coma scale. This flow chart allows one to record and score all the variables of the Glasgow coma scale with the addition of the important brain stem reflexes, right–left asymmetry, and other clinical variables that may affect the evaluation of the neurologic examination. (Reprinted from Salcman M, Schepp RS, Ducker TB: Calculated recovery rates in severe head trauma. Neurosurgery 8(3): 301, 1981.)

facts that it contains no analysis of the pupils or other brain stem reflexes, no right–left differentiation in motor response, and inadequate accountability of variables (i.e., eyes swollen shut secondary to facial trauma, or inability to verbalize secondary to endotracheal intubation). We use an alternative coma scale that contains the three variables of the Glasgow coma scale. This Maryland coma scale provides an accurate description of cranial nerve function and does not penalize trauma patients when critical data cannot be assessed due to associated injuries. This scale is, therefore, quite useful in patients with multitrauma and is more accurate in the prediction of recovery rates from severe head injury than the Glasgow coma scale. A flow chart of the Maryland coma scale is shown in Figure 31-4.

EPIDURAL HEMATOMA

The incidence[5,17,61] of epidural hematomas in all head injury patients is only about 1 percent, but in those unable to follow commands or verbalize, an 8 percent incidence of epidural hematomas is reported.[86] Since the incidence of epidural hematoma is 5 to 15 percent in fatal head injures,[5,67] the clinical importance of epidural hematoma is far greater than its overall incidence would suggest. Patients with epidural hematomas have a surgically correctable lesion, prompt treatment of which often results in the patient being neurologically normal, or having only a minor cognitive deficit. The mortality after epidural hematoma is 8 percent with early diagnosis and aggressive surgical treatment.[55]

The clinical presentation of an epidural hematoma is classically described as a loss of consciousness followed by a lucid interval as the concussion clears and a subsequent depressed level of consciousness secondary to expansion of the epidural hematoma minutes to hours later.[92] This classic clinical presentation occurs in only one third of the cases. Another one third of patients never experience a loss in consciousness and the remainder of the patients do not regain consciousness from the time of the initial injury.[55] Therefore, physicians and nurses must remain vigilant and perform repeated neurologic checks of all head-injured patients to detect the early signs of delayed deterioration. A common error in the management of epidural hematoma is to underestimate the seriousness of the delayed intracranial events caused by an apparently minor head injury. Alcohol and drugs are commonly associated with head injuries and complicate the serial neurologic assessment of these patients. Early symptoms of an intracranial mass lesion (i.e., headache, restlessness, nausea, vomiting, dizziness, and confusion) can be misinterpreted as due to alcohol or drug ingestion. Furthermore, an unrecognized CSF leak may provide intracranial decompression, delaying the onset of ICP symptoms until the epidural hematoma is quite large.

A skull fracture is associated with an epidural hematoma in 90 percent of cases.[27] This is a major reason for obtaining skull films in head trauma patients. The CT scan is the diagnositc test of choice for the detection of an epidural hematoma; the lesion is hyperdense and lentiform in shape as shown in Figure 31-5. The extent and shape of the hematoma are limited by the adhesion of the dura to the inner table of the skull. An epidural hematoma can cross the location of major venous sinuses since the sinus can be stripped from the inner table and separated from the skull with the dura. Patients without a loss of consciousness but with a skull fracture crossing either the middle meningeal artery or a major intracranial sinus require a prompt CT scan. The scan may detect a small epidural hematoma, if present, at the earliest time and thereby alert medical personnel to potential neurologic deterioration and a need for prolonged close observation. Patients with a loss of consciousness should undergo CT to examine the brain for contusions and ensure that any epidural hematoma present is diagnosed. Delayed epidural hematomas can develop even when the first CT scan shows no abnormality. A negative early CT scan does not remove the necessity for serial neurologic examination. A second CT scan is used to investigate any significant neurologic change. Patients who remain in significant neurologic depression 24 hours following the removal of an epidural hematoma must have a follow-up CT scan to assess midline shift and the surgical site. The CT should be repeated 7 to 10 days postoperatively in patients with epidural hematoma who are neurologically improving or without neurologic abnormalities. The CT scan has replaced cerebral angiograms in the diagnosis and follow-up of epidural hematomas.

An epidural hematoma in the middle fossa results from a laceration of the middle meningeal artery by a linear skull fracture in 60 to 70 percent of cases.[5,55] When a middle fossa lesion expands, the ipsilateral temporal lobe

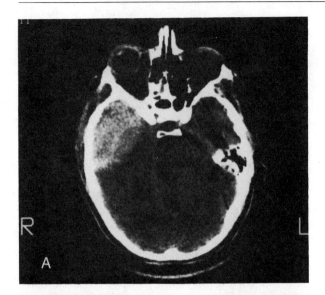

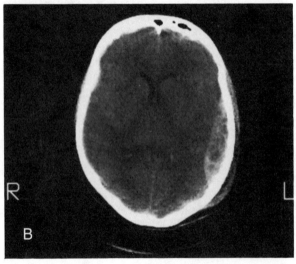

Fig. 31-5 Epidural hematomas. **(A)** A right temporal epidural hematoma. The lenticular shape of the epidural hematoma is evident. The posterior aspect of the epidural hematoma appears to make almost a right angle junction with the skull. The brain stem can be seen displaced from right to left with herniation of the temporal uncus. **(B)** An epidural hematoma in the left parietal region. Note the lenticular shape formed by the tethering of the dura to the skull.

is displaced medially and the temporal uncus and part of the hippocampal gyrus herniate past the tentorial edge. In this way, a unilateral temporal hematoma may present with uncal herination and lateral brain stem compression. The state of alertness can vary from near full wakefulness to coma. A unilateral dilated pupil is the earliest reliable sign in uncal herniation.[99] There is a pupillary abnormality in 30 to 50 percent of patients with an epidural hematoma. The clinical examination is highly predictive of the side of the epidural he-matoma.[5] In 80 to 90 percent of the cases with a size difference in pupils, the dilated pupil will be ipsilateral to the epidural hematoma.[39,79] Hemiparesis or posturing is present in 50 to 75 percent of the cases and when either is present, it is contralateral to the epidural hematoma in 95 percent of the cases.[39,55,79] Bradycardia is present in 25 percent of patients[55] and is a useful clinical sign in children and young adults.

The skull fracture causing the epidural hematoma is frequently located directly below the major force of impact and sustains the maximal swelling of soft tissue in the scalp. It is rare to have an epidural hematoma without significant soft tissue swelling and trauma of the overlying scalp.

The incidence of epidural hematoma in other locations is 11 percent in the frontal area, 6 percent in the occipital, and 12 percent into the posterior fossa.[55]

The management of an epidural hematoma over 15 cc in volume involves prompt surgical evacuation and coagulation of all bleeding vessels. When the diagnosis of an epidural hematoma is made concurrently with a deteriorating neurologic condition, 20 percent mannitol at a dosage of 0.5 g/kg body weight is given while the surgical suite is prepared. Mannitol is considered a safe drug when given immediately preoperatively to relieve brain stem compression, even though theoretically it may cause increased bleeding into the epidural hematoma due to dehydration and contraction of brain tissue. A large frontotemporoparietal trauma flap is used for the evacuation of most epidural hematomas. The temporal portion of the flap is opened first and a low temporal burr hole is placed to evacuate a portion of the epidural clot with the hope of relieving brain stem compression before the craniotomy is completed. The large trauma flap also allows access to the temporal and frontal fossae as well as to a major portion of the lateral hemisphere surface. This exposure is especially necessary for the one third of patients with epidural hematomas who also have subdural or intracerebral clots.[11]

An epidural hemorrhage located in the temporal fossa without other brain damage visualized on the CT scan can be adequately removed through a subtemporal craniectomy. After the epidural hematoma is removed, the dura is circumferentially sutured to the skull around the craniotomy site. An epidural drain is used for 24 hours if there is any question of temporal muscle or galeal bleeding.

The decision to open the dura after removal of the epidural hematoma is based on the preoperative CT scan. The dura is left closed in pure epidural hematomas and opened when a surgically significant subdural or intracerebral hematoma has been identified on the preoperative scan. When the temporal fossa is explored without a CT scan because of rapid deterioration and a unilateral dilated pupil, the dura should be opened if the dura appears blue, indicating blood beneath it.

SUBDURAL HEMATOMA

The incidence of subdural hematomas in all head injuries is only about 1 percent. However, subdural hematomas are very common in severe head injury: they occur in 26 to 63 percent of such cases.[57] An acute traumatic subdural hematoma is defined as blood in the subdural space presenting within 3 days of the trauma. Collections of blood or fluid in the subdural space on a chronic basis reflect a different disease process and are discussed elsewhere.[11] Acute subdural hematomas are divided into two types: simple and complicated. A simple subdural hematoma is a collection of blood in the subdural space without cerebral contusion or laceration. Linear or rotational acceleration–deceleration of the head produces shear forces between the brain and the skull that tear bridging vessels. Sometimes, shear forces on the surface of the brain cause disruption of cortical vessels that bleed into the subdural space. The source of a simple subdural hematoma can be either arterial or venous. Simple subdural collections form 45 percent of all acute subdural hematomas and have a 21 percent mortality.[57]

A complicated subdural hematoma occurs by the same mechanism as a simple subdural hematoma, but results from greater shear forces. These larger forces not only tear the bridging and surface vessels but also cause laceration or bursting of the brain substance with cortical vessel disruption; the cortical vessels then bleed into the subdural space. The extent of underlying injury to the cerebral cortex is often a more important determinant of mortality, elevated intracranial pressure, and the ultimate neurologic outcome of these patients than the subdural hematoma itself. Complicated subdural hematomas make up 41 percent all subdurals and have a 52.6 percent mortality.[57] Subdural hematomas are associated with 24 to 30 percent of bullet wounds or stab wounds in the cranial cavity.[7,82]

Open depressed fractures of the convexity are also associated with subdural hematomas. In these injuries, the skull fragments penetrate the dura, lacerate the brain, and damage the vessels on the cortical surface, producing the subdural hemorrhage. If a major venous sinus is involved in the fracture, the subdural hematoma may be large.

The mortality of acute subdural hematoma is in the range of 50 to 90 percent.[7,16,23,42] The presence of bilateral subdural hematomas or multiple cerebral lacerations increases the mortality rate. For example, with unilateral subdural hematoma the reported mortality ranges from 40 to 70 percent; with bilateral subdural hematomas the mortality increases to the range of 77 to 100 percent. Similarly, a single cortical laceration has a 43 percent mortality compared to a 62 percent mortality for multiple cortical lacerations.[17]

The correlation of mortality and the timing of surgical removal of subdural hematomas has been examined in two studies. In the period of 24 to 72 hours after injury, the mortality of operated patients is not statistically different.[36] However, very early surgical removal of subdural hematomas, in under 4 hours, can significantly decrease the mortality from 90 percent to 30 percent.[107] In a recent series of 44 patients with subdural hematomas of whom 19 had the subdural hematoma removed and 25 were treated with aggressive intracranial pressure management, one quarter of the patients in both groups died. This implies that surgery did not have an impressive role in changing the rate of mortality of these patients. Also, in this series another intracranial lesion in addition to the subdural hematoma was present in 84 percent of the cases.[17] The level of consciousness of a patient with a subdural hematoma on admission is a strong predictor of the ultimate outcome. Patients who are conscious at some time after the accident have a 12 percent mortality, compared to a 27 percent mortality for the flexor-unconscious patients and a 78 percent mortality for those who are decerebrate.[57]

The neurologic outcome for patients with acute subdural hematomas remains grim. In one study, only 9 percent of the survivors returned to work.[36] In another report, only 56 percent of the survivors could be managed at home.[80] The poor neurologic outcome results from the extensive concurrent brain damage associated with most subdural hematomas. This damage derives from the cerebral anoxia at the scene of the accident as well as direct cortical laceration and contusion. These primary cerebral injuries currently have no effective treatment. Poor outcomes in a majority of subdural hematomas are expected to persist pending some fundamental breakthrough in research on central nervous system regeneration.

The initial clinical presentation of subdural hematomas is often determined by the nature and magnitude of cortical and brain stem damage, and not by the mass effect of the hematoma. The typical clinical picture is a patient with a Glasgow coma score of 3 to 8 with focal neurologic signs such as hemiparesis, posturing, or pupillary abnormalities. Only occasionally is there a history of deterioration in the level of consciousness and only 13 percent of patients wtih subdural hematomas have a lucid interval.[57] Higher coma scores and the presence of a lucid interval are associated with simple rather than complicated subdural hematomas.

Ocular abnormalities are common in the clinical presentation of subdural hematomas and include pupil size inequalities, ocular muscle palsies, and retinal lesions. A pupil is enlarged, ipsilateral to the side of the subdural hematoma, in 50 to 80 percent of the cases. The sixth nerve is injured by the high intracranial pressure as it passes over the petrous ridge and, therefore, is of no localizing value. Retinal hemorrhages and enlargement of the retinal veins are often present and serve as an early clinical sign of the severity of the head injury. Localizing neurologic signs are present in about 50 percent of the patients at admission. Absent motor responses to pain stimuli or posturing on one side are contralateral to the subdural hematoma in 85 percent of the cases.[5]

The clinical presentation of subdural hematomas is variable and a large percentage of patients with this finding have additional

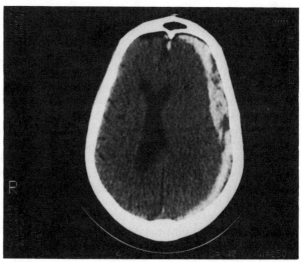

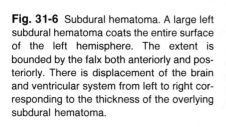

Fig. 31-6 Subdural hematoma. A large left subdural hematoma coats the entire surface of the left hemisphere. The extent is bounded by the falx both anteriorly and posteriorly. There is displacement of the brain and ventricular system from left to right corresponding to the thickness of the overlying subdural hematoma.

intracranial lesions that necessitate rapid and precise diagnosis before medical or surgical decisions are made. The size, position, degree of midline shift, ventricular displacement, basal cistern compression, and quantity of cerebral edema and contusion are visualized best on a CT scan of the head. In the acute phase, the CT scan displays blood as a hyperdense area. A subdural hematoma is a crescent-shaped lesion positioned between the cerebral hemisphere and the skull (Fig. 31-6). The crescent shape results from blood coating the cerebral hemisphere as it flows in the subdural space. The falx and the tentorium form the boundaries of the subdural space and hence define the maximum extent of a subdural hematoma. A hyperdense lesion that stops at the falx or the tentorium and covers a major portion of a cerebral hemisphere on CT scan is a subdural hematoma.

A cerebral angiogram in the presence of a subdural hematoma demonstrates an avascular lentiform mass located between the inner table of the skull and the cortex. Displacement of intracranial vessels is due to the mass effect resulting from the hematoma and the cortical contusion. A subdural hematoma is usually best visualized on the anterior–posterior projection of the angiogram. Occasionally, oblique views more accurately demonstrate the maximum thickness of the clot. The majority of sub-

dural hematomas are located in the frontotemporoparietal region; unusual locations for a subdural hematoma include the anterior fossa, interhemispheric fissure, occipital lobe, and posterior fossa.

The management of a patient with a subdural hematoma depends on the clinical presentation, the absolute volume of the hematoma, and the size of the clot relative to the swelling of the underlying cortex. Management of a head injury with a subdural hematoma is often based on treatment of the massive cerebral swelling secondary to cortical contusion and not the subdural hematoma per se. A large subdural hematoma (6 to 15 mm) with mass effect and little or no cortical damage is treated with prompt surgical evacuation. However, a small subdural hematoma (2 to 3 mm) with massive cerebral contusion and edema is treated wtih aggressive medical therapy. Controversial cases are those with moderate-sized hematomas and a moderate degree of cerebral contusion and swelling. The cerebral compliance may be so compromised by the amount of cerebral edema that even the removal of a 20 to 30 ml subdural hematoma can be beneficial in the management of the intracranial pressure. An intracranial pressure greater than 20 mmHg also influences the decision as to when to remove a moderate-sized subdural hematoma. Serial CT scans, clinical examinations, and ICP measurements are all considered in the decision to operate on these patients.

Surgical removal of a subdural hematoma can increase the risk of aggravating the brain swelling under the clot and result in herniation of brain into the craniotomy site. The traumatic injury to the cortex beneath the hematoma often includes disruption of the blood–brain barrier, and this produces vasogenic edema. Since cerebral tissue pressure under the craniotomy site is lowered by removal of the overlying skull and opening of the dura, an increase in the difference between the cerebral capillary pressure and the tissue pressure occurs. This differential pressure is the force driving the vasogenic edema. The dura may need to be closed rapidly so that surgical resection of cortex is not necessary.

Surgical removal of a subdural hematoma is performed through a large temporofrontoparietal craniotomy flap.[11] The dura is opened widely and the subdural hematoma is removed by suction and irrigation. Gentle irrigation is also used to remove the layer of clot under the edge of the craniotomy. Care is taken not to disturb the large bridging veins near the saggital sinus. Any cortical bleeding points are identified and coagulated with the bipolar cautery. The preoperative CT scan and the visual appearance of the cortical surface determine whether areas of cerebral contusion or intracerebral hematomas are surgically excised. An ICP monitoring device is inserted at the end of the removal for ICP management in the often stormy and lengthy intensive care course.

In 58 percent of the patients, the postoperative ICP is elevated over 20 mmHg. In this subgroup of subdural hematoma patients, 58 percent die.[85] In the first few days postoperatively, the CT scan may demonstrate an increased mass effect resulting from swelling of the hemisphere subjacent to the hematoma site. The ICP typically remains high normal or elevated and the brain remains in a low-compliance state for 3 to 10 days following injury. Major medical problems commonly appear in the debilitated patient in an intensive care environment over this length of time and 20 to 40 percent of the mortality after the immediate postoperative period can be attributed to medical complications. Pulmonary complications contribute to the majority of deaths.[4,37]

SKULL FRACTURES

Skull fractures[5,25] are formed during the moment of impact. The size and type of a skull fracture is determined by the kinetic energy of the striking object, the direction of the impact force, and the area of impact. Skull fractures are classified as linear, comminuted, or depressed.

Linear fractures are produced by failure of the skull to undergo elastic deformation during the impact. The fracture starts at the maximum stress point and then usually extends to the point of impact. When the impact point receives a large amount of energy, the bone locally is broken into many pieces and the fracture is referred to as being comminuted. If the impact energy is even larger, the comminuted sections of the fracture are driven inwards into the brain.[41]

The structural failure causing skull fractures is determined by the energy of impact and the ratio of the force of impact to the area of impact. When the area of impact is large, as in a patient striking the head while wearing a motorcycle helmet, no skull fracture occurs despite high-impact energies. When the area of contact is small, as in a patient struck by a hammer or the corner of a brick, skull fractures radiate from the site of impact.

Skull fractures can also be classified as being open or closed by the presence or absence of a communication between the fracture and the environment. This communication can be an overlying scalp laceration or a fracture extending into the skull base with violation of the air cavities. When either the paranasal sinus or the middle ear structures are involved in a fracture, it is potentially open. Compound fractures of the convexity and skull base have distinct clinical presentations, treatments, and complications.

The presence of a linear skull fracture serves as a marker that the skull has received an impact of considerable energy. There is controversy regarding the clinical indications for obtaining skull x-ray studies. Most authors agree that only a small number of patients have their clinical management changed by the presence or absence of a linear skull fracture.[12,33,52,98] However, one would not wish to miss a linear fracture crossing the path of the middle meningeal artery in any mild head injury. Some of these patients go on to late neurologic deterioration as a result of epidural hematoma. A number of depressed fractures, puncture wounds, and intracranial foreign objects cannot be diagnosed without skull x-ray studies. The medicolegal implications of these nondiagnosed lesions are potentially grave. In Great Britain most lawsuits involving head trauma were based on a late deterioration after a mild head injury.[58] When a complete CT scan of the head is obtained, the skull radiographs add little that affects management or ultimate neurologic outcome. Each medical facility needs to establish guidelines for obtaining skull radiographs. Clinical symptoms that merit radiologic examination include loss of consciousness, retrograde amnesia, discharge from nose or ear, ear drum discoloration, Babinski reflex, or cranial nerve abnormalities.[12] The eventual neurologic outcome of the patient is determined by the brain injury, and the presence of a linear skull fracture adds no useful information to the neurologic evaluation.

The annual incidence of depressed skull fractures is estimated[14] to be 20 per 1 million population and these occur mostly in males under the age of 30. The associated mortality is 11 percent and relates to the severity of the brain rather than bony injury. Central nervous system infections make only a small contribution to the overall mortality. Approximately 7 percent of patients with depressed skull fractures have an intracranial hematoma requiring surgical therapy. At least 11 percent of the patients have long-term neurologic sequelae after their injury.[50] Eighty-five percent of the depressed fractures are open.[13,56,87]

Surgical therapy for a depressed skull fracture should be considered when the depression is greater than the thickness of the skull. A depressed fracture is produced when the impact energy is applied over a small contact area. Typical examples include assaults with a hammer, club, or pipe; sports injuries caused by a hockey stick, golf club, or golf ball; or motor vehicle accidents when the head strikes either the interior of the car or an object outside the car while the patient is thrown from the car. A high suspicion of depressed skull frac-

ture can often be made based on the details of the injury.

Many patients with depressed skull fractures never have a loss of consciousness and skull films are not initially obtained.[59] Palpation and visual inspection of a scalp laceration are unreliable in diagnosing depressed skull fractures. The scalp may move relative to the skull at impact and hence the depression may not be directly under the scalp laceration. Furthermore, hematomas within the layers of the scalp can easily be mistaken for bony step-offs. In a depressed fracture, the inner table is typically depressed further than the outer table. In two thirds of the cases in which depressed skull fractures were initially not appreciated, skull radiographs were not obtained in the pre-CT era.[59]

The diagnosis of depressed skull fracture is made by either skull radiographs or CT scan of the head. Depressed skull fractures are usually visualized on the standard anteroposterior (AP) and lateral views of the skull, although oblique views tangential to the suspected depressed area may reveal fractures not seen in the standard views. Figure 31-7 shows a CT scan of a depressed skull fracture with bone driven into the brain.

Surgical treatment of depressed fractures has three major objectives: repairing the cosmetic defect, preventing infectious complications, and inspecting the cortex for damage.[87] In simple depressed skull fractures, the fragments are elevated when the depression is greater than the thickness of the skull. Although elevation of the fracture was once thought to reduce the incidence of late epilepsy, recent data do not support this contention.[60] The cosmetic results of elevating the fragments are generally good. In a closed fracture the chance of central nervous system infection is similar to that for elective craniotomy. Delayed repair of a closed fracture is acceptable when the CT scan of the brain discloses no underlying pathologic change.

Compound depressed skull fractures represent a neurosurgical emergency. If the dura is lacerated under the fracture site, bacteria have access to the epidural, subdural, and subarachnoid spaces, as well as the brain parenchyma. Surgical treatment includes debridement of devitalized tissue and bone with in-

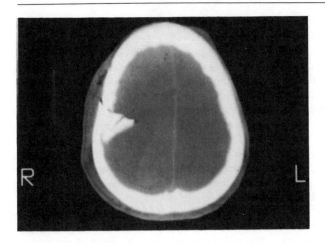

Fig. 31-7 Depressed skull fracture. A depressed skull fracture with bone fragments in the brain is demonstrated by this CT scan. The overlying traumatic scalp swelling can also be seen.

spection of the underlying dura. If the dura is intact under the fracture, it is not opened unless an underlying hematoma is visualized on CT scan and requires surgical treatment. When the dura is lacerated, the underlying brain is inspected for cortical bleeding and bone fragments. Bleeding is controlled with bipolar coagulation and the bone fragments are removed with irrigation. Devitalized brain is also resected. If the wound is not grossly contaminated, the larger fragments of bone can be soaked in antibiotic solution and replaced at the initial operation.[14,59] If the wound is considered grossly contaminated, all fragments of bone should be removed and the cranial defect repaired in 9 to 12 months with an acrylic cranioplasty.

Fractures of the base of the skull are relatively common and are reported to occur in 3.5 to 24 percent of head-injured patients.[15,31,72] The wide variance results from differences in the patient population and the difficulty in obtaining radiographic verification of the fractures.[25] Linear fractures at the base of the brain carry a risk of meningitis, unlike linear fractures over the convexity. The dura overlying the base of the skull is easily torn, placing the subarachnoid space in direct contact with the paranasal sinuses or middle ear structures. A persistent fistula with CSF leak may develop at the site of fracture. The tract is a pathway for bacteria and continually exposes the patient to the risk of meningitis.

Basal skull fractures are initially suspected by clinical signs related to the site of the fracture. Fractures in the temporal bone present with hemotympanum, blood in the external auditory canal, seventh or eighth nerve palsies, ecchymosis over the mastoid, or CSF otorrhea. Clinical signs of basilar skull fracture in the anterior skull base include bilateral periorbital ecchymosis, anosmia, and CSF rhinorrhea. A CSF leak first detected many weeks after trauma is either due to an initial missed diagnosis or the delayed development of hydrocephalus with rupture of the arachnoid at the fracture site.[95]

Basal skull fracture with CSF rhinorrhea is common after head injury and has an estimated incidence of 150,000 cases per year in the United States.[73] A watery nasal discharge containing glucose diagnoses CSF rhinorrhea clinically. A CSF leak originating in the paranasal sinuses can often be made apparent by having the patient sit on the edge of the bed in a flexed position with the head close to the knees for 2 minutes. The CSF discharged from the nose is initially mixed with blood and this may cause a diagnostic problem; however, the blood usually clears in a few days.

The management of basal skull fracture is determined by the presence or absence of a CSF leak. Patients with a basal skull fracture but no leak are managed by observation for 2 to 3 days. During this time repeated checks for rhinorrhea or otorrhea are made to verify that a CSF leak is truly absent. Monitoring of temperature, mental status, and white blood cell count provides evidence that no infectious process is developing. Prophylactic antibiotics should not be used in patients with basal skull fracture with or without a CSF leak: antibiotics are not effective in preventing meningitis and may select out resistant organisms when infections do develop.[53]

Any CSF leaks are managed initially by observing the amount of leakage and any signs of infection. A majority of cases stop without treatment within the first week.[15,70,88] If the CSF leak persists beyond 7 days, then lumbar taps are performed daily for 3 days with 40 to 60 ml spinal fluid removed each time. A large gauge needle is used and multiple holes are made in the lumbar dura at several levels to produce a CSF leak into the lumbar epidural space. Following the spinal taps, the patient is kept in a 30° head up position. A CT scan is obtained prior to puncture to rule out an intracranial mass lesion, hydrocephalus, or tight basal cisterns. If arachnoid or brain is herniated into the ethomoid sinus or the cribriform plate is fractured with a spicule of bone in the brain, then surgical repair of the anterior fossa is performed initially.

If the spinal taps fail to stop the leak, then spinal drainage may be used for 72 hours with the patient in a 30° head up position. If pneumocephalus develops during the course of CSF drainage then the drainage procedure is terminated and the dural leak is surgically closed. More persistent leaks require detailed diagnosis of the exact site of the leak by metrizamide CT scan, nuclear cisternogram, or plain film tomography. A surgical repair directed at the identified tract is then performed. Radiation cysternogram with nasal pledgets is useful in diagnosing small or questionable leaks.

A CSF otorrhea usually occurs with a fracture of the petrous bone and perforation of the tympanic membrane. Occasionally, CSF reaches the mastoid air cells by a basal skull fracture and flows directly in the external ear canal through an open fracture of the canal. If the tympanic membrane remains intact, CSF that has gained access to the middle ear can flow through the eustacian tube and present as rhinorrhea. Patients with CSF otorrhea often present with hearing loss or bleeding from the external ear canal.[51,89] Irrigation and probing of the ear in cases of suspected otorrhea have no place in the management of these patients and places the patient at risk of infection due to the manipulation. These patients are managed by placing a loose fitting sterile gauze pad over the ear; the pad is changed every nursing shift and saved as an indicator of the amount of drainage from the ear. Most cases of otorrhea stop spontaneously within the first few days. A detailed auditory and vestibular examination is performed 6 to 8 weeks following trauma to diagnose abnormalities and determine treatment. Otorrhea is more likely than rhinorrhea to resolve spontaneously.

PROTOCOL

A systematic method for evaluating and treating head-injured patients is necessary as a framework for effective and prompt treatment. Strict protocols cannot, however, be rigid. A large fraction of these patients have multitrauma that can either complicate or take precedence over the management of head injury. Optimal care requires careful coordination between many medical and trauma specialists.

As a guide, the following system of classifying head trauma patients into five major categories is useful. This system uses the Glasgow coma score as an initial assessment.

Patients with a Glasgow coma score of 3 to 5 represent those with the severest group of head injuries. These patients are intubated and hyperventilated to an arterial carbon dioxide tension of 28 to 30 mmHg. Cardiopulmonary resuscitation is completed in the emergency recovery area before the patient is transported for special radiologic tests. Mannitol is given as a drip in a dose of 0.25 to 0.5 g/kg in patients with a lateralizing pupil or motor response. Skull and cervical radiographs are obtained in the initial resuscitation area by portable equipment concurrently with the cardiopulmonary resuscitation. A thorough multiple trauma physical examination is performed. Only those systemic studies and treatments required as immediate life saving procedures should delay the neurologic evaluation and treatment. A CT scan of the head is obtained on an emergent basis once the patient demonstrates cardiopulmonary stability. Creation of emergency exploratory burr holes without CT scan is reserved for the rare patients who dilate a pupil in the resuscitation area, or for those patients whose cardiopulmonary status remains unstable and who are not transportable to CT scan facilities. Cerebral angiography is often helpful in clinical decision making when the patient is too unstable to transport for a CT scan. Mass lesions are diagnosed by vessel displacement and brain death is demonstrated by absence of blood flow beyond the carotid siphon. When the CT scan diagnoses a surgical mass lesion, it is promptly removed. Intracranial pressure monitoring is instituted in all patients by either a subarachnoid bolt or an intraventricular catheter.

The head-injured patient should also undergo full hemodynamic monitoring with an arterial line, and a thermodilution Swan-Ganz catheter so that cardiac output can be determined. Fluid administration and inotropic drugs are adjusted based on knowledge of the vascular status gained from the pulmonary wedge pressure and cardiac output. A detailed hemodynamic profile is especially crucial in multitrauma patients with large blood losses and third spacing of fluid. Intravenous fluids are adjusted to maintain a high normal plasma osmolality and a high normal stress response in cardiac output. The CT scan in all patients is repeated 24 to 48 hours following the injury or whenever the ICP is greater than 20 mmHg. The repeat CT scan often discloses increased swelling of the brain, or delayed intracranial hematomas.

Critically injured head trauma patients typically require intensive care unit management for 1 to 2 weeks and an ICP monitor for 2 to 10 days. Most of these patients need a tracheostomy; oral or nasotracheal tube complications are lessened when it is performed early in their care. These patients are often debilitated for a prolonged period and multiple medical problems can arise. Constant vigilance is required for diagnosis and therapy of medical complications. When these patients awake from their head injury, cognitive neuropsycho-metric testing is performed to evaluate their precise neurologic deficits. Cognitive retraining is begun in the acute hospital stay and continued in a rehabilitation hospital. Electrical neurometric and EEG evaluation is performed on all patients within 6 to 10 days following injury and a follow-up examination is performed every few weeks as a prognostic guide to functional brain recovery. The neurometrics evaluation is useful in predicting the clinical neurologic state of the patient at 6 months and 1 year following head trauma.[49,63,64]

Head-injured patients with an initial Glasgow coma score of 6 to 8 form a second group of patients with severe head injury but a lower mortality rate. Therapy for these patients is similar to the severely injured group with the following exception: fluid therapy is usually guided by a central venous catheter instead of a Swan-Ganz catheter, when the head injury is the major problem. However, multitrauma patients or those with concurrent cardiopulmonary disease may require a Swan-Ganz catheter for optimal fluid management.

Patients with moderately severe head injury require a shorter intensive care unit stay than those with severe injury. The ICP monitoring is usually required for 2 to 5 days. Almost all of these patients eventually wake up. Nevertheless, cognitive neuropsychometric evaluation reveals deficits in a majority of these patients. Electrical neurometric and EEG testing over a 4 to 6 month period demonstrate a progression of the coherence and frequency activity towards normal. Most of these patients require inpatient cognitive retraining at a head injury rehabilitation facility.

Patients with a Glasgow coma score of 9 to 12 are considered to have a more moderate head injury. They generally do not require intubation unless the arterial oxygen is less than 80 mmHg or the arterial carbon dioxide is greater than 45 mmHg. A CT scan is obtained on these patients on an urgent basis. Neurologic checks are continued for a minimum of 24 hours at 1 hour intervals. If these patients are not oriented with a clear sensorium by 24 to 48 hours, then a repeat CT scan is obtained to examine for any delayed intracranial pathologic change. A scan is also obtained on an urgent basis to document any neurologic deterioration. Cognitive neuropsychometric testing,

EEG, and electrical neurometric evaluation demonstrate defects in personality, thought processes, and memory. The EEG regional power spectrum often has focal abnormalities. These patients are usually discharged home and receive cognitive retraining as necessary on an outpatient basis.

Mild head injury characterizes the last two groups. Patients who present with a Glasgow coma score of 13 or 14 require close neurologic checks at least every hour for 24 hours. All of these patients should undergo skull radiographs and cervical spine films. A CT scan of the head is ordered on an urgent basis when a depressed fracture is suspected or when the patient needs clearance for a surgical procedure related to a systemic injury. The CT scan is necessary in these patients because intraoperative neurologic checks are not obtainable during anesthesia. Patients not fully awake and oriented 12 to 24 hours following head injury should also receive a CT scan to search for intracranial pathologic change. Cognitive neuropsychometric and neurometric evaluations are obtained to examine for residual deficits secondary to the head injury. A percentage of these patients are at risk for the posttraumatic concussion syndrome.[81] Early identification of the syndrome aids in counseling of patients and their families. Symptoms include headache, photophobia, personality change, sleep disturbances, and short-term memory impairment.

The mildest category of head injury patients includes those who arrive with a Glasgow coma score of 15 with a history of momentary loss of consciousness at the scene. They are clinically managed the same as those with a score of 13 to 14.

Mild head injury patients are followed up after discharge with at least one clinic visit to determine if any delayed sequelae of head injury are present and to perform a cognitive evaluation. Cognitive retraining is started and counseling given to patients with cognitive deficits and posttraumatic concussion syndrome, respectively.

Patients with mild and moderate head injury do not receive hemodynamic monitoring or endotracheal intubation except as required by other injuries. These patients do, however, require close neurologic monitoring for the onset of delayed intracranial sequelae such as epidural hematomas or increased cerebral swelling. The serial neurologic examination in this moderately and mildly injured group is essential to determine neurologic deterioration. Prompt recognition and treatment can prevent unnecessary fatality and produce a good outcome. The time from onset of neurologic change to irreversible neurologic deficit may be as short as 20 minutes in some cases. During the close observation period it is necessary to arouse the patient on an hourly basis for 24 hours to determine and record the maximum level of neurologic performance. Guidelines need to be clearly specified to the nursing service as to when the physician should be notified that a deterioration has occurred. The neurologic examination may be difficult for the staff to perform because the patient is agitated when aroused and asks to be left to sleep. Agitation and disorientation secondary to either the head injury or alcohol are treated only when severe and only after an intracranial mass lesion is excluded. A request to be left to sleep cannot be honored in the first 24 hours after head injury without risking neurologic disaster from a delayed intracranial hematoma.

MAJOR MEDICAL PROBLEMS

Dysfunction in organ systems other than the central nervous system and major medical problems are common following severe head injury. These systemic problems result from direct trauma to a specific organ, peripheral manifestations of central nervous system injury, and medical complications related to the debilitated and immobilized state of the unconscious patient.

Respiratory failure is a serious concomitant injury with head injury since the combined morbidity and mortality are greater than the expected rates for either injury separately.[38,105] This pathologic synergism results from the inability to use hyperventilation as a modality to control intracranial pressure, elevations in the PCO_2 that complicate intracranial mass effects, and the association of respiratory and brain failure with the multiple organ system failure syndrome.[91]

Support of the respiratory system starts at the scene of the accident. The paramedical personnel must provide an adequate airway as a life saving measure. This is often the single most important determinant of a good outcome. The onset or progression of anoxic brain injury can be prevented in many instances by an adequate airway, assisted ventilation, and oxygen. The continued use of assisted ventilation with high normal minute ventilation prevents excess carbon dioxide from accumulating with concomitant intracranial vasodilation and increased mass effect due to enhanced brain swelling.

The tongue of the unconscious patient may fall against the posterior pharynx and occlude the airway. The simple maneuver of the chin lift or jaw thrust often relieves the upper airway obstruction. The paramedic team may also use an esophageal obturator airway, oropharyngeal airway, or nasopharyngeal airway in the prehospital phase as required by the respiratory distress of the patient and the team's training in airway insertion.[21]

Patients with a depressed level of consciousness after head injury may aspirate at the scene of the accident, during transport, or shortly after arrival in the emergency room. Aspirated material may include the stomach contents such as food or alcohol, and foreign objects such as teeth or roadside debris. Aspiration in patients without an effective cough mechanism often begins the progression of pneumonia, respiratory failure, acute respiratory distress syndrome (ARDS), and death. The diagnosis of aspiration is made using the clinical signs of tachypnea, fever, and localized rales, evidence of hypoxemia based on arterial blood gas, and localized chest radiograph changes or diffuse infiltrates. Fiberoptic flexible bronchoscopy with removal of gross aspiration material in the emergency room is often clinically rewarding.

Intensive pulmonary therapy is required for 7 to 21 days in head trauma survivors to restore pulmonary function after aspiration. This therapy includes oxygen to correct hypoxemia, positive end-expiratory pressure (PEEP) to increase functional reserve volume and de-crease pulmonary shunt, mechanical ventilator support to relieve respiratory effort, antibiotics as indicated by culture of the broncheal secretions, and vigorous pulmonary toilet with transtracheal suctioning, bronchoscopy, and chest physiotherapy.[8,19,90] The seriousness of pulmonary complications is illustrated by the mortality rate of 41 percent for patients with ARDS found in a collaborative study of nine centers.[91] Prevention of aspiration by protecting the airway is the ideal but often unobtainable goal. A cuffed transpharyngeal airway should be utilized as soon as possible in the emergency room in all patients with a Glasgow coma score of 7 or under. This measure will lessen the pulmonary complications secondary to inadequate airway and aspiration.

Many patients with severe head injury have hypoxemia on admission without evidence of traumatic pulmonary injury or aspiration.[108] In this group, the pulmonary shunt calculated from arterial and mixed venous blood gas samples correlates with patient outcome and is an important prognostic indicator.[37] Excess autonomic discharge as a response to central nervous system injury is proposed as a cause of this early pulmonary arteriovenous shunting and the resultant arterial hypoxemia.[112,116]

Pulmonary edema can occur in head injured patients without direct pulmonary trauma. The sympathetic discharge seen in head injury produces an increase in pulmonary blood volume secondary to generalized peripheral vasoconstriction. This produces a shift of circulating blood volume from the peripheral vessels into the pulmonary vessels, an increase in the pulmonary capillary pressure, endothelial cell injury, and resultant pulmonary edema. Continued elevation of the pulmonary capillary pressure perpetuates the edema formation in areas of endothelial cell injury and can result in hypoxic respiratory failure and ARDS.[112,116]

The treatment of respiratory failure with ventilation/perfusion mismatch in head injury patients is complicated by the interaction of PEEP with cerebral pathologic conditions. This PEEP is useful in the treatment of ARDS by helping to maintain open alveoli and thus reducing the percent of pulmonary shunting. This enables one to correct the hypoxemia with a lower inspired oxygen concentration and lessens the amount of oxygen toxicity to which the lungs are exposed.[66,115] However, PEEP also indirectly affects the damaged brain by altering the cerebral perfusion, both by reducing venous return and cardiac output and by increasing the intracranial pressure secondary to an increase in the central venous pressure.

The use of PEEP in healthy volunteers shows a decreased cardiac output secondary to impairment of the venous return and an increase in the central venous pressure secondary to transmission of the airway pressure to the vena cava in the thoracic cavity. These effects are accentuated by hypotension or hypovolemia. A precipitous decrease in the cerebral perfusion pressure can occur with the onset of PEEP in head-injured patients who have high pulmonary compliance and low intracranial compliance, or in patients whose heads are not elevated. The use of PEEP remains controversial in head injury and both the timing and the amount of PEEP that should be used are unknown.[28,37,110]

We use PEEP in head-injured patients, when required by hypoxemic respiratory failure without temporally related intracranial deterioration or significant intracranial pressure elevation. The PEEP is maintained at the lowest level and always under 15 cmH$_2$O, the head of the bed is elevated at 30 to 45°, and the patient's neck is kept straight with a Philadelphia collar. Elevation of the head above the level of the PEEP with patent jugular and intracranial venous drainage assures that the brain tissues empty into a low-pressure venous system. If these measures are not successful and PEEP is required for respiratory management, then β- adrenergic inotropic support with dobutamine (1 to 3 μg/kg/min) or low dose isoproterenol (0.25 to 0.5 μg/min total dose) to increase the cardiac ejection fraction and the lower right atrial and central venous pressures is started. These measures permit the dural sinuses to continue to provide easy runoff of venous blood from the brain and ensure that cerebral edema is not enhanced by an elevation in the intracranial venous pressure. Head-injured patients on PEEP require Swan-Ganz monitoring to adjust their fluids and inotropic support so that adequate cerebral perfusion pressures and cardiac output are maintained without the use of large fluid volume.[34,66]

Respiratory failure can also be caused by fat embolism after long bone fractures. The respiratory failure can range from subclinical reductions in PaO$_2$ to ARDS. The clinical signs have a delayed onset of 1 to 3 days and the fat embolism syndrome resolves in about a week. Symptoms include mental change, cough, and dyspnea. Fat globules enter the circulation from either the marrow at a fracture site via open venous channels or by release of chylomicrons from fat stores in response to circulating catechol levels. The fat globules are filtered in the pulmonary capillaries where serum lipase hydrolyzes them. The hydrolysis products can cause direct endothelial damage and are capable of triggering the kinin cascade with additional local endothelial damage. The management of these patients is supportive and similar to the ARDS therapy outlined above[6,32,45,47] and in Chapter 19.

Pulmonary thromboembolism can occur in the unconscious patient from venous thrombus secondary to immobilization. Classic blood gas findings include a low PaO$_2$ and a respiratory alkalosis due to hyperventilation. However, in unconscious, intubated, and artificially ventilated patients only the decreased PaO$_2$ is predictable; PaCO$_2$ may mildly rise as pulmonary exchange surface is reduced. Tachycardia and fever are present in many cases of pulmonary thromboembolism. Impedance plethysmography is a highly reliable, noninvasive, readily available bedside test for the screening of patients at risk.[46] When the results of impedance plethysmography suggest pulmonary embolism, then a ventilation/perfusion lung scan is performed. In patients with a high probability of pulmonary embolism on lung scan, a pulmonary angiogram is performed for a definitive diagnosis. Anticoagulation in the first week after the injury can lead to intracranial bleeding in areas of cerebral contusion. A Greenfield filter in the inferior vena cava is the treatment of choice when the risks of anticoagulation appear high (see Chap. 23).

When intubation is required for more than 7 to 10 days, an elective tracheostomy is performed. If the patient wakes up from coma in a combative state with respiratory compromise, early tracheostomy may be performed to prevent mechanical damage to the larynx and vocal cords from the motion of the endotracheal tube. The decision to perform a tracheostomy in these patients depends on an estimate of the time required before patients can defend their airway, an assessment of the respiratory status, and the amount of sedation required to prevent agitation. The tracheostomy is removed once the patient can defend the airway and has an effective cough and adequate pulmonary function.

Abnormalities in the hematologic system are common following severe head injury. The thromboplastic activity of brain tissue is high and increased fibrinolysis is observed following trauma. Increases in the coagulation variables are present in 40 percent of cases and disseminated intravascular coagulation (DIC) is present in 8 percent of head-injured patients. The nonspecific coagulation abnormalities are correctable with fresh frozen plasma and resolve in the first days after trauma. Disseminated intravascular coagulation is a more severe abnormality: it can cause hypoxemia and can progress to ARDS. High titers of fibrin degradation products, depressed fibrinogen levels, and thrombocytopenia are present in DIC. The use of heparin has *no* place in the management of DIC in severe head injury, because the efficacy of heparin is uncertain and the risks of fatal bleeding into a contused brain are real.[22,29]

Fluid and electrolyte management in head-injured patients should encompass the abnormalities resulting from both the brain injury and its therapy. Brain injury and generalized trauma cause metabolic and endocrine changes which affect electrolyte excretion in the urine. The release of excess aldosterone in response to stress results in hypokalemia and sodium retention. Additional potassium may be excreted with the use of mannitol and other diuretics, or as a renal response to hyperventilation. The serum potassium level is maintained by the use of additional potassium chloride in the intravenous solutions. Usually, the sodium retention from aldosterone is almost exactly balanced by the excess free water accumulated by increased release of antidiuretic hormone (ADH). This results in mild hyponatremia with excess total body fluid. In some cases, severe hyponatremia can develop from the release of unbalanced ADH. The diagnosis is confirmed by the presence of urine hyperosmolarity with serum hypo-osmolarity. If hyponatremia is severe, disorientation and seizures may occur. Treatment consists of fluid restriction to 1,000 to 1,200 ml total fluid per day. On rare occasions, hypertonic saline combined with the use of a loop diuretic is required to correct severe hyponatremia with symptoms.[104,114]

Hypernatremia and hyperosmolarity are present in many head-injured patients as a consequence of the fluid restriction and hyperosmolar agents used to manage the increases in intracranial pressure. Hypothalamic dysfunction can cause diabetes insipidus with hypernatremia; this is often a grave prognostic sign in head-injured patients. The diagnosis of diabetes insipidus is confirmed by the presence of a large urine output of low specific gravity and by hypo-osmolarity with serum hyperosmolarity. Although the mild hyperosmolarity requires no specific treatment, diabetes insipidus requires exogenous ADH for fluid management. The requirements for exogenous ADH decrease after 2 to 4 weeks and the dosage in most patients can be safely tapered off. A continuous infusion of ADH (1 to 5 units/hr) is titrated to maintain an adequate urine output in critically ill patients. Stable patients are managed with 5 to 10 units of aqueous pitressin given intramuscularly every 8 to 12 hours, based on urine output.[35,100]

Cardiovascular changes also occur following head injury. Increased intracranial pressure produces a peripheral vasoconstriction with a mild increase in the cardiac output. The combined action of these two effects is to elevate the systemic blood pressure. Treatment of hypertension must be guided by the cerebral perfusion pressure and the ICP. A sustained systemic pressure elevation with a high CPP requires treatment to lessen the risk of cerebral edema. However, the systemic hypertension in response to an elevation in the intracranial pressure that maintains marginally adequate CPP is dangerous to treat for fear of causing ischemic brain damage. These two requirements can be balanced by continuous monitoring of ICP and CPP. Cardiac arrhythmias and myocardial damage are often present in patients with head injury and should be treated with inotropic and vascular unloading therapies (Chap. 8). Many of these changes are caused by a massive autonomic discharge that originates in the hypothalamus.

REFERENCES

1. Adams RA, Victor M: Principles of Neurology, 3rd Ed. McGraw-Hill, New York, 1985, p. 1184
2. Anderson DW: The National Head and Spinal Cord Injury Survey. J Neurosurg 53: 51, 1981
3. Annegers JF, Grabow JD, Groover RV et al: Seizures after head trauma: a population study. Neurology 30: 683, 1980
4. Baigelman W, O'Brian JC: Pulmonary effects of head trauma. Neurosurgery 9: 729, 1981
5. Bakay L, Glasauer FE (eds): Head Injury. Little, Brown, Boston, 1980, p. 445
6. Banyai AL: Fat embolism, Chest 69: 355, 1976
7. Barnett JC, Jr.: Hematomas associated with penetrating wounds. P. 131. In Neurological Surgery of Trauma. U.S. Army, Office of the Surgeon General, Dept. of the Army, Washington, 1965
8. Bartlett JG, Gorbach SL: The triple threat of aspiration pneumonia. Chest 68: 560, 1975
9. Becker DP, Miller JD, Greenberg RP: Prognosis after head injury. P. 2137. In Youmans (ed): Neurological Surgery, 2nd ed, Vol. IV. WB Saunders, Philadelphia, 1982
10. Becker DP, Miller JD, Ward JD et al: The outcome from severe head injury with early diagnosis and intensive management. J Neurosurg 47: 491, 1977
11. Becker DP, Miller JD, Young HG et al: Diagnosis and treatment of head injury in adults. P. 1938. In Youmans (ed): Neurological Surgery, 2nd ed, Vol. IV. WB Saunders, Philadelphia, 1982
12. Bell RS, Loop JW: The utility and futility of radiographic skull examination for trauma. N Engl J Med 284: 236, 1971
13. Braakman R: Survey and follow-up of 225 consecutive patients with a depressed skull fracture. J Neurol Neurosurg Psychiatry, 34: 106, 1971
14. Braakman R: Depressed skull fracture: Data, treatment and follow-up in 225 consecutive cases. J Neurol Neurosurg Psychiatry 35: 395, 1972
15. Brawley BW, Kelly WA: Treatment of basal skull fractures with and without cerebrospinal fluid fistulae. J Neurosurg 26: 57, 1967
16. Browder J, Turney MF: Intracerebral hemorrhage of traumatic origin. NY State J Med 42: 2230, 1942
17. Bruce DA, Gennarelli TA, Langfitt TW: Resuscitation from coma due to head injury. Crit Care Med 6: 254, 1978
18. Bruce DA, Langfitt TW, Miller JD et al: Regional cerebral blood flow, intracranial pressure, and brain metabolism in comatose patients. J Neurosurg 38: 131, 1973
19. Bynum LJ, Pierce AK: Pulmonary aspiration of gastric contents. Am Rev Respir Dis 114: 1129, 1976
20. Casson IR, Siegel O, Shan R et al: Brain damage in modern boxers. JAMA 251: 2663, 1984
21. Collicott PE (ed): Advanced Trauma Life Support Course for Physicians. Subcommittee on Advanced Trauma Life Support of the American College of Surgeons Committee on Trauma, American College of Surgeons, 1984
22. Colman RW, Robboy SJ, Minna JD: Disseminated intravascular coagulation: an approach. Am J Med, 52: 679, 1972
23. Columella F, Gaist G, Piazza G et al: Extradural hematoma at the vertex. J Neurol Neurosurg Psychiatry 31: 315, 1968
24. Cooper PJ: Epidemiology of head injury. P. 1. In Cooper PR, Fleischer AS (eds): Head Injury. Williams & Wilkins, Baltimore, 1982
25. Cooper PJ: Skull fracture and traumatic cerebrospinal fluid fistula. P. 65. In Cooper PR, Fleischer AS (eds): Head Injury. Williams & Wilkins, Baltimore, 1982
26. Cowley RA, Dunham CM: Shock Trauma/Critical Care Manual, Initial Assessment and Management. University Park Press, Baltimore, 1982
27. Dacey RG, Jane JA: Craniocerebral trauma. In Baker AB, Baker LH (eds): Clinical Neurology Harper and Row, Philadelphia, 1984
28. Demers RR, Irwin RS, Braman SS: Criteria for optimum PEEP. Respir Care, 22: 596, 1977
29. Deykin D: The clinical challenge of DIC. N Engl J Med 283: 636, 1970
30. Donegan J: Physiology and metabolism of the brain and spinal cord. In Newfield P, Cottrell JE (eds): Handbook of Neuroanesthesia: Clinical and Physiologic Essentials. Little, Brown, Boston/Toronto, 1983
31. Einhorn A, Mizrahi EM: Basilar skull fractures in children: the incidence of CNS infection and the use of antibiotics. Am J Dis Child 132: 1121, 1978
32. Evarts CM: The fat embolism syndrome: a review. Surg Clin North Am 50: 493, 1970
33. Eyes B, Evans AF: Post-traumatic skull radiographs: time for a reappraisal. Lancet 2: 85, 1978
34. Falke KJ, Pontopiddan H, Kumar H: Ventilation with end-expiratory pressure in acute lung disease. J Clin Invest 51: 2315, 1972

35. Feig PU, McCurdy DK: The hypertonic state. N Engl J Med 297: 1444, 1977

36. Fell DA, Fitzgerald S, Moiel RH et al: Acute subdural hematomas: review of 144 cases. J Neurosurg 42: 37, 1975

37. Frost EAM: Respiratory problems associated with head trauma. Neurosurgery 3: 300, 1977

38. Frost EAM, Arancibla CU, Shulman K: Pulmonary shunt as a prognostic indicator in head injury. J Neurosurg 50: 768, 1979

39. Gallagher JP, Browder EJ: Extradural hematoma. Experience with 167 patients. J Neurosurg 29: 1, 1968

40. Gennarelli TA: Cerebral concussion and diffuse brain injuries. P. 83. In Cooper PJ, Fleischer, AS (eds): Head Injury. Williams & Wilkins, Baltimore, 1982

41. Gennarelli TA, Thibault LE: Biomechanics of head injury. In Wilkins RH, Rengachary SS (eds.): Neurosurgery, Vol 2. McGraw-Hill, New York, 1985

42. Giroux JC: Hematomas of the posterior cranial fossa: a report of three cases. Can Med Assoc J 87: 59, 1962

43. Gissane W: The nature and causation of road accidents. Lancet 2: 695, 1963

44. Greenberg RP, Newlon PG, Hyatt MG et al: Prognostic implications of early multimodality evoked potentials in severely head-injured patients: a prospective study. J Neurosurg 55(2): 227, 1981

45. Guenter CA, Braun TE: Fat embolism syndrome: changing prognosis. Chest 79: 143, 1981

46. Hall R, Hirsch J, Sachett D et al: Replacement of venography in suspected venous thrombosis by impedance plethysmography and I125-fibrinogen by scanning. Ann Intern Med 94: 12, 1981

47. Hammerschmidt DE, White JG, Craddock DR: Corticosteroids inhibit complement-induced granulocyte aggregation. J Clin Invest 63: 798, 1979

48. Han JS, Kaufman B, Alfidi RJ, et al: Head trauma evaluated by magnetic resonance and computed tomography: a comparison. Radiology 150: 71, 1984

49. Harmony T: Neurometric Assessment of Brain Dysfunction in Neurological Patients. Functional Neuroscience, Vol. 3, Lawrence Erlbaum Assoc., Hillsdale, 1984

50. Harris JH, Jr.: High yield criteria and skull radiography. J Am Coll Emerg Physicians 8: 438, 1979

51. Harwood-Nash DC: Fractures of the petrous and tympanic parts of the temporal bone in children: a tomographic study of 35 cases. Am. J. Roentgenol 110: 598, 1970

52. Harwood-Nash DC, Hendrick EB, Hudson AR: The significance of skull fractures in children: a study of 1,187 patients. Radiology 101: 151, 1971

53. Ingelzi RJ, VanderArk GD: Analysis of the treatment of basilar skull fractures with and without antibiotics. J Neurosurg 43: 721, 1975

54. Jagger J, Jane JA, Rimel R: The Glasgow Coma Scale: to sum or not to sum? Lancet 2: 97, 1983

55. Jamieson KG, Yelland JDN: Extradural hematoma: report of 167 cases. J Neurosurg 29: 13, 1968

56. Jamieson KG, Yelland JDN: Depressed skull fractures in Australia. J Neurosurg 37: 150, 1972

57. Jamieson KG, Yelland JDN: Surgically treated traumatic subdural hematomas. J Neurosurg 37: 137, 1972

58. Jennett B: Some medicolegal aspects of the management of acute head injury. Br Med J 1: 1383, 1976

59. Jennett B, Miller JD: Infection after depressed fracture of skull: implications for management of nonmissile injuries. J Neurosurg 36: 333, 1972

60. Jennett B, Miller JD, Braakman R: Epilepsy after nonmissile depressed skull fracture. J Neurosurg 41: 208, 1974

61. Jennett B, Teasdale G (eds): Management of Head Injuries. FA Davis, Philadelphia, 1981

62. Jennett B, Teasdale G, Galbraith S et al: Severe head injuries in three countries. J Neurol Neurosurg Psychiatry 40: 291, 1977

63. John ER: Clinical applications of quantitative electrophysiology. Neurometrics 2: 291, 1977

64. John ER, Karmel BZ, Corning WC et al: Neurometrics. Science 196: 1393, 1977

65. Kalsbeek WD, McLaurin RL, Harris BSN et al: National Head and Spinal Cord Injury Survey: major findings. J Neurosurg [Suppl]: S19, 1980

66. Kumar A, Falke K, Griffin B et al: Continuous positive-pressure ventilation in acute respiratory failure. Effects of hemodynamics and lung function. N Engl J Med 283: 1430, 1970

67. Kvarnes TL, Trumpy JH: Extradural hematoma: report of 132 cases. Acta Neurochir (Wien) 41: 223, 1978

68. Langfitt TW: Measuring the outcome from head injuries. J Neurosurg 48: 673, 1978

69. Langfitt TW, Obrist WD: Occlusive cerebrovascular disease. P. 1167. In Wilkins RH, Rengachary SS (eds): Neurosurgery, Vol 2. McGraw-Hill, New York, 1985

70. Leech PJ, Paterson A: Conservative and operative management for cerebrospinal-fluid leakage after closed head injury. Lancet 1: 1013, 1973

71. Levin HS, Benton AI, Grossman RG (eds): Neurobehavioral Consequences of Closed Head Injury. Oxford University Press, New York, 1982

72. Lewin W, Cairns H: Fractures of the sphenoidal sinus with cerebrospinal rhinorrhea. Br Med J 1: 1, 1951

73. MacGee EE, Cauthen JC, Brackett CE: Meningitis following acute traumatic cerebrospinal fluid fistula. J Neurosurg 33: 312, 1970

74. Marshall LF, Smith RW, Shapiro HM: The outcome with aggressive treatment in severe head injuries. Part I: The significance of intracranial pressure monitoring. J Neurosurg 50: 20, 1979

75. Marmaron A, Tabaddor K: Intracranial pressure. Physiology and pathology in head injury. P. 115. In Cooper PR, Fleischer AS (eds): Head Injury. Williams & Wilkins, Baltimore, 1982

76. Matjasko J: Cardiorespiratory management in neurologic emergencies. P. 35. In Salcman M. (ed): Neurologic Emergencies. Raven Press, New York, 1980

77. McCormick WF: Pathology of closed head injury. P. 1544. In Wilkins RH, Rengachary SS (eds.): Neurosurgery, Vol 2. McGraw-Hill, New York, 1985

78. McDowell DG: Fluid dynamics of the cerebral circulation. P. 155. In CR Scurr, S Feldman (eds): Scientific Foundation of Anasthesia, 3rd ed. Heinemann, London, 1982

79. McKissock W, Richardson A, Bloom WH: Subdural hematoma: a review of 389 cases. Lancet 1: 1365, 1960

80. McKissock W, Taylor JC, Bloom WH et al: Extradural hematoma. Observation on 125 cases. Lancet 2: 167, 1960

81. McLaurin RL, Titchener JL: Post-traumatic syndrome. P. 2175. In Youmans JR (ed): Neurological Surgery, 2nd ed, Vol IV. WB Saunders, Philadelphia; 1982

82. Meirowsky AM: Penetrating Craniocerebral Trauma. Charles C Thomas, Springfield, 1984

83. Miller JD: Physiology of trauma in clinical neurosurgery. Chapter 7, Clinical Neurosurgery, Vol 29, 1982, p. 103

84. Miller JD, Becker DP: General principles and pathophysiology of head injury. P. 1896. In Youmans JR (ed): Neurological Surgery, 2nd ed. WB Saunders, Philadelphia, 1982

85. Miller JD, Becker DP, Ward JD et al: Significance of intracranial hypertension in severe head injury. J Neurosurg 47: 503, 1977

86. Miller JD, Butterworth JF, Gudeman SK et al: Farther experience in the management of severe head injury. J Neurosurg 54: 289, 1981

87. Miller JD, Jennett WB: Complications of depressed skull fracture. Lancet 2: 991, 1968

88. Mincy JE: Posttraumatic cerebrospinal fluid fistula of the frontal fossa. J Trauma 6: 618, 1966

89. Mitchell DP, Stone P: Temporal bone fractures in children. Can J Otolaryngol 2: 156, 1973

90. Murray HW: Antimicrobial therapy and pulmonary aspiration. Am J Med 66: 188, 1979

91. National Heart, Lung, and Blood Institute: Extracorporeal support for respiratory insufficiency: a collaborative study in response to RFP NHLI43–20 plo. NHLBI DLD, 1979

92. Netter FH: Nervous system. CIBA Collection of Medical Illustrations, Vol 1. CIBA Pharmaceutical Company, Summit, NJ 1953

93. O'Brist WD, Langfitt TW, Jaggi JL et al: Cerebral blood flow and Metabolism in comatose patients with acute head injury. J Neurosurg 61: 241, 1984

94. Ommaya AK: Mechanisms of cerebral concussion, contusions, and other effects of head injury. P. 1877. In Youman JR (ed): Neurological Surgery, 2nd ed, Vol. IV. WB Saunders, Philadelphia, 1982

95. Ommaya AK: Cerebrospinal fluid fistula. P. 1637. In RH Wilkins, SS Rengachary (eds): Neurosurgery, Vol 2. McGraw-Hill, New York, 1985

96. Ovegaard J, Tweed WA: Cerebral circulation after head injury Part I: Cerebral blood flow and its regulation after closed head injury with emphasis on clinical correlations. J Neurosurg 41: 531, 1974

97. Parkinson D: The biomechanics of concussion. In Weiss, MH (ed): Clinical Neurosurgery. Vol 29. Williams & Wilkins, Baltimore, 1982

98. Phillips LA: Emergency services utilization of skull radiography. Neurosurgery 4: 580, 1979

99. Plum F, Posner JR: The Diagnosis of Stupor and Coma, 3rd ed. FA Davis, Philadelphia, 1980

100. Popp AJ, Bourke RS: Pathophysiology of head injury. P. 1536. In RH Wilkins, SS Rengachary (eds): Neurosurgery, Vol 2. McGraw-Hill, New York, 1985

101. Quest DO: Increased intracranial pressure, brain herniation, and their control. P. 332. In Wilkins RH, Rengachary SS (eds.): Neuorsurgery, Vol 1. McGraw-Hill, New York, 1985

102. Rimel RW, Giordani B, Barth JR et al: Disability caused by minor head injury. Neurosurgery 9: 221, 1981

103. Rimel RW, Jane JA: Minor head injury: management and outcome. P. 1608. In Wilkens RH, Rengachary SS (eds.): Neurosurgery, Vol 2. McGraw-Hill, New York, 1985

104. Rose BD; Clinical Physiology of Acid-Base and Electrolyte Disorders. McGraw-Hill, New York, 1977

105. Rose J, Valtonen S, Jennett B: Avoidable factors contributing to death after head injury. Br Med J 2: 615, 1977

106. Ross RJ, Cole M, Thompson JS: Boxers—computed tomography, EEG, and neurological evaluation. JAMA 248: 211, 1983

106a. Saleman M (ed): Neurologic Emergencies, Raven Press, 1980

107. Seelig JM, Becker DP, Miller JD, et al: Acute subdural hematoma: major mortality reduction

in comatose patients treated within four hours. N Engl Med 304(25): 1511, 1981

108. Sinha RP, Ducker TB, Perot PL, Jr.: Arterial oxygenation. Findings and its significance in central nervous system trauma patients. JAMA 224: 1258, 1973

109. Sokoll L: Influence of functional activity on local cerebral glucose utilization. p. 385. In Ingvar DH, Lassen NA (eds.): Brain Work: The Coupling of Function. Metabolism and Blood Flow in the Brain. Academic Press, New York, 1975

110. Suter PM, Fairley HB, Isenberg MD: Optimum end-expiratory airway pressure in patients with acute pulmonary failure. N Engl J Med 292: 284, 1975

111. Teasdale G, Jennett B: Assessment of coma and impaired consciousness. A practical scale. Lancet 2:81, 1974

112. Theodore J, Robin ED: Speculations on neuro-genic pulmonary edema. Am Rev Respir Dis 113: 405, 1976

113. Toutant SM, Klauber MR, Marshall LF, et al: Absent or compressed basal cisterns on first CT scan: ominous predictors of outcome in se-Absent or compressed basal cisterns on first CT scan: ominous predictors of outcome in severe head injury. Neurosurg 61: 691, 1984

114. Valtin H: Renal function: Predictions Preserving Fluid and Solute Balance in Health. Little, Brown, Boston, 1983

115. Winter PM, MIller, JN: Oxygen toxicity. P. 218. In Shoemaker WC, Thompson WL, Holbrook PR (eds): Textbook of Critical Care. WB Saunders, Philadelphia, 1984

116. Wray NP, Nicotra MB: Pathogenesis of neurogenic pulmonary edema. Am Rev Respir Dis 118: 783, 1978

32

Spinal Cord Injury and Spinal Shock Syndrome

Mark P. Carol
Thomas B. Ducker

INTRODUCTION

Every year, approximately 9,000 young adults suffer cervical spinal cord injury. They are subject to an instantaneous and radical alteration in lifestyle that entails an overwhelming physical and emotional adjustment, and that places a tremendous financial burden on patient, family and society. To whatever extent that cervical cord injuries are remediable, constant vigilance is required to protect residual function and prevent secondary damage. For this reason, the present review is directed at initial emergency management of the spinal-cord-injured patient; its ultimate contribution to the recovery and rehabilitation of the patient with spinal cord injury is often underestimated.

To gain a fuller appreciation of the basis for the protocol followed at the Maryland Institute for Emergency Medical Services Systems, the basic pathophysiology of both spine and spinal cord trauma will be reviewed. Our protocol will then be detailed, as it relates to both

acute management and definitive treatment. Finally, some of the more important controversies in spinal cord injury treatment will be addressed. Throughout the entire discussion of treatment, it should be remembered that the treatment of spine/spinal cord injury is a rapidly changing art and science. Our recommendations are just that—recommendations—based on what we believe to be current in the science and the art that should be applied. These principles are constantly being re-evaluated, and the practitioner should be receptive to changes that may be suggested in the future or may result from his or her personal experience.

Scope of the Problem

The epidemiology of spinal cord injury has not been clearly established for three reasons: lack of centralized care for the spinal-cord-injured patient; absence of accepted standards for the evaluation of the acutely injured patient; and the lack of a centralized data bank. It has been estimated that there are 7,500 to 10,500 victims of spinal cord injury between the ages of 15 and 35 yearly in the United States.[99,146] This corresponds to an incidence of 30 to 50 patients per million per year.[126] Similar figures are cited for all industrial countries. As indicated, these figures do not include patients above the age of 35. It has also been estimated that there are 150,000 persons with significant spinal cord injuries now living in the United States.[95] The initial costs of acute care are estimated at $500 million dollars yearly with an additional $500 million dollars yearly required for chronic maintenance, care, and support. If one adds to this figure the loss in potential earnings that results from injury in this segment of the population, it can be seen that spinal cord injury is a devastating financial problem.

Causes

Motor vehicle accidents involving young men are responsible for up to 55 percent of all spinal cord injuries,[14,18] and it is estimated that 10 percent of seriously injured motor vehicle accident victims will have a spinal fracture.[21] Falls and athletic injuries account for most of the remaining injuries.[15] Tackle

football, surfing, diving, wrestling, and gymnastics are particularly perilous.[99] In particular, of those seriously injured resulting from diving accidents, more than 50 percent will have sustained a cervical spine injury.[95]

PATHOPHYSIOLOGY OF SPINAL INJURY

Anatomy

In an attempt to understand the pathophysiology of spine injury,[124,149] much research has gone into elucidating the biomechanics of the normal spine, which is an integrated unit consisting of bone, ligament, disc, and muscle. These components combine to produce a stable construct that not only supports the head but also protects the spinal cord. Functionally, these components can be examined both individually and as an integrated unit.

The seven cervical vertebrae unite to form a convex curve anteriorly, which provides for greater flexibility in the face of the need for adequate stability.[121] This curve also augments

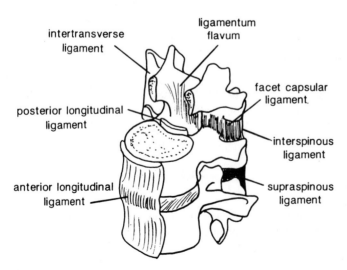

FIG. 32-1 Ligaments of the spinal column.

intertransverse ligament

ligamentum flavum

facet capsular ligament

posterior longitudinal ligament

interspinous ligament

anterior longitudinal ligament

supraspinous ligament

the spine's ability to act as a shock-absorbing structure. In addition to its structural capacity as a bony protection for the spinal cord and a support for the head, the vertebrae provide resistance to compressive forces experienced by the spine in daily and traumatic situations. The facet joints act as the major buttress resisting anterior, posterior, and translational forces. The mass of each vertebral body increases throughout the cervical segment, which is a mechanical adaptation to the progressively increasing loads to which the vertebrae are subjected. Each bone is made of both cortical and cancellous bone. The percentage of the load on the spine carried by each component varies with age. As one grows older and the cancellous core deteriorates, the cortical bone's share of the load increases.[121]

The major function of the spinal column ligaments is to resist tensile forces (Fig. 32-1). The ligaments provide no resistance to compressive forces, and buckle when the spine is subjected to axial loading forces. The ligaments combine to allow motion, but protect the spinal cord by keeping this motion within well-defined physiologic limits. The six major ligaments of the cervical spine cooperate to preserve bony alignment during movement. They are the anterior longitudinal ligament, the posterior longitudinal ligament, the interspinous and supraspinous ligaments, the ligamentous flavum, and the capsular ligaments. Injury to these ligaments may result in spinal instability irrespective of vertebral body damage.

While all of these ligaments help to stabilize the spine, the specific and proportionate contribution of each ligament to any given force has been, in the past, difficult to define. Recently, with the use of cadaver cervical spine models, a functional division of these ligaments into anterior and posterior compartments has been possible.[21,121] Anterior ligaments are all those ligaments anterior to and including the posterior longitudinal ligament. The posterior elements are defined as all structures posterior to the posterior longitudinal ligament. The anterior complex is most effective in resisting extension forces, whereas the posterior complex is basically involved in reducing flexion forces. The capsular ligaments are crucial in counteracting rotational forces.

The intervertebral disc is made up primar-ily of proteoglycans and collagen, and is comprised of three distinct parts: the annulus fibrosus, the nucleus pulposus, and the cartilaginous endplate. The centrally located pulposus is composed of a loose network of fibrin strands that lie in a mucoprotein gel. Its water content decreases with age, accounting for some of the loss in height that accompanies aging. The annulus is formed from fibrous tissue surrounding the nucleus, and is attached to the vertebral body as well as the cartilaginous endplates. The system as a whole acts as a cushion under loading conditions, with some resistance to tensile forces being provided by the annulus–endplate interface. In fact, the first component to fail under compression loading is the vertebral body endplate, not the disc.[121] Disc herniation is more likely to occur with lateral bending or torsional forces, which the disc is unable to counteract.

Mechanism of Injury

The mechanism of injury in cervical spine trauma is rarely secondary to a single force. The term *major injury vector* (MIV)[121] has been used to describe the mechanism of injury. Any injury results from a complex series of moment forces applied to a functional spinal unit consisting of two adjacent vertebrae and their interconnecting ligaments. The mechanism of injury producing this major injury vector can, in many circumstances, be identified. This should be attempted in all instances, since it will help one in deciding on the appropriate radiologic and manipulative tests needed to evaluate the stability of the cervical spine.

Six basic forces can be involved in producing a spine injury.[127] The four major ones are distraction, extension, flexion, and compression (Fig. 32-2), with two associated forces being lateral bending and rotation. Explained simply, distraction causes disruption of both anterior and posterior ligamentous structures, with compression causing bony element fractures anteriorly and posteriorly. Flexion produces posterior ligamentous injury with extension causing anterior ligamentous damage. In actuality, two or more of these forces are usu-

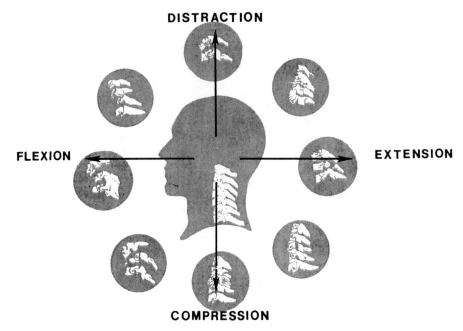

FIG. 32-2 Major forces in spinal column injury and mechanisms of injury. Very few cervical spine injuries are secondary to a single force. Most represent a combination of two or more forces in different directions. Each type of accident, (e.g., diving, motor vehicle accident, falling) usually produces a characteristic combination of forces resulting in a specific type of injury. Thus the patient's history is of definite help in treating spine-injured patients. In addition to the forces illustrated, a degree of rotational injury is often present.

ally coupled, thus producing a continuum of injuries as illustrated in Figure 32-3. The presence of rotational or lateral bending forces, although not indicated in the figure, causes the injuries to be predominantly one-sided.

It is important to remember, as will be detailed further in the discussion of treatment, that the mechanism of injury plays a major role in determining the type of definitive treatment to stabilize the fracture site. In general, injuries where bony abnormalities predominate will go on to produce a bony fusion and will often not require surgical intervention. On the other hand, injuries in which ligamentous damage predominates will not go on to fuse, and will require surgical intervention to stabilize the fracture site. Whether or not bony injury exists does not affect the fact that a spine fracture has occurred: the term still applies. In addition, significant cord injury is possible without bony or ligamentous damage being present. The most common example is a central cord syn-

drome secondary to pre-existing cervical stenosis coupled with an extension injury.

Classification of Injuries

The types of spine injuries are listed in Table 32-1.

TABLE 32-1.
Classification of
Spinal Injuries

Occipital Cl dislocation
Jefferson fracture
Odontoid fracture
Hangman's fracture
Posterior element fracture
Anterior element fracture
Lateral element fracture

STABILITY

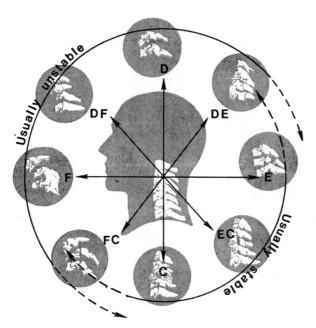

FIG. 32-3 Spinal column stability. Whether or not a fracture is stable in the long run (delayed stability) is dependent upon the relative presence of bony and ligamentous injury. Although compressive-type injuries are often acutely unstable, if bony healing is allowed to occur stability will result. This is in contrast to flexion-type injuries, where ligamentous damage predominates. These flexion fractures have the potential of being chronically unstable. An assessment of the ultimate stability of the injury will enter into any decision about the definitive therapy to be used.

OCCIPITAL C1 DISLOCATIONS

Rotation of the head with respect to the spine does not usually occur between the occiput and C1. When rotation is forced between the skull and C1, the articular processes of the skull may dislocate, either one forward and one posteriorly on the supporting lateral masses of C1, or both directly posteriorly or anteriorly. This dislocation is often fatal, due to high cord or brain stem injury, but if the patient survives, he or she is usually without major neurologic deficits. This dislocation may also be associated with a rotary subluxation or dislocation in the opposite direction of C1 or C2. Either of these conditions may be missed on routine plain films, being diagnosed only when tomograms of the area are taken.

JEFFERSON FRACTURES

Jefferson fracture is unique to the first cervical vertebrae, and is a bursting of the ring of C1 as a result of axial loading directly downward on the ring of C1. An anteroposterior (AP) film generally shows widening of the distance between the odontoid and the lateral masses of C1, and the lateral film frequently shows cracks or frank disruption of the ring of C1 posteriorly. Neurologic deficit from this type of injury is unusual and patients' injuries usually heal well after placement in a Halo brace.

ODONTOID FRACTURES

Odontoid fractures are classified into one of three types. Type 1 is an oblique fracture through the upper part of the odontoid process itself. Type 2 is a fracture at the junction of the odontoid process with the vertebral body of the second cervical vertebrae. Type 3 is really a fracture to the body of the second vertebrae with fracture line extending down into the cancellous bone of the body of the axis. Type 1 fractures are unusual and are stable injuries that have good prognosis and require only minor treatment. Type 2 fractures are the most common type. They tend to be unstable and have a high rate of nonunion when treated by conservative methods. Both Halo vests and/or surgery have been used to stabilize type 2 fractures. The particular treatment modality to be used in any given patient is dependent upon multiple factors including patient's age, skill of the surgeon, as well as socio economic factors. Type 3 fractures are more stable, and due to the large cancellous surface involved, have a good prognosis for union with conservative treatment.

TRAUMATIC SPONDYLOLISTHESIS OF THE AXIS (HANGMAN'S FRACTURE)

A hangman's fracture occurs through the pedicle of the second cervical vertebra, separating the posterior neural arch from the body of the axis. The term *hangman's fracture* is used because this is the type of fracture produced when a submental knot in the noose is used to produce death by hanging. The pathologic term for the injury is *traumatic spondylolisthesis of the axis,* and it is usually produced following a motor vehicle collision with rapid deceleration. The victim is thrown forward in the car, and the head strikes the windshield. At the moment of impact there is axial loading of the spine with extension. The cranium and C1 move as a unit producing a downward force on the posterior element of C2. A bilateral fracture of the neural arch of C2 results. Depending upon the severity of the insult, disruption of the anterior and posterior longitudinal ligaments may result. Further force will result in disc disruption at the C2-C3 interface, producing subluxation of C2 on the inferior cervical spine. Treatment decisions revolve around assessment of stability of the fracture. If the fracture is thought to be stable, then use of a cervical thoracic brace with early ambulation will

usually result in complete healing. If the fracture is unstable (i.e., subluxation is present), then prompt reduction of the dislocation is necessary. Once the fracture is satisfactorily reduced then either Halo vest fixation, in most instances, or AP fusion, in rare instances, is performed.

DISRUPTION OF THE POSTERIOR ELEMENTS OF THE LOWER CERVICAL SPINE

These include ruptured facet capsule, unilateral facet dislocation, bilateral facet dislocation, bilateral perched facets, fractured facets, ruptured interspinous ligament, spinous process fractures, laminar fractures, and pedicle fractures.

FRACTURES OF THE ANTERIOR ELEMENTS OF THE LOWER CERVICAL SPINE

These include wedge fractures, compression fractures, teardrop fractures, and disruption of the anterior longitudinal ligament. Data regarding fractures of anterior and posterior elements will be explored later in this chapter.

Spinal Stability

Clinical instability (Fig. 32-3) of the spine is defined as

the loss of the ability of the spine under physiologic loads to maintain relationships between the vertebrae in such a way that there is neither damage nor subsequent irritation to the spinal cord or nerve roots, and in addition, there is no development of incapacitating deformity or pain due to structural change.[88,121]

Experimental models suggest that stability of the cervical spine is maintained if all the anterior elements or all the posterior elements plus one additional structure are intact. A fairly universally accepted evaluation checklist for cervical spine instability has been developed by White and Punjabi.[121] This checklist is provided in detailed form in Table 32-2. If the sum

TABLE 32-2. Checklist for the Diagnosis of Clinical Instability in the Lower Cervical Spine

Element	Points
Anterior elements destroyed or unable to function	2
Posterior elements destroyed or unable to function	2
Relative sagittal plane translation > 3.5 mm	2
Relative sagittal plane rotation > 11°	2
Positive stretch test	2
Spinal cord damage	2
Nerve root damage	1
Abnormal disc narrowing	1
Dangerous loading anticipated	1

Total of 5 or more = unstable

of the points is five or more, then the spine is considered extremely unstable.

Several of these criteria require some explanation. Sagittal translation is dependent in part upon magnification factors in the radiographs. A distraction of 3.5 mm has been suggested as representing an upper limit of normal for translational factors when taking into account radiographic magnification. An 11 percent rotational factor means 11 percent greater than the amount of rotation at the motion segment above or below the segment in question. The stretch test evaluates the ability of the spine to withstand axial forces of distraction. An abnormal stretch test is indicated by either greater than 1.7 mm interspace separation, or greater than 7.5 percent change in angulation between vertebrae, when compared to pre-stretch conditions following the application of axial traction equal to one third of the body weight.[121] This test should probably not be performed in the immediate post injury period, for fear of causing further injury to the spine or spinal cord.

These criteria are used to evaluate the presence or absence of acute instability of the spine. Whether or not a fracture is stable in the long run (i.e., delayed stability) is dependent upon the relative presence of bony and ligamentous injury. Injuries with a significant amount of bony injury may be acutely unstable. However, if bony healing is allowed to ocur, stability will result. This is in sharp contrast to injuries in which ligamentous damage predominates. These fractures are chronically unstable, in most instances due to the inability of ligaments to heal. Therefore, an assessment of the ultimate stability of the injury must enter into any decision made about the mode of therapy to be used.

When a significant bony injury exists, the presence of ligamentous instability at the same level is often unimportant in determining long-term stability. Immobilization of the fracture site will help bony healing to occur and, when it does, the result will be a stable spine. However, instability may be present above or below the level of the bony fracture. In these instances, a bony fusion occurring at the site of the fracture will not result in a stable spine. It is therefore necessary to evaluate spinal ligamentous stability in all cases of cervical spine injury regardless of bone damage before choosing a definitive mode of therapy. This assessment includes the use of plain films, flexion–extension radiographs, computed tomographic (CT) scanning and tomography as well as an understanding of the mechanism of injury.

PATHOPHYSIOLOGY OF SPINAL CORD INJURY

Anatomy

The cervical portion of the spinal cord is the vital structure contained within the cervical spinal canal. Running parallel to it on each side of the spinal column are the vertebral arteries, which provide the cervical spinal cord and brain stem with their blood supply. The dura mater surrounding the spinal cord is firmly at-

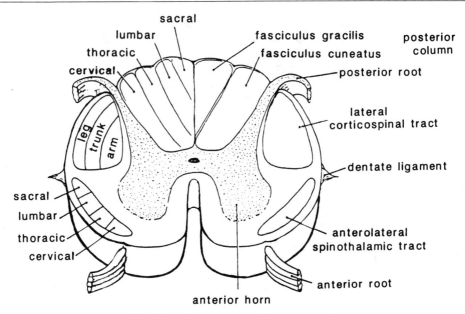

FIG. 32-4 Neuroanatomy of the spinal cord.

tached to the foramen magnum but is separated from the vertebral bodies and arches by epidural fat. Arachnoid lines the dura, the subarachnoid space being filled with cervical spinal fluid. The pia mater is closely attached to the spinal cord, and laterally forms linear folds extending longitudinally the length of the cord. These folds give rise to the dentate ligaments on either side. These ligaments extend laterally between the ventral and dorsal spinal roots, are attached to the dura, and suspend the spinal cord within the spinal fluid. This dentate ligament/spinal fluid system acts to cushion and protect the cord.

Dorsal sensory rootlets enter the spinal cord through the lateral longitudinal sulcus, with the ventral motor rootlets exiting the cord through the ventral sulcus. The ventral and dorsal rootlets merge into a single bundle as they pass through the dura, forming the nerve root at each level. Distal to the intervertebral foramen, the root splits into the dorsal and ventral branches. The nerve rootlets pass almost directly lateral at each level as they exit the foramen at the level of origin. This horizontal direction of cervical roots is in direct contast to the vertical passage of lumbar roots.

The spinal cord is made up of white and gray matter (Fig. 32-4). The gray matter is centrally located, consisting primarily of nerve cells, whereas the white matter consists primarily of myelinated nerve fibers. The white substance of the cervical cord is divided into three columns or funiculi: dorsal, lateral, and ventral. The dorsal columns contain both the fasciculus gracilis and the fasciculus cuneatus, nerve tracts that mediate proprioceptive, vibratory, and tactile sensations. The lateral and ventral funiculi contain the cortical spinal and spinothalamic tracts as well as other smaller tracts. The cortical spinal tract conveys motor impulses to the limbs, whereas the spinothalamic tract conveys impulses for pain and temperature.

The vertebral artery is the main source of blood supply for the cervical cord and the cervical spine. Just before the vertebral arteries join to form the basilar artery, they give off branches, two of which fuse and descend anteriorly on the spinal cord to form the anterior spinal artery (Fig. 32-5). The anterior spinal artery supplies 70 to 80 percent of cervical cord blood flow. Two others, the posterior spinal arteries, remain paired as they descend the length of the cervical spinal cord. These two systems do not appear to anastomose with each other to any major degree. Venous blood returns from the cord by way of a comparable

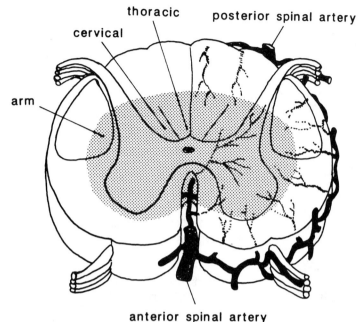

thoracic

cervical

posterior spinal artery

arm

FIG. 32-5 Arterial vascular supply of the spinal cord.

anterior spinal artery

system of anterior and posterior venous channels.

Spinal cord injury occurs secondary to mechanical insults, hemodynamic changes, and biochemical derangements. Since the treatment plan for cord injury must be aimed at these insults and changes, they will be explored here briefly.

Mechanical Insults

Mechanical insults to the spinal cord following an acute injury are of three types: (1) tissue disruption secondary to direct insult; (2) damage secondary to continued cord mobility; and (3) damage secondary to cord compression.

TISSUE DISRUPTION SECONDARY TO DIRECT INSULT

This is responsible for initial cord dysfunction. Electron micrographic (EM) studies have shown that beginning 5 minutes after trauma there is distention of the vascular structures within the cord leading to microhemorrhages and perivascular exudation.[41,42] Central ischemic and gross hemorrhagic lesions become visible within several hours, leading to gray matter necrosis.[9] Due to related direct trauma to the blood vessels, platelets and red cells infiltrate the perivascular space. Polymorphonuclear leukocytes follow[41,44] and, with fibrolytic enzymes, produce cavitation of the central gray matter. White matter pathologic change follows, including edema, distortion of perfusion, demyelination, and, ultimately, tissue necrosis.[30] Distal to the trauma, demyelination or wallerian degeneration occurs.

These changes, once they occur, cannot be altered by current therapeutic modalities. Humans can withstand the initial gray matter injury; this represents an affordable segmental loss of only a small portion of the total gray matter neuronal pool. However, humans cannot tolerate segmental loss of the peripheral white matter. This interrupts ascending and descending fibrous tracts and results in loss of distal functioning of those tracts. Neurons are rendered useless, and cord function is lost in varying degrees. Despite extensive research, there is no evidence to date to support spinal cord regeneration in humans.[131] Further damage incurred during the treatment process, however, can be altered by the therapy.

DAMAGE SECONDARY TO CONTINUED CORD MOBILITY

The principle of cord immobilization following injury dates to the time of Hypocrites, and has remained one of the few undisputed dicta in the field. Its purpose is to prevent repeated acute insults from occurring to an already injured spinal cord. That this indeed occurs, and that therapy directed at preventing these insults can improve outcome, has been demonstrated conclusively.[48] Immobilization may possibly improve the vascular perfusion of the cord, but at the least it maintains the integrity of tracts and supporting structures that survive the initial insult.

DAMAGE SECONDARY TO CORD COMPRESSION

Extra-axial compression of neural tissue, whether brain or spinal cord, causes both anatomic and physiologic changes resulting in system dysfunction. Chronic compression of the cord by bone, ligament, or disc material causes secondary changes independent of the initial insult. Histologic examination of a chronically compressed cord shows it to be edematous and soft. Meningeal vessels are collapsed and there may be white matter demyelinization. Myelin sheath and axonal cylinders may be fragmented.[53] Electrophysiologic studies have shown that evoked potentials gradually disappear with chronic compression.[46] This is thought to be due to physical injury to neural membranes.[96] Kobrine has shown alterations in spinal cord blood flow with chronic compression, which lead to increased vascular permeability, resulting in edema following release of the compression.[96] All of these responses were shown to be proportional to the duration and the severity of the compression present.

When these effects of chronic compression are added to the effects of the acute insult, the pathologic destruction and resulting clinical deficit can be far greater than those seen with the acute process alone. For this reason, much of our treatment protocol is aimed at investigating the possible presence of chronic compression, and instituting measures to relieve it. It also aims to prevent this compression from occurring later if it is not present initially. The appropriate use of plain radiographs, tomography, myelography, and CT helps to identify actual or potential spinal cord compression. The appropriate approach to removing or preventing compression is dependent upon factors discussed below.

Hemodynamic Changes

A major factor in the cause and/or evolution of spinal cord damage is the state of vascular flow to the cord. As noted earlier, the arterial supply to the spinal cord consists of one anterior and two posterior spinal arteries. These are fed by a variable number of radicular arteries. The anterior spinal artery is the largest of the three, feeding two-thirds of the cord. Central sulcal arteries arise perpendicular to this vessel and penetrate into the tissue itself. The venous drainage follows a similar pattern. The anterior and posterior systems generally do not communicate. A blood–brain barrier and autoregulation exist in spinal cord as well as in brain, and trauma may result in the loss of these protective mechanisms.[135,136,137]

An acute injury to the spinal cord produces instantaneous, as well as prolonged, systemic and local cord hemodynamic changes that have a profound effect on the pathologic outcome of the lesion. At the time of the injury, the patient may become severely hypotensive if a functional sympathectomy has occurred, resulting in decreased spinal cord blood flow. At the cord level, trauma appears to affect the penetrating central spinal arterial branches most severely. Focal areas of dilation and constriction result and changes occur on the surface of the cord causing stasis and sludging of blood. Delayed disruption of the microvascular blood flow of the cord occurs after several hours of spinal cord compression. Autoregulation is lost,[6,135] resulting in a quantitative decrease in blood flow out of proportion to any drop in blood pressure experienced.[49] The more marked the decrease in blood flow, the greater the resultant neurologic deficit. Associated with this decrease in spinal cord blood flow is a general depression of spinal cord oxygen tension. Pathologically, this alteration in blood flow correlates with the later appearance of areas of central ischemia surrounded by peripheral hyperemia, that is, loss of adequate microcirculatory perfusion.[59] The loss of autoregulation in conjuction with the postischemia hyperemia causes deleterious effects if the blood pressure rises to hypertensive levels after trauma. This may result in increased microvascular hemorrhages in the cord.[124] The risk of loss of autoregulation seems to be decreased if a normal blood pressure is maintained postinjury.[125]

Ultrastructural changes occur within spinal cord capillaries acutely after injury, with separation at the endothelial junction exposing the basil lamina to platelets.[63] Damage to the endothelium prevents the release of prostacyclins, substances that normally act to dilate vessels and prevent platelet aggregation.[114] In the absence of these prostacyclins platelet aggregation is promoted, resulting in a further decrease in blood flow at the microcirculatory level.[35,143]

In summary, following an acute injury there is a short delay before spinal cord blood flow reaches ischemic levels. The reduction in spinal cord blood flow is greater in the central gray areas than in the peripheral white matter. The loss of vasomotor responsiveness and autoregulation profoundly affects the pathologic process, with alterations in blood pressure also influencing the evolution of the lesion. Hyperemia leads to edema in the spinal cord, which is markedly affected by the time course of the rise and drop in systemic blood pressure. Local changes occur in the microcirculation causing sludging of blood flow and resulting in a decrease in tissue oxygen tension. All of these changes combine to disrupt the mirocirculation and to produce an ischemic insult to the cord. An important therapeutic implication lies in the fact that there seems to be a delay before the onset of local microcirculatory changes. These changes can be ameliorated by maintaining blood pressure and tissue oxygen tension at normal levels immediately postinjury.

Biochemical Changes

The biochemical derangements following acute cord injury are quite diverse. Initially, lactic acid accumulates in the injured tissue, presumably secondary to ischemia and its resultant anaerobic metabolism.[106] This lactic acid accumulation sets in motion what appears to be a related series of events involving liberation of membrane phospholipids and release of circulating prostaglandins, leading through platelet aggregation and thromboxane A_2 release to vasoconstriction and vasospasm.[35,38] The end result is further cord ischemia. Altered levels of epinephrine,[118,123,124] accumulation of lysosomes,[90,91] a drop in cytoxidase-activated[87] ATPase activity,[29] and other evidence indicative of altered cell membrane function have been found.[92,108] The actual cause of membrane dysfunction is not resolved, but its presence supports theories that altered membrane function is one of the major causes for the progession of neurologic deficits in acute cord injury. This membrane dysfunction may be due to the linear decrease in oxygen tension seen at the injury site. However, it is clear that the microcirculatory disturbance causes a chain reaction of events leading to further ischemia, and thus further membrane dysfunction.

Any therapeutic protocol aimed at preventing the worsening of the neurologic status following acute spinal cord injury must prevent this chain of events, beginning with tissue ischemia.

In summary, in severe spinal cord injuries, electrical conduction through the injured cord segment ceases due to direct tissue disruption from the trauma as well as from the secondary concussive effect. Vasomotor reactivity of the injured cord is lost, leading to changes in spinal cord blood flow. These local injury changes in the microcirculation may be compounded by cardiovascular instability secondary to the trauma itself. The resultant ischemia from all of these factors causes the accumulation of metabolic toxins, and sets in motion a biochemical sequence of events leading to further ischemia and irreversible damage. Inasmuch as some of these secondary events are avoidable or reversible, recovery from spinal cord injury is limited, but possible.

Functional Changes

Functionally, neurologic damage to the spinal cord can be classified into eight common syndromes (Table 32-3).

1. PHYSIOLOGICALLY COMPLETE TRANSECTION. Physiologically complete transection of the spinal cord is identified by the complete and continued absence of sensation and motor function below the level of the lesion. Complete lesions are the most devastating form of spinal cord injury and carry the poorest prognosis.

2. COMPLETE MOTOR LOSS WITH VARIABLE SENSORY SPARING.

3. PARTIAL MOTOR LOSS WITH VARIABLE SENSORY SPARING. Partial motor and sensory loss below the level of the lesion is a specific description that aids in the classification of spinal cord injury by syndrome for clinical and statistical evaluation. Prognosis is variable, but frequently is favorable for recovery of useful function in the long run.

4. BROWN-SEQUARD SYNDROME. The Brown-Sequard syndrome is characterized by *ipsilateral* motor paralysis, loss of touch and propioception (anesthesia), and *contralateral* loss of pain and temperature (analgesia) below the level of the lesion. The upper limit of analgesia is found one to two segments *below* the level of the lesion. The Brown-Sequard syndrome in pure form usu-

TABLE 32-3. Classification of Spinal Cord Injuries

Complete lesions
Complete motor loss with variable sensory sparing
Partial motor and sensory loss
Brown-Sequard syndrome
Anterior cord syndrome
Central cord syndrome
Root syndromes
Cruciate paralysis

ally occurs only after penetrating cord injuries. On the other hand, blunt trauma with primary vascular injury frequently causes a variety of asymmetrical syndromes characterized by unequal lower extremity paresis, with analgesia or hypalgesia *contralateral* to the most paretic side.

5. ANTERIOR CORD SYNDROME. The anterior cervical cord syndrome[132,133] is typically seen following hyperflexion injuries and is characterized by normesthesia in the presence of analgesia and paresis below the level of the lesion, that is, dorsal column function (proprioception, light touch, and vibration sense) is preserved in the presence of paralysis. Acutely herniated discs, thrombosis of the anterior spinal artery, or fractured, posteriorly displaced vertebral bodies can compromise anterior cord circulation and function. Since the prognosis for recovery from a vascular injury is poor, some surgeons have recommended surgery for *all* cases of anterior cord syndrome in the hope of finding a ruptured disc or some other remediable cause.[132] Others argue that immediate surgical intervention should be limited to patients with known hyperflexion and/ or axial compression injuries, in whom the suspicion of a prolapsed disc is high.[19]

6. CENTRAL CORD SYNDROME. The central cord syndrome[8,16,125,133] is characteristic of hyperextension injuries complicated by preexisting cervical spondylosis and stenosis. It is variably expressed as a paresis (weakness) or plegia (absence of motion) of the arms with relative sparing of the legs and variable sensory and bladder impairment. The cause of the central cord syndrome is uncertain; it is generally attributed to vascular injury with compromise of the penetrating branches of the anterior spinal artery.

The long tracts of the spinal cord are somatotopically organized: the central portions of the posterior column, spinothalamic and corticospinal tracts contain the supranuclear fibers supplying the neck and arms (Fig. 32-4). Because the central portion of the spinal cord is perfused by perforating endartery branches of the anterior spinal artery, the centrally located portions of the corticospinal tracts are most distally supplied, and, therefore, at greater risk from an ischemic event (Fig. 32-5). Direct injury to the anterior cord substance can also contribute to this injury.

Chances of recovery from central cord syndromes are relatively good with conservative management alone. Current studies suggest that improvement is hastened by an adequate surgical decompression.[17]

7. CRUCIATE PARALYSIS OF BELL. Bilateral upper extremity paresis disproportionately greater than the lower extremity weakness also occurs following odontoid fractures and injuries at the region of the foramen magnum.[11] Upper extremity paresis is explained by the differential involvement of decussating pyramidal fibers in the low medulla. The supranuclear fibers controlling upper extremity function cross in the lower medulla, rostral and anterior to the decussation of the leg fibers that cross at the C1/C2 level[74] (Fig. 32-4). Because of the extended rostrala–caudal decussation of the extremity fibers, a localized involvement of small areas of the caudal medulla may result in a variety of clinical findings. A cruciate paralysis may be expressed as a predominantly upper or lower extremity weakness depending upon the exact level of pathologic involvement in the midline.[11] With involvement of the more lateral portions of the pyramidal decussation, however, a fairly characteristic paralysis of the *ipsilateral* arm and the *contra-*

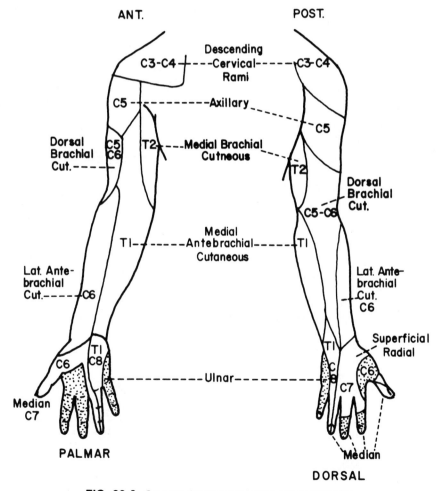

FIG. 32-6. Sensory dermatomes of the upper extremity.

lateral leg is produced by damage to the crossed arm and as yet uncrossed leg fibers.[17] This syndrome is called *hemiplegia cruciata*.

8. ROOT LESIONS. Damage to the spinal cord may result in the interruption of first-order descending pyramidal tract fibers, prior to their synapse with the anterior horn cells. Damage to upper motor neurons results in a spastic paresis, or *myelopathy*. Damage to nerve roots impairs lower motor neurons and produces a segmental sensory and motor loss, or *radiculopathy*. Radiculopathy is most typical of acutely herniated discs, or damage to the neural foramen from facet disruption. Occasionally, and especially early on, injury to the spinal cord with damage restricted to the anterior horn cells cord may mimic a radiculopathy by producing a flaccid paresis.

INITIAL EVALUATION AND TREATMENT

The need for constant vigilance to detect spinal injuries has been frequently reiterated. This diagnosis is most frequently missed in the presence of head injury and concomitant alterations of consciousness, in complicated multiply injured patients, in cases of alcoholic intoxication, and in patients who have had inadequate radiologic examination of the lower cervical spine.[14] As a consequence, ambulance crews trained in extracting patients at the site of accidents are instructed to give special attention to cervical spine immobilization, and to assume occult cervical injury. The unchallenged axiom for treating the multiple injured patient is that *one must assume that there is a cervical spine injury until proven otherwise.* Even a patient who is evaluated at the scene and found to have normal neurologic function must be presumed to have suffered a cervical injury, if there has been any loss of consciousness or if the rest of the body has not experienced axial trauma.

The initial evaluation of the patient at the scene of the accident is similar to that advised for all multiply injured patients: attention to airway, breathing, and circulation are required whatever the type of neurologic system insult. Constant monitoring of vital signs, as well as neurologic function, needs to be performed and recorded, as these may not only assist in the acute care of the patient but also help the surgeon to evaluate the type of spinal insult suffered. Blood pressure should be supported and adequate oxygenation should be insured. When the protocol of a local trauma care delivery team calls for steroids in the treatment of spine injuries, these should be administered as soon as possible *at the scene* if any effectiveness is to be obtained.

Cervical spine immobilization should be attended to with the utmost diligence. In general, a spine board that securely immobilizes the head and neck with straps is superior to cervical collars and sandbags. Where this is not available, the cervical, thoracic, and lumbar spine must be moved as a unit and no flexion or rotation of any component is to be permitted.

Therapeutic Protocol

All patients admitted to our Neurotrauma Service who are suspected of having a cervical spine injury are managed according to a rigid protocol (Table 32-4). Upon arrival, immediate immobilization of the spine is performed if this has not already been done in the field. Patients who are suspected of having sustained either a head or cervical spine injury are placed in a semirigid collar until the extent of other injuries can be ascertained. If no other major injury requires immediate treatment, they are then transferred directly to a Stryker frame for fur-

TABLE 32-4. Principles of Acute Treatment of Spinal Cord Injured Patients

Immobilize neck
Establish and support airway
Ensure adequate ventilation
Support cardiovascular system

ther management. If there is no obvious evidence or suspicion of a cervical spine injury, a cervical collar is applied and the patient is evaluated on the admitting area table. The general condition of the patient is assessed, with primary attention paid to the patient's airway, breathing, and circulation. Oxygen is given either by mask or endotracheal intubation. If intubation is necessary it is done using a protocol that assures no further cervical spine or cord injury (see Chap. 27). Our criteria for intubation on a neurologic basis is a depression of consciousness to a level of stupor (no response to verbal stimuli). Intubation may also be indicated on the basis of pulmonary or cardiac compromise, since many of the patients we see have suffered multiple system damage. When intubation is required before radiologic assessment of the cervical spine, the nasotracheal route is used.

Compromised cardiovascular function is attended to immediately. Neurogenic and hemorrhagic shock are differentiated. Neurogenic shock due to loss of central control of peripheral vascular tone is treated by elevation of the patient's extremities and use of pharmacologic agents to raise the blood pressure. Hemorrhagic shock is treated as is appropriate for the cause. We believe that treatment of neurogenic shock with high-volume fluid infusion is detrimental to the patient in the long term. Volume loading in patients with compromised central nervous system vascular permeability results in cerebral edema (in head injury) and spinal cord edema (in spinal cord and trauma), both of which may prevent the neurotrauma patient from realizing his or her full potential for improvement.

Baseline blood values are determined in all patients. Two large intravenous lines and a Foley catheter are inserted, as well as an arterial line and a Swan-Ganz line in any patient with a neurologic deficit. Steroid therapy is also begun in any such patient.

Initial evaluation includes as detailed a history as can be obtained under the circumstances. It is crucial to ascertain the mechanism of injury, if possible. The activity at the time of the accident (driving a car, falling off a roof, wrestling, diving into shallow water) should be noted. The chronology of neurologic deficit and its progression or improvement

must be made a part of the admitting history.

Careful attention should be paid to those patients who appear to have taken neurotoxic drugs or to be intoxicated at the time of arrival. It is often difficult to evaluate the presence of a head or spinal cord injury in patients presenting when intoxicated. Any neurologic deficit present at the time of admission should be assumed to be traumatic until proven otherwise. It is not acceptable to assume that a patient's inability to move or respond coherently is secondary to the presence of drugs or alcohol, even though this may subsequently be borne out.

External bruises, lacerations, and gross bony deformities are noted and used as an aid in reconstructing the mechanism of injury. Displaced or separated spinous processes may be identified as defects or tenderness on palpation of the spine. Obvious edema in the neck, bruises on the front or the back of the head, as well as signs of trauma to the shoulder girdle are of special importance, and should be recorded.

Neurologic Examination

Once the patient has been medically stabilized, a neurologic examination is performed. This consists of a concise but comprehensive neurologic assessment of spinal cord, peripheral nerve, and cerebral function (see Chapter 31). Following an evaluation of the level of consciousness, upper and lower extremity motor function, sensation to light touch and pin prick, and diaphragmatic, abdominal, and sphincteric functions are tested. The sensory examination of dermatomes for localization of cervical cord lesions is shown in Figure 32-6.

RESPIRATORY FUNCTION

This is evaluated by instructing the patient to breathe deeply while observing the chest and abdominal excursions to assess intercostal and diaphragmatic muscle functions. With major cervical cord injury, C4 paradoxical breathing may be encountered because diaphragmatic function remains intact but the in-

TABLE 32-5. Nerve Root Supply for Major Muscles

Spinal Root	Muscles Innervated	Main Action
C3,C4	Trapezius	Shoulder elevation
C4	Diaphragm	Respiration
C5	Deltoid	Arm abduction
C5,C6	Biceps, brachioradialis	Forearm flexion
C6	Extensor carpi radialis	Wrist extension
C6,C7	Flexor carpi radialis	Wrist flexion
C7	Triceps	Forearm extension
C8	Flexor digitorum profundis and superficialis	Finger flexors
T1	Interossei	Finger abduction and adduction
T4	Intercostals	Muscles of accessory respiration
T10	Abdominals	Tighten abdominal wall
L1,L2	Iliopsoas	Thigh flexion
L3,L4	Quadriceps	Leg extension
L4	Tibialis anterior	Foot dorsiflexion
L5	Extensor hallucis longus	Great toe dorsiflexion
L5,S1	Gluteus maximus	Thigh extension
S1	Semitendinosus, semimembranosus, biceps femoris (hamstrings)	Leg flexion
S1,S2	Soleus, gastrocnemius, flexor digitorum longus, flexor hallucis longus	Foot and toe plantar flexion
S2,S3,S4	Anal sphincter, bladder	Anal sphincter tone, urinary retention

Only the major spinal roots are listed with the muscles they innervate. A specific muscle is frequently supplied by multiple spinal roots. Variation is not uncommon.

tercostal muscles innervated by thoracic cord segments may be paralyzed. Concomitant loss of abdominal wall tone results in paradoxical motion of the abdominal and chest walls with each respiration.

PERIPHERAL MOTOR FUNCTION

This is tested by assessing the strength of the major muscle groups of the extremities (Table 32-5). Abduction and adduction of the fingers should be included to determine the integrity of the C8 nerve root. Special attention should be given to the relationship of the proximal and distal motor functions in the upper and lower extremities: in the central cord syndrome where significant recovery is the rule, the upper extremities are disproportionately affected, and the distal arm muscles are weakest of all. Merely asking patients to move their arms and legs may cause one to ignore the fact that they are unable to move their hands; one may thus miss the diagnosis of a central cord syndrome. Deep tendon reflexes should also be checked, as their absence may help identify root abnormalities. (Table 32-6).

SENSORY EXAMINATION

The sensory examination seeks to answer two questions: (1) Is there a sensory level (relative or absolute)? and (2) Is there an associated radicular abnormality? Here too, subtle findings are of significance. A sensory level in the region of the upper chest, for example, implies a cervical to high thoracic cord injury. The sensory dermatomes C5 through T1 are represented in the upper extremity (Fig. 32-6) and thus, the dermatomes of T2 and C4 are juxtaposed on the upper chest wall. Therefore, one must test sensation in the upper extremities in order to determine accurately where in the cervical spine a lesion may exist. Sacral sparing (sensation preserved in the sacral derma-

TABLE 32-6. Nerve Root Supply for Tendon Reflex Innervation

Spinal Root	Peripheral Nerve Innervation	Reflex
C5-C6	Musculocutaneous nerve	Biceps jerk
C7-C8	Radial nerve	Triceps jerk
C5-C6	Musculocutaneous nerve	Radial jerk
L2-L4	Femoral nerve	Knee jerk
S1	Sciatic and tibial nerves	Ankle jerk

tomes alone) may at times be the only evidence that a quadriplegic patient has an incomplete spinal cord lesion, thus offering some hope for recovery. Therefore, assessment of perineal sensation as well as anal sphincter tone must be included in the neurologic evaluation.

Mention should be made of what the patient's vital signs are at the time of arrival. Presence or absence of a complete *sympathectomy* due to the cord injury aids in determining potential for improvement. Patients with absence of neurologic function but who have not suffered a complete sympathectomy have a greater chance for improvement than those patients who have suffered sympathectomy.

An additional note should be made regarding the neurologic examination of patients who are comatose on admission. It is not sufficient to assume that the reason for their inability to move arms and legs in response to painful stimuli is secondary to their head injury. This may be the case, but the patient may also have suffered a concomitant cervical spine injury. Therefore, patients who are comatose with absence of neurologic function in the extremities should be assumed to have suffered a cervical spine injury and should be evaluated and treated as such.

Because the neurologic and hemodynamic complications of cervical spine injury may be delayed in their appearance, initial evaluation can be regarded as only the first of many sequential examinations. The stability or progression of a deficit over time defines its functional completeness. Sacral reflexes (anal wink and bulbo cavernosus reflexes) are usually the first segmental reflexes to return, often within 24 hours of injury. The return of any spinal cord reflex activity below the level of the lesion in the absence of concomitant return of voluntary motor and/or sensory function predicts an extremely poor prognosis.

Radiologic Tests

Radiologic films consisting of a lateral cervical spine film, chest film, pelvis film, and skull films are performed in that order when indicated. In our institution, upright chest films are not taken until the patient's cervical spine film has been evaluated and read as normal. Lumbar and thoracic spine films are also taken before the upright chest radiograph if the neurologic examination suggests a lesion in these regions. Should the patient have a head injury, then a computed tomographic (CT) scan is performed with the patient in traction if a cervical spine injury is suspected. If a question about pathologic findings in the cervical spine exists when the CT scan is done, the cervical spine is also included in the CT scan.

Spinal Alignment

If the patient has radiologic or neurologic evidence of a cervical spine or spinal cord injury, initial therapy aimed at control of this injury is then undertaken (Table 32-7, Fig. 32-7). This consists of alignment, decompression, and stabilization of the spine and spinal cord. Alignment is used to reduce any gross bony, or ligamentous deformities and is first attempted by closed means. Patients with minor neurologic injury (root deficit) but without bony damage are kept in a semirigid collar until the stability of the ligamentous structures of the spine can be tested. Fractures of C1 or C2 without significant displacement on flexion/extension films also require only a semirigid collar. Flexion–extension films are *only* done acutely on patients who are awake enough to perform their own study, and who are otherwise neurologically intact. Patients who have either a motor or sensory deficit or an altered level of consciousness such that they cannot flex and extend their necks by themselves and report any neurologic changes should *not* have these studies performed acutely.

TABLE 32-7. Principles of Treatment of Cord and Spine Injury

Immobilization of neck
Alignment of spinal elements
Stabilization of spine and spinal cord

INITIAL THERAPY

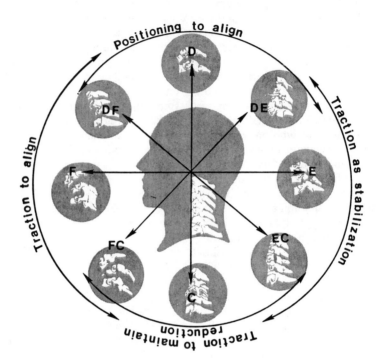

FIG. 32-7 Initial therapy of spinal column injury. Based upon an analysis of the forces involved, the appropriate initial therapy can be decided upon. The options include use of traction to: (1) align the spine only, (2) align and maintain the alignment, and (3) merely stabilize the spine to prevent further injury. In flexion injuries, a significant amount of weight is required to reduce the fracture ("locked facets"), but once reduced, the weight can be decreased to a minimal amount simply to maintain alignment. However, in *compression* injuries, weight needs to be maintained, or the involved vertebral body will recollapse. In *distraction* injuries, positioning alone will often stabilize the spine until the time of operative intervention. In *extension* injuries, traction is often used merely to prevent further movement of the spine and injury to the spinal cord.

When there is evidence of bony malalignment of the spine, or of neurologic dysfunction despite a normal cervical spine film, cervical traction is instituted. Cranial tongs or a Halo fixation device is applied and traction is begun with an amount of weight proportional to the level of injury. We usually put cranial tongs on patients whom we believe, on the basis of their spine films, will require surgical intervention at some time in their hospitalization. Patients whom we anticipate will be treated in a Halo vest at a later date have a Halo ring applied. Traction is begun with an initial weight in pounds equal to three times the cervical vertebrae level of injury (C4 lesion = 12

lbs). Once this weight has been applied, a repeat spine film and neurologic examination are performed. If reduction is not achieved, the weight is progressively increased in 5 to 10 lb stages, with a repeat film and examination performed after each increase of weight. Alternatively, this reduction can be performed under C-arm fluoroscopy with a continuous increase in weight performed and monitored.

If reduction has not been obtained with a weight equal to about 10 times the level of the injury, skilled positioning of the spine is gently performed in an attempt to achieve satisfactory reduction. Placement of rolls under the shoulder or head may help realign the spine when there has been compressive injury. Muscle relaxants may also be used to reduce any muscle spasm that may hinder satisfactory reduction. In the case of bilateral and unilateral locked facets, the patient may be intubated and paralyzed in an attempt to overcome totally any residual muscle tension present. If reduction is still not achieved, then the patient needs to be taken to the operating room for open reduction of the fracture site and ultimate stabilization.

Patients with a neurologic deficit and no bony abnormality are kept in traction with a weight equal to approximately three times the cervical level of injury pending further studies. We do this because we believe that placement of traction helps prevent small movements of the spinal column that may further damage an already injured spinal cord.

Minimyelogram

Once the patient's spine has been satisfactorily aligned either by closed or an open technique, he or she is turned to the prone position on the Stryker frame. A repeat lateral cervical spine film is taken to ensure the maintenance of adequate alignment. (If the patient cannot be aligned satisfactorily in the supine position, turning to the prone position may cause alignment to occur.) A lateral cervical puncture is then performed.[25] The head of the Stryker frame is raised so that the posterior aspect of the patient's neck is at a 20° angle with the floor. The amount of frame elevation needed will vary depending upon the degree of flexion or extension in the patient's neck. Such elevation minimizes the amount of contrast agent that may run into the head during the subsequent study and at the same time causes the agent to remain in the cervical region. Pantopaque, 3 to 6 ml, is slowly instilled in the subarachnoid space, after which a portable lateral cervical spine film is taken. Adequate visualization of the complete anterior aspect of the cervical spine may be achieved at this point. If the flow of the contrast media appears to be impeded, the head of the frame is raised further in 20° increments and serial radiographs are taken until the area of interest is visualized. If the agent fails to flow with the head of the frame elevated maximally, a complete myelographic block is assumed. At our institution the contrast media is not removed after the procedure (see Appendix for comments regarding use of metrizamide in the acute situation).

If the minimyelogram is abnormal, a decision is made as to whether the patient requires operative intervention. Any patient with a complete myelographic defect is taken to the operating room immediately. However, if the myelographic defect is minor, with only anterior compression, then an attempt is first made to reduce the compression through closed means, by either increasing the weight of traction or positioning the patient differently on the Stryker frame. Often these minor degrees of compression indicate inadequate reduction of the spine, and will disappear with the manipulations described. If they do not, however, the patient is also taken to the operating room, provided the myelographic defect is consistent with the level of injury and is presumed to be affecting the patient's level of neurologic function.

General Care

If no acute surgical intervention is required, then our patients are transferred directly to a neurologic intensive care unit following any other evaluations needed due for the systemic injury. Any medical treatment they receive in the intensive care unit is designed to optimize the conditions for spinal cord recovery. Treatment is aimed at optimizing cardiovascular and pulmonary function, nutritional support, and rehabilitation.

CARDIOVASCULAR SUPPORT

As mentioned previously, because of the loss of sympathetic control to the heart and peripheral circulation, patients with a cervical or high thoracic spinal cord injury have poor cardiovascular control and regulation. In the face of a circulating volume deficit, the spinal-cord-injured patient is unable to maintain adequate cardiac filling pressures. However, if overtransfused, the patient may develop pulmonary edema more easily. For this reason, continuous hemodynamic monitoring is performed in an effort to maintain blood pressure and blood volume in a normotensive range. This is usually accomplished with pressors, dopamine being the drug of choice. It is used because one can titrate the dose of dopamine to produce an inotropic effect at a low dose, and to improve vascular tone if given in higher α-adrenegic doses (greater than or equal to 5 μg/kg/min). The Swan-Ganz catheter, which allows one to measure cardiac output (CO) and to calculate oxygen consumption from the CO and the arteriovenous oxygen content difference, is an invaluable tool in the effort to maintain optimal tissue perfusion.

A relatively normovolemic state is maintained in the early posttraumatic period, in an effort to reduce the risk of pulmonary edema and spinal cord or cerebral edema in the region of the trauma, but at the same time maintain adequate filling pressures. Unless the heart rate is less than 50 beats/min no intervention is taken. If bradycardia becomes associated with hypotension and signs of inadequate tissue perfusion, atropine is used. A bolus of 0.5 mg atropine is given initially; if this does not raise the pulse rate, it is repeated in 0.5 mg increments, up to a total of 2.0 mg. With persistent bradycardia, an isoproterenol infusion (0.25 to 0.50 μg/min total dose) is started.[32]

A special note should be made about patients with high cervical spinal cord injury who manifest cardiovascular instability. These patients should probably not be managed on a Stryker frame because of the rapid change in cardiovascular status that turning may incur. Cardiovascular-unstable patients should be managed on a Roto-Rest bed, or in a regular bed after their spinal column is stabilized.

PULMONARY SUPPORT

Upon arrival in the intensive care unit, patients who have been intubated for reasons of spinal alignment should be extubated as soon as possible. If the patient required intubation due to an associated pulmonary injury or dysfunction, then a weaning program is started as soon as tolerated by the patient. This is usually done within the first several days. In any case, assessment of patient's ventilatory capacity is always made in all cases. Useful guidelines for assessing adequate chest mechanics are obtained by measuring the vital capacity (greater than 15 ml/kg), tidal volume (greater than 5 ml/kg), and maximum inspiratory force (less than or equal to −20 cm H_2O). Patients with high spinal cord dysfunction often lose innervation to the intercostal and abdominal musculature. This means that they are dependent on diaphragmatic innervation to generate adequate ventilatory capacities. Continued assessment of the patient's chest mechanics are therefore necessary. Chest physiotherapy is initiated as soon as possible in all patients to minimize the risk of pulmonary congestion and/or infection.

PREVENTION OF ACID PEPTIC ULCERATION

Gastric pH is controlled early in the hospitalization by the prophylactic use of antiacids on an hourly or 2-hourly basis and cimetidine (300 mg q every 12 hr) if the gastric pH is not otherwise controlled at levels greater than 4.0 whether the patient is receiving steroids or not. Peptic ulceration in the high spinal cord patient with loss of symathetic innervation is a well-described complication. Abdominal disease accounts for 10 percent of all fatalities in the spinal-cord-injured population, with perforated viscus (usually gastric or duodenal ulcer) being the most common cause. The sensory deficit present in spinal-cord-injuries makes a routine abdominal examination virtually useless. Persistent nausea and vomiting or tachycardia, or bradycardia, occurring in contrast to a pulse rate that has been previously normal, may be a sign of intrabdominal pathologic change. Pain in the shoulders or clavicular regions may be referred from diaphragmatic irritation from a peptic ulcer perforation. If these signs appear, a diagnostic work-up to rule out impending disaster should be initiated.

URINARY TRACT AND METABOLIC SUPPORT

Intermittent catherization is begun once spinal shock has resolved and the patient is stable enough to begin fluid restriction. An initial restriction of 2,400 ml a day along with catherization every 4 hr is begun. The fluids are increased and the frequency of catherization decreased as tolerated by the patient. Feeding is begun as soon as the patient arrives in the intensive care unit either via a nasogastric tube or by hyperalimentation. Regular oral intake is begun as soon as is feasible. Steroids are continued for 5 days as detailed later in this chapter. Patients do not routinely receive anticoagulation, but there is evidence that the use of an active calf compression apparatus to reduce the incidence of deep leg vein thrombosis and pulmonary embolization is of value.

ACUTE REHABILITATION THERAPY

The initial managment of all patients with cord or spinal cord injury is the use of a Stryker frame. We have seen little of the pulmonary and infectious problems described elsewhere associated with the use of the Stryker frame.[19] This most likely is due to our excellent nursing care. Patients are turned every 2 hours, and receive round-the-clock pulmonary care with the assistance of full-time respiratory therapists. Physicial therapy and occupational therapy is instituted as early as possible with our own in-house therapists, and strict attention is paid to the minutest detail to prevent decubitius ulcers.

Once the patient is stable and, if he or she has neurologic function, he or she may be transferred to a regular bed with traction at the head of the bed. These patients are still turned every 2 hours and receive frequent pulmonary toilet and respiratory care, however. Our general approach to these patients is to prevent systemic problems from occurring rather than treating them once they occur. In particular, we have found that the routine use of pulmonary toilet, even when there is no lung abnormality noted on examination or radiograph, is beneficial in the prevention of later pulmonary complications.

DEFINITIVE THERAPY

The definitive therapy to treat spine injuries depends as much on the preference of the surgeon as on the stability of the fracture site and the modalites of therapy available to the particular physician (Fig. 32-8). Inherently unstable fractures almost always require internal fixation with wire, rods, plates, bone, or acrylic to substitute for the disrupted ligaments. Inherently stable fractures can often be managed with external stabilization, although the use of specifically designed operative procedures and devices may significantly alter the duration of the convalescent period. Whether the surgical approach is posterior or anterior, or whether external stabilization involves solely traction, or incorporates the use of a Halo vest or brace, is most often determined by the physician's preference and philosophy.

External fixation with either prolonged traction or a Halo vest is useful in those instances where the fracture site is inherently stable. This is most commonly the case with compression injuries in which adequate canal decompression has been accomplished by traction. Use of external fixation will immobilize the fracture site, allowing a bony fusion to occur. Halo vests are most appropriately applied when the amount of force necessary to maintain an adequate reduction of the fracture site is less than 15 lbs. If this is not the case, redislocation or delayed angulation may occur due to the inability of the vest to maintain more than 15 lbs of distractive force. Halo vests are therefore commonly applied after a variable period of time during which the amount of traction to which the fracture site is subjected is gradually reduced. Once applied, they are usually used for anywhere from 6 weeks to 4 months depending upon the rate at which bony fusion occurs.

DEFINITIVE THERAPY

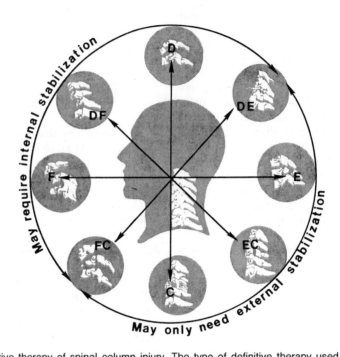

FIG. 32-8 Definitive therapy of spinal column injury. The type of definitive therapy used depends as much on the preference of the surgeon as on the stability of the fracture and the modes of therapy available. Inherently unstable fractures almost always require internal fixation with wire, acrylic, bone, or rods to substitute for disrupted ligaments. Inherently stable fractures can usually be managed with external stabilization, although the use of specifically designed operative procedures and devices may significantly reduce the time of the convalescent period and improve the outcome. Whether the surgical approach is anterior or posterior, or whether external stabilization involves solely traction or incorporates the use of a Halo vest or brace, is usually determined by the physician's surgical philosophy.

Although some encourage the use of external immobilization, including a Halo vest, to treat all cervical spine injuries regardless of the pathologic condition present,[122] we believe that prolonged external immobilization is specifically contraindicated in patients with unsatisfactorily reduced spines, and should be avoided in most instances in patients who have ligamentous instability without concurrent bony injury. Patients in this latter group have a high incidence of instability after external immobilization, due to the lack of fractured bone from the injury from which a spontaneous fusion may result. These patients should be treated with an operative fusion as the primary modality.[98] Instability is also seen in patients with both anterior and posterior ligamentous complex disruption in spite of bony fractures.[81] These patients also should not be treated in a Halo vest. The combined rate of delayed instability in the face of external immobilization, including the use of a Halo vest, has been reported in the range from 5.4 to 20 percent: most patients with delayed instability have either poorly reduced spine fracture or ligamentous instability without concurrent bony injury.[28,31] In addition, although nonoperative treatment of patients with spinal cord injuries is an acceptable management alternative in patients not included in these instability groups, operative means for stabilization may be more in the particular patient's best interest.

Our specific indications for the use of a surgical approach for the treatment of cervical spine injury are (1) to decompress the spinal canal when necessary; and (2) to provide spinal stabilization in the presence of a cervical vertebra injury likely to demonstrate delayed instability. To reiterate, this means any injury with ligamentous damage without the concurrent presence of enough bony injury to provide a stable spine once the bone fuses. We do not believe that nonsurgical treatment such as external immobilization or the use of a Halo vest is indicated in this type of patient.

Once a decision is made to operate on a patient, the type of procedure must be decided upon. There are many proponents of an entirely posterior or an entirely anterior approach for treating unstable spines. We believe, as do others, that the approach should depend upon the pathologic condition involved, including both the presence or absence of spinal cord compression and the reason for the spinal instability.

Anterior procedures are indicated acutely in patients who have persistent anterior cord compression despite *adequate* closed attempts with traction to decompress the canal (less than 5 percent of our patients). The procedure then involves removal of bone and disc fragments from the injured spinal canal space and the placement of a bone strut to maintain height and spinal alignment, as well as to produce later stability as a result of a bony fusion. However, the use of the anterior approach to produce stability in the patient without cord compression is quite controversial. Anterior cervical fusion may be indicated in extension injuries without cord compression where there is disc and ligamentous disruption. However, an anterior approach in patients with flexion injuries may acutely destabilize the spine even further than prior to surgery by disrupting a potentially intact anterior ligamentous complex in the face of already disrupted posterior ligamentous complexes.

Because of this risk, several systems for anteriorly instrumenting the spine have been devised. They all involve placement of a metal plate or rod anterior to the spine, screwed into the intact vertebral bodies above and below the level of injury after placement of a bone strut to promote bony fusion.[20,77,84,102,103] Such devices provide a force to counteract the compressive and tensial forces that cause the spine to be unstable in the first place. The use of such plates is quite controversial, in part due to experience in the past of screws working loose, causing both delayed instability as well as damage to vital structures. Several new systems have been designed to alleviate these problems, and are currently being investigated by others.[27]

Patients with flexion-type injuries that disrupt the posterior ligamentous complex where a significant anterior bony injury does not exist should be approached through a posterior operation. A posterior approach also may be necessary acutely to realign the spine in the face of unilateral or bilateral locked facets that cannot be reduced, as well as to decompress the spine when laminar fragments are causing cord compression. Such a decompressive laminectomy is only indicated in those rare instances of fracture of the posterior elements of the cervical spine with dorsal compression of the spinal cord. However, as a rule, acute laminectomy has nothing to offer to the patient with a cervical spine injury, and may cause deterioration of the patient's neurologic condition.[45] Laminectomy may be indicated on a delayed basis for those patients with a central cord syndrome due to cervical stenosis.

The goal of a posterior operation as a stabilizing procedure is to implant a substitute for the ligaments torn by the forces that produced the unstable spine. This substitute, usually wire, maintains spinal alignment until bone, which is incorporated into the wiring, forms a solid fusion. Although the posterior approaches stabilize the spine in flexion, they are not stable in extension until a bony fusion occurs. For this reason, they are not indicated in patients with an unstable spine secondary to an anterior ligamentous injury. Also, these procedures only provide resistance to tensile forces. If the spine is unstable due to an anterior bony injury, posterior wiring can not counteract the compressive forces that will cause the spine to angulate.

For this reason, alternative means of producing posterior stabilization have been developed. These include acrylic, metal plates, Harrington-type rods, clamps, and other custom devices.[6,23,52,55,73,101,115,117,121] Each of these is fraught with their own problems and they are not universally available or applicable. The goal in all internal fixation procedures is to provide a posterior "strut" capable of resisting the comprehensive forces that cause the spine to collapse or angulate when anterior bony injury exists. Acrylic is quite capable of doing so, but recent studies have shown that the bone/wire/acrylic interface deteriorates with time, introducing the possibility of delayed instability.[23,71,120,151] The use of acrylic is therefore recommended only in patients in whom bone can not be used, or who have a short life expectancy secondary to cancer.[151] We are currently investigating a posterior rodding system that creates a facet-to-facet fusion. The construct is designed to allow flexion–extension or compression–distraction forces to be countered, and will, it is hoped, provide a posterior approach in the face of anterior instability. Work on this project is underway, but remains experimental.[24]

Several types of posterior procedures using wire have been developed for stabilizing a cervical spine in cases where posterior instability alone exists. The indications for a particular technique are based upon the pathologic condition involved. Interspinous wiring is the simplest means of incorporating wire into the fusion, and is adequate for the majority of cases. It involves wiring two or more spinous processes together, producing a tension band across the fracture site. Such wiring, however, provides no resistance to rotatory forces. Thus, in cases where rotatory instability exists due to facet fractures, an alternative means of stabilization must be used. This involves wiring of the facet joints at the involved level to either the spinous process (oblique wiring; facet to spinous process wiring),[22] or to another facet joint (posterior lateral facet fusion) at a level below the injury site. This later approach is necessary when the spinous processes have been damaged by the injury, or removed prior to a laminectomy. In these cases, once the wiring has been completed, bone is incorporated into the fusion, either by actually placing it within the wire strands or by laying it over the wire at the end of the case. In this fashion a bony fusion will occur on a delayed basis and ultimately stabilize the spine.

PROGNOSIS AND SUMMARY

Several well-written articles have appeared over the past several decades exploring the prognosis for cervical spinal cord injury.[17,18,47,61,68,76,106,109,113,143,156] Improvements in outcome during this time, however, have not paralleled the introductions of new and modified modalities. Patients who have complete motor and sensory deficits at 24 to 48 hours after admission will generally remain that way. The grim statistics are that less than 10 percent will regain useful leg function at 1 year, with less than 3 percent ever ambulating (Tables 32-8 and 32-9).

This is not to suggest, however, that early intervention is not important. Patients who have some return of function within 24 to 48 hours, or who have some sensory or motor preservation at the time of admission, have a remarkably good chance of functional recov-

TABLE 32-8.   Frankel Classification of Spinal Cord Injuries

Complete	No motor or sensory function below the level of lesion
Sensory only	Complete motor paralysis below level of lesion with some preservation of sensory function—includes sacral sparing
Motor useless	Some motor function below level of lesion: these patients can move lower limbs and many can walk with or without aid
Recovery	Free of neurologic symtoms; no weakness, sensory loss, or sphincteric disturbance (abnormal reflexes may be present)

TABLE 32-9.   Prognosis in Cervical Cord Injury: Review of Retrospective Series

Study	Percentage That Regain Useful Leg Function	
	Complete Deficit	Sensory Preservation
Frankel et al.[61]	9	58
Braakman and Penning[18]	17	10
Young and Dexter[156]	2	63
Maynard et al.[109]	0	72
Ducker et al.[47]	10	80

ery. Upwards of 50 percent of those patients who have only a partial sensory loss at this time, and 90 percent of patients who have some motor function present, will ambulate.[109]

Given these statistics, it is crucial that everything possible be done to allow return of function, and to preserve all function present at admission. As detailed above, this process begins with immobilization and medical stabilization at the scene of injury, realignment on arrival at the referral center, and the use of medical adjuvants to optimize both systemic and local function. Surgical intervention, whether early or late, improves prognosis only insofar as it stabilizes the spine, realigns the canal, and decompresses viable cord tissue. The systematic application of the principles detailed in this chapter (Table 32-10) may convert an apparently complete lesion on admission to a partial lesion. If this goal is realized within 24 to 48 hours, then the patient's chances of good recovery improve dramatically.

Some 5,000 years ago the writer of the Smith papryrus, who is thought by some to be the physician pharoah Imhotep, wrote about dislocations of the cervical vertebrae, saying "when examining a man suffering from dislocation of the cervical vertebrae, he will find that he is unaware of his hands and his legs, that his penis is erect, that his urine escapes without his knowing, and that he is flatulent and his eyes are red. A disease which cannot be treated." It has taken 5,000 years to reach the point where such a conclusion may not be justified. Given proper emergency management and extended rehabilitation, not only can most patients be successfully returned to a socially acceptable existence, but on occasion functional use of limbs can also be regained.

To end on an optimistic note, modern technology is fast becoming more capable of giving hope to those individuals whom a specialized trauma center team can support through the acute spinal cord insult. Extensive research programs are underway in this country and throughout the world directed not only at the

TABLE 32-10. Treatment of Spinal Cord Injury

Spinal Cord Insult	Therapeutic Intervention
Mechnical insults	
Direct tissue disruption	Prevention only; regeneration techniques remain experimental. Immediate immobilization followed by surgical stabilization or long-term (3–6 months) skeletal traction.
Persistent extradural cord compression	Diagnostic myelography in selected cases. If compression is demonstrated, appropriate surgical decompression may be indicated. This should be accompanied by a pretreatment stabilization procedure if required (the overall efficacy of immediate myelography has not yet been clearly established).
Hemodynamic changes	
Deminished spinal cord blood flow, loss of autoregulation, and systemic vasomotor paralysis	Maintain normotensive systemic blood pressure for optimal cord perfusion.
Diminished tissue oxygen	Maintain excellent oxygenation: administer oxygen; active pulmonary therapy to avoid pneumonia atelectasis; mechanical ventilation if necessary; avoid pulmonary complications; pulmonary embolus, pneumothorax, infection, etc; reduce cord edema: steroids (generally accepted); DMSO, local hypothermic hyperbaric oxygen therapy (experimental).
Biochemical derangements	
Accumulation of norepinephrine at site of injury (controversial)	No well-accepted therapy; experimental work includes; barbiturates, DMSO, γ-hydroxybutyrate, steroids, local hypothermia, hyperbaric oxygen; α and β adrenergic blockers. Also, avoid high oxygen consumption states, fever, sepsis, agitation.
Defective blood–brain barrier	
Membrane and organelle injury	
Ancillary systemic insults	
Pulmonary complications	Meticulous, aggressive nursing care.
Urinary complications	
Skin complications	

development of automated patient-controlled artificial limbs but also towards the creation of an artificial computer-based patient-activated peripheral nervous systems. Such a creation may one day allow those who have lost limb function once again to "be aware of their arms and legs" and to use them as they were meant to be used. It is the responsibility of first line emergency medical practitioners as well as the trauma referral trauma team to give future spinal cord trauma patients the chance to benefit from this new technology.

APPENDIX: CONTROVERSIES IN MANAGEMENT

Role of Myelography

The presence of spinal cord compression has adverse effects on cord function, as documented by alterations in spinal evoked potentials, as well as in pathologic changes in neural tissue.[33,67,97] For this reason, immediate immobilization and realignment of the spine are accepted principles in the management of acute spinal injury.[131] However, even when the spine has been returned to its normal anatomic position and proper intraspinal dimensions have been reestablished, continued cord compression can exist due to extruded disc, bone, or ligamentous tissue. A routine radiograph or CT scan can demonstrate bony impingement, but cannot demonstrate soft tissue compression. Furthermore, this type of continued compression, as indicated earlier, can prevent or hinder a patient from achieving his or her full potential for neurologic recovery.

Ideally, all patients who have suffered an acute insult to the cervical spine should undergo a complete myelographic study, just as do patients who present with evidence of a chronic cervical spinal cord abnormality. This is unfortunately not usually possible, mainly due to logistics. It is simply not feasible to perform a formal cervical myelogram on an unstable patient who is in cervical traction. One cannot easily manipulate the contrast in the cervical region when traction must be maintained using currently available traction devices. In addition, many of these patients cannot tolerate such an involved procedure because of hemodynamic instability and/or multiple system injuries. These problems have prompted the development of modifications to those neuroradiologic techniques used in chronically injured patients, in an attempt to develop a universally acceptable diagnostic procedure that is a reliable means of diagnosing structural injuries to the spinal cord. Most of these modifications involve the use of smaller amounts of positive contrast medium in a myelogram performed on a patient through a C1-C2 puncture soon after the injury.

Abnormalities readily demonstrated by these minimyelographic methods include (1) a complete block of the contrast flow at the level of the bony lesion; (2) a significant anteriorly located filling defect at the level of the bony lesion, (3) a significant posterior filling defect at the level of the bony lesion. In patients found to have one of these abnormalities, an attempt should be made to improve reduction through closed means. If the defect still exists, these patients should be taken immediately to surgery for appropriate decompressive procedure, either anterior or posterior, and a simultaneous stabilizing procedure if indicated.

The theory behind the use of an emergency decompressive procedure used acutely, rather than a more elaborate procedure done when the patient is stable, is that certain patients may benefit from immediate surgical intervention. To date we have performed a minimyelogram on well over 200 consecutive patients with neurologic deficit as a result of a cervical spine injury. Although only 5 percent had an improvement in outcome as a result of an acute surgical intervention based upon the results of the myelogram, the enhanced recovery was significant with regard to their reaching full potential in their rehabilitation program. In addition, over 10 percent had defects identified which were then correctable by modifying traction. The effect that this therapy had on the eventual outcome is not known.

The use of minimyelograms in the evaluation of acute traumatic cord injury is not well established or presently widely accepted. Many people believe that a delayed complete myelographic study should be done. However, we believe that myelography loses its value in the subacute situation. We previously used myelography 2 to 6 days after the traumatic insult and demonstrated a significant block in almost 50 percent of the patients studied. However, these blocks generally failed to correlate with the level of clinical injury. As a result surgery was therefore deferred, since it was believed that the myelographic defect was secondary to swelling rather than to the acute spinal cord trauma. Our conclusion was that in the subacute period the myelographic study loses much of its diagnostic value.

Given the premise that early demonstration of a possible surgical lesion is essential, the question is whether the minimyelogram is the approach of choice. Computed tomographic scanning of the spine is an alternative means of evaluating the spine. No contrast agent is necessary, and the patient can be scanned at the same time as a cranial CT is performed, if there is associated head trauma. However, CT is not without its problems. Due to improper angling of the gantry, points of interest may be missed or misinterpreted. In addition, without the instillation of a contrast agent, it may be difficult to appreciate soft tissue compression of the cord. Transfer of a patient to the CT table while he or she is in traction is not without its hazards, and it is difficult to assess changes made by adjusting traction if a defect is found.

In conclusion, we think that immediate myelographic investigation with a positive contrast agent, once the patient is medically stable, is the diagnostic procedure of choice in cases of cervical spine injury associated with evidence of a neurologic deficit. An early study provides two valuable pieces of information.[51] It acts as an adjunct to plain cervical films in assessing the adequacy of the proposed closed and/or open techniques to be used in restoring the cervical spine to its most normal spatial configuration. It also allows identification of the 5 percent of patients who will achieve a greater rate and degree of neurologic recovery of function, if they can undergo immediate surgical decompression of the spinal cord. However, we do not think that an operation is in dicated in all patients with an abnormal myelogram. We will currently operate only if the defect seen (1) is a complete block consistent with the level of bony or neurologic injury, (2) represents significant anterior extradural compression due to a presumed disc rupture, or (3) is due to bone fragments in the canal, whether anterior or posterior. Finally, we only operate after an attempt has been made to relieve the compression defect through closed means.

The type of contrast medium to be used is the subject of debate. Pantopaque has the advantages of being universally available and extensively used over the years, both by the neurosurgeon and the technician. It can demonstrate quite adequately both anterior defects and large posterior defects when used with the proper technique. The simplest of the radiographic equipment can be used to achieve adequate examinations, but the use of a C-arm fluoroscopy unit makes studies considerably easier to perform.

Metrizamide is an alternative, as it provides a more accurate assessment of root sleeves and a more complete assessment of the posterior spaces in the upper cervical spine.[100] However, there are side effects associated with its use, such as nausea and vomiting, hypotension, and seizures, which take on major importance in a patient with an unstable cervical spine fracture.[1,2,10,12,25,33,41,79,130,138-140] Therefore, caution is recommended in its use in this setting. If used, we recommend medication with diasepam, diphenhydramine hydrochloride, and steroids to prevent CNS complications. An effort should be made to keep the patient's head above the feet at all time. For this reason CT with metrizamide is preferable to metrizamide myelography.

Adjuvant Therapies

Experimental approaches to the treatment of spinal cord injuries abound in the literature. Two new pharmacologic agents have been investigated in recent years: thyroid releasing hormone (TRH) and naloxone. Both have been shown to improve recovery in cat models of cord injury, with TRH having a more marked effect.[54,55,58,145,157] The mechanism of action of both these substances is not known. Both cause an elevation in systemic blood pressure, with an even greater increase in local spinal cord blood flow.[55,56,58,140] Since the increase in these factors is the same for the two drugs,[55,58] and since the improvements seen with TRH are greater than the naloxone, it has been suggested that something besides an increase in flow is produced by this agent. This "something" may be the drug's ability to alter local metabolic factors, or modify circulatory changes. Naloxone acts through binding to opiate receptors, TRH through an unknown mechanism (see Chap. 6).

Neither of these drugs has been tried extensively in human spinal cord injury. Two potential problems with naloxone relate to the amount of drug needed to produce this effect (up to 10 mg/kg) and its antianalgesic effect. Further recommendations regarding the clinical use of either of these drugs await more detailed studies.

The concept that improvement in microvascular perfusion is responsible for the beneficial effect of TRH and Naloxone has lead researchers to investigate a "cocktail" consisting of PGI_2, indomethacin, and heparin.[83] This combination has been used successfully to enhance brain reperfusion and functional recovery after brain ischemia.[82] Initial studies have shown that these three drugs, when used concomitantly, have as beneficial an effect on cord function as naloxone alone.[83] It is postulated that their combined mechanism of action enhances platelet antiaggregation,[104,141] thus increasing local blood flow.

Steroids

The role of glucocorticoids in the treatment of acute spinal cord injuries remains a topic of heated debate. There are a plethora of conflicting animals studies, and a paucity of controlled human studies. A major problem in the experimental assessment of any therapeutic intervention is the development of an applicable animal model of acute spinal cord injury. There is also the difficulty of interpreting megadose, high-dose, or low-dose therapy in steroid research, as well as the duration of the dosage regimens. The problems have been reviewed and addressed elsewhere.[57,69,70]

The rationale behind the use of steroids in spinal cord injury is many-faceted. It is aimed at (1) facilitation of impulse generation and conduction within the injured cord[69,153]; (2) enhancement of blood flow[7,45,60]; and (3) reduction in injury-induced lipid peroxidation and tissue degeneration.[39,40,70,116] These processes are ongoing, beginning with the injury itself. It is unclear when steroid therapy should be started to enhance these processes,[7,36] what dosages are most beneficial,[71] and for how long they should be continued.[21,64,65,112] Laboratory data indicate that a decrease in spinal cord blood flow resulting in an increase in measurable lipid peroxidation levels and decrease in synaptic transmission begins within the first 5 minutes of injury.[70] We have therefore adopted the policy that if glucocorticoids are to be administered to spinal-cord-injured patients, they should be administered as soon as possible after the insult. Given the fact that there may be an optimal window for the beneficial effects of steroids, we recommend that an initial dose be given *at the scene* in patients with suspected cord injury. The dosage we are currently using is 5 mg/kg methylprednisolone, or 1 mg/kg dexamethasone. This is continued for 3 days in divided doses and then discontinued. We believe that the side effects from this regimen are low enough,[50,53,153] with the possible gains high enough, that such an approach is warranted. However, the assessment of the role of steroids in the management of cord injury is continuing, and no definitive proof of their efficacy in humans yet exists.

Dimethyl sulfoxide (DMSO) has also been investigated as a possible tool in the treatment of cord-injured patients. Early animal studies showed that DMSO was able to accelerate return of function compared with other treatment modalities.[35-37,105,110] These studies showed that DMSO reduced tissue swelling and fluid retention, and protected the myelin sheath axon from injury. The proposed mechanism is thought to be due to its ability to inhibit platelet aggregation as a result of its interaction with prostaglandins as well as the powerful platelet aggregator thromboxane A_2. Although this is sound in theory, confirmatory patient studies have yet to be presented.

Hyperbaric Oxygen

As outlined previously, one of the factors thought to be responsible for the pathophysiologic alterations following cervical spine trauma is the profound tissue hypoxia that develops within and adjacent to injured spinal cord segments. Based upon studies by Maidia in 1965, which showed that 100 percent oxygen at 2 to 3 atmospheres of hyperbaric pressure could reverse spinal cord tissue hypoxia in a canine model of spinal cord injury,[107] hyperbaric oxygen treatment has been explored in numerous centers as an adjuvant in spinal cord injury treatment. Hortzog and co-workers[85] in 1969 reported relative improvement in recovery of spinal cord injury in baboons following treatment with 3 atmospheres of oxygen at 3, 11, and 21 hours following trauma, when compared to controls. Kelly and associates[93,94] were unable to demostrate any increase in PO_2 in injured spinal cord tissue when ventilating animals with 100 percent oxygen, but did demonstrate improved PO_2 in the tissue of the injured spinal cord when the animals were treated with 2 atmospheres of oxygen. Paraplegic animals treated with hyperbaric oxygen made neurologic recoveries equal to those receiving treatment with systemic and intrathecal steroids, as well as with hypothermia; these results were better than those for untreated controls. Similar results have been reported by Yeo and co-workers[154,155] using sheep treated 2 hours following injury, although the difference in motor function between control and treated animals was *not* statistically valid.

The therapeutic benefit of hyperbaric oxygen is thought to occur during the period immediately following impact, when secondary changes occur within the spinal cord leading to total and permanent loss of long tract conduction on the basis of local metabolic compromise. During this time hyperbaric oxygen may provide an increased substrate for oxidative metabolism in the injured segments. Hyperbaric oxygen may also act as a direct vasoconstrictor of neural blood vessels, thus leading to decreased edema formation.

Although animal studies have been generally encouraging in examining the benefit of hyperbaric oxygen treatment, human trials have been unconvincing.[34,78,80,81,89,118] In 1981 a report from our institution examined the results of 25 consecutive acute spinal cord injury patients meeting protocol requirements for receiving hyperbaric oxygen therapy and compared them to controls receiving conventional therapy.[62] Patients totally paralyzed for more than 24 hours failed to recover significant function despite receiving hyperbaric oxygen therapy. Patients with partial injuries did demonstrate significant recoveries in motor indices, although this recovery was basically the same as the recovery experienced by approximately 500 control patients. Although the two groups did not differ in their recovery, the patients receiving hyperbaric oxygen did appear to recover to their final functional levels at a quicker rate than those patients who received conventional therapy. The role of hyperbaric oxygen in therapy may therefore be important in affecting the rate of recovery, although the mechanism producing this accelerated rate of recovery is as yet unclear. Based upon this study and other isolated reports in the literature and reported at meetings, hyperbaric oxygen therapy does not appear to alter greatly the final neurologic outcome of spinal cord injury. However a careful set of prospective randomized studies are necessary to clarify what role, if any, this therapy has in the overall treatment of acute spinal cord injury.

Hypothermia

A more experimental approach to the treatment of spinal cord injury involves the use of hypothermia. The rationale for its use in patients with spinal cord injury lies in its potential ability to lower metabolic requirements of the nervous tissue, thus providing a cushion between the occurrence of total tissue destruction and the return of the normal homeostatic balance interrupted by the trauma.[150] Experimently, hypothermia has been shown to slow down the degree of swelling in the neural tissue and to vasoconstrict vessels near the site of injury, a process that may also reduce the total tissue volume.[4] The ability to vasoconstrict the spinal cord microcirculation may also prove valuable in increasing local tissue flow to the traumatized sites. Finally, local cooling of the cord may block the metabolic acidosis that results from the trauma, as well as reduce the formation of serotonin, suspected of causing microcoagulation following cord trauma.[147]

Many variables are involved in evaluating the effect of hypothermia on spinal cord injury. The first involves the speed with which it is instituted. Albin and White, the first to show the efficacy of spinal cord cooling, have demonstrated that cooling instituted within 8 hours of injury will be effective in producing beneficial results.[3,66,111] Other reports have shown that spinal cord cooling must be instituted within the first several hours following trauma.[144] The necessary duration of cooling also needs to be resolved. Most of the results seem to indicate that shorter periods of cooling are more beneficial than longer periods of cooling, perhaps because prolonged use of hypothermia eventually leads to decreased blood flow to the neural tissues and may eventually damage the cord rather than improving it.[45] The degree to which the spinal cord should be cooled is also open to investigation. Temperatures in current studies have ranged from 3° to 15°C, with varying results.[72,144]

The positive effects of hypothermia for patients with spinal cord injury found by some investigators[3,4,5,51,72,98,129] have been challenged by others who could not find any benefit from such treatment either in humans with cord trauma or in experimental animals.[13,51,86,134,142] In addition, some reports suggest that the use of hypothermia in patients with spinal cord trauma is not necessary; rather, improvement can be obtained merely by irrigating the traumatized cord with room-temperature saline solution. This may be due to the ability of the saline solution irrigation to remove metabolic toxins present in the CSF that may hinder tissue recovery.[142] Technically, local cooling of the spinal cord may not be indicated in many

patients since it requires either an anterior decompressive procedure or a posterior decompressive procedure, surgery that is not generally necessary in the majority of spinal cord injury patients.

Types of Spinal Immobilization

A wide range of devices are available for acute immobilization of the cervical spine following suspected spinal cord injury. Cervical traction is the most widely used form of acute immobilization, but is generally available only in the hospital. Of major concern is the form of cervical spine immobilization used in the field before the patient arrives at the hospital. Studies have reported the potential for neurologic deterioration during transit to be from 3 to 25 percent.[30,62,128] Proper field immobilization used should reduce the risk of neurologic deterioration.

Several studies have compared various forms of pre- and posthospital immobilization devices.[119,152] In the acute situation, sandbags and an adhesive tape across the forehand are far superior to the cervical hard collar in preventing cervical motion. However, the combined use of sandbags, tape, and a cervical hard collar best restricts flexion, extension, rotation, and lateral bending. In the chronic situation, the cervical–thoracic or Yale-type brace is very effective in controlling all but lateral bending forces.[152] This latter motion is only held in check by a Halo vest. The soft collar is of no value in either situation, since it provides no restriction to cervical motion whatsoever. Its major use is to remind the patient that he or she has suffered trauma to the neck of some degree that requires significant restraints on mobilization.

In conclusion, it is recommended that in the acute situation prior to and during transport the patient's neck be controlled with a combination of sandbags, tapes, and a hard collar, with the tape and sandbags being removed when the patient arrives at the hospital.[43] In the chronic situation, a hard collar should be used to restrain patients with a cervical strain, or following posterior procedures in the upper cervical spine. A cervical–thoracic brace is indicated as a postoperative stabilization device for flexion or extension injuries of the cervical spine when the fundamental stability potential of the procedure is not in question.[152] Where a question exists about the stability of the operative procedures performed, a Halo vest may need to be used. Halo vests should also be used in situations where instability exists and no surgical procedure has been done.[152] A Yale brace is indicated in stable hangman's fractures, or in type I odontoid fractures.

REFERENCE

1. Ahlgren P: Amipaque myelography: the side effects compared with Dimer X. Neuroradiology 9: 197, 1975
2. Ahlgren P: Amipaque myelography without late adhesive arachnoid changes. Neuroradiology 14: 231, 1978
3. Alexander E: Posterior fusions of the cervical spine. Clin Neurosurg 28: 273, 1981
4. Albin MS, White RJ, Locke GE: Treatment of spinal cord injury by selective hypothermic perfusion. Surg Forum 16: 423, 1965
5. Albin MS, White RJ, Locke GE, Kretchmer HE: Spinal cord hypothermia by localized perfusion cooling. Nature 210: 1059, 1966
6. Albin MS, White RJ, Yashon D, Harris LS: Events or localized cooling on spinal cord trauma. J Trauma 9: 1000, 1969
7. Anderson DK, Means ED, Waters TR, Green ES: Microvascular perfusion and metabolism in injured spinal cord after methylprednisolone treatment. J Neurosurg 56: 106, 1982
8. Ashford T, Palmerio C, Fine: Structure analogue in vascular muscle to the functional disorder in refractory traumatic shock and reversal by corticosteroid: electron microscopic evaluation. Ann Surg 164: 575, 1966
9. Assenmacher DR, Ducker TB: Experimental traumatic paraplegia: the vascular and pathologic changes seen in reversible and irreversible spinal cord lesions. J Bone Joint Surg 53: 671, 1971
10. Baker RA, Hillman BJ, McLennan JE et al: Sequelae of metrizamide myelography in 200 examinations. AJR 130: 499, 1978
11. Bell HS: Paralysis of both arms from injury of the upper portion of the pyramidal decussation: "cruciate paralysis." J Neurosurg 33: 376, 1970
12. Bentsen JR: Comparison of metrizamide with other myelographic agents. Clin Orthop 127: 111, 1977
13. Black P, Markowitz RS: Experimental spinal cord injury in monkeys: comparison of steroids and local hypothermia. Surg Forum 22: 409, 1971
14. Bohlman H: Traumatic fractures of upper thoracic spine with paralysis: a study of 180 cases. J Bone Joint Surg 56A: 1229, 1974
15. Bohlman H, Ducker T, Lucas J: Spine and spinal cord injuries. p. 661. In Rothman RH, Simeone FA (eds): The Spine. WB Saunders, Philadelphia, 1982
16. Bosch A, Stauffer S, Nickel V: Incomplete traumatic quadriplegia: a ten year review. JAMA 216: 473, 1971
17. Bose B, Northop BE, Osterholm JL et al: Reanalysis of central cord injury management. Neurosurgery 15: 367, 1984
18. Braakman R, Penning L: Injuries of the cervical spine. p. 227. In Vinken PJ, Bruyn GW (eds): Injuries of the Cervical Spine and Spinal Cord. Part I, Handbook of Clinical Neurology. American Elsevier, New York, 1976
19. Brockett TO, Condon N: Comparison of the wedge turning frame and kinetic treatment table in the acute cord of spinal cord injury patient. Surg Neurol 22: 53, 1984
20. Bremer AM, Nguyen TQ: Internal metal plate fixation combined with anterior interbody fusion in cases of cervical spine injury. Neurosurgery 12: 649, 1983
21. Bucy PC: Acute cervical spinal injury. Surg Neurol 20: 427, 1983
22. Cahill DW, Bellegarigue R, Ducker TB: Bilateral facet to spinous process fusion after trauma. Neurosurgery 13: 1, 1983
23. Cameron HV, Jacob R, MacNob I et al: Use of polymethylmethacrylate to enchance screw fixation in bone. J Bone Joint Surg 57A: 655, 1975
24. Carol M, Ducker T: Further development of a posterior rodding system for cervical spine fractures. Presented at 12th Annual Meeting, Cervical Spine Research Society, New Orleans, 1984
25. Carol M, Ducker TB, Byrnes DP: Mini-myelogram in cervical spinal cord trauma. Neurosurgery 7(3): 219, 1980
26. Carol M, Ducker TB, Byrnes DP: Acute care of spinal cord injury: A challenge to the emergency medicine clinician. Crit Care Q 7, 1979
27. Casper W: Anterior plate of the cervical spine. Presented at Joint Meeting, Cushey and Congress Societies, Florida, 1985
28. Chan RC, Schweigel JF, Thompson GB: Halo

thoracic brace immobilization in 188 patients with acute cervical spine injuries. J Neurosurg 58: 508, 1983

29. Clendenon NR, Allen N, Gordon WA et al: Inhibition of $N_a{}^+$-K^+ ATP-ase activity following experimental spinal cord trauma. J Neurosurg 49: 563, 1978

30. Cloward RB: Acute cervical injuries. Clin Symp 32: 15, 1980

31. Cooper PR, Maravella KR, Sklor FH et al: Halo immobilization of cervical spine fractures. Indications and results. J Neurosurg 50: 603, 1979

32. Cowely RA, Dunham CM: Shock Trauma/Critical Care Manual. University Press, Baltimore, 1983.

33. Davidson C: General pathological considerations in injuries of the spinal cord. p. 515. In Brock S (ed): Injuries of the Brain and Spinal Cord and Their Coverings. Springer Verlag, New York, 1960

34. De Jesus-Greenburg DA: Acute spinal cord injury and hyperbaric oxygen therapy: a new adjunct in management. J Neurosurg 12: 155, 1980

35. de la Torre JC: Chemotherapy of spinal cord trauma. p. 291. In Windle W (ed): The Spinal Cord and its Reaction to Traumatic Injury. Marcel Dekker, New York, 1980

36. de la Torre JC: Spinal cord injury. Review of basic and applied research. Spine 6: 315, 1981

37. de la Torre JC, Johnson CM, Goode DJ, Mullan S: Pharmologic treatment and evaluation of permanent experimental spinal cord trauma. Neurology 25: 508, 1975

38. de la Torre JC, Surgeon JW, Hill PK, Khan T: DMSO in the treatment of brain infarction: basic considerations. In Hallenbeck JM, Greenbaum L (eds): Arterial Air Embolism and Acute Stroke. Undersea Medical Society, Bethesda, Maryland, 1977

39. Demopoulos HB, Flamm ES, Poelronigro DD, Seligman ML: The free radical pathology and the microcirculation in the major central nervous system disorders. Acta Physiol Scand (Suppl). 49(2): 91, 1970

40. Demopoulos HB, Milvy P, Kakri S, Ransohoff J: Molecular aspects of membrane structure in cerebral edema. p. 29. In Reuben HJ, Schurmann K (eds): Steroids and Brain Edema. Springer Verlag, Vienna, New York, 1972

41. Dohrmann GT, Wagner FC, Bucy PC: The micro vasculature in transitory traumatic paraplegia: an electron microscopic study in the monkey. J Neurosurg 35: 263–71, 1971

42. Dohrmann GJ, Wagner FC, Bucy PC: Transitory traumatic paraplegia: electron microscopy of early alterations in myelinated nerve fibers. J Neurosurg 36: 407, 1972

43. Ducker TB: Experimental injury of the spinal cord. p. 2. In Vinlan PJ, Bryn AW (eds): Handbook of Clinical Neurology, volume 25. Elsevier, New York, 1976

44. Ducker TB, Assenmacher DR: The pathologic circulation in experimental cord injury. VA Clinic, Spinal Cord Injury Conference 18: 10, 1969

45. Ducker TB, Hamit HF: Experimental treatments of acute spinal cord injury. J Neurosurg 30: 693, 1969

46. Ducker TB, Kindt GW: The effect of trauma on the vasomotor control of spinal cord blood flow. Curr Top Surg Res 3: 163, 1971

47. Ducker TB, Russo GL, Bellagarigue R, Lucas JT: Complete sensorimotor paralysis after cord injury: mortality, recovery and therapeutics implications. J Trauma 19:837, 1979

48. Ducker TB, Salcman M, Daniell HB: Experimental cord trauma III. Therapeutic effect of immobilization and pharmacologic agents. Surg Neuro 10: 71, 1978

49. Ducker TB, Salcman M, Perot PL, Jr et al: Experimental spinal cord trauma I. Correlation of blood flow, tissue oxygen, and neurologic status in the dog. Surg Neurol 10: 60, 1978

50. Dutman RH, Lellehei RC: Circulatory collapse and shock. p. 119. In Schwartz RI (ed): Principles of Surgery. McGraw-Hill, New York, 1969

51. Eidelberg E, Statten E, Watkins LJ, Smith JS: Treatment of experimental injury in ferrets. Surg Neurol 6: 243, 1976

52. Eismont FJ, Bohlman HH: Posterior methylmethacrylate fixation for cervical spine trauma. Spine 6: 347, 1981

53. Epstein N, Hood DC, Ransohoff J: Gastrointestinal bleeding in patients with spinal cord trauma: effects of steriods. Cimetadine and mini-dose heparin. J Neurosurg 54: 16, 1981

54. Faden AI, Jacobs TP, Holaday JW: A possible pathophysiologic role for endorphine in spinal cord injury. Fed Proc 39: 762, 1980

55. Faden AI, Jacobs TP, Holaday JW: Opiate antagonist improves neurologic recovery after spinal injury. Science 211: 493, 1981

56. Faden AI, Jacobs TP, Mongey E, Holaday JW: Endorphins in experimental spinal injury: therapeutic effect of naloxone. Ann Neurol 10: 326, 1981

57. Faden AI, Jacobs TP, Patrick DH, Smith MT: Megadose corticosteroid therapy following experimental traumatic spinal injury. J Neurosurg 60: 712, 1984

58. Faden AI, Jacobs TP, Smith MT, Holaday JW: Comparison of thyrotropin releasing hormone (TRH), naloxone, and dexamethasone treatments in esperimental spinal injury. Neurology 33: 673, 1983

59. Fairholm DJ, Turnball IM: Microangiographic

study and experimental spinal cord injuries. J Neurosurg 35: 277, 1979

60. Fox JL, Yasergil MG: The relief of the intracranial vasospasm: an experimental study with methylprednisolone and cortisol. Surg Neurol 3: 214, 1975

61. Frankel HL, Hancock DO, Hystop G et al: The value of postural reduction in the initial management of closed injuries of the spine with paraplegia and tetraplegia. Paraplegia 7: 178, 1969

62. Gamache FW, Myera RAM, Ducker TB, Cowley RA: The clinical application of hyperbaric oxygen therapy in spinal cord injury: a preliminary report. Surg Neurol 15: 85, 1981

63. Goodman JH, Bingham G, Hunt WE: Platelet aggregation in spinal cord injury. Ultrastructural observations. Arch Neurol 36: 197, 1979

64. Green BA, Kahn T, Klose KJ: A comparative study of steroid therapy in acute experimental spinal cord injury. Surg Neurol 13: 91, 1980

65. Greenberg RP, Ducker TB: Evoked potential in the clinical neurosciences. J Neurosurg 56: 1, 1982

66. Griffiths IR: Spinal cord blood flow in dogs: the effect of blood pressure. J Neuro Neurosurg Psychiatry 36: 914, 1973

67. Griffiths IR: Vasogenic edema following acute and chronic spinal cord compression in the dog. J Neurosurg 42: 155, 1975

68. Gottman L: Spinal Cord Injuries Blackwell, London, 1973

69. Hall ED: Glucocorticoid effects on central nervous excitability and synaptic transmission. Int Rev Neurobiol 23: 165, 1982

70. Hall ED, Braughler JM: Glucocorticoid mechanisms in acute spinal cord injury: a review and therapeutic rationale. Surg Neurol 18(5): 320, 1982

71. Hansebout RR, Blomquist GA: Acrylic spinal fusion: a 20 year clinical series and technical note. J Neurosurg 53: 606, 1980

72. Hansebout RR, Tanner JA, Romero-Sierra C: Current status of spinal cord cooling in the treatment of acute spinal cord injury. Spine 9: 508, 1984

73. Harrington KD: Anterior cord decompression and spinal immobilization for patients with metastatic lesions of the spine. J Neurosurg 61: 107, 1984

74. Hasegawa T, Kubota T, Harahide I et al: Symptomatic duplication of the vertebral artery. Surg Neurol 20: 244, 1983

75. Hayashi N, de la Torre JC, Green BA: Regional spinal cord blood flow and tissue oxygen content after spinal cord trauma. Surg Forum 31: 461, 1980

76. Heider JS, Weiss MH, Rosenberg AW et al: Management of cervical spinal cord trauma in southern California. J Neurosurg 43: 732, 1975

77. Herrmann HD: Metal plate fixation after anterior fusion of unstable fracture dislocation of the cervical spine. Acta Neurochir (Wien) 32: 101, 1975

78. Higgins AC, Pearlstein RD, Mullen JB, Nashold BS: Effects of hyperbaric oxygen therapy on long tract neuronal conduction in the acute phase of spinal cord injury. J Neurosurg 55: 501, 1981

79. Hillal S: Reported at postgraduate course in neuroradiology, Communicate–Commentary May, 1979

80. Holback RH, Wassmann H, Hohenluchter RL et al: Clinical course of spinal lesions treated with hyperbaric oxygenation (HO). Acta Neurochir (Wien) 31: 297, 1975

81. Holdsworth F: Fractures, dislocations and fracture dislocations of the spine. J Bone Joint Surg 52: 1534

82. Hollenbeck JM, Farlow TW, Jr.: Prostaglandin I_2 and indomethacin prevent impairment of postischemic brain reperfusion in the dog. Stroke 10: 629, 1979

83. Hollenbeck JM, Jacobs TP, Faden AI: Combined PGI_2, indomethacin, and heparin improves neurological recovery after spinal trauma in cats. J Neurosurg 58: 749, 1983

84. Holness RO, Huestis WS, Howes WJ, Largilte RA: Posterior stabilization with an interlaminar clamp in cervical injuries: technical note and review of the long-term experience with method. Neurosurgery 14: 318, 1984

85. Hortzog JT, Fisher RG, Snow C: Spinal cord trauma: effect of hyperbaric oxygen therapy. Proceedings, Veterans Administration Spinal Cord Injury Conference, 17: 70, 1969

86. Howett WM, Turnbolt IM: Effects of hypothermia and methysergide on recovery from experimental paraplegia. Can J Surg 15: 179, 1972

87. Ito T, Allen M, Yashon D: A mitochondrial lesion in experimental spinal cord trauma. J Neurosurg 48: 434, 1978

88. Johnson RM, Wolf IP: Stability. In The Cervical Spine Research Editorial Subcommittee (eds): The Cervical Spine. JB Lippincott, Philadelphia, 1983

89. Jones RF, Unsworth IP, Marosszcky JE: Hyperbaric oxygen and acute spinal cord injuries in humans. Med J Aust 2: 573, 1978

90. Kao CC, Chang LW: The mechanisms of spinal cord cavilation following spinal cord transection. Part I. A correlated histochemical study. J Neurosurg 46: 197, 1977

91. Kao CC, Chang LW, Bloodworth JMDJ: The mechanism of spinal cord cavitation following

spinal cord transection. Part 2: Electron microscopic observations. J Neurosurg 46: 745, 1977

92. Kakari S, Decrescito V, Tomasula JJ et al: Distribution of biogenic amines in contused feline spinal cord. J. Histochem Cytochem 21: 408, 1973

93. Kelly D, Lassiter KRL, Calogers JA et al: Effects of hyperbaric oxygenation and tissue oxygen studies in experimental paraplegia. J Neurosurg 33: 554, 1970

94. Kelly DL, Jr., Lassiter KRL, Vongsvivut A et al: Effects of local hypothermia and tissue oxygen studies in experimental paraplegia. J Neurosurg 36: 425–429, 1972

95. Kobrine A: Injuries of the spinal cord, nerve roots and spine. In Hoff J (ed). Neurosurgery. Harper and Row, Philadelphia, 1982

96. Kobrine AI, Doyle TF, Martins AN: Local spinal cord blood flow in experimental traumatic myelopathy. J Neurosurg 42: 144, 1975

97. Kobrine AI, Evans DE, Rizzoli HV: Experimental acute balloon compression of the spinal cord: factors affecting disappearance and return of the spinal evoked response. J Neurosurg 51: 841, 1979

98. Koons DD, Gildenberg PL, Dohn DF, Henoch M: Local hypothermia in the treatment of spinal cord injuries: review of seven cases. Cleve Clin Q 39: 109, 1972

99. Leader W: Statistical reports for traumatic spinal cord injury (1975–1976). Florida Central Registry for Severely Disabled, 1976

100. Leo JS, Bergeron RT, Kricheff II, Benjamin MV: Metrizamide myelography for cervical cord injuries. Radiology 129: 707, 1978

101. Lesoin F, Bovasakao N, Cama A et al: Post-traumatic fixation of the thoracolumber spine using Roy-Camille plates. Surg Neurol 21: 581, 1984

102. Lesoin F, Cuma A, Lozes G et al: The anterior approach and plates in lower cervical post-traumatic lesions. Surg Neurol 21: 581, 1984

103. Lesoin F, Jomin M, Viaud C: Expanding bolt for anterior cervical spine osteosynthesis: technical note. Neurosurgery 12: 150, 1983

104. Levy DE, Dougherty JH, Jr., Racolinson D et al: Treatment of electrogenically induced platelet aggregation. J Cereb Blood Flow Metab 1 (Suppl): S295, 1981

105. Lim R, Mullan S: Enhancement of resistance of glial cells by dimethyl sulfoxide against sonic disruption. Ann NY Acad Sci 243: 358, 1975

106. Lucas JT, Ducker TB: Recovery in spinal cord injury. Adv Neurosurg 7: 281, 1979

107. Maeda N: Experimental studies on the effect of decompression procedures and hyperbaric oxygenation for the treatment of spinal cord injury. J of Nara Med Assoc. 16: 429, 1965

108. Markelonis G, Garbus S: Alterations of intracellular oxidative metabolism as stimuli evoking prostaglandin biosynthesis. Prostaglandins 10: 1087, 1975

109. Maynard FM, Reynolds GG, Fountain S et al: Neurologic prognosis after traumatic quadriplegia: regional spinal injury system. J Neurosurg 50: 611, 1979

110. McCallum JE, Bennett MH: DMSO as a therapeutic agent in chronic spinal cord compression. Abstract from 26th Annual Meeting, Congress of Neurological Surgeons, New Orleans, 1976

111. Meacham WF, McPherson WF: Local hypothermia in the treatment of acute injuries in the spinal cord. South Med J 6: 95, 1973

112. Means ED, Anderson DK, Waters TR, Kalaf L: Effect of methylprednisolone in compression trauma to the feline spinal cord. J Neurosurg 55: 200, 1981

113. Michaelis LS: International inquiry on neurological terminology and prognosis in paraplegia and tetraplegia. Paraplegia 7: 1, 1969

114. Moncada S, Gryglewski RJ, Bunting S, Vane JR: A lipid peroxide inhibits enzyme in blood vessel microsomes that generates from prostaglandin endoperoxides the substance (prostaglandin X) which prevents platelet aggregation. Prostaglandins 12: 715, 1976

115. Murphy MJ, Sothwick WO: Posterior approaches and fusions. In The Cervical Spine Research Editorial Subcommittee (eds): The Cervical Spine. JP Lippincott, Philadelphia, 1983

116. Naftchi NE, Demery M, Demopoulos H, Flamm E: The ameliorating effect of pharmacological agents on the traumatically injured spinal cord. p. 373. In Parvery H, Parvey S (eds): Advances in Experimental Medicine: A Centene Tribute to Claude Bernard. Elsevier North Holland, Amsterdam, New York, 1980

117. Ono K, Tada K: Metal prosthesis of the cervical vertebra. J Neurosurg 42: 562, 1975

118. Osterholm JL, Matthews GJ: Altered norepinephrine metabolism following experimental spinal cord injury, Part VI. Relationship to hemorrhagic necrosis. J Neurosurg 36: 386, 1972

119. Padolsky S, Baroff LJ, Simon RR et al: Efficacy of cervical immobilization methods. J Trauma 23(6): 461, 1983

120. Panjabi MM, Hopper W, White AA, Keggi K: Posterior spine stabilization with methylmethacrylate—biomechanical testing of a surgical specimen. Spine 2: 241, 1977

121. Panjabi M, White A: Basic biomechanics of the spine. Neurosurgery 7: 76, 1980

122. Proto DJ, Runnels JB, Jameson RM: The injured cervical spine. Immediate and long-term immobilization with the halo. JAMA 224: 591, 1973

123. Raive SE, Roth RH, Boodle-Biber M et al: Nor-

epinephrine levels in experimental spinal cord trauma. Part I. Biochemical study of hemorrhagic necrosis. J Neurosurg 46: 342, 1977

124. Raive SE, Roth RH, Collins WF: Norepinephrine levels in experimental spinal cord trauma. Part II. Histopathological study of hemorrhagic necrosis. J Neurosurg 46: 350, 1977

125. Rand RW, Crandall PH: Central spinal cord syndrome in hyperextension injuries of the cervical spine. J Bone Joint Surg 44A: 1415, 1962

126. Riggins R, Kraus J: The risk of neurological damage with fractures of the vertebrae. J Trauma 17: 126, 1977

127. Roaf R: A study of the biomechanics of spinal injuries. J Bone Joint Surg 42B: 810, 1950

128. Rogers WA: Fractures and dislocations of the cervical spine: an end result study. J Bone Joint Surg 39-A: 341, 1957

129. Rubini L, Columbo F: Modified technique for local cooling in spinal cord injuries. Spine 6: 417, 1981

130. Sackett JF, Strother CM, Quaglieri CE et al: Metrizamide-CSF contrast medium: analysis of clinical application in 215 patients. Radiology, 123: 779, 1977

131. Saul TG, Ducker TB: Treatment of spinal cord injury. In Cowley RA, Trump BF (eds): Pathology of Shock, Anoxia, and Ischemia. Williams & Willkins, Baltimore, 1982

132. Schneider RC: The syndrome of acute anterior spinal cord injury. J Neurosurg 12: 95, 1955

133. Schneider RC, Crosby EC, Russo RH et al: Traumatic spinal cord syndromes and their managements. Clin Neurosurg 20: 424, 1973

134. Selker RG: Icewater irrigation of the spinal cord. Surg Forum 22: 411, 1970

135. Senter HJ, Venes JL: Altered blood flow and secondary injury in experimental spinal cord trauma. J Neurosurg 49: 569, 1978

136. Senter HJ, Venes JL: Loss of autoregulation and posttraumatic ischemia following experimental spinal cord trauma. J Neurosurg 50: 198, 1979

137. Senter HJ, Venes JL, Kauer JL: Alteration of posttraumatic ischemia in experimental spinal cord trauma by a central vervous system depressant. J Neurosurg 50: 207, 1979

138. Skaple IO: Adhesive arachnoditis following lumbar radiculography with water soluble contrast agents: a clinical report with special reference to metrizamide. Radiology 121: 647, 1976

139. Skaple IO: Adhesive arachnoiditis following lumbar myelography. Spine 3: 61, 1978

140. Skaple IO, Amundsen P: Thoracic and cervical myelography with metrizamide: clinical experiences with a water-soluble non-ionic constrast medium. Radiology 116: 101, 1975

141. Szczklik A, Gryglewski RJ, Nizankowska E et al: Pulmonary and anti-platelet effects of intravenous and inhaled prostocyclins in man. Prostaglandins 16: 651, 1978

142. Tater CH: Acute spinal cord injury in primates produced by inflatable extradural cuff. Can J Surg 16: 22, 1973

143. Tateson JE, Moncada S, Vane JR: Effects of prostaeyclia (PGX) on cyclic AMP concentration in human platelets, Protaglandins 13: 389, 1977

144. Theirnprasit P, Bantli H, Bloedel JR, Chou SN: Effect of delay at local cooling on experimental spinal cord injury. J Neurosurg 42: 150, 1975

145. Torre JC, Johnson CM, Goode DJ, Mullan S: Pharmocologic treatment and evaluation of permanent experimental spinal cord trauma. Neurology (Minn) 25: 508, 1975

146. Trafton P: Spinal cord injury. Surg Clin North Am 62: 61, 1982

147. Tsubokawa T, Nokamura S, Taguma N et al: The circulatory disturbance of spinal cord injury and its response to local cooling therapy. Neurol Med Chir 15: 87, 1975

148. Wagner FC, Chehrazi B: Early decompression and neurological outcome in acute cervical spinal cord injuries. J Neurosurg 56: 699, 1982

149. White AA, III, Panjabe MM: Clinical Biomechanics of the Spine. JB Lippincott, Philadelphia, 1978

150. White RJ: Current status of spinal cord cooling. Clin Neurosurg 20: 400, 1973

151. Whitehill R, Reger I, Fox E et al: The use of methymethacrylate as an instantaneous fusion mass in posterior cervical fusions: a canine in vivo experimental model. Spine 9: 246, 1984

152. Wolf JW, Johnson RM: Cervical Orthoses. In Cervical Spine Research Editorial Subcommittee (eds): The Cervical Spine. JB Lippincott, Philadelphia, 1983

153. Woods JE, Anderson CF, DeWeerd JH et al: High dose intravenously administered methylprednisolone in renal transplantation. JAMA 22(3): 896, 1973

154. Yeo JD, Lowry C, McKenzie B: Preliminary report of ten patients with spinal cord injuries treated with hyperbaric oxygen. Med J Aust 2: 572, 1978

155. Yeo JD, McKenzie B, Hardwood B, Kidman A: Treatment of paraplegic sheep with hyperbaric oxygenation. Med J Aust 1: 538, 1976

156. Young J, Dexter W: Neurological recovery distal to the zone of injury in 172 cases of closed traumatic spinal cord injury. Paraplegia 16: 39, 1978

157. Young W, Flamm ES, Demopulos HB, Thomasula JJ, DeCrescito V: Effect of naloxone on posttraumatic ischemia in experimental spinal contusion. Neurosurg 55: 209, 1981

33

Maxillofacial Injuries

Paul N. Manson

Three events within the past 10 years have revolutionized the treatment of maxillofacial injuries: computed tomographic (CT) scanning, improved diagnostic abilities and supportive care for the multiply injured patient, and the technique of extended open reduction of facial bone fractures with immediate bone grafting. These three advantages have permitted a quantum leap in the functional and aesthetic results achieved from the treatment of maxillofacial injuries. The roots of the current concepts of facial injury treatment extend back to World War I, when the large number of facial and cranial injuries required the development of basic principles of maxillofacial surgery and reconstruction.[1,2] Continued improvements have been made, stimulated by the experience gained in the conflicts of World War II and the Korean and Vietnam experiences; these principles have been further refined with the knowledge gained from the management of civilian injuries. Improved knowledge of wound healing, the advent of antibiotics, critical care, safe anesthesia, and improved supportive facil-

ities have permitted the advances in the care of maxillofacial injuries.

The absolute incidence of severe facial injuries is decreasing; this is attributed to the continued efforts of legislation to improve the mechanical safety of motor vehicles.[10,11] In addition, legislation to reduce the maximum speed limit and reduce the incidence of alcohol-related traffic accidents, as well as mandatory seatbelt requirements have protected the victims of motor vehicle accidents from the more severe facial injuries.

The etiology of severe facial injuries is frequently a motor vehicle or motorcycle accident.[35] Most victims are multiply injured; those with facial injuries accompanying multiple system injuries require a simultaneous coordinated effort of multiple-injury specialty teams. Other common causes of facial injuries are assaults, altercations, bicycle accidents, athletic injuries, and home accidents such as falls.

The face is crucial to communication, nutrition, ventilation, and the perception of sen-

983

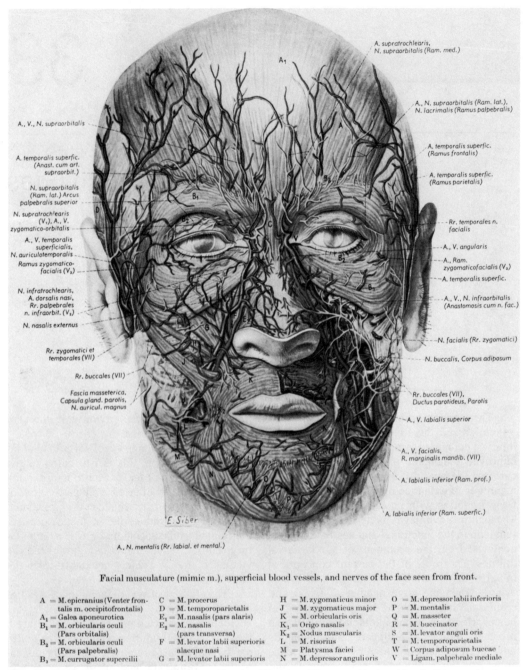

Facial musculature (mimic m.), superficial blood vessels, and nerves of the face seen from front.

A = M. epicranius (Venter frontalis m. occipitofrontalis)	C = M. procerus	H = M. zygomaticus minor	O = M. depressor labii inferioris
A₁ = Galea aponeurotica	D = M. temporoparietalis	J = M. zygomaticus major	P = M. mentalis
B₁ = M. orbicularis oculi (Pars orbitalis)	E₁ = M. nasalis (pars alaris)	K = M. orbicularis oris	Q = M. masseter
B₂ = M. orbicularis oculi (Pars palpebralis)	E₂ = M. nasalis (pars transversa)	K₁ = Origo nasalis	R = M. buccinator
B₃ = M. currugator supercilii	F = M. levator labii superioris alaeque nasi	K₂ = Nodus muscularis	S = M. levator anguli oris
	G = M. levator labii superioris	L = M. risorius	T = M. temporoparietalis
		M = Platysma faciei	W = Corpus adiposum buccae
		N = M. depressor anguli oris	V = Ligam. palpebrale mediale

FIG. 33-1 The blood supply of facial tissues. (Pernkopf E: Atlas of Topographical and Applied Human Anatomy. Urban & Schwarzenberg, Baltimore, 1980.)

sory stimuli and as the center for nonverbal communication through facial expression. Our society prizes attractiveness and the ability to communicate effectively; we recognize and judge one another with verbal and nonverbal communication initiated through facial expression. These essential functions are permanently altered by inadequate or ill-timed treatment of major facial injuries. Time and time again we have been impressed with the fact that both functional and esthetic disability may be minimized or avoided with prompt definitive diagnosis and reconstruction. The proper early treatment of maxillofacial injuries need not compromise the survival of the patient and will repay the traumatologist with superior results and grateful patients who are more fully able to return to productive roles in society.

ANATOMIC CONSIDERATIONS

The face consists of soft tissue and bone. In the soft tissue are incorporated the orifices for communication, vision, hearing, and respiration and ingestion. The skin and subcutaneous tissues have a generous blood and lymphatic supply (Fig. 33-1). Beneath the skin and subcutaneous fat are located the mimetic muscles (Fig. 33-2), which provide for facial expression. They frequently attach to the skin, and their proper realignment is an integral feature of the restoration of normal facial expression. Beneath this layer is a system of bony structural supports that enclose the oral, nasal, orbital, and cranial cavities (Fig. 33-3). This membranous facial bone is vascular and consists

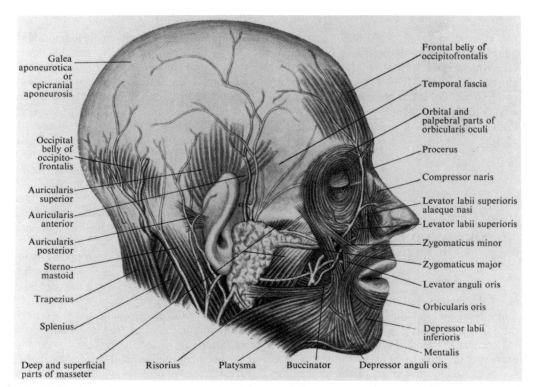

FIG. 33-2 The muscles of facial expression. (Lockhart RD: Anatomy of the Human Body, 2nd ed. Faber & Faber, Philadelphia, 1965.)

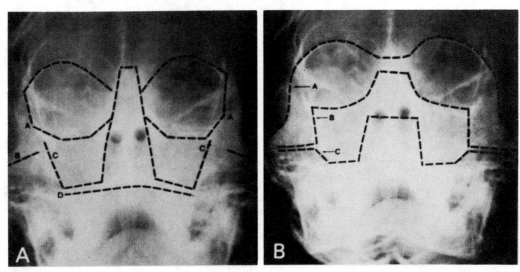

FIG. 33-3 Example of bony structural supports of the midface, which represent thicker areas of bone that reinforce the facial skeleton. These are the areas where fracture diagnosis and treatment are directed. (Ayella, RJ: Radiologic Management of the Massively Traumatized Patient. © 1979 The Williams & Wilkins Co., Baltimore.)

of alternating areas of thin and thick bone[4,28,71,107] that reinforce the facial architecture with a system of horizontal and vertical structural supports (Fig. 33-3). The diagnosis and treatment of facial bone fractures consists largely of identifying and reconstructing injury to these buttresses of the facial skeleton (Fig. 33-3).

MECHANISM OF FACIAL INJURIES

A force delivered to a portion of the bony face causes an inbending in the area in which the force is applied.[34] A reciprocal "outbending" occurs in areas of weakness. For the zygoma, for instance, a blow to the malar eminence causes an inbending of the area of the body of the zygoma, and reciprocal deformation occurs at the area of the zygomaticofrontal junction and zygomaticomaxillary junctions at the rim of the orbit. These areas along with the junction of the zygoma to the temporal bone through the arch and to the maxilla through the zygomaticomaxillary buttress and to the sphenoid in the lateral orbit are the areas in which fracture lines disconnect the zygoma from adjacent bones. The forces necessary to cause fractures are illustrated in Figure 33-4. The tolerances of the human face to impact are as follows:[66,108] nasal bones, 35 to 80 G; zygoma, 50 to 80 G; mandibular condyles, 70 to 110 G; central maxilla, 120 to 180 G; and frontal bone, 150 to 200 G. Any of these forces may result in cerebral injury with unconsciousness or cervical injury as well as the facial bone fracture.

Maxillofacial injuries are frequent and often dramatic; they easily divert attention from more occult injuries. Facial injuries almost always benefit from early appropriate consultation despite the necessity to treat in priority life-threatening injuries. The plans and recommendations provided by the facial consultant must be integrated with those formulated for the management of other injuries to form a definitive plan for patient care. Coordination of effort permits life-saving procedures to be performed simultaneous with those that achieve maximal facial functional rehabilitation. Often

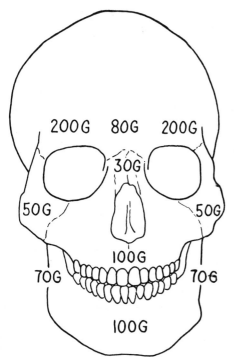

FIG. 33-4. Tolerance of the facial bones to impact. G = force equal to that of gravity at Earth surface. (Luce EA, Tubbs TD, Moore AM: Review of 1,000 major facial fractures and associated injuries. Plast Reconstr Surg 63:26, © 1979, The Williams & Wilkins Co., Baltimore.)

simultaneous operations may be performed by multiply specialty teams. Continuous monitoring of all organ systems during the resuscitation and treatment of facial injuries is an essential criterion for management; and comprehensive monitoring of all organ systems provides for the safe treatment of maxillofacial trauma.

ORGANIZATION OF TREATMENT

The organization of maxillofacial injury treatment may be conceptualized in three categories: (1) emergency treatment, (2) early treatment, and (3) elective procedures.

Emergency Treatment

The emergency treatment of facial injuries is directed toward those events that require immediate action for the prevention of life-threatening complications. These include (1) provision for an airway, (2) control of hemorrhage, (3) prevention of aspiration, (4) detection of cervical spine or cord injury, and (5) detection and evaluation of intracranial injury.

Early Maxillofacial Injury Treatment

Early treatment is that provided within 24 hours of the injury and usually consists of a clinical and radiographic examination on which are based the diagnosis and treatment plan for the maxillofacial injury. Often definitive treatment of the injury is rendered during this period. It has been our experience that better aesthetic and functional results are more easily obtained if treatment can be rendered during this period. If the general condition of the patient is appropriate and can be safely monitored on a continuous basis, most maxillofacial injuries may be definitively treated. Soft tissue wounds may be closed, arch bars for the immobilization of jaw fractures are applied, and interfragment wiring of fractures is performed.

Elective Treatment of Facial Injuries

The elective treatment of facial injuries is that performed within several weeks of the injury. It is advisable to complete diagnostic and therapeutic intervention as early as possible, and certainly within 10 to 14 days, the period during which union of facial bone fractures takes place. The advantages of delaying treatment of facial injuries have been over-emphasized in the literature on maxillofacial trauma.

The emphasis on delayed treatment originated during an era of inadequate diagnostic and support facilities. Fortunately, the accuracy of current assessment protocols now provides maxillofacial surgeons with many more options in selecting the timing of facial injury treatment. At the Maryland Institute for Emergency Medical Services Systems (MIEMSS), most patients have early definitive treatment of facial injuries. This treatment has not been accompanied by increased mortality or morbidity related to either the facial injury or the management of other organ systems.

COMPREHENSIVE EVALUATION AND MONITORING

Fifty to 70 percent of patients with facial injuries demonstrate simultaneous injury to other organ systems.[35,66,101] Patients with multiple system injuries require the systematic evaluation of all organ systems according to a protocol and continuous monitoring throughout resuscitation and operative treatment. Obviously, evaluation of head, spine, and chest trauma, the placement of arterial and venous lines, appropriate catheterization, consideration of interventricular pressure monitoring, and peritoneal lavage are essential decisions and procedures that precede the treatment of maxillofacial injury. It is important to realize that patients with gross facial trauma are sometimes rapidly assigned to maxillofacial surgery services with inadequate initial multisystem evaluation. Diagnostic failures occur in 10 percent of motor vehicle accident victims and are more frequently seen in motorcycle accident victims. These errors include problems with clinical judgment, failure to follow routine systems evaluation, false interpretation of radiographs, and inadequate radiographic or clinical examination.[35,101]

It is incumbent on the maxillofacial surgeon to confirm that a proper evaluation of all organ systems has been performed before undertaking operative intervention.

EMERGENCY TREATMENT OF MAXILLOFACIAL TRAUMA

It has not been well appreciated that maxillofacial injuries can result in early death. The mechanisms are airway obstruction, bleeding, and aspiration. Severe concomitant cervical or cranial injuries frequently prove life-threatening.

Airway Obstruction

Airway obstruction is seen in those patients with injuries that compromise the oral, tracheal, and nasal airways. Concomitant jaw and neck fractures; fractures of the nose and jaws; fractures of the larynx; injuries that result in significant swelling of the floor of the mouth, pharynx, or soft palate area; and burns all may result in swelling with inability to breathe. The multiply fractured mandible, for instance, will cause the tongue to fall back against the pharynx obstructing the airway. Simply holding the jaw forward with the fingers or with a towel clip in the tongue or positioning the patient in the prone position (if safe for other injuries) will improve the airway obstruction from this mechanism. Airway obstruction may be caused by foreign objects such as fractured teeth, denture segments, or bridgework. Only a short period of time exists between the onset of blatant symptoms of respiratory obstruction (noisy respiration, stridor, hoarseness, retraction, drooling, inability to swallow) and the cyanosis that indicates almost complete inability to breathe and impending death. The alert clinician must anticipate respiratory emergency and secure the airway by prophylactic intubation or tracheostomy before complete respiratory obstruction demands a chaotic "crash" intubation or tracheostomy.

It has been difficult to demonstrate a difference between tracheostomy or endotracheal intubation as far as laryngeal damage is concerned. The indications for tracheostomy relate more to the ease of managing the facial fracture than to considerations of laryngeal or tracheal damage. Tracheostomy is usually performed on the following injuries: panfacial fractures (combined maxillary, mandibular, and nasal fractures); the multiply fractured mandible (where the floor of the mouth, tongue, and neck are grossly swollen and intermaxillary fixation is required; maxillary fractures where intermaxillary fixation cannot be delayed); massive soft tissue swelling from blunt injury or burns; and cases in which rigid external fixation would prevent easy reintubation (the use of a headframe or complex internal suspension wires). In patients with jaw fractures, a decision must first be made as to the necessity of placing the patient in intermaxillary fixation during the immediate postoperative period. These patients require either tracheostomy, nasotracheal intubation until full awake, or alert postoperative monitoring for airway management in the emetic stage of anesthesia recovery. Patients with swelling who require immediate intermaxillary fixation are best managed with a tracheostomy. It has been our experience that patients who require intermaxillary fixation, who are comatose, or who have significant chest pathology will not be able to manage their airway satisfactorily within 1 week and are best managed with a tracheostomy at the time of treatment for the facial fracture.

Life-Threatening Hemorrhage

Bleeding from facial lacerations may result in significant hemorrhage, particularly if the temporal artery or other major branches of the external carotid system have been partially transsected. This bleeding may be controlled with digital pressure until precise identification of only the vessel may be accomplished. Blind probing with clamps in the presence of important cranial nerves such as facial nerve branches (Fig. 33-5) must be avoided.[27] It is rare that significant bleeding cannot be controlled with digital pressure.

Major hemorrhage from closed maxillofacial injuries usually results from lacerations of arteries and veins within the walls of fractured sinuses; it presents from the nose and mouth. Nasal bleeding may result from nasal, zygo-matic, orbital, frontal sinus, nasoethmoid, or anterior cranial fossa (dural venous sinus) fractures. Most significant hemorrhage accompanies either LeFort or nasoethmoid fractures. Profuse hemorrhage can be controlled by any of several mechanisms:

MANUAL REDUCTION OF FRACTURE FRAGMENTS

It has been well appreciated that gross malposition of facial bone fractures contributes to brisk facial bleeding. The manual repositioning of fracture fragments (closed reduction) may significantly reduce the hemorrhage observed. This is particularly true of fracture fragments involving sinuses. Intermaxillary fixation of LeFort fractures or of fractures of the mandible frequently reduces the bleeding.

ANTERIOR-POSTERIOR NASAL PACKING

The most important measure for the control of profuse nasopharyngeal bleeding is anterior-posterior packing of the nose. The efficient control of nasal bleeding is accomplished by placing a posterior obturator in the nasopharynx. This may either be a posterior pack or two inflated Foley catheter balloons (Fig.33-6). Many feel that the gauze posterior pack more accurately fits the posterior choanae. The nasal cavity is then packed tightly with antibiotic impregnated gauze against this posterior obturator. The technique is as follows: a catheter is inserted in each nostril and retrieved from the pharynx and brought through the open mouth. A 4 × 4-inch gauze sheet may be tied into a roll with ties; two ties are then individually secured to one of the Foley catheters and the pack is led into the nasopharynx in this fashion. Alternatively, two #30-cc balloon Foley catheters are passed into the pharynx and pulled (after being inflated) to occlude the posterior choanae on each side. Either mechanism establishes a posterior obturator and is adequate. If the gauze is used, a third (center) tie is brought back through the mouth so that it can be used to retrieve the packing when the

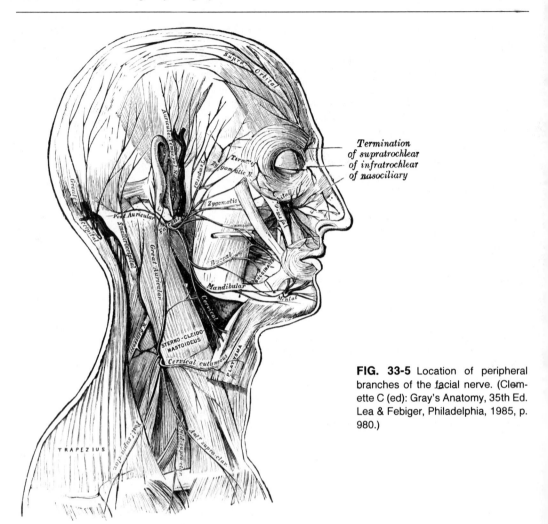

FIG. 33-5 Location of peripheral branches of the facial nerve. (Clemette C (ed): Gray's Anatomy, 35th Ed. Lea & Febiger, Philadelphia, 1985, p. 980.)

pack can be discontinued. Teramycin-soaked Vaseline gauze is then carefully packed into each nasal cavity. The recesses of the nose should be carefully filled to occlude the entire nasal cavity with some pressure. If areas are omitted or if too much emphasis is placed on packing of only the anterior nose, the packing will not function properly to decrease hemorrhage. If nasopharyngeal bleeding continues after packing, the anterior pack should be taken out and replaced, as it is probably not packed tightly enough. The catheters or ties from the posterior packing may be ligated to each other beneath the nasal columella to produce more tension. Any such tie must be relaxed periodically to avoid excessive pressure on the columella and subsequent columella necrosis (Fig. 33-7). In this regard, any tube placed in the nose may necrose the nasal ala if not taped judiciously (Fig. 33-8). Excessive pressure from the packing or from a hematoma may damage the nasal septum. It is usually our habit to relax any ties across the columella after several hours. Nasal packing may be removed after 24 to 72 hours, especially if a CSF leak is present.

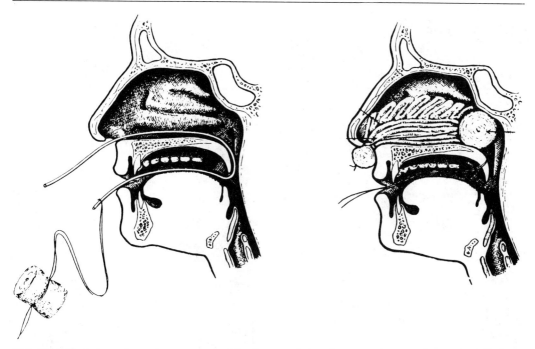

FIG. 33-6 Technique of anterior-posterior packing for control of profuse nasopharyngeal bleeding by pressure of the packing material.

EXTERNAL COMPRESSION DRESSING

A soft circumferential external facial compression dressing may provide additional pressure to soft tissues overlying facial fractures. These external compression dressings may assist in achieving hemostasis but are rarely necessary. Their temporary use has been thought to reduce bleeding in those patients who have not responded to manual reduction of fractures and anterior-posterior nasal packing. Again, excessive pressure on soft tissues over bony prominences may cause soft tissue necrosis.

SELECTIVE ARTERIAL LIGATION

In uncontrolled severe maxillofacial hemorrhage that has not responded to the above maneuvers, arterial ligation may control bleeding. Arterial ligation generally includes the bilateral external carotid and superficial tempo-

ral arteries. This reduces the blood flow through the areas of the internal maxillary artery in LeFort fracture by approximately 80 percent. Although the external carotid arteries themselves may be ligated, such ligation is only associated with a 60 percent blood flow reduction; the addition of the superficial temporal artery ligation further decreases the flow. More selective arterial ligations such as the internal maxillary or ethmoid artery may be performed; however, in the face of acute profuse hemorrhage, these procedures are technically difficult and frequently may be disappointing in reducing blood flow.

COAGULATION FACTORS

Appropriate blood replacement by transfusion and hourly assessment of depleted coagulation factors is imperative in patients with continuing significant blood loss and those receiving multiple transfusions. Coagulation ab-

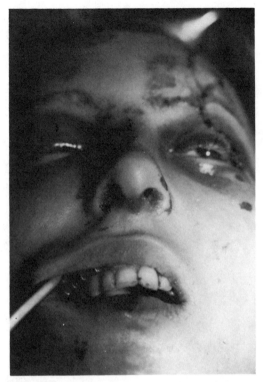

FIG. 33-7 Ties for an anterior-posterior pack that are tied under the columella should be relaxed after several hours or columella necrosis will result.

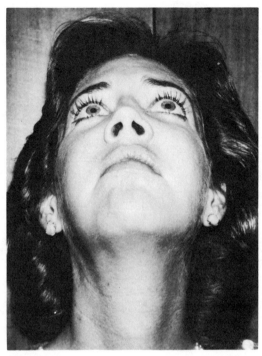

FIG. 33-8 Nasal alar "notch" from an injudiciously taped NG tube that created excessive pressure on the nasal alae.

normalities are commonly noted in patients with massive bleeding. When cerebral injuries exist with major maxillofacial injuries, coagulation abnormalities are noted to occur with surprising repidity.

ASPIRATION

Pulmonary aspiration of oral secretions, gastric contents, or blood frequently accompanies major maxillofacial injury. Patients with cerebral injury are especially susceptible to aspiration. Patients with LeFort or mandibular fractures frequently aspirate a surprising amount of blood. Endotracheal intubation or tracheostomy prevents aspiration in these patients. Aspirated material can be quite toxic to tracheal and pulmonary alveolar lining. Noisy respirations, low arterial oxygen content, and decreased lung compliance accom-

pany an abnormal chest radiograph. Tracheal suction removes and identifies the aspirated material. Therapy depends on the quantity and character of the aspirate.

CERVICAL SPINE INJURIES

Cervical spine injuries frequently accompany maxillofacial trauma.[5,40] Patients with major maxillofacial trauma should be assumed to have a cervical spine injury until proved otherwise. Twenty percent of patients with maxillofacial trauma have a cervical spine injury and 10 percent of patients with cervical spine fractures have an accompanying facial injury.[64] A study of 1,000 patients has shown an association between mandibular fractures and high cervical fractures (Fig. 33-9). Frontal bone injuries (hyperextension injuries) were associated with cervical injuries at all levels. Locations of cervical spine injury that were most frequently missed were high and low cer-

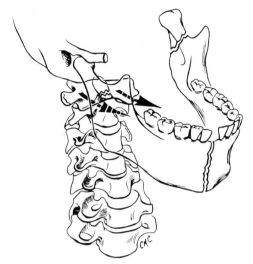

FIG. 33-9 There is an association between mandible fractures and high cervical fractures. The presence of one should alert the surgeon to look for the other.

Fort fractures. Accompanying intracranial injury should be assumed to exist in these patients, and a thorough craniofacial CT scan is mandatory. If patients with significant intracranial injuries require a prolonged general anesthetic, a device that can monitor intracranial pressure such as a Richman screw is inserted as a first step in the operation so that intracranial pressure can be continuously monitored and provide proper notification of deterioration of the intracerebral condition. The combination of intracranial pressure monitoring and thorough CT examination of the skull and brain has permitted proper diagnosis of patients with intracranial injuries and safe anesthesia despite prolonged operative intervention for other injuries.[76] CSF leaks, pneumocephalus, and open skull fractures are discussed in later sections. The prognosis for many brain injuries is surprisingly good.[63,67]

vical fractures. The absence of head or facial trauma does not exclude a significant cervical injury. If the entire cervical spine cannot be visualized, the patient should be managed as if an unstable cervical fracture were present by suitable protection from movement and proper immobilization of the spine. Facial fracture management may vary depending on the kind of cervical fracture present and its immobilization. Some approaches to fractures may not be technically possible if the head cannot be rotated and alternate means of mandibular immobilization employed.

INTRACRANIAL INJURIES

Intracranial injuries frequently accompany maxillofacial trauma.[63] Symptoms produced by anterior intracranial injuries are sometimes few and easily overlooked. Injuries of the frontal lobes, frontal skull, or anterior cranial fossa frequently accompany fractures of the frontal sinus, superior orbit, nasoethmoid, or high Le-

EARLY TREATMENT OF MAXILLOFACIAL TRAUMA

The definitive diagnosis and treatment of the maxillofacial injury is begun once the management of emergent conditions has been accomplished. The first priority is a thorough clinical examination, which is performed as soon as emergency resuscitation measures are complete. The diagnosis of most facial injuries is accomplished by this thorough clinical examination. In most cases, radiographs serve to confirm the diagnosis and perhaps add additional information. The importance of a thorough clinical examination cannot be overemphasized. Facial injuries should be suspected in any patient who has contusions, bruises, lacerations, or evidence of blunt or open injuries to the craniofacial region. The presence of a laceration suggests injury to underlying soft tissue or bone structures. One should assume that there is a fracture under any laceration or bruise until proved otherwise.

An orderly examination of facial structures should be accomplished progressing from either superior to inferior or inferior to superior. The same orderly examination should be conducted when reviewing radiographs of patients with facial injuries. Symptoms produced by facial injuries include pain or localized tenderness, crepitation from areas of underlying bony fracture, numbness in the distribution of a specific nerve, paralysis in the distribution of a specific nerve, malocclusion (an abnormal relationship of the dentition), visual disturbance, facial asymmetry, deformity, obstructed respiration, and bleeding.

The clinical examination begins with an evaluation for symmetry and deformity. Visual inspection of the face permits comparison of one side with the other. Palpation of all bony surfaces follows in an orderly fashion. The orbital rims, the nose, the brows, the zygomatic arches, the malar prominences, the border of the mandible, and the intraoral (put on gloves!) maxillary and mandibular dentition are carefully palpated and visualized to detect bony irregularity, bruise, hematoma, and swelling. Tenderness and crepitation indicate underlying fracture. Next, evaluation of the sensory and motor nerve function in the facial area is

performed. The presence of hypesthesia or anesthesia in the distribution of the sensory areas supplied by the supraorbital, infraorbital, or mental nerve areas should suggest a fracture somewhere along the paths of these sensory nerves. Extraocular movements (C.N. III, IV, VI) and the muscles of facial expression (C.N. VII) must be examined in the cooperative patient. Pupillary size and symmetry, eyelid excursion, and the presence of double vision or visual loss are noted. The excursion and deviation of the jaws, the presence of pain when opening the jaw, the relationship of the teeth and the symmetry of the dental arch, and the ability to bring the teeth into maximum intercuspation are important keys to the diagnosis of patients with fractures involving the dentition. A finger in the ear canal can detect condylar movement. The presence of fractured or missing teeth should imply more significant maxillary or mandibular injury, which must be confirmed with further examination and appropriate radiographs. Patients with dentures or bridge work should have these items removed to permit accurate evaluation. The presence of hyphema or visual abnormalities such as

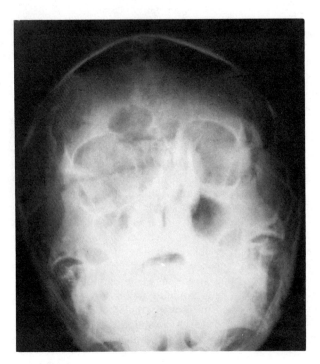

FIG. 33-10 Water's view of the skull. The inferior orbit and maxillary sinus areas are well visualized. A nasoethmoidal and a right zygomatic fracture with pneumocephalus are seen.

field defect, double vision, decreased vision, or absent vision should be noted as well as globe turgor and extraocular motion. A penetrating ocular injury or globe rupture should be suspected with any injury to the eye or periorbital area. The presence of a periorbital hematoma with the "eye swollen shut" should not deter the clinician from an examination of the globe. Indeed, some have suggested that the examination be performed with a determination inversely proportional to the difficulty, although care must be exercised to avoid extrusion of globe contents through a laceration. It is only with this kind of thorough examination that globe ruptures or penetrating globe injuries will not be missed.

RADIOGRAPHIC DIAGNOSIS OF FACIAL INJURIES

Patients with serious or multiple injuries should not be sent unmonitored for extensive radiographic evaluation of facial injuries. Simple bedside radiographs combined with a thorough clinical examination provide much of the information necessary for emergency diagnosis and treatment. At centers where appropriate patient screening exists, patients may be properly monitored and all necessary diagnostic studies such as CT scans obtained.

Plain radiographs have largely been replaced in most units with a craniofacial CT scan. Plain radiographs are reviewed here to familiarize the traumatologist with their interpretation. A careful radiologic technician may take these plain facial films in the emergency area. Here they are often reversed from their usual projection, but the quality may be surprisingly good if there is cooperation between the examining clinician and radiologic technician and if the clinician carefully explains to the technician what information is necessary. Emergency plain radiographics include

1. *Water's view of the skull* (Fig. 33-10) is the single most informative plain radiograph

and shows frontal, supraorbital areas, the orbital floor, the lateral and inferiolateral orbital rim, and the nasal arch. The maxillary sinuses are well visualized, including their lateral and medial walls.
2. *Towne's view of the skull* (Fig. 33-11) demonstrates condylar and subcondylar areas of the mandible and the floor of the orbit.
3. *Caldwell posterior-anterior skull film* (Fig. 33-12) demonstrates the zygomaticofrontal junctions, the frontal sinus, the frontal bone and roofs of the orbits, the medial orbit, and nasoethmoid area; the ramus of the mandible can often be visualized.
4. *Lateral skull film* (Fig. 33-13) demonstrates frontal skull, the roofs of the orbits, the frontal sinus, and a lateral view of the facial bones such as the zygoma.

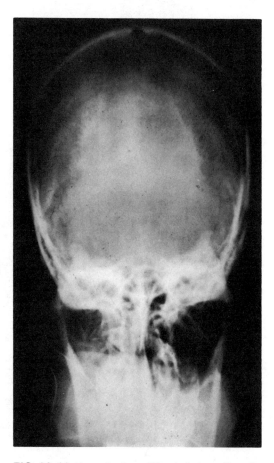

FIG. 33-11 Towne's view of the skull shows the subcondylar areas of the mandible.

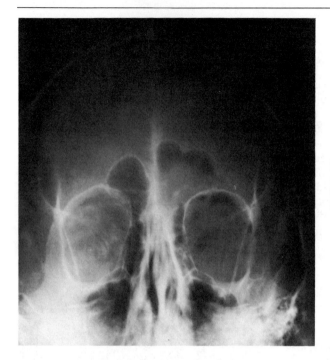

FIG. 33-12 Caldwell skull. The frontal and supraorbital areas are well visualized. A frontal sinus fracture and air fluid level on the left are seen.

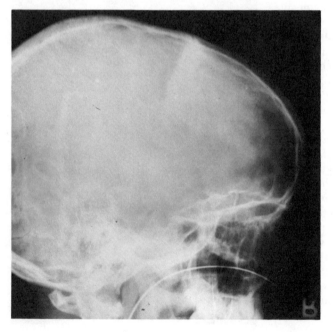

FIG. 33-13 Lateral skull demonstrates the frontal sinus, roof of the orbit and a lateral view of the facial bones. Pneumocephalus, frontal, and orbital roof fractures are seen.

FIG. 33-14 Computed tomography of patients with mandibular, LeFort, and higher facial fractures. **(A)** Parasymphysis
mandible fracture.

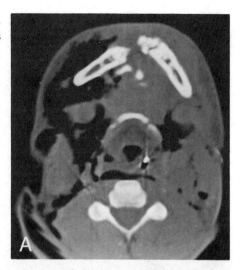

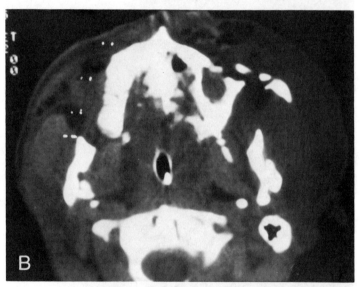

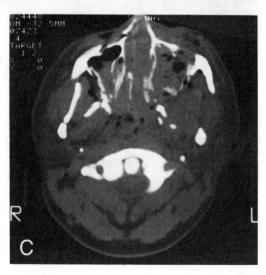

FIG. 33-14 (*Continued*) **(B)** Subcondylar fracture. **(C)**
LeFort maxillary fracture.

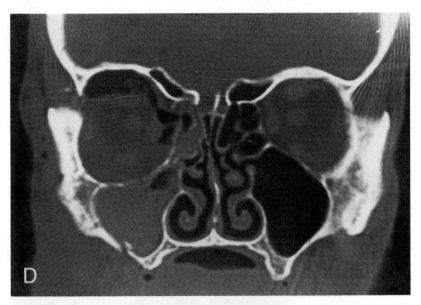

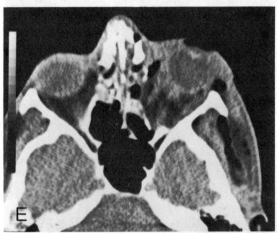

FIG. 33-14 (*Continued*) (**D**) Coronal view of zygomatic fracture and fracture of medial orbit and floor. (**E**) Nasoethmoidal fracture. (**F**) Frontal sinus fractures.

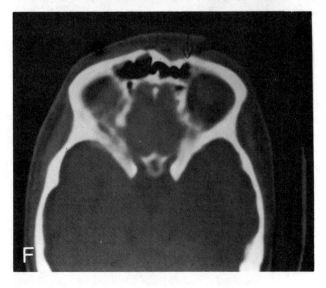

5. *PA and lateral oblique mandible films* are specialized films that show the body, symphysis, ramus, condylar, angle, and coronoid mandibular areas.

Computed Tomography

A CT scan is required for treatment of any concomittant craniofacial injury.[28,94,95] These injuries include those of the frontal sinus, orbital and supraorbital areas, nasoethmoid, and high LeFort (II and III) fractures. The examination should be performed with thin (at least 4 mm) cuts through the orbit for accurate definition of the areas of injury.[28,68] This examination must precede the operative treatment of any patient with extensive upper facial injuries (Fig. 33-14).

RECONSTRUCTIVE AIDS

Dental Models

Alginate impressions[44] of the maxillary and mandibular dental arches are obtained when jaw fractures are complex or may require treatment with plastic splints to hold the dentition in a particular occlusal relationship. These impressions are taken soon after admission, and plaster models are prepared from the alginate impressions within the first 24 hours. The plaster models obtained are used to provide a patient record, to study occlusion between fracture fragments containing teeth, and sometimes to construct plastic splints to maintain fracture reduction. These dental impressions are best taken at the time of the initial evaluation, especially if an anesthetic is necessary for the performance of another procedure.

Old Photographs

Wallet photographs or those provided by the family often assist in comparing the pre- and postinjury condition of facial structures. They help visualize the result to be achieved by fracture reduction and can provide accurate information on preexisting facial asymmetry as well as a clue to preexisting abnormal dental relationships.

Manual Reduction of Fractures

Grossly displaced fracture fragments can be reduced to their approximate position.

APPLICATION OF INTERMAXILLARY FIXATION

Early immobilization of fractures involving the upper or lower jaws is desirable in most cases and mandatory in cases in which the fragments are grossly unstable. Movement between fragments is reduced, contributing to patient comfort and reducing the tendency for bleeding or aggravation of CSF leaks to occur. Intermaxillary fixation is accomplished by ligating soft metal arch bars to the maxillary and mandibular teeth (Fig. 33-15). These bars are then united either by wires or by elastic bands (Fig. 33-15) between the lugs, fixing the jaws in a proper dental relationship. Arch bars may be ligated to the molar, premolar, and cuspid teeth under local anesthesia or general anesthesia. Frequently they may be placed at the same time as the definitive treatment of an abdominal chest or lower extremity injury is being delivered in the operating room. Simultaneous procedures reduce the length of time the patient will spend under general anesthesia. In patients who may vomit or who may require observation of respiratory status, intermaxil-

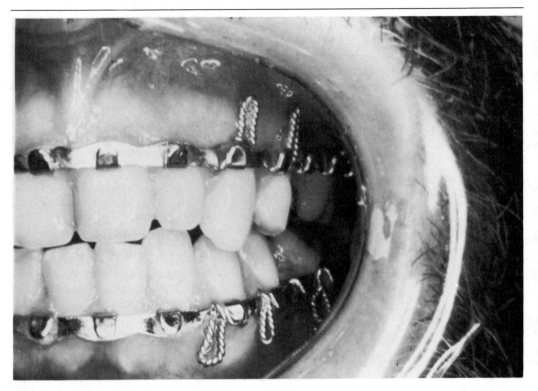

FIG. 33-15 Intermaxillary fixation by ligating arch bars to the teeth and uniting the arch bars with wires or elastic bands.

lary fixation of the arch bars by wires or elastics may be omitted until the danger of vomiting or respiratory obstruction has passed. When the control of fracture fragments makes intermaxillary fixation mandatory, consideration should be given to either leaving the nasotracheal tube in place or to performing a tracheostomy.

CUTANEOUS WOUNDS

The results of the improper management of soft tissue injuries may be disastrous and permanent; therefore, prompt evaluation and proper initial management are essential. A definitive plan for appropriate debridement, wound care, and closure will maximize the rehabilitation of the facial injury.

Cutaneous wounds of major magnitude are frequently associated with other life-threatening injuries. Management of these injuries will often postpone definitive management of the open wound. Because of this unavoidable delay, it is mandatory that an initial thorough inspection, cleansing, and removal of foreign materials be performed. Definitive debridement of nonviable tissue may be delayed. The initial cleansing and subsequent protection of the wound with a sterile dressing is carried out early in the course of events following arrival in the emergency room. Open wounds must be protected with a sterile dressing following the cleansing until definitive treatment and therapy is undertaken. A culture will provide information as to the initial bacteria inoculated into the wound.

Primary closure of soft tissue wounds is preferable. However, the age of the wound, degree of contamination, the extent of sheering, avulsive and crushing forces, and the amount of tissue lost will indicate the timing and method of wound closure. Fortunately, wounds of the face without significant tissue loss may be closed literally at any time following the injury because the excellent blood and lymphatic supply in facial soft tissues protects the tissue from infections. In general, soft tissue lacerations are closed following fracture reduction and the application of intermaxillary fixation devices to prevent disruption of the wound closure. Procedures such as the application of arch bars and circumdental wires strain soft tissue closures. Generally, there is little justification not to treat soft tissue wounds definitively within 6 to 12 hours of the injury—if untreated within this period, they may be closed following a judicious debridement of the wound edges.

wound. Removal of this damaged tissue improves the appearance of the scar that will be formed. About 1 or 2 mm of tissue may easily be debrided in areas such as the forehead or cheek and usually may be spared in any area. Alternatively, if sufficient soft tissue exists, areas of ragged scarring may be converted into more desirable clean linear lacerations. Debridement is best performed with an #11 blade or with sharp (iris suture) scissors. Aggressive debridement requires considerable judgment and is generally not indicated at the time of primary repair. Debridement must be especially conservative in regions such as the vermilion border of the lip, the oral commissure, the eyelids, and the distal portion of the nose. Deformity created by soft tissue excision in these areas is frequently unable to be reconstructed satisfactorily. Apparently devitalized tissue in these areas often survives; the ultimate result is frequently improved by having additional tissue to work with on a secondary basis.

Inspection

Cutaneous wounds should be inspected for foreign bodies and for depth. The presence of a cutaneous wound should signal the possibility of injury to underlying deep structures such as facial bone fractures, divided nerves, ducts, blood vessels, or penetrating injuries into a body cavity or structures such as the globe. Appropriate examination of the functions of organs adjacent to the area of injury should be performed with diligence to detect hidden injuries.

Debridement

Devitalized tissue should be conservatively debrided. There is generally a rim of contused devitalized tissue along the edge of a

Pressure Irrigation

Pressure irrigation of wounds may be performed with a jet lavage or with a #22 needle attached to a 30-cc Luer-Lok syringe; the Luer-Lok prevents the needle from becoming a missile. The pressure irrigation of wounds helps dislodge dirt, foreign material, and bacteria from the surfaces of the wound. Within 6 to 8 hours, bacteria become lodged in the wound in a protein-fibrin coagulum. This coagulum may be disrupted with proper pressure irrigation, resulting in a cleaner wound that will require less soft tissue debridement. Irrigation with a topical antibiotic or antiseptic seems to afford protective action against infection and may be used for moderate or severe contamination. Large volumes of fluid are frequently used for irrigation according to the maxim: "dilution is the solution to pollution." Pressure irrigation of wounds may be harmful if excess pressure is used, as it will drive bacteria into the wound surfaces, making them inaccessible to anything but sharp debridement.

Foreign Material

"Tattoo" or "road dirt" (foreign material) must be removed at the time of the initial treatment. These particles contaminate the wound, increase the incidence of infection, and result in permanent colored areas that are unsightly. They cannot be satisfactorily removed after cutaneous healing and present a permanent deformity that is impossible to treat effectively (Fig. 33-16A,B). The removal of this foreign material should be accomplished by a light scrubbing or by physically grasping and removing embedded material. A small accurate forceps, such as a jeweler forceps or splinter forceps, may be helpful. Alternatively, the use of a small (dermatology) curete may be used for curetting foreign material from the surface of small lacerations. The tip of a #11 scalpel blade is also useful. Occasionally, a light dermabrasion will remove embedded material.

Soft Tissue Closure

The approximation and alignment of most facial wounds is accomplished with a layered closure involving a combination of subcutaneous and dermal sutures. For wounds such as the forehead, brow, or cheek, an interrupted layer of inverted dermal stitches such as 4-0 Vicryl or Dexon is first placed. These stitches alone should result in reasonably accurate skin alignment. Fine alignment of the skin is achieved by dermal suture of 6-0 nylon. Care should be taken to align landmarks such as the eyebrow to preserve facial features. Generally, a single layer of 6-0 nylon sutures is appropriate for eyelid lacerations not involving the lid margin (subcutaneous sutures are not placed in eyelid skin in the area from the medial to the lateral canthus). Care should be taken to align structures properly such as the columella or nasal ala. Brilliant green can be used for marking key landmarks before injection of an anesthetic agent (which is deforming). It is often more difficult to align structures

properly once a local anesthetic has been injected. This is especially true in areas such as the vermilion border, which blanch with the injection of an anesthetic agent containing epinephrine.

Suture Removal

Cutaneous facial sutures are usually removed at intervals from the third to fifth postoperative days. Removal of alternate sutures at intervals enables one to confirm wound closure and yet to remove as many sutures as possible. In patients on steroids, a delay in wound healing may be anticipated and suture removal appropriately delayed.

Prophylactic Antibiotics

Systemic antibiotics are generally not administered for uncomplicated facial lacerations. Topical antibiotic irrigation has been shown to be of value for moderate or severe contamination.[37,65] Dog or cat bites and contaminated wounds through the oral cavity or through a sinus have classically been treated with prophylactic penicillin. The antibiotic is probably not as necessary as was believed in the past and is never a substitute for proper surgical debridement and cleansing of the wound. Too frequently, reliance is placed on the administration of an antibiotic rather than on a thorough surgical examination, debridement, and cleansing of the wound surfaces. To be effective, antibiotics must be given before wound closure is performed; otherwise, they are not truly prophylactic. It has been difficult to determine the value of prophylactic antibiotics in the treatment of most facial injuries. Antibiotics are indicated when (1) wound closure has been delayed, (2) contamination is excessive, (3) a surgically clean wound cannot be established, and (3) there is ischemic tissue.

FIG. 33-16 (A) Foreign material ground into lacerations must be removed at the time of initial cleansing. It cannot be removed satisfactorily once healing has occurred. (B) Result after removing material with scrubbing a #11 blade and small curette. After the foreign material is removed, the lacerations are repaired.

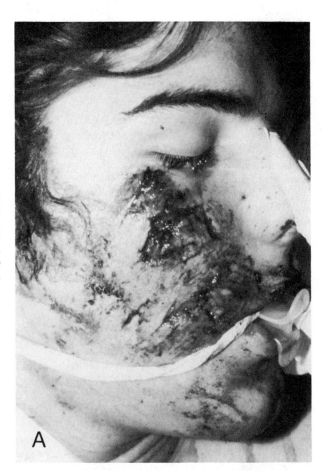

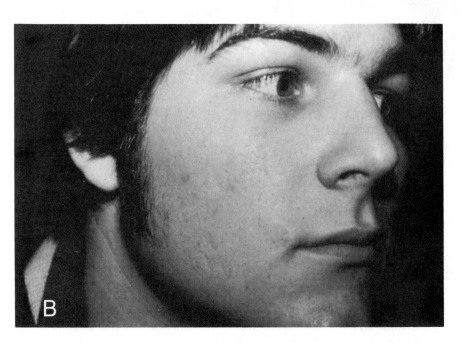

Malalignment of Facial Wounds

Meticulous alignment of facial tissues with a layered repair yields the most satisfactory appearance and minimizes the need for secondary procedures. Late reconstructions or revisions are seldom as satisfactory as proper initial treatment. If significant malalignment of facial landmarks is detected during the first few days, a revision can be accomplished within this period.

Postoperative Wound Hygiene

All suture lines are cleansed several times a day with a 50:50 peroxide saline mixture on cotton-tip applicators. Bacitracin is used for application to facial sutures; ophthalmic ointment (an ointment that is pH corrected for use in the eye) is used on periorbital suture lines. These ointments, applied to the sutures after cleansing, prevent excessive drying and crust formation. They lubricate the suture line during the period of healing and decrease bacterial proliferation around the sutures. Periodic cleansing of the suture line decreases inflammation and crust formation and ultimately reduces the amount of cutaneous scarring observed.

Post-operative Wound Hygiene of Intraoral Wounds

Intraoral hygiene is performed at regular intervals with irrigations of either a suitable mouthwash or half-strength peroxide saline. The teeth should be brushed gently several times daily.

Late Scarring from Wounds

Scars mature over a 1- to 3-year period. A prominent raised, red scar often displays soft tissue contracture initially.[97] Scar revisions are not performed during the early maturation period of a wound unless there is gross malalignment of tissues or contracture of the type that will cause functional symptoms, such as ectropion and cornea exposure. Many scars that have a startling appearance initially will improve sufficiently to obviate the need for revisional surgery. A frank discussion with the patient regarding the time course of scar maturation helps the patient understand the healing process and encourages patience during the period of healing. Cosmetics can be appropriately used to mask the appearance of facial scarring during the period of maturation.

Specialized Wounds

The presence of an eyelid or periorbital hematoma, laceration, or contusion should prompt a thorough examination of the globe for possible penetration, hyphema, retinal injury, or orbital fracture. Small, apparently superficial lacerations may be the only visible evidence of a penetrating wound of the globe or retained intraocular foreign body. The early detection of such injuries is crucial and is accomplished by thorough examination. Unfortunately, the presence of lid edema often makes the examination of the globe difficult. Rough manipulation may cause extrusion of ocular contents through a globe laceration.

Eyelid Margin Lacerations

Lacerations of the eyelid margin (involving the tarsal plate) are managed by a precise repair performed with meticulous alignment of the lid margin. Three or four sutures at the lid margin facilitate alignment of the cilia, gray line, and internal lid margin. Alignment of the internal lid margin is the most important feature, since its surface rests against the cornea. Generally, complex repairs such as the "halving" repair are unnecessary, and simple approximation with slight eversion suffices. The wound repair is begun with a layer of conjunctival sutures and tarsal plate sutures with the knots on the inside of the wound. The lid margin is then approximated and the skin closed. A temporary suture uniting the eyelids (one stitch temporary tarsorrhaphy with rubber bolster to prevent its tearing the lid margin) is useful to prevent corneal irritation and exposure.

Deep eyelid lacerations often expose orbital fat. In these lacerations, one should suspect a penetrating injury to the globe. Involvement of the lacrimal gland should be suspected if a deep laceration is present in the outer portion of the upper lid. Injuries of the cornea frequently occur from exposure when lid lacerations are present. This must be prevented with proper lubrication with large quantities of a protective eye ointment and a patch dressing, until a definitive repair is performed.

Lacrimal System

Lacrimal canalicular injury should be suspected when lacerations occur in the medial canthal area. Injury to the lacrimal system may be caused either by soft tissue lacerations or by fractures involving the bones adjacent to the nasolacrimal duct. Lacerations may transect the lacrimal system in the area of the medial canthus, whereas fractures tear or compress the lacrimal system by bone displacement or the product of callus of fracture healing. The integrity of the lacrimal system may be assessed by placing fluorescein on the eye and observing its passage to an applicator placed in the nose under the inferior turbinate. A more rapid and precise evaluation of lacrimal integrity is obtained with a #22 angiocath sleeve by injecting yellow fluorescein solution through the lacrimal punctum after it has been gently dilated. Light finger pressure is used to obstruct the opposing punctum. The presence of fluorescein either in the wound or in the nose indicates lacrimal system transection or patency, respectively. The lower lacrimal canaliculus should always be repaired, since the upper canaliculis alone is inadequate for satisfactory tear drainage. Repair of the canalicular system should be performed with a precise microsurgical plastic repair with fine sutures over silicone tubing threaded into the nose. Both cannuliculi are intubated.

Windshield Lacerations

Multiple small avulsive flap lacerations are commonly seen. They are managed by meticulous cleansing of road dirt and embedded foreign body. The small flaps can either be debrided and the lacerations closed, or they might be trimmed and reapproximated to adjacent tissue with fine sutures (Fig. 33-16). An alternative technique of dermabrasion of the superficial portions of the flap is rarely practiced. Generally, meticulous realignment of the small avulsed flaps with fine sutures results in the best aesthetic appearance.

Facial Nerve Injury

Lacerations may transect branches of the facial nerve, while contusions or temporal bone fractures are a common cause of temporary or permanent paralysis from a blunt injury. Facial nerve injury should be suspected when lacerations are present over facial nerve branches. The diagnosis is confirmed by comparing motor activity on both sides of the face. If a patient is unable to be examined, appropriate careful exploration of the wound should confirm the depth of penetration. The facial nerves travel underneath the mimetic muscles and may be damaged if penetration has reached this level. The major branches of the facial nerve are (1) temporal, located on a line between the tragus and 1 cm. superior to the eyebrow; (2) orbital-zygomatic, located on a line between the tragus and the lateral canthus; (3) buccal, located on a line between the tragus and the floor of the nostril traveling with the parotid duct; (4) marginal mandibular, which parallels the lower mandibular border; and (5) cervical, which runs approximately at the level of the hyoid crease and does not require repair (see Fig. 33-5).

Lacerations of the facial nerve should be repaired at the time of soft tissue closure. Magnification is used with fine (8–0 or 9–0) suture material. The distal nerve segment will not respond to stimulation after 48 hours, making identification more difficult if a delayed repair is elected. Repair of branches need not be performed in the distal portion of the buccal branches. It is our recommendation that any branches be repaired where they are able to be identified. Temporal bone fractures are a frequent cause of traumatic facial paralysis and should be considered in the differential diagnosis of a facial nerve palsy.

Eyelid Dressings

A firm compression dressing is important in controlling postoperative edema in the eyelid area. The dressing also prevents eyelid displacement, resulting in corneal exposure. A closed eyelid with the application of ointment is ideal treatment for corneal abrasions secondary to injury. Pressure dressings should be well padded and a layer of Xeroform gauze placed between the eye ointment and the dressing. Following removal of dressings at 48 to 72 hours, the patient may use cool compresses to cleanse secretions around the eyelid area. Elevation of the head during this period helps minimize edema.

Losses of Portions of the Nose

Injuries to the nose may involve full-thickness losses of tip or nasal ala. For major losses, a skin to mucosa closure is accomplished and delayed reconstruction performed. Loss of a portion of the nasal tip, for instance, may be repaired with a composite graft or local flap depending on the age of the patient. Loss of a portion of the nostril rim can be replaced with a composite graft of ear skin and cartilage that resurfaces both the external and internal lining and provides cartilage support. An ideal wound bed and painstaking care are necessary for the survival of composite grafts. They are generally performed in an elective rather than an emergent situation.

Lacerations of the Ear

Complex lacerations of the ear are frequent. The landmarks of the ear serve as a guide for proper reapproximation of structures. Small portions of the cartilage may be debrided to faciliate accurate skin alignment. Generally, no cartilage sutures are used; the skin on the anterior and posterior surface of the helix is closed with fine interrupted absorbable sutures. Portions of the ear helix that have very small remaining pedicles will often survive because of the excellent blood supply of the ear. Avulsed tissue may be returned as a composite graft and debrided if it does not survive. When larger losses of the helix have occurred, exposed underlying cartilage may be salvaged by coverage with a local flap. Avulsion of the ear will frequently require secondary reconstruction in the same manner as congenital absence of the ear.

Lacerations of the Lips and Cheeks

Vertical lacerations of the lip margin are quite common. The repair should approximate the mucosa and vermilion surfaces, care being taken for accurate alignment of both the anterior and posterior edges of the vermilion border and for the "white role" adjacent to the anterior edge of the vermillion. This is most accurately identified before the installation of local anesthetic solution. The muscle layer of the lip is approximated with a layer of absorbable sutures and the cutaneous laceration closed with subcutaneous and cuticular sutures.

The lips are commonly lacerated by teeth, and the wounds produced must be surgically clean if closure of the mucosal layer is to be performed. Many surgeons leave the mucosal surface of these puncture wounds open, debriding and closing the cutaneous surface. The closure of the mucosal portion depends on the ability to establish a surgically clean wound by debridement and irrigation. The oral flora invariably contaminates these puncture wounds, and infection will follow inadequate cleansing or inappropriate closure without debridement.

Lacerations of the Parotid Gland or Duct

Deep lacerations in the posterior portion of the cheek may involve the parotid gland, facial nerve, or parotid duct. Drainage from lacerations of the gland without major duct injury will cease if regular wound closure is performed and a drain is utilized. Permanent fistula from glandular lacerations without major duct system injury has not been observed. Some clear drainage with a high amylase may persist from the wound for several weeks. Subcutaneous fluid collections need not be aspirated or drained in the absence of fever or in-

flammatory or skin changes, which signify impending fistulization or skin breakdown.

Duct Lacerations

Stenson's duct extends from the anterior margin of the parotid gland (1 inch anterior to the tragus on a line between the tragus and floor of the nostril) to the intraoral buccal surface opposite the second maxillary bicuspid. Ductal lacerations are nearly always accompanied by buccal branch facial paralysis since the two structures travel adjacent to each other. Ductal injuries are managed by a repair with fine sutures over a Stent tube left in place for 1 to 2 weeks. Creation of a fistula into the mouth by relocating the proximal duct stump into the oral cavity has been described but has not been necessary in our experience. Ligation

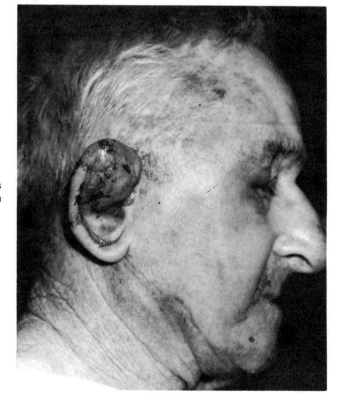

FIG. 33-17 Auricular hematoma. This blood must be evacuated to prevent skin necrosis or cartilage deformity.

of the duct is another acceptable method of management but again has not been used in our experience. Considerable temporary swelling accompanies duct ligation and the obstruction produced predisposes to infection. Duct repair is favored in most situations.

Auricular Hematoma

Significant hematomas (Fig. 33-17) involving the ear should be drained and a light but bulky pressure dressing consisting of mineral oil soaked cotton carefully applied into the crevices of the auricle to prevent recurrence. The drain is removed in 24 to 48 hours. If the hematoma is not evacuated, it serves as a focus for cartilage proliferation or necrosis and resultant "cauliflower ear" deformity.

SPECIALIZED RADIOGRAPHIC EXAMINATION OF MAXILLOFACIAL INJURIES (FACIAL SERIES)

This series consists of plain radiographs using the Water's, Caldwell, lateral skull, submentovertex, and Towne skull views described earlier.

Anteroposterior and Lateral Tomograms

Polytomography was formerly frequently used to evaluate fractures involving the thin portions of bone in the frontal sinus, orbit, mandibular condylar, frontobasilar, and nasoethmoid region. CT scans have replaced tomograms because of the better definition of soft tissue and bone structures and the reduced X-ray exposure required.

Computed Tomography

This examination is the standard examination for facial bone fractures. Seldom are plain films obtained for the purpose of evaluating facial injuries at our institution.

Xeroradiography

This examination is infrequently used. It may disclose foreign bodies, soft tissue densities or fractures within the thin bones of the facial skeleton. Because of the increased X-ray exposure required and its inferiority to CT scans, it is seldom obtained.

Fractures Involving the Dentition

Specific films are ordered for additional views of the mandible, maxilla, and the teeth:

1. *PA mandible* view demonstrates the symphysis and parasymphysis region of the mandible; the angle and ramus are visible as well.
2. *Lateral oblique mandible view* demonstrates the body, angle, ramus, condyle and sucondylar area. Two views are required, one for each side of the mandible.
3. *Caldwell view* demonstrates the ramus and the angle of the mandible from another perspective than seen in the PA mandible.
4. *Panorex examination* demonstrates the entire lower maxilla and mandible and is obtained with the patient standing with a specialized rotating X-ray machine (Fig. 33-18). Frequently, this view cannot be obtained in patients with multiple injuries who are unable to stand or travel to the appropriate facility. The view demonstrates the entire maxilla and mandible on one plain film and is quite helpful where its performance may be accomplished without jeopardizing the care of the patient.
5. *Bite wing, occlusal, palatal, and apical views* of the teeth are helpful in visualizing

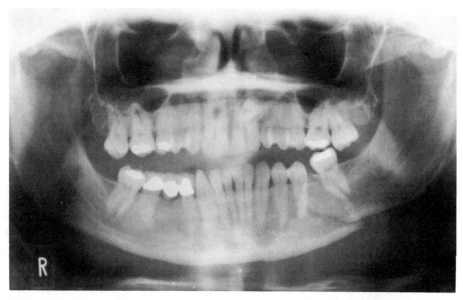

FIG. 33-18 Panorex examination of the mandible demonstrates the entire mandible and lower maxilla. A body fracture is visualized.

fractures of the symphysis and in examining the course of the fractures adjacent to the roots of teeth involved in the fracture line. Sometimes these views are helpful in determining whether teeth should be extracted or salvaged. A palatal film is helpful in detecting fractures that divide the upper jaw sagittally. Again, these views generally require that the patient be sent to an appropriate X-ray facility where these dental films are available. Frequently, decisions must be made without views of these radiographic examinations.

GROSS LOSS OF SOFT TISSUE STRUCTURE OF THE FACE

Large losses of soft tissue generally occur from severe avulsive injuries or from wounds such as a shotgun wound. The loss is replaced by local or distant flap reconstruction. Skin to mucosa closure may be accomplished as a temporary mechanism to prevent contracture and close the wound. Underlying bony structures are repaired or stabilized in external fixation in that area of injury and appropriate internal or external stabilization of the rest of the bony skeleton performed. Soft tissue reconstruction is then accomplished over this bony repair.

LOCAL ANESTHESIA IN THE TREATMENT OF MAXILLOFACIAL INJURIES

Local anesthesia may be established by local infiltration or the performance of a regional block (Fig. 33-19). The administration of a local anesthetic is subject to the same general rules that apply for its use in other areas of the body. Although multiple local anesthetic agents are available, lidocaine (Xylocaine) has remained the standard local anesthetic for general use. Frequently, a vasoconstrictor such as epinephrine is used with an anesthetic in the head and neck area. The use of a vasoconstrictor decreases bleeding and prolongs the effectiveness of the anesthetic agent. Usually, 1 percent Xylocaine with 1/100,000 epinephrine or 0.5 percent Xylocaine with 1/200,000 epinephrine is used for local anesthesia. The regional

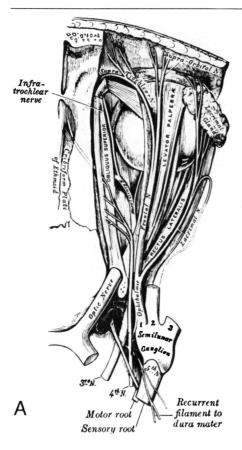

A

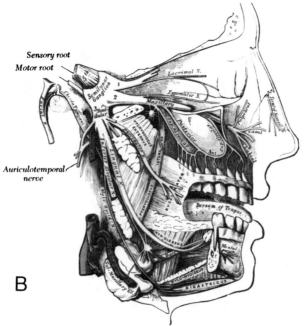

B

FIG. 33-19 Sensory branches of the trigeminal nerve of the face. **(A)** Frontal and orbital. Nerves of the orbit. Seen from above. **(B)** Maxillary and mandibular. (Clemette C (ed): Gray's Anatomy, 35th Ed. Lea & Febiger, Philadelphia, 1985.)

blocks are effective in 10 to 15 minutes and will provide satisfactory anesthesia for 1 to 2 hours. The maximum dose of Xylocaine should not exceed a total of 500 mg (50 ml of 1 percent or 100 ml of 0.5 percent) for the average healthy patient; modifications are possible depending on the time of administration and the patient's general condition.

NERVE SUPPLY OF THE SCALP

The primary sensory supply to the scalp comes from branches of the trigeminal nerve anteriorly and the cervical nerves posteriorly. In the forehead, the frontal nerve divides into the supraorbital and supratrochear nerves to supply the greater portion of the forehead. The zygomaticotemporal nerve exits through the lateral portion of the orbit and innervates some skin in the temple region. The area of the temple is also supplied by branches of the trigeminal nerve: the temporoalar branch and auriculotemporal branch. In the posterior region of the scalp the greater and lesser occipital nerves divide to supply nearly the entire posterior portion of the occiput. The scalp may be anesthetized by the subcutaneous infiltration of an anesthetic agent from the glabella to the external occipital protuberance parallelling the top of the ear. This provides anesthesia of the entire superior portion of the scalp on the ipsilateral side.

SENSORY INNERVATION TO THE FACE

Regional facial blocks may be established by anesthetizing divisions of the trigeminal nerve (Fig. 33-19). In the superior portion of the orbit, the supraorbital and supratrochelar nerves exit at the roof of the orbit on to the anteriomedial orbital rim and are easily anesthetized at the rim area. The supraorbital

notch is a palpable landmark in the superior orbital rim which allows identification of the supraorbital foramen. The foramen is generally located between the pupil and the medial limbus with the patient looking straight ahead. The anterolateral portion of the supraorbital rim area is supplied by branches of the lacrimal nerve. Regional block of the infraorbital nerve, a terminal division of the maxillary nerve that exists from the infraorbital foramen below the anteroinferior orbital rim, provides anesthesia to the side of the nose, upper lip, and upper anterior teeth. Portions of the lower eyelid are anesthetized as well. The foramen is located 8 to 10 mm below the inferior orbital rim and is at the limbus of the cornea with the patient looking straight ahead. Approaching it from an inferior direction facilitates location of the area of the foramen. It is unnecessary to enter the foramen. The lateral portion of the cheek is supplied by a penetrating branch of the maxillary division of the trigeminal nerve, the zygomaticofacial nerve. It exits through a small canal in the body of the zygoma just below the area of the inferior lateral orbital rim.

NOSE

Anesthesia of the nose requires bilateral infraorbital nerve blocks, installation of anesthetic over the glabella (supratrochlear and infratrochlear), and at the anterior nasal spine area (anterior superior dental alveolar). Occasionally this may be supplemented by blocking the external nasal branches over the dorsum of the nose.

THE LOWER FACE

The mandibular division of the trigeminal nerve supplies the lower facial area. This division of the trigeminal nerve divides into the lingual and inferior aveolar nerves. The inferior alveolar nerve supplies the lower jaw and emerges from the mental foramen to supply the skin of the lower lip anteriorly. Anesthesia of the lower anterior lip may be established with a mental nerve block. The needle is inserted into the area between the bicuspids and anesthetic solution is injected. The foramen for the mental nerve is usually located about 1 cm below the gingival border. In patients who are edentulous, this foramen may lie on the superior surface of the remaining portion of the bone of the mandible, the alveolus having atrophied.

Anesthetizing the mandibular nerve produces anesthesia of the lower jaw area. The nerve may be approached intraorally by inserting the anesthetic needle lateral to the pterygomandibular raphe, advancing it along the medial surface of the ramus. This block anesthetizes the temporal region, the anterior two-thirds of the tongue, as well as the associated mucous membrane, the lower lip, and temporomandibular joint areas.

Anesthetizing the maxillary nerve produces anesthesia of the mid-face area. Inserting a needle through the sigmoid notch area of the mandible with the patient's jaw open, the needle is advanced several centimeters until the pterygoid plate is encountered. The needle is then slightly withdrawn and then advanced superiorly and anteriorly for another 1 to 2 cm. This locates the area of the maxillary division of the trigeminal nerve as the nerve enters the posterior portion of the orbit.

Sensory Innervation of the Nasal Cavity

The sensory supply of the nasal cavity is from branches of the olfactory, nasopalatine, and ethmoidal nerves. Superiorly, branches of the olfactory nerve enter through the cribriform plate area. Anteriorly, nasal branches of the ethmoidal nerves supply the anterosuperior nasal cavity. The posterior and the inferior portions of the nasal cavity are supplied by branches of the nasopalatine nerves from the sphenopalatine ganglion. These are generally anesthetized by solutions of cocaine combined with Xylocaine and norepinephrine. Generally, 300 mg cocaine flakes is placed on cotton-tip applicators moistened with a solution of Xylocaine 1 percent with 1/100,000 norepinephrine. Placing these applicators in the general distribution of the superior portion of the nose (cribriform plate area) and the inferior turbinate posteriorly anesthetizes the entire nasal cavity.

Nerve Supply to the External Ear

Sensory innervation of the auricle is provided by branches of the occipital nerves, greater auricular, and auriculotemporal nerves. They approach the ear from inferiorly and anteriorly so that an effective regional block of the auricle may be performed by field block.

DEFINITIVE FRACTURE DIAGNOSIS AND MANAGEMENT BY REGION

Nasal Fractures

By virtue of its projection and delicate structure of its bones, the nose is the most frequently encountered facial fracture. The nose may be fractured by forces from a lateral or frontal direction. Laterally directed forces produce nasal injuries that are deviated laterally. Forces approaching the nose from an anterior direction produce frontal impact injuries that crush the nasal pyramid and drive it between the orbits. These frontal impact injuries are the most severe and result in true fractures involving not only the nose but the medial portions of the orbit (nasoethmoidal–orbital injury). The patient with a nasal fracture has a history of an injury and almost always presents with some swelling over the external surface of the nose. The area of swelling identifies the area of maximal injury. Almost all nasal fractures are accompanied by bleeding from the nose presenting from one or both nasal cavities. In the absence of bleeding through a nostril, one should question the diagnosis of a nasal fracture. The diagnosis of the nasal fracture is confirmed by localized tenderness or bruising over a portion of the nasal pyramid. The pyramid should be inspected for deviation laterally or for flattening in an anteroposterior direction. The interior of the nasal cavity should be inspected for mucosal lacerations, swelling, or hematoma along the septum or turbinate structures. If this swelling or hematoma is sufficiently prominent, obstruction to breathing on the affected side will result. In addition, if the septum has been dislocated, it will partially obstruct the airway. Frequently, there will be small lacerations over the nasal bridge.

Radiographic evaluation of the nose consists of views of the nasal bones, a lateral view of the nose, and a Water's view. Sometimes sinus films are indicated. Nasal films seldom assist the surgeon in treating a nasal fracture; however, they may disclose fractures in adjacent bones such as the maxilla and orbit. Although a CT scan can demonstrate a nasal fracture, the procedure is not necessary for the diagnosis or treatment of an isolated nasal injury. A CT scan should be obtained in any case in which a nasoethmoidal orbital injury is suspected.

Treatment of a nasal fracture depends on the clinical examination. If the nasal pyramid is straight and there is no significant septal dislocation or deviation, surgical reduction is not required. Generally, surgical reduction is postponed until the presence of swelling and edema have subsided. This generally requires 5 to 7 days. The fracture may be treated acutely depending on the judgment of the surgeon. Early treatment of a displaced nasal fracture is recommended. Nasal fractures that have healed in malalignment require a total rhinoplasty. Frequently, a nasal injury will require some secondary correction. The septum is the area that usually requires secondary surgical treatment for airway obstruction. Generally, the amount of secondary surgery required is reduced by proper primary treatment.

Displaced nasal fractures are managed by closed reduction. Local anesthesia of the external nose and the nasal cavity is established. Alternatively, general anesthesia can be used in anxious patients or those undergoing other surgical procedures. A closed reduction of the septum is performed, placing it in the midline, accomplished with a septal forceps. Any significant septal hematomas may be drained. The septum is encouraged to remain in the midline by the use of a terramycin-impregnated nasal pack placed to either side of the septum. The closed repositioning of the nasal pyramid is then performed by first outfracturing the pyramid and then molding it in the proper position through infracture. This completes the nasal fracture, many of which are greensticked, and allows the fracture to remain stable in the midline. If the distal portion of the nose is depressed, it may be held in place by inserting some packing between the septum and the distal portion of the nose intranasally. A light nasal splint is applied. This consists of either plaster or metal. Open nasal injuries may be treated by interfragment wiring of bone fragments. Most nasal fractures are compounded into the nose, and some are compounded through the skin. Small lacerations are closed with the timing similar to that used in the closure of cutaneous wounds. Intranasal lacerations need not be sutured. An area of torn mucous membrane may be gently replaced into its proper position with light packing saturated with terramycin ointment. Bony healing in most nasal injuries takes 1 to 2 weeks. The nasal packing is generally removed on the third or fourth postoperative day and the nasal splint removed within 7 to 10 days. Patients should be cautioned to restrict activity because of the possibility of nasal bleeding. They should not blow their nose forcefully but should gently wipe it, as blowing the nose forcefully drives intranasal secretions through mucosal lacerations and increases the potential for infection. The patient should be cautioned to avoid sports or situations in which physical contact might secondarily damage the nose for 4 to 6 weeks until solid, pain-free healing has occurred.

Nasal fractures in children are of particular importance because of the early treatment required and the potential for late deformity of growth disturbance. It is important to treat nasal fractures early in children, as they heal within several days and are difficult to reposition. A dislocated nasal fracture that has healed in malalignment requires a formal rhinoplasty. Most surgeons are hesitant to perform this procedure in children who have not completed a major portion of their facial growth. The effect of rhinoplasty on subsequent nasal growth is unknown. Thus, a child in whom a nasal fracture is suspected should be appropriately examined and treated even if that diagnosis and treatment requires a general anesthetic. Although growth disturbance following nasal injury has been reported in children, it is not a common occurrence.

TECHNIQUE OF NASAL FRACTURE CLOSED REDUCTION

If local anesthesia is to be administered, the external nose is anesthetized with a field block consisting of the bilateral infraorbital, supratrochlear, infratrochlear, and anterior superior dental alveolar branches of the tri geminal nerve. The external nasal branches over the dorsum of the nose may require a separate injection. The interior of the nose is anesthetized with a mixture of cocaine, Xylocaine, and epinephrine. After this mixture takes effect, the interior of the nose can be visualized and the extent of damage and the requirements of adequate treatment evaluated. Frquently, the septum is dislocated from the volmerine groove. In addition, "septal buckling," areas of overlap, or "telescoping" are identified. The handle of a #3 scalpel may be used to elevate and outfracture depressed or greensticked nasal bone fragments. Following the outfracture, they are molded back into proper position with thumb pressure over a gauze sponge. It is important to complete the fracture similar to the requirement in forearm bones in order for the alignment to remain stable. The septal cartilage should be moved into position with an Asch forceps and checked again after the nasal pyramid has been reduced. The nasal bones and the septum should be able to be freely placed in the proper position. If packing or a splint is required to hold them, it is unlikely that they will remain in this position. The concept of completing the fracture so that the nose can freely deviate to either direction cannot be overemphasized as the basis for control of nasal fracture fragments. Fixation is accomplished by a combination of nasal packing with antibiotic-impregnated gauze and the application of a plaster or metal splint onto the nose. The nose is first painted with a layer of benzoin; ½-inch steri-strips are then placed transversely across the nasal dorsum. The nasal dorsum is then covered with a layer of ½-inch regular adhesive tape, after which a metal or plaster nasal splint is applied. Metal splints should be suitably trimmed to prevent any sharp edges from pressing directly into nasal skin. The interior gauze packing is removed as early as practical with the requirement of fixation of the bony and cartilaginous injury. The interior of the nose can then be cleansed with saline and the nares cleansed with peroxide on cotton-tip applicators. The external nasal splint is generally removed 7 to 10 days after the injury.

NASAL BONES

The nasal bones are paired, thin membranous bones that articulate superiorly with the nasal process of the frontal bone and laterally with the frontal process of the maxilla. The superior third of the nose consists of bone and the lower two-thirds cartilage. The middle third of the nose consists of the upper lateral cartilages that join the bony septum. The lower third consists of the lower lateral cartilages and the septum.

Fractures of the Zygoma

The zygoma forms a central structure of the midface. It consists of a prominent dense section of bone that forms the eminence of the cheek. The zygoma forms the lateral portion of the orbit articulating with the greater wing of the sphenoid and the inferior portion of the orbit and articulates with the ethmoid and lacrimal bones. At the superior orbital rim it articulates with the zygomatic process of the frontal bone and with the maxilla at the medial third of the inferior orbital rim. In the floor of the orbit, the infraorbital nerve travels from the posterior portion of the inferior orbital fissure diagonally across the orbit in a medial direction. Several millimeters from the rim, the infraorbital nerve turns inferiorly into the dense bone of the orbital rim. It then exits 8 to 10 mm below the orbital rim parallel to the limbus of the cornea in straightforward gaze. The zygomatic arch extends from the body of the zygoma posteriorly to articulate with the temporal bone adjacent to the ear canal. Inferiorly, the zygoma articulates with the maxillary alveolus; thus, the zygoma forms a portion of the roof of the maxillary sinus. Fractures of the zygoma account for most midface injuries, if nasal fractures are excluded. Several types of zygomatic fractures are observed. The fracture can only involve the zygomatic arch (Fig. 33-20) and is usually the result of a lateral blow. Depression of the arch may be masked by swelling but is later visible as a hollow in the lateral portion of the cheek anterior to the auri-

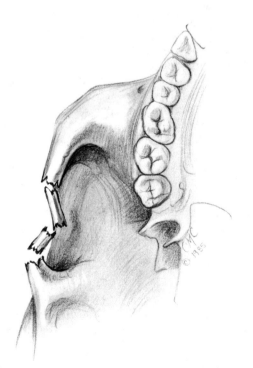

FIG. 33-20 An isolated fracture of the zygomatic arch. Impingement of the coronoid process of the mandible may occur.

cle. The depressed zygomatic arch may impinge on the coronoid process of the mandible and limit mandibular excursion. Malocclusion or decreased range of mandibular excursion may both be produced by fractures of the zygomatic arch. Treatment of a zygomatic arch fractures involves elevation of the arch by passing an elevator underneath the depressed fracture segments and pushing them outward. The procedure is generally accomplished under general anesthesia and involves making an incision in the hairline down through the temporal fascia over the temporalis muscle. When the temporal muscle is reached, an elevator may then be passed beneath the layer of fascia behind the arch and used to push the fractured segments outward. The strong periosteal and fascial attachments at the arch prevent the fracture fragments from severe displacement. The arch is usually stable following closed reduction. The fracture pattern is generally a W-shaped deformity (Fig. 33-20). Elevating the central limbs of the W stabilizes the arch. Frequently, some protection is placed over the cheek (a bent metal finger splint may be used) and taped to the forehead and cheek areas to prevent re-injury and displacement.

Alternative methods of reduction employ a towel clamp that can be inserted percutaneously around the arch and used to pull it outward. Another possible means of reduction involves placement of a large suture around the arch, which then can be used to pull the arch outward. This suture can be ligated to the bent metal finger splint to provide outward traction if necessary. Alternatively, percutaneous K-wire fixation of the arch has been described.

UNDISPLACED FRACTURES OF THE BODY OF THE ZYGOMA

At least one fourth of zygomatic injuries involve nondisplaced fractures of the zygoma. The clinical signs of infraorbital nerve anesthesia—periorbital and subconjunctival hematoma—may be present. Radiographs will demonstrate fractures at the zygomaticofrontal–zygomaticomaxillary junctions and inferiorly at the zygomatic buttress, where it joins the maxillary alveolus. The radiographs will not confirm any displacement. The undisplaced zygoma fracture is generally stable through intact periosteal attachments despite the bone fracture and no operative treatment needs to be performed. The floor of the orbit should be visualized with a CT scan to confirm the integrity of the thin portion of the orbital floor.

DISPLACED FRACTURES OF BODY OF THE ZYGOMA

Displaced fractures of the body of the zygoma (Fig. 33-21) are classified by both the direction of rotation and comminution.[114] The zygoma, when fractured, breaks at the rim at the zygomaticofrontal junction and at the medial portion of the inferior orbital rim where it joints the maxilla (Fig. 33-22). Occasionally, the entire frontal process of the zygoma is a separate fragment. Within the orbit, the fracture usually travels along the junction of the lateral orbital wall (junction of the zygoma with the greater wing of the sphenoid), across the inferior orbital fissure then paralells the canal for the infraorbital nerve anteriorly to reach the rim. The zygomaticomaxillary buttress is fractured just above the maxillary alveolus. The zygomatic arch is fractured in displaced fractures of the body of the zygoma and fractures adjacent to the body and the junction with the temporal bone. Several types of zygomatic displacement are described: lateral rotation, medial rotation, inferior depression, and posterior depression.[52,62]

CLINICAL SYMPTOMS

The pathognomonic sign of an orbital fracture is a combination of a periorbital and subconjunctival hematoma (Fig. 33-21). Many of these fractures will be zygomatic or cheek bone injuries. These fractures tear the lining of the maxillary sinus and, as do orbital floor fractures, cause ipsilateral epistaxis. Displacement of the zygoma will displace the attachment of the lateral eyelids because of the attachment of the lateral palpebral ligament to Whitnall's tubricle about 1 cm below the zygomaticofrontal junction. A downward depression of the palpebral fissure is produced that is quite noticeable. The displacement of the canthus may contribute to a sagging of the lower eyelid with improper flow of tears producing epiphora and lower lid ectropion. The palpebral fissure is wider on that side. Posterior depression of the zygoma is accompanied by flattening of the cheek once sufficient swelling has resolved for it to be noticeable. Palpable "step" deformities of the orbital rim may be identified and signal zygomatic displacement. Anesthesia of the ipsilateral upper lip, medial cheek, ipsilateral nose and anterior ipsilateral maxillary teeth is pathognomonic of a fracture involving the infraorbital nerve. Indeed, the diagnosis should be questioned if the combination of anesthesia in the distribution of the infraorbital nerve and the periorbital and subconjunctival hematoma are not present. Displacement of the arch may contribute to poor range of mandibular excursion and to a minor malocclusion caused by pain and swelling. Intraorally a hematoma is observed in a buccal sulcus. A finger placed

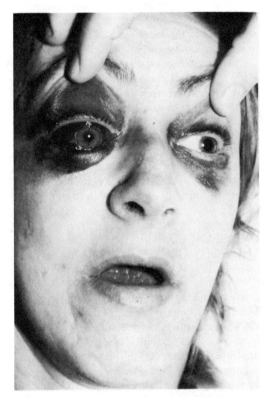

FIG. 33-21 The pathognomonic sign of an orbital fracture is the combination of a subconjunctival and periorbital hematoma.

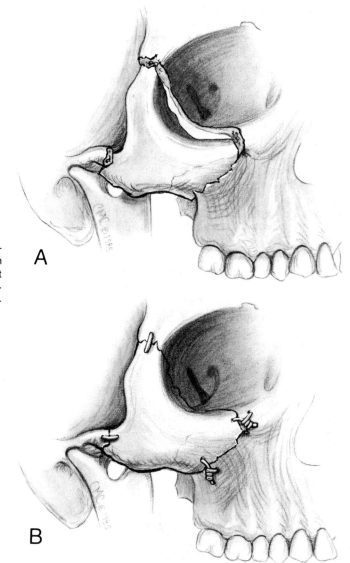

FIG. 33-22 **(A)** Zygomatic fracture. **(B)** Repositioning with open reduction and internal fixation at the zygomaticofrontal, lower orbital rim, arch, and zygomaticomaxillary buttresses.

A

B

intraorally can palpate the fracture where the zygoma attaches to the maxillary alveolus.

RADIOGRAPHIC EVALUATION OF THE ZYGOMA FRACTURES

Zygomatic fractures may be identified on plain facial roentgenograms or CT scan. Although plain roentgenograms are no longer used in our unit for the identification of fractures involving the orbit, the fracture pattern may be easily confirmed with plain facial films. A Caldwell view is necessary for assessment of displacement at the zygomaticofrontal junction. The Water's view shows displacement at the inferior orbital rim and displacement at the zygomaticomaxillary buttress. The submentovertex view is necessary to define the arch fracture and can be used to assess posterior displacement of the body of the zygoma. A hematoma in the maxillary sinus is frequently seen. Plain films are of limited value in assessment of the thin bones of the internal orbit. It is our practice to obtain a CT scan with at least 4-mm cuts through the orbit for definition of the zygoma and thin portions of the orbit, providing unexcelled documentation of both the bone and soft tissue injury.

The indications for open reduction are displacement and the resultant clinical deformity and functional symptoms of anesthesia or orbital symptoms. Loss of cheek prominence, enophthalmos (retrusion of the globe), vertical malpostion of the globe, and anesthesia of the infraorbital nerve accompany displaced fractures of the zygoma. The mechanaism for the globe displacement involves loss of the globe support and enlargement of the orbit, permitting the orbital soft tissue to sink posteriorly and inferiorly. The infraorbital nerve may be compressed between fracture fragments and frequently the anesthesia does not resolve if decompression is not achieved. Displaced fractures may be treated with either closed or open reduction techniques. We have been dissatisfied with closed reduction techniques as late displacement occurs, resulting in a return of the deformity. Closed reduction techniques are suitable for fractures treated early or for frac-

tures which show no displacement at the zygomaticofrontal junction. The fracture should not be comminuted. The fracture may be pushed back into position by placing an elevator behind the body of the zygoma either through an exposure into the maxillary antrum or with an incision adjacent to the zygomaticofrontal junction. The elevator is placed behind the body of the zygoma in the temporal fossa and the body of the zygoma pushed back to position. If reduction is satisfactory a "click" will often be obtained. The treatment of zygomatic fractures by open reduction (Fig. 33-22) involves an exposure of the fracture sites along the orbital rim utilizing upper lid or brow incision at the zygomaticofrontal junction and exposure of the lower orbital rim and orbital floor with an incision in the lower eyelid. The entire floor should be explored to detect missing areas of bone or enlargement of the orbit produced by bone displacement. The integrity of the orbital rim is restored by interfragment wiring; the integrity of the thin internal portion of the orbit is restored by either bone grafting, packing the displaced fragments into position with a combined maxillary sinus and orbital floor exposure, or placing a plastic sheet such as 6 or 8 mm supramid in the orbital floor. The zygomatic arch fracture is usually treated as for isolated arch fractures. The zygomatico-

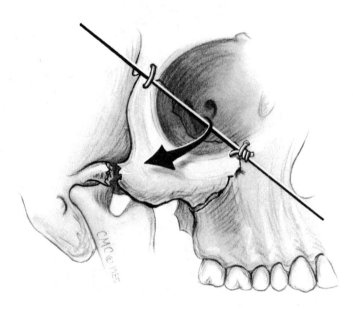

FIG. 33-23 Rotation of the zygoma may occur following a two point fixation alone.

maxillary buttress adjacent to the maxillary alveolus may be exposed and wired through a gingival buccal sulcus incision. A drain is placed in the maxillary antrum.

Occasionally an arch fracture requires support by means of open reduction and K-wire fixation or packing. A protective guard taped to the skin is used postoperatively to prevent accidental displacement.

Open reduction of zygomatic fractures is employed for the following indications: entrapment, vertical dystopia, enophthamos, trismus, contour deformity and numbness. Late sequelae of residual enophthalmos, double vision, loss of malar prominence, and hypesthesia or anesthesia in the distribution of the infraorbital nerve are not uncommon and may sometimes be improved by secondary surgical treatment.

Blepharoplasty incisions (a lower subciliary with skin muscle flap and lateral limb of upper lid blepharoplasty) provide a superior cosmetic result in patients requiring open reduction of zygomaticomaxillary fractures. These two incisions enable one to expose virtually the entire orbital rim and to complete interfragment wiring joining the zygoma to intact adjacent bones. Reconstruction of the orbital rim involves wiring to the zygomaticofrontal and zygomaticomaxillary junctions, and between these two points as necessary. Three-dimensional stability is achieved by an intra-oral incision in the gingival–buccal sulcus to expose the junction of the zygoma with the maxilla. This third point of fixation is routinely secured intraorally to prevent retrusion or rotation of the zygoma, which is easily missed in the presence of edema (Fig. 33-23). This retrusion results in clinical flattening of the malar eminence. An additional means of fixation involves packing the maxillary antrum or K-wire fixation with a transfacial K-wire to stabilize the zygomatic body.

Orbital Fractures

The internal orbit is commonly fractured either by itself or accompanying fractures of adjacent facial bones such as the supraorbital area, zygoma, and nasoethmoidal orbital area. The orbital rim can be divided into three sections as far as the patterns of commonly produced fractures are concerned. The supraorbital area, the nasoethmoidal area, and the zygoma (Fig. 33-24). The internal orbit is commonly fractured as an extension of the fractures in adjacent bones. The weakest area in the walls of the internal orbit is the medial wall or the lamina papyracea over the thin ethmoid bones (Fig. 33-25). The next weakest section is the floor medial and adjacent to the infraorbital nerve. The floor is usually fractured in its posterior inclined section which is immediately behind the globe.[12-14,50] This area is in direct continuity with the thin lamina papyracea; thus, fractures of the thin portions of the medial wall and the floor often occur concomitantly. The orbital floor fracture may occur through indirect means and the mechanism for these fractures involves either hydraulic pressure[103] or a blow to the rim, which causes a remote fracture of the floor by the creation of a "buckling" force[26,86] (Fig. 33-26). Pure blowout fractures are usually produced by a concomitant blow to the rim with a buckling force on the orbital floor; hydraulic pressure then forces the orbital contents into the fracture site[13,50] (Fig. 33-27).

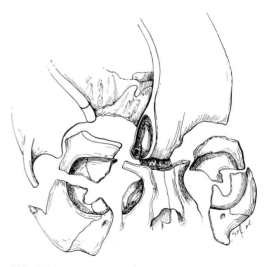

FIG. 33-24 Division of the orbital rim into zygomatic, nasoethmoidal, and supraorbital areas.

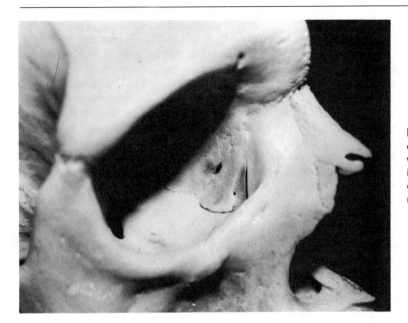

FIG. 33-25 Thin sections of the orbit are the medial wall, floor adjacent to the infraorbital nerve, and medial portion of the orbital roof.

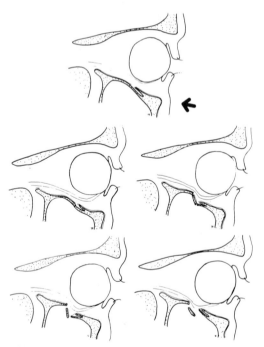

FIG. 33-26 Fracture of the orbital floor produced by a buckling force to the rim. (Fujino T, Makino K: Entrapment mechanisms and ocular injury in orbital blowout fracture. Plast Reconstr Surg 65:571, © 1980, The Williams & Wilkins Co., Baltimore.)

ANATOMIC CONSIDERATIONS

The orbit is a pyramidal or cone-shaped cavity containing the globe, the extraocular muscles, fat, and cranial nerves. Posteriorly, the optic nerve enters the orbit through the optic foramen. Within the optic canal, the nerve is enclosed in a dural sheath and this area is vulnerable to compression. The optic foramen is located about 40 mm posterior to the orbital rim, a fact that must be constantly kept in mind when performing orbital explorations. Safe orbital exploration must involve a knowledge of the location of the superior and inferior orbital fissures as well as the contents of these fissures. The extraocular muscle cone begins adjacent to the optic foramen. Five of the extraocular muscles begin their course at this muscle cone. The four external rectus muscles (superior, inferior, medial, and inferior) extend from this area forward to attach to the globe. The superior oblique muscle courses forward to the trochlea and then turns at a acute angle to attach to the globe. The inferior oblique muscle takes its origin immediately behind the infraorbital rim lateral to the lacrimal sac. It then travels posterolaterally to attach to the globe. Each

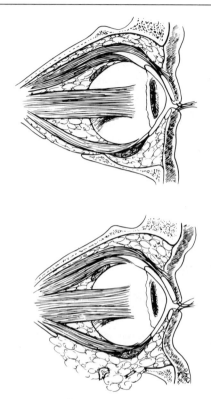

FIG. 33-27 Hydraulic compression forces the soft tissue orbital contents into the fracture site, entrapping extraocular soft tissue and restricting muscle movement.

of these muscles has a dominent field of action that may be identified in examination (Fig. 33-28A).

Orbital fractures have a significant (at least 10 to 25 percent) incidence of associated ocular injury.[21,24,45,89] Although many of these injuries are minor, a significant number are not; thus, any periorbital injury demands precise evaluation of the globe to rule out such conditions as globe penetration, retinal dettachment, orbital foreign body. A diagnostic eye evaluation is essential and consists of a thorough visual examination.

This visual examination should include visual acuity (a card may be used), confrontation fields, determination of intraocular pressure, and a forced duction test.[6] Visual acuity may be obtained by simply holding a visual examination card in front of the patient and checking each eye individually. Confrontation fields may be performed by having the patient look directly at the examiner's nose; the patient signals when he or she sees a finger entering a peripheral field of gaze. A fundoscopic examination should be performed. Intraocular pressure can be determined by taking a tonometer and placing it on the cornea, which has been anesthetized with a drop of topical anesthetic. Low pressures suggest globe rupture. A forced duction test is performed in patients with double vision or fracture of the internal portions of the orbit by placing a drop of anesthetic within the conjunctival sac. A small fine-tooth forceps is used to grasp the insertion of the inferior rectus or medial rectus as appropriate and rotate the globe upward detecting any increase in pressure required to accomplish globe excursion.

RADIOGRAPHS

Routine radiographs will show most orbital fractures but do not permit sufficient definition of bone and soft tissue detail required for evaluation for surgical correction.[25] Formerly, tomograms were the examination used, whereas CT scans are currently used. Orbital fractures will be seen on the Water's view on plain film as a bulge of the orbital contents into the superior antrum. Clouding of the antrum is usually noted on the ipsilateral side. Medial blowout fractures produce clouding of the ethmoid area and air in the superior portion of the orbit. Precise evaluation of an orbital blowout fracture uses CT scan. Orbital fractures are best evaluated radiographically by means of CT scan with axial cuts and coronal reconstruction (Fig. 33-28B). Multiplanar reconstructions may be required.

CLINICAL EXAMINATION

The clinical examination is still the most important diagnostic measure available and identifies the patient who would benefit from a CT scan. The most reliable signs of an orbital fracture are the presence of a palpebral and subconjunctival hematoma (combination) and the presence of hypesthesia in the infraorbital

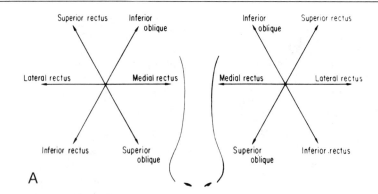

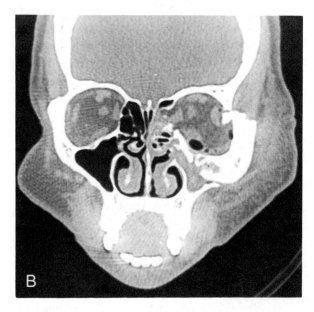

FIG. 33-28 **(A)** Dominant field of action of each of the extraocular muscles. Diplopia when looking into a particular direction is associated with lesions involving that muscle. (Reprinted with permission from Richards RD (ed): Ophthalmologic Disorders. Medical Examination Publishing Co., Flushing, NY, 1973.) **(B)** Fracture of the medial wall and floor of the orbit accompanying a nasoethmoidal fracture.

nerve distribution. These are the most consistent clinical findings in fractures of the internal portion of the orbit. Other findings include vertical or horizontal muscle entrapment in fracture fragments (inferior oblique, inferior rectus; medial rectus) vertical or horizontal globe dystopia (position change), ipsilateral epistaxis, and enophthalmos.[90] The globe positional change is produced by the loss of posterior and medial support of the orbit allowing the orbital contents to sink backward, downward, and slightly medially. This produces enophthalmos once the swelling has resolved. The enophthalmos may be measured by placing a Hertel exophthalmometer on the lateral orbital rim and measuring the position of the cornea relative

to the lateral orbital rim. Another technique involves measuring the position of the globe relative to the inferior orbital rim. Ipsilateral epistaxis is produced by fractures involving the maxillary or ethmoid sinuses with blood exiting the ipsilateral nares. Medial wall fractures may exist as an isolated injury or coexist with floor fractures (50 percent). The physical findings in isolated medial blowout fractures include subcutaneous emphysema, orbital emphysema, epistaxis, horizontal diplopia, the retraction syndrome, enophthalmos, and proptosis, depending on the amount of hemorrhage or swelling present. Patients with medial blowout fractures often have a downward and forward globe positional change caused by air in the superior portion of the orbit. The patient may demonstrate retraction of the globe on looking in the field of the medial rectus muscle, which demonstrates muscle incarceration. The forced duction test may also detect incarceration of the muscle as opposed to contusion or cranial nerve damage. Many isolated orbital floor and most isolated medial blowout fractures do not require surgical correction.[91]

TREATMENT

Isolated minimally symptomatic fractures of the orbital floor and medial wall present difficult value judgments in terms of the indications for open reduction and floor replacement.[91] Several indications for operation are usually offered[110]: persistent entrapment, enophthalmos, and vertical globe dystopia. Massive bone loss in the orbital floor is usually an indication for open reduction, as these patients generally develop severe (cosmetically deforming) enophthalmos and globe dystopia. The presence of a sensory deficit alone is not an indication for reduction as the sensory deficits produced by isolated internal orbital fractures almost always resolve completely without treatment. Our usual plan is to perform a surgical exploration if the floor defect is large enough or if enophthalmos or vertical dystopia of the globe exists. If entrapment persists beyond a short period of observation (5 to 7 days), or in the presence of a positive forced duction test, surgical treatment is advised. During this short period of observation, entrapment symptoms will resolve significantly and not require open reduction, in one-half of cases. Saccadic velocities measure the change in the acceleration developed over time when the globe moves in a specific direction. The acceleration velocities can differentiate muscle contusion and paralysis from muscle entrapment. The differentiation becomes quite important in deciding which patients should be treated surgically.

The goal of treatment is to obtain orthophoric vision in the primary field of gaze and not necessarily total normal eye movement to the full extent of excursion. This goal can often be accomplished with nonoperative treatment in minor orbital floor fractures. Nonoperative treatment of blowout fractures prevailed for

several years, but most surgeons who deal with a significant number of orbital fractures now prefer surgery for the conditions described. The surgery consists of an exploration of the entire area of the floor fracture, release of any entrapped periorbital contents, and reconstruction of the floor with either a plastic plate or a bone graft tailored to support the orbital contents while healing occurs. The superior–inferior muscle balance and diplopia generally result from entrapment of fat and fascia, which are linked with fine ligaments to the inferior rectus inferior oblique muscle system. This musculofibrous aponeurotic system was described by Koorneef[55] and accounts for the usual mechanism of muscle entrapment rather than actual incarceration of the muscle.

COMPLICATIONS FROM SURGERY

Complications from surgery occur in 10 to 15 percent of cases and include infection, hematoma, and cosmetic deformities of the eyelid secondary to the surgical approach utilized (such as scleral show and ectropion). Damage to vision has been reported and in most large series consists of 2 percent of patients submitted to surgical exploration.[24,79,87] Occasionally some hypesthesia persists in the inferior infraorbital nerve distribution. Additional complications can include undercorrection, overcorrection, and damage to eye muscles at the time of surgery. Blindness is usually produced by blind packing of the maxillary antrum. Concomitant visualization of the floor is necessary if any packing is used. Thorough knowledge of the optic nerve is important in orbital exploration. Implants should be tailored to avoid pressure on the nerve and rough manipulation of other fractures such as the zygoma should be discouraged because fractures may extend to the optic canal and produce compression of the optic nerve by swelling and hematoma formation. In addition, vigorous manipulation may precipitate a retinal detachment or create excess global pressure. It is not unusual for late visual problems to occur unrelated to any surgical manipulation; this mechanism of late visual loss should be recalled in patients who have those symptoms. Orbital floor exploration may produce a retrobulbar hemorrhage with proptosis of the globe. In some series, the incidence of this problem approaches 3 percent.

BONE GRAFTING

Orbital bone grafting restores the integrity of the orbital floor; a thin piece of iliac crest, calvarial bone, or split rib is used.[32,33,66,111] The split rib is the easiest to contour and may be molded with a Tessier rib forcep to approximate the dimensions of the orbit. It is used when support of the orbital floor or wall reconstruction is necessary (Fig. 33-29). The donor site morbidity seems to be the lowest with cranial bone but again the bone is more difficult to contour to the thin dimensions of the orbit than is split rib. In practical applications, these bone grafts are often exposed to the orbital, nasal, and oral cavities; curiously, this does not prevent their "take." An alternative to the use of bone grafts involves alloplastic material such as a thin (0.8 mm) piece of supramid. This should be wired into place to prevent late displacement. Figures on long-term infection and extrusion of this material approach 5 to 10 percent in some series. Alloplastics are the most common material used to provide orbital structure support; they have done well despite free communication between the orbit and maxillary sinuses.

Nasoethmoidal Orbital Fractures

Nasoethmoidal orbital fractures involve the entire nose, medial and inferior portion of the orbit, and frontal process of the maxilla.[32,72,75,106] By virtue of their extension, these fractures often involve the orbital roof, frontal sinus, and frontal bone. They result from a direct blow to the nasofrontal or glabellar area and can accompany LeFort II or III fractures. These are injuries of significance and are surprisingly easily missed in the presence of swelling. One should suspect a nasoethmoid fracture when there are nasal fractures, lacerations of the frontal or nasal area and bilateral

periorbital ecchymosis (spectacle hematoma). A spectacle hematoma should signal the possible presence of a fracture involving the anterior cranial fossa. Nasoethmoid fractures are frequently unilateral (one-third) and may occur as an isolated central midface fracture or coexist with LeFort II or III fractures. Dural fistulae are invariably present and are easily missed. The dural fistula may manifest itself as either a CSF leak or as pneumocephalus. The CSF leak is easily obscured by the presence of bloody nasal secretion and often a period of 2 to 3 days must elapse before it can be confirmed with certainty. Many CSF leaks close during this short time interval, and the benefit of prophylactic antibiotics has been questioned.[37,48,53,60,66,85,92] Injury to the nasolacrimal duct is invariable by its passage through the frontal process of the maxilla. Fractures of the medial wall, floor of the orbit, and the medial orbital rim are invariably present.

The diagnosis is suggested by the presence of epistaxis, depression or comminution of the nasal dorsum, pain and tenderness in the area of the nose, and bilateral eyelid hematoma. Fractures surrounding the lower two-thirds of the medial orbital rim are the sine qua non of the nasoethmoid injury. This central fragment provides canthal ligament attachment. The diagnosis is established by a CT scan that demonstrates fractures surrounding this fragment. The canthal ligament is usually not detached in the absence of external lacerations. One of the more reliable clinical signs of nasoethmoid fracture is movement on direct finger pressure over the medial canthal ligament, which signals instability of the lower two-thirds of the medial orbital rim. Traumatic telecanthus (increase in the distance between the medial canthal ligaments) may be observed either immediately postinjury in fractures that are extremely unstable, or this sign may occur slowly over a period of several days with resolution of swelling. Nasal bleeding is often profuse with fractures of the ethmoid and frontal sinuses. In fractures that are grossly unstable, lateral movement of the canthus can sometimes be detected if lateral traction is applied to the medial portion of the eyelids (eyelid traction test). Nasoethmoid fractures commonly accompany depressed comminuted nasal fractures. Finger pressure over the nose can detect

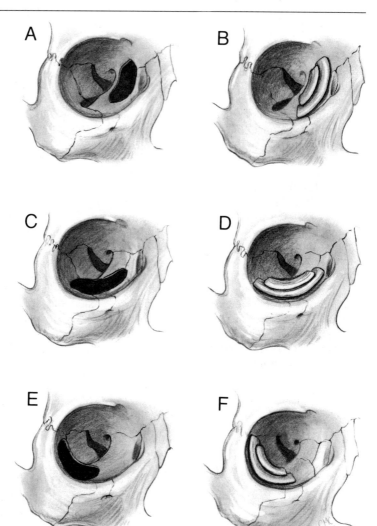

FIG. 33-29 **(A)** Medial orbital blow-out fracture. **(B)** Repair with bone graft. **(C)** Floor "blow-out" fracture. **(D)** Repair with bone graft. **(E)** Lateral orbital "blow-out." **(F)** Repair with bone graft.

these depressed fractures and identify the loss of septal and bone support. A CT scan confirms the impression. One should suspect injury to the structures in the anterior cranial fossa as well, since these often accompany nasoethmoid fractures. A CT scan is thus mandatory and must be performed before operative treatment.

RADIOGRAPHIC EVALUATION

Nasoethmoid fractures are difficult to evaluate radiographically and, although the injury may be suggested on Water's, Caldwell, and lateral skull films, the CT scan is the proper diagnostic radiographic modality. The craniofacial CT scan should include the brain and frontal cranium and thin orbital cuts done at 3- to 4-mm intervals with the appropriate coronal reconstructions. Reconstructions in the longitudinal axis of the orbit are also preferred. Emergency plastic surgery consultation is recommended for these injuries. These injuries are commonly misdiagnosed as severe nasal fractures. Because of the associated potential for severe late deformity and menigitis, these patients should be treated early if the maximal rehabilitation is to be accomplished.

TREATMENT

These injuries require a definitive open reduction with interfragment wiring linking all the fragments together (Fig. 33-30). A transnasal reduction of the medial orbital rims is required to ensure stability and to narrow the intercanthal distance. Bone grafts are usually required in the reconstruction of the injury of the medial wall of the orbit and the orbital floor. The nose may require an onlay nasal bone graft to preserve dorsal height and nasal contour. The CSF leak does not require definitive closure in the absence of other neurosurgical indications for exploration such as lacerations of the frontal lobe, depressed or open frontal skull fractures and severe brain contusion or hematoma. The frontal sinus is invariably injured; however, treatment is not performed unless displacement of the anterior or posterior walls requires frontal sinus reconstruction or treatment of the depressed posterior wall fracture. The lacrimal system is always involved in nasoethmoidal fractures; at this stage, however, only bone replacement

and fixation are required. Late lacrimal system obstruction occurs commonly but is only symptomatic in 5 to 10 percent of patients. These patients should have a late dacryocystorrhinostomy (surgical creation of a channel from the obstructed lacrimal sac into the nose) for relief of the obstruction. Transsection of the intracannulicular portion of the lacrimal system is rare in the absence of canthal ligament avulsion or detachment.

Lacrimal System

The lacrimal system is frequently injured in lacerations involving the medial portion of the eyelids and is also injured when the bony canals for the lacrimal system are fractured.[49] The most frequent fracture of this type is the nasoethmoid fracture. Evaluation and management of the lacrimal system following trauma may include a fluorescein irrigation or dacryocystography. Fluorescein irrigation involves

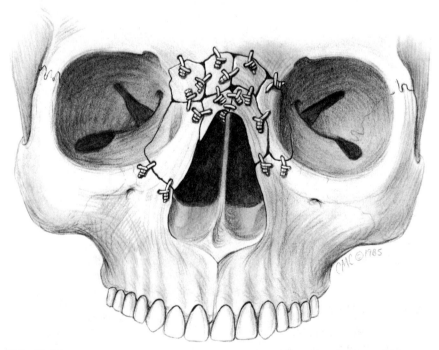

FIG. 33-30 Scheme of interfragment wiring for reconstruction of a nasoethmoidal fracture.

the use of a dye (fluorescein) placed in the conjunctival sac. If it passes into the nose, the lacrimal system is assumed to be patent. The dye is detected as it flows under the inferior turbinate at the orifice of the nasolacrimal duct, which is 2 cm posterior to the nares. If dye does not pass freely into the nose, the lacrimal puncta can be dilated with a pediatric punctum dilator and a #22 angiocath sleeve used to irrigate dye through the lacrimal system. The appearance of the dye in the nose indicates incomplete obstruction or a patent system, which perhaps is temporarily functionally obstructed from swelling and edema. In the late evaluation of lacrimal injuries, a radiopaque dye may be used to perform a dacryocystogram which identifies the area of obstruction. In practice, these are rarely necessary.

In lacerations involving the lacrimal system, the lacrimal system is intubated with fine tubes of silicone [these should be small (0.025 inch outside diameter) and the upper and lower punctum are both intubated]. The tubes are then brought into the nose where they are tied together and remain until no tears are noted on the cheek. This indicates the patency of the system. The lacrimal ducts or intracanalicular portion of the lacrimal system are repaired with fine sutures over this silicone tube stint.

Supraorbital Fractures

Supraorbital fractures occur as an extension of fractures of the orbital roof.[15,80,93,102,105] Patients displaying the symptoms of supraorbital fractures have a characteristic downward and outward projection of the globe. Lid closure is often incomplete. Anesthesia in the distribution of the supraorbital nerve may occur. Dural or cerebral injuries frequently coexist with supraorbital fractures, and the frontal sinus is commonly fractured as it forms the medial portion of the roof of the orbit. Symptoms such as ptosis and ocular muscle palsies or anesthesia in the distribution of the first division of the trigeminal nerve are common. Blindness occurs if the fractures extend to the orbital apex and produce pressure on the optic nerve.

Superior Orbital Fissure Syndrome

Fractures involving the superior orbital fissure can produce a combination of cranial nerve palsies known as a superior orbital fissure syndrome.[57] The syndrome, if complete, involves ptosis of the eyelid, proptosis of the globe, ocular muscle palsies of the third, fourth, and sixth cranial nerves, and anesthesia in the distribution of the first division of the trigeminal nerve (Fig. 33-31). If accompanied by blindness,[113] it is termed the orbital apex syndrome and involves concomitant injury to structures in the superior orbital fissure and the optic foramen. A CT scan should demonstrate the fractures involved.[68] If blindness occurs at the onset of the injury, optic nerve decompression[54] is not believed to be of benefit. If blindness occurs late after a period of intact vision, optic nerve decompression should be considered,[27] however, the value of this maneuver is open to question. Supraorbital fractures are diagnosed radiographically by means of a thorough craniofacial CT scan.

TREATMENT

Displaced fractures require open reduction (Fig. 33-32). Interfragment wiring is used to reconstruct the integrity of the orbital rim. Frequently, this reconstructs the proper position of the orbital roof. Defects or missing bone of the orbital roof area are managed by a split-rib graft.

Carotid Cavernous Sinus Fistula

Severe fractures may produce a fistula between the carotid artery and the cavernous sinus. The symptoms often involve visual loss, proptosis, and pulsation of the globe. The symptom of a pulsating globe may be due to either loss of the orbital roof through fracture with transmission of cerebral pulsation or the

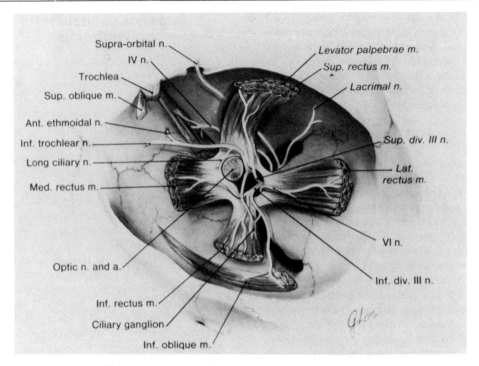

FIG. 33-31 The contents of the superior orbital fissure.

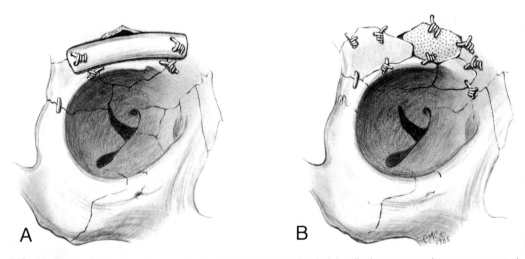

FIG. 33-32 Supraorbital fractures produce downward and forward globe displacement and are reconstructed by open reduction and bone grafting (**A**), or interfragment wiring (**B**).

carotid–cavernous sinus fistula. The condition can only be diagnosed by angiogram if suspected; it is corrected by radiographic techniques that clot or balloon occlude the abnormal communication.

Frontobasilar Fractures

These injuries, which consist of injuries to the frontal bone or anterior cranial fossa, involve fractures of the nasoethmoid, supraorbital, zygomatic, frontal sinus, or frontal bone area, which extend to the anterior cranial fossa[109,112] (Fig. 33-33). They are easily overlooked and must be suspected. There is often minimal evidence of underlying brain injury owing to the silent nature of frontal lobe symptoms.

RADIOGRAPHIC DIAGNOSIS

The diagnosis of a frontobasilar fracture is suspected when injuries to adjacent structures exist. The symptoms present for each of the regional categories of facial fractures adjacent to the anterior cranial fossa described are present. The patients often have frontal lobe contusions or lacerations present with periorbital hematoma or swelling (Fig. 33-34). CSF rhinorrhea,[62] pneumocephalus,[46] or orbital emphysema is frequently seen. Traumatic epistaxis is usually present. The radiographic evaluation consists of CT. CSF leaks may be identified clinically by the presence of rhinorrhea or confirmed by metrizamide CT scanning.[99]

TREATMENT

The treatment of frontobasilar fractures is individualized depending on the presence of associated lacerations and damage to the orbit, frontal sinus, and frontal skull areas. The indications for operations involve an integration of the indications for each of the subcategories of fractures described. A diagnosis must be suspected in patients with forehead bruises or hematoma if the diagnosis is not to be missed. For instance, it is not unusual to detect segments of extruded frontal lobe in the nasal cav-

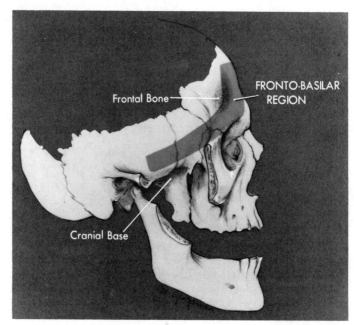

FIG. 33-33 Fractures involving the frontobasilar region also involve the anterior cranial fossae.

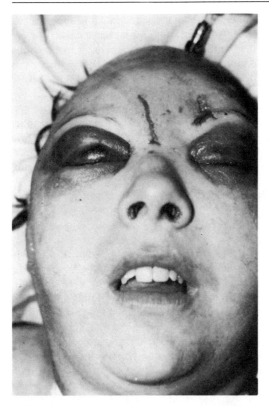

FIG. 33-34 Spectacle hematoma is one of the signs of an anterior cranial fossae fracture.

ity. This finding is often detected by an alert physician performing a careful examination of the nose.

Frontal Sinus Fractures

The frontal sinus develops between the ages of 5 to 10 and forms a pneumatized cavity in the lower central portion of the frontal bone, which communicates by the nasofrontal duct with the middle meatus of the nose. The duct passes through the ethmoid sinus area. The extent of the frontal sinus is variable and asymmetric. It is frequently larger on one side than on the other and is separated by an intrasinus septum. Two nasofrontal ducts extend from the posterior inferior recesses of the frontal sinus through the ethmoids down into the nose. A frontal sinus fracture should be suspected when contusions, bruises, or lacerations occur in the central area of the forehead. Once the swelling has resolved, a depression may be present in the glabellar area. Associated fractures such as supraorbital, nasoethmoid, or frontal bone are commonly extended into the frontal sinus area. CSF leak or pneumocephalus may be present as a symptom of a dural laceration as the posterior wall of the frontal sinus forms the boundary between the cranial cavity and sinus cavities. Epistaxis may be present.

RADIOGRAPHIC EVALUATION

Plain films such as the Caldwell and Water's films permit visualization of the area and may show linear fractures, spintering, or comminution of the anterior wall of the frontal sinus or hematoma. The floor of the frontal sinus may be visualized as the superomedial portion of the roof of the orbit. Again, these plain films have largely been replaced by the use of a facial CT scan. The CT scan is taken in the axial plane with 3- to 4-mm cuts and reconstructed as appropriate to document the extent of the injury. Accurate evaluation of the injury involves assessment of involvement of the anterior and posterior tables and the floor of the frontal sinus. The involvement of the posterior table (Fig. 33-35) is most significant, as it indicates underlying dural laceration with the potential for dural fistula with its symptoms of CSF leak and pneumocephalus. If the floor of the frontal sinus is comminuted, obstruction of the nasofrontal duct is usually present; generally, operative treatment is required to prevent abscess formation.

TREATMENT

The treatment of frontal sinus fractures includes a wide variety of operative procedures.[3,18,19,23,42,43,58,84,88,98] No procedure is clearly superior to any other. For the acute injury involving only the anterior wall, fragments may be elevated; if stable, this maneuver is sufficient. If unstable, they should be wired into place. Assessment of the patency of the nasofrontal duct is important, and a fluid level in

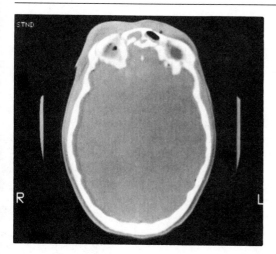

FIG. 33-35 Depressed fracture of the anterior and posterior tables of the frontal sinus.

nated areas of mucosa, and invaginating the duct mucosa into the nasofrontal duct to provide a seal between the nose and the frontal sinus. The patient should not blow the nose for a 6-week period. The anterior frontal sinus wall may be reconstructed with interfragment wiring or bone grafts to limit deformity. Acute reconstructions of this type are accompanied by a higher incidence of infection than delayed reconstructions. Patients selected for delayed reconstruction should wait for a period of 6 to 12 months, after which frontal cranioplasty can be performed. It has been shown that the cavity of the frontal sinus following "cranializations" obliterates with a combination of a fibrous-bony scar material over a 1-year period, a process called osteoneogenesis.

the sinus implies obstruction. Some workers believe that a rubber catheter may be placed down through a fractured nasofrontal duct and ensure patency during the period of healing. The catheter acts as a stent for the nasofrontal duct. Late problems occur in up to 50 percent of cases because of restenosis of the duct with late mucocele (retention cyst), obstruction, and infection. In fractures displaying more severe comminution and displacement of the anterior and posterior walls, bone fragments may be debrided and the mucosa stripped with closure of the duct by mucosal invagination or plugging with bone, fascia, or muscle. This converts the frontal sinus to a closed cavity and in effect "cranializes" the sinus. Alternatively, the sinus may be exenterated, which involves removal of both the anterior and posterior walls of the frontal sinus, removal of the entire mucous membrane and collapse of the skin against the dura.[48] This eliminates the potential space described in the cranialization procedure and is the safest procedure in terms of the subsequent incidence of infection. It is cosmetically severely deforming and so is seldom used. In the presence of established infection, it does control "dead space" and infection. Our preferred procedure in those frontal sinus injuries with fractures of the anterior and posterior walls involves stripping the mucosa, lightly burring the residual bony surface to eliminate invagi-

Frontal Bone Fractures

Frontal bone fractures may be classified and treated in various risk groups.[25,38,46] These groups include fractures of the frontal bones alone; fracture of the frontal bone extending into the frontal sinus area or the orbit; open depressed fractures; and open, depressed fractures where resection of brain and dural patch are required. Fractures displaying comminution of the frontal bones alone are reconstructed by interosseous wiring with a 5 percent risk of infection. If the fracture is open, the forehead skin is damaged, treatment is delayed, and a brain resection and dural patch have been necessary,[48] immediate bone reconstruction has been accompanied by increased risk of infection. It is often deferred in these patients and reconstructed by secondary frontal cranioplasty. These patients usually have extensive forehead skin damage with large areas of abraded and contused skin. After frontal lobe resection, the potential space existing between the reconstructed dura and the reconstructed frontal bone provides an environment conducive to infection. Meningitis and brain abscess may follow epidural infection. Our practice in these injuries is to complete the reconstruction of the roots of the orbits and the nasoethmoid area and to discard the multiple devitalized segments of frontal bone in these massive open injuries.

Infraorbital Rim Fractures

The diagnosis is suggested by a palpable step deformity of the rim with tenderness. Signs of an orbital floor or medial orbital wall fracture may or may not be present. Anesthesia in the distribution of the infraorbital nerve is present if the nerve is involved in the fracture site.

The radiographic examination consists of a Water's view and Caldwell view on plain films. Again, CT scan is superior to plain films.

Maxillary Sinus Fractures

The diagnosis of a maxillary sinus fracture is suggested by the presence of a blunt injury to the sinus with swelling in the cheek area and the presence of epistaxis. Nasal, orbital, or maxillary fractures are often present. Isolated maxillary sinus fractures occur but generally do not require treatment. The radiographic evaluation performed is a sinus series. Treatment consists of administration of decongestants and follow-up radiographs to evaluate whether the sinus congestion has satisfactorily resolved. The presence of an air–fluid level in a fractured sinus does not mean that drainage is indicated; however, it does mean that that patient should be followed to make sure that the air fluid level resolves. Fever in the presence of a facial injury that cannot otherwise be identified as to the source should prompt a diagnostic sinus aspiration. Aspiration of the sinus can yield valuable diagnostic information from Gram stain and culture. Adequate surgical drainage is indicated if infection is confirmed by analysis of the aspirated material.

LeFort Fractures

LeFort fractures involve injury to the maxilla and adjacent bones in the orbit, nose, and zygomatic areas.[16,56] Using cadaver experiments, Rene LeFort[61] published an accurate analysis of the fracture patterns that has yet to be surpassed. He described fractures occurring at three levels within the facial skeleton and identified these lines of weakness occurring in the areas of the thin bones of sinuses or of the orbits. The patterns are as follows (Fig. 33-36):

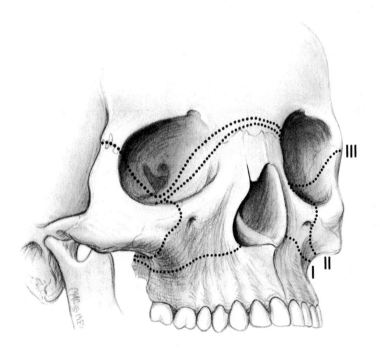

FIG. 33-36 LeFort I, II, and III levels of midfacial fractures.

LEFORT I FRACTURE

A LeFort I fracture or horizontal fracture of the maxilla separates the entire maxillary alveolus from the upper facial skeleton. The fracture lines run from the pterygoid plates, which are transsected at their inferior portions across the lower portion of the maxillary sinus to the pyriform aperature. The fracture created is thus horizontal or transverse and separates the entire maxillary alveolus as a unit from the remainder of the midface. Occasionally with any LeFort fracture, the palate can be split in the midline or a lateral segments of the maxillary alveolus fractured involving either the molar or the molar and bicuspid teeth. The latter are tuberosity fractures of the maxillary alveolus and should be diligently searched for, as their presence is often not accompanied by a mucosal laceration. They are detected as a disturbance of occlusion that generally appears after initial fracture treatment.

LEFORT II FRACTURE

The LeFort II or pyramidal fracture separates a central pyramidal or triangularly shaped nasomaxillary segment from the adjacent zygomas and upper portions of the facial skeleton. The fracture line runs from the base of the pterygoid plates diagonally up through the maxilla, separating the maxilla from the zygoma. The fracture line traverses the infraorbital foramen or travels near it, goes across the infraorbital rim traveling in the thin portion of the orbital floor, and then goes up the medial portion of the orbit to separate a portion of the nose from the nasal process of the frontal bone. The segment thus sectioned is a central fragment involving the maxillary alveolus, portions of the medial orbit and the nose.

LEFORT III FRACTURE

The LeFort III fracture is a disjunction of the entire facial bones from the cranial skeleton. The facial bones are separated through the upper orbits. LeFort III fractures are rarely a single fragment but exist as comminuted combinations of the lesser LeFort fragments. Rarely an isolated LeFort III fracture is a single fragment and presents with bilateral eyelid hema-

tomas and an occlusal abnormality of minor severity. Minimal mobility is present. The periorbital swelling is the clue to the presence of the upper facial fracture. The usual LeFort fracture is more severe on one side than the other, and it is common to observe a LeFort III level injury on one side with a LeFort II level injury on the other side. The other fragments isolated by the fractures include a zygomatic fracture on the LeFort III side, an orbital fracture on this side, a unilateral or bilateral fracture of the nasoethmoid area and a lower fragment of a LeFort I or LeFort II type.[71,104]

LEFORT IV FRACTURES

These fractures were not described by LeFort, but the classification has been extended to include the supraorbital area.[107] The supraorbital fracture may coexist with other facial fractures; its presence implies that stabilization must include the supraorbital injury.

DIAGNOSTIC CONSIDERATIONS

The diagnosis of a LeFort fracture is confirmed by a mobile maxilla. This is the hallmark of the maxillary fracture. Mobility may be minimal in an impacted or green-sticked fracture but an occlusal disturbance should be present with malocclusion or an open bite anteriorly or anteriolaterally. Uncommonly, LeFort fractures may present with little maxillary mobility and minor disturbances of occlusion. Zygomatic, orbital, nasal, and nasoethmoid fractures are commonly associated components of the upper LeFort fractures and the symptoms described under these regional fractures should be present. Hematomas are present in the buccal sulcus area; again, a careful evaluation of the maxillary alveolus for sagittal fractures of the palate or alveolar fractures should be performed. Classically, mid-face elongation and retrusion are the associated deformities of LeFort fractures. These are observed after a several day period has elapsed if the patient has not been placed in intermaxillary fixation. The maxilla drops downward and posteriorly, with premature occlusion occurring in the molar area. This opens the bite anteriorly. Profuse nasopharyngeal bleeding usually accompanies LeFort fractures. Facial swelling may be massive. CSF leaks and pneumocephalus occur in the LeFort II and III fracture patterns especially if a nasoethmoidal fracture is present.

RADIOGRAPHIC EVALUATION

The radiographic evaluation consists of a thorough cranial facial CT scan continued through the entire face. Alternatively, plain skull films demonstrate fractures at the various LeFort levels.

TREATMENT

Treatment consists of placing the patient in intermaxillary fixation in occlusion for 6 to 8 weeks. This stabilizes the lower (occlusal) fragment of the maxilla which contains the teeth. The stabilization of the maxillary alveolus thus depends on its relationship with the mandible and an intact relationship of the mandible with the cranial base. Any associated mandibular fractures should be stabilized either in vertical (ramus) height dimension or in horizontal dimension in the mandibular alveolus to preserve the proper relation of the maxillary alveolus to the cranial base. Reconstruction of maxillary fractures involves reconstructing the "structual pillars" of the facial skeleton (Fig. 33-37).[32,33,69-71,73,77,78,104] The heavier areas of bone are traced with arrows.

These thicker areas, the nasofrontal and zygomaticomaxillary buttresses, are stabilized by interfragment wiring replacing unusable or missing bone with bone grafts (Fig. 33-38).

Intermaxillary fixation is the principal treatment used to restore the projection of the lower midface and proper occlusion.[44,83,96] The projection of the upper mid-face is restored by open reduction and internal fixation of the component parts. Structural support is provided up to the frontal cranium. Stabilization of the upper portion of the LeFort fracture is accomplished by open reduction of zygomatic or nasoethmoid fractures as appropriate. Supraorbital and frontal sinus fractures are also treated in the same manner as for regional fractures. The reconstruction thus proceeds from stable bone to stable bone. Intermaxillary fixation should be applied as soon after the injury as possible. This limits the deformity of midface elongation and retrusion, which are symptoms of the untreated LeFort fracture (where the alveolar segment of the maxilla is not placed intermaxillary fixation). Suspension wires (which extend from the arch bar to the frontal cranium) were once a component of LeFort fracture treatment but are now seldom used. They were utilized when the treatment involved closed reduction and fracture fixation by compression with suspension wires. The open reduction technique described obviates the need for suspension wires.

Any sagittal (anteroposterior) fracture of

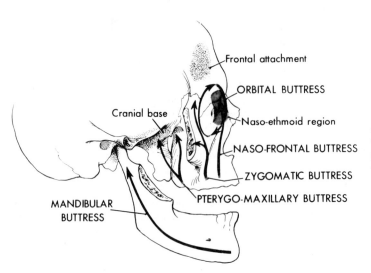

Frontal attachment

ORBITAL BUTTRESS

Cranial base

Naso-ethmoid region

NASO-FRONTAL BUTTRESS

ZYGOMATIC BUTTRESS

PTERYGO-MAXILLARY BUTTRESS

MANDIBULAR BUTTRESS

FIG. 33-37 Structural pillars of the facial skeleton: Anterior vertical nasomaxillary, lateral zygomaticomaxillary, and posterior pterygoid pillars.

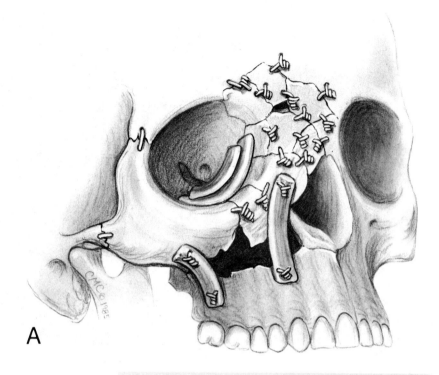

A

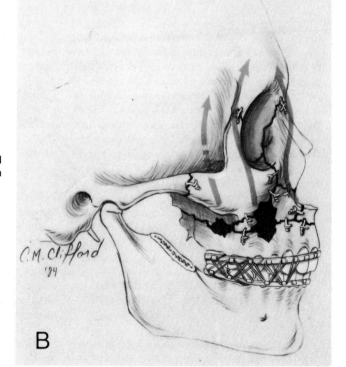

B

FIG. 33-38 Stabilizing the structural pillars with interfragment wiring with (**A**) or without (**B**) bone grafts.

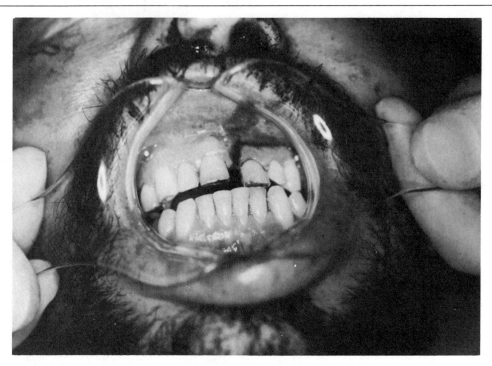

FIG. 33-39 Split palate accompanying a midfacial LeFort fracture.

the maxillary alveolus[70] or palatoalveolar fractures (Fig. 33-39) require a dental splint on the palatal surface of the teeth to prevent rotation of maxillary segments. Occlusal "stops" may be incorporated into the splint to compensate for critical missing teeth. This prevents telescoping of dental segments. Routine drainage of the maxillary sinuses is preferred by either Caldwell-Luc antrostomy or nasal antrostomy. Otherwise, unexplained temperature elevations following fractures that involve the sinuses should prompt sinus radiographs and aspiration. Late follow-up radiographs should detect clear sinuses to assess sinus obstruction.

The Mandible as a Basis for LeFort Fracture Treatment

The mandible, unless altered by fractures, usually assumes a position of "rest" between centric rest and centric occlusion because of a balance of muscular forces. This position serves as a guide to maxillary fracture reduction.

External Fixation in the Use of Headframes

Headframes may be used in patients with loss of frontal cranial support and comminuted maxillary or mandibular fractures, especially those with bone loss, where stabilization of remaining fragments is necessary (Fig. 33-40). Retrusion of zygomatic or nasal fractures despite open reduction techniques is another indication for the use of external traction. If the position of the mandible relative to the cranial base (such as reduced facial height in concomitant subcondylar and LeFort fractures) cannot be stabilized with open reduction and internal fixation, the use of a headframe from the cranium to the mandible might allow one to cor-

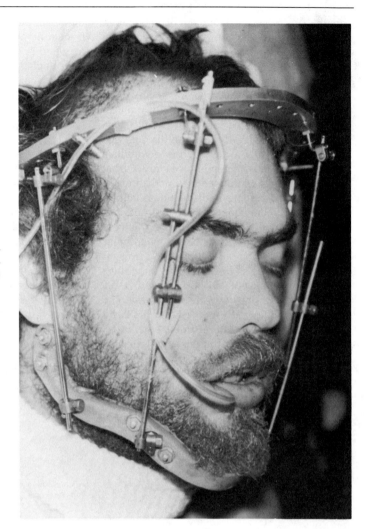

FIG. 33-40 Headframe from cranium to mandible to stabilize position of mandible relative to cranial base.

rect this position (Fig. 33-40). Headframes are generally employed for a 6- to 10-week period. Some headframes, such as the Georgiade,[29] provide only simple external traction whereas others provide rigid spacial fixation of fracture fragments (University of Tennessee). The principal means of external fixation of the mandible is with the Joe Hall Morris biphasic appliance. This involves the use of bone screws, two per fragment, placed in each segment of the mandible. The screws are then connected with an acrylic connector. A temporary stabilizing device is useful in the initial reduction, which consists of rods with clamps connecting and stabilizing the screws during the application of the acrylic connector. Patients find external fixation uncomfortable; these devices are used less frequently as open reduction techniques improve.

Mandibular Fractures

The mandibular fracture is a common facial injury in the multiply injured patient. Mandibular fractures often coexist with cervical spine injuries or injuries to the brain. Mandibular fractures are usually compounded into the mouth and less commonly compounded through the skin. The sites of mandibular fracture vary with the age of the patient and with the state of the dentition. Generally, mandibular fractures occur in structurally weak areas such as the subcondylar area, the angle, or the cuspid region (Fig. 33-41). In the angle and cuspid areas, the roots of the teeth extend close to the inferior border of the mandible, and this area is structurally weak. In the edentulous mandible, the most common area to be fractured is the junction between the body and the angle. In both dentulous and edentulous mandible fractures, the subcondylar area is frequently involved. Many mandibular fractures are multiple; thus, the presence of a mandibular fracture should prompt a thorough search for a second fracture.[36,47] In edentulous mandibles the most common area to be fractured is the junction between the body and angle area. The loss of the molar teeth creates a particularly weak section; most fractures in the edentulous mandible will be present in this area. The second most common area to be fractured in the edentulous mandible is the subcondylar area. In dentulous mandibles, the subcondylar area is the most frequently fractured followed by

the angle and parasymphysis area. The "most frequently observed" fracture varies according to whether one is considering only single or both single and multiple fractures of the mandible. The goal in treating mandibular fractures is to re-establish the preinjury occlusion and less optimally to achieve a result which can be corrected by occlusal grinding or orthodontics (one-half a cusp change or tilting of the teeth).

The mandible has vertical and horizontal segments (Fig. 33-41). The horizontal segment contains the body and parasymphysis area; these segments constitute the basal bone of the horizontal segment. The superior portion of the horizontal segment consists of alveolar bone structure containing the teeth. Teeth are numbered from right to left in the maxilla and from left to right in the mandible. The numbering progresses from 1 to 32, as illustrated. The normal adult mandible has three molars per side, two bicuspid teeth per side, a cuspid and two central incisors. Thus, there are 16 teeth in the lower dental arch. The vertical portion of the mandible is characterized by an angle, the ramus, coronoid, condylar, and condylar neck (subcondylar) areas. The thin subcondy-

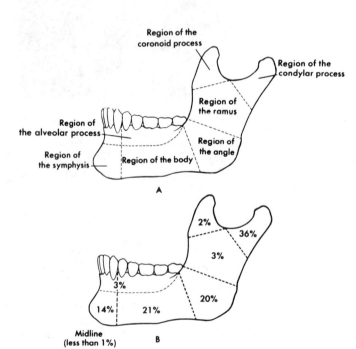

FIG. 33-41 Common sites of mandible fractures and relative frequency (dentulous mandible). (Dingman R, Natvig P: Surgery of Facial Fractures. WB Saunders Co, Philadelphia, 1964.)

lar area of the ramus is a frequent area for fracture.

DIAGNOSIS

The diagnosis of mandibular fractures is suggested by pain, swelling, tenderness, malocclusion, fractured teeth, gaps, or level discrepancy in the dentition, asymmetry of dental arch form, intraoral laceration or hematoma, and localized pain. Often the patient volunteers that the teeth do not feel that they are coming together properly. Numbness in the distribution of the mental nerve may accompany fractures of the body, angle, or ramus area. Swelling, bruising, and extraoral or intraoral lacerations frequently occur. Bleeding may be observed from a tooth socket, indicating that the fracture involves the bone adjacent to that tooth. Fractured or missing teeth are frequently present, and trismus or pain on moving the jaw are noted. The patient frequently cannot bring the jaws into proper occlusal relationship. An open bite deformity may occur with inability to close the jaws either anteriorly, laterally, or bilaterally. There may be abnormality or irregularity in the dental arch form on inspection and the patient may not be able to bring the teeth into full intercuspation. Irregularity along the mandibular border or a gap or level discrepancy in the dentition may signal a fracture. Condylar fractures or dislocations may cause a laceration of the ear canal, since the condyle is positioned adjacent to the anterior wall of the canal. Such patients present with bleeding from the ear canal which, of course, may be caused by either simple laceration or by middle cranial fossa fractures. Fractures of only the alveolar segment produce an instability of a section of mandibular dentition. Alveolar fractures involve a separation from the tooth-bearing alveolus from the lower (basal) bone of the mandible.

RADIOGRAPHIC EVALUATION

Radiographic evaluation consists of lateral oblique mandible, posterior–anterior mandible, and Towne's skull views. The lateral oblique views of the mandible visualize the body, angle and subcondylar area. The PA view visualizes the mandibular symphysis and the angles. The Towne view demonstrates the condyle and subcondylar area. If the patient is unable to cooperate for these films, they may be taken "reversed" and still provide adequate diagnostic information. The Panorex examination requires considerable patient cooperation and usually travel to a dental facility. This circumferential picture of the mandible and lower maxilla is taken with the patient standing, which displays the interrelationship of the teeth. It is a good examination if it can be obtained without risk to the patient. Specialized dental films such as occlusal, palatal, or apical films demonstrate the mandibular symphysis and the palate and show the roots of the teeth involved in the fracture line. Generally, these films also involve travel to a specialized dental facility.

INTERMAXILLARY FIXATION

Intermaxillary fixation remains a standard treatment for most fractures of the jaw and generally is accomplished with Eric arch bars ligated to the teeth with #24 to #28 wires.[20] These arch bars are interconnected and provide intermaxillary fixation for a 4- to 8-week period. Prolonged intermaxillary fixation has been shown to cause degenerative changes in temporal mandibular joint cartilage; therefore, intermaxillary fixation is released as soon as appropriate depending on the healing and anatomical site of the fracture. Intermaxillary fixation is hazardous in patients with loose teeth and periodontal disease, as it usually results in extraction of the teeth. Such patients might be considered for plate and screw fixation of the mandible, a stable fixation system that avoids the necessity to place the patient in intermaxillary fixation.[100] Proper occlusion is observed by confirming the relationships of the first molar, cuspid, and central incisor teeth. Intercuspation of the teeth should be maximal and should fit a reasonable pattern. Deviation from normal occlusion is due either to a preexisting skeletal abnormality, to extractions or absence of teeth, or to failure to achieve a satisfactory reduction. Patients placed in intermaxillary fixation for 6 weeks will average a 10-

to 15-lb weight loss. A liquid diet with adequate calorie and vitamin supplement is taken during this period. Patients unable to consume a liquid diet should either be fed intravenously or with a nasogastric tube as appropriate.

Healing of mandibular fractures is assessed by absence of pain and mobility at fracture sites. Radiographic evidence of union may not be present, as facial bones in the area of fracture do not calcify completely. The patient must be observed for deviation of occlusal relationship once the intermaxillary fixation is released. Appropriate oral hygiene must be similar to cutaneous wound care and consists of frequent brushing and mouthwash irrigation. A Waterpick or pressure irrigation device is useful.

Fracture displacement is determined by the nature and direction of the fractures and the pull of mandibular muscles on the fracture fragments. The muscles that elevate the mandible are the masseter, temporal, and medial pterygoid. Those that depress it are the digastric, mylohyoid, genioglossus, hyoglossus, and lateral pterygoid. Forward movements of the mandible are produced by the lateral pterygoid, anterior fibers of the temporal and some fibers of the masseter. Retraction is produced by the posterior fibers of the temporal, the deep layer of the masseter, and the medial pterygoid. Grinding motions are produced by the pterygoid muscles acting alternatively. The designation "favorable" or "unfavorable" is determined by the direction of the pull of the muscles on the fragment and the direction of the fracture line. If the direction of the fracture line opposes the displacement from muscular force, the fracture is considered favorable. The presence or absence of opposed teeth must be considered in this designation of favorable or unfavorable fracture.

ANATOMIC LOCATIONS OF MANDIBULAR FRACTURES

Symphysis and parasymphysis fracture usually require both intermaxillary fixation and open reduction at the inferior border. To achieve maximum stability, a plate is used. An interosseous wire can suffice but does not provide the same degree of stability. A lingual splint may be necessary to prevent lingual rotation of segments (Fig. 33-42). Body fractures

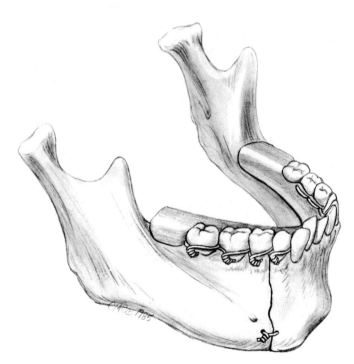

FIG. 33-42 Lingual splint and inferior border wire used to reduce a mandibular fracture.

generally require intermaxillary fixation and frequently require open reduction at the inferior border. Angle fractures generally require open reduction at the inferior border and intermaxillary fixation. Ramus, coronoid, subcondylar, and condylar fractures can generally be treated with intermaxillary fixation alone.

The complications of treatment of mandibular fractures include infection, nonunion, malocclusion, pain, hypesthesia, or anesthesia. Complications are most frequent in angle fractures, comminuted fractures, and fractures in the edentulous mandible, which display decreased bone height and ability to heal. Teeth present in the line of fracture or fractures with poor immobilization or delayed treatment where significant periodontal disease is present are susceptible to infection. The teeth in the line of fracture are generally retained unless they are grossly loose. An antibiotic is recommended. The complication rate for these teeth is approximately 30 percent, and many require late extraction. During the immediate postfracture period, however, they can provide a source of stability for intermaxillary fixation. Third molars in the fracture line generally require extraction as do grossly mobile teeth or teeth with significant periodontal involvement. Multiple root fractures are an additional indication for removal. Open reduction of mandibular fractures may be accomplished either extraorally or intraorally. Intraoral reduction is accomplished for symphysis and parasymphysis fractures and for some angle fractures.

DELAYED UNION AND NONUNION

A delayed union occurs when a mandibular fracture is not united after 8 to 12 weeks of fixation. Mobility is demonstrable but not necessarily in all planes. There is often a radiolucency at the fracture site. Nonunion is defined by mobility in multiple planes of the fracture fragments with "rounding" or sclerosis of the fractured bone ends. It is present from 2 to 6 months after initial reduction. Conservative debridement and further stabilization may result in bone healing. Alternatively, bone grafting is indicated with additional means of stabilization if increased immobilization does not suffice.

CHILDREN'S FRACTURES

The incidence of children's fractures is quite low, with those in the 0- to 5-year age group accounting for 1 percent of facial fractures observed and those in the 5- to 12-year age group accounting for between 3 and 5 percent of the fractures observed. The actual numbers of patients in these age groups by numerical frequency is 25 to 30 percent of the population. Children are thus protected both by environmental and anatomic factors. They are protected by their parents. Small forces are generated in the usual child's injuries and thus lacerations are common but facial fractures are uncommon. The face is small compared with the head size and thus the large frontal cranium is subjected to injuries whereas the face is protected. The face is small, the bones are elastic, and the sinuses are undeveloped; therefore, the facial bones are not as easily fractured. Fractures in the upper face are managed as in adults, but early treatment is important. Healing is especially rapid in children, and healing in malalignment occurs if an early reduction is not performed. It is difficult to accomplish revisional surgery when healing in malalignment of a nasal or LeFort fracture has occurred. It is mandatory that these patients receive early proper reduction and fixation.

Many mandibular fractures in children may be treated with more conservative techniques. In addition, one must be careful to avoid injury of the tooth buds and supplement open reduction techniques with closed reduction and splinting maneuvers to prevent injury to tooth buds.

In patients who are less than 10 years old, approximately two-thirds of the mandibular fractures observed are subcondylar fractures. If the child can bring himself or herself into satisfactory intercuspation, it is not necessary to place this patient in intermaxillary fixation. Alternatively, intermaxillary fixation is used when the patient cannot bring the teeth into proper occlusal relationship. Fractures of the mandible may thus be managed by soft diet alone or with intermaxillary fixation and a liquid diet. The period of intermaxillary fixation is short, as children heal with considerable rapidity. The root structure of children's teeth is shallow, especially during the period of mixed dentition. Thus, intermaxillary fixation devices are difficult to apply and are not well tolerated. Tooth extraction may be common, and other kinds of immobilization may be preferred. Growth disturbances after facial fractures in children are rare and are usually seen in patients sustaining comminuted fractures of the condylar head (growth center of the mandible) or nasoethmoid area. Patients displaying problems with nasal or mid-face growth have generally had a significant nasal or midfacial injury at an early age.

Mandibular Reconstruction

Mandibular reconstruction for missing bone segments is accomplished by bone grafting with the iliac crest as the usual bone source. Some type of fixation either internal or external is used to stabilize the remaining segments of the mandible while the bone graft is healing. Generally, patients are placed in intermaxillary fixation as well which preserves proper dental relationships.

Facial Fractures with Soft Tissue Loss (Gunshot and Shotgun Wounds)

Gunshot and shotgun wounds are a frequent cause of civilian injury.[9,39] The usual civilian gunshot wounds seen in the emergency room are produced by low-velocity weapons. The injury delivered to tissue is proportional to the formula

$$KE = \frac{MV^2}{2g}$$

where the energy imparted by the missile is proportional to the square of the velocity. Low-velocity gunshot wounds are managed as facial fractures in the manner described for regional injuries. The gunshot entry and exit wound are managed as overlying lacerations and may be excised and closed. This method of manage-

ment has been quite successful in the treatment in most low-velocity gunshot injuries, as soft tissue injury is minimal. Gunshot injuries fall into patterns and generally involve either the mandible and tongue, the lower mid-face, the orbits, or the frontal cranium and orbits. It is surprising how many are similar to these patterns (Fig. 33-43).

Shotgun wounds are characterized by both injury and loss of bone and soft tissue.[74,82] They may be evaluated most accurately by determining the area of soft tissue and bone loss. Treatment involves identification of the areas of injury and of bone and soft tissue loss.[22] Conservative soft tissue debridement is then performed. Early or immediate soft tissue closure or skin to mucosal closure in areas of soft tissue loss is then performed to limit contracture. Immediate rigid skeletal fixation[29] is performed in the areas of bone injury, and external fixation compensates for bone loss in the areas in which it has occurred. Fractures in the zone of injury are managed as described in the regional treatment of facial fractures. It has been helpful to use a nonabsorbable intraoral closure, which prevents the wound breakdown observed with absorbable intraoral closures. Flap or bone graft reconstruction is performed during an interval dictated by the state of healing of the wounds. Delayed bone graft reconstruction is sometimes necessary for mandibular, maxillary, or orbital defects after completion of soft tissue reconstruction. The fixation of the bone fragments must be maintained during the entire period to ensure stability of the bone reconstruction and to prevent soft tissue contracture. Certain patterns of injury can be observed in shotgun wounds:

1. *Central mandibular and maxillary loss* involves the mandible, the upper and lower lips, and the base of the nose.
2. *Lateral mandibular wounds* involve lateral lower face soft tissue and the lateral mandible. There is generally bone loss in the lateral portion of the mandible. The maxilla and zygoma are frequently injured, but little tissue is missing in this area.
3. *Lateral maxillary wounds* are subject to significant infection and wound breakdown when primary closure is performed by advancement of skin over significant maxillary

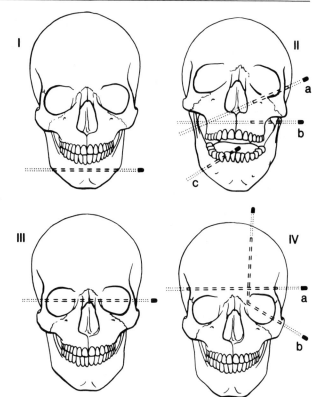

FIG. 33-43 Common patterns of low velocity gunshot wounds through facial tissues.

sinus damage (dead space). Generally, initial treatment involves stabilization and skin to mucosal closure with early soft tissue reconstruction with the provision of flap obliteration of the maxillary sinus. The skin can then be closed over the flap reconstruction.

4. *Central mid-face wounds* require fixation of the zygomas by transfacial K-wire fixation or headframe and maintaining the intercanthal distance with canthopexy. Flap and bone graft reconstruction are later provided. Brain injuries accompanying shotgun injuries are extremely lethal and demand adequate debridement.

Reconstruction of self-inflicted injuries has been worthwhile.[30,31,41] In 30 patients presenting with shotgun wounds in suicide attempts, one repeat suicide gesture proved fatal. Late deformity is principally proportional to the orbital and maxillary deformity, as mandibular reconstruction is cosmetically and functionally successful.

REFERENCES

1. Adams WM: Internal wiring fixation of facial fractures. Surgery 12: 523, 1942
2. Adams WM, Adam LH: Internal wire fixation of facial fractures: A 15 year follow-up report. Am J Surg 92: 12, 1956
3. Adkins WY, Cassone RD, Putney FJ: Solitary Frontal sinus fractures. Laryngoscope 89: 1099, 1979
4. Ayella RJ: The face. p. 33. In Radiologic Management of the Massively Traumatized Patient. Williams & Wilkins, Baltimore, 1978
5. Babcock JL: Cervical spine injuries: Diagnosis and classification. Arch Surg 111: 646, 1976
6. Barton FE, and Berry WL: Evaluation of the acutely injured orbit. In Aston S, Hornblass A, Rees T, Meltzer M (eds): Third International Symposium of Plastic and Reconstructive Surgery of the Eye and Adnexae. Williams & Wilkins, Baltimore, 1982
7. Becker DP, Miller JD, Ward JD et al: The outcome from severe head injury with early diagno-

sis and intensive management. J Neurosurg 47: 491, 1977

8. Brawley BW, Kelly WA: Treatment of basal skull fractures with and without cerebrospinal fluid fistulae. J Neurosurg 26: 57, 1967
9. Broadbent TR, Woolf RM: Gunshot wounds of the face, initial care. J Trauma 12: 229, 1972
10. Bucholz RW, Burkhead WZ, Graham W et al: Occult cervical spine injuries in fatal traffic accidents. J trauma 19: 768, 1979
11. Christian MS: Non-fatal injuries sustained by seatbelt wearers: A comparative study. Br Med J 2: 1310, 1976
12. Converse JM, Smith B: Enophthalmos and diplopia in fracture of the orbital floor. Br J Plast Surg 9: 265, 1957
13. Converse JM, Smith B, O'Bear MF, Wood-Smith D: Orbital blow-out fractures: A ten year study. Plast Reconstr Surg 39: 20, 1967
14. Cramer LM, Tooze FM, Lerman S: Blow-out fractures of the orbit. Br J Plast Surg 18: 171, 1965
15. Curtin HD, Wolfe P, Schramm V: Orbital roof blow-out fractures. AJR 139: 969, 1981
16. Dawson RL, Fordyce GL: Complex fractures of the middle third of the face and this early treatment. Br J Surg 41: 25, 1953
17. Dingman RO, Grabb WC: Surgical anatomy of the mandibular ramus of the facial nerve based on the dissection of 100 facial halves. Plast Reconstr Surg 29: 266, 1962
18. Donald PJ, Bernstein L: Compound frontal sinus injuries with intracranial penetration. Laryngoscope 88: 225, 1978
19. Donald PJ: Frontal sinus ablation by cranialization. Arch Otolaryngol 108: 142, 1982
20. Eid K, Lynch OJ, Whitaker LA: Mandibular fractures: The problem patient. J Trauma 16: 658, 1976
21. Emery JM, von Noorden GK, Schlernitzauer DA: Orbital floor fractures: Long-term follow-up of cases with and without surgical repair. Trans Am Acad Ophthalmol Oto-Laryngol 75: 802, 1971
22. Finch DR, Dibbell DG: Immediate reconstruction of gunshot injuries to the face. J Trauma 19: 965, 1979
23. Finney LA, Reynolds DH, Yates BM: Comminuted subfrontal fractures. J Trauma 4: 711, 1964
24. Fradkin AH: Orbital floor fractures and ocular complications. Am J Ophthalmol 72: 699, 1971
25. Fueger GF, Bright J, Milauskas A: The roentgenological anatomy of the floor and of the orbit. p. 28. In Bleeker GM, Lyle TK (eds): Fractures of the Orbit. Williams & Wilkins, Baltimore, 1970
26. Fujino T, Makino K: Entrapment mechanisms and ocular injury in orbital blow-out fracture. Plast Reconstr Surg 65: 571, 1980
27. Fukado Y: Results in 400 cases of surgical decompression of the optic nerve. p. 474. In Proceedings of the Second Symposium on Orbital Disorders, Amsterdam, 1973. Modern Problems in Ophthalmology. Vol. 14. Karger, Basel, 1975
28. Gentry LR, Manor WF, Turski PA, Strother CM: High resolution analysis of struts in facial trauma: 1. Normal anatomy; 2. Osseous and soft tissue complications. AJR 140: 523; 542, 1983
29. Georgiade N, Nash T: An external cranial fixation apparatus for severe maxillofacial injuries. Plast Reconst Surg 38: 142, 1966
30. Goodman JM, Kalsbeck J: Outcome of self-inflicted gunshot wounds of the head. J Trauma 5: 636, 1965
31. Goodstein WA, Stryker A, Weiner LJ: Primary treatment of shotgun injuries to the face. J Trauma 19: 961, 1979
32. Gruss JS: Naso-ethmoid-orbital fractures: Classification and role of primary bone grafting. Plast Reconstr Surg 75: 303, 1985
33. Gruss JS, MacKinnon SE, Kassel EE, Cooper PW: The role of primary bone grafting in complex craniomaxillofacial trauma. Plast Reconstr Surg 75: 17, 1985
34. Gurdjian E, Webster J: Mechanism of head injury. p. 58. In Head Injury. Little, Brown, Boston, 1958
35. Gwyn PP, Carraway JM, Horton CE et al: Facial fractures—Associated injuries and complications. Plast Reconstr Surg 47: 225, 1971
36. Hagan EH, Huelke DF: An analysis of 319 case reports of mandibular fractures. J Oral Surg 19: 93, 1961
37. Haines SJ: Topical antibiotic prophylaxis in neurosurgery. Neurosurgery 11: 250, 1982
38. Hambager CA, Wiesall J: Disorders of the Skull Base Region. Wiley, New York, 1968
39. Hubschmann O, Shapiro K, Baden M et al: Craniocerebral gunshot injuries in civilian practice—Prognostic criteria and surgical management: Experience with 82 cases. J Trauma 19: 6, 1979
40. Huelke DF, O'Day J, Mendelsohn RA: Cervical injuries suffered in automobile crashes. J Neurosurg 54: 316, 1981
41. Hutcherson RR, Kreuger DW: Accidents masking suicide attempts. J Trauma 20: 800, 1980
42. Hybels RC, Newman MH: Posterior table fractures of the frontal sinus: 1. An experimental study. Laryngoscope 87: 171, 1977
43. Hybels RC: Posterior table fractures of the frontal sinus: Clinical aspects. Laryngoscope 87: 1740, 1977

44. Irby WB: Facial Trauma and Concomitant Problems. 2nd ed. CV Mosby, St. Louis, 1979

45. Jabaley ME, Lerman M, Sanders HJ: Ocular injuries in orbital fractures. A review of 119 cases. Plast Reconstr Surg 56: 410, 1975

46. Jacobs JB, Pusky MS: Traumatic pneumocephalus. Laryngoscope 90: 515, 1980

47. James RB, Fredericks C, Kent JM: Prospective study of mandibular fractures. J Oral Surg 39: 275, 1981

48. Jefferson A, Reilly G: Fractures of the floor of the anterior cranial fossa: The skeleton of patients for dural repair. Br J Surg 59: 585, 1972

49. Jones LT, Wobig JL: Surgery of the Eyelids and Lacrimal System. Aesculapius Birmingham, AL, 1976

50. Jones DEP, Evans JNG: "Blow-out" fractures of the orbit: An investigation into their anatomical basis. J Laryngol Otol 81: 1109, 1967

51. Jones WD, Whitaker LA, Murtagh F: Application of reconstructive cranio-facial techniques to acute craniofacial trauma. J Trauma 17: 339, 1977

52. Karlan MS, Cassisi NJ: Fractures of the zygoma—A geometric, biomechanical and surgical analysis. Arch Otolaryngol 105: 320, 1979

53. Klastersky J, Sadeghi M, Brihaye J: Antimicrobial prophylaxis in patients with rhinorrhea or otorrhea: A double blind study. Surg Neurol 6: 111, 1976

54. Kline LB, Morawtz RB, Swaid SN: Indirect injury of optic nerve. Neurosurgery 14: 756, 1984

55. Koorneef L: Spatial Aspects of the Orbital Musculo-Fibrous Tissue in Man. Swets and Zeitlinger, B.V., Amsterdam and Lisse, 1977

56. Kuepper RC, Harrigan WF: Treatment of midfacial fractures at Bellevue Hospital Center, 1955–1976. J Oral Surg 35: 420, 1977

57. Kurza A, Patel M: Superior orbital fissure syndrome associated with fractures of the zygoma and orbit. Plast Reconstr Surg 64: 715, 1979

58. Larrabee WF Jr, Travis LW, Tabb HG: Frontal sinus fractures—their suppurative complications and surgical management. Laryngoscope 90: 1810, 1980

59. Larsen OD, Thomasen M: Zygomatic fractures. I. A simplified classification for practical use. Scand J Plast Reconstr Surg 12: 55, 1978

60. Leech P: Cerebrospinal fluid leakage, dural fistula and meningitis after basal skull fractures. Injury 6: 141, 1974

61. LeFort R: Etude experimental sur les fractures de la machoire supérieure. I, II, III. Rev Chir Paris 23: 201; 360; 479, 1901

62. Lewin W: Cerebrospinal fluid rhinorrhea in closed head injuries. Br J Surg 42: 1, 1954

63. Lewin W, Marshall TF, Roberts AH: Long-term outcome after severe head injury. Br Med J 2: 1533, 1979

64. Lewis VL, Manson PN, Morgan RF, et al: Facial injuries associated with cervical fractures: Recognition, patterns, and management. J Trauma 25: 90, 1985

65. Lindsey D, Nava C, Marti M: Effectiveness of Penicillin irrigation in control of infection in sutured lacerations. J Trauma 22: 186, 1982

66. Luce EA, Tubbs TD, Moore AM: Review of 1,000 major facial fractures and associated injuries. Plast Reconstr Surg 63: 26, 1979

67. McCoy FJ, Chandler RA, Magnan CG Jr, et al: An analysis of facial fractures and their complications. Plast Reconstr Surg 29: 381, 1962

68. McDonald JV: The surgical management of severe open brain injuries with consideration of the long-term results. J Trauma 20: 842, 1980

69. Manfredi SJ, Raji MR, Sprinkle PM et al: Computerized tomographic scan findings in facial fractures associated with blindness. Plast Reconstr Surg 68: 479, 1981

70. Manson PN, Crawley WA, Yaremchuk MJ, et al: Midface fractures: Advantages of extended open reduction and immediate bone grafting. Plast Reconstr Surg 76: 1, 1985

71. Manson PN, Shack RB, Leonard LG et al: Sagittal fractures of the maxilla and palate. Plast Reconstr Surg, 72: 484, 1983

72. Manson PN, Su CT, Hoopes JE: Structural pillars of the facial skeleton. Plast Reconstr Surg 66: 54, 1980

73. Manson PN, Sargent L, Rochman G et al: 162 Nasoethmoidal-orbital fractures: Technical considerations in immediate reconstruction. Plast Reconstr Surg (submitted for publication)

74. Matras H, Juderna H: Combined craniofacial fractures. J Maxillofac Surg 8: 52, 1980

75. May M, West JW, Heeneman H et al: Shotgun wounds to the head and neck. Arch Otolaryngol 98: 373, 1973

76. May M: Nasofrontal ethmoidal injuries. Laryngoscope 87: 948, 1977

77. Mektubjian SR: Operative policy in severe facial trauma in combination with other severe trauma. J Maxillofac Surg 10: 14, 1982

78. Merville L: Multiple dislocations of the facial skeleton. J Maxillofac Surg 2: 187, 1979

79. Merville LC, Derome P: Concomitant dislocation of the face and skull. J Maxillofac Surg 6: 2, 1978

80. Milauskas AI, Fueger GF: Serious ocular complications associated with blow-out fractures of the orbit. Am J Ophthalmol 62: 670, 1966

81. Miller SH, Lung RJ, Davis TS, et al: Management

of fractures of the supraorbital rim. J Trauma 18: 507, 1978

82. Mincy J: Post traumatic spinal fluid fistula of the frontal fossa. J Trauma 6: 618, 1966

83. Mladick RA, Georgiade NG, Royer J: Immediate flap reconstruction for massive shotgun wound of face. Plast Reconstr Surg 45: 186, 1970

84. Morgan BDG, Madan DK, Bergerot JPC: Fractures of the middle third of the face—A review of 300 cases. Br J Plast Surg 25: 147, 1972

85. Morgan PR, Morrison WU: Complications of frontal and ethmoid sinusitis. Laryngoscope 90: 661, 1980

86. Morley TP, Hetherington RF: Traumatic CSF rhinorrhea and otorrhea, pneumocephalus and meningitis. Surg Gynecol Obstet 104: 88, 1957

87. Nahum AM: The biomechanics of maxillofacial trauma. Clin Plast Surg 2: 59, 1975

88. Nicholson LT, Guzak BF: Blindness after blowout fractures of the orbit. Arch Ophthalmol 86: 369, 1971

89. Peri G, Chabannes J, Menes R et al: Fractures of the frontal sinus. J Maxillofac Surg 9: 73, 1981

90. Petro J, Tooze FM, Bales CR, Baker G: Ocular injuries associated with periorbital fractures. Trauma 19: 730, 1970

91. Pfeiffer RL: Traumatic enophthalmos. Arch Ophthalmol 30: 718, 1943

92. Putterman AM, Stevens T, Vrist MF: Nonsurgical management of blow-out fractures of the orbital floor. Am J Ophthalmol 77: 232, 1974

93. Raaf J: Post traumatic cerebrospinal fluid leaks. Arch Surg 95: 648, 1957

94. Rougier J, Freidel C, Freidel M: Fractures of the orbital roof and ethmoid region. In Bleeker GM, Lyle TK (eds): Proceedings of the Symposium on Orbital Fractures, Excerpta Medica Amsterdam, 1969

95. Rowe LD, Miller E, Brandt-Zawadzki M: Computed tomography in maxillofacial trauma. Laryngoscope 91: 745, 1981

96. Rowe L: Spacial analysis of midfacial fractures with multidirectional and computed tomography: Clinicopathologic correlates in 44 cases. Otolaryngol Head Neck Surg 90: 651, 1982

97. Rowe NL, Killey HC: Fractures of the Facial Skeleton. 2nd ed. Churchill Livingstone, Edinburgh, 1968

98. Rubin LR: Langer's lines and facial scars. Plast Reconstr Surg 3: 147, 1948

99. Sataloff ST, Sariego J, Myers DL, Rechter HJ: Surgical management of the frontal sinus. Neurosurgery 15: 593, 1984

100. Schaefer S, Diehl J, Briggs W: The diagnosis of CSF rhinorrhea by metrizamide CT scanning. Laryngoscope 90: 871, 1980

101. Schilli W: Compression osteosynthesis. J Oral Surg 35: 802, 1977

102. Schultz RC: Facial injuries from automobile accidents: A study of 400 consecutive cases. Plast Reconstr Surg 40: 415, 1967

103. Schultz RC: Supra-orbital and glabellar fractures. Plast Reconstr Surg 45: 227, 1970

104. Smith B, Regan WF Sr: Blow-out fracture of the orbit: Mechanism and correction of internal orbital fractures. Am J Ophthalmol 44: 733, 1957

105. Sofferman RA, Danielson PA, Quatela V, Reed R: Retrospective analysis of surgically treated LeFort fractures. Arch Otolaryngol 109: 446, 1983

106. Stranc MF, Gustafson EH: Primary treatment of fractures of the orbital roof. Proc Soc Med 66: 303, 1973

107. Stranc MF: Primary treatment of nasoethmoid injuries. Br J Plast Surg 23: 8, 1970

108. Sturla F, Absi D, Buquet J: Anatomical and mechanical considerations of craniofacial fractures: An experimental study. Plast Reconstr Surg 66: 815, 1980

109. Swearingen JJ: Tolerances of the human face to crash impact. Report from the Office of Aviation Medicine, Federal Aviation Agency, July 1965

110. Tajisma S, Nakjuina H: The treatment of fractures involving the frontobasal region. Clin Plast Surg 7: 525, 1980

111. Tajima S, Sugimoto C, Tanino R et al: Surgical treatment of malunited fractures of zygoma with diplopia and with comments on blow-out fracture. J Maxillofac Surg 2: 201, 1974

112. Tessier P, Hervovet F, Lekieffer M et al: Plastic Surgery of the Orbit and Eyelids. Wolfe SA (transl). Masson USA, New York, 1977

113. Vondra J: Fractures of the Base of the Skull. Charles C Thomas, Springfield IL, 1965

114. Weymuller EA Jr: Blindness and LeFort III fractures. Ann Otol Rhinol Laryngol 93: 2, 1984

115. Yanagisawa E: Pitfalls in the management of zygomatic fractures. Laryngoscope 83: 527, 1973

SUGGESTED READINGS

Andreasen JO: Traumatic Injuries of the Teeth. 2nd ed. WB Saunders, Philadelphia, 1981

Archer WH: Oral and Maxillofacial Surgery. WB Saunders, Philadelphia, 1975

Aston S, Hornblass A, Meltzer M, Rees T: Third International Symposium on Plastic and Reconstructive Surgery of the Eye and Adnexae. Williams & Wilkins, Baltimore, 1982

Converse JM: Surgical Treatment of Facial Injuries. Williams & Wilkins, Baltimore, 1974

Dingman R, Natvig P: Surgery of Facial Fractures. WB Saunders, Philadelphia, 1964

DuBrul EL: Sicher's Oral Anatomy. CV Mosby, St. Louis, 1980

Foster CA, Sherman JE: Surgery of Facial Bone Fractures. Churchill Livingstone, New York, 1986

Georgiade NG: Plastic and Maxillofacial Trauma Symposium. CV Mosby, St. Louis, 1969

Irby WB: Facial Trauma and Concommitant Problems. CV Mosby, St. Louis, 1979

Kawamoto HK Jr, Wolfe SA (eds): Maxillofacial Surgery. Clinics in Plastic Surgery. WB Saunders, Philadelphia, 1982

Kelly J: Management of War Injuries to the Jaws and Related Structures. U.S. Government Printing Office, Washington, DC: 008–045–0018–6

Kruger GO: Oral Surgery. CV Mosby, St. Louis, 1979

Rowe N, Killey H: Fractures of the Facial Skeleton. Churchill Livingstone, London, 1968

Rowe N, Williams J Li: Maxillofacial Injuries. Churchill Livingstone, Edinburgh, 1985

Tessier P, et al: Symposium on Plastic Surgery in the Orbital Region. CV Mosby, St. Louis, 1976

34

Acute Orthopedic Injuries

Andrew R. Burgess
Bert R. Mandelbaum

INTRODUCTION

The comprehensive care of the critically injured patient demands early and aggressive attention to orthopedic injuries. Therefore, to provide optimal care to the multiply injured trauma patient, each trauma team member must become familiar not only with the pathophysiology of high-energy trauma and the systemic effects of such bone and soft tissue insults, but also with the various orthopedic options and their timing, risks, and benefits.

Most trauma specialists now acknowledge that the management of orthopedic injuries is an integral part of the early overall treatment of multiply injured patients; however, controversy still exists about the exact timing of each intervention. Experience indicates that this timing directly affects pulmonary physiology, neuroendocrine response, risk of sepsis, nutri-

tional status, and eventual musculoskeletal function. Various studies[7,11,15,27,28,46,59,60] also show that in terms of patient morbidity and mortality, early fracture fixation combined with aggressive ventilatory support provides maximal patient benefit.

The authors have designed a schema to illustrate the value of early orthopedic intervention in the management of the multiply injured patient. This schema depends on five factors: (1) collection of a pertinent data base; (2) fundamental knowledge of the pathophysiology of trauma; (3) logical determination of the goals of therapy; (4) knowledge of available orthopedic options (based on existing surgical/institutional limits) and their optimal timing; and (5) clinical judgment for integrating this information into a comprehensive, therapeutic plan for managing a critically, multiply injured patient.

CLINICAL DATA BASE

Formulating a therapeutic plan depends on establishing a relevant data base (accounting for both specifics of the injury and the patient's status preinjury) by obtaining answers to the following questions: who? when? where? and how? The answers to these questions will influence the selection of orthopedic therapy.

Who Is This Individual?

The clinician should make every effort to determine the patient's age, past medical history, occupation, and life goals; all these factors have a bearing on the choice of therapy. For example, a severe injury in a young patient might justify the risk of an extensive attempt at limb salvage, whereas an elderly patient might be better served by a definitive amputation.

Past medical history is important, not only to determine premorbid conditions, but also with reference to drug or alcohol abuse, psychiatric history, and medication history. Cumulative demographic data on patients admitted with multiple trauma injuries indicate that the typical trauma patient is young, male, and frequently under the influence of alcohol or drugs.

Some traditional concepts about selecting appropriate recipients for major orthopedic intervention must be modified when considering the critically injured patient. Advanced age or extreme severity of injuries become reasons for aggressive orthopedic treatment rather than indications for conservative methods. For the physiologically compromised patient, the systemic benefits of early fracture fixation and mobilization generally will offset the perioperative risk.

When Did the Injury Occur and When Should Therapy Begin?

Knowledge of the timing of events responsible for the patient's injury, the sequence of events, and the elapsed time since injury forms part of the data base and, as such, influences the therapeutic plans. The second question concerns the timing of the patient's orthopedic treatment once he or she is admitted to the medical system. Setting treatment priorities often depends on the answers to the following questions: How much time elapsed from injury to admission to the treatment facility? How long was the patient in shock? How long did wounds remain open before they were cleaned and debrided? How long were compromised extremities ischemic before the return of circulation? For example, a patient in shock for 2 hours who is then transported in antishock trousers to the receiving facility needs early examination for evidence of elevated compartment pressures in the involved extremities.

Where Did the Injury Occur?

Many treatment decisions depend on knowledge of the physical surroundings at the injury scene, particularly the potential for and type of contamination. For example, the contamination involved in a household injury differs from that of a barnyard or industrial injury. Military wounds often have gross contamination, and high-velocity missile wounds almost always require debridement beyond the initial surgery.

How Did the Injury Occur?

The data collected to answer the question how, that is, the details of the trauma itself, are as important as the other who, when, and where data. In particular, knowledge about the type and degree of energy that produced the injury plays a vital role. Recent works corroborate the clinical impression that the harder the fracture impact is, the more systemic sequelae can be expected.[68] Although, upon first inspection, a high-energy pedestrian injury may resemble a low-energy fracture occurring at home, the high-energy fracture presents a greater threat to the patient because it releases more marrow products into the blood,[8,29,64] generally compromises more soft tissue and bone viability, and presents a higher risk of late sepsis, myoglobulinemia, and other complications.

TRAUMA PATHOPHYSIOLOGY

Injury Evaluation

Although the initial physical exam generally forms the cornerstone of the patient's data base, it often produces less than ideal results when performed on a multiply injured patient because of the patient's potential inability to comply with directions, the need for acute respiratory intervention, and other complicating factors. Ideally, a physical examination (keeping the history of injury in mind) should be performed immediately when the patient arrives in the emergency department; data from this exam may be correlated with information from the field providers. Although not primarily involved in the patient's *initial* resuscitation and stabilization, the orthopedic surgeon should ascertain several pieces of information prior to formulating an orthopedic plan: the total amount of blood loss, the presence of other injuries (specifically chest, abdominal, or head), and whether or not the patient is in shock.

The evaluation of orthopedic injuries, particularly those to the pelvis and extremities, begins with assessment of limb viability. After visual inspection, the orthopedist assesses vascular integrity by manual examination and noninvasive methods if possible, interpreting the physical exam based on the history of the traumatic incident. Knowing such history might indicate the need for invasive assessment if the examination results suggest a more serious injury than is immediately obvious. For example, since many critically injured patients cannot cooperate with sensory or motor examinations immediately after the injury, the orthopedist must actively consider the possibility of compartment syndrome. Open injuries do not obviate the need to search for elevated soft tissue pressures, and the orthopedist

should test the extremity for this syndrome before and after fracture reduction.

Neurologic assessment of pelvic and extremity injuries is generally difficult in the critically injured patient. Many patients are in altered states of consciousness or have a drug- or alcohol-altered sensorium. Orthopedically, one must direct attention to areas that require detailed neurologic examinations. For instance, the orthopedist should carefully examine a patient with a posterior hip dislocation for sciatic nerve function. Similarly, a humeral fracture leads the examiner to document the neurologic integrity of the upper extremity distal to the injury.

The orthopedist must use other diagnostic modalities (see discussion below) judiciously in the critically ill patient. The timing and priorities of investigative studies depend on their relation to the treatment program for the injuries under investigation.

VASCULAR ASSESSMENT

Vascular tree injuries from high-energy external forces result in a spectrum of changes in the blood vessels, ranging from vessel wall contusion and intimal or adventitial tears to rupture of a particular blood vessel.[40] The vascular injury directly affects the blood vessel and indirectly affects the respective limb, which may become ischemic as a result of treatment delays caused by transport, resuscitation, stabilization, and diagnosis. During this ischemic time, a series of humoral mediators are released from the ischemic limb as well as from the injured blood vessel, producing local, regional, and systemic effects[5] (see below).

As the first step in the physical evaluation, the orthopedist must note pulses and capillary filling. In addition to this physical examination, we rely strongly on the noninvasive Doppler ultrasound probe to document pulses and quantify limb occlusion pressures; we also advocate aggressive use of peripheral vessel angiography for the multiply injured patient with limbs at risk or for the patient with severe pelvic injuries and hemodynamic instability (Fig. 34-1).

The clinician must be aware of the ability of his or her institution to perform angiographic tests quickly and with minimal risk to the patient; the clinician must also be cognizant of

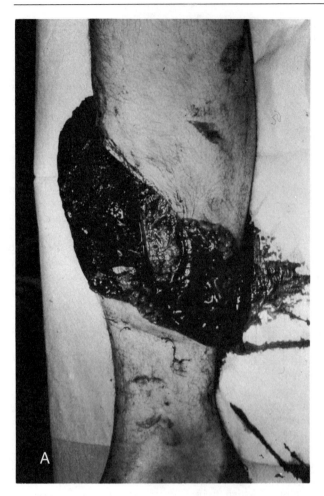

FIG. 34-1 (**A**) Clinical presentation of a 25-year-old victim of a motorcycle accident. On admission, lower limb was pulseless. (*Figure continues.*)

the effects of angiographic dye loads on kidney function and circulatory volume in the injured patient. If assessment of organ injuries requires central, large-vessel angiography, indication of the extremities at risk will permit evaluation of pelvic and/or extremity injury at the time of central angiography. This will yield valuable information about distal injuries with minimal additional risk to the patient. Selective intraoperative angiograms are also valuable in the subset of patients who demonstrate potentially fatal distal hemorrhage in the wake of postresuscitation blood pressure increases or in whom concurrent coagulopathy occurs. For example, a study demonstrating a two- or three-vessel transection associated with extensive soft tissue damage may indicate the need for a life-saving amputation for control of hemorrhage, whereas a study demonstrating single vessel transection, distal to the trifurcation in the leg, may suggest a less drastic procedure to control hemorrhage.

SOFT TISSUE ASSESSMENT

The orthopedist must realize that contiguous injuries to soft tissue and bone, including open fractures, will most likely accompany arterial injuries in the multiply injured patient. Assessment of viability therefore continues with assessment of the musculoskeletal soft tissue injuries. One must consider a soft tissue injury in terms of the "zone of injury." Using

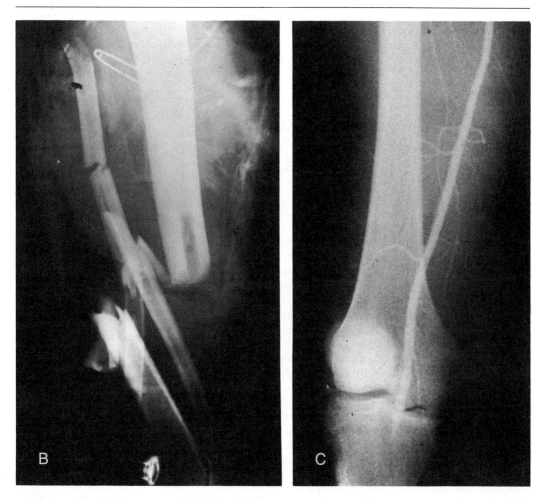

FIG. 34-1 (B) Radiographic evaluation of compound-comminuted fractures. **(C)** Arteriogram showed arterial injury at popliteal trifurcation far above the area of open fractures. Exploration revealed avulsion of arterial trunks from popliteal artery. Only the posterior tibial artery could be reconstructed. The limb survived and the fracture healed in 8 months. (Bosse MJ, Burgess AR, Brumback RJ: Evaluation and treatment of the high-energy open fracture. Adv Orthop Surg 7:3, 1984.)

this concept, and in the light of the history, an isolated sharp wound usually injures tissue over a minimal area, whereas blunt wounds or twisting wounds to extremities often disperse their energy over a greater area than first indicated by either visual examination or radiographs. Consequently, the skin must be assessed to: determine the direction, size, and orientation of the lacerations; identify the skin bridges that remain; evaluate any degloving component or separation from fascial planes; and consider the effect of abrasions or gross contamination.

Muscle is assessed with regard to its color, bleeding, contractility, connection to bony tissues, and overall contamination. Fascia, periosteum, tendons, and ligaments are evaluated in terms of blood supply, bony attachment, and contamination. When evaluating periosteum and soft tissue, one must pay attention to their intimate relationships to bone. Have the soft tissues been stripped from the bone, thus compromising both the hard and soft tissues? Do the remaining soft tissues, including muscle, skin, and fascia, provide enough coverage for compromised neurovascular structures?

Early assessment of these structures often directs the initial therapy and indicates its realistic, long-term goals.

NEUROLOGIC ASSESSMENT

If possible, neurologic assessment follows vascular and soft tissue evaluation. Many trauma patients, however, have associated injuries that produce altered states of consciousness or have serious central nervous system injuries that preclude an accurate neurologic examination. As part of the soft tissue assessment at the time of surgery, visualization of the neurovascular bundles in the area of injury will give an indication of peripheral nerve supply. Since examination of peripheral nerve and nerve root injuries in the multiply injured patient often proves difficult, the clinician should document any and all neurologic findings as completely as possible (for both medical and legal reasons), particularly those in the high-risk areas. The peripheral neurologic exam might dictate some extremity procedures that would be beneficial and without risk for the cooperative, neurologically intact patient but less than optimal for the patient with neurologic deficits. A totally insensate foot, for example, may be less suitable for a salvage procedure than one that is as severely injured but has a sensate plantar surface. Even if a foot survives insensate, it will be of little or no benefit to the patient; therefore, the quicker surgical alternative of a primary or delayed secondary amputation would be more beneficial to the multiply injured patient, allowing more rapid recovery and rehabilitation.

BONE AND JOINT ASSESSMENT

Orthopedic decisions are based on the physical examination of the bony injuries. Only after assessing the overall viability of the extremity, including the vasculature, soft tissue, and neurologic status, can one direct attention to the status of the bone and other structural elements of the involved extremity.

Any discussion of open fractures must include a classification schema, such as that devised by Gustilo and Anderson,[31] which relates the severity of injury energy to the amount of

blood-vessel, soft-tissue, and bone devitalization. In this schema, a *grade I fracture,* caused by a low-energy force, results in minimal displacement and causes a small (usually < 1 cm) puncture in the soft tissue integument; soft tissue penetration usually proceeds from the inside out. A *grade II fracture,* caused by an external force that first produces soft tissue injury and then bone fracture, is characterized by soft tissue lacerations (approximately 1 cm) with minimal soft tissue damage. A *grade III fracture,* an open injury resulting from a high-velocity external force, has bony comminution, displacement, and devascularization, accompanied by extensive soft tissue damage, overall contamination, and devitalized skin, subcutaneous tissue, nerve, tendon, and artery. This classification system provides a mechanism for relating impact energy to nonunion and infection rates.

It is important to know how to "read" the radiographic pattern of limb or pelvic fractures. An orthopedist experienced in treating high-energy injuries can often gain information about the energy involved in the initial impact by correctly interpreting the radiographs. Torsional injuries manifest as spiral fractures and higher-energy fractures tend to be extensively comminuted. Injuries showing segmental fracture patterns often indicate a wide area of impact. Patterns of air dissection along fascial and hard/soft tissue interfaces indicate that some devitalization of tissues has occurred and, with an associated break in the skin, may indicate possible contamination of tissue planes.

Fracture patterns indicating injury in the functional area of a joint will also influence overall patient treatment. Simple shaft fractures of long bones do not necessarily require perfect anatomic reduction for good, long-term function. Fractures closer to the joints (or other surfaces where complex motion occurs) require more anatomic reconstruction. Knowledge of the difference between these two types of injuries enables the orthopedist to plan immediate surgery to immobilize the long bone fracture (which would benefit a critically injured patient) or postpone the complex, taxing, anatomic reconstruction of an intra-articular fracture until the critically injured patient becomes more stable. When an open wound accompanies an orthopedic injury, visualization of bone is essential in the patient examination but, as noted above, other diagnostic modalities are often of greater value in assessing the implications of hard tissue injury to outcome.

Pathomechanics of Orthopedic Injury

To care for the critically ill, multiply injured patient in the intensive care unit, the surgeon and critical care specialist must understand the implications of the pathomechanical and pathophysiologic details that contribute to the patient's overall status at any specific time. A comprehensive understanding of these details enables the entire team to facilitate the overall systemic stabilization and resuscitation of the patient by interpreting the polytraumatic injury as a condition with local, regional, and systemic effects.[1,67]

In the critical evaluation of the mechanisms of injury, one must understand a basic principle of physics: the force applied is equal to the mass times the velocity at impact. The amount of injury, devitalization, and destruction of blood vessels, nerves, soft tissue, and bone is directly related to the dissipation of this force into the tissues at the time of injury.[31] The orthopedist must understand the magnitude, duration, and direction of the forces on bone, as well as the rate at which the bone is loaded.

In biomechanical terminology, *stress* is the internal resistance to deformation, that is, the load divided by the area on which the load acts. *Strain* is the change in linear dimension resulting from an externally applied force.

Strain energy is the energy a structure is capable of absorbing. The more rapidly a bone is loaded, the greater will be the energy absorption prior to fracture. Rapid loading infuses enormous amounts of strain energy and, as the bone is loaded, it begins to deform (elastic strain energy). As the energy dissipates, the fracture occurs in the form of an explosion (plastic strain energy). The importance of this stress–strain biomechanical relationship becomes obvious when one is discerning the changes that occur during and shortly after the bone fractures.

Sauter and Klopper[65] have shown that when rabbit femurs are fractured with different strain rates, the quantity of fat emboli is directly related to *strain* rate and occurs at the moment of fracture, not when the bone is being compressed. These animal studies[65] obviously indicate that the critical factors in the explosive disorganization of bone and injection of marrow into the circulation are the pressure and duration of external forces. Thus, high pressures and prolonged durations of bone loading produce more emboli than shorter durations of loading. Understanding this concept is a crucial step in understanding the correlation between the local changes and some of the regional and systemic reactions to local phenomena.[2,53,67]

LOCAL CHANGES

Since no high-energy fracture occurs in a completely isolated, self-contained state, a contiguous area around the wound (the zone of injury noted earlier) will initiate a series of inflammatory cascade reactions. These changes reflect the magnitude of tissue damage and are directly related to several factors that determine the quality and quantity of eventual tissue necrosis, including increased oxygen consumption postinjury and hypoxemia related to hypoxia, both of which may perpetuate the progression of tissue necrosis.[48] These changes are mediated by the release of various inflammatory substances (including proteases, prostaglandins, leucotrienes, kinins, thromboxanes, and thromboplastins;[34,35] see Chapter 3) that produce myriad regional and systemic, in addition to local, effects (see below).

Under normal physiologic circumstances of minimal injury, these local factors have a very efficient rapid metabolism and clearance time. However, in circulatory disturbances such as traumatic hemorrhagic shock, these substances persist, thus producing prolonged local, regional, and systemic effects.[67] The ramifications of this distant mediation are important in the interpretation of the multiply injured patient's progress.

REGIONAL CHANGES

As part of the initial regional response to trauma, the blood flow to the injured limb increases,[37] affecting the significant relationship of the circulation from the periosteal and medullary circulation to injured bone.[57] A rapid rise of local oxygen consumption during the early posttraumatic period further potentiates tissue hypoxia and secondary ischemia.[37] In addition, the hemorrhagic shock associated with polytraumatic injuries requires transfusions, utilizing banked blood with an inherent average of 70 percent less 2,3-diphosphoglycerate per hemoglobin molecule than does fresh blood.[10] This factor alone increases the affinity of oxygen for the hemoglobin molecule and decreases the tendency for tissue oxygen release by shifting the oxyhemoglobin dissociation curve to the left. This complex interaction is physiologically mediated by local factors in which prostaglandins may play a significant role.[29,49]

SYSTEMIC CHANGES

Severe polytrauma and associated hemorrhagic shock with significant blood loss results in a cascade of systemic changes that allow the body to maintain perfusion in the acute setting. In the severely injured patient, various systemic phenomena interact in a continuum, often progressing in a "downhill" direction unless aggressive intervention is undertaken to break the cycle. In this attempt to maintain systemic integrity, body systems initiate a series of events that may prove detrimental to the host organism, such as excessive protein catabolism and decreased functioning of cell-mediated and humoral immune systems either primarily or secondarily related to corticosteroid release.[35] Lastly, possible inadequate detoxification and clearance of metabolic byproducts may potentiate posttraumatic pulmonary insufficiency (see Chapter 19).

Successful treatment for the multiply injured patient depends on an understanding of these systemic phenomena.

Neuroendocrine System. In the period after injury, the organism's first priority is to maintain perfusion, which depends on a complex, interlocking, neuroendocrine negative feedback system on the local and systemic levels. The restoration of a normal neuroendocrine functional system is best achieved by preventing systemic organ failure through prompt restoration of blood volume, relief of pain, good nutrition, adequate surgical debridement, and stabilization of all fractures.

The body's major concern during hypovolemic hemorrhagic shock is the perfusion of the brain and heart; consequently it diverts the blood flow to these ischemia-intolerant organs.[77] In severe shock, however, the compensatory mechanisms that allow this diversion fail, so that blood flow in localized areas of tissue often stops and thrombosis occludes the microcirculation. In addition, on the microvascular level, capillary permeability increases, and fluid and proteins extravasate into the interstitium throughout the body. Metabolic waste products, toxic substances, and microaggregates of platelets, white blood cells, and clot accumulate in the traumatized tissue. As the patient is resuscitated, these waste products and microaggregates are washed into the venous circulation and find their way to the pulmonary circulation. The neuroendocrine axis directs the modulation of these responses.[29] Epinephrine, secreted by the adrenal gland as long as the patient is stressed, is the principal and dominant hormone in the shock state.[42] An increase in heart rate, myocardial contractility, and constriction of the venules and small veins are principally responsible for shunting to the ischemia-intolerant organs. In addition, epinephrine stimulates glycolysis and lipolysis.[42]

Cortisol peaks during the early stages in response to trauma, further increasing blood glucose concentration by adding to the interleukin-1-stimulated proteolysis of skeletal muscle protein into amino acids, and by potentiating the conversion of these amino acids into glucose. Cortisol also stimulates lipolysis by facilitating catecholamine activation of hormone-sensitive adipose tissue lipoprotein lipase, thus providing free fatty acid substrates for aerobic metabolism (see Chapters 15 and 17).

Aldosterone, a mineralocorticoid, is also present at high levels after trauma, as determined by the conversion of angiotensin I to angiotensin II in the pulmonary circulation.[70]

Angiotensin II then stimulates the adrenal cortex to synthesize and release aldoterone, which provides renal conservation of sodium and water, thus increasing systemic blood pressure.[70] [In disease states such as the adult respiratory distress syndrome (ARDS) there is less conversion of angiotensin I to angiotensin II[70] thus possibly potentiating the tendency to hypotension.]

The pituitary gland releases the opiate peptides endorphin and enkephalin during hypovolemia, shock, and periods of increased pain; these peptides are thought to modulate overall sympathetic activity[23] and their opiate-like properties may contribute to an already present hypotensive state.[3] Arachidonic acid and its metabolites are also at very high levels during the acute response to shock. The two major products from arachadonic acid and its metabolites are prostacycline (PGI$_2$) and thromboxane A$_2$ (TXA$_2$). Thromboxane A$_2$ is synthesized by white cells as well as by platelets and is responsible for vasoconstriction and platelet aggregation. Prostacycline, produced by the vascular endothelial cell, is a vasodilator and platelet disaggregator, which constitutes its major functional value.[33-35,49] This neuroendocrine system may represent an important mechanism for local vascular control in injured extremities (see Chapters 3 and 6). In essence, the neuroendocrine response is directed towards maintaining tissue perfusion and metabolism in response to acute stress. If cardiopulmonary instability, blood loss, and pain persist in the ensuing days secondary to multisystem injuries, this integrated system ensures systemic viability at the expense of potentiating the catabolic state. The goals in therapeutic intervention should be to prevent and inhibit destabilizing states.

Immune System. Traumatic injury is associated with functional impairment of the immune system that may contribute to morbidity and mortality from infectious complications. Goris and Draaisma[26] have shown that in the first posttraumatic week, nervous system injury and hemorrhage are the leading causes of death; after 1 week, however, respiratory failure and remote organ failure associated with sepsis become the leading causes of death. The immune system response ordinarily includes (1) efficient phagocytosis by neutro-

phils and macrophages as well as (2) cell-mediated immunity and (3) humoral immunity. Trauma causes changes in each of these three immune systems.

The phagocytotic mechanism is depressed through the suppression of the reticuloendothelial system[1,17] (see Chapter 14). Saba and colleagues[63] have shown that levels of the opsonic protein, fibronectin, an α-2 opsonic glycoprotein thought to be responsible for increasing the affinity phagocytotic cells for circulating microcomplexes, are also depressed.

Humoral immunity is also depressed secondary to decreased serum immunoglobulins[61] and complement; this mechanism's details, however, have not been fully elucidated (see Chapters 3 and 14).

Traumatic injury affects cell-mediated immunity through the thymus-dependent T-cell lymphocyte population.[6,36,43,56] Multiple causes, including activation of a suppressor cell system[74] and the depression of lymphocyte reactivity in the response to mitogenic stimulation,[56,76] have been postulated for this phenomenon. Immune competency is based on maintenance of the functional integrity and integration of all three systems. Thus, it appears that trauma causes the patient to become an immunocompromised host. This information, therefore, has a critical bearing on the selection of surgical orthopedic priorities for the multiply injured patient.

Hematologic System. The hematologic system's response to injury is characterized by the loss of the red and white cell populations and platelets, and by a reduction in the quantity of coagulation cofactors (see Chapter 23). Resuscitation measures are designed to replenish these blood components with banked blood, citrate-stored blood, fresh frozen plasma, and platelets. The traumatic orthopedic injury activates the coagulation system by releasing cellular materials and thromboplastins and by forming thromboxane A$_2$, producing further platelet activation.[64] In addition to the increase in platelet function, there may also be inhibition of the fibrinolytic system. Together, these changes result in increasing numbers of platelets and fibrin complexes that may filter into pulmonary circulation.[31] As a result of inhibition of fibrinolysis, these microaggregates become localized in the pulmonary microcirculation and may play a major role in the initiation of the posttraumatic ARDS syndrome (see Chapters 18 and 19).

Pulmonary System. In the healthy physiologic state, the lung acts as a filter for all aggregates; through phagocytosis and activation of fibrinolysis, it is 80 percent effective in clearing such material. However, the multiply injured patient's compromised neuroendocrine, immune, and hematologic systems decrease the lung's effectiveness, resulting in one of the consistent findings of the posttraumatic period: respiratory insufficiency occurring in the first 72 hours.

In a series of patients reported by Trunkey and his co-workers,[72] one-third of the patients who sustained blunt trauma died of primary trauma to the heart, brain, and kidney, another third died of infection and sepsis, and the last third died from progressive respiratory insufficiency. Goris and Draaisma[26] confirm respiratory failure (despite aggressive blood gas monitoring and aggressive respiratory support) as the third most common cause of death in the first week after severe trauma. Trunkey et al.[72] conclude that after the initial resuscitation and stabilization phase, acute respiratory insufficiency syndrome ranks as the leading cause of death.

In addition to the coagulation- and prostaglandin-induced microaggregates, polytraumatic orthopedic injuries (including extremity and pelvic fractures) seem to release fat microglobules, reticuloendothelial system fragments, and connective tissue, which enter the venous circulation, reach the pulmonary circulation, and may contribute to pulmonary insufficiency syndrome.[39] The ineffective clearance of these complexes by the reticulendothelial system potentiates this problem.[64] Factors impeding the reticuloendothelial system include an increased load of microaggregates, ischemic injury, collagenous debris, and a low flow state that depresses microvascular flow.

Animal model studies have shown that when femurs are fractured, fat emboli move to the lungs in 100 percent of the animals.[38,45] When these materials reach the pulmonary microcirculation, they cause a mechanical obstruction at the level of the pulmonary ateriole. Since the fibrinolytic pathway is often impaired

after polytrauma, the fibrin and platelet aggregates may stimulate a intravascular coagulation process that further obstructs pulmonary blood flow at the microcirculatory level (see Chapter 18).

Although clinical fat embolism occurs rarely as a complication of large bone injury, trauma causes a release of neutral fats from bone marrow. Watson[75] showed that fat and bone marrow emboli originate from the site of the trauma. Fat released from ruptured fat cells gains access to the circulation through torn venules as a result of a local shift between extravascular flow and pressures; subsequently, fat may be located in the pulmonary microcirculation.[71] Studies of aircraft accident victims by Bierre and Koelmeyer[9] revealed that pulmonary fat embolism occurs very rapidly after severe injury and may be followed by bone marrow emboli, depending on the nature of other injuries. Using the quality and quantity of fat in the lung as an index, the clinician can make a postmortem determination of the severity of the overall injury. One must assume that many of these postmortem pulmonary findings occur in the blunt trauma victim with fractured long bones.

Kerstell[39] has demonstrated that the fatty acid profiles of pulmonary embolic fat most closely resemble those of depot marrow fat rather than albumin-bound free fatty acids in circulating lipoproteins and chylomicra. In addition, Rayfer et al.[55] showed that 25 to 50 times more neutral fat appeared in the pulmonary circulation of dogs with bilateral femoral fractures than in that of the uninjured control animals. Postmortem examination of the dogs with fractures revealed that embolic material was very closely related to that of marrow fat. Using ^{14}C-labeled free fatty acids injected into marrow cavities before fracture, Rayfer et al.[55] confirmed that the embolic fat to the lung did originate in the marrow.

In summary, the interactions among fat emboli, microglobules, and free fatty acids (as well as peripheral circulation of arachidonic acid and prostaglandin metabolites, decrease in tissue fibronectin, activation of complement system, and sequestration of leukocytes with release of their lysosomal and protease enzymes) may cause both mechanical obstruction and an increase in pulmonary vascular permeability.[73] These interactions also result in an increase in interstitial edema and hemor-rhagic changes around the capillary–alveolar membrane level. Concomitantly, a decrease in surfactant occurs, which causes a further de-crease in the number of open alveoli and in the dynamic compliance of the lung.[24,25,69] Other physiologic changes include a ventila-tion–perfusion mismatch, a right-to-left shunt, an increase in pulmonary vascular resistance, a decrease in functional residual capacity, and a potentiation of an already present metabolic acidosis through the production of respiratory retention of carbon dioxide.[12,20]

There appears to be a close relationship between the severity of trauma (the amount of injury to bone and soft tissue) and the overall quantity of materials sequestered in the pulmo-nary arterioles. Temporally, it should be recog-nized that there is a constant embolization from unstable extremity and pelvic injuries; one justification for early orthopedic surgical intervention is based on stopping this persis-tent embolization.[27,28] Thus, there is a strong interaction between local changes with regard to soft tissue and bone injury, the tissue factors that are released from the zone of injury, and the humoral and metabolic interactions at the systemic level. These factors pathologically alter the pulmonary circulation, resulting in post-traumatic respiratory insufficiency.[4,9,12,16,18–21,25,54,65,66] Modig[48] postulates that any delay in the treatment of multiple fractures or the de-bridement of ischemic soft tissues may result in a progression to the "delayed microembo-lism syndrome."

Thus, early traumatic respiratory insuffi-ciency, due to its common pathophysiologic pathway, necessitates aggressive intervention to inhibit a further dangerous progression of events.

Summary

In conclusion, the pathophysiology of trauma originates as a dissipation of energy from external forces exerted on the patient, and it is directly related to the biomechanical prin-ciples exemplified by the stress and strain rela-tionships and to the magnitude of energy im-parted by the injury. The consequences of

injuries to the vascular tree, soft tissues, nerves, and bones can be divided into local, regional, and systemic changes that interact in a progressive pathologic cycle. Although the injury may be localized in the extremity, criti-cal care in the posttraumatic period must focus on minimizing lung injury and preventing multi-system organ failure. Thus, early stabilization of major fractures and debridement of devital-ized tissue become physiologic principles for care of the multiply injured patient.

MANAGEMENT GOALS FOR THE MULTIPLY INJURED PATIENT

During and after the initial resuscitation and stabilization of the patient, the trauma team (including general surgeons, orthopedic surgeons, and critical care physicians) must es-tablish realistic goals as a framework for pa-tient care. Some goals address short-term ob-jectives and some are directed to long-term functional or "quality of life" objectives. The short-term goals include early fracture stabili-zation, achievement of the vertical chest, mini-mization of infection and nonunion, and estab-lishment and maintenance of an effective nutritional support program.

Early Stabilization

Early fracture stabilization benefits local, regional, and systemic systems. According to Olerud,[52] early fixation provides an optimal en-vironment for wound and fracture, thus pro-moting extremity healing. In addition, local fracture stabilization decreases ischemia and tissue necrosis by providing adequate perfu-sion to the fracture site. It also enhances re-moval of particulate matter from the fracture by allowing efficient lymphatic flow and ve-nous return. Most importantly, the metabolism of local humoral mediators (including prosta-glandins, bradykinins, serotonin, and histamines) may be increased, thereby having less effect on the overall systemic pathophysiologic changes. The regional changes that occur with early stabilization include a decrease of tissue hypoxia through effective oxygen and substrate delivery and enhancement of the injured tissue's oxygen consumption. Thus, orthopedic care should be directed at minimizing the total release of toxic substances from the extremity that may have deleterious consequences for the other organ systems.

Early stable fixation appears to improve regional venous return, which may facilitate systemic venous return and thereby permit an increase in cardiac output. Stable fracture fixation decreases blood loss through fragment immobilization; stable fixation also minimizes hematoma formation and, consequently, reduces compartment pressures. Thus, fixation reduces the need for blood transfusion, thereby minimizing tissue hypoxia and decreasing the overall numbers of microaggregates that result from using banked blood.[10] This action may, in turn, decrease the infusion of microaggregates that eventually would find their way to the pulmonary microcirculation. Goris et al.[27,28] showed that early osteosynthesis and mechanical ventilation decreased overall mortality rates. These interventions were most significant in the most severely injured patients; there appeared to be a corresponding decrease in the number of late deaths from sepsis. Early stabilization may also reduce the evolution of the "fat embolism syndrome," as suggested by a retrospective Finnish study of multiply injured patients, which demonstrated that 22 percent of patients without early fixation developed this fat embolism syndrome, as opposed to 1.4 percent of those who underwent early skeletal stabilization.[27,28] Other systemic benefits associated with early stabilization include reduction of the neuroendocrine response by decreasing the overall pain level.

Vertical Chest

Rigidly stabilized fractures make the patient more comfortable and permit participation in physical therapy because the patient can be mobilized effectively and turned frequently. It is well documented that (along with chest physiotherapy, including postural drainage and percussion) the turning movement, in and of itself, will minimize the ventilation–perfusion mismatch, thereby improving respiratory function. Combining early mechanical ventilation with internal fracture fixation and patient mobilization also decreases the incidence of deep vein thromboses and decubitus ulcers.[27] The timing of fracture fixation and stabilization is critical to reducing the morbidity and mortality of the multiply injured patient. Goris et al.[28] and Riska et al.[58-60] have shown that early fixation results in improved patient outcome.

Infection and Nonunion

The classic rationale for early surgical fixation is minimizing deterioration of extremities, based on minimizing fracture instability and the consequent damage to the extremity soft tissues. Early operative repair is also justifiable in terms of microbial flora: on admission, the patient has not yet acquired the nosocomial, resistant flora present in most intensive care units. Furthermore, compared with the results of later surgical therapy, early operative intervention does not increase the frequency of acute infections or chronic osteomyelitis. Thus, it appears that the optimal time for fracture fixation is shortly after initial resuscitation and stabilization so that maximal local, regional, and systemic benefits can result, influencing healing, fracture union, and overall morbidity and mortality.[41]

Nutrition

Early fracture fixation also takes advantage of the patient's nutritional status: when first admitted, most multiply injured patients are well nourished; with time, however, most undergo proteolysis. Because of the magnitude of this posttrauma proteolysis and catabolism, it is essential to maintain nutritional integrity as part of the orthopedic management, from the early postinjury period through discharge. The profound catabolic state initiated by the traumatic injury results in a negative nitrogen balance. Multiply injured patients require 1,500 to 2,000 calories/m² surface area and 14 to 20 g nitrogen as amino acids or proteins per day to minimize trauma's effects: impaired immune competence, decreased muscle mass, and inhibited wound healing (see Chapter 15).

ORTHOPEDIC TREATMENT OPTIONS

If the orthopedist and other trauma team members have a thorough understanding of the pathophysiology of blunt trauma and its systemic effects, they formulate an individualized treatment plan based on the collected data base, knowledge of the therapeutic goals for the specific patient, and a full understanding of the implications of various operative and nonoperative treatment options. Technologic evolution of biomechanical engineering and its application to orthopedic trauma has resulted in many treatment options. Each option must be selected and tailored to fit the individual patient's specific set of pathologic indications, the nature of the blunt trauma involved, the diagnostic and surgical limitations of the institution, and the capability of the orthopedic surgical team.

Any given option has advantages and disadvantages for any individual setting (Table 34-1). Some are well suited to certain parts of the musculoskeletal system but become second- or third-choice options in other anatomic areas. Before choosing any option, the orthopedist should establish the nature of wounding, the energy involved in impact, and the preinjury status of the patient.

TABLE 34-1. Orthopedic Options

Option	Advantages	Disadvantages
Traction	Quick No surgery "Gold standard"	Patient often immobile Not rigid fixation
Neufeld's traction	Increased patient mobility	Not rigid fixation
Casts	Quick "Gold standard"	Hidden area of injury "Fracture disease" Constrictive Not rigid fixation Open wounds difficult to treat
External fixation	Open wound management simplified Nonconstricting Good wound observation Stable fixation Minimal metal Joints remain free Patient mobilization	Pin tract problems Heavy, cumbersome "Nonunion machine"
Internal fixation (plates, etc.)	Most stable Patient mobilization Adjacent joints free	Large surgical wound "Foreign body" Prolonged operative time Skill-dependent Load-sharing
Intramedullary fixation (closed)	Stable Minimal blood loss Minimal devitalization Fracture site unviolated Increased patient mobilization Adjacent joints free	Requires image intensification and skilled team

Standard Traction

For treating long bone fractures, traction is the gold standard against which all other modalities are judged. Its advantages include speed of application, the lack of need for major surgery, and the fact that most hospital personnel are familiar with its use. The disadvantages of traction are primarily related to the need for patient immobilization. In the classic splint and suspension traction, the patient is often forced to lie recumbent and cannot be turned easily from side to side. In addition, the nonrigid fixation of the long bone may cause the release of additional marrow products into the circulation (see section on pathophysiology above). The lack of complete fracture immobilization may also require additional narcotics for pain control. Traction, because it involves patient immobilization, patient recumbency, additional marrow by-product release, and increased narcotic medication, therefore inevitably compromises the patient's respiratory system. Also, since the use of traction often requires relative immobility for the joints proximal and distal to the fractured bone, it can result in impaired or extended recovery to full limb use.

Neufeld's Traction

As described by Browner et al.,[14] Neufeld's traction used for the multiply injured patient corrects some of the disadvantages of standard traction: it permits side-to-side patient mobilization for additional pulmonary toilet and it enables some patients to sit upright in bedside chairs while maintaining lower extremity traction. These great advantages minimize some of the respiratory complications of prolonged recumbency. However, Neufeld's traction still does not rigidly immobilize the bone, and the patient therefore does not gain the full benefits of joint usage, still has an increased need for narcotics, and is compromised by the continued release of marrow products into the circulation.

Cast Immobilization

Cast immobilization of long bone fractures is another standard against which other options are judged. It is quick and can be applied by most surgeons with a basic knowledge of orthopedic principles. However, for the multiply injured patient, it has several disadvantages. Blunt trauma results from high-energy impact, and casts hide both wounds and crush injuries, preventing the clinician caring for the patient from regularly examining the wound and giving full sensory examination to document changes in neurovascular status. To immobilize a long bone completely, the cast must also immobilize the joints above and below the fracture site, leading to additional posthealing stiffness, muscle atrophy, and osteoporosis.[50] Finally, because fixation is not rigid, additional marrow products may be released into the circulation, and the patient may need more pain medication than would be required with rigid fixation.

External Fixation

As a method of treating open fractures in high-energy crush injuries, external fixation has gained acceptance over the last decade.[13] However, because of its inherent disadvantages, it should be considered primarily a treatment for soft tissue wounds. Its advantages in high-energy injuries center around wound management and the good access it gives to open wounds. The external fixator, a nonconstricting type of immobilization, permits observation of the wound or crush injury on a regular basis. Because this type of fixation is extremely stable, a minimal amount of foreign material is placed into the bone and soft tissue, and the joints above and below the injury remain free. Using external fixation to stabilize a long bone fracture allows complete patient mobilization, maximizing the patient's pulmonary toilet and general skin care. The disadvantages of external fixation are based on the neurologic and biomechanical limits of the fixator itself: (1)

the fixator is often heavy and cumbersome; (2) the pin tracts, if they do not receive proper care, may present drainage problems and produce long-term infection and osteomyelitis; and (3) the fixator does not allow the bone to load and, therefore, does not promote bone healing. Because of this last disadvantage, some orthopedists consider it a "nonunion" machine. We emphasize that to permit full physiologic loading of the healing fracture, the device should be unloaded or removed as quickly as possible (unless there is a grossly unstable fracture construct or missing bone) when the soft tissues are healed or are clean enough to permit skin grafting or flap reconstruction.

Internal Fixation

PLATES AND SCREWS

The European literature reported the use of plates and screws as early as the turn of the century, but acceptance of this method has been slow in North America.[50] Plates and screws provide the most stable of all types of fixation, often achieving that most important anatomic reduction near joints. As such, plates and screws provide patient mobility and immediate mobilization of the adjacent joints, both cephalad and caudad to the long bone injury. With the bone firmly fixed, the nearby soft tissues recover rapidly from the trauma of impact and that of the surgery necessary to place the devices. Edema resolves quickly and the rigid fixation minimizes pain. Of equal importance, rigid fixation reduces the overall systemic effects of the skeletal injury as it minimizes the systemic sequelae secondary to the release of bone marrow by-products; pulmonary function and physiology also improve as a result of increased patient mobility[15] and decreased pain medication. Although a patient may be able to tolerate a nonanatomic reduction in long bone shaft fractures, perfect anatomic reduction is critical to full return of function when joint mechanisms are involved. In general, accomplishing this latter goal necessitates internal fixation using plates and screws.

Internal fixation with plates and screws does have some disadvantages. First, open reduction and internal fixation using hardware generally require relatively long operative times and surgeons and nurses familiar with both the equipment and techniques. Second, these procedures add direct surgical insult to sites already compromised by blunt trauma. Third, to gain access to the fractured bone for stabilization, soft tissue and periosteum damaged in the initial injury must undergo additional surgical trauma. Fourth, these procedures place foreign material (metal plates and screws) in the wound and directly violate the injury hematoma. Therefore, open reduction methods result in higher infection risks than do closed techniques.

In summary, the orthopedic surgeon must consider the risks of open reduction and internal fixation (the necessity for surgical intervention, perioperative surgical complications, and the length of time involved in such complex surgery) before choosing this method.

INTRAMEDULLARY FIXATION

Intramedullary (IM) fixation, a recently developed treatment for long bone fractures, involves placing a fixation device in the IM marrow cavity of the fractured long bone, spanning the fracture site, and achieving stability. The advent of image intensification and newer radiographic techniques has made possible IM splinting by "closed" techniques: the surgeon can gain access, reduce, and then splint a fracture by IM rods inserted through a site remote from the original injury area. The advantage of remote IM rod insertion is obvious: the internal splint can stabilize the bone without additional soft tissue trauma at the initial injury site. This procedure minimizes further soft tissue dissection and devitalization of both periosteum and bone, eliminates the additional bleeding that a surgical procedure in the injured area could cause, reduces the risk of infection, and has the advantage of skeletal stabilization without risking additional trauma to an injured area.[22]

Although the resulting reduction may not be as exactly anatomic as could be achieved by internal plate and screw fixation, exact anatomic reductions are not necessary for shaft fractures, and the benefits of this closed technique far outweigh this slight disadvantage. The primary disadvantage of closed IM fixation is that it requires a surgical team familiar with both the instrumentation and the radiographic techniques.

CHOOSING THE BEST OPTION

Table 34-1 charts the advantages and disadvantages of the various therapeutic options for traumatic fractures. The orthopedic surgeon must base his or her treatment choice on the requirements for anatomic stabilization at a given level of injury severity (the primary concern) and on the ease of application and the complications of the hardware (the secondary concern) (Table 34-2).

Pelvic Fractures

Severe pelvic fractures are best managed by the immediate application of a simple anterior frame (external fixator), placed percutane-ously into the iliac crest, for partial stabilization (Fig. 34-2). Later (2 to 21 days postinjury), when the coagulation profile is normal and when fluid replacement volumes, cardiac and inotropic measures, and respiratory support have rendered the patient hemodynamically stable, the orthopedic surgeon can fully address any posterior instability. Timely and proper treatment of a pelvic fracture with stabilization of the pelvic ring will limit the acute hemorrhage from the fracture site by reducing the volume of retroperitoneal space; closing down the displaced and widened pelvis reduces the volume of hemorrhage required to produce a tamponade effect.[13]

The pelvic fixator reduces blood loss by a second method: stabilizing the pelvis against shear effects that occur secondary to patient motion. These shearing forces tend to disrupt clots that may have formed earlier during the resuscitation process. In addition, an external fixator contributes to good nursing care and pulmonary toilet by permitting patient mobilization rather than causing confinement with pelvic slings or traction. Pelvic fixation also reduces the amount of narcotics and other pain medications required by the patient with a pelvic fracture.

The orthopedic literature describes other, more complex pelvic frames; however, these take longer to apply and do not control posterior pelvic instability.

Internal pelvic fixation techniques are only rarely indicated for breaks in the anterior pel-

TABLE 34-2. Indications for Various Orthopedic Options

Option	Indications
Traction	Temporizing; skilled team unavailable; occasionally for an isolated injury
Neufeld's traction	Temporizing, especially with moderate open wounds that may become amenable to rodding, yet in a patient who needs full chest mobilization
Cast	Minimally displaced closed fractures near wrist or ankle; suitable for low-energy closed injuries
External fixation	Severe soft tissue injuries associated with fractures; acute pelvic stabilization; missing bone; fast, gross stabilization in salvage situations
Internal fixation (plates)	Intra-articular fractures; forearm fractures; proximal femur fractures; "floating joints"
Intramedullary fixation (closed rodding)	Long bone fractures (femur, humerus, tibia)

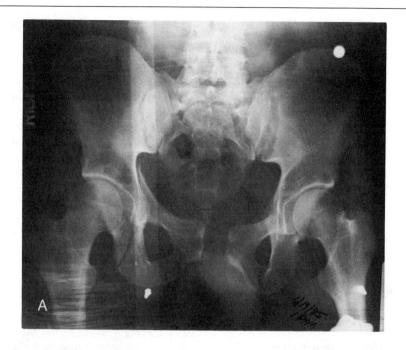

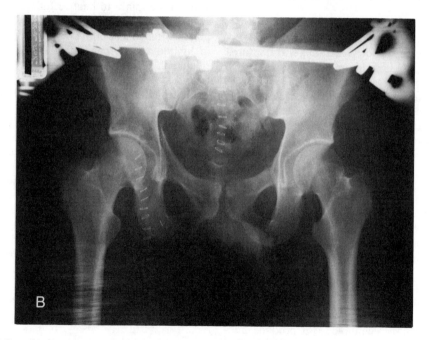

FIG. 34-2 (A) Pelvic fractures with pubic separation and posterior instability are due to separation at left sacroiliac articulation. **(B)** Stabilization of previously shown pelvic fractures (Fig. 34-2A) by anterior external fixation device. This preoperative therapy allowed control of retroperitoneal hemorrhage and, by allowing circulatory stability, facilitated abdominal exploration and vein graft repairs of vascular injury to the lower extremity. Radiograph was taken in postoperative period, after general surgical procedures were performed.

vic ring. When fractures near the sacroiliac joint, sacrum, or iliac wing require such fixation to achieve posterior stability, these difficult techniques should be reserved for the experienced surgical team familiar with the anatomic considerations, the surgical approaches, and the specific application techniques.

Basically, the concept of pelvic fracture treatment for the critically injured patient involves two steps. First, the orthopedist must provide gross resuscitative stabilization, that is, stabilize (with a simple anterior external fixator) disruptive skeletal elements, to minimize hemorrhage (by stabilizing posterior hematomas and closing the potential pelvic retroperitoneal space) and hasten the tamponade effect. Second, the orthopedist must use definitive treatment to improve long-term musculoskeletal function.

Femoral Fractures

In general, IM nailing[22,30,32] represents the best management for closed femoral fractures in the multiply injured patient. As advantages, this procedure uses a surgical approach remote from the trauma site, results in minimal soft tissue dissection and blood loss, and affords patients additional mobility since they are not "tied" to traction. New locking rod systems[32] permit closed method treatment even of comminuted femur shaft fractures (Fig. 34-3). The orthopedic surgeon, however, can consider other methods: open IM nailing, plating, traction, cast bracing, and external fixation.

Open IM nailing gives the patient additional mobility and improved pulmonary toilet, but it requires direct access to the injury site, thereby further devitalizing damaged tissue and increasing nonunion and infection.

As noted above, traction is the gold standard of treatment for fractures; however, although traction techniques can produce adequate results, they usually require prolonged bed rest (often in recumbency), which increases the risk of complications from pulmonary, urinary, and integumental problems.[62] Neufelds' traction is a good alternative to normal balanced traction for femoral fracture management in the multiply injured patient be-

cause it affords the patient full mobility in bed and access to a bedside chair without losing the benefit of adequate femoral traction.

External fixation of femoral fractures is best saved for salvage procedures when massive soft tissue wounds accompany the fracture. The advantages of this fixation method include fast application and good wound access for further debridement, dressing changes, and/or reconstructive procedures.[13] Femoral external fixation, however, is often heavy and cumbersome.

The European surgical community popularized internal femoral fracture fixation using plates.[44,50] This technique allows full mobility after surgery (although weight bearing is often not permitted). However, like open IM nailing, it requires a direct assault on the already damaged injury site, increasing the risk of infection and additional blood loss. Long bone plating also has a second disadvantage: it does not allow the bone to sense the full load placed upon it and, thereby, does not allow the bone beneath the plate to heal to full strength.[45] In addition, the "stress shielding" effect of such plates often necessitates a prolonged period of limited weight bearing after the device is removed. As a third disadvantage, plating requires a skilled surgical team well practiced in the techniques necessary for this demanding procedure.[45] Anatomic bone reconstruction (possible with open reduction and internal fixation using plates) is not a relative benefit when dealing with shaft fractures of long bones such as the femur. Anatomic reconstruction using plates should be reserved for periarticular and articular fractures of the proximal and distal end of the femur, where the extremely accurate reduction afforded by plating offsets the added risk of prolonged surgical intervention.[50] (It is often unnecessary to fix these latter two types of fractures during initial management; they may be treated on a delayed basis from 2 days to 2 weeks postinjury.)

Tibial Fractures

Much debate exists about the choice of tibial fracture treatment because additional soft tissue wounds frequently accompany these

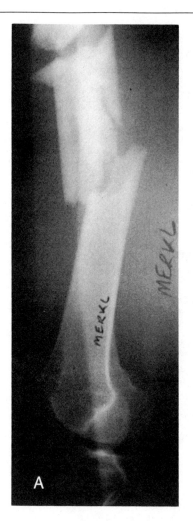 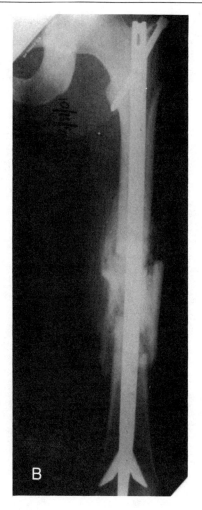

FIG. 34-3 **(A)** Comminuted midshaft femoral fracture. **(B)** Closed reduction of comminuted femoral fracture using locking rod system inserted remote from fracture site.

injuries. Techniques valid for the treatment of isolated tibial injuries, such as a sports-related injury or one caused by a domestic, low-energy accident, may not be appropriate for a tibia injured in a high-energy accident, such as a motorcycle or motor vehicle/pedestrian accident. An isolated tibial fracture in an otherwise mobile, healthy patient is not likely to lead to posttraumatic complications based on prolonged recumbency, lung function, fluid or blood replacement problems, and pulmonary embolization. However, a tibial shaft fracture in a multiply injured patient, most likely the result of high-energy trauma, becomes part of a complex of systemic injuries that compromise

pulmonary, hemodynamic, and neurologic functions in conjunction with musculoskeletal injuries to other parts of the body.

Casting techniques, if they do not hinder the patient's overall mobility, can manage some tibial fractures in the multiply injured patient, but most tibial fractures require immobilization of the knee above and the ankle below the injury, a fact that the trauma team must consider in overall patient planning. Casting, therefore, does have a place in the management of tibial fractures even in the multiply injured patient.

Because of the tibia's superficial location, and because the subcutaneous border often re-

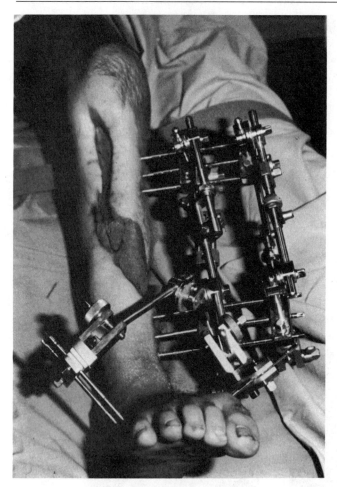

FIG. 34-4 Use of external fixation device in patient with compound comminuted tibial and fibular fractures, with loss of soft tissue in region of fractures. External fixator permits dressing and debridement. A critical feature of external fixation in this type of injury is the immobilization of the foot to prevent motion at fracture sites, especially when vascular repair is also done.

ceives high-energy open injuries, most trauma centers[13] prefer the external fixator for treating open tibial fractures. This device can be applied quickly, it adds minimal surgical insult because the hardware is applied away from the injury site, and, most importantly, it permits full dressing and debridement access to the soft tissue wounds that often accompany tibial fractures in the multiply injured patient (Fig. 34-4). Judicious use of the external fixator can completely stabilize the tibial bone injury, minimizing any additional release of fat and other microembolic particles into the blood stream.

Open reduction and internal fixation of the tibia using plates and screws have the advantage of rigid immobilization of the tibial fracture and the accompanying stabilization of soft tissue, minimizing further soft tissue trauma.[49-52]

However, these procedures are technically demanding to apply, require an additional surgical approach within the injury site, and necessitate the application of a large foreign body to an already compromised and injured area. For these reasons, their use in closed fractures often prompt debate and their use in open tibial fractures has generally been confined to salvage procedures for a leg at high risk.[50]

The IM nailing of tibial fractures also has the advantage of rigid fixation,[38,50] but it is technically difficult and best applied through a site remote from the fracture to avoid a double insult to both the periosteal and intraosteal blood supply of the tibia. Since its use necessitates familiarity with the techniques and the skillful use and interpretation of either plain radiographs or image intensification for proper anatomic reduction, it is primarily valuable for closed tibial fractures, although some grade I open fractures can benefit from this treatment. The secondary advantages of internal or external fixation with hardware include the fact that the ankle and/or knee joint often remains free of the shaft immobilization. Although this is not important in the initial management of the multiply injured patient, allowing the ankle and knee to remain free minimizes the problems of long-term joint stiffness above and below the tibial shaft and also minimizes leg muscle atrophy.[50]

Humeral Fractures

Humeral fractures usually receive classic conservative treatment unless they involve intra-articular fractures of the proximal humeral head or distal humerus. However, this conservative treatment may not be applicable to the multiply injured patient since it requires that the patient remain erect during waking hours and semierect during sleep. In addition, conservative treatment of a humeral fracture often does not permit full access for chest ther-

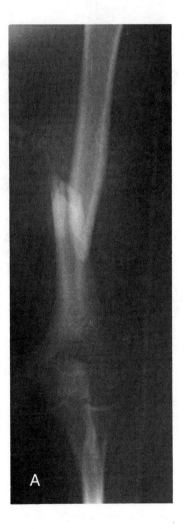 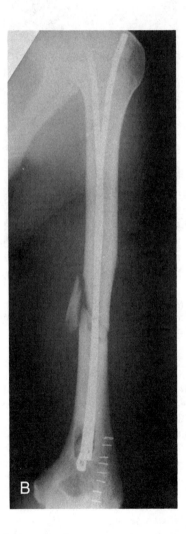

FIG. 34-5 **(A)** Midshaft fracture of humerus. **(B)** Internal fixation of humeral fractures by use of intramedullary rods. This permits the patient to receive better pulmonary toilet and allows more rapid complete mobilization.

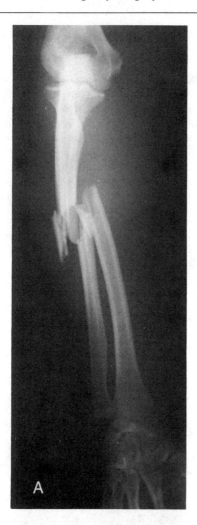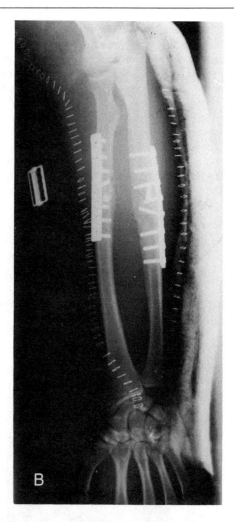

FIG. 34-6 (A) Fractures of both radius and ulna in a multiply injured patient. (B) Use of plate and screw fixation to achieve early anatomic reconstruction and full mobility of hand and wrist by allowing normal motion of forearm bones.

apy (including postural drainage and percussion). Therefore, a fractured humerus in a multiply injured patient often receives operative treatment that permits full mobility of the humerus, ensuring maximum patient mobility and access for full pulmonary toilet.

Orthopedists most often use one of two open fracture treatment methods for the humerus: open reduction using plates and screws[50] or IM fixation. Each method's advantages and disadvantages parallel those for other long bones (such as the femur and tibia). Plating the humerus results in rigid fixation, rotational control, and complete mobility of the

joints above and below the injury. Its disadvantages include the need for a surgical incision in the already traumatized area around the fracture site and the fact that it is a technically demanding procedure.[50] The IM techniques of humeral fixation, in use for many years, permit immobilization of the fracture through a remote site (Fig. 34-5).

Humeral fracture stabilization occasionally requires external fixation because associated soft tissue injury necessitates access to the wound.

Salvaging a severely injured upper extremity may require a combination of internal and external techniques; such combinations should be tailored to the individual patient as well as to the injuries.

Forearm Fractures

Forearm fractures in the multiply injured patient often require internal fixation using plates and screws.[50] Because full mobility of the hand and wrist demands the use of both bones of the forearm, repair of the forearm's long bone shaft necessitates a relatively anatomic reduction. Plate and screw fixation techniques tend to accomplish this goal best (Fig. 34-6). The disadvantages of plate and screw fixation (see above) are relatively less important in treating forearm fractures because of this necessity for the anatomic reapproximation of bony fragments. The orthopedic surgeon should avoid less anatomic methods, such as IM nailing and external fixation, unless grossly contaminated wounds or loss of soft tissue/bone continuity dictate such an application.

Most importantly, forearm fractures in the unstable multiply injured patient do not require treatment at admission. Unlike most lower extremity long bone fractures and fractures of the humerus, forearm fractures may be splinted or temporarily held in external fixation devices without severely compromising the patient's sytemic function, chances of resuscitation, mobility, pulmonary function, or eventual return to function.

Articular Fractures

The orthopedic surgeon should acutely reduce and immobilize articular fractures to gain additional mobility for the patient for overall body positioning, pulmonary toilet and other procedures. However, the orthopedist should delay the time-consuming and taxing repair necessary to obtain anatomic reduction until after the initial resuscitation and stabilization period. (Because of the need to rehabilitate the patient to long-term musculoskeletal function, intra-articular fractures deserve anatomic re-

duction when possible.[46,47,50]) The benefits of performing this prolonged surgery in the acute stage do not offset its risks and added morbidity.

Dislocations

When appropriate, the orthopedist should treat dislocations of the body's major joints (shoulder, elbow, hip, and knee) in the patient's early treatment stage. Although the proximal dislocations (i.e., shoulder and hip) should be reduced as soon as possible, they usually do not present the potential threat to limb viability that elbow and knee dislocations do.

Elbow dislocations can often present with vascular compromise of the arm below the elbow; if the vascular examination discloses a deficit distal to the dislocation, the orthopedist should reduce the elbow dislocation as soon as possible.

Knee dislocations have an extremely high incidence of vascular compromise, probably because it takes an extreme amount of energy to tear all the ligamentous structures of the knee. This high energy, plus the fact that the popliteal artery is the neurovascular structure closest to the knee joint (tethered in that position by adjacent structures), makes the arterial supply distal to the knee extremely susceptible to either gross vascular interruption or intimal damage. For these reasons, the orthopedist should accomplish joint reductions quickly and, for a knee dislocation, should request a definitive angiographic assessment (either by comparative Doppler pulse measurements or an angiographic study with contrast medium) distal to the dislocation.

CONCLUSION

Successful orthopedic treatment for the multiply injured patient requires that each member of the trauma team (the critical care physician, the general surgeon, the anesthesiologist, and the orthopedic surgeon) have a comprehensive understanding of the pathomechanical and pathophysiologic details of musculoskeletal injury. The critical care physician must be able to visualize the mechanisms of injury, the details of transport, and the methods of resuscitation and stabilization, as well as the needs and requirements of the multiply injured patient. Optimal management involves a five-step process: (1) establishing the patient's data base; (2) reviewing the pathophysiology of the traumatic insult; (3) determining individualized, realistic therapeutic goals; (4) selecting the best procedural option and timing for accomplishing those goals; and (5) exercising clinical judgment to meld those goals and options into a comprehensive therapeutic plan that maximizes overall results and minimizes the morbidity of the injuries.

REFERENCES

1. Alexander JW, Hegg M, Altmeirer WA: Neutrophil functions in selected disorders. Ann Surg 168: 447, 1968
2. Allardyce DB, Meek RN, Woodruff B et al: Increasing our knowledge of the pathogenesis of fat embolism. A prospective study of 43 patients with fractured femoral shafts. J Trauma 14: 955, 1974
3. Almqvist P, Kuenzig M, Schwartz SI: The effect of naloxone and cyproheptadine on pulmonary platelet trapping, hypotension, and platelet aggregability in traumatized dogs. J Trauma 23(5): 405, 1983
4. Amundsen E: Posttraumatic pulmonary insufficiency. Acta Chir Scand 499(suppl): 3, 1980
5. Avikainen V, Willman K, Rokkan P: Stress hormones, lipids, and factors of hemostasis in trauma patients with and without fat embolism syndrome: a comparative study at least one year after severe trauma. J Trauma 20(2): 148, 1980
6. Baker CC, Miller CL, Trunkey DD, Lim RC: Identity of mononuclear cells which compromise the resistance of trauma patients. J Surg Res 26: 478, 1979
7. Baker CC, Oppenheimer L, Stephens B et al: Epidemiology of trauma deaths. Am J Surg 140: 144, 1980
8. Balk R, Bone RC: The adult respiratory distress syndrome. Med Clin North Am 67(3): 685, 1983
9. Bierre A, Koelmeyer TD: Pulmonary fat and bone marrow embolism in aircraft accident victims. Pathology 15: 131, 1983
10. Booji LHDJ: Pitfalls in anesthesia for multiply injured patients (symposium paper). Injury 14: 81, 1982
11. Borzotta AP, Polk HC: Multiple system organ failure. Surg Clin North Am 63(2): 315, 1983
12. Brigham KL: Mechanisms of lung injury. Clin Chest Med 3: 9, 1982
13. Brooker A, Edwards C: External Fixation: The Current State of the Art. Williams & Wilkins, Baltimore, 1979
14. Browner BD, Kenzora JE, Edwards CC: The use of modified Neufeld traction in the management of femoral fractures in polytrauma. J Trauma 21(9): 779, 1981
15. Burri C, Kreuzer U, Limmer J: Principles and practice of fracture treatment in the multiply injured patient (symposium paper). Injury 14: 44, 1982
16. Chow SP, Hoaglund FT, Ma A, Mok CK: Fat embolism in Hong Kong Chinese. J Bone Joint Surg 62A(7): 1138, 1980
17. Christou NV, Meakins JL: Neutrophil function in surgical patients: two inhibitors of granulocyte chemotaxis associated with sepsis. J Surg Res 26: 355, 1979
18. Crivello MS, Walker Smith GJ, Morris DK: Prevention of pulmonary pathologic changes of trauma by indomethacin. Surg Forum 31: 179, 1980
19. Czer LSC, Appel P, Shoemaker WC: Pathogenesis of respiratory failure (ARDS) after hemorrhage and trauma. II: Cardiorespiratory patterns after development of ARDS. Crit Care Med 8(9): 513, 1980
20. Dantzker DR: Gas exchange in the adult respiratory distress syndrome. Clin Chest Med 3: 57, 1982
21. Demling RH: The pathogenesis of respiratory failure after trauma and sepsis. Surg Clin North Am 60(6): 1373, 1980
22. Esser MP, Cloke JH, Hart JA: Closed Kuntscher nailing. A clinical review after twenty years. Injury 13: 455, 1981
23. Faden AI, Holaday, JW: Experimental endotoxin shock: the pathophysiological function of endorphins and treatment with opiate antagonists. J Infect Dis 140: 229, 1980
24. Gilmore JP, Zucker JH: The contribution of neural pathways to blood volume hemostasis in the subhuman primate. Basic Respir Contr 75: 281, 1980

25. Gong H: Positive pressure ventilation in adult respiratory distress syndrome. Clin Chest Med 3: 69, 1982

26. Goris RJA, Draaisma J: Causes of death after blunt trauma. J Trauma 22(2): 141, 1982

27. Goris RJA, Gimbrere JSF, Van Niekerk JLM et al: Early osteosynthesis and prophylactic mechanical ventilation in the multitrauma patient. J Trauma 22(11): 895, 1982

28. Goris RJA, Gimbrere JSF, Van Niekerk JLM et al: Improved survival of multiply injured patients by early external fixation and prophylactic mechanical ventilation (symposium paper). Injury 14: 39, 1982

29. Gossling HR, Pellegrini VD: Fat embolism syndrome: a review of the pathophysiology and physiological basis of treatment. Clin Orthop Rel Res 165: 68, 1982

30. Grosse A: Grosse-Kempf locking nailing. In Browner B, Edwards C (eds): The Science and Practice of Intramedullary Nailing. Lea and Febiger, Philadelphia, 1985

31. Gustilo RR, Anderson JT: Prevention of infection in the treatment of 1,025 open fractures of long bones. J Bone Joint Surg 584: 453, 1976

32. Hansen ST, Winquist RA: Closed intramedullary nailing of the femur. Clin Orthop 138: 56, 1979

33. Harlan JM, Harker LA: Hemostasis, thrombosis, and thromboembolic disorders: the role of arachidonic acid metabolites in platelet vessel wall interactions. Med Clin North Am 65: 855, 1981

34. Hechtman HB, Utsonomiya T, Krauz MM et al: The management of cardiorespiratory failure in surgical patients. Adv Surg 15: 123, 1981

35. Holcroft JW, Trunkey DD: Pathophysiology of shock and adult respiratory distress syndrome. Surg Ann 15: 1, 1983

36. Howard RJ: Effect of burn injury, mechanical trauma, and operation on immune defenses. Surg Clin North Am 59(2): 199, 1979

37. Jacobs RR, McClain OM: Effects of fracture stabilization by internal fixation. Injury 12: 194, 1980

38. Karlstom G, Olerud S: Fractures of the tibial shaft; a critical evaluation of treatment alternatives. Clin Orthop 105: 82, 1974

39. Kerstell J: The pathogenesis of the fat embolism syndrome. Am J Surg 121: 712, 1971

40. Kieley SB, Snyder WH, Weigelt JA: Arterial injuries below the knee: 50 patients with 82 injuries. J Trauma 23: 285, 1983

41. Laduca JN, Boone LL, Seibel RW, Border JR: Primary open reduction and internal fixation of open fractures. J Trauma 20(7): 580, 1980

42. Liddell MJ, Daniel AM, Maclean LD et al: The role of stress hormones in the catabolic metabolism of shock. Surg Gynecol Obstet 149: 822, 1979

43. Lundy J, Ford CM: Surgery, trauma, and immune suppression: evolving the mechanism. Ann Surg 194(4): 434, 1983

44. Magerl F, Wyssa A, Brunner C, Binder W: Plate osteosynthesis of femoral shaft fractures. Clin Orthop 138: 62, 1979

45. Manning JB, Bach AW, Herman CM, Carrico CJ: Fat release after femur nailing in the dog. J Trauma 23(4): 322, 1983

46. Merriam WF, Misfud RP: Internal fixation in patients with multiple injuries. Injury 15: 78, 1983

47. Miller J: Fractures involving joints. Instructional Course Lectures, AAOS 30: 94, 1981

48. Modig J: Posttraumatic pulmonary insufficiency caused by the microembolism syndrome. Acta Chir Scand 499(suppl): 57, 1980

49. Moncada S, Vane JR: Arachidonic acid metabolites and the interaction between platelets and blood vessel walls. N Engl J Med 300: 1142, 1979

50. Muller ME, Allgower M, Willeneger H: Manual of Internal Fixation. Springer Verlag, Berlin, 1970

51. Nicoll EA: Closed and open treatment of tibial fractures. Clin Orthop 105: 144, 1974

52. Olerud S, Larkstrom G: Tibial fractures treated by AO compression osteosynthesis. Acta Orthop Scand 3: 140, 1972

53. Palmovic AC: Fat embolism in trauma. Arch Pathol 80: 650, 1965

54. Pingleton SK: Complications of acute respiratory failure. Med Clin North Am 67(3): 7252, 1983

55. Rayfer PK, Montemurno R, Scudese V, Sherr S: Experimental production of and recovery of pulmonary fat embolism in dogs: the origin of fat. Surg Forum 22: 446, 1971

56. Rank CM, Long CL, Blakemore WS: Comparison between *in vitro* lymphocyte activity and metabolic changes in trauma patients. J Trauma 22(2): 134, 1982

57. Rhinelander F: The normal microcirculation of the diaphyseal cortex and its response to fracture. J Bone Joint Surg 50A: 789, 1968

58. Riska EB, Myllynen P: Fat embolism in patients with multiple injuries. J Trauma 22(11): 891, 1982

59. Riska EB, Von Bonsdorff H, Hakkinen S et al: Prevention of fat embolism by early internal fixation of fractures in patients with multiple injuries. Injury 18: 110, 1976

60. Riska EB, Von Bonsdorff H, Hakkinen S et al: Primary operative fixation of long bone fractures in patients with multiple injuries. J Trauma 17(2): 111, 1977

61. Ritzmann SE, Larson DL, McClung C et al: Immunoglobulin levels in burned patients. Lancet 1: 1152, 1969

62. Rokkanen P, Slatis P, Vankka E: Closed or open intramedullary nailing femoral shaft fractures: a comparison with conservatively treated cases. J Bone Joint Surg 51: 313, 1969

63. Saba TM, Jaffe E: Plasma fibronectin: its synthesis by vascular endothelial cells and roles in cardiopulmonary integrity after trauma as related to reticuloendothelial function. Am J Med 68: 577, 1980

64. Saldeen T: Trends in microvascular research: the microembolism syndrome. Microvasc Res 11: 227, 1976

65. Sauter AJM, Klopper PJ: Fat embolism after static and dynamic loads: an experimental investigation. Acta Orthop Scand 54: 94, 1983

66. Schonfeld SA, Ploysongsang Y, DiLisio R et al: Fat embolism prophylaxis with corticosteroids. Ann Intern Med 99: 438, 1983

67. Sevitt S: Reflections on pathology in trauma. Injury 14(4): 297, 1982

68. Sheikh MA: Respiratory changes after fractures and surgical skeletal injury. Injury 13: 489, 1981

69. Shoemaker WC, Appel P, Czer LSC et al: Pathogenesis of respiratory failure (ARDS) after hemorrhage and trauma. II. Cardiorespiratory patterns preceding the development of ARDS. Crit Care Med 8(9): 504, 1980

70. Skillman JJ, Lancer DP, Hickler RB et al: Hemorrhage in normal men: effect on renin cortisol, aldosterone, and urine composition. Ann Surg 166: 865, 1967

71. Talucci RC, Manning J, Lampard S, Bach CJ: Early intramedullary nailing of femoral shaft fractures: a cause of fat embolism syndrome. Am J Surg 146: 107, 1983

72. Trunkey DD, Chapman MW, Lim RC, Dunphy E: Management of pelvic fractures in blunt injury. J Trauma 14: 912, 1974

73. Vaage J: The role of platelets in posttraumatic pulmonary insufficiency. Acta Chir Scand 499(suppl): 141, 1980

74. Wang BS, Heacock EH, Wu AVO, Mannick JA: Generation of suppressor cells in mice after surgical trauma. J Clin Invest 66: 200, 1980

75. Watson AJ: Genesis of fat emboli. J Clin Pathol 23(suppl): 132, 1970

76. Wolfe JHN, Wu AVO, O'Connor NE et al: Anergy, immunosuppressive serum, and impaired lymphocyte blastogenesis in burn patients. Arch Surg 117: 1266, 1982

77. Zaricznyj B, Rockwood CA, Jr., O'Donoghue DH, Ridings GR: Relationship between trauma to the extremities and stomach motility. J Trauma 17(12): 920, 1977

35

Management of the Obstetric Patient After Trauma

Lindsay Staubus Alger
M. Carlyle Crenshaw, Jr.

INTRODUCTION

Pregnancy no longer is considered an illness. The majority of women in their childbearing years work outside the home and continue to do so during pregnancy. Consequently, with increasing frequency pregnant women are being exposed to the hazards of the workplace as they are employed in more dangerous jobs and commute longer distances in smaller cars. The pregnant woman is likely to continue her participation in sports, remodeling of the nursery, or a variety of household chores, all of which expose her to potential injury. Accidents are the leading cause of death among women under the age of 35 in the United States.[56] Motor vehicle accidents, falls, burns, drownings, and firearm injuries are the most frequent causes.[43] Each time an injured woman is evaluated, the possibility that she is pregnant must be considered.

An obstetrician is unlikely to be immedi-

ately available in the emergency or critical care admitting areas during the initial evaluation and management of the seriously injured pregnant woman. Therefore, it is incumbent upon the surgeon to be sufficiently familiar with the anatomic and physiologic changes of pregnancy, detection of fetal distress, and fundamentals of delivery, whether vaginal or operative, to avoid the diagnostic and therapeutic hesitancy that can impede the critical care team in this situation.

Maternal outcome is primarily dependent upon the severity of maternal injury. Pregnancy generally does not adversely affect the outcome but may delay appropriate diagnosis and prompt institution of therapy. In the absence of fetal distress or uterine injury, obstetric intervention is rarely indicated and might further compromise the mother and infant. Only when the patient is moribund or it becomes necessary to reduce the uterine mass to provide exposure to the retroperitoneum is obstetric intervention warranted.

Fetal outcome is related to maternal outcome. Certainly maternal death, shock, or sepsis will compromise the fetus. Maternal shock is associated with an 80 percent fetal mortality.[64] Fetal outcome also is related to uterine, placental, and umbilical cord injuries and, less commonly, to direct fetal trauma. Skull fractures and intracerebral hemorrhage are the most common causes of fetal death in this event.[7,64] The guiding principle in the management of the fetus is that maternal well-being comes first.

The first trimester fetus is well protected from injury within the bony confines of the pelvis. Only catastrophic trauma is likely to damage the fetus at this stage. In combined series of over 3,000 spontaneous abortions, trauma occasionally preceded the pregnancy loss but could be implicated as a cause in none.[40,44] During the second half of pregnancy the uterus, and hence the fetus, is much more vulnerable to trauma. Most fetal injuries occur in late pregnancy. The ratio of amniotic fluid to fetal size is reduced and the head is relatively fixed in the pelvis while the remainder of the fetus lies above its protective walls. In this setting fetal injury has been reported following seemingly trivial accidents.

PHYSIOLOGIC CHANGES AFFECTING MATERNAL RESPONSE TO TRAUMA

The types of injuries sustained and the maternal response to trauma are influenced by the physiologic and anatomic changes accompanying pregnancy. Although these changes are essential to permit proper growth and development of the fetus as well as to prepare the woman for delivery, the resultant alterations may mimic pathologic conditions of the nongravid patient and confuse the diagnosis. Almost every organ system undergoes substantial changes. Not only are physiologic parameters altered but laboratory values also vary secondary to hormonal effects. In addition, it will be necessary to modify treatment regimens

in order to maintain homeostasis of the pregnancy.

Cardiovascular System

Beginning in the first trimester, the maternal blood volume increases until, at 30 weeks' gestation, it plateaus at 50 percent above prepregnancy levels.[65] This physiologic hypervolemia improves maternal tolerance of hemorrhage but may mask signs of the severity of the blood loss. The pregnant patient can maintain stable vital signs and adequate perfusion of vital organs with a 10 to 20 percent acute blood loss or even a 30 to 35 percent gradual blood loss.[52] However, marked uterine artery vasoconstriction occurs in the effort to maintain maternal homeostasis, thus potentially sacrificing the fetus. When nearly exsanguinated, the gravida will suddenly show signs of shock and her blood pressure and pulse become unobtainable. Unless treated immediately, reversal may be impossible.

Cardiac output also increases by 40 percent early in pregnancy but is extremely sensitive to maternal position.[73] Near term the inferior vena cava is almost completely occluded in the supine position by the compressive weight of the gravid uterus.[46] The decrease in venous return will cause cardiac output to fall below nonpregnant values. The normal pregnant woman is able to compensate for this and maintain her blood pressure by increasing peripheral vascular resistance and, in fact, arterial blood pressure is usually slightly higher in the supine than the lateral recumbent position.[72] However, the injured patient who is already maximally vasoconstricted may become profoundly hypotensive in the supine position. In addition, animal studies suggest that placental abruption also is more likely to occur in the supine position secondary to increased venous pressure in the intervillous space.[42] This mechanism could theoretically potentiate trauma-induced placental separation. Conclusive evidence for this in humans is lacking.

Since vascular resistance dramatically decreases during pregnancy, as evidenced by the palmar erythema and spider telangiectasia that frequently develop, there is a reduction in the

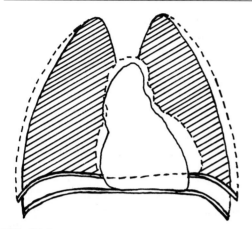

FIG. 35-1 Elevation of the diaphragm by the enlarging uterus shifts the cardiac axis counterclockwise and reduces the functional residual capacity of the lungs.

When evaluating the acutely injured patient, the relative tachycardia associated with pregnancy must be considered. The heart rate increases by 15 to 20 beats/min by the third trimester although the resting pulse remains[75] less than 100 beats/min. On cardiac auscultation a third heart sound is commonly heard, as are systolic flow murmurs of grade I or II intensity.[54] The elevation of the diaphragm that causes counterclockwise rotation of the heart results in a progressive left axis deviation on the electrocardiogram (Fig. 35-1). Additionally, T waves become flattened or inverted in leads III, V_1, and V_2.

Hematopoietic System

Although red blood cell volume increases by approximately 25 percent, plasma volume increases[60] by 50 percent. The resultant hemodilution is known as "the physiologic anemia of pregnancy" and must not be mistakenly assumed to represent blood loss. Hemoglobin levels as low as 10 g/100 ml are observed in normal pregnant women not receiving iron supplements.[26] A white blood cell count up to 18,000/mm^3 can be expected during the second and third trimesters and is not indicative of infection.[29,59] In the nonpregnant individual counts over 15,000/mm^3 suggest liver or splenic injury but this cannot be relied upon as a sign during pregnancy. Labor results in a further increase, with counts reaching 25,000/mm^3 at times. Since the increase is largely attributable to greater numbers of neutrophils, and occasional immature forms may be seen on the peripheral smear, the differential count may appear to be shifted slightly to the left although a true left shift with toxic granulations is not seen.[48] Platelet counts may be depressed slightly but significant thrombocytopenia is abnormal and most likely indicates a consumptive coagulopathy.[59,70] Increased concentrations of fibrinogen and other clotting factors accompanied by a decrease in circulating plasminogen activator are physiologic changes that prepare the gravida for delivery, but predispose to thromboembolic complications following trauma, surgery, or prolonged bed rest.[10,57] When anticoagulation is required, heparin is the drug of choice since it does not cross the

mean arterial pressure (diastolic fall greater than systolic) of 5 to 15 mmHg during the second trimester.[51] As term approaches, blood pressure returns toward nonpregnant levels. The effect of pregnancy on central venous pressure (CVP) is less clear. In the supine position there is a progressive fall in the CVP to values less than half of nonpregnant controls by the third trimester.[18] However, the normal pregnant patient will respond to a fluid challenge with a rise in CVP similar to that seen in nonpregnant individuals.[77] Peripheral venous pressure, although unchanged by pregnancy in the upper extremities, is elevated in the lower extremities, thereby potentiating bleeding from leg wounds.[53]

Peripheral blood flow is greatly increased. Augmented pelvic vascularity increases the risk of maternal hemorrhage and hematoma formation with abdominal injuries. During the first two trimesters the pregnant woman paradoxically responds to stress with vasodilation.[27] Consequently, a patient may be in shock without displaying the characteristic findings of cold and clammy skin. Circumstantial evidence indicates that sex steroids may produce structural changes in blood vessels. Ruptures of splenic artery aneurysms occurring before the age of 45 are most likely to occur in women, usually between the seventh and ninth months of pregnancy.[1] Dissecting aortic aneurysms and aortic valve leaflet rupture also occur more frequently during pregnancy.[68]

placenta. Injury to the placenta, which contains large amounts of thromboplastin, or to the uterus, a major source of plasminogen activator, may precipitate disseminated intravascular coagulation.[7] Since low levels of intravascular coagulation occur routinely, elevated levels of fibrin degradation products are expected. It is their absence that is noteworthy.[33]

Pulmonary System

The majority of pregnant women experience dyspnea at some time during the course of their pregnancy. Because of a decreased functional residual capacity (FRC) hypoventilation produces hypoxia and hypercarbia more readily than in nonpregnant women.[3,23] Under the stimulatory influence of progesterone, physiologic hyperventilation (increased tidal volume) causes the arterial PCO_2 to fall to between 27 and 32 mmHg and the mean PO_2 to rise[4,50] to 100 to 108 mmHg. The PO_2 is influenced by maternal position and length of gestation; it decreases in the supine position and as pregnancy advances.[5] Renal bicarbonate excretion compensates so that the pH remains almost unchanged while plasma bicarbonate falls[4,30] on average to 18 to 21 mEq. Although still uncommon, pulmonary embolism associated with a PO_2 greater than 80 mmHg is seen more often during pregnancy.[63] As pregnancy advances, elevation of the diaphragm resulting from an enlarging uterus makes the gravida more susceptible to postoperative atelectasis and pneumonia.

Gastrointestinal System

Pregnancy reduces lower esophageal sphincteric function, placing the acutely injured patient at greater risk for regurgitating gastric contents and, hence, for aspiration.[32,41] Gastric emptying and intestinal motility are slowed and if emergency surgery is indicated it should be assumed that the patient has a full stomach.[25] Placement of a nasogastric tube should be considered prior to induction of anesthesia.

Rupture of the spleen may be encountered more frequently associated with blunt abdominal trauma, as compressive forces are transmitted through the increased abdominal contents to the spleen. The liver is not enlarged during pregnancy[19] and hepatic blood flow is unaltered.[38] Therefore, it is not particularly predisposed to traumatic injury. However, total serum alkaline phosphatase levels rise to two to four times normal by the late third trimester because of placental production.[78] Levels of serum lactic dehydrogenase also may be elevated but serum glutamic oxaloacetic transaminase and pyruvic transaminase (SGOT, SGPT) values remain within normal limits.[16,69] Total serum protein concentrations decline largely due to a reduction in the albumin levels of 1.0 g/dl.

Diagnosis of intra-abdominal injury is complicated by the changing anatomic relationships as pregnancy progresses. The uterus may interfere with palpation of other viscera or the detection of intraperitoneal blood. The small bowel is displaced superiorly by the enlarging uterus, which in turn may protect it from penetrating injury. However, with the bowel confined to the upper abdomen, injuries to this area may involve multiple loops of bowel. Pain originating from displaced viscera may be referred to an uncharacteristic area of the abdomen. Typical physical findings of guarding, rigidity, and rebound that suggest intraperitoneal injury are diminished in the pregnant patient with a stretched and lax abdominal wall. Nausea and vomiting may accompany otherwise uncomplicated pregnancies.

Urogenital System

The renal collecting system is dilated from the time of early pregnancy.[31] This physiologic hydronephrosis is more pronounced on the right than the left. The bladder is elevated out of the pelvis and is compressed between the uterus and abdominal wall, where traumatic injury may cause it to rupture. Renal plasma flow rises early in pregnancy resulting in an increase in creatinine clearance rate (greater than 150 ml/min) and a fall in blood urea nitrogen (BUN) and creatinine levels.[22] A BUN value greater than 10 mg/dl or a creatinine level above 0.8 mg/dl is not normal.

Musculoskeletal System

Under the influence of the hormone relaxin, the ligaments of the pubic symphysis and sacroiliac joints become increasingly lax.[39] This facilitates delivery and makes the pelvis less susceptible to fracture. However, the increased joint instability, additional weight, and shift of the center of gravity during pregnancy make the pregnant woman more likely to fall than at any other time during her adult life.[34]

Nervous System

Little is known about the effects of pregnancy on the nervous system. Vascular headaches, at times accompanied by paresthesias and visual changes, are seen more frequently, particularly during the first half of gestation. During the third trimester eclampsia, a complication confined to pregnancy, may be mistaken for seizures secondary to head trauma. A patient presenting with seizures late in pregnancy should be presumed to be eclamptic and should

be treated as such with magnesium sulfate and delivery until the presence of other intracranial pathology has been established.

Physiologic changes of pregnancy are outlined in Table 35-1. Laboratory values commonly altered by pregnancy are summarized in Table 35-2.

EVALUATION OF THE INJURED PREGNANT WOMAN

Initial evaluation of the acutely injured pregnant woman is directed towards determining the maternal status, specifically, the nature and extent of her injuries. Although there is always a second patient at risk, the fetus, the best chance of ensuring fetal survival is to ensure maternal survival. Proper acute management of the injured gravida varies only minorly from that of any other seriously injuried individual. For life-threatening injuries, the fetus can essentially be ignored.

TABLE 35-1. Physiologic Changes of Pregnancy

System	Alteration
Cardiovascular	↑Blood volume ↑Cardiovascular output ↑Heart rate ↓Peripheral resistance (spider telangiectasia) ↓Mean arterial pressure ↓Venous return in supine position ↓CVP in supine position ↑Peripheral blood flow Grade I–II/VI systolic flow murmur Left axis deviation on electrocardiogram
Hematopoietic	Hemodilution Low-grade intravascular coagulation ↑Risk of thromboembolism
Pulmonary	Dyspnea ↑Tidal volume and physiologic hyperventilation ↓Functional residual capacity ↑Risk of atelectasis
Gastrointestinal	↑Gastric emptying time ↓Lower esophageal sphincteric function ↑Risk of aspiration ↑Risk of splenic rupture Small bowel displaced superiorly
Urogenital system	Physiologic hydronephrosis (right greater than left) Bladder elevated out of pelvis ↑Renal plasma flow

TABLE 35-2.   Selected Laboratory Values in Pregnancy

Value	Nonpregnant Level	Pregnant Level
Hematocrit (%)	38–43	33–41
WBC (per mm³)	4,750–9,600	5,000–16,000
Platelet count (thousands/mm³)	150–400	134–400
ESR (whole blood; mm/hr)	20	44–114
Fibrinogen (mg/dl)	300	425
Fibrin degradation products	6.5 ± 2.1	14.0 ± 6.9
Total protein (mg/dl)	7.0	6.0
Albumin (mg/dl)	3.5–4.5	2.5–3.5
Alkaline phosphatase (Bodansky; IV/L)	20.6	82
BUN (mg/dl)	13	8.7
Creatinine (mg/dl)	0.67	0.46
Creatine clearance (mg/min)	120	150–200
PO_2 (mmHg)	95	100–108
PCO_2 (mmHg)	40	27–32
HCO_3 (mmol)	25	18–21

General Considerations

In the absence of vital signs, even when a pupillary response is unobtainable, resuscitation should be begun immediately to allow for a possible postmortem cesarean section. The patient is maintained in the left lateral tilt position whenever possible. A rolled blanket or towel placed under the right hip and back will accomplish this. Since the gravida is normally hypervolemic it may be necessary to administer enormous quantities of blood and fluid to the patient in shock before vital signs return to normal.[9] The pregnant trauma victim will always require greater blood volume replacement than a similarily sized nonpregnant woman. Vasopressors other than dopamine and ephedrine should not be used to treat hypovolemic shock since these drugs can further reduce uterine blood flow and aggrevate fetal hypoxia.[9,35] An initial baseline arterial blood gas determination is particularly useful in the gravida to avoid unnecessary fetal hypoxia. Oxygen by mask should be used liberally if there is any suspicion of diminution of circulation or oxygen saturation until the maternal status is established. The goal is to maintain the maternal PO_2 above 80 mmHg at all times.

Radiologic Evaluation

Radiologic studies should be performed when indicated. Reluctance to obtain such valuable diagnostic information due to concern for potential fetal damage is unwarranted and could result in a delayed or missed diagnosis. Chest, abdominal, and skeletal films as well as a limited intravenous pyelogram are frequently necessary and are unlikely to adversely affect the fetus at any time in gestation, although there is less concern after the first trimester. However, only those films that would alter management should be ordered. The uterus should be shielded when possible and duplication of films avoided. If the injuries are severe, a fetal monitor should accompany the patient to the radiology department. Uterine blood flow can be reduced by 20 percent following acute hemorrhage while the maternal blood pressure remains stable.[35] Abnormalities in the fetal heart rate tracing may alert the physician not only to fetal distress but also to maternal decompensation. Whenever possible, ultrasonography should be substituted for radiologic studies.

Diagnosing Intraperitoneal Hemorrhage

The patient should be evaluated for possible visceral trauma by palpating for pain over the spleen, liver, or uterus. Pregnancy may mimic or mask the signs of intraperitoneal bleeding and make diagnosis difficult. Buchsbaum noted a 15.4 percent maternal mortality rate following splenic rupture, contributed to in part by the failure to make the diagnosis.[12]

During a vehicular accident, the uterus is subject to inertial forces that can cause lacerations, rupture, and even complete avulsion.

Prior to 14 weeks' gestation, laparoscopy can be safe and useful in the assessment of lower intra-abdominal injury. Throughout pregnancy peritoneal lavage can establish the presence of intra-abdominal bleeding or prevent an unnecessary exploratory laparotomy.[49] Pregnancy reduces the effectiveness and increases the risks of needle paracentesis and culdocentesis as diagnostic techniques. Lavage can be performed accurately even in advanced pregnancy using the "mini-lap" or open technique (Chapter 26). Return of blood, amniotic fluid, or bowel contents mandates immediate laparotomy. Alternatively, if the patient's status permits, the presence of intra-abdominal blood can be identified by computed tomography (CT), due to its high attenuation as compared to soft tissue. Although this exposes the fetus to low-dose radiation, CT is less invasive and is superior in evaluating retroperitoneal injuries.[37]

Surgical Intervention

The fetus can tolerate the stress of surgery and anesthesia. Certainly, alterations in maternal homeostasis such as hypovolemia or hypoxia have a far greater effect on the course of pregnancy. During laparotomy the uterus may be packed or retracted out of the field provided that blood flow through the uterine vessels is not compromised. The risk of precipitating premature labor by diagnostic laparotomy is minimal.[66] Should uterine contractions ensue in a preterm gestation, a tocolytic agent such as ritodrine may be used to inhibit uterine activity once the patient has been stabilized and her vital signs have returned to normal. Cesarean section should be reserved for the usual obstetric indications and only rarely to provide exposure to the operating field. The pediatric staff should be notified well in advance if an operative delivery is contemplated. A laparotomy is not an indication for a cesarean section even if the patient is already in labor. Labor and vaginal delivery are well tolerated within a few hours postoperatively.[28] The additional operating time required for cesarean delivery will only increase the operative risk and a uterine scar will enhance the likelihood of uterine rupture in a subsequent pregnancy. Death of the fetus from prematurity following an ill-advised cesarean section has been documented too often.[12] If the fetus is known to be dead, labor can be induced once the mother's condition is stable. Although pelvic fracture on occasion may injure the fetus and obstruct the birth canal, there is no indication for routine cesarean section when undisplaced pelvic fractures are recognized in the trauma victim in labor. A trial of labor is warranted but regional anesthesia may be required to treat severe musculoskeletal pain.

Use of Antibiotics

The indications for antibiotic use in the trauma victim are unchanged by pregnancy. Tetanus prophylaxis should be administered in routine fashion. Although the use of prophylatic antibiotics is generally condemned, the use of "preventative antibiotics," for example following bowel injury, may have value. An increase in the dose may be necessary due to pregnancy-induced changes in excretion rates and the volume of distribution. However, therapeutic tissue levels are unlikely to be found in the fetus, while low circulating antibiotic levels may obscure the pediatrician's search for sepsis should delivery occur. Tetracycline and chloramphenicol should not be administered to pregnant women.

Initial Obstetric Evaluation

Once the maternal condition has been stabilized, attention is directed towards establishing whether the uterus and its contents are intact. Initial assessment for uterine or fetal injury requires determining (1) the gestational age of the fetus, (2) whether the fetus is alive or in distress, and (3) whether the patient has suffered trauma to the genital tract or is in labor. Since the patient may be unable to provide any information and the family initially may be unavailable, the critical care physician must rely upon clinical evaluation.

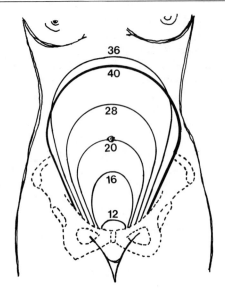

FIG. 35-2 Increase in uterine size with advancing gestational age. The 12 weeks gestation is just palpable at the pubic symphysis. At 20 weeks of gestation, the top of the fundus is at the umbilicus.

Abdominal palpation of the uterus serves the dual purpose of detecting uterine trauma as well as estimating gestational age. The uterus is not palpable abdominally until approximately 12 to 13 weeks gestation (Fig. 35-2). By 20 weeks' gestation, the top of the fundus has reached the umbilicus. Thereafter until 32 weeks' gestation, fetal age in weeks is approximately equal to the distance in cen-timeters from the top of the symphysis pubis to the top of the fundus[45] (Fig. 35-3). If the fundal height is more than 27 cm the fetus may survive if delivered and must be considered potentially salvageable. Even when the patient can provide the date of her last menstrual period it is still advisable to confirm gestational age by physical examination. Marking the top of the fundus on the abdominal skin with a pen permits serial assessment of possible changes in uterine size that may indicate intrauterine or retroplacental bleeding.

A localized area of uterine tenderness is suggestive of injury or abruption since labor pains are experienced bilaterally, involve a major portion of the uterus, and resolve at the end of a contraction. An exception is round ligament pain. Sudden stretching of these supporting ligaments of the uterus can result in unilateral or bilateral pain localized to the upper lateral portion of the fundus. This is particularly likely in gestations between 16 and 18 weeks. This benign condition may be treated symptomatically with local heat and mild analgesics.

Fetal Monitoring

A Doppler sonographic device usually will permit auscultation of the fetal heart tones by 12 weeks' gestation. Once the fundus is palpa-

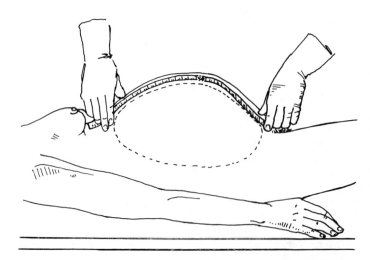

FIG. 35-3 Measuring fundal height in centimeters from the pubic symphysis to the dome of the uterus.

ble above the umbilicus it should be possible to auscultate the fetal heart with a conventional stethoscope or, preferably, a fetoscope. Whenever feasible, the third trimester fetus should be continuously monitored with an external fetal heart rate monitor. In the absence of fetal heart sounds a complete ultrasonographic evaluation of the fetal thoracic cavity to demonstrate absence of cardiac motion is indicated before fetal death can be declared.

The normal fetal heart rate is 120 to 160 beats/min. Tachycardia may occur as a response to maternal drug administration, exogenous or endogenous catecholamines, maternal fever, or early fetal asphyxia. Fetal bradycardia, particularly when less than 100 beats/min, is ominous and usually indicates fetal hypoxia secondary to inadequate uteroplacental perfusion. It may alert the physician to a possible placental separation but more likely represents inadequacy of the maternal circulation or oxygenation. To avoid mistaking the maternal heart rate for the fetal heart rate, the two should be obtained simultaneously and com-

pared. Persistent bradycardia despite efforts to improve oxygenation is an indication for immediate delivery of the near-term fetus.

Decelerations occurring with uterine contractions indicate fetal stress (Fig. 35-4). They may be secondary to uteroplacental insufficiency resulting from impaired perfusion or oxygenation of the placenta or to direct umbilical cord compression as seen with a prolapsed cord. An immediate attempt should be made to resuscitate the fetus in utero. This is accomplished by placing the patient in slight Trendelenburg position and avoiding the dorsal supine position. Oxygen is administered by mask or, if necessary, via an endotracheal tube. An adequate circulating blood volume must be restored using salt solutions and blood products as indicated. In addition to fluid administration, maternal hypotension may be corrected by the use of ephedrine, 10 mg by IV push. This agent does not cause uterine artery constriction and therefore increases placental perfusion.[71] Should decelerations persist despite these maneuvers, the fetus is likely to

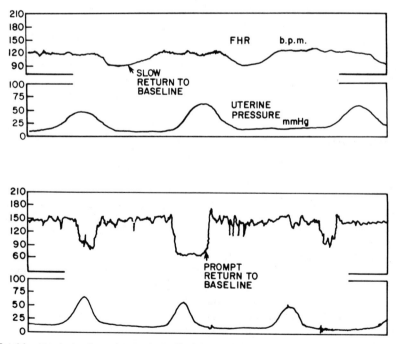

FIG. 35-4 Fetal heart rate tracings demonstrate (top) late decelerations and reduced beat-to-beat variability suggesting fetal distress, and (bottom) variable decelerations with prompt return to baseline heart rate, suggesting umbilical cord compression.

be in distress. Obstetric consultation is essential to determine whether the situation warrants immediate delivery and, if so, whether this can be accomplished vaginally or will require surgery.

Speculum Examination

A sterile speculum examination should be performed whenever the maternal condition permits her to assume the lithotomy position. This enables the examiner to determine the degree of cervical dilatation, the source of vaginal bleeding, and whether there is leakage of amniotic fluid. Bleeding per cervical os suggests placental separation or uterine injury. The amniotic sac may be ruptured with blunt or penetrating trauma resulting in possible premature labor or prolapse of the umbilical cord. In the absence of blood, ruptured membranes are probable if fluid from the posterior vaginal fornix causes pH-sensitive nitrazine paper to turn dark blue. To discourage ascending infection in such patients a bimanual examination is avoided unless genital tract trauma or advanced labor is present. Cervical cultures for group B streptococci, *Neisseria gonorrhea,* and *Chlamydia trachomatis* are indicated if the membranes are no longer intact.

Premature Labor

The presence and frequency of uterine contractions are best documented by monitoring the patient with a tocodynamometer. This can also be accomplished manually by placing a hand on the fundus and palpating for episodic increases in uterine tone. Contractions, as opposed to uterine irritability, last at least 40 seconds and generally must occur regularly at intervals of less than 8 minutes to cause cervical effacement and dilatation. When, in a pregnancy of less than 36 weeks' gestation, contractions occur with sufficient frequency and intensity to produce cervical change, a diagnosis of premature labor is made. As initial manage-

ment, factors such as hypovolemia and hypoxia, which predispose a patient to premature labor, should be corrected. The possibility of uterine injury, placental abruption, or intra-abdominal bleeding with peritoneal irritation should be investigated. In the absence of cervical change, nothing further need be done. However, when accompanied by progressive ripening, contractions that persist despite maternal hydration and bed rest are an indication for tocolytic therapy once maternal cardiovascular stability has been achieved. Because of the associated risks, it is essential that the use of tocolytic agents be restricted to patients with documented cervical change.

Intravenous ritodrine, although usually the drug of choice, must be used with extreme caution in the acutely injured patient. Tachycardia, hypokalemia, a widened pulse pressure, and hemodilution, side effects normally well-tolerated by the pregnant woman, may be life-threatening in the hemodynamically unstable gravida.[58] Maternal tachycardia greater than 120 beats/min, hypotension, significant bleeding, and fetal distress are contraindications to its use. Magnesium sulfate, although possibly less effective, has fewer cardiovascular side effects and may therefore be preferable when a tocolytic agent must be used in an injured patient to maintain the pregnancy. Once the cervix is 4 cm dilated such drugs are unlikely to be effective and the risks associated with their use warrant discontinuation of tocolytic therapy.

LABOR AND DELIVERY OF INJURED PATIENTS

Rarely, a trauma victim may arrive at a critical care facility already in advanced labor. Subsequent to admission, labor triggered by an occult placental abruption, uterine injury, or peritoneal irritation, whether traumatically or operatively induced, may go unrecognized in a seriously injured, sedated, or marginally responsive pregnant woman. If delivery is imminent a pediatrician should be notified immediately. The patient may be delivered satisfactorily in bed; hurried attempts to move her to a delivery suite may result in an unattended delivery in the corridor.

The lateral Sims's position, with an assistant supporting the superior leg, allows the patient to rest comfortably on her side, facilitates delivery of the shoulders, and is less likely to result in perineal tears when an episiotomy is not used (Fig. 35-5). Unlike the usual operative procedure, a simple vaginal delivery does not require sterile technique until after delivery of the fetus, although, when time permits, sterile technique is always preferable. Wearing surgical gloves serves to protect the surgeon more than the patient and a cap and mask are unnecessary. A quick cleaning of the perineum with a povidone–iodine scrub solution is recommended but not essential. As the fetal head distends the introitus, the operator supports the perineum with one hand while the other hand maintains pressure against the occiput to allow gradual distention of the introitus and a controlled delivery of the fetal head (Fig. 35-6). The sudden decompresion that occurs when the head is allowed to pop out may cause shearing of intracerebral blood vessels and is particularly hazardous for the premature infant. The patient whose second stage of labor is too rapid to permit an obstetrician to be summoned for the delivery is unlikely to require an episiotomy.

To prevent aspiration of amniotic fluid or meconium, the fetal nares and oropharynx are suctioned with a bulb syringe. A finger is then passed along the neck to determine whether an encircling loop of umbilical cord is present. If a loop is detected an attempt should be made to slip the loop over the fetal head before delivering the rest of the infant. If the cord is not sufficiently loose to permit this, it should be severed between two clamps. The shoulder in apposition to the symphysis is delivered first. The sides of the fetal head are grasped between the operator's hands and steady, gentle traction is applied towards the sacrum until the shoulder becomes visible under the pubic arch (Fig. 35-7). The direction of traction is then reversed towards the symphysis and the posterior shoulder delivered. The remainder of the fetus will follow without difficulty as traction is applied along the long axis of the infant. The neonate may be suctioned once more, particularly in the presence of meconium, taking care to keep the body below the level of the

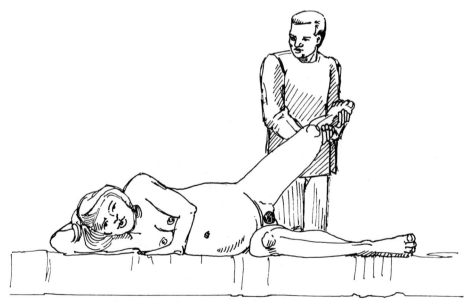

FIG. 35-5 Lateral Sims's position for vaginal delivery.

introitus at all times to encourage placental blood flow to the newborn. The cord is then cut between two clamps and the infant immediately wrapped in a warm towel. As long as there is no active bleeding, watchful waiting for spontaneous separation of the placenta is indicated and, therefore, attention can be directed towards resuscitating the infant.

Neonatal Resuscitation

If the infant's heart rate is above 100 beats/min and there is good respiratory effort with crying, nothing more than a thorough drying followed by wrapping in a warm blanket is required. The newborn, particularly if premature, has limited capacity for autoregulating temperature and these maneuvers will prevent evaporative heat loss. If breathing efforts are depressed the neonate should be stimulated by rubbing its back up and down along the spine. This encourages the infant to gasp and cry. Concomitantly, 100 percent oxygen can be delivered by free flow to the face. If the heart rate is less than 60 beats/min, external cardiac compression is indicated using two fingertips

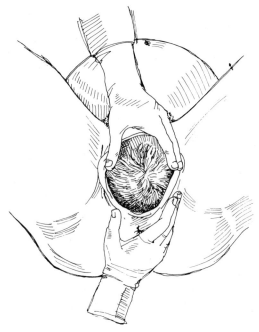

FIG. 35-6 Crowning of fetal head. The perineum is supported with one hand while the other permits controlled expulsion of the occiput.

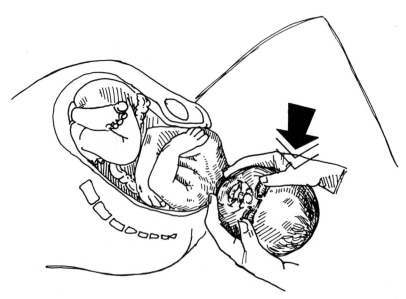

FIG. 35-7 The anterior shoulder of the fetus is delivered from behind the pubic symphysis by applying gentle traction to the head directed towards the maternal sacrum.

over the midsternum at the rate of 120 compressions/min. If possible, the infant should be ventilated with 100 percent oxygen by bag and a well-fitting mask at 40 to 60 inflations/min. However, neonatal equipment may not be immediately available and adult equipment is inappropriate and may cause a pneumothorax. In the interim, mouth-to-mouth ventilation should be instituted with the resuscitator's mouth placed over the infant's mouth and nose. Gentle puffs just sufficient to inflate the lungs at about 40/min are used. The respiratory status is re-evaluated after 1 or 2 minutes. Continued depression is an indication for intubation.

Placental Delivery

The parturient must not be left alone and requires intermittent assessment for evidence of hemorrhage or placental separation. Placental separation is heralded by increased vaginal bleeding and lengthening of the visible portion of the umbilical cord. Gentle traction on the cord along with expulsive efforts by the mother generally result in an uneventful delivery of the placenta. Massaging the uterine fundus at this time should result in a prompt reduction in vaginal blood loss.

INJURIES SPECIFIC TO PREGNANCY

Uterine Rupture

Traumatic uterine rupture is uncommon because of the elastic properies of the myometrium. Although exceedingly rare in the nonpregnant state, rupture has been reported as early as 3 months' gestation. The point of rupture is frequently at the placental implantation site where the increased vascularity weakens this portion of the uterine wall.

Approximately 1 percent of pregnant victims of severe automobile collisions will sustain a uterine rupture, frequently as a result of a passing vehicle running over the abdomen of the ejected gravida.[21] Use of seat belts decreases the frequency of maternal injury. A properly applied shoulder restraint system will improve fetal outcome as well. Experimental work on pregnant baboons that compared lap belts to a shoulder harness demonstrated a reduction in fetal mortality from 50 to 8 percent.[22] Ideally, the pregnant woman should use a three-point restraint system with the belt placed across the lap over a soft pillow. Use of a lap belt alone allows sufficient forward flexion and uterine compression to rupture the uterus. Similarly, wearing the belt too high will transmit the force of impact directly to the uterus, potentially leading to rupture.

DIAGNOSIS

In addition to the usual signs and symptoms of intra-abdominal bleeding with shock, following a major uterine rupture an abdominal mass may be palpated in which fetal parts are often easily identified. The contracted uterus may be distinguished as a separate, firm mass. The fetal heart tones are frequently absent. Vaginal bleeding may be present but is more likely when the laceration involves the lower uterine segment and cervix. Peritoneal lavage is always positive and may yield a liter of amniotic fluid. When the uterine defect is minor, localized uterine tenderness may be the only finding initially.

MANAGEMENT

Uterine rupture is a true emergency and demands immediate laparotomy even in the presence of shock. Type-specific whole blood should be administered until cross-matched blood becomes available. If, upon opening the abdomen, rapid bleeding obscures visualization, direct aortic compression should be applied. When the fetus has been extruded through the rent in the uterus, it is first removed. The uterine defect should be repaired, when possible, since this will preserve the patient's childbearing capacity and is usually quicker and safer than hysterectomy.

Bilateral internal iliac artery ligation may reduce the hemorrhage significantly while repair is attempted. In milder forms of uterine wall separation repair can usually be accomplished without emptying the uterus, although cesarean section is recommended for delivery. Longitudinal tears involving the uterine artery or its major branches may make salvage impossible and necessitate a hysterectomy. Although total hysterectomy is usually the procedure of choice, a subtotal hysterectomy can be performed more quickly and with less bleeding if the patient's condition remains unstable.

Uterine Penetration

INCIDENCE

Penetrating abdominal injuries may involve the uterus, and particularly in the case of gunshot wounds, the fetus as well. The uterus is the most likely organ to be injured in gunshot wounds of the abdomen, as it acts as a shield for the mother. Only 19 percent of women injured by gunshots have other associated visceral injuries.[13] There have been no reported maternal deaths resulting from gunshot wounds of the uterus since 1912. Fetal injuries occur in the majority of cases, however, and can prove fatal. Perinatal mortality ranges from 41 to 71 percent, with more recent series reporting the lowest rates.[64] Stab wounds have a better prognosis and are less common than bullet wounds. Visceral injury is also less common since an organ can slide away from the advancing knife point. Half of patients who receive knife wounds sustain an injury that does not require surgical repair.[55]

MANAGEMENT

Since the gravid patient is slow to manifest evidence of shock or peritonitis, penetrating gunshot wounds require surgical exploration. The fetus generally tolerates the stress of an-

esthesis and surgery uneventfully. Standard surgical techniques are used. If the uterus is not involved and does not hinder exploration and repair of injuries, the pregnancy should be left intact. If the bullet has penetrated the uterus it is likely that the fetus has been injured. Preoperative radiographs may suggest fetal involvement but are of little help in determining the severity of the injury.

The surgeon must weigh the risks of leaving a fetal injury untreated against those of premature delivery. Even when amniotic fluid is found in the peritoneal cavity, the membranes may subsequently seal by regeneration. Injured infants have also been delivered alive vaginally. Fetal wounds do undergo slow healing in utero.[10] Although, theoretically, amnionitis is a possible sequela of entry of a nonsterile bullet, this has not proved to be a problem. Buchsbaum and Caruso, investigating the cause of fetal death following gunshot wounds, found that only half of the infants had sustained injuries that could have contributed to their death while the other half, uninjured but delivered by cesarean section, died due to prematurity.[14] Since the perinatal mortality rate for the fetus of at least 34 weeks' gestation is less than 3 percent, suspected fetal injury warrants immediate delivery by cesarean section. For gestations less than 34 weeks, each case must be evaluated individually. If the fetus is dead and other injuries have been successfully repaired, cesarean section is not indicated.

Stab wounds do not necessarily mandate exploratory laparotomy. A fistulogram performed with Hypaque is useful for excluding peritoneal penetration. If peritoneal entry is suspected, peritoneal lavage along with a retrograde cystogram can generally rule out pelvic visceral injury in lower abdominal wounds. If the uterus has been penetrated, as evidenced by intraperitoneal amniotic fluid or bleeding, repair of the defect is indicated. Since the rent in the amniotic membranes is not exposed to bacterial contamination from the vagina, chorioamnitis is unlikely. The membranes frequently reseal and the pregnancy may continue until term. Transperitoneal stab wounds to the upper abdomen are likely to involve multiple loops of bowel and, therefore, will usually require surgical exploration.

It is impossible to assess the extent of fetal injuries while the conceptus remains in utero. Although the fetus is likely to be affected, injuries are frequently superficial. Even with more serious wounds the relative benefits of early repair must be weighed against the risks of prematurity. If the infant has survived the initial insult, it is less likely to be in immediate danger and may well tolerate a subsequent vaginal delivery even with injuries as severe as laceration of the abdominal wall with evisceration of the bowel.

The hypertrophied veins of the broad ligament and pelvis are particularly susceptible to injury. In the presence of torn uterine vessels and a potentially viable fetus, immediate cesarean section is indicated both to salvage the fetus and to provide exposure. Life-threatening maternal hemorrhage may occasionally require hysterotomy and delivery of a previable fetus in order to gain adequate visualization for repair. When a broad ligament hematoma occurs it may be impossible to isolate the bleeding vessel. The internal iliac artery on the affected side should be ligated first (but not severed). Since there is extensive collateral circulation, particularly from the ovarian vessels, this is unlikely to be sufficient and bilateral internal iliac as well as ovarian artery ligations may be necessary. This will not impair future reproductive capacity. If these maneuvers fail hysterectomy should be performed.

Retroperitoneal bleeding is frequently difficult to control but in the pregnant trauma victim it can be life threatening. A nonexpanding retroperitoneal hematoma found at laparotomy should be left alone. If continued, expansion and bleeding necessitate intervention, the clot should be evacuated and identifiable bleeding vessels ligated. However, solid packing with later removal may be the only way of controlling hemorrhage from multiple venous plexuses.

PLACENTAL ABRUPTION

Premature separation of the normally implanted placenta with resultant retroplacental bleeding after the 20th week of pregnancy is known as abruptio placentae. It occurs in about 1 in 120 deliveries but is seen more commonly in trauma victims.[44] Inertial forces in vehicular accidents, penetrating injuries, and even shock have been implicated. Crosby and Castiloe found that 3.4 percent of seriously injured gravidas sustained a clinically apparent placental separation.[21] This was much more common than uterine rupture. The majority of patients with identifiable pelvic fractures also had placental separation. Excluding maternal death, placental abruption was the most common cause of fetal death.

DIAGNOSIS

The pregnant trauma victim should be examined for evidence of vaginal bleeding, uterine tenderness, increased uterine tone or hypercontractility, increasing uterine size, and signs of fetal distress. In mild cases the only evidence of abruption may be vaginal bleeding as blood insinuates its way between the membranes and uterus and escapes through the cervix. The amount of uterine blood loss which can be seen externally is indicative of the patient's general condition. Uterine hypertonicity and tenderness are not prominent features. However, these patients remain at risk for premature labor or subsequent extension of the area of placental separation.

Since vaginal bleeding in the absence of other symptoms may also occur when the placenta is implanted over the internal cervical os, it is best to defer the pelvic examination in this situation until a placenta previa has been ruled out by sonogram. If necessary, a gentle sterile speculum examination can be performed: advance the speculum blades under direct visualization to detect cervical dilatation or genital tract trauma. Although ultrasonography is extremely useful for determing placental location it is frequently misleading when used to diagnose abruption. For a retroplacental clot to form of sufficient size to permit sonographic diagnosis, blockage of the blood's egress is required. More commonly an escape route is present as evidenced by vaginal bleeding.

It is possible for a woman to have an

abruption without demonstrating vaginal bleeding. In concealed hemorrhage there is uterine tetany and tenderness, fetal distress or death, and possible maternal shock. Localized uterine tenderness may become generalized as further retroplacental bleeding occurs. The extent of the maternal blood loss is frequently underestimated in this situation. Patients with these findings are at particular risk for a hypofibrinogenemic coagulopathy because thromboplastin from decidua and placenta enters the maternal circulation, triggering intravascular coagulation. In most patients there is an element of both revealed and concealed hemorrhage. Although, blood is predominantly maternal in origin, there may be fetal blood loss, at times into the maternal circulation, as well. A Kleihauer-Betke stain of maternal blood may reveal unexpected fetomaternal hemorrhage. This will require the administration of Rh D_o immunoglobulin to the previously unsensitized Rh negative patient to prevent maternal Rh sensitization. Unless more than half the placental surface has separated, the fetal heart tones can still be detected although the rate may be abnormal.

Disseminated intravascular coagulation (DIC) occurs in about 30 percent of abruptions that are severe enough to kill the fetus but is very uncommon when the fetus survives.[61] When DIC develops, it generally does so within 6 hours and most often is evident by the time the woman is hospitalized. Hypofibrinogenemia is a common concomitant of DIC but a severe defibrination syndrome may be present even with a fibrinogen level above 200 mg/dl due to the effects of fibrin split products. Observation of a red-topped tube of blood for evidence of clotting provides a quick screening test while one awaits laboratory results. Measurements of a prothrombin time, partial thromboplastin time, fibrin split products, fibrinogen level, and platelet count are reliable indices of the severity of the coagulopathy and the response to therapy but provide little additional useful information in the initial management of the patient.

TREATMENT

Minor degrees of placental abruption require only careful observation of maternal and fetal vital signs, blood loss, uterine size, and manifestations of labor. This is accomplished using an external fetal heart rate monitor and tocodynamometer. The fundal height is noted with a marking pen. More severe cases demand prompt restoration of an effective circulation followed by delivery if there is evidence of fetal distress or a coagulopathy. Additional measures include (1) administration of oxygen by face mask, (2) monitoring fluid intake and urinary output, and (3) replacement of blood through a large-bore cannula based upon hematocrit and central venous pressure monitoring. Whole blood (as much as 20 units) and a balanced salt solution are administered in quantities to maintain a hematocrit of at least 30 percent, although the patient and fetus generally will tolerate a hematocrit of 25 once the mother's condition has been stabilized.

If a coagulation defect is present, give fresh frozen plasma or cryoprecipitate. To supply 4 g fibrinogen will require 15 to 20 bags of cryoprecipitate. Fibrinogen administration carries a risk of hepatitis B and is best avoided except when operative delivery is planned in the presence of a fibrinogen level less than 100 mg/dl. Fibrinogen, 2 to 6 g, along with platelets and fresh blood can be life-saving. Although considerable debate surrounds the use of heparin in this setting, we do not recommend its use since it is a potent anticoagulant that may potentiate hemorrhage and since prompt delivery is a more effective means of disrupting the coagulation cascade.

Definitive treatment requires delivery. If the fetus is dead the vaginal route is preferable unless the rate of hemorrhage exceeds the rate at which blood can reasonably be replaced. Cesarean section is indicated if the cervix is unfavorable, or other obstetric considerations contraindicate vaginal delivery. Women with severe placental abruption transfused for 18 hours or more at the University of Virginia Hospital did not experience more complications than those delivered sooner.[61] If the fetus is alive with no manifestations of distress on the monitor, the obstetric service may follow the patient expectantly depending upon the gestational age. In the presence of fetal distress in the third-trimester fetus, immediate operative delivery is indicated if the maternal status permits.

Placental or Cord Laceration

Isolated traumatic laceration of the placenta or cord is extremely rare following blunt abdominal trauma. However, it can occur without major maternal injury. VanSante[73] reported a case of fetal death from a placental laceration at the area of insertion of the umbilical cord subsequent to the mother falling off a stepladder. Placental laceration is not uncommon with penetrating uterine injuries but does not uniformly necessitate delivery. Although amniocentesis can be used to diagnosis fetal bleeding in utero, this complication is not sufficiently common to warrant routine use of this diagnostic procedure.

Amniotic Fluid Embolism

As a consequence of traumatic injury, a partial separation of the placenta or interruption of the amniotic membrane and continuity of the uterine wall may allow entry of amniotic fluid into the maternal circulation through subplacental sinusoids. The particulate matter is quickly filtered out in the distal pulmonary circulation, causing mechanical obstruction. Pulmonary hypertension rapidly ensues with a reduction in the flow of blood to the left side of the heart, fall in cardiac output, and consequent hypotension. There is reflex bronchospasm and further hypoxia. Although this is a rare complication, the mortality is extremely high. Approximately 50 percent of patients die at the time of embolization and an additional 25 percent die subsequently.[15] An adverse outcome is particularly likely if the fluid contains particulate material such as meconium, while it is uncommon prior to the third trimester.

DIAGNOSIS

The syndrome is characterized by the abrupt onset of dyspnea, cyanosis, cardiovascular collapse, hemorrhage, coma, and seizures. Death may occur within 10 minutes of the onset of symptoms. If the patient survives the initial shocklike episode, severe bleeding secondary to a consumptive and fibrinolytic coagulopathy develops. Marked thrombocytopenia and hypofibrinogenemia result. There is little time for confirmatory tests although aspiration of blood from the right ventricle may demonstrate amniotic debris floating over the buffy coat of white cells.[36]

MANAGEMENT

Treatment is frequently unsatisfactory but is directed toward supporting the cardiovascular system and controlling the coagulopathy. Since death is usually secondary to cor pulmonale, the blood volume should be maintained to ensure a sustained, elevated right-sided heart filling pressure. Cardiac inotropic support is indicated and mechanical ventilation is usually required. Although administration of heparin immediately upon clinical diagnosis of amniotic fluid embolism has been recommended to prevent or control the coagulopathy,[17] there are not enough reports to allow proper evaluation of its efficacy. The mainstay of therapy continues to be blood replacement therapy, including platelets and fibrinogen if necessary.

Eclampsia

The most frequent cause of de novo seizures and coma during late pregnancy is eclampsia. Therefore, this possibility must be considered even in the presence of head trauma. An eclamptic gravida may sustain head injury as a direct consequence of a seizure. When initially evaluated in her postictal, obtunded state, it may be difficult to determine the cause of the observed CNS disturbance. The hallmarks of eclampsia are hypertension and proteinuria. The combination of a diastolic blood pressure greater than 90 mmHg and at least 1+ proteinuria is adequate to make a preliminary diagnosis of eclampsia.

The cause of eclampsia is unknown. Vasospasm as well as increased pressor responses are basic to the disease. The end result is uteroplacental hypoperfusion and impaired function of other organ systems. The most serious complications of eclampsia are cerebral vascular accident, cardiac failure, pulmonary edema, acute renal failure, and fetal distress, often due to placental abruption. Although thrombocytopenia is frequent, severe thrombocytopenia (less than 50,000 platelets/mm³) or a coagulopathy occur in less than 3 percent of patients. Eclampsia is a leading cause of maternal death in the United States.

Although definitive treatment requires delivery of the fetus, intravenous magnesium sulfate is the cornerstone of management and is sufficiently benign to warrant prompt institution while the remainder of the neurologic work-up proceeds. This treatment has depressive effects on both the neuromuscular junction and cortical neuronal burst firing in the primate model.[11] It is administered as a 4 g loading dose over 5 minutes, immediately followed by a maintenance infusion of 1 to 2 g/hr, depending upon urine output. Significant hypertension as manifested by a diastolic blood pressure greater than 110 mmHg is managed with intravenous hydralazine, 5 to 10 mg as necessary to maintain the diastolic pressure between 90 and 110 mmHg. This may be best accomplished using a continuous, low dose hydralazine infusion.

The patient's fluid intake and urinary output through an indwelling catheter should be carefully monitored. Oliguria that persists despite a fluid challenge is an indication for placement of a central line, preferably a Swan-Ganz.[8] Diuretics are contraindicated unless there is documented left heart failure. Baseline clotting and renal function studies are performed.

These measures should not hinder the neurologic evaluation of the patient and will prevent irreparable damage in the interim. It is equally important that the possibility of a nonobstetric cerebral complication be entertained in every apparent case of eclampsia.

Sepsis

Despite the availability of effective antibiotic regimens, sepsis remains a major cause of obstetric deaths. Pelvic endometritis–salpingitis–peritonitis is uncommon during pregnancy and extremely rare after the first trimester because the cervical mucus plug forms an effective barrier to the ascent of microorganisms. The uterine cavity is filled with amniotic fluid that has intrinsic antibacterial activity which becomes increasingly effective as pregnancy progresses.[67] However, direct hematogenous spread to the pelvic organs is possible.

Septic abortion, amnionitis with or without ruptured membranes, postpartum endometritis, and pyelonephritis are the entities most frequently encountered, but sepsis may follow trauma as well. Postabortal trauma victims and those with fecally contaminated wounds are especially at risk for developing septic shock and require prompt treatment with appropriate antibiotics.

The major threat is septic shock. The fetus tolerates the initial stages of maternal septic hypovolemia quite well but in the terminal phase the adverse effects on the fetal cardiovascular system secondary to uterine hypoperfusion become apparent. Fetal tachycardia secondary to pyrexia and early asphyxia are followed by bradycardia and, finally, fetal death. Treatment is designed to (1) improve maternal perfusion, (2) identify the infectious source, and (3) eliminate the infection. Maternal volume expansion and cardiovascular support directed at establishing an adequate urine output are accomplished as in the nonpregnant patient. The goal is to achieve a urine output greater than 30 ml/hr, while maintaining a CVP of less than 10 cm H_2O. When the infection does not involve the uterine cavity or its contents (e.g., pyelonephritis, pelvic peritonitis, or a ruptured appendiceal or ovarian abscess), it is usually possible to conserve the pregnancy by administering antibiotics and performing any indicated surgical drainage or excision.

In contrast, proper treatment of chorioamnionitis or septic abortion requires immediate evacuation of the uterine contents, no matter what the duration of the pregnancy, in addition to antibiotic therapy. The fetal age and maternal status will determine the best method of emptying the uterus. If the uterus is less than 15 weeks' size, a careful suction curettage is performed once a loading dose of antibiotics has been administered. The septic uterus is particularly vulnerable to perforation and therefore uterine sounding is avoided. In later gestations, infection may impair myometrial contractility so as to preclude vaginal delivery, necessitating a hysterotomy or cesarean section even in the presence of fetal death.

It is essential that the antibiotic regimen selected include coverage for anaerobic organisms. *Peptostreptococcus, peptococcus,* and bacteroides are common infecting organisms. Clindamycin, 900 mg intravenously every 8 hours in conjunction with an aminoglycoside is a good choice. The increased volume of distribution during pregnancy requires that large doses be used in the absence of renal failure. Peak and trough aminoglycoside levels will aid in selecting the appropriate dosage. In general, a loading dose of tobramycin/gentamycin, 1.7 mg/kg is administered intravenously followed by a maintenance dose of 1.5 mg/kg at 8 hour intervals. Although this regimen does not provide coverage for the enterococcus, this organism is rarely a primary pathogen in obstetric infection.

POSTMORTEM CESAREAN SECTION

Maternal injuries may be so severe as to prove fatal despite aggressive efforts at resuscitation. The physician must decide whether to initiate resuscitative measures in the moribund patient in an effort to save the infant and at what point to shift the emphasis from maternal salvage to immediate operative delivery of the infant. Although postmortem cesarean section is sufficiently uncommon that an obstetrician is unlikely to perform one during his or her professional lifetime, the increased exposure of working women to the hazards of the workplace and highway, combined with rapid transport to medical facilities, make it likely that the critical care surgeon will.

The requisites for performing a perimortem cesarean section are (1) a viable fetus, (2) certainty of an unfavorable maternal outcome so that an operative delivery will not itself prejudice her chances of survival, and (3) a basic knowledge of the operative technique. If the mother is brain dead but her vital functions are maintained by cardiopulmonary mechanical support, it should be possible to obtain obstetric and pediatric assistance. In certain situations consideration may be given to attempting to continue the pregnancy for prolonged periods using mechanical support in an effort to gain further fetal maturation.[2] It is also helpful to consult with the family regarding their wishes, but the rights of the unborn infant take priority. No physician in this country has ever been found liable for performing a postmortem cesarean section, even when the decision to proceed was in direct conflict with the expressed wishes of the family.[6,62] As of publication the legal department of the American College of Obstetricians and Gynecologists has no record of any adverse ruling. Precious time should never be wasted attempting to obtain consent if it is not immediately available.

In the truly emergent situation, where the patient is already dead or dying, immediate action is imperative. Postmortem cesarean section can be justified if any fetal heart activity is detectable, regardless of the rate. Even after maternal resuscitation has proven unsuccessful, continued cardiac massage, ventilation, and bicarbonate administration until delivery will improve the chances of fetal survival. The likelihood of a successful outcome as evidenced by a live infant without residual impairment, depends upon (1) the gestational age, (2) the time elapsed from maternal death to delivery, (3) the cause of maternal death, (4) the duration of fetal compromise prior to maternal death, (5) the effectiveness of interval maternal resuscitation, and (6) the adequacy of the neonatal resuscitation.

Gestational Age

The infant's chances of survival are directly related to its age. Although a fetus less than 28 weeks' gestation might survive, such a premature infant is unlikely to tolerate the twin insults of antepartum hypoxic stress as well as postpartum respiratory distress and remain intact. Antepartum asphyxia increases the severity of newborn respiratory distress as well as the risk of intracerebral bleeding or necrotizing enterocolitis. The urgency of the situation and frequent unavailability of information do not generally permit one to determine the fetal age using standard criteria, such as the date of the last menstrual period, quickening, or sonographic evaluation. Instead the surgeon must rely on determination of the fundal height. If the fundal height measures at least 28 cm or, if a tape is unavailable, extends more than four fingerbreadths above the umbilicus, the surgeon should assume the fetus is potentially salvageable.

Interval from Death to Delivery

A previously uncompromised fetus can be expected to tolerate 10 minutes of total anoxia. Although it is stated that survival is possible up to 20 minutes following maternal death, intact survival is rare after 10 to 15 minutes have elapsed.[76] To insure optimal outcome, delivery should be accomplished within 5 minutes of maternal death.

Cause of Maternal Death

The prognosis is further jeopardized when death follows a protracted respiratory, metabolic, or malignant illness in which case the fetal reserves are diminished as a result of chronic hypoxia or acidosis. An acute insult such as head trauma or electrocution in a previously healthy woman is more likely to allow delivery of a healthy infant than an injury complicated by hemorrhage and shock. In the latter situation, the infant is deprived of adequate placental perfusion for a period of time prior to maternal death. An asphyxic maternal death, such as by drowning or smoke inhalation, does not generally warrant attempts to salvage the fetus.

Technique

The only instrument necessary is a scalpel. Suction and retractors to improve visualization of the operative field and a clamp for the umbilical cord are desirable but not essential. An assistant is useful to provide exposure.

The patient is placed in the dorsal supine position and requires no preparation. Traditionally the right-handed operator stands on the right side of the table thus freeing the right hand for lifting the fetal presenting part out of the pelvis and through the uterine incision. Since the fetal pole is unlikely to be engaged, it is more important that the surgeon work from whichever side he or she feels most comfortable. A vertical midline abdominal incision is made, extending from the umbilicus to the sym-

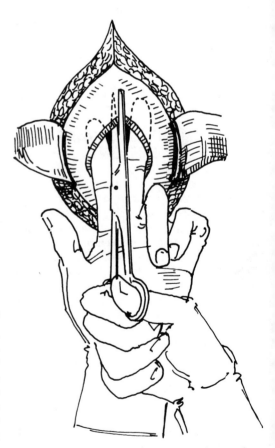

FIG. 35-8 The uterine wall is elevated away from the fetus as the uterine incision is extended vertically with a scalpel or scissors.

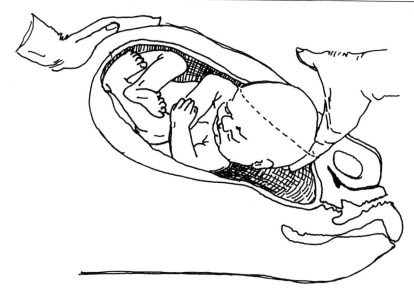

FIG. 35-9 The surgeon's palm is used to lift the fetal occiput through the incision while fundal pressure is applied simultaneously.

physis. All layers of the abdominal wall are incised until the peritoneal cavity is entered. The peritoneal incision may be extended superiorly and inferiorly either bluntly or using the scalpel. The lower uterine segment is quickly palpated to confirm the identity of the presenting fetal part and degree of uterine rotation. The myometrium is incised vertically in the midline for 1 to 2 inches just superior to the bladder reflection. Entry at a point as low as possible on the uterine wall minimizes the thickness of the myometrium traversed and reduces the likelihood of encountering an anteriorly located placenta. The scalpel handle or a finger can be used to separate the last few myometrial fibers bluntly to avoid accidently cutting the fetus. Using the separated fingers of one hand to elevate the uterine wall away from the underlying fetus, one then extends the uterine incision superiorly between two fingers for a total distance of approximately 4 to 5 inches (Fig. 35-8). Since the lower uterine segment is generally poorly developed and the fetus often in a nonvertex presentation prior to term, this classic incision has the advantage of enabling the surgeon to extend the incision length should it become necessary. If the placenta is discovered in the line of the incision, it must either be detached or incised. Prompt clamping of the umbilical cord will prevent fetal exsanguination.

If the vertex is presenting, slip a hand between the symphysis and the fetal head and then lift the head through the uterine incision using the fingers and palm, aided by the application of transabdominal fundal pressure (Fig. 35-9). Aspirate the nasopharynx with a bulb syringe, if available, to minimize fetal aspiration of amniotic fluid. Deliver the shoulders in the anteroposterior diameter using gentle traction alternating upwards and downwards as an assistant applies fundal pressure. The remainder of the fetus follows easily. Hold the fetus at the level of the maternal abdomen tilted with its head down. Clamp the cord and then sever it distally with the scalpel blade.

While awaiting the arrival of a pediatrician, initiate resuscitation of the neonate as previously described.

CONCLUSION

The initial medical contact for the acutely injured pregnant women will involve a member of the critical care team. Familiarity with the anatomic and physiologic changes accompanying pregnancy and its complications is essential during these first crucial minutes of patient management. The actions taken prior to obstetric consultation may prove pivotal to two lives.

REFERENCES

1. Abramovich DR, Francis W, Helsby CR: Two cases of ruptured aneurysm of splanchnic arteries in pregnancy with comment on the lesser sac syndrome. J Obstet Gynaecol Br Commonw 76: 1037, 1969

2. Aderet NB, Cohen I, Abramowicz JS: Traumatic coma during pregnancy with persistent vegetative state. Case report. Br J Obstet Gynaecol 91: 939, 1984

3. Alaily AB, Carrol KB: Pulmonary ventilation in pregnancy. Br J Obstet Gynaecol 85: 518, 1978

4. Anderson GJ, James GB, Mathers NP et al: The maternal oxygen tension and acid base status during pregnancy. J Obstet Gynaecol Br Commonw 76: 16, 1969

5. Ang CK, Tan TH, Waters WAW, Wood C: Postural influence on maternal capillary oxygen and carbon dioxide tension. Br Med J 4: 201, 1969

6. Arthur RK: Postmortem cesarean section. Am J Obstet Gynecol 132: 175, 1978

7. Baker DP: Trauma in the pregnant patient. Surg Clin North Am 62: 275, 1982

8. Berkowitz RL, Rafferty TD: Invasive hemodynamic monitoring in critically ill pregnant patients: role of Swan-Ganz catheterization. Am J Obstet Gynecol 137: 127, 1980

9. Boba A, Linkie DM, Plotz EJ: Effects of vasopressor administration and fluid replacement on fetal bradycardia and hypoxia induced by maternal hemorrhage. Obstet Gynecol 27: 408, 1966

10. Bonnar J, McNicol GP, Douglas AS: Coagulation and fibrinolytic mechanisms during and after normal childbirth. Br Med J 2: 200, 1970

11. Borges LF, Gücer G: Effect of magnesium on epileptic foci. Epilepsia 19: 81, 1978

12. Buchsbaum HJ: Accidental injury complicating pregnancy. Am J Obstet Gynecol 102: 752, 1968

13. Buchsbaum HJ: Penetrating injury of the abdomen. p.82. In Buchsbaum HJ (ed): Trauma in Pregnancy. WB Saunders, Philadelphia, 1979

14. Buchsbaum HJ, Caruso PA: Gunshot wounds of the pregnant uterus. Obstet Gynecol 33: 673, 1969

15. Cavanagh D: Shock. p.37. In Cavanagh D, Woods RE, O'Connor TCF (eds): Obstetric Emergencies. Harper & Row, Hagerstown, Maryland, 1978

16. Cerruti R, Fenari S, Grella P et al: Behavior of serum enzymes in pregnancy. Clin Exp Obstet Gynecol 3: 22, 1976

17. Chung AF, Merkatz IR: Survival following amniotic fluid embolism with early heparinization. Obstet Gynecol 42: 809, 1973

18. Colditz RB, Josey WE: Central venous pressure in supine position during normal pregnancy. Obstet Gynecol 36: 769, 1970

19. Coombes B, Shibata J, Adams R et al: Alterations in sulfobromophthalein sodium-removal mechanisms from blood during normal pregnancy. J Clin Invest 42: 1431, 1963

20. Crosby WM: Trauma during pregnancy: maternal and fetal injury. Obstet Gynecol Surv 29: 683, 1974

21. Crosby WM, Costiloe JP: Safety of lap belt restraint for pregnant victims of automobile collisions. N Engl J Med 284: 632, 1977

22. Crosby WM, King AI, Stout LC: Fetal survival following impact: improvement with shoulder harness restraint. Am J Obstet Gynecol 112: 1101, 1972

23. Cugell DW, Frank NR, Gaensler EA, Badger TL: Pulmonary function in pregnancy. I. Serial observations in normal women. Am Rev Tuberc 67: 568, 1953

24. Davidson JM: Changes in renal function and other aspects of homeostasis in early pregnancy. J Obstet Gynaecol Br Commonw 81: 1003, 1974

25. Davison JS, Davison MC, Hay DM: Gastric emptying time in late pregnancy and labour. J Obstet Gynaecol Br Commonw 77: 37, 1970

26. DeLeeuw NKM, Lowenstein L, Hsieh YS: Iron deficiency and hydremia of normal pregnancy. Medicine 45: 291, 1966

27. Dolezal A, Figor S: The phenomenon of reactive vasodilatation in pregnancy. Am J Obstet Gynecol 83: 907, 1962

28. Dyer I, Barclay DL: Accidental trauma complicating pregnancy and delivery. Am J Obstet Gynecol 83: 907, 1962

29. Efrati P, Presentey B, Margolith M, Rosenszajn L: Leukocytes of normal pregnant women. Obstet Gynecol 23: 429, 1964

30. Fadel HE, Northrop G, Misenhimer HR, Harp RJ: Normal pregnancy: a model of sustained respiratory alkalosis. J Perinat Med 3: 195, 1979

31. Fainstat T: Ureteral dilatation in pregnancy: a review. Obstet Gynecol Surv 18: 845, 1963

32. Fisher RS, Roberts GS, Grabowski CJ et al: Altered lower esophageal sphincter functioning during early pregnancy. Gastroenterology 74: 1233, 1978

33. Fletcher AP, Alkjaersig NK, Burstein R: The influ-

ence of pregnancy upon blood coagulation and plasma fibrinolytic enzyme function. Am J Obstet Gynecol 134: 743, 1979

34. Fort AJ, Harlin RS: Pregnancy outcome after non-catastrophic maternal trauma during pregnancy. Obstet Gynecol 35: 912, 1970
35. Greiss FC: Uterine vascular response to hemorrhage during pregnancy. Obstet Gynecol 27: 549, 1966
36. Gross P, Benz EJ: Pulmonary embolism by amniotic fluid: report of 3 cases with new diagnostic procedure. Surg Gynecol Obstet 85: 315, 1947
37. Grumbach K, Mechlin MB, Mintz MC: Computed tomography and ultrasound of the traumatized and acutely ill patient. Emerg Med Clin North Am 3: 607, 1985
38. Haemmerli UP: Jaundice during pregnancy with special emphasis on recurrent jaundice during pregnancy and its differential diagnosis. Acta Med Scand 444(suppl): 1, 1960
39. Hall K: Relaxin. J Reprod Fertil 1: 368, 1960
40. Hertig AT, Shelton WH: Minimal criteria required to prove primafacie case of abortion. Ann Surg 117: 596, 1943
41. Hey VMF, Cowley DS, Ganguli PC et al: Gastroesophageal reflux in late pregnancy. Anesthesia 32: 372, 1977
42. Howard BK, Goodson JH: Experimental placental abruption. Obstet Gynecol 2: 442, 1953
43. Jackson FC: Accidental injury—the problem and the initiatives. p.1. In Buchsbaum HJ (ed): Trauma in Pregnancy. WB Saunders, Philadelphia, 1979
44. Javert CT: Role of the patient's activities in the occurrence of spontaneous abortion. Fertil Steril 11: 550, 1960
45. Jiminez JM, Tyson JE, Santos-Ramos R, Duenhoelter JH: Comparison of obstetric and pediatric evaluation of gestational age. Pediatr Res 13: 498, 1979
46. Kerr MG: The mechanical effects of the gravid uterus in late pregnancy. J Obstet Gynaecol Br Commonw 72: 513, 1965
47. Knab DR: Abruptio placentae. Obstet Gynecol 52: 625, 1978
48. Kuvin SF, Brecher G: Differential neutrophil counts in pregnancy. N Engl J Med 266: 877, 1962
49. Lazarus HM, Nelson JA: Refining the technique of diagnostic peritoneal lavage. ER Rep 1: 111, 1980
50. Lyons HA, Antonio R: The sensitivity of the respiratory center in pregnancy and after the administration of progesterone. Trans Assoc Am Physicians 72: 173, 1959
51. MacGillivray I, Rose GA, Rowe B: Blood pressure survey in pregnancy. Clin Sci 37: 395, 1969
52. Marx G: Shock in the obstetric patient. Anesthesiology 26: 423, 1965

53. McLennan CE: Antecubital and femoral venous pressure in normal and toxemic pregnancies. Am J Obstet Gynecol 45: 568, 1943
54. Mendelson CL: Cardiac Disease in Pregnancy: Medical Care, Cardiovascular Surgery and Obstetric Management as Related to Maternal and Fetal Welfare. FA Davis, Philadelphia, 1960
55. Nance FC, Cohn I, Jr.: Surgical judgement in the management of stab wounds: a retrospective and prospective analysis based on a study of 600 stab wounds. Ann Surg 170: 569, 1969
56. National Safety Council: Accident Facts. National Safety Council, Chicago, 1975
57. Nilsson IM, Kullander S: Coagulation and fibrinolytic studies during pregnancy. Acta Obstet Gynecol Scand 46: 273, 1967
58. Osler M: Side effects and metabolic changes during treatment with betamimetics (ritodrine). Dan Med Bull 26: 119, 1979
59. Pitkin RM, Witte DL: Platelet and leukocyte counts in pregnancy. JAMA 242: 2696, 1979
60. Pritchard JA: Hematologic aspects of pregnancy. Clin Obstet Gynecol 3: 378, 1960
61. Pritchard JA, MacDonald PC: Williams Obstetrics, 16th Ed. Appleton-Century-Crofts, New York, 1980
62. Ritter J: Postmortem cesarean section. JAMA 175: 715, 1961
63. Robin ED: Overdiagnosis and overtreatment of pulmonary embolism: the emperor may have no clothes. Ann Intern Med 87: 775, 1977
64. Rothenberger D, Quattlebaum FW, Perry JF et al: Blunt maternal trauma: a review of 103 cases. J Trauma 18: 173, 1978
65. Rovinsky JJ, Jaffin H: Cardiovascular hemodynamics in pregnancy. I. Blood and plasma volumes in multiple pregnancy. Am J Obstet Gynecol 93: 1, 1965
66. Saunders P, Milton PJD: Laparotomy during pregnancy: an assessment of diagnostic accuracy and fetal wastage. Br Med J 3: 165, 1973
67. Schlievert P, Johnson W, Galask RP: Bacterial growth inhibition by amniotic fluid. VI. Evidence for a zinc-peptide antibacterial system. Am J Obstet Gynecol 125: 906, 1976
68. Schnitker MA, Bayer CA: Dissecting aneurysm of the aorta in young individuals, particularly in association with pregnancy. With report of a case. Ann Intern Med 20: 486, 1944
69. Scholtes G: Liver function and liver disease during pregnancy. J Perinat Med 7: 55, 1979
70. Shaper AG, Kear J, MacIntosh DM et al: The platelet count, platelet adhesiveness, and aggregation and the mechanism of fibrinolytic inhibition in pregnancy and the puerperium. J Obstet Gynaecol Br Commonw 75: 433, 1968
71. Shnider S, deLorimier AA, Holl JW et al: Vaso-

pressors in obstetrics. I. Correction of fetal acidosis with ephedrine during spinal hypotension. Am J Obstet Gynecol 102: 911, 1968

72. Trower R, Walters WAW: Brachial artery blood pressure in the lateral recumbent position during pregnancy. Aust NZJ Obstet Gynaecol 8: 146, 1968

73. Ueland K, Novy MJ, Peterson EN, Metcalfe J: Maternal cardiovascular dynamics. IV. The influence of gestational age on the maternal cardiovascular response to posture and exercise. Am J Obstet Gynecol 104: 856, 1969

74. VanSante TJ: En geval van intra-uterine placentaverscheuring door ietsel. Ned Tijdschr Geneeskd 86: 2848, 1942

75. Walters WAW, MacGregor WG, Hills M: Cardiac output at rest during pregnancy and the puerperium. Clin Sci 30: 1, 1966

76. Weber CE: Postmortem cesarean section: review of the literature and case reports. Am J Obstet Gynecol 110: 158, 1971

77. Wilson JN: Rational approach to management of clinical shock. Arch Surg 91: 92, 1965

78. Zuckerman H: Serum alkaline phosphatase in pregnancy and puerperium. Obstet Gynecol 25: 819, 1965

36

The Acute Burn Patient*

Basil A. Pruitt, Jr.

INTRODUCTION

An extensive burn evokes a systemic response, the magnitude and duration of which are proportional to the extent of body surface injured. Since the resulting multisystem dysfunction assumes a pattern of initial hypofunction succeeded by hyperfunction, monitoring and therapy are guided by both the extent of burn and the time postinjury.[107] In the immediate postburn period, prevention and correction of hemodynamic and pulmonary insufficiency take precedence while later in the course the prevention and correction of variable degrees of dysfunction of specific organ systems can influence wound closure, the incidence of infec-

tion and other complications, and the rapidity and quality of recovery.

The relationship between burn size and physiologic change determines the intensity of care required and the optimal treatment site where the necessary care can be provided.[3] Patients with minor burns, that is, second-degree burns involving less than 15 percent of the total body surface area in adults or less than 10 percent of the total body surface area in children and third-degree burns of less than 2 percent of the body surface area not involving the hands, face, eyes, ears, feet, or perineum, can be cared for on an outpatient basis after initial treatment in an emergency room or a physician's office. Those patients in this category with full-thickness burns may require subsequent hospitalization for skin graft closure of the wound, but minor grafting procedures can also be carried out on an outpatient basis. Patients with moderate burn injuries, that is, second-degree burns of 15 to 25 percent of the body surface in adults or 10 to 20 percent of

* The opinions or assertions contained herein are the private views of the author and are not to be construed as official or as reflecting the views of the Department of the Army or the Department of Defense.

1099

the body surface area in children and those with third-degree burns of less than 10 percent of the body surface area not involving the hands, face, eyes, ears, feet, or perineum, can be cared for in a general hospital by personnel experienced in burn care. Patients with major burn injury, which include those with second-degree burns of more than 25 percent of the body surface area in adults or 20 percent in children, third-degree burns of 10 percent or more of the total body surface, and significant burns involving hands, face, eyes, ears, feet, and perineum, significant associated inhalation injury, significant electrical burns, and burn injury complicated by associated mechanical trauma as well as all poor-risk patients, are best cared for in a hospital with specialized facilities. Here, multidisciplinary health professionals are available to provide care ranging from resuscitation through wound care and eventual rehabilitation.

SYSTEMIC AND LOCAL EFFECTS OF BURN INJURY

The earliest manifestations of the systemic effects of thermal injury involve the cardiovascular system, in which a marked increase in peripheral vascular resistance is accompanied by a decrease in cardiac output.[124] These initial changes have been attributed to neurogenic and hormonal influences and occur prior to significant decrease in blood volume. As edema

occurs in injured tissues, blood volume decreases and cardiac output falls, with the compensatory vascular response maintaining the increase in peripheral vascular resistance. All of these pathophysiologic changes result in a diminution of tissue blood flow. Although some investigators have attributed the early depression of cardiac output to a circulating myocardial depressant factor,[12,136] such a factor has never been characterized. In recent physiologic studies of patients with less than predicted normal cardiac output during the resuscitation period, an observed decrease in left ventricular filling consistent with a volume deficit appears to explain the depression of cardiac output[44] (Table 36-1).

The initial pulmonary response to an extensive burn is characterized by an increase in respiratory rate with an initial decrease in tidal volume. This rapid shallow breathing is typically adequate to maintain arterial oxygen tension but may produce a respiratory alkalosis associated with hypocarbia. If blood volume loss is either persistent or profound, ventilatory rate may decrease and hypoxemia supervene. Following resuscitation, hyperventilation represents the pulmonary manifestation of postinjury hypermetabolism and results from an increase in both ventilatory rate and tidal volume with modest, if any, parenchymal change (work of breathing is often at the upper limit of predicted normal and may be slightly elevated)[116] (Fig. 36-1).

Elevated circulating levels of vasoactive hormones and the liberation of various pharmacologically active materials from the wound may alter the hydrostatic pressure balance across the pulmonary capillary and pulmonary capillary permeability, respectively,[38] but in the uncomplicated burn patient, the increased

TABLE 36-1. Early Postburn Echocardiographic Hemodynamic Indices in Patients with Decreased Cardiac Output[a]

	Time Postburn in Hours		
	0–12	12–24	24–48
Stroke index (ml/m²)	35 ± 11	27 ± 11[b]	37 ± 11
Left ventricular ejection fraction	0.79 ± 0.09	0.74 ± 0.07	0.75 ± 0.07
Velocity of internal fiber shortening (circ/sec)	1.77 ± 0.52	1.73 ± 0.14	1.60 ± 0.28
Left ventricular end-diastolic volume index (ml/m²)	44 ± 15	37 ± 16[b]	50 ± 16

[a] All values = mean ± one standard deviation.
[b] Significantly decreased compared to burn patients with predicted normal cardiac output.

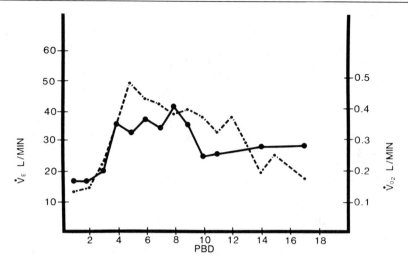

FIG. 36-1 The marked elevation of minute ventilation that occurs in burn patients following resuscitation parallels the hypermetabolic changes in oxygen consumption. Note changes in both physiologic indices across time. (--•--) $\dot{V}_E$, minute ventilation L/min; (—•—) $\dot{V}_{O_2}$, oxygen consumption L/min.

lung lymph flow is not associated with an increase in extravascular lung water.[141]

The pathophysiologic changes that affect the kidney and the gastrointestinal tract appear to be most closely related to alterations in organ blood flow. Initial postburn oliguria is a reflection of decreased glomerular filtration rate and renal blood flow as a result of hypovolemia and diminution of cardiac output. Following resuscitation, glomerular filtration rate is commonly elevated as a reflection of the hyperdynamic circulatory state that persists until the wounds are healed.[98] To ensure adequate circulating levels of drugs excreted by the kidney, the dosage of such agents must take into account this increase in renal blood flow. Morphologic studies and assessment of gastroduodenal mucosal blood flow, using radiolabeled microspheres, indicate that focal ischemia of the mucosa of the upper gastrointestinal tract is the most important factor in the pathogenesis of stress ulcers.[37,67] Similar changes may occur in the gastrointestinal tract in association with hypotension due to blood loss or sepsis later in the postburn course.

Phasic changes in the hematologic system may also occur. The initial red cell destruction that occurs in areas of burn produces a red cell mass deficit[71,124] (Table 36-2). The anticipated effect of the subsequent increase in erythropoietin levels is often nullified by blood sampling and operation.[4] An immediate elevation of the white blood cell count is followed by an absolute or relative leukopenia, which may be exaggerated by gram-negative sepsis.[79] The lymphocyte populations change across time with a relative prominence of B cells and emergence of suppressor cells following resuscitation.[78] Circulating immunoglobulin levels are initially depressed but return to normal in the patient with an uncomplicated burn following resuscitation.[93] The observed changes in the levels of clotting factors are con-

TABLE 36-2. Changes in Red Cell Mass in Severely Burned Patients

Time Postburn in Hours	Mean Red Cell Mass (ml/kg)
0–12	31
13–24	25
25–36	24
37–48	22
49–60	20
61–72	17
73–84	15
85–96	16

sistent with an early postburn consumption and subsequent increased production[32] (Table 36-3). Secondary decreases in clotting factors occur in association with supervening sepsis and other complications inducing intravascular coagulation.

Alterations in central nervous system function also assume a biphasic pattern. In the early postburn period, mild agitation may accompany either hypovolemia or hypoxemia but, if hypotension is severe or prolonged, obtundation may occur. Following resuscitation, sensory deprivation, electrolyte and metabolic imbalances, and sepsis exert variable effects upon central nervous system function with obtundation commonly associated with severe abnormalities. Neural and endocrine regulatory mechanisms sited in the hypothalmus are also altered, with the degree of disturbance showing a general relationship to the extent of burn.[15]

The severity of the local effects of thermal injury is determined by both the temperature to which the tissues are exposed and the duration of exposure. Sufficient thermal energy will cause protein coagulation and cell death, as is characteristically seen in areas of full-thickness burn.[86] The vessels in such tissue are thrombosed and the nerves coagulated. Adjacent to the frankly nonviable tissue is a variable volume of tissue in which cells are injured and blood flow reduced.[55] The amount of this tissue that ultimately survives is dependent upon prompt and adequate resuscitation to restore blood flow, protection of exposed tissue from desiccation, and prevention of infection.

Edema forms in the dead and injured tissue with the edema volume reaching its maximum in the second postburn day (Fig. 36-2). Following this, with proper fluid management, it recedes as evaporative water loss from the wound surface and renal excretion reduce the resuscitation-induced water and salt loading.

TABLE 36-3. Selected Coagulation Factor Changes in Burn Patients

	Maximum Change	Time Postburn in Days
Platelets	608,000/ml	10–20
Fibrinogen	1044 mg/dl	6–9
Factor V	150–400% of control	1–120
Factor VIII	80 times normal	1–49

The administration of excessive volumes of resuscitation fluid may exaggerate edema formation and further compromise the local blood supply and delivery of nutrients.[129] During the resuscitation period copious serous drainage occurs from the burn wound surface[9] and following resuscitation extensive evaporative water and mineral loss can occur from the burn surface, depending upon the method of wound care employed and the environmental conditions. The avascularity of a full-thickness burn renders it susceptible to infection by the organisms that invariably colonize its surface. Moreover, pharmacologically active materials liberated from the injured tissue or by resident microorganisms may exert deleterious effects upon various organ systems, such as the production of suppressor cells by the immune system and injury to the pulmonary capillary bed related to activation of complement.[95,142]

FLUID RESUSCITATION

The fluid loss due to burn injury was first appreciated and repletion thereof attempted by oral administration of fluids in the 19th century.[22] Intravenous infusions of saline solution were utilized by Parascondolo[99] of Naples in 1901 and Haldore Sneve[137] in the United States in 1905. It remained for Underhill[143] to demonstrate the plasmalike composition of burn blister fluid in 1930. Harkins and Evans et al. subsequently quantified the blood volume changes that occurred following burn injury.[42,47] Those studies verified the relationship between the magnitude of blood and plasma volume losses and the extent of burn injury and led directly to the development of formulas by which the fluid needs of a burn patient could be estimated.

The increase in capillary permeability caused by burn injury is greatest in the immediate postburn period and the resulting decrease in blood and plasma volume is most rapid at that time.[124] If a patient with an extensive burn is untreated, the hypovolemia that occurs can

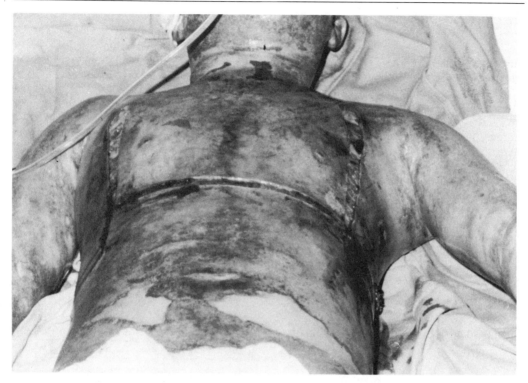

FIG. 36-2 The edema that forms in burn-injured tissue is at a maximum during the second 24 hours. Note distortion of left axillary anatomy by swelling. Limitation of chest wall motion due to the third-degree burn and underlying edema necessitated performance of bilateral anterior axillary line and costal margin escharotomies in this patient.

be sufficient to produce shock and organ failure, most commonly acute renal failure. A secure intravenous pathway must therefore be promptly established. Ideally a large-caliber cannula should be placed in an appropriately sized peripheral vein underlying unburned skin. If such a site is not available, the cannula can be placed in a high flow central vein or in a peripheral vein underlying burned skin. Resuscitation is begun by infusing a physiologic electrolyte solution at a rate of 300 to 500 ml/hr and subsequently modified according to the patient's needs as calculated by the resuscitation formula of choice.

Since the resuscitation fluid needs of the burn patient are proportional to the severity of the injury, the percentage of the body surface burned should be estimated using any of several commonly available burn diagrams or the Rule of Nines, which permits assessment of the extent of involvement of various body parts. The Rule of Nines expresses the fact that in the adult the surface area of various body parts represents 9 percent or a multiple of 9 percent of the total body surface: head and neck 9 percent, each upper extremity 9 percent, each lower extremity 18 percent, anterior trunk 18 percent, posterior trunk 18 percent, and the perineum and genitalia 1 percent. Fluid needs are also related to body size and it is necessary to determine the patient's preinjury weight in order to calculate resuscitation fluid requirements. The resuscitation fluid requirements are then calculated on the basis of extent of burn and body weight using the fluid formula of choice. Following estimation of fluid needs, the fluid infusion rate is adjusted so that one-half of the estimated volume will be administered in the first 8 hours postburn, the period when intravascular volume decreases most rapidly. The remaining half of the estimated volume is scheduled for administration over the subsequent 16 hours of the first postburn day. The adequacy of resuscitation should be monitored as described below and the volume of fluid infused adjusted according to the patient's response to injury and treatment.

Functional capillary integrity is largely restored by the second postburn day and capillary permeability appears to return towards normal during the latter half of the first postburn day. Recent studies indicate that even though transcapillary albumin loss in the area of injury remains elevated for several days, increased return of extravasated protein reestablishes transvascular albumin equilibrium between 24 and 48 hours postburn.[21] As a result of these changes, the amount of fluid required per unit time to maintain blood volume in the second 24 hours postburn is less than in the first 24 hours postburn, and colloid-containing fluids can then be utilized to keep volume load-

ing at a minimum. These changes in transcapillary fluid movement are recognized by the formulas' recommendations for estimating lesser fluid needs for the second 24 hours postburn.

Several formulas have been advocated for estimating the fluid needs of burn patients (Table 36-4).[14,31,42,82,111,128] Although the composition and amount of fluids recommended by the various formulae vary markedly, each formula has been reported to be effective in resuscitating large numbers of burn patients. The clinical success of the various formulas is indicative of the physiologic elasticity of the majority of burn patients and speaks against unique specificity or precision of any one formula in preventing or correcting blood volume deficits in burn patients as a group.

Resuscitation, guided by the Brooke formula, permits a modest (approximately 20 percent) decrease in blood and plasma volume,

TABLE 36-4. Commonly Used Formulas for Estimating Fluid Needs of Adult Burn Patients

Formula	Crystalloid Fluid	Colloid Fluid	Glucose in Water
First 24 Hours			
"Burn budget" of Cope and Moore	Lactated Ringer's: 1000–4000 ml 0.5 Normal saline: 1,200 ml	7.5% of body weight	1,500–5,000 ml
Evans	Normal saline: 1.0 ml/kg/% burn	1.0 ml/kg/% burn	2,000 ml
Brooke	Lactated Ringer's: 1.5 ml/kg/% burn	0.5 ml/kg/% burn	2,000 ml
Parkland	Lactated Ringer's: 4 ml/kg/% burn		
"Hypertonic saline" (250 mEq Na/L)	Volume to maintain urine output of 30 ml/hr		
Modified Brooke	Lactated Ringer's: 2 ml/kg/% burn[a]		
Second 24 Hours			
"Burn budget" of Cope and Moore	Lactated Ringer's: 1,000–4,000 ml 0.5 Normal saline: 1,200 ml	2.5% of body weight	1,500–5,000 ml
Evans	½ of first 24 hour requirement	½ of first 24 hour requirement	2,000 ml
Brooke	½ to ¾ of first 24 hour requirement	½ to ¾ of first 24 hour requirement	2,000 ml
Parkland		20% to 60% of calculated plasma volume	To maintain adequate urinary output
"Hypertonic saline"	Up to 3,500 ml of ⅓ isotonic salt solution		
Modified Brooke		0.3 to 0.5 ml/kg/% burn[b]	To maintain adequate urinary output

[a] 3 ml/kg/% burn in pediatric age group.
[b] Albumin diluted to physiologic concentration in normal saline.

defends against further loss, and restores plasma volume to predicted normal levels by the end of the second postburn day. Cardiac output, which is initially depressed, increases as resuscitation proceeds even during a time of modest progressive decrease in blood and plasma volume. The cardiac output returns to predicted normal levels between the 12th and 18th postburn hours and rises to supranormal levels, two to two and one half times predicted normal, as plasma volume returns toward normal during the second 24 hours postburn[124] (Fig. 36-3). The majority of formulas recommend a total volume of crystalloid and colloid containing fluids of approximately 2 ml/kg body weight/percent burn for the first 24 hours. The one formula that recommends a total volume dose of 4 ml/kg body weight/percent burn was originally proposed for use in those patients, usually older and with extensive burns, who did not respond to resuscitation in the anticipated manner.[14] The proponents of that formula considered a circulating myocardial depressant factor to be responsible for the impaired cardiac response to fluid infusion in such patients but, as noted earlier, in one group of patients with depressed cardiac output during the initial 24 hours postburn, the myocardium was hyperdynamic.[44]

The composition of the resuscitation fluids in the first 24 hours appears to be less important than in the second 24 hours postburn. As-sessment of transcapillary fluid dynamics in the first 24 hours postburn indicates that colloid-containing fluids are retained within the circulation to no greater extent than an equal volume of crystalloid fluid.[123] Other studies have indicated that capillary integrity is progressively restored during the first postburn day[19] and that colloid-containing fluids exert a greater augmentative effect on intravascular volume during the latter half of the first 24 hours postburn. Whatever formula is used to estimate resuscitation needs, one must keep in mind that it is merely a first approximation of fluid needs. The actual volume administered should be varied in accordance with the individual patient's response, and fluid should be added or withheld as necessary.

Even with the infusion of amounts of resuscitation fluid far in excess of formula estimates, acute pulmonary edema is infrequent in the first 48 hours postburn in patients with uncomplicated burns. Laboratory studies indicate that the immediate postburn elevation of pulmonary vascular resistance is greater and persists longer than elevation of peripheral vascular resistance and appears to minimize loss of fluid through the pulmonary capillary[6] (Table 36-5). When the pulmonary vascular status returns towards normal and the edema in the areas of injury is resorbed, the consequences of excessive volume infusion may be realized and pulmonary edema is most commonly ob-

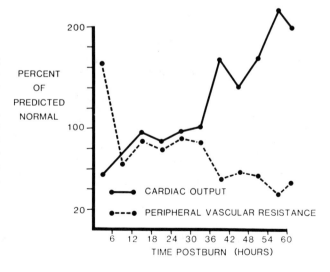

FIG. 36-3 Changes in cardiac output and peripheral resistance in burn patients during resuscitation. Cardiac output, which is depressed on admission, increases as soon as resuscitation is begun, returns to predicted normal in the latter half of the first postburn day, and rises to supranormal hypermetabolic levels as plasma volume returns to predicted normal levels in the second 24 hours postburn. Note reciprocal movement of peripheral vascular resistance.

PERCENT OF PREDICTED NORMAL

CARDIAC OUTPUT
PERIPHERAL VASCULAR RESISTANCE

TIME POSTBURN (HOURS)

TABLE 36-5.   Effect of Burn Injury on Vascular Resistance in Canine Model of 40–45 Percent Burn

	Maximum Increase (% of Preburn Value)	Time of Return to Preburn Value in Hours
Mean systemic vascular resistance	181	18–24
Mean pulmonary vascular resistance	211	42

served in such patients on the third to sixth postburn days. The current predominant use of crystalloid fluids for volume replacement in the first 24 hours postburn has been implicated as a significant etiologic factor in the development of pulmonary edema. However, recent studies by Goodwin et al. as well as others have indicated that lung water is little changed during the first 24 hours postburn and is little influenced by plasma colloid oncotic pressure.[44,61,141] Following resuscitation, in uncomplicated burn patients, extravascular lung water increases modestly in concert with pulmonary capillary blood flow as the edema fluid is reprocessed through the circulation and excreted. Moreover, in a controlled randomized comparison, those patients who received only crystalloid-containing fluids in the first 24 hours showed no change in lung water during the first 7 postburn days, while those who received resuscitation fluids containing colloids in the first 24 hours showed a progressive rise in extravascular lung water during that period (Table 36-6). The patients in the group receiving colloid in the first 24 hours had a greater incidence of pulmonary edema evident radiographically and had a higher mortality.

TABLE 36-6.   Lung Water Changes Following Burn Injury Related to Composition of Resuscitation Fluid

Postburn Day	Lung Water (ml/ml)[b]	
	Crystalloid Only in First 24 Hours[a]	Colloid and Crystalloid in First 24 Hours[a]
0.5	0.13 ± 0.005	0.13 ± 0.007
1.0	0.123 ± 0.004	0.125 ± 0.006
2.0	0.138 ± 0.007	0.123 ± 0.006
3.0	0.140 ± 0.007	0.145 ± 0.009
5.0	0.149 ± 0.006	0.167 ± 0.011
7.0	0.137 ± 0.011	0.173 ± 0.015

[a] Mean ± Standard error of the mean.
[b] ml/ml, alveolar volume.

Several investigators have proposed the use of hypertonic saline solutions to minimize fluid loading during resuscitation of those patients who can be classified as being volume-sensitive: the very young, the very old, and those with pre-existing cardiopulmonary disease.[25,82] The advocates of hypertonic resuscitation have claimed that such fluids reduce the need for escharotomy and the occurrence of ileus and induce higher urinary outputs and a lesser fractional retention of the administered sodium dose. Laboratory studies of hypertonic resuscitation have verified a natriuresis and a mild kaliuresis but have failed to confirm a significant diuretic effect of hypertonic fluids.[91] Studies in humans have indicated that in patients given hypertonic salt solutions, elevation of the serum sodium concentration above 165 mEq/L resulted in a marked drop of urinary output necessitating infusion of more dilute solutions to continue resuscitation.[134] Additionally, the plasma volume augmentative effect of hypertonic fluids implies transfer of intracellular volume to the extracellular compartment and cellular dehydration in excess of 15 percent has been associated with impairment of cell function. These limits of serum sodium elevation and cell dehydration appear to define the physiologic tolerance to hypertonic resuscitation. Other studies indicate that 1 mEq of sodium has the restorative effect upon cardiac output equivalent to that of 13 ml salt-free volume.[90] Substitution of salt dose for volume dose can be made in that ratio in those patients with limited cardiopulmonary reserve susceptible to volume overload. Even in those patients, postresuscitation fluid management must be meticulous since the patient will perceive thirst and, if permitted, will avidly imbibe water and produce delayed-onset edema.

Following resuscitation, the burn patient's physiologic milieu is such that electrolyte-free water loss is accelerated and salt excretion is retarded. Evaporative water loss from the burn wound is prodigious and elevated circulating levels of renin, angiotensin, and aldosterone limit renal salt excretion. These factors promote the development of hypernatremia and limit the ability of the burn patient to offload the salt administered during resuscitation.[145] This physiologic state complicates the postresuscitation fluid management of patients who have received hypertonic fluids. Hypertonic fluids appear to have little applicability to the resuscitation of the majority of even extensively burned patients and their use is best limited to those patients judged to have limited cardiopulmonary reserve.

A number of physiologic indices are useful in monitoring the burn patient's response to resuscitation. The hourly urinary output is the most readily available and generally reliable index of resuscitation adequacy. An indwelling urethral catheter should be placed and the resuscitation fluids infused to obtain 30 to 50 ml urine/hr in the adult (1 ml/kg/hr in patients weighing less than 30 kg). Urinary output that falls below or exceeds those limits by more than one third mandates appropriate adjustment of the fluid infusion rate. A need for more than twice the estimated resuscitation volume that persists into the latter half of the first postburn day is an indication for the administration of colloid-containing fluid to reduce volume needs. In such patients, placement of a Swan-Ganz catheter to measure pulmonary capillary wedge pressure is indicated to permit assessment of intravascular volume status and myocardial function. An inotropic agent can be utilized to improve myocardial function in those patients who have received more than estimated fluid needs and in whom no significant volume deficit exists.[1] In such patients, persistent oliguria in association with a pulmonary capillary wedge pressure within or above the physiologic range can be used as an indication for administration of an inotropic agent such as dopamine.

Oliguria is commonly associated with elevation of systemic vascular resistance and reduction in cardiac output, both of which customarily respond to increased fluid administration. Infrequently, elevation of systemic vascular resistance may persist or occur secondarily in patients who have even received

fluids in excess of estimated needs. In such patients, the administration of hydralazine in a dosage of 0.5 mg/kg has reduced systemic vascular resistance, resulting in an increase in cardiac output and hourly urinary output[124] (Table 36-7). The importance of adequate fluid loading prior to the initiation of such treatment is indicated by the further depression of cardiac output that occurred in hydralazine-treated patients who had received inadequate volume replacement.

In the second 24 hours, colloid-containing fluids (we prefer albumin diluted to plasma equivalency in saline) are commonly utilized to keep both volume and salt loading at a minimum. Electrolyte-free water is also administered to maintain an adequate urinary output. During this second 24 hours, volume loading can be further minimized by planned 50 percent reduction of the fluid infusion rate. Maintenance of hourly output at desired levels for 3 hours thereafter can be followed by further stepwise reduction of fluid administration.

The patient's general condition should be assessed on a regularly scheduled basis. Restlessness and anxiety are early signs of hypoxemia and hypovolemia and their appearance should prompt the appropriate therapeutic response. Monitoring of the blood pressure by sphygmomanometric technique can be misleading, particularly in a burned limb that is the site of progressive edema formation. As edema forms, the auditory signal may be progressively attenuated and lead the unwary to infuse more fluid, which results in even greater edema formation and further impairment of the ability to assess the blood pressure accurately. This sequence of events can lead to massive

TABLE 36-7. Effect of Hydralazine 0.5 mg/kg on Hemodynamic Indices in Five Burn Patients with Persistent Depression of Cardiac Output and Elevation of Peripheral Resistance

	Fraction of Predicted Normal (Mean Values)	
	Before Hydralazine	After Hydralazine
Peripheral resistance	0.98	0.52
Cardiac output	0.77	1.10
Mean blood pressure	0.82	0.61

fluid overload. The marked elevation of vasoactive humoral factors, such as the catecholamines, makes even intra-arterial monitoring of the blood pressure unreliable in patients with massive burns. If repeated arterial blood sampling is deemed necessary, for example, in burn patients with severe inhalation injury, an artery in the forearm should be cannulated to reduce the risk of complications related to repetitive arterial puncture. This is an important consideration in the very young and the elderly, in some of whom repeated arterial sampling at the groin level has been associated with femoral artery thrombosis and limb ischemia.

Other indices of the physiologic status of the burn patient that should be monitored on a scheduled basis include serum chemical values and arterial blood gases, which should be measured at least daily during resuscitation and the postresuscitation diuretic phase and as indicated thereafter. The electrocardiogram should be monitored in those patients with pre-existing cardiovascular disease and, as described below, in patients with high-voltage electric injury. A chest radiograph should be obtained daily for the first 5 to 7 days postburn and thereafter as indicated by the patient's respiratory status.

MONITORING AND MAINTENANCE OF THE PERIPHERAL CIRCULATION

Circumferential third-degree burns of an extremity may compromise the blood supply of underlying or distal unburned tissue. As edema forms beneath an unyielding eschar, tissue pressure progressively increases. When tissue pressure exceeds venous pressure, transcapillary extravasation of fluid increases further. As tissue pressure approaches arteriolar pressure, nutrient blood flow of unburned tissue is compromised and tissue hypoxia may result in cell death. As a general rule, even extensive partial-thickness burns of a limb do not produce vascular impairment but occasionally marked edema formation, as a result of excessive administration of resuscitation fluid to a patient with circumferential deep dermal burns, may impair tissue blood flow. The accumulation of edema in a burned limb can be minimized and the need for escharotomy reduced by continual elevation of the limb and active exercise of the extremity for 5 minutes every hour.[132]

The clinical signs of circulatory compromise in a burned limb include cyanosis of distal unburned skin (swelling and coolness, normal accompaniments of thermal injury, are not signs of circulatory embarrassment), impaired capillary refilling, and neurologic abnormalities, particularly progressive paresthesias and relentless deep tissue pain. All of the clinical signs are imprecise indices of circulatory compromise in the burn patient. Assessment of blood flow using the Doppler ultrasound flowmeter is the most reliable means to confirm that the patient requires an escharotomy to maintain or restore blood flow to unburned tissues.[89] The ultrasound probe is used to detect pulsatile flow in the distal palmar arch vessels in the upper limb and the posterior tibial artery in the lower limb. The probe can also be used to assess flow in individual digital vessels of fingers or toes. Absence of pulsatile flow in the examined vessel or progressive diminution of the auditory signal in sequential examinations is an indication for escharotomy.

Escharotomy is performed as a bedside procedure that requires neither general nor local anesthesia since the incisions are placed in insensate full-thickness burn.[114] A scalpel is used to incise the eschar in the midlateral or midmedial line of the limb with the excision extending from the distal to the proximal limit of the encircling burn. The escharotomy incision should extend only through the eschar and the immediately underlying superficial fascia. An incision of that depth will permit the cut edges of the eschar to separate and will avoid the bleeding that commonly occurs if the escharotomy is unnecessarily extended more deeply into unburned subcutaneous tissues. The bleeding associated with a properly performed escharotomy can be controlled by electrocautery or brief application of a pressure dressing. In an extensively burned limb, the incisions must be carried across involved joints, sites where the vessels and nerves are most easily compressed by subeschar edema. In the regions of the knee and elbow, care must be taken to avoid injury to the peroneal or ulnar nerves, respectively, by inappropriately deep or misplaced incisions.

Edema beneath an encircling truncal burn may, in similar fashion, restrict the ventilatory excursion of the thoracic cage. The patient with such an injury may complain of anxiety and shortness of breath and have evidence of a restrictive ventilatory defect.[103] Chest wall escharotomies should be placed in the anterior axillary lines extending from the clavicles to the costal margins. If the full-thickness burn involves the anterior abdominal wall to significant degree, the anterior axillary line escharotomies should be connected inferiorly by an escharotomy that follows the contour of the costal margin (Fig. 36-2). If digital escharotomies are required, those incisions are placed in the midlateral line of the involved digit; take care to avoid the neurovascular bundles. Circumferential full-thickness burns of the neck and of the penis may necessitate placement of escharotomy incisions in the midlateral lines of the neck or the middorsal line of the penis.

In the vast majority of patients with circumferential limb burns, escharotomy will suffice to restore blood flow to unburned tissues. But in patients in whom edema occurs in tissues below the investing fascia (patients with high-voltage electric injury, or associated mechanical trauma, and those with direct thermal injury of subfascial tissue) fasciotomy may be required. Stony hardness to palpation of a fascial compartment underlying a limb burn wound is an indication for fasciotomy. In the lower limb, the anterior tibial compartment is most frequently involved. Signs of ischemia of those tissues include impaired sensation over the dorsal aspect of the first plantar web space and foot drop, but the latter sign occurs relatively late and customarily signifies necrosis of the tibialis anterior.[5] Needle manometers, wick catheters, slit catheters, and washout of injected [133]xenon have all been used to monitor the status of muscle blood flow in a variety of patients including those with burns.[29] The increase in sensitivity of such techniques (compromised in hypovolemic hypotensive patients)

compared to noninvasive methodology does not offset the risk of microbial seeding of deep tissues associated with the need to traverse the invariably contaminated burn wound.

Fasciotomy should be performed in the operating room with the patient under general anesthesia. Separate incisions are used to gain access to specific fascial compartments or a partial fibulectomy is formed to gain access to all fascial compartments of the calf. The high incidence of ischemic necrosis of the intrinsic muscles of the hand in patients with full-thickness burns of both the palm and dorsum justifies the performance of interosseous fasciotomies in such patients.[133] The wounds produced by either escharotomy or fasciotomy should be covered at all times by a generous application of the topical antimicrobial agent used on the burn wound to prevent infection of the exposed unburned tissues.

MANAGEMENT OF GASTROINTESTINAL CHANGES

The gastrointestinal tract is also involved in the systemic response to burn injury. The ileus that occurs immediately postburn in virtually all patients with burns of more than 25 percent of the total body surface precludes oral intake and necessitates nasogastric intubation to prevent emesis and aspiration.[59] Gastrointestinal motility commonly returns following resuscitation when hemodynamic stability has been restored and tissue edema is reabsorbed. At that time, the nasogastric tube can be removed and the enteral administration of fluids and food begun. Specific burn-related changes in the upper gastrointestinal tract have also been noted. Gastric and duodenal mucosal erosions, which appear to be related to mucosal ischemia, have been observed as early as 5 hours postburn.[35] Such lesions are rare in patients with burns of less than 30 percent of the body surface and almost universal in patients with burns of more than 50 percent of the total body surface.[37] Progression of these early lesions to frank ulceration is related to gastric acid production, and although disruption of the gastric mucosal barrier has not been correlated with the initial gastritic and duodenitic changes, it has been associated with progression of the mucosal disease[36,76] (Table 36-8).

Intragastric administration of antacid solutions or the administration of the H_2 histamine receptor antagonist cimetidine prevents the progression of the mucosal disease and has essentially eliminated perforation and hemorrhage as life-threatening complications of stress ulcers in burn patients.[121] Sufficient antacids should be instilled every hour or 2 hours to maintain the pH of the gastric contents above 5.0 as assessed by hourly monitoring. Alternatively, 400 mg cimetidine can be administered intravenously every 4 hours until gastrointestinal motility is restored, following which the dosage is changed to 300 mg by the oral route every 4 to 6 hours until the burns have healed or have been closed by grafting. A comparison of antacid therapy and H_2 receptor antagonist therapy has revealed equal effectiveness of the two treatments in terms of preventing hemorrhage and perforation, although cimetidine was associated with more complete gastroduodenal mucosal healing at 10 days postburn.[77] Advantages of the H_2 histamine receptor antagonist include its availability for parenteral use and its freedom from the risk of medication-induced bezoar formation, which may occur with large-volume antacid therapy. In any patient in whom either antacid or cimetidine prophylaxis fails to control intragastric pH, combined treatment should be used to prevent progression of mucosal damage.

TABLE 36-8. Postburn Gastroduodenal Disease Related to Gastric Acid Production

	Gastric Acid Output mEq/hr; Mean ± Standard Deviation
Normal stomach and duodenum (n = 3)	1.42 ± 0.48
Gastric lesions only (n = 14)	2.58 ± 3.31
Gastric and duodenal lesions (n = 17)	5.01 ± 2.09
Major complications (n = 9)	5.37 ± 2.53
Hemorrhage (n = 8)	5.22 ± 2.67
Perforation (n = 1)	6.56

INHALATION INJURY

Respiratory insufficiency in the immediate postburn period is most commonly due to inhalation injury, which can be noninflammatory due to carbon monoxide poisoning or inflammatory due to the inhalation of smoke or other irritative products of incomplete combustion. Both forms of inhalation injury occur most commonly in patients burned in a closed space, particularly those patients with mental obtundation due to either intoxication or mechanical trauma.[40] Inhalation injury may also be present in patients burned outdoors by ignited petroleum products.

Since the clinical signs of carbon monoxide poisoning are imprecise, nonspecific treatment by administration of 100 percent oxygen using a securely fitting nonrebreathing mask should be begun by the first responder for any patient suspected of having this form of inhalation injury. In the hospital setting, a blood sample should be obtained to determine the carboxyhemoglobin level and the necessary ventilatory support should be provided. Carbon monoxide impairs tissue oxygenation by avidly binding to hemoglobin and reducing its oxygen-carrying capacity, by shifting the oxygen–hemoglobin dissociation curve to the left, and by binding to the terminal cytochrome oxidase. The administration of 100 percent oxygen accelerates the dissociation of carbon monoxide from hemoglobin so that the carboxyhemoglobin level is reduced by 50 percent in less than 1 hour compared to almost 4 hours using room air.[157] Such treatment should be continued until carboxyhemoglobin levels are below 20 percent.[155] Hyperbaric oxygen treatment has been advocated for the treatment of severe carbon monoxide poisoning, but even though carboxyhemoglobin levels were rapidly reduced survival appeared to be little influenced by such treatment.[97] A secondary rise in carboxyhemoglobin levels reflecting release from peripheral tissues has been described following hyperbaric oxygen treatment (see Chapter 37).

The inflammatory form of inhalation injury may involve all of the tracheobronchial tree or segments thereof. The distribution of such chemically induced changes is related to the size of the aerosol particles carrying the irritative materials, while the severity of the inflammatory reaction is related to the duration of exposure as well as the type and concentration of the irritative agents.[17] Direct thermal injury of the airway is rare as a clinical problem because of the low heat-carrying capacity of air but the inhalation of steam, which has a much greater heat content, can damage the upper airway and glottic structures. Instillation of hot liquids into the oropharynx can also cause direct thermal injury of the oropharynx.

The clinical signs of inhalation injury are quite variable and include wheezing, dyspnea, bronchorrhea, hoarseness, and brassy coughing.[40] The most reliable clinical sign of inhalation injury is the production of carbonaceous sputum but the associated bronchorrhea and coughing may rapidly clear the airway and that sign may be evident for only a few hours following injury. Singeing of the nasal vibrissae may occur whenever the face is burned and is not a reliable index of inhalation injury. Inflammatory change evident on direct examination of the oropharynx is a much more reliable index of the presence of inhalation injury in the more distal portions of the airway.

The clinical signs of inhalation injury, which appear as the inflammatory changes in the airway develop and increase in severity, are commonly absent immediately after burning and are usually first evident on the second or third postinjury day. Reliance on clinical signs may thus result in a delay in diagnosis and treatment of inhalation injury. This delay can be avoided by the use of three diagnostic modalities that facilitate early diagnosis: endoscopic examination, ventilation–perfusion scintiphotography, and pulmonary function testing.

Direct examination of the airway (following application of a topical anesthetic) using the fiberoptic bronchoscope permits identification of inflammatory changes in both the supraglottic and infraglottic airway.[50] Edema and erythema of the airway mucosa as well as mucosal erosions and the presence of carbonaceous material are all signs of inhalation injury that can be identified at the time of endoscopic examination. An appropriately sized endotracheal tube should be placed over the endoscope before one begins the examination. If obstruction at the glottic level appears imminent, the endotracheal tube should be placed and the examination of the lower airway carried out by passing the endoscope through the endotracheal tube, which is left in place following examination. In patients with lesser edema of the glottic structures, the need for intubation may be reduced by the insufflation, every 2 to 4 hours, of an aerosol of 0.5 ml 2.25 percent racemic epinephrine diluted to 2 ml in normal saline. Endoscopic examination can result in a falsely positive assessment in patients with pre-existing bronchitis and a falsely negative assessment when the endoscopic examination is carried out in a hypotensive patient in whom the bronchial circulation is so reduced that the inflammatory changes are inapparent. A falsely negative assessment can also occur when the aerosol particles containing the irritative material are so small that the principal site of deposition is in the terminal bronchioles and alveoli and little of the aerosol is deposited in the larger airways.

^{133}Xenon ventilation–perfusion scans are also effective in identifying inhalation injury, particularly that principally involving the distal airway.[92] Scintiphotography is carried out following the injection of 10 μCi radioactive gas into a peripheral vein. The gas should be equally distributed throughout the lungs and rapidly cleared. Positive findings include a clearing pattern showing unequal density of radioactivity and retention of the radioactive gas within the parenchyma beyond 90 seconds following injection. Falsely positive determinations (8 percent of scans) can result from associated mechanical trauma such as lung contusion and pre-existing bronchitis. Falsely negative determinations (5 percent of scans) can occur when the test is performed after the third day postburn, when the hyperventilation characteristic of postburn hypermetabolism has become established.

A variety of pulmonary function tests are also helpful in identifying patients with inhalation injury.[101] Arterial oxygen tension, peak flow, and flow at various fractions of vital capacity are all significantly decreased in patients with inhalation injury compared to burn patients without inhalation injury. Conversely, pulmonary resistance, the ventilation–perfusion gradient, and the percent rise of nitrogen washout slope are all significantly elevated in patients with inhalation injury (Table 36-9). The maximum expiratory flow volume loop is the most useful pulmonary function test, since it allows one to verify depression of peak flow rate and, when performed serially, permits assessment of the effectiveness of pharmacologic interventions and provides prognostic information. The hyperventilation characteristic of postburn hypermetabolism may confound interpretation of pulmonary function testing as may lack of cooperation in an obtunded, disoriented, or agitated patient. The accuracy of the three diagnostic modalities in identifying inhalation injury is 91 percent for pulmonary function testing alone, 87 percent for [133]xenon scintiphotography alone, and 86 percent for endoscopic examination alone. In combination, all three modalities enable one to diagnose inhalation injury with 96 percent accuracy, with the residual 4 percent error accounted for by falsely positive assessments.[2]

The treatment of respiratory insufficiency due to inhalation injury takes the form of a graduated therapeutic response keyed to the severity of pulmonary insufficiency. In patients with mild disease, coughing is encouraged, warm humidified oxygen is administered, and incentive spirometry is employed on a scheduled basis. Endotracheal toilet is carried out in all patients with inhalation injury. Catheter aspiration of the airway is generally adequate to clear bronchorrhea and moderate amounts of particulate debris. In patients with extensive mucosal sloughing, particularly those in whom large cylindrical bronchial casts form, bronchoscopy using the rigid bronchoscope may be required to clear the airway on a daily or even more frequent basis. In patients with significant bronchospasm, the administration of bronchodilators such as Isuprel may improve ventilation. Endotracheal intubation may be re-quired to prevent obstruction due to upper airway edema or to provide prolonged access to the lower tracheobronchial tree in patients with severe lower airway injury. The indications for mechanical ventilation are the same in burn patients with inhalation injury as in other patients. High levels of minute ventilation may be needed to meet the elevated peripheral oxygen needs of the hypermetabolic burn patient.

Upper airway sequelae (stenosis and granuloma formation) in burn patients requiring endotracheal intubation are directly related to duration of intubation, presence of a tracheal stoma, and severity of pulmonary injury. Accordingly, a nasotracheal tube is the preferred initial route of access to the tracheobronchial tree in burn patients. Tracheostomy can be performed later to reduce nasopharyngeal and laryngeal trauma and the risk of sinusitis and to facilitate lower airway toilet in those patients in whom access to the lower airway will be required for more than 3 weeks. Follow-up fiberoptic bronchoscopy should be carried out to document sequelae of airway injury in any patient in whom intubation was necessary for more than 10 days. Xeroradiographic examination is useful in assessing the severity of compromise in those patients with tracheal stenosis.[74] To minimize the duration of endotracheal intubation, frequent scheduled assessment of pulmonary function, such as, inspiratory force, vital capacity, and dead space/tidal volume ratio instituted at the time of intubation, should be used to match the patient's pulmonary status to the level of ventilator support and thus expedite removal of the endotracheal tube.

Systemic administration of steroids as a prophylactic measure has been shown to have no significant effect on the incidence of pul-

TABLE 36-9. Pulmonary Function Tests Altered by Inhalation Injury

	Burn Patients with Inhalation Injury (n = 7)	Burn Patients without Inhalation Injury (n = 8)
Resistance (cmH_2O/L/sec)	4.85	3.05
Ventilation perfusion gradient (mmHg)	37.4	27.2
Nitrogen washout slope (% rise)	3.1	1.6
Arterial PO_2 (mmHg)	69.4	85.5
Peak flow (% of predicted)	61.9	99.1
Flow at 75% of vital capacity (% of predicted)	47.7	120.1

monary complications, mortality within the first 10 days postburn, or overall mortality[66] and actually to increase the risk of septic complications.[88] Even so, systemic steroids may be used to control the intractable bronchospasm that occurs in a few patients with inhalation injury. Prophylactic systemic antibiotics appear to have little beneficial effect. Even aerosolized gentamicin administered prophylactically to a group of burn patients three times a day had no effect on the incidence of pulmonary infiltrates, requirement for mechanical ventilation, occurrence of sepsis, time of death, occurrence of pulmonary complications as a cause of death, or overall mortality as compared to those receiving placebo treatment.[66] Antibiotics are reserved for the treatment of pulmonary infections, such as suppurative tracheobronchitis or pneumonia, documented by radiographic changes and recovery of specific organisms from the endobronchial secretions.

Pulmonary edema infrequently occurs in burn patients during the resuscitation period and is usually a reflection of cardiac insufficiency. In such patients, a Swan-Ganz catheter should be inserted with subsequent adjustment of fluid therapy, diuretic therapy, and inotropic support guided by measurements of pulmonary capillary wedge pressure and cardiac output. Later in the postburn period, pulmonary edema may occur as a result of failure to reduce postoperative fluid administration following the intraoperative subcutaneous infiltration of large volumes of saline to improve graft harvest or following extensive grafting that markedly reduces evaporative water loss. Other pulmonary and chest wall complications, such as lung contusion, rib fractures, pneumothorax, pulmonary embolus, aspiration, and atelectasis, are treated as in other surgical patients.[117]

Hyperventilation is a characteristic of the hypermetabolic response to injury in patients with burns involving more than 40 percent of the body surface.[116] This hyperventilation can be accentuated by the use of mafenide acetate as the topical antimicrobial applied to the burn wounds. The ventilatory response to mafenide acetate is a result of carbonic anhydrase inhibition, which increases the arteriolar–alveolar carbon dioxide gradient and also causes renal bicarbonate wasting.[102] The renal effects of carbonic anhydrase inhibition appear to be time-limited and seldom persist for more than 10 days. In the majority of patients the exaggeration of postinjury hyperventilation associated with mafenide acetate treatment is tolerated. If pulmonary complications, such as pneumonia, supervene, it may be necessary to administer sodium bicarbonate and reduce the frequency or even discontinue the application of mafenide acetate burn cream and use another topical antimicrobial.

PARTICULAR BURNS

Chemical Burns

The severity of tissue injury due to chemical agents is related to the concentration and amount of the chemical in contact with the tissue and the duration of contact. Consequently, treatment of the burn wound of patients with chemical injuries takes immediate priority. Copious water lavage of the involved areas should be promptly instituted and all clothing removed (Fig. 36-4). Time should not be wasted searching for a specific neutralizing agent, the use of which may only produce an exothermic reaction and further damage tissue. Irrigation of the wound should be continued until all of the offending agent has been removed. Skin burned by strong acids may be misinterpreted as an area of suntan because of its bronzed appearance and soft leatherlike texture. Failure to recognize such an area as a burn wound can result in underestimation of the fluid needs of such a patient and the development of oliguria during resuscitation.

Some treatment modifications may be necessary for burns caused by specific chemical agents. Alkali powders, such as lime, should be quickly brushed from the skin before water lavage is begun. Following initial water lavage, phenol burns should be washed with a solvent such as polyethylene glycol, propylene glycol,

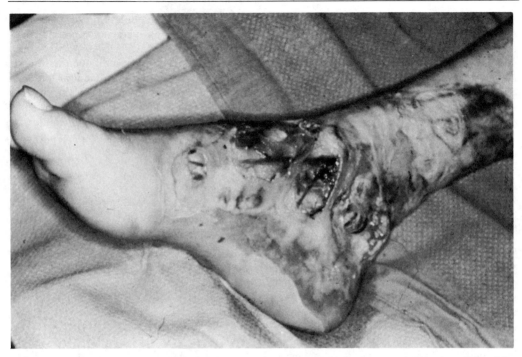

FIG. 36-4 Failure to remove the shoes of this patient and to lavage the area resulted in deep tissue injury by continued contact with concentrated alkali solution. Note the thrombosed vessels and the discoloration and edema of the exposed extensor tendons at midfoot level.

or glycerol to remove residual phenol, which is only minimally soluble in water.[100] In patients with extensive burns due to phenol, systemic toxicity may produce hypothermia that requires but responds poorly to external warming. As treatment for patients with persistent or progressive deep tissue pain due to hydrofluoric acid burns, calcium gluconate may be injected locally.[54] The effectiveness of such treatment has been questioned[60] and local excision of the involved tissue with immediate grafting is presently recommended.

Immediate irrigation of chemically injured eyes using water, saline, or phosphate buffer is mandatory. Extended irrigation by means of small cannulae secured in the conjunctival sulci or a scleral contact lens adapted for irrigation has been recommended for the treatment of eyes with extensive conjunctival and subconjunctival injury due to concentrated alkali. Following irrigation, 1 percent atropine or another cycloplegic should be instilled to counteract the effects of iritis. Simultaneous applica-

tion of a miotic agent may further minimize the consequences of iritis. Subconjunctival injection of autologous serum, local instillation of cysteine or edetic acid sodium, and even excision of necrotic conjunctiva and application of a variety of mucosal grafts have all been recommended to inactivate or remove the tissue collagenase activated by the alkali.[10,64] Xerophthalmia and symblepharon formation that may result from severe alkali injury respond poorly to treatment and may cause persistent disability.[65]

Bitumen Burns

Burns due to bitumen and hot tar may be extensive but most commonly are of limited extent and often involve the hands and face. The bitumen should be cooled by water lavage to limit tissue damage and prevent further spread. The cooling should be carried out only until the bitumen has hardened and cooled and systemic hypothermia should be avoided. Bitumen adherent to skin blisters after cooling should be removed with the blister epithelium in the course of initial cleansing and debridement. Bitumen adherent to unblistered tissue should be left in place and covered with a liberal application of a petrolatum or animal-fat material, such as petrolatum, lanolin, mineral oil, or antibacterial ointments. The burn with adherent bitumen should then be dressed and the dressing removed on a daily or more frequent basis. Such dressing changes with repeated ointment application result in bitumen emulsification and effect removal within 24 to 72 hours. The burn wound is thereafter treated as any other burn. The use of solvents to remove adherent bitumen that themselves may cause secondary tissue injury and systemic toxicity is proscribed.[115]

Electric Injury

Injury due to electricity results from the heat generated as the current passes through tissue of variable resistance. Although different tissues offer variable resistance to current passage, such differences are unimportant with application of high voltage, in which case body parts act as volume conductors.[51] Following cessation of current flow the body part acts as a volume radiator in dissipating tissue heat. At the points of contact, charring of the skin commonly occurs to produce severe local tissue destruction and arcing may produce similar severe cutaneous damage on the flexor surfaces of joints (Fig. 36-5). These characteristics of high-voltage electric injury explain the differences in clinical characteristics and the specific treatment needs of patients with high-voltage electric injury compared to patients with conventional thermal injury.

The occurrence of cardiopulmonary arrest in the immediate postinjury period requires immediate application of cardiopulmonary resuscitation. Thereafter, electrocardiographic (ECG) monitoring of such patients is necessary for 48 hours even in the absence of arrhythmias or for 48 hours beyond the last occurrence of an arrhythmia. The limited cutaneous injury evident at contact sites and the inapparent but extensive deep tissue injury account for the greater susceptibility to acute renal failure in

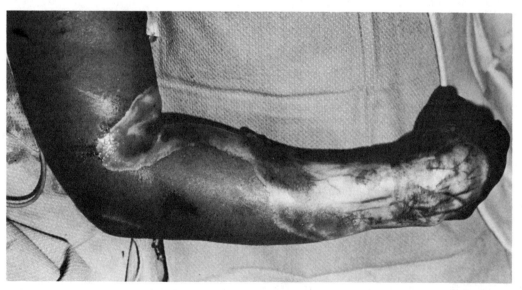

FIG. 36-5 The marked flexion deformity of digits and wrist is characteristic of high-voltage electric injury. Note charring of skin in antecubital space and burns of opposing flexor surfaces about the elbow, typical of current arcing at joints.

patients with electric injury because their fluid needs are underestimated and hemochromagens are liberated from damaged muscle and other tissue.[39] Resuscitation fluids should be administered to patients with high-voltage electric injury and significant hemochromagen loads in their urine at a rate to maintain an hourly urine output of 75 to 100 ml. If an hourly urinary output of 75 ml or more cannot be maintained by reasonable rates of fluid infusion, 12.5 g mannitol should be added to each liter of resuscitation fluid until the desired urinary output has been achieved and it is apparent that the hemochromagen levels are decreasing.

Edema in injured tissues beneath the investing fascia of a limb may increase tissue pressure to a sufficient level to impair nutrient blood flow or interrupt flow to distal unburned tissue. As noted previously, fasciotomy is required in such a situation. The extent and depth of tissue injury due to electric current may necessitate early surgical debridement and even amputation. If there are indications of deep tissue injury but large vessel pulses are intact, arteriography may be helpful in determining both the need for operative debridement and the extent of debridement necessary.[52] Both [133]xenon washout curves and technetium 99m pyrophosphate scanning have been used to assess muscle viability following electric injury, but both have been applied to such a small number of patients that it is difficult to determine the reliability, accuracy, or clinical usefulness of either.[28,53]

As soon as the patient is hemodynamically stable, operative exploration of severely damaged tissue should be carried out with the patient under general anesthesia. Explore the involved muscle thoroughly, keeping in mind that nonviable periosseous tissue may be present beneath superficial tissues that appear viable. All nonviable tissue must be surgically debrided to reduce the risk of infection and remove the source of postinjury hyperkalemia. Severe injury of the upper limb often involves the pectoral muscles and edema in the pectoral area mandates exploration of that area and excision of any nonviable muscle identified. All surgical wounds are packed open and the patient returned to the operating room in 24 to 48 hours for further debridement if necessary or wound closure by grafting or suture tech-

nique if possible. Progressive continuing tissue necrosis as a characteristic of electric injury has been implicated as the reason for the frequent need for further debridement in such patients. In general, the need for debridement at the time of reoperation appears to be related to imprecision of muscle viability assessment at the time of initial debridement. However, recent studies by Robson et al. have implicated local elevation of tissue thromboxane levels as a cause of the progressive tissue loss observed in some patients with electric injury.[130]

Although the large cross-sectional area of the thorax and abdomen make visceral injury uncommon, instances of intestinal perforation, focal necrosis of gallbladder and pancreas, and direct liver injury have been reported.[94] Delayed dysfunction of the gastrointestinal tract may also occur, such as the development of cholelithiasis as reported in approximately one third of one group of 45 patients within 2 years of high-voltage electric injury.[11]

Electric injury may also produce neurologic deficits of either immediate or delayed onset. Peripheral motor nerves more commonly show deficits than do sensory nerves, and recovery is rare if such damage is apparent immediately after injury. Late-appearing neurologic deficits may involve nerves far removed from the points of electric contact and may occur as part of a polyneuritic syndrome with highly variable functional recovery. Direct neuronal injury is considered to be the cause of immediate postinjury spinal cord deficits, which more commonly clear than do spinal cord deficits of delayed onset.[27] Delayed-onset spinal cord deficits are highly variable and range from localized nerve deficits associated with signs of ascending paralysis, transverse myelitis, or a syndrome similar to amyotrophic lateral sclerosis to paraplegia and quadriplegia.[68]

An arteritis caused by electric injury has been implicated as the cause of significant hemorrhage from large vessels occurring at variable times postinjury.[104] In most such cases, the hemorrhage has appeared to be a consequence of inadequate initial debridement or desiccation and necrosis of a vessel wall exposed following debridement. Tetanic contractions of the paraspinus muscles induced by electric current may cause compression fractures of the vertebrae[63] and vertebral injuries as well as long bone fractures may occur in patients who fall from a height following electric shock. Such fractures are diagnosed and treated as in other patients. In any patient who has sustained high voltage injury, especially those with a contact point on the head or neck, cataracts may form during the initial hospital period or as late as 3 or more years after injury.[131] An ophthalmologic evaluation should be obtained for all such patients before they are discharged from the hospital and they should be informed of the possibility of cataract formation.

POSTRESUSCITATION FLUID AND ELECTROLYTE DISTURBANCES

Fluid and electrolyte management following resuscitation must take into account not only the fluids previously administered but also the movement of fluid and electrolytes across the burn surface and the renal response to injury and sepsis. The destruction of the water vapor barrier of the skin by thermal injury results in prodigious evaporative water losses which, if unreplaced, can lead to dehydration.[154] Hypernatremia, as a manifestation of dehydration, is the most frequent electrolyte disturbance of burn patients and is most often due to inadequate replacement of total body water loss, which ranges from 2 to 3.1 ml/kg/percent burn/day.[144] Total insensible water loss in the burn patient can be estimated using the formula: water loss (ml/hr) = (25 + % of body surface area burned) × total body surface (m²). This provides an estimate at the low end of the range of observed losses and one must evaluate the adequacy of hydration by monitoring body weight, serum sodium concentration, and serum osmolality on at least a daily basis and adjust fluid therapy accordingly.

The administration of resuscitation fluid produces a gain in weight that may exceed 20 percent of preburn weight in patients with extensive burns. Postresuscitation fluid management should therefore permit gradual loss of the excess fluid so that the patient returns to preinjury weight between the third and tenth postburn days.[46] The increase in urinary output characteristic of postresuscitation diuresis should not be replaced volumetrically. A daily weight loss of 2 to 3 percent should be permitted until the patient returns to his or her preburn weight.

Other causes of hypernatremia in the burn patient include osmolar-induced diuresis, sepsis, and defects in osmotic regulation (Table 36-10). An osmotic diuresis can be induced by an increase in either urinary glucose or urinary nitrogen excretion and should be treated by reduction in administration of the respective nutrient and, in the case of glucose intolerance, administration of insulin. The hypernatremia of sepsis appears to be multifactorial and related to nutrient intolerance, increased metabolic rate and body temperature, and an increase in renal blood flow and renal water loss. The source of infection should be identified and controlled by surgical means and the administration of antimicrobial agents and fluids adjusted as necessary. Osmotic regulatory defects are rare but have been identified in a small number of patients based on appropriate response to administration of vasopressin.

Hyponatremia is most often encountered in the latter half of the resuscitation period, particularly in children with extensive burns who receive hypotonic fluids rapidly or in large volume. Studies by McManus et al. found that 42 percent of seizures in burned children could be related to hyponatremia and that the seizures in all but three of such patients occurred within the first 48 hours postburn.[81] Such seizures may progress to obtundation and computer tomographic studies have shown evidence of cerebral edema in such patients. Signs of cerebral edema during resuscitation should

TABLE 36-10. Causes of Hypernatremia in 51 Burn Patients

Osmolar-induced diuresis	2
Defect in osmotic regulation	2
Sepsis	16
Inadequate replacement of evaporative water loss	31

prompt reduction in the volume of fluid administered, the administration of a diuretic, and use of hyperventilation to induce hypocarbia. In patients whose wounds are treated with 0.5 percent silver nitrate soaks, significant trans-eschar leaching of electrolytes may occur and necessitate administration of supplemental sodium, potassium, and calcium. The amount of sodium needed by such patients is related to the extent of burn: 10 g sodium chloride and 30 to 50 ml molar sodium lactate per day are recommended for patients with burns of up to 50 percent of the total body surface, and 15 to 30 g sodium chloride and 50 to 80 ml molar sodium lactate per day have been recommended for patients with more extensive burns.[87] Hyponatremia has also been associated with sepsis and related to an observed reduction in free water clearance.[16]

Recent studies have identified a subset of burn patients with persistent hyponatremia following resuscitation in whom there was no evidence of a blood volume deficit. In those patients, inappropriately high levels of antidiuretic hormone (ADH) were measured and the nature of ADH responsiveness to either water or salt loading was consistent with a resetting of threshold values of water balance regulating mechanisms.[135] Water restriction may be required if symptoms or signs of water intoxication develop. Hyponatremia has also been considered to be a manifestation of the "sick-cell" syndrome in certain patients with extensive burns.[48] Curreri et al. have identified increases in erythrocyte sodium concentration in burn patients receiving less than their estimated nutritional needs.[34] These investigators found that administration of sufficient carbohydrate to meet measured energy needs returned red cell sodium to normal levels. Other investigators have reported that administration of insulin and 50 percent glucose corrected the "sick-cell" syndrome.[49]

Hyperkalemia may occur in the immediate postburn period as a result of red cell and other tissue injury and may be accentuated by acidosis. Metabolic acidosis as a manifestation of hypovolemia due to inadequate resuscitation customarily responds to increased fluid administration. Mechanical ventilation should be used to reduce the hypercarbia of respiratory acidosis. If serum potassium rises to levels associated with cardiac dysfunction, ion ex-

change resins should be administered and glucose and insulin infused. Following resuscitation, elevated renal potassium losses may cause hypokalemia, which can be further accentuated by alkalosis, the renal effects of mafenide acetate,[146] and the effects of topical application of 0.5 percent silver nitrate soaks.[87] Monitoring of serum potassium levels and urinary potassium losses will permit appropriate potassium supplementation.

Modest hypocalcemia is a frequent finding in patients with burns of more than 30 percent of the total body surface and, as previously noted, may be accentuated by the use of topical 0.5 percent silver nitrate soaks.[87] The decrease in total serum calcium appears to be consistent with the decrease in calcium-binding proteins; ionized calcium levels appear to be little influenced. Other investigators have measured low levels of ionized calcium in association with low levels of phosphate and have related this to increased circulating levels of calcitonin and elevated levels of catecholamines in the early postinjury period.[73] Marked depression of phosphate levels later in the hospital course was observed in some burn patients who died.[96] The hypophosphatemia observed in patients receiving large volumes of antacids as prophylaxis for Curling's ulcer commonly responds to reduction in antacid dosage and, if necessary, phosphate replacement. Decreased serum levels of zinc have been observed in burn patients and related to early postburn impairment of taste and appetite and late disturbances of wound healing.[30,62] Zinc deficiency appears to be uncommon and a regular diet customarily maintains zinc levels within the normal range. Magnesium deficiency has also been reported as the cause of muscle cramps and psychiatric signs that cleared with magnesium supplementation.[18]

WOUND CARE

When the immediate postinjury hemodynamic and ventilatory needs of the burn patient have been addressed, initial wound care can be carried out. Tetanus prophylaxis using toxoid and hyperimmune globulin or toxoid alone is dictated by the patient's tetanus immunization status. The burn wound should be gently cleansed with any available surgical detergent and adherent debris and nonviable epithelium removed. Body hair should be shaved from the burn and a generous margin of unburned skin. Bullae less than 2 cm in diameter can be left intact, but larger bullae should be debrided lest they rupture and their protein-rich contents serve as a pabulum for microbial proliferation. The topical antimicrobial of choice is then applied to the surface of all burn wounds and the wound care regimen continued following resuscitation as described below.

Both patient and microbial factors influence the occurrence of infection in the burn wound (Table 36-11). The severity of injury as indexed by extent of burn is the single most important patient factor. Burn wound infections are rare in patients with burns of less than 30 percent of the body surface but increase in incidence as the extent of burn increases above that level.[110] The incidence of infection is also related to patient age, being least in the young adult (15 to 40 years of age), greatest in burned children less than 15 years, and intermediate in the elderly.[113] Other host factors include coexisting diseases such as diabetes mellitus, which increases the risk of fungal infection.[20] The local blood supply is also an important factor, as indicated by the higher incidence of wound infection in avascular third-degree burns and the increased risk of infection in partial-thickness burns and even split-thickness skin graft donor sites in patients

who develop systemic hypotension. The immunosuppression of burn injury, related to burn size, which affects all limbs of the immune system, permits the rapid spread and systemic dissemination of wound infections in extensively burned patients and explains, at least in part, the high incidence of infections in sites other than the burn wound in such patients.[109]

The burn wound is not sterile even immediately following injury, but few microorganisms can be recovered from the burn surface at that time. The flora of the burn wound subsequently changes, both in terms of microbial density and predominant organisms. Gram-positive organisms initially predominate but gram-negative organisms can be recovered from the majority of burn wounds by the end of the first postburn week. Such organisms become the predominant flora during the second week postburn.[122] In untreated burn wounds, the microbial density increases across time and invasive infection is commonly associated with microbial densities greater than 10^5 organisms/g tissue.[84] Other microbial factors that influence the occurrence of wound infection include toxin production, enzyme production, bacterial motility, and antimicrobial resistance.[108] Prior to the development of topical antimicrobial therapy in the mid-1960s, imbalance between the impaired host defense capacity and microbial invasive capacity in patients with extensive burns frequently resulted in invasive burn wound infection, which was the principal cause of death in 60 percent of burn patients who died.[126]

TABLE 36-11. Important Factors in Burn Wound Infection

Patient Factors	Microbial Factors
Extent of burn	Time-related changes in
Age	flora
Sources of contamination	Microbial density
Local blood supply	Metabolic products
Wound environment	Endotoxins
Coexisting disease	Exotoxins
Presence of foreign	Vascular permeability
bodies	factor
Effects of therapeutic	Enzymes
agents	Motility
	Antibiotic resistance
	Intrinsic
	Therapy-induced

Topical Chemotherapy

The proliferation of bacteria in the nonviable eschar can be controlled and the incidence of invasive infection reduced by the use of topical chemotherapeutic agents. Although the author and many others no longer recommend prophylactic use of penicillin for burn patients, those clinicians caring for pediatric burn patients feel that the frequent presence of beta streptococci in the nasopharynges of children justifies administration of penicillin for 3 to 5 days postburn to all burned children. There are three widely used topical agents of verified effectiveness: mafenide acetate burn cream, 0.5 percent silver nitrate soaks, and silver sulfadiazine burn cream.[43,85,87] Knowledge of the advantages and limitations of each of those agents, listed in Table 36-12, will enable the physician to individualize topical therapy. If the use of one agent is attended by significant side effects, topical therapy should be continued using one of the other agents.

All of the agents appear to be equally effective when applied to burn wounds early postinjury before a significant degree of microbial proliferation has occurred within the eschar. Mafenide acetate burn cream is specifically indicated for use in patients in whom delayed institution of topical therapy has permitted significant microbial proliferation within the eschar. Mafenide acetate diffuses freely into nonviable burned tissue and will limit further intraeschar microbial proliferation and reduce the risk of invasive infection. We apply mafenide acetate burn cream to all burned surfaces following the daily cleansing and 12 hours later, in the evening, apply silver sulfadiazine burn cream (Fig. 36-6). This program of alternate application of the two topical agents achieves optimal antimicrobial coverage and appears to reduce the incidence of side effects from both agents.

Monitoring the Burn Wound with Biopsies

In the vast majority of burn patients, topical chemotherapy maintains the microbial population of the burn wound below levels associated with invasive infection, but none of the agents sterilize the eschar.[70] Consequently, burn wound infection may occur in certain patients (most commonly those with burns of more than 30 percent of the total body surface) and the wounds of every patient should be examined closely at least daily to identify signs of wound infection (Fig. 36-7). This examination is best carried out at the daily wound cleansing when all dressings and topical agent have been removed from the wound surface. Identification of any of the local signs of burn wound infection listed in Table 36-13 is an indication to biopsy the area of the burn showing the most pronounced changes to confirm a diagnosis of wound infection.

Focal and even generalized changes in the color of the wound that mimic those of infection may occur as the eschar matures or as a result of local trauma. Unexpectedly rapid eschar separation, which can be caused by infection, may occur independent of infection in areas where deep thermal injury has caused fat liquifaction. The uncertainty of clinical signs

TABLE 36-12. Advantages and Limitations of Topical Antimicrobial Agents

Mafenide Acetate	Silver Sulfadiazine	0.5% Silver Nitrate Soaks
	Advantages	
Diffuses into nonviable eschar	Painless upon application	Painless upon application
Wound visible	Wound visible	No patient hypersensitivity
Ease of use	Ease of use	Reduction of heat loss
Sensitivity of gram-negative organisms	Controls proliferation of yeasts	Sensitivity of gram-negative organisms
Joint motion maintained	Joint motion maintained	Dressings assist in debridement
	Limitations	
Painful when applied to second-degree burns	Patient hypersensitivity	No tissue penetration
Accentuates postburn hyperventilation	Plasmid-mediated sulfonamide—multiple antibiotic resistance	Electrolyte deficits: Na^+, K^+, and Ca^{++}
Increases renal bicarbonate losses	Bone marrow suppression (usually transient)	Methemoglobinemia (rare)
Patient hypersensitivity $\approx$ 7%	Resistance of certain gram-negative organisms	Dressings limit joint motion
	Low tissue diffusibility	Discolors unburned skin and environment

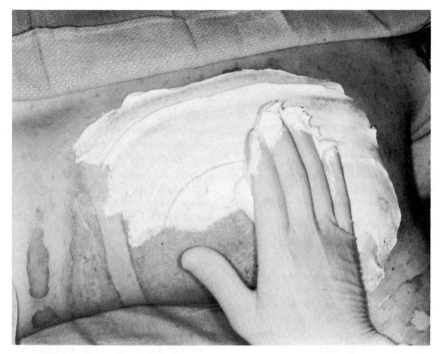

FIG. 36-6 Topical chemotherapy of the burn wound limits microbial proliferation and maintains the bacterial density at levels not associated with invasive infection. After the daily wound cleansing and inspection, the topical agent, mafenide acetate cream in this patient, is applied with the sterile gloved hand as shown.

necessitates that other techniques be used to differentiate between microbial invasion of viable tissue underlying the burn wound and microbial colonization of the burn eschar. Standardized quantitative surface cultures provide information about the microbial population of the wound surface but may not accurately reflect the microbial status at the viable/nonvia-

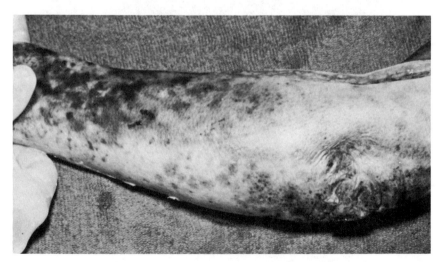

FIG. 36-7 The multifocal areas of wound discoloration evident in the arm burns of this patient are characteristic of burn wound infection.

TABLE 36-13. Local Signs of Burn Wound Infection

Conversion of partial-thickness injury to full-thickness necrosis
Dark brown, black or violaceous discoloration (can be unifocal, multifocal, or generalized)
Hemorrhagic discoloration of tissue beneath eschar
Edema and/or violaceous discoloration of unburned skin at wound margins
Green pigment visible in subcutaneous tissue[a]
Erythematous nodular lesions (ecthyma gangrenosa) in unburned skin[a]
Unexpectedly rapid eschar separation[b]
Rapid centrifugal advance of subcutaneous edema with central necrosis[b]
Punctate vesicular lesions in healing or healed partial-thickness burn[c]
Crusted serrated margins of partial-thickness burns (usually burns of face)[c]

[a] Characteristic of *Pseudomonas* infection
[b] Characteristic of fungal infection
[c] Characteristic of herpetic infection

ble tissue interface, which is best assessed by wound biopsy. A 500 mg lenticular sample of eschar and underlying unburned tissue should be obtained, using a scalpel, from that area

of the wound showing the most pronounced signs of wound infection (Fig. 36-8). Local anesthetic, if needed, is injected at the periphery of the biopsy site to avoid distorting the sample.

The biopsy specimen is bisected and one portion is submitted for quantitative culture. A report of 10^5 organisms/g tissue is consistent with but, because of the limitations of quantitative cultures, not diagnostic of burn wound infection.[69,156] The other half of the specimen is processed by either rapid or frozen section technique (requiring 4 hours or 30 minutes, respectively)[57,58] for histologic examination, which is the most accurate means of differentiating microbial colonization from microbial invasion.[106] The pathologist examines the prepared sections to identify the histologic signs of invasive burn wound infection. The diagnosis of invasive burn wound infection can only be made if microorganisms are identified in unburned tissue.[119] Other histologic findings indicative of burn wound infection are listed in Table 36-14. Burn wound biopsy findings must

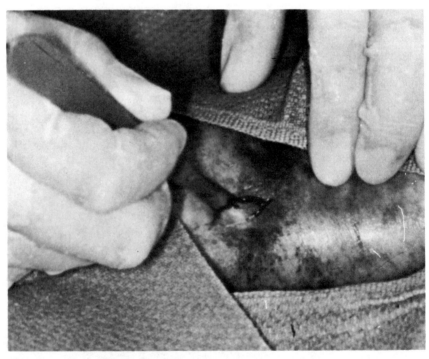

FIG. 36-8 A biopsy is the most reliable technique for assessing the microbial status of a burn wound. As shown here, a lenticular specimen, which must include underlying unburned tissue, is harvested from that area of the wound showing the tinctorial changes characteristic of infection.

TABLE 36-14. Histologic Signs of Burn Wound Infection

Microorganisms in unburned tissue
Heightened inflammatory reaction in unburned tissue
Small vessel thrombosis and ischemic necrosis of
  unburned tissue
Hemorrhage in unburned tissue
Dense microbial growth
  Intraeschar
  Along hair follicles and sweat glands
  At viable–nonviable tissue interface
Intracellular inclusions
  Light microscopy: Type A Cowdry bodies, owl's
    eye inclusions
  Electron microscopy: intracellular virions

always be interpreted in light of the patient's general condition. A negative biopsy report in a patient with systemic signs of sepsis mandates a repeat biopsy as well as an avid search for another source of infection.

Treatment of Burn Wound Infection

The diagnosis of invasive burn wound infection necessitates changes in both local and systemic treatment. If a nonabsorbable topical agent is being used, that should be stopped and treatment with mafenide acetate burn cream begun. Systemic administration of an antibiotic active against the invading organism should be begun and necessary therapy used to support blood volume, cardiac output, and pulmonary function. If the burn wound infection is limited to the subcutaneous tissue and is unifocal or even multifocal but involves less than 2 percent of the total body surface, twice-daily subeschar infusion of a β-lactam antibiotic solution should be begun.[13] Ten grams of the antibiotic should be dissolved in 150 ml saline and infused into the subcutaneous tissue underlying all areas of infection using a no. 20 spinal needle to limit the number of injection sites. A therapeutic response to the subeschar infusions is indicated by stabilization of lesion size and desiccation of the eschar surface overlying the area of infection. It is important to adjust fluid management to account for the sodium content of the antibiotic solution.

In patients with more extensive burn wound infections or infections involving the investing fascia or tissues beneath the investing fascia, subeschar antibiotic infusion should be carried out immediately and again 6 hours later, after which the patient should be taken to the operating room for surgical removal of all infected tissue. In patients with extensive subfascial involvement of a limb, as may occur with invasive fungal infection, amputation may be necessary. The excised wounds must be covered with a biologic dressing or skin substitute to prevent desiccation of the exposed tissue and formation of a neoeschar. If the adequacy of the excision is uncertain, the wounds should be dressed with 0.5 percent silver nitrate soaks or 5 percent mafenide acetate solution and the patient returned to the operating room 24 to 48 hours later for inspection of the wounds and further debridement if necessary. When control of the wound infection is certain, definitive closure of the wounds is obtained by skin grafting.

The survival of patients with generalized burn wound infection, particularly those with systemic sepsis and hematogenous involvement of other organs, is quite low. However, the survival of patients with focal burn wound infection without positive blood cultures following subeschar antibiotic infusion and surgical excision of the infected tissue emphasizes the importance of early diagnosis and prompt treatment of this complication.[80]

Burn Wound Excision

In an attempt to reduce, if not eliminate, the occurrence of invasive burn wound infections, early (within the first week postburn) excision of the burned tissue is carried out with increasing frequency. Such excisions are carried out using the scalpel to remove all tissue superficial to the investing fascia (Fig. 36-9) or by what is termed the tangential technique, with the plane of excision at a variable depth within the dermis or the subcutaneous tissue.[56,75] The surprisingly large blood loss associated with burn wound excision dictates that no more than 20 percent of the total body surface be excised at a single sitting.[26,138] To pre-

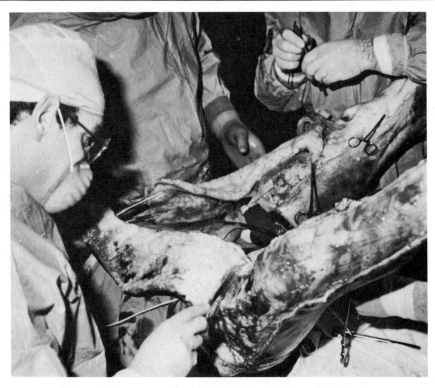

FIG. 36-9 Deep unequivocally full-thickness burns are most rapidly removed by scalpel excision at the level of the investing fascia. The use of the tourniquets on both thighs at the upper limits of excision minimizes operative blood loss. A biologic dressing was applied at this sitting to prevent desiccation of surgically exposed tissue.

vent desiccation of the wounds produced by the excision, they must be covered with the patient's own skin if donor sites are available or with a biologic dressing or a skin substitute if sufficient skin graft donor sites are not available.

Although burn wounds are often excised today, a beneficial effect of the procedure upon mortality remains unconfirmed. Those studies in which improved survival has been attributed to burn wound excision have either used historic controls or failed to randomize patients.[24,83] Recent evaluations of burn wound excision in patients with burns of less than 20 percent of the total body surface have shown only that hospital stay is reduced and return to work is hastened.[41] In patients with more extensive burns, excision has been credited with decreasing the occurrence of burn wound infection but the infections were defined on the basis of quantitative biopsy cultures and no improvement in mortality was ob-

served.[45,139] Even though a beneficial effect of excision upon survival has not been verified, surgical removal of the burned tissue should be begun during the first postburn week in those patients who have stabilized following resuscitation. This will reduce the risk of infection, preserve viable tissue, maintain function, and reduce stresses related to burn size by early wound closure.

DIAGNOSIS AND TREATMENT OF OTHER INFECTIONS

Effective topical chemotherapy and current techniques of burn wound management have significantly decreased the occurrence of invasive burn wound infection.[106] However, infections in sites other than the burn wound remain the most frequent cause of morbidity and mortality in the extensively burned patient and are a reflection of injury-related immunosuppression[109] (Table 36-15). The systemic response to an extensive burn characterized by hyperthermia, tachycardia, hyperventilation, and leukocytosis, as well as disorientation and even obtundation in some patients, confounds the diagnosis of sepsis and necessitates a scheduled program of infection surveillance.

The most frequent sites of infection in burn patients treated with topical antimicrobial therapy are the lungs and previously cannulated veins. The prevalent form of pneumonia has changed from hematogenous due to dissemination of bacteria from an infected burn wound or an infected vein to airborne or bronchopneumonia.[118] Bronchopneumonia in the burn patient is treated as in any other patient by the administration of specific antibiotics and ventilatory support as required. Hematogenous pneumonia is also treated by systemic administration of specific antibiotics, but the primary focus of infection must be identified and treated as well. In patients with radiographic signs of hematogenous pneumonia or patients with a positive blood culture and no other identifiable focus of infection, all previously cannulated veins should be examined for the presence of suppurative thrombophlebitis.[125] If an area of intraluminal sepsis is identified, the involved segment of vein must be excised. In patients with systemic signs of sepsis with or without an identifiable focus of infection, blood cultures showing growth of multiple organisms or sequential blood cultures showing growth of different organisms reflect the immunologic impairment of the patient and should not be interpreted as technical errors. Those patients, invariably critically ill, require systemic administration of multiple antibiotics to provide coverage of all the recovered organisms, and even so, survival rates are low.

METABOLIC CHANGES AND NUTRITIONAL SUPPORT

Burn injury elicits the stereotypic byphasic metabolic response of all injured patients. The hypometabolic "ebb" phase present during the resuscitation period is succeeded by the hypermetabolic "flow" phase in which metabolic rate is elevated in proportion to the extent of the burn. It rises in curvilinear fashion to levels of two to two and one half times predicted normal in patients with burns of more than 50 percent of the total body surface.[148] Contrary to earlier belief, this hypermetabolism is not primarily a response to external cooling due to evaporative water loss from the burn surface, but appears to be due to increased heat production related to a resetting of thermal regulatory mechanisms.[151] The hypermetabolism observed in burn patients is not temperature-dependent, but is temperature-sensitive.[7] Maintaining a warm environmental temperature of comfort can reduce metabolic rate by up to 10 percent in patients with burns of more than 50 percent of the total body surface. Maintaining a warm (30 to 32° C) environmental temperature will prevent the imposition of cold stress on extensively burned patients, reduce energy expenditure, and decrease the level of nutritional support required to maintain energy equilibrium.[152]

Multiple, apparently interrelated, alterations of neuroendocrine function, which are related to both extent of burn and time postburn, are associated with the hypermetabolic response to burn injury. The catecholamine and glucagon levels are elevated immediately

TABLE 36-15. Infections in 40 Fatal Burns (1983)

Infection		Number of Patients
Pneumonia		23
Burn wound infections		17
Aerobic bacterial infections	5	
Clostridial infection	1	
Candidal and fungal infections	14	
Viral infections	2	
Suppurative thrombophylebitis		5
Bacterial endocarditis		5
Peritonitis		2
Prostatic abscess		1
Acute sinusitis		1
Septicemia		23

postburn, while circulating levels of the thyroid hormones are depressed and levels of insulin are either absolutely or relatively low.[150,151] In the patient with an uncomplicated burn, the abnormal levels of circulating hormones slowly return toward normal as wound healing occurs and reach preinjury levels when the wounds are closed and convalescence begins. Supervening infection is associated with persistence of or reversion to the neurohormonal pattern of the early postresuscitation catabolic period.[120] The additional metabolic stress of sepsis can be avoided by the prevention of infection and minimized by the early diagnosis and prompt treatment of septic complications.

The hormonal changes that orchestrate the metabolic response to injury also influence the distribution and utilization of nutrients. Increased proteolysis of lean body mass, which appears to be related to increased hepatic gluconeogenesis, and elevated total body glucose flow, are indices of the increased needs of severely injured burn patients for both protein and carbohydrate.[8,149] Fat metabolism is also disturbed following burn injury.[140] The rapid development of essential fatty acid deficiencies in burn patients receiving fat-free parenteral diets indicates the importance of including fatty acids in the nutritional support regimen of such patients.[153]

Increased levels of nutritional support are not required during resuscitation and may only exaggerate the usually transient hyperglycemia and elevation of blood urea nitrogen that reflect the glycogenolytic and organ blood flow effects of the catabolic hormones. Following resuscitation and re-establishment of fluid compartment equilibrium, nutritional support should be matched to energy and nitrogen needs. The calorie expenditure of the burn patient can be measured by indirect calorimetry or estimated according to a variety of formulas or nomograms. The nitrogen needs can be estimated on the basis of urinary nitrogen excretion.[147] The curvilinear relationship of burn size and metabolic rate, which plateaus at a maximum rate of two to two and one half times normal, can be used for a simplified estimate of daily calorie and nitrogen needs in patients with burns of 50 percent or more of the total body surface: 2,000 to 2,200 calories/m² body surface and 12 to 18 g nitrogen/m² body surface.[120]

The enteral route should be used to feed all patients with adequate gastrointestinal function. Since spontaneous food intake is "fixed" at preinjury levels, nutritional balance can only be achieved by the use of between-meal supplements administered every 2 to 4 hours around the clock.[112] In patients with a functioning gastrointestinal tract who either cannot or will not eat, tube feedings should be administered with gastric residual measured before each intragastric instillation to prevent aspiration. In patients with gastrointestinal dysfunction or in whom enteral support does not meet nutritional needs, parenteral alimentation should be instituted by infusing a solution of synthetic amino acids and hypertonic glucose through a separate intravenous line placed in a high-flow central vein. The increased amount of electrolyte-free water needed by the burn patient to replace large evaporative water losses will often permit the administration of the necessary nutrients in less concentrated solutions and facilitate the patient's adaptation to the nutritional regimen.

Even though the measured respiratory quotient of burn patients is consistent with preferential utilization of fat as an energy source, the administration of fat emulsions is associated with less nitrogen-sparing than an equal amount of carbohydrate in severely hypermetabolic burn patients.[72] Nevertheless, it is important to provide 500 to 1,000 ml (depending upon the extent of burn and size of the patient) of a fat emulsion twice each week in the nutritional support regimen of burn patients to prevent essential fatty acid deficiencies.

Scheduled monitoring of a variety of clinical and laboratory variables is an essential part of the nutritional management of the severely burned patient (Table 36-16). Weight change as well as intake and output records should be reviewed on a daily basis. An increase in body weight of more than 200 to 400 g per day (the apparent maximum tissue increase achievable in the absence of pharmacological manipulation) is an indication of excess fluid retention that requires reduction in the volume of administered fluid.[112,125] Excessive urinary glucose and urea may induce an osmotic diuresis and are treated by reduction in the administered nutrient load or, in the case of glucosuria, by the administration of insulin.

TABLE 36-16. Monitoring Nutritional Management

Variable	Frequency of Monitoring[a]
Blood	
Hematocrit	Daily
pH and blood gases	Daily
Electrolytes	Daily
Blood urea nitrogen	Daily
Glucose	Daily
Calcium and phosphorus	3 × week
Transaminases and bilirubin	2 × week
Total protein albumin and globulin	2 × week
Magnesium	2 × week
Trace metals	As indicated
Ammonia	As indicated
Urine	
Sodium	Daily
Potassium	Daily
Specific gravity	2–4 × day
Glucose	4–8 × day
Adequacy of hydration	
Intake and output review	Daily
Body weight	Daily
Serum osmolality	Daily
Pulmonary function	As indicated
Cardiac function	As indicated

[a] A higher or lower frequency may be indicated by the patient's condition.

The sudden appearance of hyperglycemia in a patient who has tolerated a given carbohydrate load is often an early sign of sepsis. This should prompt a thorough search for a site of infection while the level of blood glucose is controlled by the administration of insulin or reduction in the amount of carbohydrate administered.

The muscle wasting associated with inactivity can be minimized by institution of a program of physical therapy immediately following resuscitation. The level of activity should be progressively increased as tolerated by the patient. Analgesics should also be used judiciously to prevent the additional stress associated with pain related to wound manipulation and activity. It is unrealistic to expect nutritional support to effect significant gain in lean body mass in profoundly hypermetabolic critically ill patients. However, this program of metabolic support will maintain lean body mass, support wound healing, and prevent the development of the secondary immunosuppression and other organ system complications that may occur in patients receiving inadequate metabolic support.

ASSESSMENT OF OUTCOME

Raw mortality data are of little value in assessing treatment outcome in burn patients because of the many variables that affect mortality. The sigmoid dose–response relationship between burn size and mortality requires a technique of data transformation to establish a straight line relationship and generate an error term that permits comparison of outcomes.[23] The effect of age on burn injury outcome also requires stratification of patient groups by age to make meaningful comparisons of outcome.[127] Patients with associated injuries should be excluded from burn mortality analyses since inhalation injury and mechanical trauma exert a burn-independent mortality effect.[2,158] Moreover, since the death rate of burn patients is related to time postburn (i.e., relatively high in the first 10 days postburn and markedly lower thereafter), outcome analyses should be confined to those patients seen within the first 10 days postburn. The distribution of burn size within the population being analyzed is also important since a mortality curve based on experience with only small burns can be unwarrantedly biased in an upward direction. When those factors are taken into account, analyses of burn-specific mortality reveal that significant improvement in survival as expressed by the LA_{50} (that extent of burn associated with a 50 percent mortality) has occurred over the past four decades.[33,105] At the U.S. Army Institute of Surgical Research, prompt physiologically guided resuscitation, up-to-date burn wound care, and improvements in general supportive measures have resulted in an LA_{50} in percent body surface area burned of 45.21 for the pediatric (<15 years) age group, 60.81 for young adults (15 to 40 years), and 39.19 for burn patients older than 40 years.

REFERENCES

1. Agarwal N, Petro J, Salisbury RE: Physiologic profile monitoring in burned patients. J Trauma 23: 577, 1983

2. Agee RN, Long JM, Hunt JL et al: Use of [133]xenon in early diagnosis of inhalation injury. J Trauma 16: 218, 1976

3. American Burn Association: Specific Optimal Criteria for Hospital Resources for Care of Patients with Burn Injury. p 1, 1976

4. Andes WA, Rogers PW, Beason JW et al: Erythropoietin response to the anemia of thermal injury. J Lab Clin Med 88: 584, 1976

5. Asch MJ, Flemma RJ, Pruitt BA, Jr.: Ischemic necrosis of tibialis anterior muscle in burn patients: report of three cases. Surgery 66: 846, 1969

6. Asch MJ, Feldman RJ, Walker HL et al: Systemic and pulmonary hemodynamic changes accompanying thermal injury. Ann Surg 178: 218, 1973

7. Aulick LH, Hander EH, Wilmore DW et al: The relative significance of thermal and metabolic demands on burn hypermetabolism. J Trauma 19: 559, 1979

8. Aulick LH, Wilmore DW: Increased peripheral amino acid release following burn injury. Surgery 85: 560, 1979

9. Baar S: Serum and plasma proteins in thermally injured patients treated with plasma, its admixture with albumin or serum alone. Ann Surg 161: 112, 1965

10. Ballen P: Mucous membrane grafts in chemical (lye) burns. Am J Ophthalmol 55: 302, 1963

11. Baxter CR: Present concepts in the management of major electrical injury. Surg Clin North Am 50: 1401, 1970

12. Baxter CR, Cook WA, Shires GT: Serum myocardial depressant factor of burn shock. Surg Forum 17: 1, 1966

13. Baxter CR, Curreri PW, Marvin JA: The control of burn wound sepsis by the use of quantitative bacteriologic studies and subeschar clysis with antibiotics. Surg Clin North Am 53: 1509, 1973

14. Baxter CR, Shires T: Physiologic response to crystalloid resuscitation of severe burns. Ann NY Acad Sci 150: 874, 1968

15. Becker RA, Vaughan GM, Ziegler MG et al: Hypermetabolic low triiodothyronine syndrome of burn injury. Crit Care Med 10: 870, 1982

16. Bilbrey GL, Beisel WR: Depression of free water clearance during pneumococcal bacteremia. Ann Surg 177: 112, 1973

17. Brain JD, Valberg PA: Models of lung retention based on ICRP task group report. Arch Environ Health 28: 1, 1974

18. Broughton A, Anderson IRM, Bowden CH: Magnesium-deficiency syndrome in burns. Lancet 2: 1156, 1968

19. Brouhard BH, Carvajal HF, Linares HA: Burn edema and protein leakage in the rat. I. Relationship to time of injury. Microvasc Res 15: 221, 1978

20. Bruck HM, Nash G, Foley FD et al: Opportunistic fungal infection of the burn wound with phycomycetes and aspergillus. Arch Surg 102: 476, 1971

21. Brown WL, Bowler EG, Mason AD, Jr., et al: Edema formation in burned rats. Am J Physiol (in press) 1986

22. Buhl: Mittheilungen aus der Pfeufer'schen Klinik. Epidemische Cholera. Z Rationelle Med 6: 1, 1855

23. Bull JP, Squire JR: A study of mortality in a burns unit: standards for the evaluation of alternative methods of treatment. Ann Surg 130: 160, 1949

24. Burke JF, Bondoc CC, Quinby WC et al: Primary burn excision and immediate grafting: a method shortening illness. J Trauma 14: 389, 1974

25. Caldwell FT, Bowser BH: Critical evaluation of hypertonic and hypotonic solutions to resuscitate severely burned children: a prospective study. Ann Surg 189: 546, 1979

26. Canizaro PC, Sawyer RB, Switzer WE: Blood loss during excision of third degree burns. Arch Surg 88: 800, 1964

27. Christensen JA, Sherman RT, Balis GA et al: Delayed neurologic injury secondary to high-voltage current, with recovery. J Trauma 20: 166, 1980

28. Clayton JM, Hayes AC, Hammel J et al: [133]Xenon determination of muscle blood flow in electrical injury. J Trauma 17: 293, 1977

29. Clayton JM, Russell HE, Hartford CE et al: Sequential circulatory changes in the circumferentially burned limb. Ann Surg 185: 391, 1977

30. Cohen IK, Schechter PJ, Henkin RI: Hypogeusia, anorexia, and altered zinc metabolism following thermal burn. JAMA 223: 914, 1973

31. Cope O, Moore FD: The redistribution of body water and the fluid therapy of the burn patient. Ann Surg 126: 1010, 1947

32. Curreri PW, Katz AJ, Dotin LN et al: Coagulation abnormalities in the thermally injured patient. Curr Top Surg Res 2: 401, 1970

33. Curreri PW, Luterman A, Braun DW, Jr., et al: Burn injury: analysis of survival and hospitalization time for 937 patients. Ann Surg 192: 472, 1980

34. Curreri PW, Wilmore DW, Mason AD, Jr., et al: Intracellular cation alterations following major trauma: effect of supranormal caloric intake. J Trauma 11: 390, 1971

35. Czaja AJ, McAlhaney JC, Jr., Andes WA: Acute gastric disease after cutaneous thermal injury. Arch Surg 110: 600, 1975
36. Czaja AJ, McAlhaney JC, Pruitt BA, Jr.: Gastric acid secretion and acute gastroduodenal disease after burns. Arch Surg 111: 243, 1976
37. Czaja AJ, McAlhany JC, Pruitt BA, Jr.: Acute gastroduodenal disease after thermal injury. N Engl J Med 291: 925, 1974
38. Demling RH, Wong C: Early lung dysfunction after major burns (role of edema and vasoactive mediators). J Trauma 25: 959, 1985
39. DiVicenti FC, Moncrief JA, Pruitt BA, Jr.: Electrical injuries: a review of 65 cases. J Trauma 9: 497, 1969
40. DiVincenti FC, Pruitt BA, Jr., Reckler JM: Inhalation injuries. J Trauma 11: 109, 1971
41. Engrav LH, Heimbach DM, Reus JL et al: Early excision and grafting vs. nonoperative treatment of burns of indeterminant depth: a randomized prospective study. J Trauma 23: 1001, 1983
42. Evans EI, Purnell OJ, Robinette PW et al: Fluid and electrolyte requirements in severe burns. Ann Surg 135: 804, 1952
43. Fox CL, Jr., Rappole BW, Stanford W: Control of Pseudomonas infection in burns by silver sulfadiazine. Surg Gynecol Obstet 128: 1021, 1969
44. Goodwin CW, Dorethy J, Lam V et al: Randomized trial of efficacy of crystalloid and colloid resuscitation on hemodynamic response and lung water following thermal injury. Ann Surg 197: 520, 1983
45. Gray DT, Pine RW, Harnar TJ et al: Early surgical excision versus conventional therapy in patients with 20 to 40 percent burns. Am J Surg 144: 76, 1982
46. Gump FE, Kinney JM: Energy balance and weight loss in burned patients. Arch Surg 103: 442, 1971
47. Harkins HN: The Treatment of Burns, Charles C Thomas, Springfield, IL, 1942
48. Hinton P, Allison SP, Littlejohn S et al: Electrolyte changes after burn injury and effect of treatment. Lancet 2: 218, 1973
49. Hinton P, Allison SP, Littlejohn S et al: Insulin and glucose to rec ,ce catabolic response to injury in burn patients. Lancet 1: 767, 1971
50. Hunt JL, Agee RN, Pruitt BA, Jr.: Fiberoptic bronchoscopy in acute inhalation injury. J Trauma 15: 641, 1975
51. Hunt JL, Mason AD, Jr., Masterson TS et al: The pathophysiology of acute electric injuries. J Trauma 16: 335, 1976
52. Hunt JL, McManus WF, Haney WB et al: Vascular lesions in acute electric injuries. J Trauma 14: 461, 1974
53. Hunt JL, Sato RM, Baxter CR: Acute electric burns: current diagnostic and therapeutic approaches to management. Arch Surg 115: 434, 1980
54. Iverson RE, Laub DR, Madison MS: Hydrofluoric acid burns. Plast Reconstr Surg 48: 107, 1971
55. Jackson DM: Second thoughts on the burn wound. J Trauma 9: 839, 1969
56. Janzekovic Z: The burn wound from the surgical point of view. J Trauma 15: 42, 1975
57. Kim SH, Hubbard GB, McManus WF et al: Frozen section technique to evaluate early burn wound biopsy: a comparison with the rapid section technique. J Trauma 25: 1134, 1986
58. Kim SH, Hubbard GB, Worley BL et al: The rapid section technique for burn wound biopsy. J Burn Care Rehab 6: 433, 1985
59. Kirksey TD, Moncrief JA, Pruitt BA, Jr., et al: Gastrointestinal complications in burns. Am J Surg 116: 627, 1968
60. Kohnlein HE, Merkle P, Springorum HW: Hydrogen fluoride burns: experiments and treatment. Surg Forum 24: 50, 1973
61. Lam V, Goodwin CW, Jr., Treat RC et al: Does pulmonary extravascular water vary with colloid oncotic pressure after burn injury. Am Rev Respir Dis 119(4): 139, 1979
62. Larson DL, Maxwell R, Abston S et al: Zinc deficiency in burned children. Plast Reconstr Surg 46: 13, 1970
63. Layton TR, McMurtry JM, McClain EJ et al: Multiple spine fractures from electric injury. J Burn Care Rehab 5: 373, 1984
64. Lemp MA: Cornea and sclera. Arch Ophthalmol 92: 158, 1974
65. Lemp MA: Artificial tear solutions. Int Ophthalmol Clin 13: 221, 1973
66. Levine BA, Petroff PA, Slade CL et al: Prospective trials of dexamethasone and aerosolized gentamicin in the treatment of inhalation injury in the burned patient. J Trauma 18: 188, 1978
67. Levine BA, Schwesinger WH, Sirinek KR et al: Cimetidine prevents reduction in gastric mucosal blood flow during shock. Surgery 84: 113, 1978
68. Levine NS, Atkins A, McKeel DW, Jr., et al: Spinal cord injury following electrical accidents: case reports. J Trauma 15: 459, 1975
69. Lindberg RB, Moncrief JA, and Mason AD, Jr.: Control of experimental and clinical burn wound sepsis by topical application of sulfamylon compounds. Ann NY Acad Sci 150: 950, 1968
70. Lindberg RB, Moncrief JA, Switzer WE et al: The successful control of burn wound sepsis. J Trauma 5: 601, 1965
71. Loebl EC, Baxter CR, Curreri PW: The mecha-

nism of erythrocyte destruction in the early post-burn period. Ann Surg 178: 681, 1973

72. Long JM, Wilmore DW, Mason AD et al: Effect of carbohydrate and fat intake on nitrogen excretion during total feeding. Ann Surg 185: 417, 1977

73. Loven L, Nordstrom H, Lennquist S: Changes in calcium and phosphate and their regulating hormones in patients with severe burn injuries. Scand J Plast Reconstr Surg 18: 49, 1984

74. Lund T, Goodwin CW, McManus WF et al: Upper airway sequelae in burn patients requiring endotracheal intubation or tracheostomy. Ann Surg 201: 374, 1985

75. MacMillan BG, Artz CP: A planned evaluation of early excision of more than twenty-five per cent of the body surface in burns. Surg Forum 7: 88, 1957

76. McAlhaney JC, Jr., Czaja AJ, Villareal Y et al: The gastric mucosal barrier in thermally injured patients: correlation with gastroduodenal endoscopy. Surg Forum 25: 414, 1974

77. McElwee HP, Sirinek KR, Levine BA: Cimetidine affords protection equal to antacids in prevention of stress ulceration following thermal injury. Surgery 86: 620, 1979

78. McIrvine AJ, O'Mahony JB, Saporoschetz I et al: Depressed immune response in burn patients: use of monoclonal antibodies and functional assays to define the role of suppressor cells. Ann Surg 196: 297, 1982

79. McManus AT: Examination of neutrophil function in a rat model of decreased host resistance following burn trauma. Rev Infect Dis 5(Suppl 5): S898, 1983

80. McManus WF, Goodwin CW, Pruitt BA Jr: Subeschar treatment of burn wound infection. Arch Surg 118: 291, 1983

81. McManus WF, Hunt JL, Pruitt BA Jr: Postburn convulsive disorders in children. J Trauma 14: 396, 1974

82. Monafo WW: The treatment of burn shock by the intravenous and oral administration of hypertonic lactated saline solution. J Trauma 10: 575, 1970

83. Monafo WW, Aulenbacher CE, Pappalardo C: Early tangential excision of the eschars of major burns. Arch Surg 104: 503, 1972

84. Moncrief JA, Lindberg RB, Switzer WE et al: Use of topical antibacterial therapy in the treatment of the burn wound. Arch Surg 92: 558, 1966

85. Moncrief JA, Lindberg RB, Switzer WE et al: The use of a topical sulfonamide in the control of burn wound sepsis. J Trauma 6: 407, 1966

86. Moritz AR, Henriques FC, Jr.: Studies of thermal injury. II. The relative importance of time and surface temperature in causation of cutaneous burns. Am J Pathol 23: 695, 1947

87. Moyer CA, Brentano L, Gravens DL et al: Treatment of large human burns with 0.5% silver nitrate solution. Arch Surg 90: 812, 1965

88. Moylan JA, Chan CK: Inhalation injury—an increasing problem. Ann Surg 188: 34, 1978

89. Moylan JA, Inge WW, Jr., Pruitt BA, Jr.: Circulatory changes following circumferential extremity burns evaluated by the ultrasonic flowmeter: an analysis of 60 thermally injured limbs. J Trauma 11: 763, 1971

90. Moylan JA, Mason AD, Jr., Rogers PW: Postburn shock: a critical evaluation of resuscitation. J Trauma 13: 354, 1973

91. Moylan JA, Reckler JM, Mason AD, Jr.: Resuscitation with hypertonic lactate saline in thermal injury. Am J Surg 125: 580, 1973

92. Moylan JA, Jr., Wilmore DW, Mouton DE, et al: Early diagnosis of inhalation injury using [133]xenon lung scan. Ann Surg 176: 477, 1972

93. Munster AM, Hoagland HC, Pruitt BA, Jr.: The effect of thermal injury on serum immunoglobulins. Ann Surg 172: 965, 1970

94. Newsome TW, Curreri PW, Eurenius K: Visceral injuries: an unusual complication of an electrical burn. Arch Surg 105: 494, 1972

95. Ninnemann JL, Stein MD: Bacterial endotoxin and the generation of suppressor T cells following thermal injury. J Trauma 20: 959, 1980

96. Nordstrom H, Lennquist S, Lindell B et al: Hypophosphataemia in severe burns. Acta Chir Scand 143: 395, 1977

97. Ogawa M, Tamura H, Katsurada K et al: Respiratory changes in carbon monoxide poisoning with reference to hyperbaric oxygenation. Med J Osaka Univ 22: 251, 1972

98. O'Neill JA, Jr., Pruitt BA, Jr., Moncrief JA: Studies of renal function during the early postburn period. p. 95. In Matter P, Barclay TL, Konickova Z (eds): Research in Burns, Hans Huber, Bern, 1971

99. Parascandolo K: Experimentelle untersuchungen uber verbrennung. Wein Med Wochnschr 54: 575–579, 1904; Cited by Harkins HN: Treatment of Burns, Charles C Thomas, Springfield, IL, 1942

100. Pardoe R, Minami RT, Sato RM et al: Phenol burns. Burns 3: 29, 1976

101. Petroff PA, Hander EW, Clayton WH et al: Pulmonary function studies after smoke inhalation. Am J Surg 132: 346, 1976

102. Petroff PA, Hander EW, Mason AD, Jr.: Ventilatory patterns following burn injury and effect of sulfamylon. J Trauma 15: 650, 1975

103. Petroff PA, Pruitt BA, Jr.: Pulmonary disease in the burn patient. p. 95. In Artz CP, Moncrief JA and Pruitt BA, Jr. (eds): Burns: A Team Approach. WB Saunders, Philadelphia, 1979

104. Ponten B, Erikson U, Johansson SH et al: New

orbservations on tissue changes along the pathway of the current in an electrical injury. Scand J Plast Reconstr Surg 4: 75, 1970

105. Pruitt BA: The universal trauma model. 1984 Scudder Oration. Bull Am Coll Surg 70: 2, 1985 198x

106. Pruitt BA, Jr.: The diagnosis and treatment of infection in the burn patient. Burns 11(2): 79, 1984

107. Pruitt BA, Jr.: The universal trauma model. 1984 Scudder Oration, Bull Am Coll Surg 70: 2, 1985 198x

108. Pruitt BA, Jr.: Infections of burns and other wounds caused by *Pseudomonas aeruginosa*. p. 55. In Sabath LD (ed): *Pseudomonas aeruginosa; the Organism, Diseases it Causes, and Their Treatment*. Hans Huber, Berne, 1980

109. Pruitt BA, Jr.: The burn patient. II. Later care and complications of thermal injury. Curr Probl Surg 16, (5): 45, 1979

110. Pruitt BA, Jr.: The burn patient. II. Later care and complications of thermal injury. Curr Probl Surg 16, (5): 12, 1979

111. Pruitt BA, Jr.: Multidisciplinary care and research for burn injury. J Trauma 17: 263, 1977

112. Pruitt BA, Jr.: Postburn hypermetabolism and nutrition of the burn patient. p. 396. In Ballinger WF, Collins JA, Drucker WR, et al (eds): Manual of Surgical Nutrition. WB Saunders, Philadelphia, 1975

113. Pruitt BA, Jr., Curreri PW: The burn wound and its care. Arch Surg 103: 461, 1971

114. Pruitt BA, Jr., Dowling JA, Moncrief JA: Escharotomy in early burn care. Arch Surg 96: 502, 1963

115. Pruitt BA, Jr., Edlich RF: Treatment of bitumen burns. JAMA 247: 1565, 1982

116. Pruitt BA, Jr., Erickson DR, Morris: Progressive pulmonary insufficiency and other pulmonary complications of thermal injury. J Trauma 15: 369, 1975

117. Pruitt BA, Jr., Flemma RJ, DiVincenti FC et al: Pulmonary complications in burn patients. J Thorac Cardiovasc Surg 59: 7, 1970

118. Pruitt BA, Jr., Flemma RJ, DiVincenti FC et al: Pulmonary complications in burn patients: a comparative study of 697 patients. J Thorac Cardiovasc Surg 59: 7, 1970

119. Pruitt BA, Jr., Foley FD: The use of biopsies in burn patient care. Surgery 73: 887, 1973

120. Pruitt BA, Jr., Goodwin CW, Jr.: Nutritional management of the seriously ill burned patient. p. 63. In Winters RW (ed): Nutritional Support of the Seriously Ill Patient. Academic Press, New York, 1983

121. Pruitt BA, Jr., Goodwin CW, Jr.: Stress ulcer disease in the burned patient. World J Surg 5: 209, 1981

122. Pruitt BA, Jr., Lindberg RB: *Pseudomonas aeruginosa* infections in burn patients. p. 339. In Doggett RG (ed): *Pseudomonas aeruginosa*. Academic Press, New York, 1979

123. Pruitt BA, Jr., Mason AD, Jr.: Hemodynamic studies of burned patients during resuscitation. p. 83. In Matter P, Barclay TL, Konickova Z (eds): Research in Burns. Hans Huber, Bern, 1971

124. Pruitt BA, Jr., Mason AD, Jr., Moncrief JA: Hemodynamic changes in the early postburn patient: the influence of fluid administration and of a vasodilator (hydralazine). J Trauma 11: 36, 1971

125. Pruitt BA, Jr., McManus WF, Kim SH et al: Diagnosis and treatment of cannula-related intravenous sepsis in burn patients. Ann Surg 191: 546, 1980

126. Pruitt BA, Jr., O'Neill JA, Jr., Moncrief JA et al: Successful control of burn wound sepsis. JAMA 203: 1054, 1968

127. Pruitt BA, Jr., Tumbusch WT, Mason AD, Jr., et al: Mortality in 1100 consecutive burns treated at a burns unit. Ann Surg 159: 396, 1964

128. Reiss E, Stirman JA, Artz CP et al: Fluid and electrolyte balance in burns. JAMA 152: 1309, 1953

129. Remensnyder JP: Topography of tissue oxygen tension changes in acute burn edema. Arch Surg 105: 477, 1972

130. Robson MC, Murphy RC, Heggers JP: A new explanation for the progressive tissue loss in electrical injuries. Plast Reconstr Surg 73: 431, 1984

131. Saffle JR, Crandall A, Warden GD: Cataracts: a long-term complication of electrical injury. J Trauma 25: 17, 1985

132. Salisbury RE, Loveless S, Silverstein P et al: Postburn edema of the upper extremity: evaluation of present treatment. J Trauma 13: 857, 1973

133. Salisbury RE, McKeel DW, Mason AD, Jr.: Ischemic necrosis of the intrinsic muscles of the hand after thermal injuries. J Bone Joint Surg 56A: 1701, 1974

134. Shimazaki S, Yoshioka T, Tanaka N et al: Body fluid changes during hypertonic lactated saline solution therapy for burn shock. J Trauma 17: 38, 1977

135. Shirani KZ, Vaughan GM, Robertson GL et al: Inappropriate vasopressin secretion (SIADH) in burned patients. J Trauma 23: 217, 1983

136. Shoemaker WC, Vladeck BC, Bassin R et al: Burn pathophysiology in man. I. Sequential hemodynamic alterations. J Surg Res 14: 64, 1973

137. Sneve H: The treatment of burns and skin grafting. JAMA 45: 1, 1905

138. Snelling CF, Shaw K: The effect of topical epinephrine hydrocholoride in saline on blood loss

following tangential excision of burn wounds. Plast Reconstr Surg 72: 830, 1983

139. Sorensen B, Fisker MP, Steensen JP et al: Acute excision or exposure treatment? Final results of a three year randomized controlled clinical trial. Scand J Plast Reconstr Surg 18: 87, 1984

140. Strome DR, Newman JJ, Goodwin CW, Jr., et al: Mechanisms of reduced lipolytic response in rat adipocytes following thermal injury. Surg Forum 34: 103, 1983

141. Tranbaugh RF, Lewis FR, Christensen JM et al: Lung water changes after thermal injury: the effects of crystalloid resuscitation and sepsis. Ann Surg 192: 479, 1980

142. Tvedten HW, Till GO, Ward PA: Mediators of lung injury in mice following systemic activation of complement. Am J Pathol 119: 92, 1985

143. Underhill FP: The significance of anhydremia in extensive superficial burns. JAMA 95: 852, 1930

144. Warden GD, Wilmore DW, Rogers PW et al: Hypernatremic state in hypermetabolic burn patients. Arch Surg 106: 420, 1973

145. Warden GD, Wilmore DW, Rogers PW et al: Hypernatremic state in hypermetabolic burn patients. Arch Surg 106: 420, 1973

146. White MG, Asch MJ: Acid-base effects of topical mafenide acetate in the burn patient. N Engl J Med 284: 1281, 1971

147. Wilmore DW: The Metabolic Management of the Critically Ill. Plenum Press, New York, 1977

148. Wilmore DW: Hormonal responses and their effect on metabolism. Surg Clin North Am 56: 999, 1976

149. Wilmore DW: Carbohydrate metabolism in trauma. Clin Endocrinol Metabol 5: 731, 1976

150. Wilmore DW, Lindsey CA, Moylan JA et al: Hyperglucagonemia after burns. Lancet 1: 73, 1974

151. Wilmore DW, Long JM, Mason AD, Jr., et al: Catecholamines: mediator of the hypermetabolic response to thermal injury. Ann Surg 180: 653, 1974

152. Wilmore DW, Mason AD, Jr., Johnson DW et al: Effect of ambient temperature on heat production and heat loss in burn patients. J Appl Physiol 38: 593, 1975

153. Wilmore DW, Moylan JA, Helmkamp GM et al: Clinical evaluation of a 10% intravenous fat emulsion for parenteral nutrition in thermally injured patients. Ann Surg 178: 503, 1973

154. Wilson JS, Moncrief JA: Vapor pressure of normal and burned skin. Ann Surg 162: 130, 1965

155. Winter PM, Miller JN: Carbon monoxide poisoning. JAMA 236: 1502, 1976

156. Woolfrey BF, Fox JM, Quall CO: An evaluation of burn wound quantitative microbiology. I. Quantitative eschar cultures. Am J Clin Pathol 75: 532, 1981

157. Zarem HA, Rattenborg CC, Harmel MH: Carbon monoxide toxicity in human fire victims. Arch Surg 107: 851, 1973

158. Zawacki BE, Azen SP, Imbus SH et al: Multifactorial probit analysis of mortality in burned patients. Ann Surg 189: 1, 1979

37

Hyperbaric Oxygen Therapy for Gas Gangrene and Carbon Monoxide Poisoning

Roy A.M. Myers

GAS GANGRENE

Gas gangrene classically relates to the clinical picture of gas in the tissues produced by a clostridial infection, detectable by palpation and radiography. The disease is associated with rapid deterioration and a high mortality/morbidity ratio. In reality, the diagnosis of gas gangrene reflects a series of clinical conditions relating to both clostridial and nonclostridial organisms. In our experience, the nonclostridial types of infection are far more common. A major problem exists in differentiating among entities.

The first description of gas gangrene was probably reported by Hippocrates (ca. 470 to 400 B.C.). He described a rapidly progressing disease involving swelling of the foot, a reddishness about the ankle, and the development of small black blisters; this was followed by a high fever and madness and by death on the second day of the illness.[35] In 1562, Paré described the wounded at the Seige of Rouen, and one suspects that gas gangrene was being described.[55]

Fabricius Hildanus,[42] in a letter written in 1607, detailed a classic description of gas gangrene. His patient had intense pain with edema, skin discoloration, and crepitus in the tissues, with the early formation of bullae and rapid spread from the lower to upper leg, scrotum, and trunk; the outcome was fatal. He described a number of other patients with very similar conditions and noted crepitus and escape of air when incising the tissue. In 1829, Larrey[50] vividly described traumatic gangrene with a rapidly fatal outcome (in less than 10 hours) during the Napoleonic wars. Malgaigne[52] described the gas liberated from the wound as being inflammable and determined that it was hydrogen sulfide (H_2S).

Clostridium perfringens, or *C. welchii*, was first isolated in 1892 by Welch and Nuttall[78] from gas gangrene infections. Other species were then described, including *C. novyi*

(C. oedematiens) and *C. septicum.*[55] For clarification, it is best to regard gas gangrene as the invasive anaerobic infection specifically involving muscle, profound toxemia, massive tissue destruction, edema, variable gas production in the tissues, and death. The muscle lesion is necrosis rather than inflammation and is a consequence of toxin liberation in an anaerobic environment. Robb-Smith[67] was the first to describe the muscle lesion as a myonecrosis. Because the lesion is not isolated in muscle and has components of severe necrotizing cellulitis, it can be confused with similar clinical presentations caused by other anaerobic organisms. The latter types of infections are particularly common in diabetics.[10,58] A different therapeutic approach is required in this condition; in essence, a more aggressive surgical approach to the removal of infection and infected material is needed.

Gas gangrene has commonly been associated with combat injuries. The documented incidence of clostridial infections during World War I was 12 percent.[17] This fell to less than 1 percent in World War II[51] and to under 0.1 percent in the Korean War.[38] These falling incidences are attributable to a multiplicity of factors, particularly improved methods of local wound care, nonclosure of wounds, and improved evacuation from the front line. These lessons appear not to have been understood in the civilian conflict situation: 27 cases of gas gangrene were reported in Miami, Florida, over a 10-year period compared with 22 cases during the 8 years of the Vietnam conflict.[11]

Because of the ubiquitous nature of clostridial organisms and the ease with which they contaminate wounds, it is surprising that the incidence of clostridial infections appears to be diminishing. It is readily understood when one realizes that open wound treatment results in exposure of the wound to an ambient oxygen concentration in the air of more than 140 mmHg. This relatively high level of oxygen inhibits the organisms from becoming a problem. Wounds that are immediately closed provide an anaerobic environment in which the organisms proliferate; thus, the contamination becomes the infection. Primary wound closure is greatly favored in civilian practice and is responsible for the increased incidence of the infection. In the front-line situation, quick and adequate debridement is undertaken; delayed wound closure follows because of the urgent need to evacuate the patients.[11]

The major factors associated with the development of clostridial infection in a traumatized wound relate to (1) the presence of foreign material in the wound; (2) ischemia as a consequence of damaged blood supply; and (3) swelling, edema, and occlusive effects from plaster dressings with fractures.

Accidental trauma remains the commonest associated factor, accounting for up to 66 percent of all clinical cases.[32] More commonly, the disease is associated with puncture wounds, open fractures, drug addiction resulting in intravenous injection sites and indurated tissue around the sites, prolonged tourniquet applications or immobilization casts, foreign bodies in wounds with hemorrhagic or necrotic tissue as a consequence of trauma, high-velocity missile wounds, prolonged delay of surgery, traumatic or surgical interruption of blood supply, and criminal abortion. The net result of these factors is the development of a hypoxic environment, with the reduced oxidation–reduction (redox) potential necessary for the development of bacterial proliferation. The clostridial organism is a common wound contaminant and requires only an anaerobic environment in which to proliferate. Thus, one is facing a specific set of circumstances in addition to the presence of the organisms.

There are two other situations in which clostridial infection may develop: after some surgical procedures and spontaneously in an immune-deficient host. The condition has been reported after amputation for peripheral vascular disease; after intramuscular injections and femoral venipuncture; following surgery to gallbladder, common bile duct, appendix, small bowel, and stomach; and after hernia repairs. It has also been noted in patients with perforations of the esophagus, with retroperitoneal rupture of the duodenum, after hip nailing, with thermal burns, following endoscopy, and after vaginal delivery.[32] Because of the late diagnosis in these situations, the condition is extensive and far advanced at the time of discovery and has a higher mortality compared with that in patients who develop gas gangrene after trauma.[36] In patients with altered immunologic status such as carcinomatosis and diabetes, spontaneous metastatic clostridial gas gangrene can occur (Fig. 37-1). There is no relation-

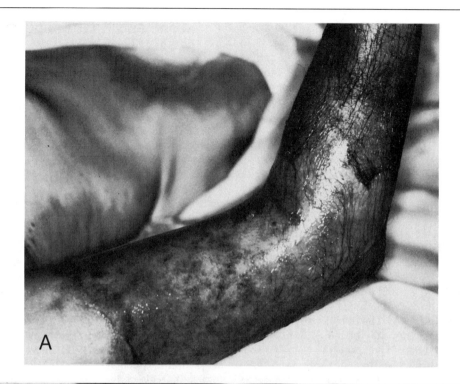

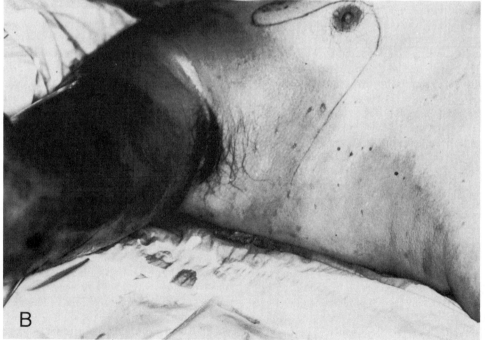

FIG. 37–1 (A) Classic clostridial myonecrosis originating in elbow region. Proximal and distal gas extension and tissue involvement. **(B)** Two hours later, massive extension of inflammatory process: from arm to shoulder, axilla to hip.

ship to major trauma, and the condition has a rapid and usually fulminating outcome.[47] In all these situations, a lowered oxygen reduction potential results from circulatory failure in the local tissues; thus, they become hypoxic, providing the organism with the appropriate milieu for proliferation.

Bacteriology

The clostridial organism is a large gram-positive anaerobic bacillus with a central or subterminal spore, as seen in growth on an artificial medium. It is a ubiquitous organism and is found in soil, dust, water, and the intestinal tract of humans and animals. In humans, it is particularly evident in the large bowel and diseased gallbladders. The bacilli are of the genus *Clostridium*. They may be motile or nonmotile depending on the species. More than 100 species have been described, but only six of these are reported to cause clinical clostridium gas gangrene in humans. *Clostridium perfringens*, occurring in 80 percent of described cases, is the most common cause of the condition. It is found worldwide except in the North African desert. Most of the *Clostridium* species are strictly anaerobic and are unable to multiply in living tissues. However, *C. perfringens* is not a strict anerobe and may grow freely in oxygen tensions up to 30 mmHg and with restricted growth in up to 70 mmHg of oxygen. Seldom is only one of the clostridial organisms isolated from a wound: invariably, the wound is infected with many clostridial organisms, such as *C. novyi* (40 percent), *C. septicum* (20 percent), and other species (less than 10 percent).[13,51] In a review of 34 patients, Caplan[13] found 29 patients having more than one organism in their wound. *Enterococcus* (in 50 percent), *Escherichia coli* (in 32 percent), *Staphylococcus* (in 29 percent), and *Enterobacter* (in 23 percent) as well as clostridial organisms were found in wounds.[13] A major difficulty exists in making the diagnosis of clostridial infection rather than clostridial contamination. A similar experience was reported by Niinikoski and Aho[59] with the same type of mixed flora.

Toxins and Host Response

More than 20 different exotoxins are produced by the clostridial organisms. Of these, nine are responsible for the local and systemic effects of gas gangrene. The major presentation is an inflammatory response with the production of a nonpurulent drainage. Included in the many exotoxins are the α-, θ-, κ-, μ-, and ν-toxins, fibrinolysin, neuraminidase, circulating factor, and bursting factor.[36,51] The α-toxin is an oxygen-stable lecithinase-c; it has hemolytic and necrotizing effects and is lethal.[27,48,60] It is able to hydrolyze intact lecithin, producing phosphatidylcholine and a water-insoluble diglyceride. Its action is synergistic with the hyaluronidase hemolysins and elastases, resulting in a rapidly spreading liquefactive necrosis characteristic of the condition. The other clostridial species are responsible for producing several toxins, including fetortoxin, which is cardiotoxic and produces hemolysis and necrosis; κ-toxin, which lyses protease; and other toxins that affect the immunologic receptors on erythrocytes and inhibit phagocytosis.[36] With constant production of these toxins, the clostridial infection is progressive, dependent on the production and liberation of these toxins, which are detoxified in the liver and kidneys and also become tissue fixed. In general, the total clinical picture of hemolysis, anemia, jaundice, renal failure with hemoglobinuria, tissue necrosis, cardiotoxicity, and brain dysfunction is believed to be a direct result of the production of various toxins.

Incidence

The estimated incidence of gas gangrene varies greatly from between 900 and 1,000 patients per year[36] to 3,000 per year.[29] In reviewing 187,936 major open wounds, Altemeier and Furste[2] determined the incidence to be between 0.03 percent and 5.2 percent, depending on wound type and treatment. In postabortion clostridial gangrene, the reported incidence was 0.5 to 1 percent.[73]

The Maryland Institute for Emergency

Medical Services Systems (MIEMSS), a tertiary referral center for trauma, has a hyperbaric chamber facility. Over the past 14 years, more than 145 patients have been referred to MIEMSS with clostridial infections. In addition to these, more than 400 patients with nonclostridial gas gangrene have been treated.

Clinical Manifestations

The incubation time varies greatly, from 1 hour[53] to as much as 41 days.[3] In general, it is short and, depending on the situation in which it develops (i.e., war or peace), the period may be shorter or longer. Studying the infection in Bulgaria, Kiranov[45] determined that during war, 87 percent of cases involved an incubation period of 4 days; in peace time, the same percentage was achieved at day 11. Antibiotic prophylaxis does not guarantee prevention of clostridial infections.[62] In essence, a high degree of suspicion is essential if one is to make an early diagnosis, at which time the treatment of the condition is much easier and a more satisfactory outcome can be achieved.

MacLennan[51] divided the histotoxic clostridial infections into three forms: simple contamination, anaerobic cellulitis, and myonecrosis or gangrene. It must be stressed that the full range of clostridial soft tissue infections is far more complex.

SIMPLE CONTAMINATION OF SOFT TISSUE

In this situation, there are no clinical signs of sepsis. This forms the most common setting in which clostridial organisms can be isolated from clinical specimens. Clostridia can be cultured from 10 percent to 30 percent of traumatic wounds in civilians and up to 80 percent of war wounds. There is no difference in the frequency of isolation of clostridia from well-healing posttraumatic open wounds or from suppurative wounds. It is thus imperative that the diagnosis of clostridial infection be made on clinical grounds, not on bacteriologic isolation.

SUPPURATIVE INFECTION WITHOUT SIGNS OF MYONECROSIS OR TOXEMIA

This is the most common form of clostridial disease. Organisms have been isolated from about one in four intra-abdominal infections. Finegold et al.[26] isolated clostridia in 6 percent of female patients with suppurative infections of the genital tract; clostridial organisms have been obtained from transtracheal aspirates or empyema fluid in 10 percent of patients with anaerobic pleuropulmonary infections. The clostridial organisms are part of a mixed anaerobic flora. Clinically, the patients do not present with clostridial toxemia, and it is not possible to differentiate the role of clostridia from that of any other organism in the same wound.

CLOSTRIDIAL CELLULITIS WITHOUT TOXICITY

This condition involves a localized infection of the skin and soft tissue with no systemic signs of toxicity. There may be invasion and local necrosis, which is idolent and spreads slowly to contiguous areas. These are seen in stump infections of amputees, perirectal abscesses, diabetic foot ulcers, and decubitus ulcers. By progressive contiguous advancement and suppurative destruction, the muscles may become involved, but there is no myonecrosis.

CLOSTRIDIAL CELLULITIS WITH TOXICITY

This type of infection may be seen in heroin addicts who present with localized pain and tenderness and develop fluctuation in the area, indicating a collection of fluid requiring surgical drainage. These lesions are commonly on thighs and forearms; in some patients, they are not related to trauma or heroin injections. There may be subcutaneous abscesses, purulent myocytis, and fasciitis. On culture, pure clostridia or mixed infections with aerobes and anaerobes may be found. Crepitus may be present but does not necessarily indicate a poor prognosis. The lesions are commonly seen in the feet of diabetic patients and may progress, with development of extension and further toxicity.

DIFFUSE SPREADING CELLULITIS WITH FASCIITIS

This form may rapidly spread through fascial planes, with production of gas, suppuration, and systemic signs similar to those of overwhelming clostridial toxemia. On palpation, there is diffuse subcutaneous crepitus but relatively little pain. Evidence of systemic spread includes shock, renal failure, and intravascular hemolysis. The major difference between this condition and true clostridial myonecrosis is the absence of myonecrosis. However, there may be mild inflammatory reaction in the muscle groups adjacent to the affected fascia or subcutaneous tissue. This condition may occur in association with silent carcinoma of the large bowel, in which it is devastating. It may present as a spontaneous nontraumatic clostridial infection and may arise from subcutaneous and intramuscular injections of contaminated material. With the use of vasoconstrictor drugs such as epinephrine, minor trauma may provide a route of entry for the pathogen. It must be emphasized that, except for the absence of myonecrosis, the disease is very similar to classic clostridial gas gangrene. The general clinical picture of this type of infection is rapid spread of crepitus via the fascial planes over a period of hours, with overwhelming toxemia and death.

TRUE CLOSTRIDIAL MYONECROSIS OR GAS GANGRENE

Indications of this condition are muscle involvement with destruction, local crepitus, and systemic signs of toxemia. The incubation period varies from hours to weeks but is usually 2 to 3 days. The onset of the disease is acute, with pain being the earliest and most severe symptom. This increases in severity and extends beyond the original borders over the next few hours (Fig. 37-1B). Systemic toxicity rapidly ensues. The skin becomes edematous and tense; it is initially pale and then becomes magenta blue. Accompanying this are large hemorrhagic bullae teeming with organisms. The hallmark of the condition is now apparent: abundant gram-positive rods but very few inflammatory cells in the smear. The patients become ill, pale, and sweaty. Mentally, the patient is oriented to time and place but has a flattening of affect, *la belle indifference.* There may be heightened alertness and awareness of surroundings, with a sense of impending doom. The patient lapses into toxic delirium and coma prior to death. The skin of the involved limb shows characteristic changes with an initial profuse serous or serosanguineous discharge having a sweet, mousey odor. The skin becomes red, yellow, brown, green, or black and is covered by blebs and bullae, which may develop very rapidly into the fulminant type of the disease. Examination of the muscles at this stage shows at first a pale muscle with edema; progression of the infection leads to a loss of contractility, absence of bleeding, and a change to a brick red color, with gas bubbles between the muscle fibers. The muscle is frankly gangrenous black and friable just before death (Fig. 37-2). Systemic shock is associated with renal failure and jaundice. The brain, eye, and liver may be involved with hemorrhages. The lungs may show pulmonary infarction, and gas-containing pleural fluid may be present in the pleural cavity. Radiographically, gas bubbles are seen in the lines of the muscle fibers. The presence or absence of gas is, however, of little diagnostic significance because more than 50 percent of the patients have no gas. Organisms associated with the infection may be responsible for the gas production.

The uterus is an important site of clostridial infection. An acute necrotizing endometritis can develop, which most commonly follows septic abortion, but can occasionally complicate normal deliveries, particularly if the membranes have been ruptured for some time. Bloodstream invasion by toxigenic clostridia rarely occurs as a complication of myonecrosis. It may follow endometrial or intestinal tract involvement. Organisms in the circulation do not always manifest clinically or in the lethal form.[65] As a result of the activity of the lecithinases, there may be rapid and massive hemolysis with clostridial bacteremia. This may lead

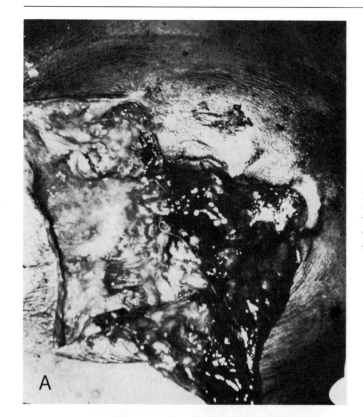

FIG. 37–2 (A) Postgallbladder surgery, right subcostal incision. Presented on postoperative day 5 as wound dehiscence. **(B)** Adequate debridement with excision of all necrotic skin, fat, fascia, and muscle.

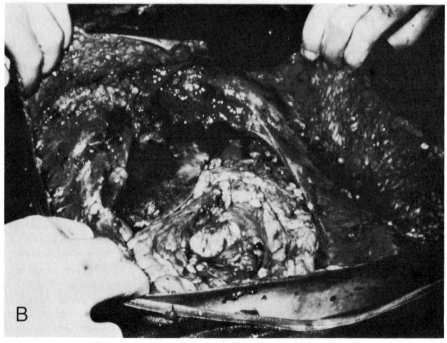

TABLE 37-1. Classification of Clostridial Infections

Category	Type	Subtype	Example
I	Simple clostridial contamination		Traumatic wound
II	Clostridial cellulitis	Suppurative	Intra-abdominal infections (1 in 4)
			Female genital tract
			Anaerobic pleuropulmonary infections
		Without toxicity	Infected stumps; diabetic foot ulcers
		With toxicity	Heroin addicts' injection sites
		Diffuse spreading with fasciitis	Metastatic clostridial infection from silent carcinoma
			IM, SC injections of contaminated material
III	Clostridial myonecrosis; true gas gangrene	Spreading	Classic gas gangrene
IV	Primary organ involvement		Uterus
			Gallbladder

(Modified from Altemeier WA, Fullen WD: Prevention and treatment of gas gangrene. JAMA 217: 806, 1971.)

to severe intoxication or renal shutdown from acute tubular necrosis.

A classification of clostridial infections is presented in Table 37-1. This is the author's modification of Altemeier and Fullen's[1] table as modified by Hart et al.[29] in an endeavor to describe clinical indications for surgery verses strictly medical and hyperbaric treatments. According to this classification, types IIC, IID, III, and IV require primary surgery with the addition of antibiotics and hyperbaric therapy, as suggested by Hart et al.[29]

NONCLOSTRIDIAL LESIONS SIMULATING GAS GANGRENE (NECROTIZING SOFT TISSUE INFECTIONS)

Symptomatology resembling that of clostridial gas gangrene is produced by many other organisms. Significant diagnostic skill is necessary to differentiate these conditions, and great confusion exists regarding the definition of these various conditions in the literature. Part of the confusion results from the location of the infection, whether it is necrotizing subcutaneous tissue, fascia, muscles, or a skin lesion. In many situations, more than one level of tissue is involved; thus, the clinical entities are quite blurred. A variety of names have been given to these conditions, including acute nonclostridial crepitant cellulitis, nonclostridial gas gangrene, synergistic necrotizing cellulitis, necrotizing cellulitis, bacterial synergistic gangrene, gangreous or necrotizing erysipelas, hemolytic streptococcal gangrene, necrotizing fasciitis, and Fournier's gangrene. Further complicating these presentations are the facts that some of them are associated with traumatic wound infections and others with nontraumatic wound infections such as those of vascular gangrene or idiopathic origin.

Other causes of gas in tissues may result from traumatic wounds from punctures, shotguns, or knives penetrating subcutaneous tissues. Wounds of the lungs, bronchi, esophagus, and gut, with gas escaping into the soft tissues and peritoneal cavity, may also allow air in the tissues. Gases injected under high pressure, blast injuries, iatrogenic causes, and jet irrigation of wounds can all produce soft tissue gas. In most of these situations, the clinical presentation is a relatively benign condition in the face of large amounts of gas. Chemicals may also be responsible for causing gas in soft tissues, for example, wound contamination with benzol or magnesium. Tissue or wound irrigation with hydrogen peroxide may similarly produce gas in the soft tissues.

A useful clinical division of soft tissue infections is as follows: (1) crepitant anaerobic cellulitis, (2) necrotizing fasciitis, (3) nonclostridial myonecrosis, (4) clostridial myonecrosis, (5) fungal necrotizing cellulitis, and (6) miscellaneous necrotizing infections in the immunocompromised host. This latter type of infection occurs in patients with wounds from trauma or surgery contaminated with foreign bodies and in patients who are diabetic and/or have vascular insufficiency. There is local tissue hypoxia and a decreased oxidation reduction potential, which promotes the growth of the anaerobic organisms. In general, these are endogenous organisms arising from the microflora of mucous membranes. Under hypoxic conditions, there is proliferation of both facultative aerobic and anaerobic organisms. The latter develop as a result of the growth of the aerobic organisms changing the oxidation reduction potential in the area, permitting the anerobic organisms to become established and grow more rapidly. Clinically, the soft tissue infections appear as tender, red, hard, swollen wounds with ecchymoses, blisters, dermal gangrene, crepitus, and edema without clear margins. There is marked tissue necrosis, a putrid discharge, and production of gas (usually hydrogen). The spread is through soft tissues and fascial planes (Fig. 37-2A). In some situations, the classic signs of tissue inflammation are absent. A wide range of systemic responses occurs, including fever, tachycardia, hypovolemia and hypocalcemia, hypoalbuminurea, and severely edematous wounds with ecchymoses, blisters, and crepitus, indicating a far advanced clinical problem. The edema, necrosis, and liquefaction of soft tissues may or may not involve the deep fascia.[10,54,74,80] With spread of the infection through the subcutaneous planes, the vessels are involved by the inflammatory process with secondary thrombosis, overlying skin infarction, and secondary infection. If the fascia is initially involved with progression of the process, the infection may penetrate anatomic planes deep to the fascia and thus extend around muscle groups, with compromise of the blood supply and secondary infection. The mid-sized arteries and veins may be surrounded by acute inflammatory processes, with subsequent thrombosis of arterioles and venules. When the muscles become involved, the condition is termed "necrotizing myositis."

CREPITANT ANAEROBIC CELLULITIS

This condition manifests as a necrotic soft tissue infection with abundant connective tissue gas. It often occurs in patients who have experienced local trauma and who have a com-

promised vascular supply, such as peripheral vascular insufficiency of the lower limbs. The infection is composed of multiple aerobic and anaerobic organisms, including *Bacteroides, Peptostreptococcus, Clostridia,* and Enterobacter. There is often a lack of marked systemic toxicity, gradule onset in the condition, and less severe pain. There is no muscle involvement, and the condition is essentially a cellulitis.

NECROTIZING FASCIITIS

This condition carries a high mortality rate, ranging up to 40 percent. First described by Meleney,[54] it consists of a hemolytic streptococcal gangrene. Meleney's clinical assessment was excellent but, in his time, the culturing techniques were inadequate to demonstrate the other organisms present, which specifically include *Streptococcus pyogenes.* In this condition, there is extensive necrosis of the superficial and deep fascia, with extensive dissection of the infection along the fascial planes. There is significant systemic toxicity. Necrosis of the overlying skin occurs as a result of thrombosis of subcutaneous blood vessels. Initially there is severe pain, but necrosis of the overlying skin through involvement of cutaneous nerves creates analgesia. The patient usually has had minor trauma or surgery, and the condition is most commonly seen in patients exhibiting small vessel disease such as diabetes. Multiple organisms have been isolated: *Peptostreptococcus, Bacteroides,* and *Fusobacterium* species. In addition to these anaerobic organisms, aerobic organisms have also been found: *Streptococcus* sp., *Staphylococcus aureus,* and Enterobacter.

NONCLOSTRIDIAL MYONECROSIS

Stone and Martin[74] described a nonclostridial myonecrosis that results from a synergistic necrotizing cellulitis with an aggressive soft tissue invasion. The infection is similar to clostridial myonecrosis with a propensity for involvement of the muscle tissue. This muscle tissue involvement differentiates it from the traditional necrotizing fasciitis. Skin and subcutaneous tissue may be involved as well. There is significant local tenderness with minimal skin changes except for the drainage of a foul-smelling dishwater pus from ulcers that may be present on the skin. There is significant systemic toxicity. The condition most commonly involves the perineal region with extensions from perirectal abscesses in a person with a compromised peripheral vascular supply. Again, multiple organisms have been isolated from this type of infection and include *Peptostreptococcus, Bacteroides,* Enterobacter, and *Peptococcus* sp. The mortality rate is very high, ranging from 50 to 75 percent.

Diagnosis

The diagnosis of clostridial gas gangrene must be made on the basis of both clinical and bacteriologic findings. A high degree of suspicion must be entertained, and one must not wait for culture confirmation of the infection. Such delay often results in the patient's death. Myositis and myonecrosis are the fundamental clinical signs of the condition. Gas visualization on radiographic examination is also a typical sign, and the skin findings of discoloration are also classic. A Gram's stain from the blister secretions must be undertaken immediately. When the gram-positive club-shaped rod is found, occasionally with the terminal spore and a lack of leukocytes on the smear, one must consider this case diagnosed as clostridial infection. At this time of suspicion of the diagnosis, one must adopt an aggressive therapeutic approach (Fig. 37-2B). Samples for bacteriology must be taken from deep muscle tissue and superficial smears. In this situation, a needle aspiration may be undertaken.

Prophylaxis

Prevention of the infection can be achieved by proper wound management and care. Adequate early and meticulous debride-

ment of all wounds is essential, particularly in higher-risk patients with compromised vascular supply, extensive trauma, and high-velocity trauma. Hemostatis must be meticulous and deep wounds should be left widely open and adequately drained to be closed at a secondary procedure. Tight dressings and plaster casts must be avoided. In patients with deep penetrating wounds in the perineum and pelvis, buttocks, or upper legs or with decubitus ulcers or perianal and ischiorectal abscesses, the aggressive use of colostomies should be undertaken. In patients particularly at risk with peripheral vascular disease or diabetes, delayed closure of traumatic wounds or lower limb amputations is important. Open fractures should be carefully treated; internal fixation and closure should be avoided in the early stages. It is essential that a high degree of suspicion be entertained in any patient with a wound at risk. When there is any possibility of gas gangrene development, wound care should be meticulous.

PROPHYLACTIC ANTIBIOTICS

Penicillin is the antibiotic of choice; however, the prophylactic application of penicillin may not be possible because of drug allergy. In this situation, chloramphenicol[25] and erythromycin[31] have been used. Tetracycline and clindamycin are not recommended because of the relative resistance of clostridial organisms to these drugs. Penicillin should be given as early as possible and in the dose of 10 million IU/day, either IV or IM.[25]

POLYVALENT ANTITOXIN

The effectiveness of polyvalent antitoxin has not been proved. Altemeier and Fullen[1] describe the lack of effectiveness of prophylactic administration of gas gangrene antitoxin at the time of injury. This antitoxin has been discontinued in their surgical service since 1943. The National Research Council and U.S. Department of Defense do not give gas gangrene antitoxin prophylactically. However, Altemeier[1] does state that polyvalent gas gangrene antitoxin is given before and after operation (50,000 units every 4 to 6 hours for 24 to 48 hours). This has been given particularly to patients with profound toxemia and hypotension. Many surgeons doubt the efficacy of this antitoxin and express concern about the development of anaphylactic reaction to the serum.[66,72,76,77]

Treatment

In a critique of gas gangrene therapy, Pierce[64] pointed out that "the modern treatment of gas gangrene involves the simultaneous use of antibiotics, surgical debridement, and hyperbaric oxygen." None is rightly primary and none is merely an adjunct. All should be used together with knowledge and skill to save lives and reduce limb loss. A major influence on surgeons' approach to treatment has been the work of Altemeier and Fullen,[1] who noted in 1971 that, until well-controlled studies have been undertaken, hyperbaric oxygen therapy should be considered experimental. They stated that no other therapy has replaced good surgery. However, their review of the literature was incomplete; a reference to Irvine et al.[40] indicated that even in animal experimentation, hyperbaric oxygen had not been shown to be useful. Consequently, many surgeons were prejudiced in favor of operation and equally prejudiced against hyperbaric oxygen. An interesting sideline is that it is apparently irrelevant that there have been no controlled operative studies showing the value of surgery above other forms of therapy in clostridial gas gangrene.

RATIONALE FOR HYPERBARIC OXYGEN THERAPY

Bert,[7] in 1878, was the first to demonstrate the inhibition of growth of anaerobic organisms by exposing them to high-pressure oxygen. Ozorio De Almeida and Pacheco[61] unsuccessfully used oxygen in experimentally induced gas gangrene in 1941. This was followed in 1961 by Brummelkamp et al.[12] using guinea pigs inoculated with clostridial organisms and treated with and without high-pressure oxygen.

Three experiments were conducted with four control animals and four treated animals in each; the treated animals were exposed to 3 atm of absolute pressure (ATA) of hyperbaric oxygen. The first group was inoculated with 0.25 ml clostridial inoculum subcutaneously; all four control animals became ill (ulceration developed in two). The hyperbaric oxygen-treated animals had no illness or ulceration. In the second group, 0.5 ml inoculum was given subcutaneously. All four control animals became ill and showed the development of ulceration, whereas in only one of the hyperbaric oxygen-treated animals did ulceration develop. In the final experiment, 0.5 ml clostridial organisms was inoculated intramuscularly. All four control animals became ill and showed ulceration, and two died. In the hyperbaric oxygen-treated group, ulceration occurred in only two cases. In a second experiment, broth cultures of *C. perfringens* were exposed to varying degrees of high-pressure oxygen. With an exposure for 1½ hours at a pressure of 2 ATA, the toxin production was normal. At 3 ATA, however, there was no further toxin production. The measured partial pressure of oxygen in this broth at 3 ATA was 250 mmHg.

Using a Beckman electrode and measuring 5 cm deep in the phlegmon of a patient with clinical gas gangrene, Schoemaker[70] was able to determine that, at 2 ATA of oxygen pressure, the partial pressure of oxygen in the gangrenous area was 250 mmHg of oxygen. However, at 3 ATA, the partial pressure of oxygen was 330 mmHg. At 3 ATA even in the gangrenous phlegmon, the toxin is fixed and thus inhibited. Once the toxin production is halted, the disease cycle is broken and tissue death ceases.

Van Unnik[75] was able to demonstrate in 1965 that α-toxin production was inhibited by exposure of the clostridial organism to 3 ATA oxygen pressure. The toxin already elaborated and fixed in the tissues was not detoxified by this oxygen. Once the cycle of toxin elaboration and symptom production has been broken, residual toxin is fixed and destroyed by the tissues, with a rapid clinical improvement. There is, however, a cyclical phase to production and, as new organisms develop from spores, they will then produce new toxin. It is for this theoretical reason that hyperbaric oxygen is instituted on a repetitive basis.

In 1966, Hunt et al.[39] were able to create a dead space within the tissue of rabbits, which they could infect and sample at will. Hyperbaric oxygen at 2 ATA did not modify the bacterial count or duration of infection in the rabbits. The oxygen tension in the model was a maximum of 178 mmHg. Repeating the experiments at 3 ATA, there was reduction in the bacterial count and in the type of infection in the rabbit, showing the need for at least 3 ATA pressure for sufficient oxygen toxicity on the clostridial organism.[39]

In both in vitro and in vivo studies, Hill and Osterhout[33] showed that high oxygen concentrations were able to overcome the catalase effects in necrotizing tissue. In plain trypticase soy agar, oxygen under increased pressure appeared to be bactericidal. Two percent whole human blood and, to a lesser extent, muscle tissue protected against this inactivation. This protective action was due to catalase elaborated by the organism. Kaye,[41] in 1967, was able to demonstrate both in vitro and in vivo a bactericidal effect of hyperbaric oxygen on clostridial organisms. In 1970, Demello et al.[20] showed that hyperbaric oxygen reduced the germination rate of heat-activated spores of *C. perfringens.*

The rationale for the use of hyperbaric oxygen in the treatment of gas gangrene lies in the principle that progress of the disease is stopped by maintaining a pharmacologic barrier to its advancement. The high oxygen tension gradient at the advancing edge of the infection prevents progression of the infection.

Using implanted Silastic TM tonometers in the subcutaneous layer adjacent to the toxic clostridial cellulitis and measuring tissue oxygen and carbon dioxide tensions, Kivisaari and Niinikoski[46] were able to show that the tissue levels were significantly elevated during hyperbaric oxygenation therapy to levels of 500 mmHg O_2. This tension remained above the baseline for at least 30 minutes after decompression to normal air.

The mechanism whereby hyperbaric oxygen is able to elevate tissue oxygen levels significantly relates to the solubility of oxygen in plasma. In the normal situation with 97 percent saturation of the hemoglobin (Hb), 19.8 vol percent of oxygen is carried by Hb. In persons breathing 21 percent oxygen (as represented by air), 0.3 vol percent of oxygen is carried in simple solution in the plasma. When breathing 100 percent oxygen, this is increased to 2.1 vol percent of plasma carriage. With hyperbaric pressure, the amount of transported plasma oxygen increases by 2.3 vol percent per absolute pressure of atmosphere increase (for each 33 feet of seawater pressure equivalent, there is a 1 ATA increase). At 3 ATA, the plasma carriage of oxygen is 6.7 vol percent, which is able to provide the body with sufficient oxygen for total body oxygen needs without any red blood cell (RBC) carriage. The arterial and alveolar oxygen concentration at 3 ATA is 2,193 mmHg.

Animal Studies. Many animals have been used, ranging from mice and guinea pigs to dogs and rabbits. However, guinea pigs are particularly sensitive to pulmonary oxygen toxicity, which may obscure any therapeutic beneficial effects of hyperbaric oxygen. In the single negative animal experiment relating to hyperbaric oxygen and clostridial infections, Irvine used the guinea pig model. In his studies, a number of guinea pigs died from oxygen toxicity, which clouded the outcome. In other studies, mice, rabbits, and dogs have been shown to be far more suitable, particularly in relationship to oxygen toxicity. In numerous animal models,[19,21,34,40,41,43] a great variation of experimental methodology was undertaken, resulting in different outcomes. In general, a culture of clostridial organisms was injected into crushed muscle tissue of the hamstring muscle in various animal models. Epinephrine, sterile dirt, and calcium were used to simulate the types of infections in the human situation. Mortalities in the control animals ranged from 41 to 100 percent. When hyperbaric oxygen was used as the sole therapy, mortality was substantially reduced, even when hyperbaric therapy was delayed up to 18 hours. Delays of over 18 hours created no change from the control situation.[34,43] In trials conducted by Irvine et al.[40] and Demello et al.[19,21] antibiotics were used. In Demello's trials, surgical debridement was added to the protocol. In all the experiments, there was significant reduction in mortality when hyperbaric oxygen was used. The one exception to this was Irvine's experiments, in which a number of the guinea pigs died from oxygen toxicity. In Demello's experimentation with the use of hyperbaric oxygen, antibiotics, and debridement together, the mortality rate was reduced from 50 to 5 percent in dogs and somewhat less in rabbits and guinea pigs. In addition to the decrease in mortality, tissue loss was reduced with the use of hyperbaric oxygen. Hill and Osterhout[34] showed that control mice inoculated with clostridial organisms in a lower extremity became emaciated and deformed. Fifty percent of the survivors sloughed the entire extremity, in sharp contrast to the hyperbaric-treated survivors, in which major tissue loss did not occur. This large volume of animal experimentation shows that the initial statements by Altemeier[1] may need modification in light of recent scientific knowledge. There seems to be little doubt that hyperbaric oxygen has a dramatic effect in tissue and life salvage in the animal studies. It is now incumbent on surgeons to prove, in a randomized trial, that extensive surgery alone is as effective as hyperbaric oxygen followed by lesser surgery.

Major Clinical Series. The first human case of clostridial gas gangrene treated with hyperbaric oxygen was attempted by Brummelkamp et al. in Amsterdam in 1960.[12] The major problems experienced in trying to determine the effectivity of specific therapies in the treatment of clostridial gas gangrene have been due to the sporadic nature of the disease and the fact that very few investigators have any extensive experience with this condition. There are multiple variables: (1) the type of receiving center (i.e., whether a tertiary referral center or a primary receiving center); (2) the types of antibiotics used; (3) whether surgery has been used initially or after the addition of antibiotics and hyperbaric therapy; (4) what time in the disease phase the patients presented; and (5) at what stage in the presentation the mortalities occurred. The amount of tissue ablation and limb amputation is not clearly stated in most series.

In Altemeier and Fullen's series,[1] hyperbaric oxygen was specifically excluded. It is difficult to compare this group with hyperbaric oxygen-treated groups because most of the patients in that series developed clostridial gas gangrene while in the hospital and were thus treated early with high amputations. Most patients treated with hyperbaric oxygen come to a hyperbaric facility through a referral system; patients come from a wide geographic area and thus there are considerable delays in treatment with hyperbaric oxygen. In addition, most cases were referred for hyperbaric oxygen when all other forms of treatment had failed, which inevitably included extensive surgery and antibiotics.

The major clinical series reported[1,9,18,24, 28–30,32,36,37,62,76] vary significantly in their descriptions of the severity of the illness, the distribution of the illness, what types of treatment were given, whether there were amputations or no amputations, and, ultimately, the mortality rate. Altemeier's series of 54 cases[1] shows that primary surgery was the major form of therapy, with many high amputations and a mortality rate of 14.8 percent. From this information, it is very difficult to determine the actual severity of illness; because all patients in the series were in a primary system without being referred, one must assume that the disease was identified early and treated aggressively. In other series, the distribution ranges from unknown to posttraumatic, postoperative, or occult; involving trunk, neck, or pelvis; treated within 24 hours of onset or 24 hours or more after onset; and treated with hyperbaric oxygen, surgery, and antibiotics. In other reports,[37,62] the primary treatment is unknown.

The mortality rate varies considerably with posttrauma, postoperative, or occult onset, with the latter having the highest mortality rate. In the review by Heimbach et al.,[32] the mortality rate was 5.1 percent when hyperbaric oxygen was begun within 24 hours of onset. This is the lowest mortality rate reported and reflects the experiences of the Air Force in San Antonio.[31] The experience of Boerema and Brummelkamp[8] in Europe was reported and updated by Bakker.[4] Their experience with 341 cases of clostridial gas gangrene confirmed clinically and bacteriologically is one of the largest reported series in the world. Most of their patients developed the disease as a result of accidents, with 225 patients being involved in traffic, industrial, agricultural, or sports accidents. Their second group of cases, 93 in number, occurred after acute or elective operation; amputation for arteriosclerotic and/or diabetic

TABLE 37-2. Clinical Series of Clostridial Gas Gangrene

Reference	No. of Cases	Distribution	Primary Treatment	Amputations	Mortality (%)	Morbidity and Mortality (%)
Altemeier and Fullen (1971)[1]	54	Unknown	Surgery	Many high	14.8	—
Boerema and Groeneveld (1970)[9]	118	All severe	HBO, no radical surg	27 of 85 involving lower extremities	22.2	—
Davis and Dunn (1973)[18]	23 (267 cited)	Unknown	HBO	Unknown	21.7	—
Eraklis et al. (1969)[24]	15	Posttrauma 6 Postop 5 Occult 4	HBO	Some tissue saved	46.6	—
Guidi et al. (1981)[28]	21	Trunk, neck, and pelvis	Surg and HBO equal	10, no amputation	20	—
Hart et al. (1974)[30]	44	Posttrauma 27 Postop 11 Occult 6	HBO, debridement after HBO	6 of 28	7.4 27.2 83.5	— 22.7 —
Hart et al. (1983)[29]	139	Posttrauma Head and trunk 15 Extremity 58	HBO + antib + surg	1.7 (25%)	20 5	— 32
		Postop Head and trunk 21 Extremity 8	HBO + antib + surg	2 (17%)	19 38	— 31
		Spontaneous Head and trunk 24 Extremity 13	HBO + antib + surg	5 (33%)	46 23	— 50
Heimbach et al. (1977)[32]	58	Treatment within 24 hr	HBO	Unknown	5.1	—
Hitchcock et al. (1975)[36]	44	Unknown	Surg + antib	Unknown	45	—
	89	Posttrauma 45 Postop 45 Occult 2	HBO	Unknown	5.8 35 50	— 21.8
Holland et al. (1975)[37]	49	Extremity 26 Trunk 8 Combined 15	Unknown	Unknown	7.7 47 50	— 26.5
Parker (1969)[62]	56	Postop	Unknown	Unknown	51.3	—
VanZyl (1966)[76]	170	Posttrauma 156 Postop 23 No trauma 14	HBO	Much tissue saved	25	—

HBO, hyperbaric oxygen; surg, surgery; antib, antibiotics.

gangrene was the commonest postoperative cause. Other relatively common causes were colon surgery and cholecystectomy. The final group of patients, numbering 23, acquired the disease after intramuscular injections, ergotamine injections, and injection of other compounds given to patients with rheumatoid arthritis, diabetes, or leukemia. There were also three cases following criminal abortion and two following insect stings. The mortality rates were 11.5 percent in group 1, 32.3 percent in group 2, and 60.9 percent in group 3, for a combined overall mortality rate of 20.2 percent. These figures include patients dying 4 or more days after therapy as a result of pulmonary embolism, cardiac infarction, metastatic colonic carcinoma, and manifest gas gangrene. In all, 10.6 percent of the total mortality was a direct result of clostridial infection. Analysis of the patients who died, a total of 36 of 341 cases, showed that all 36 patients had died within 26 hours after the start of hyperbaric oxygen therapy, that is, before the fourth session. This dramatically demonstrates the importance of initiating therapy within the first 24 hours after onset. Where this did occur, there was complete salvage of all patients.

The other important feature in the work from Amsterdam is the effect of hyperbaric oxygen therapy on reducing the amputation rate. Of 254 patients with gas gangrene of the extremities, 54 had already undergone amputations elsewhere before receiving hyperbaric oxygen. Of the remaining 200, 24 percent (48 of 200) required amputation after completion of hyperbaric therapy. In 11 of these cases, re-amputational stump correction was carried out in the primary amputated group, and in 19 cases, ablation was undertaken in an extremity that was already considered lost at the time of admission. In the remaining 18 cases (9 percent), amputation had to be undertaken despite hyperbaric oxygen therapy. From this, it can be seen that the amputation rate using hyperbaric therapy was far lower than was achieved after primary surgery, 50 percent[14] and 55 percent.[28] Hart et al.[29] reported a 17 percent amputation rate with combined therapeutic management. As a result of their experiences, the Amsterdam group "postulated that primary surgery in the case of clostridial gas gangrene of the extremities is contraindicated."

The work of Hitchcock et al.[36] supports these findings: 44 patients were treated by wide surgical debridement and antibiotics and had a mortality rate of 45 percent; a second group of 89 patients had hyperbaric oxygen added to the approach of debridement and antibiotics and the mortality rate was reduced to 22 percent. The experience of Holland et al.[37] again supports this, with an overall mortality rate of 26.5 percent in 49 patients. Where the infection was limited to the extremity, the mortality rate was 7.7 percent, but where there was spread to the trunk prior to admission, the mortality rate was 47 percent. In the cases of combined trunk and limb involvement, the mortality rate was 50 percent. In reporting of the work in the Air Force with 58 patients, Heimbach et al.[32] showed that when hyperbaric oxygen was begun within 24 hours of onset, the mortality rate was 5.1 percent. In addition, when no amputations had been performed before referral, 59 percent left the hospital with functional limbs. In a questionnaire to treaters of clostridial infections, VanZyl[76] was able to estimate the amount of tissues saved by not making conventional surgical decisions initially and only doing so after hyperbaric oxygen had been undertaken. Of the 47 cases analyzed, 23 saved between 90 and 100 percent of tissue, 4 between 60 and 80 percent, and 16 between 20 and 40 percent. The remaining 4 were under 10 to 20 percent[76] (Table 37-2).

It is thus evident that the weight of the clinical literature is in favor of the use of hyperbaric oxygen to reduce mortality and increase the amount of actual tissue salvage, including reduced amputations.

Application of Hyperbaric Oxygen Therapy

The initial work by Boerema[8] indicating the effectiveness of hyperbaric oxygen therapy and the associated reduction in surgical ablative techniques has created a dilemma for the surgical field and the hyperbaric physician. Heimbach[31] reviewed 116 case reports and commentaries on the efficacy of hyperbaric oxygen in the treatment of clostridial gas gangrene. From this he determined that the cumulative mortality of the series is approximately

25 percent and that the disease-specific fatality rate is 15 percent. When treatment was begun within 24 hours of presumptive diagnosis of gas gangrene, the disease-specific fatality rate was 5 percent.

Many referrals to hyperbaric units are done at a late stage in the disease, after all other therapy has been offered. Our own experience shows similar results: of 110 patients treated, the condition had developed in only 2 cases in MIEMSS; the rest had been transferred from other hospitals. It must be stressed that hyperbaric therapy is used as an adjunct to surgery and antibiotic therapy. Where all three are being used, the maximal treatment effect was noted by Demello et al.[20] Slack et al.[72] are very positive about the effects of combination of hyperbaric oxygen with antibiotics and surgery. Physicians in hyperbaric oxygen facilities have no doubt of the effectiveness of all three modalities combined, whereas persons without chambers, having no experience with the use of oxygen, continue ablative aggressive surgical therapy with high amputation rates and maintain the need for removal of all necrotic tissue in accordance with general surgical principles. A major problem with this approach is the lack of understanding of the mechanism of spread of intoxication and the specific oxygen action on the α-lecithinase and clostridial organism.

Pickleman[63] characterized the problem experienced by most surgeons in treating gas gangrene. He states that the use of hyperbaric oxygen in recent years has been extensively recommended but that no controlled studies have been carried out. Since facilities for the administration of hyperbaric oxygen are not widely available, radical debridement remains the definitive treatment for the patient with gas gangrene, with the adjunctive use of hyperbaric oxygen if it is conveniently available. Altemeier and Fullen[1] in 1971 also discussed the use of hyperbaric oxygen but felt that it was experimental and difficult to obtain. Their appreciation of the toxic effects of oxygen was somewhat exaggerated, and they too felt that hyperbaric oxygen therapy could not replace good surgery in the treatment of established gas gangrene.

However, there have been numerous changes in the field of hyperbaric medicine,

particularly over the last 3 years. In 1977, there were 37 functional hyperbaric units throughout the country; in June 1984, this number had grown to 200.[57,69] With this increase in hyperbaric chambers throughout the country, it is evident that the availability of this therapy is much greater than in earlier years. It now becomes feasible to transport a patient with known clostridial infection to a local hyperbaric chamber for combined therapy. With increased experience in clinical hyperbaric medicine, the considered dangers of oxygen have been notably reduced: The addition of air breaks during the oxygen breathing periods has greatly reduced the incidence of cerebral oxygen toxicity and convulsions. Limiting oxygen therapy to 90 minutes per dive has reduced the long-term pulmonary toxic effects as well. Thus, the objections to the general use of hyperbaric oxygen therapy in the treatment of gas gangrene have been considerably reduced. Whether a controlled clinical trial can be undertaken is difficult to determine because of the small numbers of patients seen by the various units. It is conceivable that pooling of the results may be a second means of comparing effectiveness.

Side Effects. Safe dose limits of oxygen exposure have been developed,[5,6,22] and a review of oxygen toxicity has been published by Clark and Lambertsen.[15,16] At sea level, 100 percent oxygen can be given continuously for up to 12 hours; however, prolongation beyond that may produce pulmonary oxygen toxicity.[49] A decrease in vital capacity is seen after 6 hours on 100 percent oxygen at 2 ATA. By 10 hours, severe pulmonary irritation is evident.[16] By mixing normoxic breathing with hyperbaric oxygen, this safe period of hyperbaric oxygen at 2 atm can be extended significantly.[79] Consequently, the hyperbaric routine that has been developed consists of 20-minute oxygen-breathing periods with 5-minute air breaks in order to enhance the safe time for oxygen breathing. At greater depths or pressures, central nervous system (CNS) manifestations of oxygen toxicity occur and culminate in a motor seizure. CNS oxygen toxicity should appear before pulmonary changes at 2.5 atm of 100 percent oxygen.[49] Because of concern for oxygen toxicity manifested by CNS symptoms, the maximum depth for 100 percent oxygen has been set at 66 feet of seawater or 3.0 ATA. In practice, 2 percent of patients treated at this depth for 90 minutes may go into oxygen convulsions. The treatment of this is rapid cessation of treatment with 100 percent oxygen and allowing the patient to breathe normoxic 3.0 ATA pressure air. Signs and symptoms rapidly reverse and no permanent damage has been noted. Animal experimentation work has been undertaken at extremes of pressure and 100 percent oxygen; permanent nerve tissue damage has occurred in the spinal cord in these cases. However, these depths are not used in the current clinical treatment schedules.

Pulmonary overpressure accidents can occur in any situation where breath-holding occurs during ascent after compressed gas breathing. In essence, the same type of lesion develops as in a patient on a ventilator who struggles against the machine and thus increases the intraalveolar pressures to the bursting point. These problems can be readily avoided by not decompressing a convulsing patient in whom the danger of breath-holding is present and by performing a predive evaluation of the patient to rule out bronchial asthma and pulmonary air-containing cysts or bullae. Provided the patient has an open airway and breathes normally during chamber decompression, there should be no pulmonary overpressure accidents.

Critical Care. Patients requiring critical care can receive hyperbaric oxygen therapy in a monoplace or multiplace chamber (see Fig. 37-3). Monoplace chambers have the ability for electroencephalographic (EEG), electrocardiographic (ECG), and intracranial pressure monitoring. Ventilator support is also available and intravenous infusions and medications can be continued with standard pump equipment. However, it is easier to provide this critical care in a multiplace chamber, where a nurse or physician can be with the patient. In the multiplace chamber, the same monitoring as in a critical care unit can be given in the chamber environment. The only modification is a pressure or volume-cycle ventilator. Attendants in the chamber can perform routine endotracheal intubation, defibrillation, intravenous or intracardiac drug administration, and general clinical assessment of patients. Blood samples can be undertaken during the treatment and sent through a pressure lock to the exterior, where they will then be analyzed in a regular laboratory. Suctioning can be undertaken in the multiplace chamber, and misadventures such as convulsions or pneumothorax can be readily controlled. In essence, it is important to have a specially trained staff to provide routine critical care treatment in the chamber. Attendant personnel should be adequately trained to equalize middle ear pressures during a dive.

Compressed air nitrogen narcosis, or rapture of the deep, usually occurs with deeper treatments than those normally carried out in the clinical field. This condition results from the high partial pressure of nitrogen, which produces symptoms of alcoholic intoxication and normally occurs at 100 feet of seawater, although occasionally at 50 feet. Other than these minor problems, there is very little difference between the requirements and ability of a person to function in a hyperbaric chamber as an inside tender compared with their normal function in a critical care unit. Thus, with careful planning, training, and teamwork, a seriously ill patient who would benefit from hyperbaric oxygen can safely be placed in a hyperbaric chamber with intensive care and critical care therapy being maintained at depth.

SURGERY

The dictim that "prevention is better than cure" is best demonstrated in the condition of clostridial gas gangrene. Aggressive local wound debridement, nonclosure of contaminated or potentially contaminated wounds, and removal of all foreign bodies and necrotic tissue have done much to prevent the development of the condition. Inevitably, where cases do develop, basic surgical principles have not been followed. Early diagnosis and aggressive treatment allow the disease to be more easily controlled. Simple treatment techniques such as removal of plaster casts, occlusive dressings, sutures, clips, and, in general, agents producing localized edema, compartment syndromes, and anoxia, which all may further spread the infection, are beneficial.

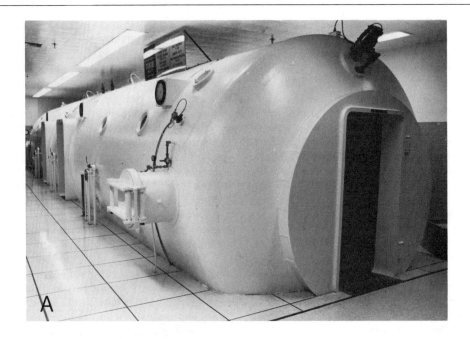

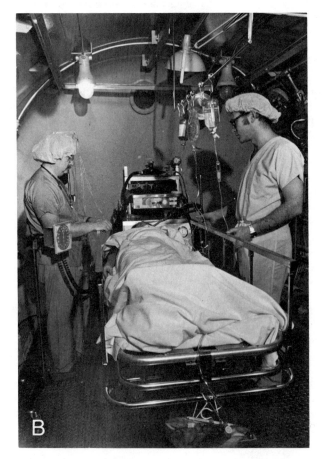

FIG.   37–3 (A) Multiplace   hyperbaric chamber. **(B)** Hyperbaric treatment of intubated and ventilated patient with smoke inhalation and carbon monoxide poisoning.

Where there is only contamination, local wound care and routine management of infected wounds are necessary. For localized cellulitis with clostridial organisms, incision and drainage may be the appropriate surgical technique. Spreading cellulitis or classical myonecrosis requires the triple approach of surgery, antibiotics, and hyperbaric oxygen.

There are two schools of thought regarding the appropriate time for surgical intervention. One supports aggressive ablative surgery, in which, in the face of a clostridial infection, aggressive debridement and even amputation are undertaken immediately.[44] The second school is that of Boerema and Groeneveld,[9] recommending a conservative surgical approach. In one series, 11 of 16 patients had primary or subsequent amputation.[56] Although these clinicians were aware of the effectiveness of hyperbaric oxygen therapy, that treatment was not available in their facility. In another report, four patients were treated with high-dose antibiotics and amputation and survived.[23] Emergency operative treatment is advocated, following Altemeier and Fullen's advice[1]; it is the most important therapy, with excision of a single muscle group being attempted wherever possible. When irreversible change has occurred in the muscle, guillotine-type open amputation is necessary. The surgery-only approach was generally used during the late 1960s and early 1970s.

As more experience is gained with the addition of hyperbaric oxygen therapy to the therapeutic armamentarium, there is mounting evidence that combined therapy is more appropriate for the treatment of clostridial gas gangrene. Hyperbarists and surgeons are fully in agreement about the need for fasciotomy and reduction of the compartmentlike syndrome (edema, inflammation, and toxemia of the spreading clostridial infection). There is fair debate as to the timing of the fasciotomy and debridement. Hyperbarists strongly advocate that fasiotomy be done initially, either before or after the first hyperbaric treatment, and that debridement be held until at least two hyperbaric oxygen treatments have been undertaken. The spread of the disease has generally been arrested by this time and a less toxic patient is then operated on, where demarcation lines are now evident as a result of the oxygen effect on the organisms and toxins.

Rodeing et al.[68] recommend the late use of surgery in the quiescent phase in patients in whom there has been complete demarcation of the wound. In their experience, surgery was delayed until hyperbaric oxygen had been completed and clear demarcation of necrotic tissue was evident.

On the basis of our experience, we fall between these two camps, strongly recommending early fasciotomy followed by hyperbaric oxygen therapy and subsequent debridement. Occasionally, toxicity persists; in such cases, surgery may need to be undertaken earlier, particularly if there is no response to hyperbaric oxygen therapy, or if a limb is obviously dead. At this stage, early amputation is essential to remove the mass of toxic tissue. Where ablative surgery is undertaken, the limb stump must be left open for secondary closure once complete control of the infection has been obtained and there are no further signs of toxicity in the patient. A positive culture in a clean wound does not necessarily indicate clostridial infection; spores may be found for months after successful treatment of a wound. At surgery, it is essential that minute attention be given to control of bleeding at the amputation or surgical site; otherwise, excessive bleeding may result, complicating the septic shock. Obviously, necrotic tissue can be excised, but it may be difficult to differentiate viable and nonviable tissue.

ANTIBIOTICS

In patients with true clostridial myonecrosis with no other associated organisms, penicillin is the drug of choice. Penicillin is given in large doses, between 6 and 20 million units every 24 hours, in divided doses.[14,31,37] The clostridial organism is exquisitely sensitive to this.[68] However, the American literature indicates that the usual clostridial infection is actually a mixed infection with numerous clostridia and other organisms.[13] In light of this, it is essential that other antibiotics be given. Patients who are allergic to penicillin can be given erythromycin as a second drug of choice in a dose of 4 g/day. Equally useful for adults and children is chloramphenicol in a dose of 50 to 100 mg/kg/day IV, in four divided doses. Particularly in view of the mixed infections, clindamycin (600 mg IV every 4 hours in adults and 5 mg/kg every 6 hours in children) and gentamycin (1.5 mg/kg in adults and 2.5 mg/kg in children are given every 8 hours) can be used. Metronidazole[71] has been used successfully in the treatment of clostridial and other anaerobic infections. Sodium penicillin should be used in place of potassium penicillin because these patients often show shock and poor renal function and have extensive tissue destruction with production of increased amounts of potassium and consequent electrolyte imbalance that would be exacerbated by potassium in the penicillin.

TETANUS PROPHYLAXIS

All patients with gas gangrene are at increased risk for the development of tetanus. They have the tissue milieu for clostridial growth and should have aggressive prophylaxis against tetanus. This should include both 500 units of tetanus immunoglobulin and 0.5 ml of tetanus toxoid injected intramuscularly at a different site. It is important to determine the patient's tetanus prophylactic status.

Summary of Management of Clostridial Myonecrosis

First, in establishing the diagnosis, the physician must consider the patient's history and be suspicious and particularly aware of pain and toxicity. The local wound should be examined for erythema, odor, discharge, bullae, and crepitus. The diagnosis is confirmed by gram-positive rods on a smear of the discharge and by the intramuscular vesicular gas pattern.

Second, once the diagnosis has been made, sutures are removed and wounds are opened when necessary. As part of the initial management, antibiotic coverage and umbrella are provided with a triple approach of penicillin, aminoglycoside, and clindamycin. The patient is resuscitated with fluids and blood as required. This is aimed specifically at treating shock.

Blood samples for laboratory investigations (Hb, Hct, leukocyte count, electrolytes,

renal and liver function tests, and ABGs) are obtained on admission. Roentgenograms are also taken of the affected limb.

Third, the patient is transferred to a medical facility with a hyperbaric unit.

Fourth, surgical debridement and hyperbaric oxygen therapy are started. Adequate monitoring is necessary, which is accomplished by placement of arterial lines and subclavian and Swan-Ganz catheters. At this stage, an intense combination of medical (fluids and antibiotics), surgical (wound care and debridement), and hyperbaric oxygen therapy is undertaken. Myringotomies should be performed, particularly in patients who are intubated, to prevent barotrauma to the ears consequent to increased pressure. This may be done rapidly. At a later stage, pressure-equalizing tubes can be inserted. The hyperbaric oxygen protocol developed by Boerema and Brummelkamp[8] involves three sessions of 2 hours each during the first 24 hours, followed by two sessions during the next 24 hours for the next 2 days, for a total of seven treatments in 72 hours.

Dressings are changed at 4-hour intervals or more frequently as necessary; a physiologic solution such as Ringer's lactate should be used to dilute the toxic exudate from the organism. Disinfectants are dangerous because they compromise tissue and wound margins. Hemostatis must be established to prevent catalase release from RBCs. All nonviable tissue should be excised to prevent the development of the appropriate milieu for anaerobic organisms. It usually takes 3 to 4 days of hyperbaric oxygen therapy to produce a clean, clear wound with no toxicity or hemolysis.

The final treatment phase is reconstructive. Administration of antibiotics, oxygen therapy, and grafting are complete, and skin closure is effected by whatever means possible.

CARBON MONOXIDE POISONING

Carbon monoxide is one of the oldest and most common agents of poisoning; it has been with us since humans first used fire for warmth, cooking, and defense. More than one half of the yearly poison deaths in this country are due to carbon monoxide.[156] The major causes of deaths from carbon monoxide are the incomplete combustion of organic material and smoke from fires of all kinds.[145] Automobile exhaust is a common source, with exposure occurring accidentally on the roads when rusted manifolds permit exhaust fumes to enter the driving cabin or intentionally, with an engine running in a closed garage.

Exhaust fumes occur both in home and in industrial situations. The propane forklift used in many industries for transporting and storing materials is a prolific producer of carbon monoxide, as is the machinery used to clear the ice rink during a hockey game intermission. Significantly increased levels have been observed in workers using these types of equipment. Improperly maintained heating systems are a common source, causing the more difficult to diagnose chronic type of poisoning; large numbers of people have been simultaneously poisoned in this situation. Improperly ventilated charcoal or Sterno fires also produce significant amounts of carbon monoxide.[117] Methylene chloride, a hydrocarbon solvent used in household and industrial aerosols and paint strippers, is converted in vivo to carbon monoxide.[143] As a result of economic changes and increased electricity rates, many Americans are returning to the use of wood and gas for cooking food and heating their homes. Inadequate or improper ventilation of these heaters and stoves readily results in carbon monoxide poisoning.[120] Significant problems of carbon monoxide poisoning may occur in the foundry industry, when green sand molds are heated during the pouring and casting phase.[73]

Pathophysiology

One mechanism of carbon monoxide poisoning has been known since 1857, when Claude Bernard reported that it caused a hypoxic death by its reversible combination with hemoglobin.[88] Haldane, in 1895, clearly described the equilibrium reactions.[114]

The effects of carbon monoxide in concentrations encountered clinically are based on a number of reactions. These include the combination with hemoglobin, displacement of oxygen, and subsequent disruption of oxygen transport systems. The laws governing the combination of hemoglobin with carbon monoxide and oxygen were established in the classic in vitro experiments on human blood by Douglas et al.,[98] during the early 1900s, who determined that the relative ratio of carboxyhemoglobin (COHb) to oxyhemoglobin is dependent on the relative partial pressures of oxygen and carbon monoxide in the immediate environment. It is thus not the partial pressure of carbon monoxide alone that affects the COHb concentration.

The affinity of carbon monoxide for hemoglobin is 230 to 270 times as great as that of oxygen. Haldane's first law is stated as follows:

$$M \cdot PCO/PO_2 = COHb/O_2Hb$$

where COHb is the concentration of COHb and O_2Hb represents the oxyhemoglobin concentration; M is the affinity constant, estimated at between 230 and 270; and PCO and PO_2 are the partial pressures of carbon monoxide and oxygen to which the hemoglobin molecule is exposed.

Other factors involved in the percentage saturation of COHb relate to workload, which is a measure of heart rate and ventilation during the exercise, or a reflection of the activity and of the varying oxygen partial pressures at the time of the exposure. The rate of carbon monoxide uptake is inversely proportional to the partial pressure of oxygen at the time of exposure.[143]

HYPOXIA

Carbon monoxide is rapidly absorbed through the lungs and readily combines with hemoglobin with greater affinity than does oxygen. Inspired concentrations of 0.01 percent can result in a COHb equilibrium concentration of 14 percent. Where this concentration increases to 0.05 percent, 44 percent COHb levels are noted. Several minutes of 0.1 percent carbon monoxide level will result in a 60 percent COHb level.[120] Further increases in carbon monoxide concentrations result in a dramatic increase in carbon monoxide saturation. At fire scenes, 10 percent levels of carbon monoxide in the smoke have been recorded. When firefighters do not use face masks, the strenuous activity and increased carbon monoxide levels can result in COHb levels of 75 percent in less than 1 minute.[152] Cigarette smoking produces COHb levels of more than 10 percent. Automobile exhausts contain carbon monoxide levels of up to 9 percent, whereas coal gas combustion produces 10 to 18 percent carbon monoxide levels.

The hypoxia is explained by the displacement of oxygen from hemoglobin by carbon monoxide. In the normal person, 20 ml oxygen per 100 ml of whole blood (20 vol percent) is measured. Normal cellular function requires the delivery of some 5 vol percent of oxygen, which is essentially the arteriovenous oxygen difference (a–vDO$_2$). With the hemoglobin sites occupied by carbon monoxide, a relative hypoxemia is produced, and the delivery of 5 vol percent oxygen at the tissue level only occurs at lower than normal cellular PO$_2$ level. The explanation of this reduction of mean cellular PO$_2$ in carbon monoxide poisoning stems from partial saturation of each hemoglobin molecule with carbon monoxide. This in turn results in a tighter binding of the remaining oxygen to the hemoglobin and produces a leftward shift of the oxyhemoglobin dissociation curve, where tissue oxygen is further lowered in order to release oxygen from the COHb molecule. The net result of these two components is a hypoxia of the tissues.

In addition to the combination of carbon monoxide with hemoglobin, it has an affinity for other iron-containing hemoproteins, such as myoglobin and cytochromes. Most of the carbon monoxide in the body is combined with hemoglobin. However, Coburn[94] calculated that some 10 to 15 percent carbon monoxide present in the extravascular tissues is combined with myoglobin and possibly with cytochrome. Myoglobin, acting as an oxygen reservoir, is part of the oxygen transport mechanism, delivering this oxygen when needed.[105] Oxygen has a greater affinity for myoglobin than for hemoglobin; the oxymyoglobin dissociation curve shows that affinity is present for a PO$_2$ of less than 60 mmHg. Like COHb, myoglobin also exhibits a leftward shift of the oxygen dissociation curve in the presence of carbon monoxide. Carbon monoxide has a greater affinity for cardiac than for skeletal muscle and will shift from the blood into the muscle under hypoxic conditions.[94] When tissue oxygen levels are restored to normal, the carbon monoxide from the myoglobin will reappear in the blood.

Low levels of carbon monoxide poisoning also may be a significant public health hazard. Several investigators[85,100,102] showed that increased COHb levels of the magnitude found after smoking or heavy atmospheric pollution impair exercise performance even in clinically normal subjects. Patients dying as a result of exposure to smoke inhalation, where the level of COHb poisoning was under 50 percent,[115] may in fact have died from a cardiac dysrhythmia as a result of this COHb union.[102] Acute circulatory failure and myocardial damages have occurred in 45 percent of some 270 cases dying from carbon monoxide poisoning. At autopsy, dilatation of the heart, pulmonary edema, and diminished potassium levels in the myocardium were evident, as were histologic lesions of the myocardial cells.[95] These dysrhythmias and hypotension of cardiac arrests produce further problems in survivors with the genesis of neurologic injuries as a result of anoxia. It then becomes difficult to determine the precise effects of carbon monoxide poisoning versus those of severe anoxia. Angina patients are particularly sensitive to carbon monoxide exposure, and the onset during physical exertion is accelerated by elevating COHb levels.[84] A wide range of cardiac changes have been seen, ranging from conduction defects to dysrhythmias, including ventricular fibrillation, low voltages, and depressed ST segments.[97,124] The precise mechanism is not fully understood.[116,129]

CELLULAR ASPHYXIA

The affinity of carbon monoxide for cellular cytochrome oxidase is lower than that for hemoglobin. Caughey[92] postulated a direct cellular function effect rather than an indirect one from carbon monoxide poisoning. Chance et al.[93] and Estabrook et al.[104] found that carbon monoxide inhibits the actions of the cytochrome system directly, by binding to these iron-containing proteins. Tissues with the highest metabolic rates, such as the CNS and heart, are more susceptible to the effects. It has been postulated that there is a direct carbon monoxide inhibition effect on cellular respiration where the carbon monoxide competes with oxygen for receptors on the cytochrome chain; the primary effect seems to be cytochrome a_3 and P450. Goldbaum et al.[111] showed that the physically dissolved carbon monoxide in the plasma is more important than the absolute COHb level, which only reflects a RBC-bound carbon monoxide. He postulates that the toxic action of carbon monoxide is on cellular respiration occurring in the mitochondria, where carbon monoxide competes with oxygen for cytochrome a_3. In experimental studies, neither the transfusion of erythrocytes containing 80 percent COHb nor the intraperitoneal ingestion of carbon monoxide gas produced toxic symptoms in dogs.[111] However, inhalation of carbon monoxide to levels similar to the above two forms and resulting in COHb levels of 65 percent or more was fatal within 15 to 65 minutes in all dogs. COHb is thus an indicator to the total-body carbon monoxide burden, but not the specific measurer of this level. The partially dissolved carbon monoxide in the plasma is not measured in the normal COHb assessment. The resolution of the actual role at the cellular level with cytochrome a_3 and P450 involvement is one of great controversy; in a review, Coburn[3,94] disputes the cytochrome story, maintaining that the coefficient of diffusion of carbon monoxide is such that when a low or zero level is registered on the RBC there should be a low or zero level at the tissue cellular level.

A major problem exists in relationship to the cause of the symptomatology as it relates to COHb levels. Geyer[108] replaced the blood of rats with perfluorochemical-type blood substitutes. The animals all survived indefinitely in a breathing mixture containing 10 percent carbon monoxide, which proved rapidly fatal to the normal rats with normal blood constituents. He mistakenly claimed that this showed the role of the COHb in producing hypoxia. The use of fluorohydrocarbon, however, allows for oxygen transport of some 7.04 vol percent in the dissolved solution. This exceeds the normally required 5 to 6 vol percent oxygen extracted from the arterial blood by the tissues

for normal function ($a-vDO_2$). The cytochrome oxidase system of myoglobin has a preference for oxygen nine times that of carbon monoxide[85] and the relatively high level of oxygen available in the fluorocarbon solution prevented carbon monoxide uptake by the tissues. Thus no tissue poisoning occurred, and all the rats survived. The actual mechanism of carbon monoxide poisoning is partly resolved, but much more needs to be determined, particularly whether there are raised levels in the brain and myocardium.

An indication that tissue carbon monoxide levels may have a far more significant role than has been previously accepted is evident in a report by Cramer,[96] relating to fetal death as a result of accidental maternal carbon monoxide poisoning. In this particular case, the mother and father were admitted to an emergency room after exposure to carbon monoxide from incomplete combustion in a natural gas kitchen stove used to heat the house at night. When they awoke, they experienced headaches and vomiting and were unable to leave the house. In the local emergency room the mother's COHb level was 23.7 percent and the father's 45 percent. Both patients were treated with 100 percent oxygen by nonrebreathing mask for 8 hours, by which time their COHb levels were below 3 percent. The following day, both were discharged home. Within 48 hours, the mother returned, having noted no fetal movements. Sonography confirmed the absence of fetal heart tones, and labor was induced with prostaglandin E_2 (PGE$_2$). A stillborn male infant was delivered. Blood from the infant, who showed the classic signs of cherry-red lips, pink nail beds, and pink skin in the nonmacerated areas as well as a right ventricular blood sample of 25 percent COHb, nevertheless was found to have a COHb level of 35.1 percent, on analysis of the liver and spleen tissue samples. The difference in levels of COHb between the right ventricle and the tissue preparations of spleen and liver must represent the intracellular deposition of carbon monoxide.

It is not surprising that the fetal levels were higher than the maternal levels, as there is usually a 10 to 15 percent greater fetal level than maternal level. Carbon monoxide crosses the placenta by simple diffusion[126] or by a carrier-mediated mechanism[108] and enters the fetal blood.[109,126] In addition, the placental carbon monoxide diffusion ability increases with gestational age in proportion to the weight of the fetus.[90] There is a slow, steady state of diffusion of carbon monoxide across the placenta, so that at about 10 hours exposure, the fetal COHb level exceeds the maternal level. Thus the degree of fetal hemoglobin saturation is dependent on the concentration of carbon monoxide and the length of exposure to inhalation by the mother.[127]

It is important to realize that the fetal PaO_2 level is normally 20 to 30 mmHg lower than the normal adult levels of 100 mmHg. The PaO_2 level in fetal blood decreases in proportion to the increasing COHb concentrations in the fetal and maternal blood. In the fetus, the oxyhemoglobin dissociation curve is normally to the left of the adult, which permits the discharge of oxygen at normally lower oxygen tensions in the fetal tissues. COHb poisoning causes a further shift to the left of both maternal and fetal oxyhemoglobin curves, substantially impairing the release of oxygen from the mother to the fetus and from fetal hemoglobin to fetal tissue. One of the earliest reports of fetal death with maternal survival was in 1924, by Philips, where the classic red tinging to the skin was found and appeared to have modified the process of maceration.[139] In reviewing the literature, Muller and Graham[130] found eight further cases in which maternal carbon monoxide intoxication had resulted in neonates showing a variety of psychomotor disturbances ranging from mental retardation to idiocy, and with hypotonia of extremities and necks. Fifteen more cases were discussed in which death of the fetus occurred.

Neuropathologic Lesions of Carbon Monoxide Poisoning

The precise mechanism of carbon monoxide effects on the CNS system is unknown. One of the principal carbon monoxide actions is that of competing with oxygen for binding sites on the hemoglobin molecule, thereby limiting the tissue oxygen supply.[114,144] It could be inferred that the cerebral metabolic effects will be similar to those seen in arterial hypoxemia.[150] Another proposed mechanism of symptomatology and neuropathologic lesions of carbon monoxide poisoning is a direct cellular action of carbon monoxide,[93,118,121] or this may be due to carbon monoxide-induced reduction of cerebral blood flow.[103,142] Thus, the basic mechanism(s) by which carbon monoxide causes cerebral damage remains undefined. In attempting to determine the metabolic effects of carbon monoxide intoxication on the rat brain using varying concentrations of carbon monoxide from 0.5 to 2 percent with 30-minute exposure, MacMillian[128] measured that the cerebral energy homeostasis was maintained until levels of 2 percent carbon monoxide intoxication were reached. At this level, there were significant decreases in systemic blood pressure, decreases in cerebral adenosine triphosphate (ATP), increases in adenosine diphosphate (ADP) and adenosine monophosphate (AMP), plus early depletion of tissue citrate and α-oxyglutarate. This pattern is very similar to that previously documented for various cerebral oligemic states, suggesting a possible modifying role for altered cerebral perfusion in the production of symptoms and pathology.

In the unanesthetized animal exposed to 1 percent carbon monoxide for 30 and 60 minutes, consciousness was retained, and a correlation was suggested between conscious behavior and cerebral energy state. Those animals exposed to 2 percent carbon monoxide for 30 minutes became unresponsive later on during exposure. In comparing carbon monoxide-induced changes in intermediary metabolites, energy phosphates, intracellular pH, and cytoplasmic redoxidates with those seen in hypoxemia, no basic qualitative or quantitative differences in the metabolic responses of brain tissue to the two conditions are indicated. Moderately advanced carbon monoxide exposure is associated with a high degree of resistance of the cerebral energy homeostasis. When this energy homeostasis is disrupted, it is partly related to hypotension and imminent cardiovascular collapse. Thus, the carbon monoxide-induced cardiovascular depression with limitation of cerebral blood flow may be one of the important modifying factors leading to cellular damage in carbon monoxide poisoning.[128]

Computed tomography (CT) has been used to investigate the degenerative changes induced in the brain by acute carbon monoxide poisoning[147] in patients who had been comatose for at least 6 hours. These patients were intubated on admission, and CT scan was done as early as possible before hyperbaric oxygen therapy, which was given at 3 ATA for 1 hour and repeated as the patient's condition required. The number of repeats ranged from 3 to 23 times. The CT scans were repeated from 2 to 8 times per person in the 21 patients assessed during the year following admission.

Two groups of patients were discerned from this study. One group showed no abnormalities; blood gases were found to have a pH more in the normal range, as well as a smaller base excess and larger bicarbonate levels. Their COHb levels were also higher, in the range of 40 percent. Nine of the 10 patients had good recoveries, and one had moderate disability. The second group of 11 patients showed abnormalities of reduced tissue density present in the globus pallidus after 2 weeks that remained after 3 months. One year later, repeat CT scan showed marked ventricular dilatation with cortical atrophy. The low-density areas remained in the globus pallidus. The outcome in this group was poor, with severe disability in three patients, vegatative state in five, and death in two. The low-density area changes were thought not to be due to cyst formation, breakdown of cellular structures from infarction, infection or massive coagulative necrosis as occurring in malignant tumors, or degenerative alterations, but that the direct effect of carbon monoxide poisoning could be brain edema leading to softening and necrosis, with the degenerative demyelination changes. Contradicting this, however, is the fact that these areas of low density are seldom demonstrated in the globus pallidus or other parts of the brain as a result of hypoxic disease. For this reason, Sawada et al.[147] suggested that carbon monoxide may have a specific cytotoxic action. Gray matter, with its many nerve cells, has a higher rate of oxygen consumption than white matter, and should thus be more susceptible to hypoxia. In acute carbon monoxide poisoning, however, the white matter is most severely affected, and very little associated gray matter damage is noted. The edema that occurs in the brain may be of a vasogenic origin due to the increase in extracellular fluid from increased vascular permeability. Thus, the detection of diffuse brain edema by CT scan in the early stages of carbon monoxide poisoning may be an indicator of a poor prognosis.[119]

Clinical Presentation

Clinical manifestations of carbon monoxide poisoning vary greatly and depend on a number of factors, including the level of concentration to which that patient was exposed, duration of the exposure, rate and depth of breathing, and the heart rate at the time. An essential component that has been underplayed is the time relationship between the exposure, the discovery of the patient, and the delay in time to get the patient from the scene to the hospital. Added to this are the problems of obtaining COHb results in every hospital, and the physician's awareness of the entity of carbon monoxide poisoning. Many of the early writings relating to carbon monoxide poisoning show classic symptoms found in emergency rooms, with long intervals between discovery and hospitalization reflecting a poor EMS delivery system, and a poorly developed resuscitation system where oxygen was not applied until the patient was hospitalized.

Classic symptomatology as described by Sayers and Davenport[148] in 1930 indicates very few symptoms with concentrations of COHb of less than 10 percent. Between 10 and 20 percent, the patient experiences tightness across the forehead and headache. Twenty to 30 percent saturation results in more pronounced symptomatology, with throbbing in the temple regions; from 30 to 40 percent, the patient has a very severe headache with generalized weakness, dizziness, dimness of vision, nausea, and vomiting and ultimately collapses. With levels approaching the 40 to 50 percent saturation, there may be syncope in addition to the previous symptoms, and increases in both pulse and respiratory rate. Concentrations of over 50 percent can lead to coma and intermittent convulsions, and at 60 percent saturation or above, death may accompany the depressed cardiac and respiratory function.

There is significant overlap of symptomatology with varying levels of carbon monoxide poisoning. The major problem is that one is only measuring a red cell load of carbon monoxide, and not the tissue load, which may be causing the symptoms. In our experience, the COHb level is only an indicator that the patient has been exposed to carbon monoxide poisoning but does not necessarily tell us the severity of poisoning. We have had many patients admitted to us in coma after exposure to carbon monoxide. Because of either a long delay between discovery and cessation of the generation of carbon monoxide or intervening treatment with normobaric oxygen, patients with low or zero levels of carbon monoxide have presented in a comatose state.[55] Other patients with levels of carbon monoxide poisoning above 50 percent have presented to our admitting area in an oriented, conscious state with minimal symptomatology. This wide discrepancy of clinical presentation in COHb level is unfortunately very common in our experience, indicating the need for the development of better means of determining CNS involvement with carbon monoxide poisoning.[133] There are no pathopneumonic symptoms, and carbon monoxide poisoning has been known to be an imitator of other illnesses, resulting in further delays in diagnosis and treatment.[113]

Physical findings in assessment of these patients vary greatly, dependent on the time relationship between discovery and treatment and the concentration of exposure. The most common include tachycardia and tachypnea. There are varied levels of blood pressure relating to whether or not shock is present. There may be mild hypotension with a systolic blood pressure in the range of 100 mmHg; however, hypertension has been reported.[158] The classic description of a cherry-red color is, in fact, exceptionally rare and most likely represents a true soaking with carbon monoxide caused by a significant length of exposure to carbon monoxide poisoning. The associated findings of exposure to smoke or toxic gas inhalation with soot in the nasal and upper airways, singed nasal hair, and voice changes with trachitis must also be considered as indicating the likelihood of exposure to carbon monoxide poisoning.

The most important clinical component of exposure relates to the cardiac and neurologic status. In our experience, the severe cardiac involvement presenting with hypotension, arrhythmias, and severe impairment of tissue perfusion is uncommon and usually fatal. The presence of heart disease in a patient with carbon monoxide poisoning results in severer symptomatology at lower COHb levels.

The nervous system is the other main symptom-producing system to be involved with carbon monoxide poisoning.[107] The major problem with attempts to correlate clinical carbon monoxide poisoning with animal model research is the lack of correlation of morbidity with COHb levels versus mortality and these levels. There is no animal research indicating morbidity. In a 3-year follow-up evaluation of unconscious carbon monoxide victims, Smith and Brandon[151] showed a 33 percent personality deterioration and a 43 percent memory impairment correlating directly with the level of consciousness on admission. In addition, 8 of the 71 patients showed gross neuropsychiatric damage. The one recent study indicating mortality and COHb levels is that by Halpin et al.,[115] in which some 37 percent of victims dying from smoke inhalation were found to have COHb levels below 50 percent. These victims died exclusively from smoke inhalation within 6 hours of exposure. Central nervous system morbidity is often subtle and overlooked in the normal situation.[122]

Our methodology of assessing normality is that relating to the Glasgow Coma Scale as well as to the general orientation of the patient. The questions asked of the patient are usually those of age, name, and address. Without corroboration from family members or the rescuers, these cannot be checked for accuracy in the emergency room. An attempt to be more specific will often include the question of what day it is. Where an error occurs, the physician often tends to overlook the mistake in favor of the patient, in the belief that it was a mistake that could have been made by anyone, but this error may, instead, be part of the abnormal neurologic presentation in the patient. In order to overcome this problem, we have developed and tested and are now routinely using a short psychometric screening battery that includes well-established psychometric tests. They were selected on the basis of two criteria: (1) they must have well-defined normal values and be amenable to administration in an emergency setting and (2) they must assess functions cited in the literature as vulnerable to the effects of carbon monoxide.[133]

The Maryland Institute for Emergency Medical Services Systems (MIEMSS) uses the following battery of tests[81,87,154,157]:

General orientation: to establish rapport with the patient and provide an informal assessment of mental status

Digit span: to assess short-term memory and ability to focus and maintain attention

Trail making: to test visual discrimination and temporospatial orientation

Digit symbol: to sample visuomotor coordination and visual discrimination (to determine the effects of toxic substances on neuropsychologic functioning)

Aphasia screening: to evaluate a variety of language and praxic functions (useful in detecting lateralized effects of disturbances of cerebral functioning)

Block design: to assess visuospatial functioning (especially vulnerable to right cerebral hemisphere dysfunctions)

We have succeeded in determining an 86 percent predictability of carbon monoxide poisoning versus normality from the use of our test battery and have found it a most appropriate method to determine diffuse cerebral dysfunction. The test has further been used to assess improvement; thus we have a tool with which to measure the effects of carbon monoxide poisoning without using the COHb level.

Diagnosis

Appropriate equipment is required to make the diagnosis of carbon monoxide poisoning. The possibility of carbon monoxide poisoning must be considered when there is suspicion of smoke, exhaust fumes, or substances related to carbon monoxide poisoning, and the clinical presentation is one of nausea, vomiting, mental confusion, dizziness, or unconsciousness. The picture may be clouded by the prior ingestion of alcohol; there is a high incidence of correlation between fires and alcohol, hence carbon monoxide poisoning problems. The tentative diagnosis should be verified as soon as possible by the direct measurement of blood COHb saturation in either arterial or venous blood or by analysis of the victim's exhaled air for carbon monoxide.

It is essential, however, that rapid initial treatment be based on clinical appearances, even before COHb levels are available for confirmation. It must also be stressed that the COHb measurement only measures RBC-loaded carbon monoxide; there are no tissue measurements for carbon monoxide. Should there have been a sufficient amount of time between the exposure completion or therapy recommencement and the drawing of blood samples, the COHb level may be within normal limits, and thus not represent the true insult, as a large portion of carbon monoxide has been off-gassed from the RBC.

Other parameters have been used in an endeavor to measure carbon monoxide effects, and these are nonspecific for carbon monoxide poisoning. The arterial blood gases may be deceptively normal, as the PO_2 level is a measure of oxygen dissolved in plasma and is not affected by changes in hemoglobin saturation. The blood-gas analyzer commonly uses this PO_2 value to calculate the total oxygen content and hemoglobin saturations, and these then appear normal. The specific measure of blood COHb should thus be obtained by carbon monoxide-oximetric determinations. Nonspecific changes in the arterial blood gases with a metabolic acidosis, and ECG abnormalities with nonspecific ST-wave changes and dysrhythmias, have been used in the past for evidence of carbon monoxide poisoning.[82,125] Computed tomography may also show nonspecific changes.[119,147] Electroencephalography has shown evidence of a diffuse frontal slow-wave activity consistent with metabolic encephalopathy and has been used to indicate carbon monoxide poisoning.[107,136] There are major problems with these tests in that they are nonspecific and not always readily available in the emergency situation when the diagnosis needs to be made. The diagnosis is made on the basis of detecting carbon monoxide in the blood and in the expired alveolar air. With a high index of suspicion, we believe a clinically effective way of assessing the severity of carbon monoxide toxicity would be to measure by psychometric testing, realizing that drugs may also alter these test results. However, this system is far more sensitive than the generally accepted medical history and assessment of orientation.

Prognostic Factors

It is apparent that there are no specific prognostic indicators as to the outcome of the patient suffering from carbon monoxide poisoning. The severely affected persons with coma do manifest CT-scan abnormalities of the basal ganglion region, which would appear to indicate a poorer outcome.[119,147] However, none of our other diagnostic indicators can be used for an effective prognostication of the outcome. The major problem is that no specific comparative trials have been used to compare the various treatments. The major literature reports on long-term and severe neuropsychiatric sequelae of carbon monoxide are those of earlier writings before aggressive oxygen therapy with normobaric or hyperbaric oxygen were used. Today's literature reviews would not appear to show the same incidence of severe neuropsychiatric distrubances. The milder types of disturbance have not been aggressively pursued as predictors of outcome; many of these subtle deficits have been ignored. The actual COHb level on admission is equally ineffective, as are abnormal blood gas, ECG, and EEG findings in prognostication of outcome. To further complicate the problem, there are no patients available with preexposure psychometric tests which can be compared to the postexposure tests. It is thus not possible to compare any preexposure neurologic situation with that of a patient postexposure, and therefore the ability to prognosticate and measure improvement on therapy is not available.

Treatment of Carbon Monoxide Poisoning

The transfer of carbon monoxide into cells is regulated by the PO_2 level of blood and body tissues. With PO_2 values of below 60 mmHg in the tissues, there is a relatively greater transfer of oxygen and carbon monoxide from hemoglobin to myoglobin, due to the nature of the oxyhemoglobin and oxymyoglobin dissociation curves. Higher-than-normal tissue concentrations of oxygen should halt the movement of carbon monoxide from hemoglobin to myoglobin and the cytochrome enzymes and also physically dilute the carbon monoxide tissue and blood levels. The use of high oxygen levels has been shown to reduce effectively the carbon monoxide half-life ($t\frac{1}{2}$). In 1942, End and Long[102] succeeded in demonstrating a dramatic reduction in half-life of carbon monoxide under hyperbaric conditions at 3 ATA, which was far more rapid than that of oxygen (95 percent), carbon dioxide (5 percent), or 100 percent oxygen alone at atmospheric pressure. The slowest half-life was that in air. They also showed a species difference, with dogs eliminating carbon monoxide far more rapidly than guinea pigs under similar conditions.[102] Review of the carbon monoxide half-life shows great variations from 3 to 5 hours in air to 30 to 80 minutes in 100 percent oxygen, and 20 to 30 minutes in hyperbaric oxygen.[120,123,138,148] Douglas et al.[98] showed that by using 95 percent oxygen and 5 percent carbogen the half-life clearance was faster than with 100 percent oxygen alone.

In assessing carbon monoxide half-life by using blood samples taken in the field and repeat samples from our admitting and treatment areas, we were able to reconfirm these wide variations under all aspects of treatment, that is, air, 100 percent oxygen, and hyperbaric oxygen.[132] However, wide individual differences as well as differences in the actual groups were evident (see Tables 37-3 and 37-4). Normobaric 100 percent oxygen ranges of 31.5 to 149.7 minutes and hyperbaric oxygen ranges of 4.2 to 86.4 minutes were found. The shortest half-times were found in one patient in whom the normobaric oxygen half-life was 31.5 minutes, and 4.2 minutes in hyperbaric ox-

TABLE 37-3. Patients Treated First with 100 Percent Oxygen at Surface and Then at 66 Feet[a] Seawater Pressure (3 ATA)

Patient	Initial CO Percent (Level)	Rate Constant (1/min)		Half-time (minute)	
		Surface	66 FSW (3 ATA)	Surface	66 FSW (3 ATA)
1	45	0.0222	0.1657	31.5	4.2
2	49	0.00463	0.00802	149.7	86.4
3	55	0.00912	0.01514	76.0	45.8
4	54	0.0060	0.01438	115.5	48.2
5	44	0.0200	0.0292	34.7	23.7
6	44	0.0134	0.0294	51.7	23.6
7	18.4	0.00763	0.00928	90.8	74.7

[a] Rate constants and half-times for carbon monoxide elimination for patients with carbon monoxide poisoning, treated initially with 100 percent oxygen "at the surface" and subsequently at 66 feet seawater pressure on 100 percent oxygen.

ygen. Another patient's times were 34.7 minutes in 100 percent oxygen and 23.7 minutes in hyperbaric oxygen; yet a further patient had a 90.8-minute normobaric oxygen versus a 74.7-minute hyperbaric oxygen time. It would appear that patients coming from fires with short but high concentration exposures had high initial levels of carbon monoxide, which then rapidly fell off. Other patients coming from long exposures (soaking) but lower carbon monoxide concentrations had lower initial COHb levels but also had longer carbon monoxide half-lives.[132]

In 1895, Haldane[114] kept a mouse alive in oxygen under 2 atm of pressure after its hemoglobin had been saturated wtih carbon monoxide. The major deterrent against the use of hyperbaric oxygen occurred as a result of Paul Bert's work.[89] Bert used oxygen inhalation for the treatment of compressed air sickness to accelerate nitrogen elimination but showed that excessive pressures and 100 percent oxygen produced pneumonia and convulsions in his animals. Oxygen was then described as being a "toxic poison." In 1935, Shilling and Adams[149] succeeded in defining safe levels of oxygen usage under hyperbaric conditions. It was found that 3 atm of absolute pressure for as long as 3 hours was safe and could be used for longer periods at lower pressures. Bean[86] was able to show that a fall in blood pH occurred with oxygen inhalation under pressure and that this favored dissociation of COHb oxyhemoglobin and carbon monoxide.

In the field or at the scene of the carbon monoxide exposure, the patient must be removed from the source of carbon monoxide and placed on as high an oxygen concentration as possible. Major problems exist in the field deliverance of oxygen. A number of different modalities for oxygen delivery exist, including nasal cannulae providing approximately 23 percent oxygen concentration in the nasopharynx to a plastic face mask with a rebreathing system and a reservoir supply of oxygen close to the face in-line from the oxygen supply. This

TABLE 37-4. Patients Treated with 100 Percent Oxygen at Surface Only[a]

Patient	Initial CO Level	CO Elimination	
		Rate Constant (1/min)	Half-time (min)
1	5.1	0.0115	60.3
2	15	0.0139	49.9
3	6.2	0.00445	155.8
4	6.4	0.00438	158.3
5	14	0.00151	459.0
6	24	0.0118	58.7
7	27	0.00150	462.1
8	17	0.00762	91.0
9	60.5	0.01817	38.1
10	48	0.0256	27.1
11	26.6	0.00237	292.5
12	20	0.00900	77.0

[a] Rate constants and half-times for carbon monoxide elimination for patients with carbon monoxide poisoning, treated initially with 100 percent oxygen "at the surface."

could provide up to 70 to 80 percent oxygen levels.

In order to achieve 100 percent oxygen by face mask, it is essential to use an aviator-type or anesthesia-type face mask with a soft face fit so the mask may fit the contour of the face snugly. Without this type of face mask, it is impossible to obtain 100 percent oxygen. In collapsed patients, it is necessary to perform cardiopulmonary resuscitation and whichever form of airway intubation is possible, ranging from the esophageal airway, or esophagogastric airway, to an endotracheal airway. The choice of airways depends on the paramedic skills and the legal status of paramedic endotracheal intubation in the particular area. On reaching the hospital, these patients should be placed on ventilators, so that the oxygen source can be ensured and 100 percent oxygen administered. Where there is a concern for smoke inhalation in association with carbon monoxide poisoning, this must obviously be attended to, and the presence of facial and oral burns must be sought. An IV line is established in order to sample the blood for COHb levels and provide IV fluids and an access line for medications. The cornerstone of treatment, however, is oxygen.

Controversy exists regarding who should be referred to a hyperbaric center and who remains in the emergency room. Hyperbaric chambers should act as the triage source for carbon monoxide poisoning. All patients suspected of carbon monoxide poisoning who are unconscious in the hospital should be transferred to a hyperbaric facility for hyperbaric oxygen treatment. Any patient who has been unconscious, and who has received 4 hours or more of 100 percent oxygen by face mask or endotracheal intubation with no change in the level of consciousness, must be referred to a hyperbaric facility for aggressive hyperbaric therapy which may necessitate more than one hyperbaric exposure. We would recommend this even if the exposure was more than 72 hours earlier. In our own experience, excellent results have been achieved with exposures up to 48 hours earlier.[135] There is a significant likelihood of permanent brain sequelae following this type of poisoning when the patient is in coma and unresponsive to normobaric treatment. These patients may require intensive

care monitoring and treatment. They should be advised to seek long-term follow-up evaluation over several years, with psychometric testing and rehabilitation, when indicated. With this approach, we will learn more about the long-term effects of carbon monoxide poisoning.

Protocol for Hyperbaric Treatment of Carbon Monoxide Poisoning

The incidence of post-carbon monoxide sequelae ranges between 10 and 40 percent. Plum et al.[141] reported five cases of delayed encephalopathy following a period of apparently full recovery. Gordon[112] described a patient's attempt at suicide with coal gas poisoning, followed at 21 days by the development of lack of concentration, inappropriate behavior resulting in psychiatric disturbance, a parkinsonian gait, and loss of time and place orientation. The patient required help in feeding and dressing; later, his condition deteriorated, and the patient died. Autopsy revealed diffuse demyelinization of the white matter and softening of the left globus pallidus. Bour et al.[91] described 20 delayed deaths from carbon monoxide poisoning. Autopsies in the group showed initial neurologic improvement, then deterioration. They also showed diffuse demyelinization of white matter. None of these patients was treated with hyperbaric oxygen, and the recurrence of symptoms was ascribed to the demyelinization process.

In our own work, we have noted, in 213 cases observed over a 3½-year period, a 10 percent recurrence of symptom rate in patients not treated with hyperbaric oxygen. A group of 84 patients considered to be the less seriously involved of the two groups, with carbon monoxide levels under 25 percent, normal response to our psychometric test, and minimal symptomatology were treated with normobaric oxygen for more than 4 hours and ultimately discharged home. The second group of 131 patients was determined to be seriously impaired, with carbon monoxide levels of over 40 percent, abnormal psychometric testing, and severe symptoms. This group was treated in the hyperbaric chamber with dramatic response and no recurrence of symptoms on follow-up. The recurrence of symptoms in the first group occurred between 2 and 21 days after initial treatment. In a third group, six unconscious patients were referred to our department for hyperbaric oxygen treatment after being treated with 100 percent normobaric oxygen for 4 to 6 hours at the primary hospital; these patients showed no change in their neurologic status. They were treated with hyperbaric oxygen at 3 ATA (66 ft seawater pressure equivalent) and showed dramatic recovery in the hyperbaric environment. From this experience, we have become very aggressive in our treatment of neurologic sequelae from carbon monoxide poisoning[131] (Tables 37-3 and 37-4).

MIEMSS has a multiplace hyperbaric chamber (Fig. 37-3A) and is the regional center for the referral of patients involved with smoke inhalation and carbon monoxide poisoning. All patients meeting the criteria of unconsciousness or showing clouded mentation in the field consequent to carbon monoxide exposure are referred directly to us. Often this results in by-passing local hospitals. En route to the hospital, oxygen is administered by a plastic face mask with a rebreathing system and oxygen reservoir bag in line. Blood samples are taken at the scene of the accident, at the time of the first IV line insertion, and then repetitively in the admitting area of MIEMSS. We have thus been able to determine the treatment effect. The next step is to determine the severity of carbon monoxide effects; this is done by the use of psychometric tests.[133] Unconsciousness or an abnormal result on psychometric tests, irrespective of the carbon monoxide level, are indications for hyperbaric oxygen treatment. In addition to these, a COHb level at hospital admission of above 40 percent irrespective of neurologic status is treated with hyperbaric oxygen.

Where there are normal psychometric tests and the patient has levels of carbon monoxide below 40 percent, the patient is treated with normobaric oxygen until the COHb level is below 5 percent on two consecutive tests 1 hour apart. Using this approach to the treatment of carbon monoxide poisoning, we have found that symptomatic patients receiving hyperbaric oxygen respond rapidly and dramatically. The psychometric testing returns to normal, and the COHb level rapidly falls to below 5 percent.

A patient with a COHb level of 40 percent at a primary receiving hospital should still be referred to a hyperbaric facility for further treatment. This is done to reduce the incidence of recurrent symptomatology and possible mitochondrial cellular damage as a result of carbon monoxide toxic action on the individual cells, rather than on the RBC.

Conclusion

It is often stated that there are very few hyperbaric facilities in the country[137] and that the costs of treatment are exorbitantly high. From our registry and survey on hyperbaric facilities,[134] we have ascertained that since 1977, the number of hyperbaric chambers in the country has grown from 37 to more than 200 functional units. There are more monoplace chambers (100) than multiplace chambers (86). Monoplace chambers are treating twice as many patients as the multiplace chambers. The actual cost per treatment now ranges from $100 to $250 nationwide, with variations within each state and across the nation. It is evident that most hospitals throughout the country are within easy reach of a hyperbaric facility; the major problem is lack of awareness that these chambers exist.

Concern is expressed for transferring unstable cardiac patients to other hospitals.[137] This is unfounded in our experiences over the past 5 years with more than 400 victims of carbon monoxide poisoning. The only patients who succumbed from cardiac carbon monoxide effects were those whose treatment was delayed by great and lengthy debate centered around the importance of stabilizing the patient with adequate monitoring and cardiotonic drugs, before treatment with hyperbaric oxygen. Commonly this type of patient dies en route to the hospital or succumbs at the scene with a cardiac arrest. Once the patient reaches the hospital and is placed on oxygen treatment, the major problem of the cardiac dysrhythmia is averted. With a good hospital delivery system and meticulous detail paid to the form of oxygen delivery, use of a tight fitting face mask versus nasal catheter, en route to the hospital the patient can be receiving as high an oxygen concentration as is given in the hospital. Obviously, when one is talking of great distances (over 20 to 30 miles), one must ensure a stable patient before transport, a prerequisite for any transportation of patients to tertiary referral centers.

We do not recommend the use of other forms of therapy. Hypothermia[140] has been used in an attempt to reduce oxygen consumption by the brain. This was undertaken in the experimental model and led to a higher fatality rate. Corticosteroids for brain edema are now being found to have minimal benefit[106] in the anoxic or ischemic brain, and thus have no value in carbon monoxide poisoning treatment.

Fluosol, an oxygen-carrying blood substitute receiving fairly wide attention in the research laboratories of both Japan and the United States, is being considered in carbon monoxide poisoning. The major problems relating to this are the large volumes that would be required to reduce effectively the carbon monoxide half-life and the fact that it is a research protocol at the present time. The half-life of carbon monoxide in perfluorochemical emulsions[159] is 15 to 20 minutes. Other work, however, indicates that the actual volume of oxygen carried in the fluosol is only 5 to 6 vol percent. Thus, some 3 L or more of fluid may be required to reduce the half-life.[155] The use of carbogen (93 to 97 percent oxygen with 3 to 7 percent carbon dioxide) has not found favor. Although the carbon monoxide half-life has been greatly reduced using this technique, it is not recommended[148]; oxygen is far more readily available and easier to administer.

The most important factors in the treatment of carbon monoxide poisoning are to administer as high a concentration of oxygen as is possible, maintain fluid and electrolyte balance, and give careful attention to the vital signs and response to therapy. The acidosis which often accompanies a hypoxic exposure is generally not treated pharmacologically, and the deliverance of high oxygen concentrations will rapidly resolve this acidosis. It should be noted that acidosis in itself shifts the oxyhemoglobin dissociation curve to the right and thus helps in the delivery of oxygen to the tissues.

Because of the involvement of the central nervous system with carbon monoxide poisoning, it is essential that a detailed neurologic assessment be made, which may require psychometric testing and psychological or psychiatric follow-up within 1 week of discharge from the hospital.

Carbon monoxide poisoning is a far more complex problem than has generally been accepted; due to the lack of a means of closely diagnosing neurologic involvement, and the late and long-term sequelae, the subject has been poorly understood. With our improving awareness and the potential for using psychometric testing to help establish neurologic involvement, one will be in a better position to measure treatment effects on carbon monoxide poisoning. The psychometric test is a tool for measuring the degree of involvement that will enable us to assess the response to therapy. It will permit controlled and randomized trials to compare 100 percent oxygen with hyperbaric oxygen as treatment modalities.

REFERENCES

Gas Gangrene

1. Altemeier WA, and Fullen WD: Prevention and treatment of gas gangrene. JAMA 217: 806, 1971
2. Altemeier WA, and Furste WL: Collective review: Gas gangrene. Surg Gynecol Obstet (Int Abstr Surg) 84: 507, 1947
3. Arapov DA: Die anaerobie Infektion. p. 1130. Grosse Med Enzyklopaedie. Medgis, Moskow, 1956
4. Bakker DJ: The use of hyperbaric oxygen in the treatment of certain infectious diseases especially gas gangrene and acute dermal gangrene. Academisch Proefschrift, Donderdag 20 December 1984. Drukkerij Veenman B.V., Wageningen, The Netherlands, 1984
5. Bean JW: Effects of oxygen at high pressure. Physiol Rev 5: 1, 1945

6. Behnke AR, Forbes HS, and Motley EP: Circulatory and visual effects of oxygen at 3 atmospheres pressure. Am J Physiol 114: 436, 1935
7. Bert P: La pression barometrique. Recherches de physiologie experimentale. Masson, Paris, 1878
8. Boerema I, and Brummelkamp WH: Traitement des infections à germes anaerobies par l'inhalation d'oxygene en hyperpression. Presse Med 69: 439, 1961
9. Boerema I, and Groeneveld PHA: Gas gangrene treated with hyperbaric oxygenation. p. 255. In Wada J, Iwa T (eds): Proceedings of the Fourth International Conference on Hyperbaric Oxygen. Igaku Shoin, Tokyo, 1970
10. Bressman AN, Wagner W: Nonclostridial gas gangrene: Report of 48 cases and review of the literature. JAMA 233: 958, 1975
11. Brown PM, and Kinman PB: Gas gangrene in a metropolitan community. J Bone Joint Surg 56A: 1445, 1974
12. Brummelkamp WH, Hogendijk J, and Boerema I: Treatment of anaerobic infections (clostridial myositis) by drenching the tissues with oxygen under high atmospheric pressure. Surgery 49: 299, 1961
13. Caplan ES, and Kluge RM: Gas gangrene. Arch Intern Med 136: 788, 1976
14. Chauveau A, and Arloing S: Etude experimentale sur la septicemie gangréneuse. Bull Acad Med (Paris) 12: 604, 1884
15. Clark JM: Oxygen toxicity. p. 200. In Bennett PB, Elliott DH (eds): The Physiology and Medicine of Diving. 3rd ed. Baillière Tindall, London, 1982
16. Clark JM, and Lambertsen CJ: Rate of development of pulmonary oxygen toxicity in man during oxygen breathing at 2.0 ATA. J Appl Physiol 30: 739, 1971
17. Committee Upon Anaerobic Bacteria and Infections. Special Report Series. Medical Research Council, No. 39. His Majesty's Stationery Office, London, 1919
18. Davis JD, and Dunn JM: Hyperbaric medicine in the United States air force. JAMA 2224: 205, 1973
19. Demello FJ, Hahlin JJ, and Hitchcock CR: Comparative study of experimental Clostridium perfringens infection in dogs treated with antibiotics, surgery and hyperbaric oxygen. Surgery 73: 936, 1973
20. Demello FJ, Hashimoto T, Hitchcock CR, and Haglin JJ: The effect of hyperbaric oxygen on the germination and toxin production of clostridium perfringens spores. p. 276. In Wada J, Iwa T (eds): Proceedings of the Fourth International Congress on Hyperbaric Medicine. Igaku Shoin, Tokyo, 1970
21. Demello FJ, Hitchcock CR, and Haglin JJ: Evaluation of hyperbaric oxygen, antibiotics, and surgery in experimental gas gangrene. p. 554. In Proceedings of the Fifth International Hyperbaric Conference. Simon Fraser University, Burnaby, Canada, 1974
22. Donald KW: Oxygen poisoning in man, I and II. Br Med J 1: 667, 1947
23. Edlich RF, Spengler M, and Rodeheaver GT: Gas forming infections. Curr Concepts Trauma Care p. 18, Summer, 1982
24. Eraklis AJ, Filler RM, Pappas AM, Bernhard WF: Evaluation of hyperbaric oxygen as an adjunct in the treatment of anaerobic infections. Am J Surg 117: 485, 1969
25. Finegold SM: Anaerobic Bacteria in Human Disease. Academic Press, New York, 1977
26. Finegold SM, Bartlett JG, Chow AW, et al: Management of anaerobic infections, UCLA Conference. Ann Intern Med 83: 375, 1975
27. Glenny AT, Llewellyn-Jones M, and Mason JH: The intracutaneous method of testing the toxins and antitoxins of the "gas gangrene" organisms. J Pathol 34: 201, 1931
28. Guidi ML, Proietti R, et al: The combined use of hyperbaric oxygen, antibiotics, and surgery in the treatment of gas gangrene. Resuscitation 9: 267, 1981
29. Hart GB, Lamb RC, and Strauss MB: Gas gangrene: I. A collective review. J Trauma 23: 11, 1983
30. Hart GB, O'Reilly RR, Cave RH, Broussard ND: The treatment of clostridial myonecrosis with hyperbaric oxygen. J Trauma 14: 712, 1974
31. Heimbach RD: Gas gangrene: Review and update. HBO Rev 1: 41, 1980
32. Heimbach RD, Boerema I, Brummelkamp WH, and Wolfe WG: Current therapy of gas gangrene. p. 153. In Davis JC, Hunt TK (eds): Hyperbaric Oxygen Therapy. Undersea Medical Society, Bethesda, MD, 1977
33. Hill GB, and Osterhout S: In vitro and in vivo experimental effects of hyperbaric oxygen on Clostridium perfringens. p. 538. In Brown IW, Cox BG (eds): Proceedings of the Third International Conference on Hyperbaric Medicine. National Research Council Publication 1404. National Academy of Science, Washington, DC, 1966
34. Hill GB, and Osterhout S: Experimental effects of hyperbaric oxygen on selected clostridial species. I. In-vitro studies. J Infect Dis 125: 17, 1972
35. Hippocrates: Hippocratic writings. p. 18. In Lloyd GER (ed): Epidemics. Book I. (trans.) Penguin Classics, Middlesex, England, 1983
36. Hitchcock CR, Demello FJ, and Haglin JJ: Gas

infection: New approaches to an old disease. Surg Clin North Am 55: 1403, 1975

37. Holland JA, Hill GB, Wolfe WG, et al: Experimental and clinical experience with hyperbaric oxygen in the treatment of clostridial myonecrosis. Surgery 77: 75, 1975

38. Howard JM, and Inui KK: Clostridial myositis-gas gangrene. Observations of battle casualties in Korea. Surgery 36: 1115, 1954

39. Hunt TK, Ledingham IMCA, and Hutchison JPG: Effect of hyperbaric oxygen on experimental infections in rabbits. p. 572. In Brown IW Jr, Cox BG (eds): Proceedings of the Third International Conference on Hyperbaric Medicine. National Research Council Publication 1404. National Academy of Science, Washington, DC, 1966

40. Irvine TT, Moir ERS, and Smith G: Treatment of clostridium welchii infection with hyperbaric oxygen. Surg Gynecol Obstet 127: 1058, 1968

41. Kaye D: Effect of hyperbaric oxygen on clostridia in vitro and in vivo. Proc Soc Exp Biol Med 124: 360, 1967

42. Kellett CE: The early history of gas gangrene. Ann Med Hist 1: 452, 1939

43. Kelley HG, and Page WG: Treatment of anaerobic infections in mice with hyperpressure oxygen. Surg Forum 14: 63, 1963

44. Kerner M, Meakins JL, Wilson WE, and McLean P: Gas gangrene complicating limb trauma. J Trauma 16: 106, 1976

45. Kiranov IG: Inkubationsperiode der anaeroben Gasbrandinfektion. Unfallheilk 83: 76, 1980

46. Kivisaari J, and Niinikoski J: Use of silastic tube and capillary sampling technic in the measurement of tissue PO_2 and PCO_2. Am J Surg 125: 623, 1973

47. Kizer KEW, and Ogle LC: Occult clostridial myonecrosis—case report. Ann Emerg Med 6: 307, 1981

48. Klose F: Ein Beitrag zur Kenntnis der durch die Gruppe der Gas-Oedem-Bazillen erzeugten anaeroben Wundinfektion. MMW 9: 295, 1917

49. Lambertsen CJ: Effects of excessive pressures of oxygen, nitrogen, helium, carbon dioxide and carbon monoxide. p. 1901. In Mountcastle VB (ed): Medical Physiology. 14th ed. CV Mosby, St. Louis, 1980

50. Larrey DJ: Clinique chirurgicale, exercée, particulièrement dans les camps et les hôpitaux militaires, depuis 1792 jusqu'en 1829. Paris, 1829

51. MacLennan JD: The histotoxic clostridial infections of man. Bacteriol Rev 26: 177, 1962

52. Malgaigne JF: Sur la nature et la gravité de l'emphysème traumatique. Rev Med Chir 3: 1815

53. Martin PGC: A case illustrating the early onset of gas gangrene. J R Nav Med Serv 28: 388, 1942

54. Meleney FL: Hemolytic streptococcus gangrene. Arch Surg 9: 317, 1924

55. Millar WM: Gas gangrene in civil life. Surg Gynecol Obstet 54: 232, 1932

56. Mohr JA, Griffiths W, Holm R, et al: Clostridial myonecrosis (gas gangrene) during kefalosporin prophylaxis. JAMA 239: 847, 1978

57. Myers RAM, and Schnitzer BM: Hyperbaric oxygen use—Update 1984. Postgrad Med 76: 83, 1984

58. Nichols RL, and Smith JW: Gas in the wound: What does it mean? Surg Clin North Am 55: 1289, 1975

59. Niinikoski J, and Aho AJ: Combination of hyperbaric oxygen, surgery and antibiotics: The treatment of clostridial gas gangrene. Infect Surg 2: 23, 1983

60. Nora PF, Mousavipour M, and Laufman H: Mechanism of action of high pressure oxygen in Clostridium perfringens toxicity. p. 565. In Brown IW Jr, Cox BG (eds): Proceedings of the Third International Conference on Hyperbaric Medicine. National Research Council Publication 1404. Washington, DC, National Academy of Science, 1966

61. Ozorio De Almeida A, and Pacheco G: Ensaios de tratemento das gangrenas gagosas experimentais pelo oxigenio em altas pressoes e pelo oxigenio em estado nascente. Rev Bras Bio 1: 1, 1941

62. Parker MT: Postoperative clostridial infection in Britain. Br Med J 3: 671, 1969

63. Pickleman J: Diagnosing and treating gas gangrene. Surg Rounds 9: 38, 1980

64. Pierce EC: Gas gangrene: A critique of therapy. Surg Rounds 8: 15, 1984

65. Rathbun HK: Clostridial bacteremia without hemolysis. Arch Intern Med 122: 496, 1968

66. Rifkind D: The diagnosis and treatment of gas gangrene. Surg Clin North Am 43: 511, 1963

67. Robb-Smith AHT: Tissue changes induced by Cl. welchii type A filtrates. Lancet 2: 362, 1945

68. Rodeing B, Groeneveld PH, and Boerema I: Ten years of experience in the treatment of gas gangrene with hyperbaric oxygen. Surg Gynecol Obstet 134: 579, 1972

69. Schnitzer B, Myers RAM, Britten G, et al: Hyperbaric Chambers: U.S. and Canada. Undersea Medical Society, McGregor and Werner, Hollywood, MD, 1983

70. Schoemaker G: Oxygen tension measurements under hyperbaric conditions. p. 330. In Boerema I, Brummelkamp WH, Meijne NG (eds): Clinical Application of Hyperbaric Oxygen. Elsevier, Amsterdam, 1964

71. Serota AJ, and Finegold SM: Necrotizing soft tissue infections following abdominal surgery. Infect Surg 1: 50, 1982

72. Slack WK, Hanson GC, and Chew HER: Hyperbaric oxygen in the treatment of gas gangrene and clostridial infection—Report of 40 patients treated in a single person hyperbaric oxygen chamber. Br J Surg 56: 505, 1969

73. Smith LP, McLean AP, and Maughan GB: Clostridium welchii septicotoxemia: A review and report of 3 cases. Am J Obstet Gynecol 110: 135, 1971

74. Stone HH, and Martin JG Jr: Synergistic necrotizing cellulitis. Ann Surg 175: 702, 1972

75. van Unnik AJM: Inhibition of toxin production in Clostridium perfringens in-vitro by hyperbaric oxygen. Antonie v Leeuwenhoek 31: 181, 1965

76. VanZyl JJW: Discussion of hyperbaric oxygen. p. 552. In Brown IW Jr, Cox BG (eds): Proceedings of the Third International Conference on Hyperbaric Medicine. National Research Council Publication 1401. National Academy of Science, Washington, DC, 1966

77. Weinstein L, and Braga MA: Current concepts gas gangrene, medical intelligence. N Engl J Med 289: 1129, 1972

78. Welch WH, and Nuttall GH: A gas producing bacillus capable of rapid development in the blood vessels after death. Bull Johns Hopkins Hosp 3: 81, 1892

79. Widell PJ, Bennett PB, Kivlin P, and Gray W: Pulmonary oxygen toxicity in man at 22 ATA with intermittent air breathing. Aerospace Med 45: 407, 1974

80. Wilson B: Necrotizing fasciitis. Am Surg 18: 426, 1952

86. Bean JW: Effects of high oxygen pressure on carbon monoxide transport, on blood and tissue acidity, and on oxygen consumption and pulmonary ventilation. J Physiol (Lond) 72: 27, 1931

87. Benton AL: Benton Visual Retention Test: Clinical and Experimental Applications. 4th ed. The Psychological Corp., New York, 1974

88. Bernard C: Leçons sur les effects des substances toxiques et medicamentenses. Baillière, Paris, 1857

89. Bert P: La pression barometrique. Masson, Paris, 1878

90. Bissonnette JM, Wickham WK, and Drummond WH: Placental diffusing capacities at various carbon monoxide tensions. J Clin Invest 59: 1038, 1977

91. Bour H, Tuten M, and Pasquier P: The central nervous system and carbon monoxide poisoning. 1. Clinical data with reference to 20 fatal cases. Prog Brain Res 24: 1, 1967

92. Caughey WS: Carbon monoxide bonding in hemoproteins. Ann NY Acad Sci 174: 148, 1970

93. Chance B, Erecinska M, Wagner M: Mitochondrial responses to carbon monoxide toxicity. Ann NY Acad Sci 174: 193, 1970

94. Coburn RF: The carbon monoxide body stores. Ann NY Acad Sci 174: 11, 1970

95. Cosby RS, Bergeron M: Electrocardiographic changes in carbon monoxide poisoning. Am J Cardiol 11: 93, 1963

96. Cramer CR: Fetal death due to accidental maternal carbon monoxide poisoning. J Toxicol Clin Toxicol 19(3): 297, 1982

97. DeBias DA, Banerjee CM, Birkhead NC, et al: Effects of carbon monoxide inhalation on ventricular fibrillation. Arch Environ Health 31: 38, 1976

98. Douglas CG, Haldane JS, and Haldane JBS: The laws of combustion of hemoglobin with carbon monoxide and oxygen. J Physiol (Lond) 44: 275, 1912

99. Douglas TA, and Lawson DD: Carbon monoxide poisoning. Lancet 1: 68, 1962

100. Drinkwater BL, Raven PB, Horvath et al: Air pollution, exercise and heat stress. Arch Environ Health 28: 177, 1974

101. Ekblony B, and Huot R: Response to submaximal and maximal exercise at different levels of carboxyhemoglobin. Acta Physiol Scand 86: 474, 1972

102. End E, and Long CW: Oxygen under pressure in carbon monoxide poisoning. J Indust Hyg 24 (10): 302, 1942

103. Eos G, and Priestman G: Cerebral vascular changes in carbon monoxide poisoning. J Neuropathol Exp Neurol 1: 158, 1942

104. Estabrook RW, Franklin MR, and Hildebrandt AG: Factors influencing the inhibitory effect of

Carbon Monoxide Poisoning

81. Adjutant General's Office: The Trail Making Test. Parts A and B. U.S. Army War Department, Washington, DC, 1944

82. Anderson RF, Allensworth DC, DeGroot WJ: Myocardial toxicity from carbon monoxide poisoning. Ann Intern Med 67: 1172, 1967

83. Aronow WS, and Cassidy J: Effect of carbon monoxide on maximal treadmill exercise. A study in normal persons. Ann Intern Med 83: 496, 1975

84. Aronow WS, and Isbell MW: Carbon monoxide effect on exercise-induced angina pectoris. Ann Intern Med 79: 392, 1973

85. Ball EG, Strittmatter CF, Cooper O: The reaction of cytochrome oxidase with carbon monoxide. J Biol Chem 193: 635, 1951

carbon monoxide on cytochrome P-450-catalyzed mixed function oxidation reactions. Ann NY Acad Sci 174: 218, 1970

105. Fabel H: Normal and critical O_2—supply of the heart. p. 159. In Lubbers DW, et al (eds): Oxygen Transport in Blood and Tissues. Grune & Stratton, New York, 1968

106. Fishman RA: Steroids in the treatment of brain edema. N Engl J Med 306: 359, 1982

107. Garland A, and Pearce J: Neurological complications of carbon monoxide poisoning. Q J Med 36(144): 445, 1967

108. Geyer RP: Review of perfluorochemical-type blood substitutes. p. 3. In Proceedings of the Tenth International Congress for Nutrition: Symposium on Perfluorochemical Artificial Blood, Kyoto 1975. Igakushobo, Osaka, Japan, 1975

109. Ginsberg MD, and Myers RE: Fetal brain damage following maternal carbon monoxide intoxication: An experimental study. Acta Obstet Gynaecol Scand 53: 309, 1974

110. Ginsberg R, and Romano J: Carbon monoxide encephalopathy. Need for appropriate treatment. Am J Psychiatry 133: 317, 1976

111. Goldbaum LR, Orellano T, Degal E: Mechanism of the toxic action of carbon monoxide. Ann Clin Lab Sci 6: 372, 1976

112. Gordon EB: Carbon monoxide encephalopathy. Br Med J 1: 1232, 1965

113. Grace TW, and Platt FW: Subacute carbon monoxide poisoning: Another great imitator. JAMA 246: 1698, 1981

114. Haldane J: The relation of the action of carbonic oxide to oxygen tension. J Physiol (Lond) 18: 201, 1895

115. Halpin B, Fisher RS, and Caplan YH: Fire Fatality Study, International Symposium on Toxicity and Physiology of Combustion Products. University of Utah, Salt Lake City, Utah, March 22–26, 1976

116. Hayes JM, and Hall GV: The myocardial toxicity of carbon monoxide. Med J Aust 1: 865, 1964

117. Hovath SM, Dahms TE, and O'Hanlon JF: Carbon monoxide and human vigilance. Arch Environ Health 23: 343, 1971

118. Hsu YK, and Cheng YL: Cerebral subcortical myelinopathy in carbon monoxide poisoning. Brain 61: 384, 1938

119. Ikeda T, Kondo T, Mogami H, et al: Computerized tomography in cases of acute carbon monoxide poisoning. Med J Osaka Univ 29 (3–4): 253, 1978

120. Jackson DL, and Menges H: Accidental carbon monoxide poisoning. JAMA 243: 772, 1980

121. Jakob H: Uber die diffuse hemispharen markerkraukung nach kohlenoxydvergiftung bei fallen nut klinisch intervallarer verlaufsform. 2. Neurol Psychiatry 167: 161, 1939

122. Jefferson J: Subtle neuropsychiatric sequelae of carbon monoxide intoxication. Two case reports. Am J Psychiatry 133 (8): 961, 1976

123. Kindwall E: Carbon monoxide poisoning. p. 177. In Dairs JC, Hunt TK (eds): Hyperbaric Oxygen Therapy. Undersea Medical Society, Bethesda, MD, 1977

124. Komatsu F: Dig Sci Labour 10: 315, 1955

125. Larkin JM, Brahos GJ, and Moylan JA: Treatment of carbon monoxide poisoning: Prognostic factors. J Trauma 16: 111, 1976

126. Longo LD: The biological effects of carbon monoxide on the pregnant woman, fetus and newborn infant. Am J Obstet Gynecol 129: 69, 1977

127. Longo LD, and Ching KS: Placental diffusing capacity for carbon monoxide and oxygen in unanesthetized sheep. J Appl Physiol 43: 885, 1977

128. MacMillian V: The effects of acute carbon monoxide intoxication on the cerebral energy metabolism of the rat. Can J Pharmacol 53: 354, 1975

129. Marek Z, and Piejko M: Circulatory failure in acute carbon monoxide poisoning. Forensic Sci 1: 419, 1972

130. Muller GL, and Graham S: Intrauterine death of the fetus due to accidental carbon monoxide poisoning. N Engl J Med 252: 1075, 1955

131. Myers RAM, Emhoff TA, and Snyder SK: Subacute sequelae of carbon monoxide poisoning. Presented at the Eighth International Congress on Hyperbaric Medicine, Long Beach, CA, September, 1984

132. Myers RAM, Jones DW, and Britten JS: Carbon monoxide half-life. Presented at the Eighth International Congress on Hyperbaric Medicine, Long Beach, CA, September, 1984

133. Myers RAM, Messier LD, Jones DW, and Cowley RA: New direction in the research and treatment of carbon monoxide exposure. Am J Emerg Med 2: 226, 1983

134. Myers RAM, and Schnitzer BM: Hyperbaric oxygen use. Postgrad Med J 76: 5, 1984

135. Myers RAM, Snyder SK, Linberg S, and Cowley RA: Value of hyperbaric oxygen in suspected carbon monoxide poisoning. JAMA 246: 2478, 1981

136. Neufeld MY, Swanson JW, and Klass DW: Localized EEG abnormalities in acute carbon monoxide poisoning. Arch Neurol 38: 524, 1981

137. Olson KR: Carbon monoxide poisoning: Mechanisms, presentation, and controversies in management. Presented at the Clinical Pharmacology and Toxicology Service, San Francisco General Hospital, San Francisco, CA, 1983

138. Peterson JE, Stewart RD: Absorption and elimination of carbon monoxide by inactive young men. Arch Environ Health 21: 165, 1970

139. Phillips P: Carbon monoxide poisoning during pregnancy. Br Med J 1: 14, 1924

140. Pierce EC, Zacharias A, Alday JM et al: Carbon monoxide poisoning: Experimental hypothermic and hyperbaric studies. Surgery 72: 229, 1972

141. Plum F, Posner JB, Hain RF: Delayed neurological deterioration after anoxia. Arch Intern Med 110: 18, 1962

142. Preziosi TJ, Lindenberg R, Levy D, Christenson M: An experimental investigation in animals of the functional and morphologic effects of single and repeated exposures to high and low concentrations of carbon monoxide. Ann NY Acad Sci 174: 369, 1970

143. Ratney RS, Wegman DH, Elkins HB: In vivo conversion of methylene chloride to carbon monoxide. Arch Environ Health 28: 223, 1974

144. Root WS: Respiration, Handbook of Physiology, Section 3, p. 1087 Vol. II. American Physiological Society, Washington, DC, 1965

145. Sammons JH, Coleman RL: Firefighters' occupational exposure to carbon monoxide. J Occup Med 16: 543, 1974

146. Sasaki T: On half-clearance time of CO-hemoglobin in blood during hyperbaric oxygen therapy. Bull Tokyo Med Dent Univ 22: 63, 1975

147. Sawada Y. Ohashi N. Maemura K et al: Computerized tomography as an indication of long-term outcome after acute carbon monoxide poisoning. Lancet 1: 783, 1980

148. Sayers PR, Davenport SJ: Review of carbon monoxide poisoning. Public Health Bulletin 195. U.S. Government Printing Office, Washington, DC, 1930

149. Shilling CW, Adams BH: A study of the convulsive seizures caused by breathing oxygen at high pressures. U.S. Naval Med Bull 33: 327, 1935

150. Siesjo BK, Nilsson L: The influence of arterial hypoxemia upon labile phosphates and upon extracellular lactate and pyruvate concentrations in the rat brain. Scand J Clin Lab Invest 27: 83, 1971

151. Smith JS, Brandon S: Morbidity from acute carbon monoxide poisoning at three year follow up. Br Med J 1: 318, 1973

152. Stewart RD, Hake CL: Paint-remover hazard. JAMA 235: 398, 1976

153. Stewart RD, Stewart RS, Stamm W et al: Rapid estimation of carboxyhemoglobin level in fire fighters. JAMA 235: 390, 1976

154. Strub RL, Black WF: The Mental Status Examination in Neurology. FA Davis, Philadelphia, 1977

155. Tremper KK, Friedman AE, Levine EM et al: The preoperative treatment of severely anemic patients with a perfluorochemical oxygen-transport fluid, fluosol-DA. N Engl J Med 307: 277, 1982

156. Vital Statistics of the United States: U.S. Public Health Service, Government Printing Office, Washington, DC, 1976

157. Wechsler D: The Wechsler Adult Intelligence Scale. The Psychological Corp., New York, 1955

158. Whorton MD: Carbon monoxide intoxication: A review of 14 patients. J Am Coll Emerg Physicians 5: 505, 1976

159. Yokoyama K: Effect of perfluorochemical (PFC) emulsion on acute carbon monoxide poisoning in rats. Jpn J Surg 8: 342, 1978

Appendix: The Critical Care Record

Among the organizing modalities that have been most useful in the care of the critically injured patient is the use of a critical care record form, which enables the integration of physiologic cardiovascular and respiratory parameters with estimates of fluid balance and neurologic metabolic status. Such a record needs to establish the temporal relationship between changes in vital signs, altered intake and output, critical blood chemistries, and the medications, treatments, and nursing observations that define a change in patient status. There are many such forms in existence. Some of the functions presented on these forms have already been computerized for ease of care.[1] However, we feel that it is useful to present the Maryland Institute for Emergency Medical Services Systems Critical Care Daily Record form on which physical and physiologic data can be related on a common time base, to assist in the organization of care and the recognition of pathophysiologic changes in the patient that may require an alteration in therapy. Figure A-1 in this section is taken from the two sides of the critical care daily record form. On the front side are shown the physiological vital signs (Fig. A-1A), the intake and output form (Fig. A-1B), and the medication report (Fig. A-1C), all on a common shift-by-shift time base. Figure A-1D, which is from the reverse side of the form, shows the nursing observations. In addition, there is a similar format for routine nursing treatments, culture reports, and special procedures, and a summary of the physiologic observations, all of which also can be recorded on the same time base.

From the time of admission, through the acute clinical course, the form is filled out daily. The intensity and frequency of observations may vary, depending on the stage of illness. In some instances, such as during operative surgery, special forms may expand a given time segment. However, all the data is concatenated and summarized on this form, which has proven useful to both the physician and nursing staff at MIEMSS. In addition, special computer-based data outputs are shown in several of the preceding chapters relating to the application of newer quantitative methodologies to care of cardiovascular, metabolic, and respiratory instability in critically ill patients. Chapters 9, 15, and 19 deal with these subjects. In these chapters are shown a standardized format for the presentation of cardiovascular and metabolic data. Chapter 19 also shows examples of the use of computer outputs for the evaluation of respiratory function. These types of computer outputs as replacement for paper documents such as the Critical Care Daily Record will inevitably continue with the evolution of this technology.

The critical care physician and surgeon will need to become conversant with computer techniques and must learn how to achieve the integration of multivariable patient data into patterns that provide information relevant to the care of the critically ill injured patient. It seems clear that the future of critical care lies in this direction and that the critical care specialist of the future whether a surgeon, internist, emergency medical physician, or anesthesiologist will need to become comfortable with these new technologies and to readily accept the novel ways of thinking inherent in their use. However, the future is upon us today and the critical care doctor must learn from the lessons of the past and adapt his or her physiologic care to be able to implement the knowledge of tomorrow. To echo the words of Dante Alighieri from *la Divina Commedia* [*Purgatorio;* Canto XXVI, lines 143 and 144]: "I see in thought all past folly, I see with joy the day for which I hope before me."

Bibliography

1. Siegel JH, Coleman B: Computers in the care of critically ill patient. Urol Clin North Am 13(1): 101, 1986

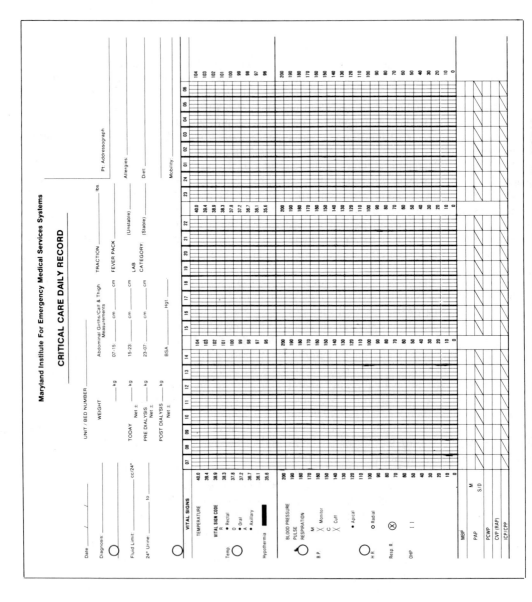

FIG. A-1A CRITICAL CARE DAILY RECORD: VITAL SIGN FORM.

1172

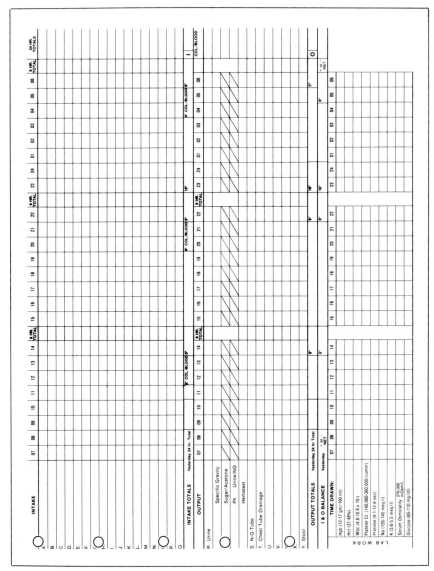

FIG. A-1B CRITICAL CARE DAILY RECORD: FLUID BALANCE FORM.

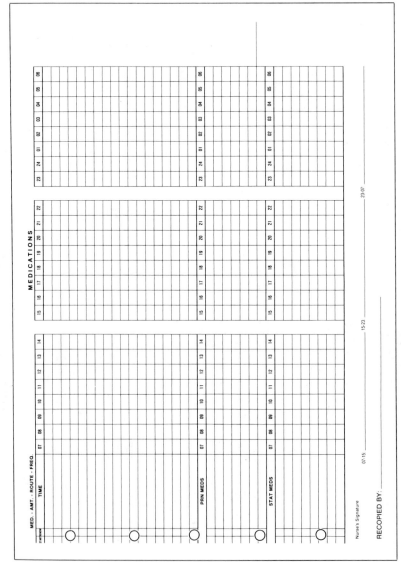

FIG. A-1C CRITICAL CARE DAILY RECORD: MEDICATION FORM.

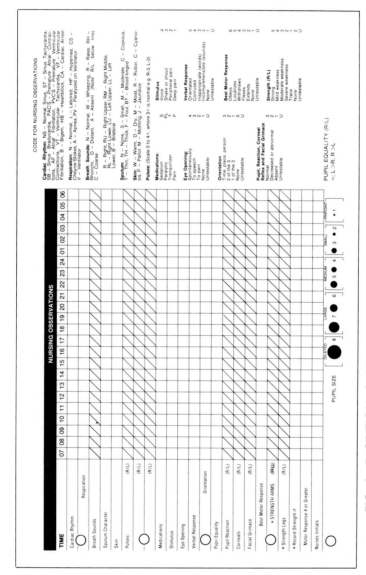

FIG. A-1D CRITICAL CARE DAILY RECORD: NURSING OBSERVATION FORM.

Index

The letter f refers to figures and the letter t refers to tables.